Minimally Invasive Dental Implant Surgery

Minimally Invasive Dental Implant Surgery

Edited by

Daniel R. Cullum DDS
Oral and Maxillofacial Surgeon
Private Practice
Coeur d'Alene, ID, USA
Guest Lecturer
Loma Linda University Department of OMS
Loma Linda, CA, USA
Guest Lecturer
UCLA Department of OMS
Los Angeles, CA, USA

Douglas Deporter DDS, Dipl Perio, PhD
Discipline of Periodontics
Faculty of Dentistry
University of Toronto
Toronto, ON, Canada

WILEY Blackwell

Published by John Wiley & Sons, Inc., Hoboken, New Jersey
Published simultaneously in Canada

For general information on our other products and services or for technical support, please contact our Customer Care Department within the United States at (800) 762-2974, outside the United States at (317) 572-3993 or fax (317) 572-4002.

Wiley also publishes its books in a variety of electronic formats. Some content that appears in print may not be available in electronic formats. For more information about Wiley products, visit our web site at www.wiley.com.

Library of Congress Cataloging-in-Publication Data:
Minimally invasive dental implant surgery / edited by Daniel R. Cullum, Douglas Deporter.
p. ; cm.
Includes bibliographical references and index.
ISBN 978-0-8138-1452-0 (cloth)
I. Cullum, Daniel R. (Daniel Ray), editor. II. Deporter, Douglas, editor.
[DNLM: 1. Dental Implantation—methods. 2. Minimally Invasive Surgical Procedures—methods. 3. Patient Care Planning. WU 640]
RK667.I45
617.6'93—dc23

2015025339

Cover images courtesy of Daniel R. Cullum.

Contents

Contributors, vii
Memorial, viii
Foreword, ix
Preface, x
Acknowledgments, xi
Copyright note, xii

Section I: Technology, Diagnosis, and Treatment Planning

1. Diagnosis and Treatment Planning for Minimally Invasive Dental Implant Treatment, 3
Jean-Francois Bedard & Daniel R. Cullum

2. Diagnostic Imaging for Patient Evaluation and Minimally Invasive Treatment Planning, 28
Scott D. Ganz

3. Risk Assessment and Avoiding Complications, 51
David Dara Yarmand, Douglas Deporter, & Daniel R. Cullum

4. The Provisional Restoration: A Diagnostic, Functional, and Esthetic Template, 66
Aldo Leopardi & Daniel R. Cullum

Section II: Technology and Surgery

5. Extraction Site Management for Ridge Preservation and Implant Site Development, 89
Barry Bartee & Daniel R. Cullum

6. Engineering Biologic Width and Tissue Levels with Implant and Abutment Surface Preparation, 107
Myron Nevins, Cary A. Shapoff, Khalid Al Hezaimi, & David M. Kim

7. Recombinant Human Bone Morphogenetic Protein-2 or Recombinant Human Platelet-Derived Growth Factor BB in Extraction Site Preservation and Bone Augmentation, 119
Craig M. Misch, Marc L. Nevins, & Jason A. Boch

8. Periodontal and Peri-implant Soft Tissue Surgery, 137
Giles Horrocks, Christine Cole, & Daniel R. Cullum

9. Minimally Invasive Implant Surgery Using Computer-Guided Technology, 169
Gary Orentlicher, Andrew Horowitz, & Marcus Abboud

Section III: Optimizing Anatomical Limits with Short, Narrow and Angled Implants

10. Short Implants, 193
Douglas Deporter

11. Narrow Implants, 208
Joerg Neugebauer, Douglas Deporter, & Daniel R. Cullum

12. Minimally Invasive Complete Arch Treatment: The Versatility of Angled Implants, 219
Ole T. Jensen & Daniel R. Cullum

13. Wedge Implants and Piezoelectric Surgery: A Minimally Invasive Implant Concept for the Treatment of Narrow Alveolar Ridges, 227
Tomaso Vercellotti & Claudio Stacchi

Section IV: Implant Site Development

14. Single-Stage Implant Placement and Simultaneous Grafting: The "Esthetic Contour Graft", 241
Bach T. Le & Sze Wing Cynthia Au Yeung

15. Trans-Alveolar Sinus Elevation and Contiguous Sinus Floor Elevation, 251
Daniel R. Cullum & Douglas Deporter

16. Ridge Expansion, 285
Daniel R. Cullum

17. Ridge Expansion Combined with Trans-Alveolar Sinus Elevation, 311
Daniel R. Cullum

Section V: Immediate Implant Reconstruction

18. Immediate Implant Placement for Single- and Multi-Rooted Teeth, 337
Daniel R. Cullum & Douglas Deporter

19. Immediate Esthetic Zone Tooth Replacement, 367
Daniel R. Cullum & Howard Park

Section VI: Comprehensive Applications of Minimally Invasive Surgery

20. Skeletal Anchorage and Orthodontics in Implant Site Development, 387
Michael P. Chaffee & Daniel R. Cullum

21. Minimally Invasive Comprehensive Treatment: Case Studies, 412
Daniel R. Cullum & Earl Ness

Index, 443

Contributors

Marcus Abboud, DMD
Associate Professor and Founding Chair
Department of Prosthodontics and Digital Technology
Stony Brook University
Stony Brook, NY, USA

Khalid Al Hezaimi, BDS, MSc
Research Chair for Growth Factors and Bone Regeneration
King Saud University
Riyadh, Saudi Arabia

Sze Wing Cynthia Au Yeung, BDS, DDS, MD
Assistant Professor
Division of Oral & Maxillofacial Surgery
The Herman Ostrow School of Dentistry of USC
Los Angeles County/USC Medical Center
Los Angeles, CA, USA;
Private Practice
Los Angeles, CA, USA

Barry Bartee, DDS, MD
Osteogenics Biomedical, Inc.
Private Practice
Restorative and Implant Dentistry
Lubbock, TX, USA

Jean-Francois Bedard, DMD (deceased)
Private Practice, Prosthodontics
Denver, CO, USA

Jason A. Boch, DMD DMSc
Instructor, Harvard School of Dental Medicine
Department of Oral Medicine, Infection, and Immunity
Boston, MA, USA;
Private Practice
Wayland, MA, USA

Michael P. Chaffee, DDS, MS
Orthodontist, Private Practice
Coeur d'Alene, ID, USA

Christine Cole, DDS, MHS
Private Practice, Periodontics
Boulder, CO, USA

Daniel R. Cullum, DDS
Private Practice, Oral/Maxillofacial Surgery
Implants Northwest
Coeur d'Alene, ID, USA
Guest Lecturer
Loma Linda University Department of OMS
Loma Linda, CA
Guest Lecturer
UCLA Department of OMS
Los Angeles, CA, USA

Douglas Deporter, DDS, Dipl Perio, PhD
Discipline of Periodontics
Faculty of Dentistry
University of Toronto
Toronto, ON, Canada

Scott D. Ganz, DMD
Department Restorative Dentistry and Department of Diagnostic Imaging
Rutgers School of Dental Medicine
Newark, NJ, USA;
Private Practice
Maxillofacial Prosthodontics and Implant Dentistry
Fort Lee, NJ, USA

Andrew Horowitz, DMD, MD
Private Practice
New York Oral, Maxillofacial and Implant Surgery
Scarsdale, NY, USA;
Associate Attending
Division of Oral and Maxillofacial Surgery
White Plains Hospital
White Plains, NY, USA

Giles Horrocks, DDS, MS
Private Practice, Periodontics
Boulder, CO, USA

Ole T. Jensen, DDS, MS
Adjunct Professor
University of Utah, School of Dentistry
Salt Lake City, UT, USA

David M. Kim, DDS, DMSc
Assistant Professor
Division of Periodontology, Department of Oral Medicine, Infection and Immunity
Harvard School of Dental Medicine
Boston, MA, USA

Bach T. Le, DDS, MD, FICD, FACD
Clinical Associate Professor
Division of Oral & Maxillofacial Surgery
The Herman Ostrow School of Dentistry of USC
Los Angeles County/USC Medical Center
Los Angeles, CA, USA

Aldo Leopardi, BDS, DDS, MS
Private Practice, Prosthodontist
Greenwood Village, CO, USA

Craig M. Misch, DDS, MDS
Oral & Maxillofacial Surgery and Prosthodontics
Sarasota, FL, USA;
Clinical Associate Professor
Department of Implant Dentistry
New York University
New York, NY, USA

Earl Ness, DDS, MSD
Private Practice Prosthodontics
Spokane, WA, USA

Joerg Neugebauer, DDS, PhD
Department for Oral Surgery and Implantology
University of Cologne
Cologne, Germany
Private office for dentistry, Landsberg am Lech, Germany

Marc L. Nevins, DMD, MMSc
Boston Periodontics & Dental Implants
Boston, MA, USA

Myron Nevins, DDS
Associate Clinical Professor
Division of Periodontology, Department of Oral Medicine, Infection and Immunity
Harvard School of Dental Medicine
Boston, MA, USA

Gary Orentlicher, DMD
Private Practice
New York Oral, Maxillofacial and Implant Surgery
Scarsdale, NY, USA;
Chief, Division of Oral and Maxillofacial Surgery
White Plains Hospital
White Plains, NY, USA

Howard Park, DMD, MD
Guest Lecturer
UCLA Department of OMS
Los Angeles, CA, USA

Cary A. Shapoff, DDS
Private Practice
Fairfield, CT, USA

Claudio Stacchi, DDS, MSc
Department of Medical, Surgical and Health Sciences
University of Trieste
Trieste, Italy

Tomaso Vercellotti, MD, DDS
Private Practice
Genoa, Italy;
Honorary Professor of University College of London
Eastman Dental Institute
London, UK

David Dara Yarmand, DDS, MD
Private Practice, OMS
Toronto, ON, Canada

Memorial to Jean-Francois Bedard

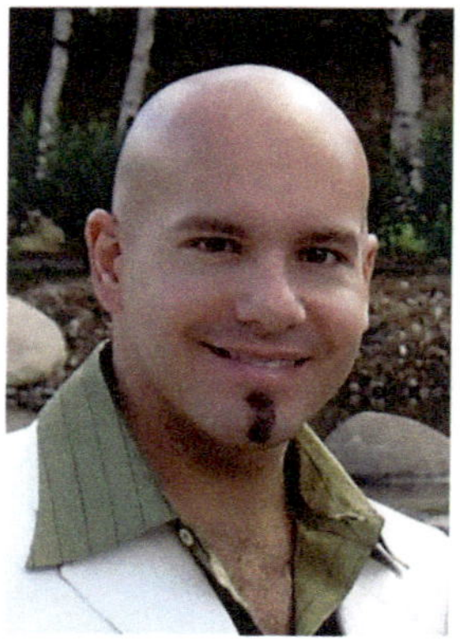

Remembering a great son, husband, father, and friend ... To Deanna and all the family, words cannot describe your loss and sorrow. Any time spent with this special man was both a joy and privilege. Jean was and will always be the unique fun-loving soul that we all loved to be with. His love for you and the kids was both obvious and spoken. He treasured you greatly in his heart, and when he was away you were always on his mind. We shared with Jean many outstanding moments on the mountain, at meetings, at great restaurants, even in the Starbucks' line ... that will not be forgotten. Jean was kind hearted, passionate, exacting, and highly skilled. He truly enjoyed life to the fullest! Please accept our deepest sympathies, you will remain in our thoughts and prayers as you move forward through this tragedy.

Dan and Spring Cullum

Foreword

It has been a joy and privilege to be asked to write a *Foreword* for this beautiful book *Minimally Invasive Dental Implant Surgery,* edited by two eminent, world-renowned colleagues, Drs. Cullum and Deporter.

In the past years there has been an exponential increase in scientific information in implant dentistry, and it is really important that what is learned from basic and clinical research should flow in a clear and direct way to the practicing professional. In the field of biomedicine there is an ever increasing demand for minimally invasive procedures (e.g. robotic surgery) in order to decrease the biological costs for patients. Professional communities must be kept up to date on the most current findings and developments in diverse scientific areas.

Drs. Cullum and Deporter together with many outstanding contributors have provided, in this first-rate book, a comprehensive update of knowledge on many different facets of implant dentistry. This book is sorely needed, and provides an important resource to implant dentistry which covers the field thoroughly focusing on specific issues that confront the dental implant professional every day. All the most relevant aspects of today's implant dentistry have been covered in this book, and all the material is presented with a rigorous scientific approach. The information, such as the basic principles, the most recent advances, and practical applications, are presented in a well-integrated way. Beautiful illustrated case reports complete the book.

This book is a milestone contribution in implant dentistry, and will set a new standard for many years to come.

Prof. Adriano Piattelli, MD DDS
Professor of Oral Pathology and Medicine
Department of Medical, Oral and Biotechnological Sciences
School of Dentistry
University "Gabriele D'Annunzio", Chieti-Pescara, Chieti, Italy

Preface

Developing a minimally invasive mindset ...

A new paradigm in dentistry began with the introduction of osseointegration and the predictable replacement of teeth with dental implants. Innovation and research have helped to refine the associated techniques such that today with careful planning and execution we are able to provide predictable and pleasing esthetic and functional implant treatments for our patients. Minimally invasive surgery is the next step ... using the "least invasive" procedure, with the fewest number of steps and smallest cost. Surgery ... simple, fast, and clean **... when less is more.**

Advances in technology now allow unprecedented diagnostic and planning capability. Following evidence-based protocols allows ideal implant placement even, where appropriate, with immediate implantation and immediate function. Choosing to utilize site preservation grafting at the time of tooth extraction lessens the later need for dedicated ridge augmentation grafting with its associated trauma and protracted treatment times. Combining or "stacking" multiple bone manipulation and soft tissue grafting procedures permits shorter treatment times, and using truly short implants helps to avoid complications in posterior jaw sites.

With surgery there is always risk. Flapless surgery can minimize surgical trauma, but comes with limited visibility and the potential for complications and unfavorable outcomes without adequate training and experience. Using computer-guided surgery also comes with risks and requires considerable time and investment to achieve competence. Technology is not a substitute for surgical training, experience or judgment, and significant perils often await its misapplication **... when more is less.**

The focus of this book is to provide a reference for predictable and minimally invasive surgical techniques that can be progressively applied within a construct of advancing skills. The contributors were carefully chosen with the purpose of exploring the field from different perspectives but with a common philosophy. As in other surgical disciplines, developing a minimally invasive mindset in implant dentistry requires a clear understanding of bone and soft tissue biology, wound healing, dental implant design, and the required surgical and/or prosthodontic skills to achieve predictable and optimal treatment outcomes. It is our hope that this book helps the practicing clinician to achieve these lofty goals.

Thank you to the team at Wiley Blackwell for their efforts and assistance.

Daniel R. Cullum DDS

Acknowledgments

Undertaking a comprehensive textbook is an ominous project. The time demand is more than one could ever have imagined. To that end I wish to thank my family and friends for the time we missed together: my wife Spring in particular has been outstanding in her support and love, my parents for teaching me to work, my dad for instilling a love for dentistry, my office staff and manager Lincoln, for the extra demands of business and busyness. A special thank you to Doug for his contribution and interaction, and to all of the contributors for their efforts and expertise. I want to also thank the many teachers and mentors who have influenced my career and praise God for gifting me with the strength, energy and skill to complete this project! Minimally invasive surgery is more demanding in time, skill and judgment, however, it has changed the way I practice and we want to share the many benefits for our patients.

Dan Cullum

I would like to thank Dan for giving me the opportunity to participate in this project. For over 25 years, I have striven to deliver minimally invasive dental implant treatment using short implants and the OSFE and BAOSFE approaches to sinus floor elevation. This book has been a challenging project. In the end I enjoyed the work and interacting with Dan, contributed a bit myself, and learned a lot from the contributors. Producing a comprehensive book like this one is a group effort. I would like to express my appreciation to all who contributed and wish them continued success and good health in future.

Douglas Deporter

Copyright note

SECTION I

Technology, Diagnosis, and Treatment Planning

CHAPTER 1

Diagnosis and Treatment Planning for Minimally Invasive Dental Implant Treatment

Jean-Francois Bedard[1] **& Daniel R. Cullum**[2]

[1]Private Practice, Prosthodontics, Denver, CO, USA

[2]Private Practice, Coeur d'Alene, ID; Loma Linda University Department of OMS, Loma Linda, CA; UCLA Department of OMS, Los Angeles, CA, USA

Introduction

While the recent trend in dental implantology has been toward less invasive surgical procedures, an argument can be made that the prosthetic phase has become more complex. Our desire to provide patients with minimally invasive treatment options requires that the diagnostic aspects be completed comprehensively. There is no "minimally invasive" diagnosis. Treatment options may be more or less invasive, but the diagnosis needs to be thorough and complete. Despite significant advances in dental implant technology, implants remain endosseous anchorage devices intended for prosthetic reconstruction of missing teeth.[1]

Many diagnostic tools, including cone beam computed tomography (CBCT) imaging and dental implant planning software (see also Chapters 2 and 9), have been developed to provide clinicians with user-friendly and precise methodology to examine and virtually plan possible therapeutic interventions.[2] These technologies greatly facilitate communication with the patient and treatment team members.[3] Clinicians should, however, use caution when applying these technologies and develop an understanding of their advantages and limitations. Restorative management of dental implants requires a clear understanding of the final restoration design, planning for the phases of treatment and anticipating contingency plans.[4]

In addition, it is important to realize that minimally invasive surgery does not imply less complexity or that less skill and judgment are necessary. On the contrary, often more skill and judgment are required with minimally invasive approaches, and clinicians should be trained and competent in both minimally invasive and traditional approaches. Clinicians providing surgical care also should be competent in anticipating, preventing, and managing potential surgical and prosthetic complications. Thus, the skills and judgments of the treatment team remain paramount.

For successful implant treatment outcomes, there must be sufficient quality and quantity of supporting hard and soft tissues, the implants must be in the proper number, location, and orientation, and the prosthesis must be fabricated with detailed attention to esthetics, phonetics, occlusal function, and access for oral hygiene.[5] This chapter will address principles for the diagnosis and treatment planning for prosthetic reconstruction of commonly encountered clinical situations in the context of employing minimally invasive procedures.

The diagnostic process

Developing an accurate diagnosis is best achieved using a systematic process. Initial patient evaluation should begin with a subjective assessment, including chief complaint, history of the present illness or problem, and past dental and medical histories. A full discussion of the patient's immediate concern (chief complaint), expectations, goals, and desires (immediate, short and long term) regarding treatment can prevent misunderstandings and help to avoid disappointments. While it is important to pay attention to the chief complaint, it is equally important not to let the chief complaint prevent a comprehensive approach in the clinical decision-making process. For example, patients presenting for single tooth replacement may not appreciate the need for a full diagnostic work-up and any additional treatment that might be required to achieve an optimal result. Consultation or referral to a more experienced clinician or implant team may be indicated if there is any discrepancy between the alignment of treatment goals and expectations and the clinical reality.

Following a thorough subjective assessment, the collection of objective diagnostic data begins. A focused head and neck examination and dental/oral examination are completed, with special attention given to teeth opposing and adjacent to potential implant sites. A complete periodontal examination, including probing, should be a part of the diagnostic record. The periodontal evaluation also should include an esthetic evaluation of the gingiva, including gingival display, symmetry, and biotype. An occlusal evaluation is necessary, with special attention afforded to vertical space relationships, interdental spaces, attrition, deep bite, cross-bite, and any other issues that might potentially impact the prosthetic outcome.

Radiographic evaluation may include any or all of periapical radiography, panoramic radiography, and CBCT 3-D imaging of the affected jaw(s) and proposed implant site(s).[2] Following the initial diagnostic examination, more sophisticated planning may be required with the use of surgical guides or templates fabricated from diagnostic wax-ups and/or tooth set-ups and 3-D planning.[6] A record of the bite relationship should be taken in wax or a suitable elastomeric material, and diagnostic casts prepared. Mounting of these casts with a facebow transfer is ideal, especially if a diagnostic wax-up is being done.

Digital photographs are an important aspect in diagnosis to help communicate clinical and technical information to patients, dental

Minimally Invasive Dental Implant Surgery, First Edition. Edited by Daniel R. Cullum and Douglas Deporter.

colleagues, and laboratory technicians. Referring to a digital photograph will help to answer questions that can arise in the treatment after teeth have been removed or otherwise altered. Extraoral photographs should be taken from both lateral and frontal views with the lips in repose as well as during a full smile. Intraoral photographs should include an occlusal view of each arch, a frontal view with the teeth in full contact, and right and left lateral views. The camera system need not be elaborate or complex; however; a modern digital single-lens reflex camera with macro lens and a dedicated macro flash system will give the best results. In addition, it is suggested that a high-quality set of intraoral mirrors and lip retractors be available, and that both the dentist and clinical staff be trained in their proper use.

Following a thorough review of the findings and, if need be, consultation with specialists, a set of treatment options is developed. The clinician is required to put all the findings together and come up with possible solutions. As a part of the diagnosis, a risk assessment is completed, including the demands of the case and whether or not a minimally invasive treatment approach is appropriate and/or involvement of other experienced colleagues is indicated.

This process must be purposeful and lead to a plan with the patient's full understanding and support. A plan is rarely a single option, but rather a discussion encompassing multiple possibilities even though some options may be eliminated quickly based on a patient's desires (for example, a reluctance to accept a removable prosthesis). Some treatment options may require additions to the basic plan (for example, a patient requiring multiple implants to be placed in order to secure a prosthesis may require bone augmentation or reduction procedures prior to implant placement). The final plan should include an indication of advantages and disadvantages, expected prognosis, costs, and possible complications in order to adequately inform the patient prior to their consent.

Informed consent

Informed consent involves more than simply presenting a few treatment alternatives. The patient should fully understand the associated risks, benefits, and limitations, including possible complications and alternatives for any treatment proposal. The first treatment option should always be "no treatment," and the implications of that decision should be considered and discussed. Many patients will be concerned regarding the anticipated esthetic outcome, and this should be discussed and documented fully in advance. There is no substitute for a set of mounted models with a diagnostic wax-up to directly visualize the proposed treatment. Digital photographs, 3-D imaging and planning, and a wax try-in or mock-up of the proposed treatment are important aspects of planning and informed consent. Patients should have an opportunity to have all of their questions answered, preferably with a friend or loved one in attendance, and this will often require more than one interaction. Diligence at this phase of treatment is critical to developing trust and rapport with the patient for those inevitable challenges that can occur.

Comprehensive evaluation and risk assessment

Comprehensive examination begins before the patient is seated in the dental operatory. Evaluation of the patient begins with interactions while standing and sitting upright during normal conversation. This is best facilitated in a consultation room with a home living room environment. Most patients begin adaptive responses and compensations when placed in the dental operatory and in a reclined position. The patient and clinician will benefit from a systematic approach and review of the findings.

Facial analysis

Evaluation of facial dimension includes inspection of facial symmetry from the frontal (Figure 1.1a), lateral, and three-quarter views. This inspection will allow confirmation that the facial thirds are harmonious (Figure 1.1b) and determination of the skeletal classification (Class I, II, or III).[7] Diagnosis of the facial type (braciocephalic versus dolicocepahlic) can have significant implications with the amount of bite force generated on posterior teeth and the importance of anterior guidance (deep bite versus open bite). Further examination and palpation of the head and neck include the muscles of mastication to evaluate for hyperactivity or myospasm, temporomandibular joint disorders affecting mandibular range of motion or discomfort, and to rule out the presence of any masses, suspicious lymphadenopathies, or sinus issues.

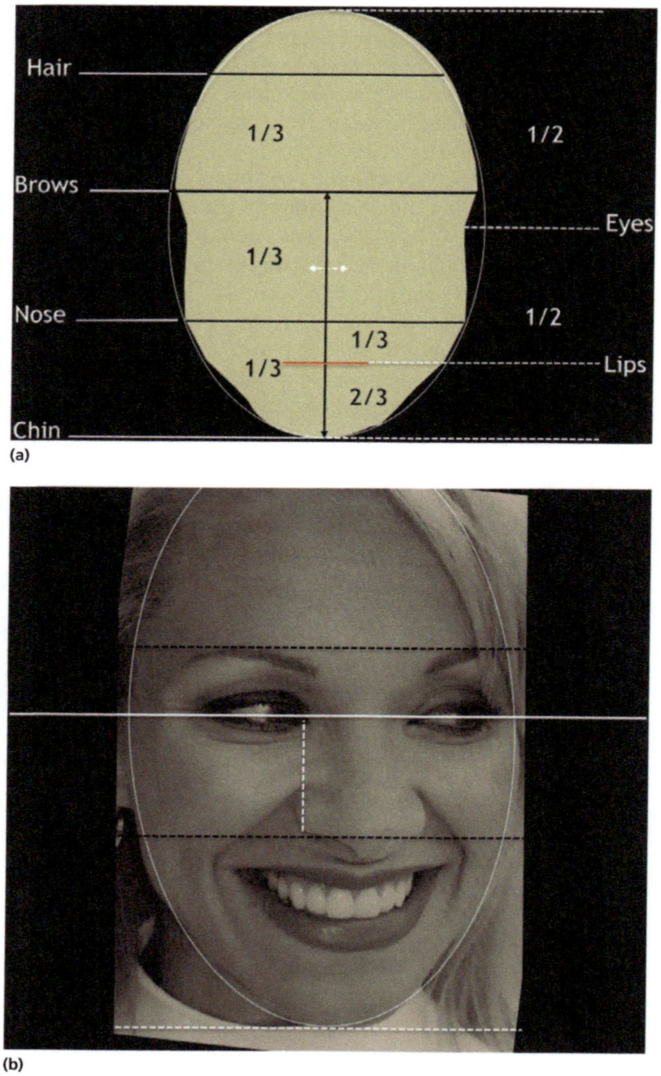

Figure 1.1 (a) Facial perspectives and proportions. (b) Facial perspectives and proportions projected over face.

Dento-facial analysis

Evaluation of the esthetic zone – *incisal plane, plane of occlusion, incisal edge position, dental/facial midlines, lip support,* and *gingival display* – is included in the dento-facial analysis[8] (Figure 1.2a). Digital photography is indispensable for this pretreatment evaluation. Careful and systematic investigation of these features may change what appears initially to be a simple, single-tooth case into a complex interdisciplinary restorative challenge with increased treatment risk. On frontal evaluation, the anterior incisal plane should be parallel to the interpupillary plane and curve upwards in the canine region to follow the contours of the lower lip and the Frankfort horizontal plane[9] (Figure 1.2b). The plane of occlusion should follow the interpupillary line, the curve of Spee, the curve of Wilson, and the curve of Monson[10] (Figure 1.3).

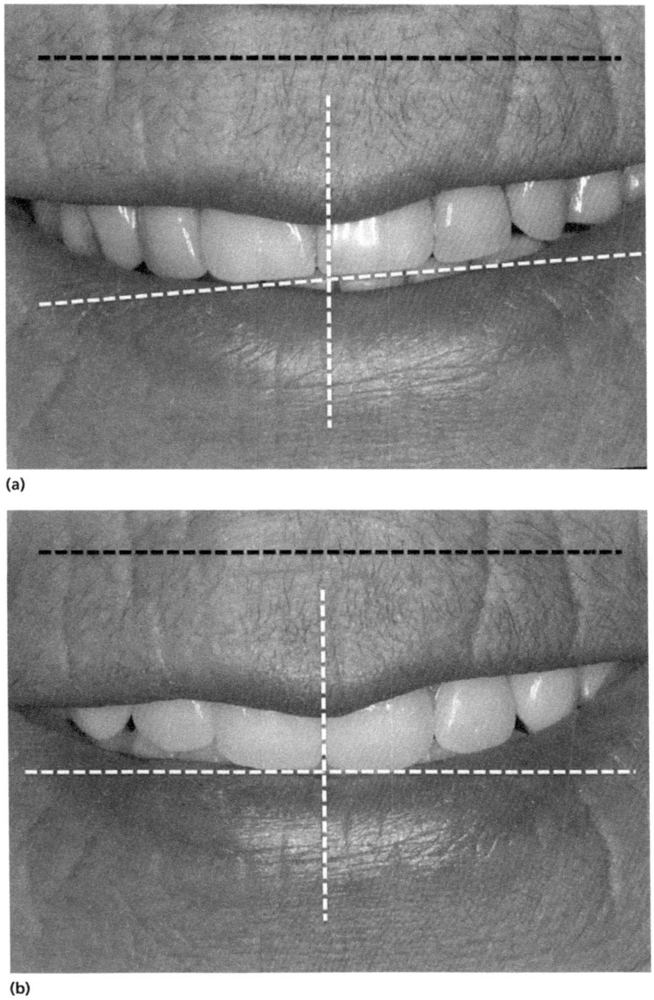

Figure 1.3 (a) Midline and anterior incisal plane discrepancies. (b) New midline and anterior incisal plane after correction.

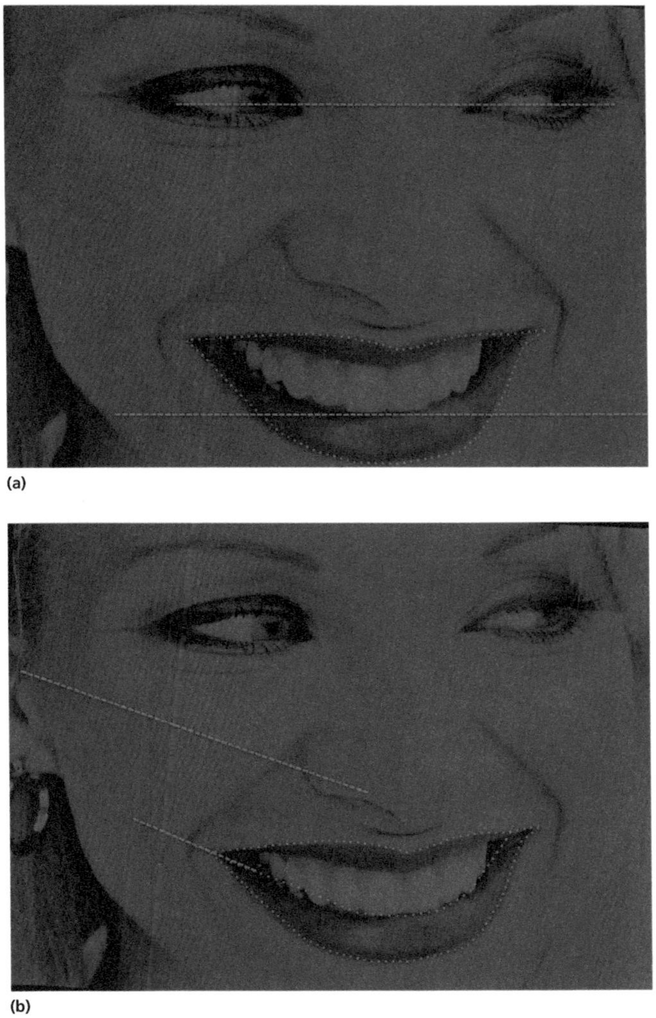

Figure 1.2 (a) Parallelism between interpupillary plane and overall anterior incisal plane. (b) Parallelism between Frankfort plane and posterior occlusal plane.

Incisal edge position and tooth display at rest are patient-specific. Consideration of empirically determined norms can be helpful as the amount of display is age and gender dependent, excluding other variables such as lip length and lip movement on animation.[11] Accepted guidelines for the position of the maxillary central incisal edge at rest is 3.4 mm in females and 1.9 mm in males "below the lip". If the patient has a "short" upper lip, then exposure can be as much as 3.65 mm; with a "long" upper lip exposure can be as little as 0.59 mm.[10] With aging, tooth exposure generally decreases due to lip laxity and decreased animation, and can be further reduced with incisal edge wear (see "Dento-gingival analysis" section). The accepted guidelines range from 3.37 mm of exposure for patients younger than 29 years of age to as little as 1.26 mm for those up to 50 years of age.

Assessment of the *facial and dento-facial midlines* for alignment will reveal any significant horizontal or vertical asymmetry, and any orthodontic, orthognathic, and/or facial plastic surgical treatment that may be indicated[12] (see Chapter 20). If significant dental asymmetry is found, orthodontic treatment (see Chapter 20) and/or prosthetic restoration of adjacent or opposing teeth may be required (Figure 1.4).

A key determinant of esthetic risk in implant therapy is the amount of *gingival display* exhibited during a full smile.[7] If there is no exposure of the dento-gingival margin, the primary esthetic considerations are limited to tooth shade, tooth width, and incisal edge anatomy.[13] Conversely, if there is full exposure of the gingival margin, then the entire dento-gingival complex must be considered, and the esthetic demands of the case will increase exponentially. If it is

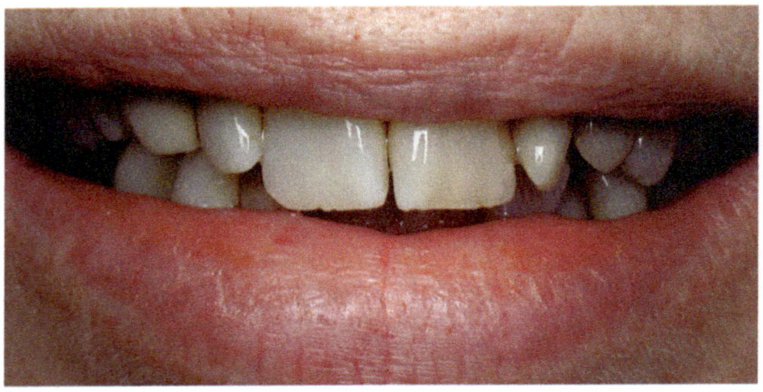

(a)

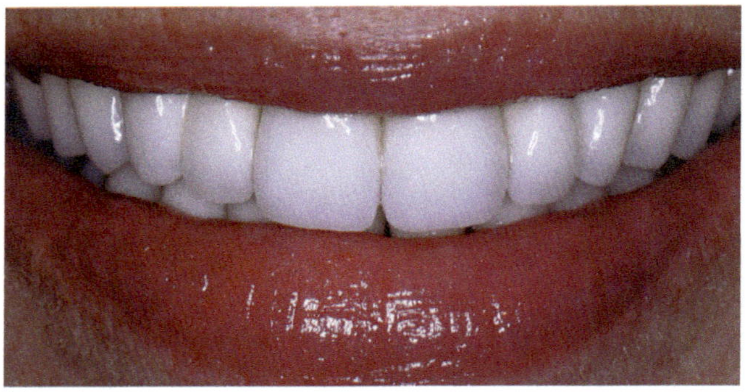

(b)

Figure 1.4 (a) Anterior smile view of preoperative disharmony. (b) Anterior smile view after camouflage of disharmony harmony.

determined that there is altered passive eruption, vertical maxillary excess, or excessive gingival display due to hypermobility of the lip, then periodontal crown lengthening, fixed prosthetic enhancement, surgical, or orthodontic treatment options are best addressed preoperatively along with anticipated limitations in treatment outcome.

Dento-gingival analysis

Gingival plane

Generally, a patient's maxillary anterior teeth display similar gingival length and proportions. The maxillary canines and central incisors may have slightly longer gingival contours than the lateral incisors with relatively more tooth exposure. (Figure 1.5a–c) The maxillary anterior teeth are progressively inclined to the distal, placing the gingival zeniths slightly distal to the midpoint of the tooth width. Tooth shape, tooth positions, and loss of bone or soft tissue support will cause discrepancies in gingival and/or papilla height. Generally, the closer to the midline these discrepancies occur, the more significant their impact will be. Facial angulation or positioning moves the gingival margin apically. Schematics representing tissue defects and gingival levels can aid diagnosis and risk assessment in treatment planning (Figure 1.5b–g) Options to manage gingival height discrepancy include orthodontic treatment, prosthetic soft tissue manipulation with long-term provisional restorations, and/or gingival surgery.

Modification of the gingival levels is often desirable and should be considered during the treatment planning process.[14] Figure 1.6a and b shows a young female patient who presented with a significant asymmetry in the esthetic zone. On dento-facial and dento-gingival evaluation of her smile, the proportions of the maxillary right canines and lateral incisors became the focus of the treatment objectives. Because the left canine and lateral incisor presented with pleasing proportions, a reasonable approach was to reproduce them to the degree possible on the right side (Figure 1.6c and d). The treatment plan in this case consisted of gingivoplasty to increase the length of the right crowns relative to the contralateral teeth. Restorative treatment included narrowing the width of the right lateral incisor and increasing the width of the cuspid to achieve more pleasing proportions (Figure 1.6e). These changes were first evaluated by digital superimposition of a mirror image of the left cuspid and lateral incisor teeth onto the right side. Thereafter, the teeth were prepared and restored with provisional restorations (Figure 1.6f).

Lip support

In addition to support from alveolar bone and soft tissue, the upper lip is mainly supported by the gingival two-thirds of the anterior maxillary teeth, not the incisal one-third. The shape and volume of the anterior maxillary alveolus (relative undercut and proclination) and the effects of aging with altered muscle tone also will effect labial position and mobility on animation.[11]

Gingival biotype

Gingival biotype is another key determinant in esthetic risk.[15] Patients exhibiting a thin, scalloped gingival biotype are more likely to have translucency of the underlying restorative material and/or buccal soft tissue recession over time and, as a result, may show exposed implant components.[16] (See also Chapter 3.) The possible need for modification of the gingival biotype (see also Chapter 8), either preoperatively or following completion of the treatment, is best discussed before treatment begins.

Interdental papilla

Normal interdental papilla reformation following implant restoration is one of the most challenging outcomes in implant dentistry. The height and symmetry of interdental papillae following implant restoration are determined by the height of the interproximal bone crest of the adjacent tooth or implant.[17] A single tooth implant placed between two healthy natural teeth has the best prognosis for reforming esthetically pleasing papillae. In such situations, papillae with 4.0–4.5 mm of soft tissue height can be anticipated (see further discussion in "Planning for ideal implant position" section). Tooth shape is also an important factor in predicting the presence or absence of esthetically pleasing interdental papillae. Square crown forms typically have shorter, thicker papillae and interproximal contacts, which may extend into the middle third of the clinical crown.[13] Conversely, teeth with long, tapered crown shapes have thinner and more delicate papillae, and the interproximal contact zone may be limited to the incisal third of the crown. In this latter situation, when an extraction is done even in a minimally traumatic fashion, recession of papillae and incomplete soft tissue fill between crowns is a common finding.

Maxillary central incisor position

This is the key to anterior esthetics, and is the foundation for the diagnostic and treatment processes. Concepts such as dominance (relative size/shade), symmetry, proportions, and incisal edge position must be understood and applied if esthetic success is to be achieved.[5]

Tooth proportion

Tooth proportion may ultimately be influenced by factors beyond the control of the implant surgeon, such as orthodontic positioning and tooth migration. Guidelines for ideal proportions include a

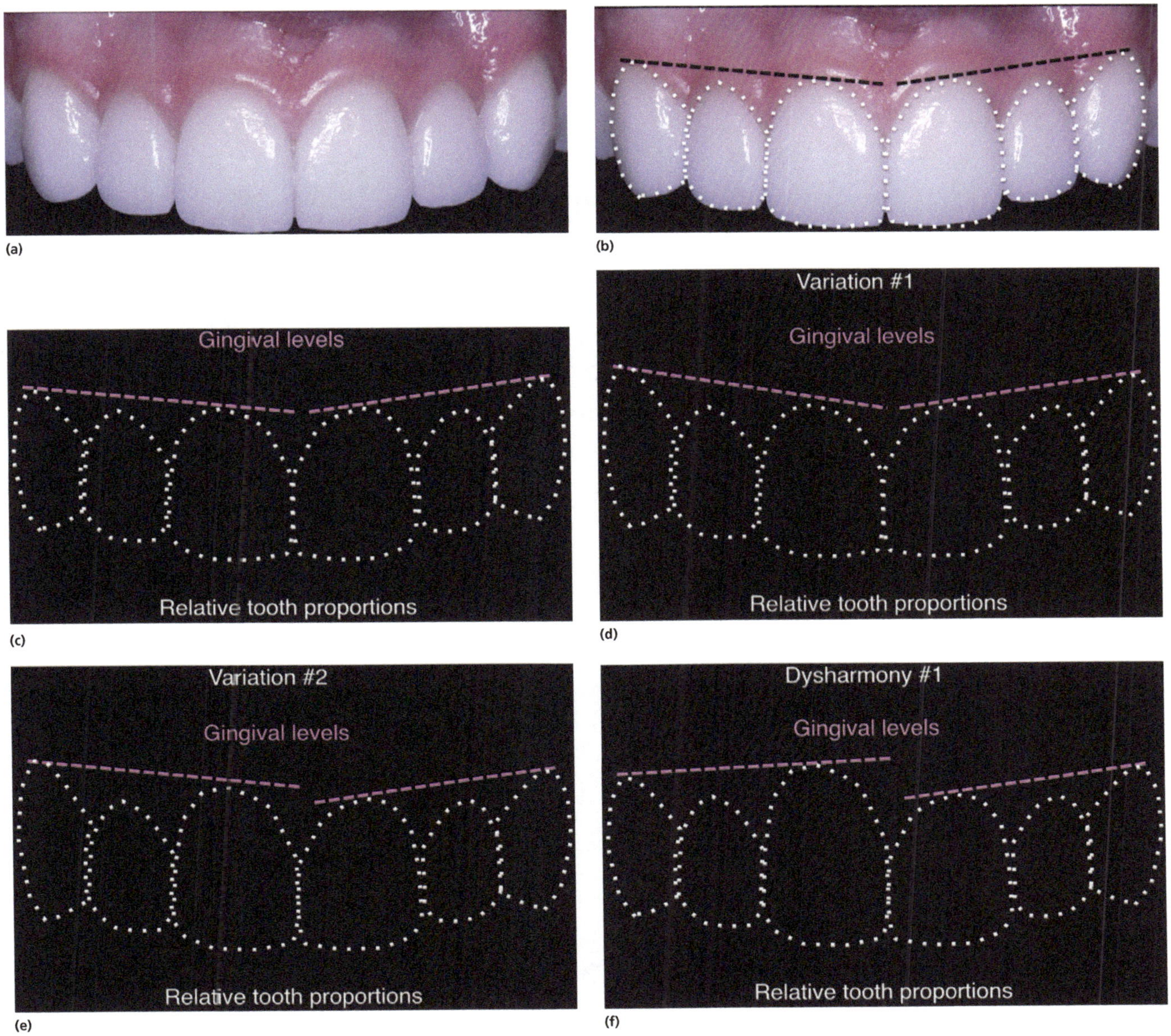

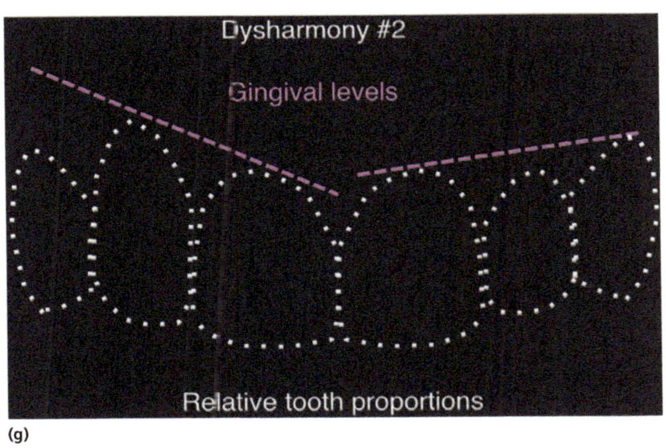

Figure 1.5 (a) Esthetic dento-gingival presentation demonstrating the free gingival margin of maxillary anterior dentition. (b) Same as (a) with teeth outlines drawn. Imaginary lines joining gingival margins of canines to centrals; laterals should ideally be shorter or even with this line. Note that the planes slope downward towards the midline. (c) Diagrammatic representation of (b). (d) Variation #1 (of gingival levels): the right canine is longer gingivally, but perspective is maintained. (e) Variation #2: the right canine and central incisor are longer gingivally, but the gingival plane remains in relative harmony as it slants downward. (f) Dysharmony #1: the right central incisor is significantly longer than in (c), creating a more significant unilateral asymmetry because of the upward plane toward midline. (g) Dysharmony #2: right central incisor is very long gingivally creating visual tension away from ideal plane.

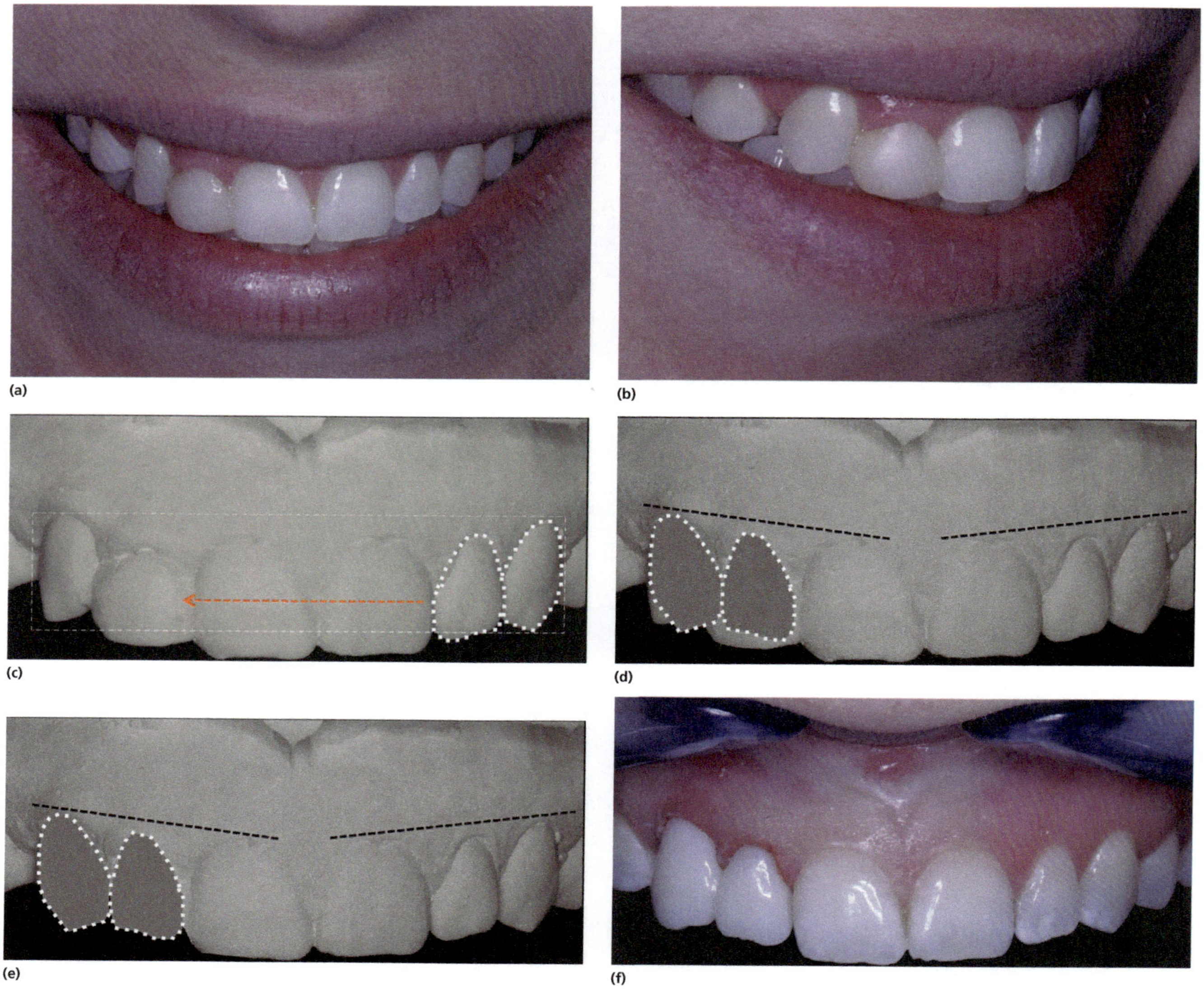

Figure 1.6 (a) Anterior smile view demonstrating significant white and pink disproportions of the right lateral incisor. (b) Right lateral smile view. (c) Esthetic analysis on laboratory study cast. (d) Esthetic superimposition of the left canine and lateral incisor mirror images over the right canine and lateral incisor sites. (e) Same as (d) but with preoperative right canine and lateral incisor teeth eliminated. (f) Anterior retracted dentition of provisional crowns immediately post-insertion; note slight tissue recontouring with diamond gingivoplasty at the right lateral incisor.

width : length (W : L) ratio of 75–80% (Figure 1.7a). For diagnostic purposes, a W : L ratio greater than 85% is indicative of a "short, square" tooth form, while a W : L ratio less than 75% is indicative of a "long, narrow" tooth form (Figure 1.7b and c).

Tooth shape

Tooth shape includes considerable variations in form: round/ovoid, square, or tapered. The shape influences the position of the contact point with the adjacent teeth and embrasure depth. Restoration with a square-shaped crown form fills the embrasure space with restorative material and moves the interproximal contact point apically. As noted previously, tooth shape plays a role in the dimensions of interdental papillae.[13] Patients with a square tooth form typically have a "high crest" bone anatomy, whereas triangular-shaped or ovoid crown forms are more likely to have a "low crest" bone anatomy with a longer zone of soft tissue attachment, and are at higher risk of unfavorable papilla reformation and recession.[13]

Axial inclination

The axial inclination of the maxillary anterior teeth tends to be progressively distal, and this fact will influence the contours of the gingival soft tissue, with the gingival zeniths of the anterior maxillary teeth slightly distal to the mid-tooth width (as discussed previously). This outcome may be difficult to achieve with a dental implant due to size, shape, and proximity limitations. Soft tissue manipulation with long-term provisional restorations (see also Chapter 4), and/or gingival surgery (see also Chapter 8), may be helpful in this regard and should be considered in the initial restorative treatment plan.

Incisal embrasure anatomy

Incisal embrasure anatomy also can influence tooth proportion and shape. The relative angles and depth of a youthful adult incisal embrasure anatomy are shown in Figure 1.8a. With aging and incisal wear, the incisal embrasure depth becomes reduced, and it may even disappear with extreme wear (Figure 1.8b). If lengthening the tooth

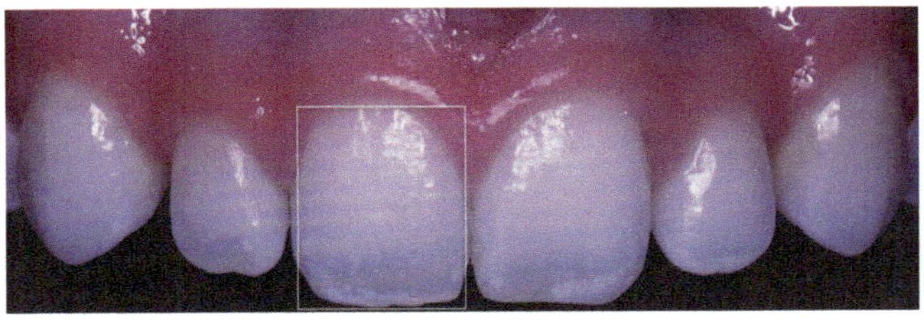
(a)

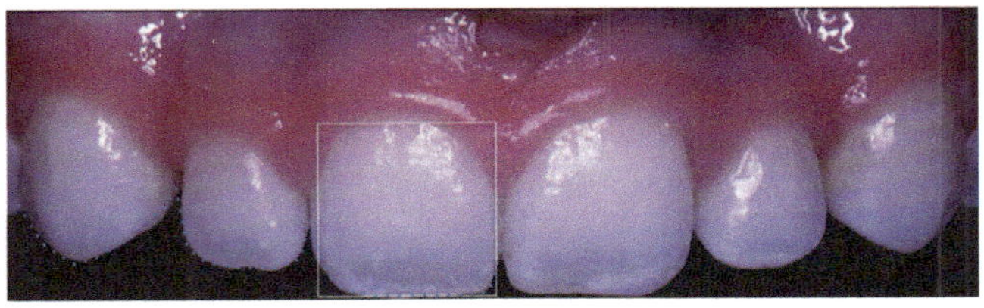
(b)

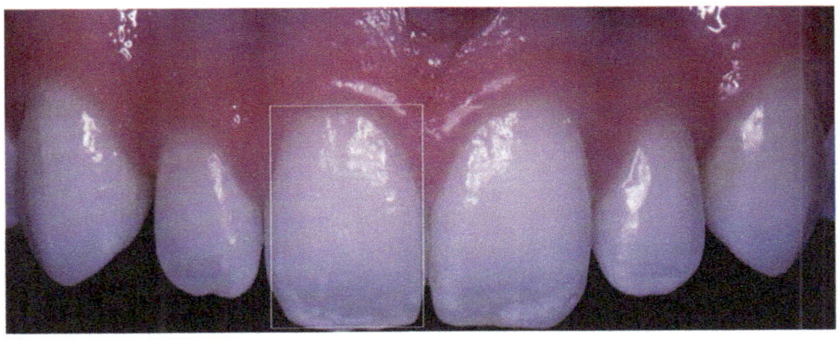
(c)

Figure 1.7 (a) Ideal width-to-length ratio of maxillary central incisors (75–80%). (b) Short tooth width-to-length ratio (larger than 75–80%). (c) Long tooth width-to-length ratio (smaller than 75–80%).

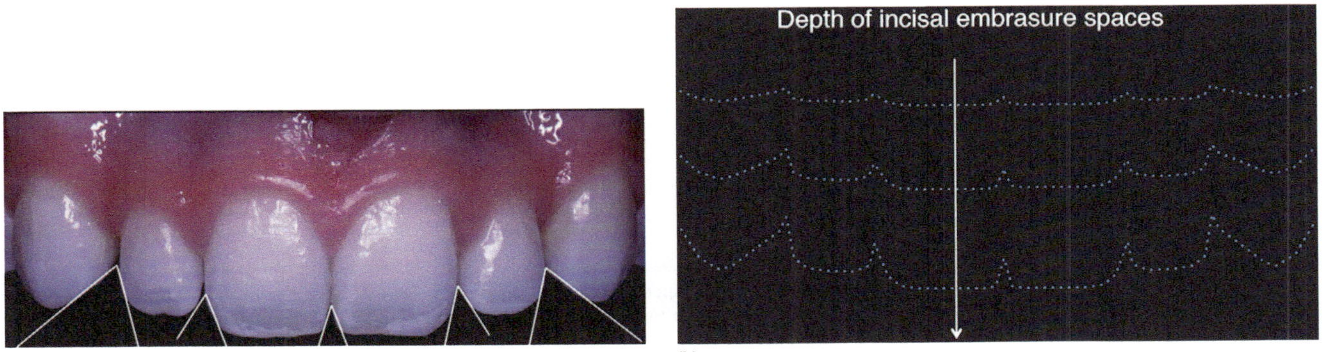

(a) (b)

Figure 1.8 (a) A youthful incisal embrasure anatomy. (b) Variation in incisal embrasure anatomy and depth of incisal planes; the flatter the embrasures (top of figure), the more worn/aged teeth will look. The deeper the embrasures (bottom of figure), the younger the dentition will appear.

is not an option, a simple and effective way to provide a more youthful appearance is to deepen the existing incisal embrasures interproximally. For a more natural appearance, the incisal embrasure of the maxillary lateral incisor should be more pronounced.

Prosthetic modifications of contour and illusion can be used to improve harmony and solve width and/or height imbalances at single or adjacent tooth/implant sites.[7] Moving the facial height of contours inward will "round" a tooth, making it look "narrower"; accentuating the labial planes will also "round" a tooth, making it look "shorter" (Figure 1.9). While these techniques often can help rescue a challenging treatment scenario, the patient should be advised in advance as to the possible limitations of therapy.

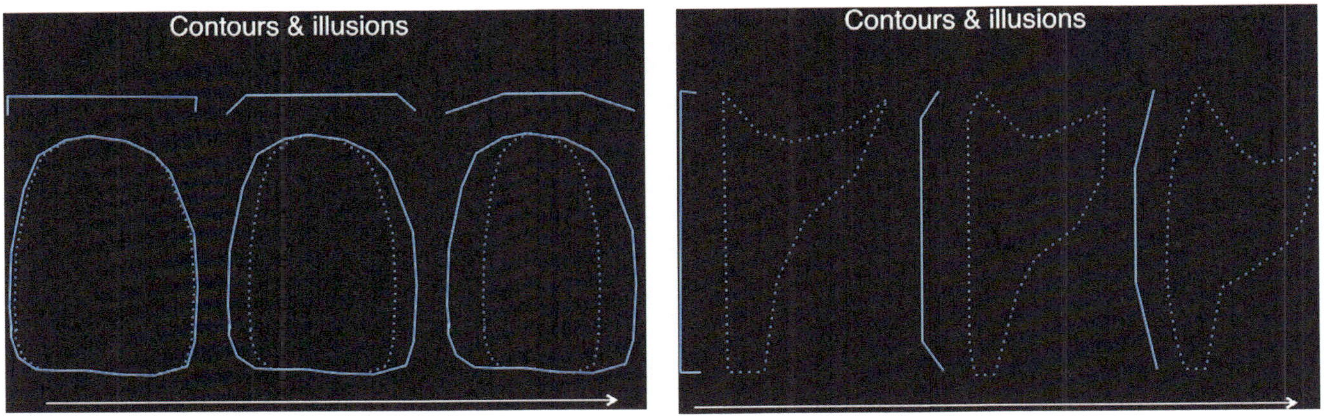

(a) (b)

Figure 1.9 (a) Mesio-distal contours: given a particular width for a tooth to occupy a desired space, moving the facial height of contours inward will "round" a tooth, making it look "narrower" (and vice versa). (b) Gingivo-incisal contours: given a particular length for a tooth to occupy a desired space, accentuating the labial planes will also "round" a tooth, making it look "shorter" (and vice versa).

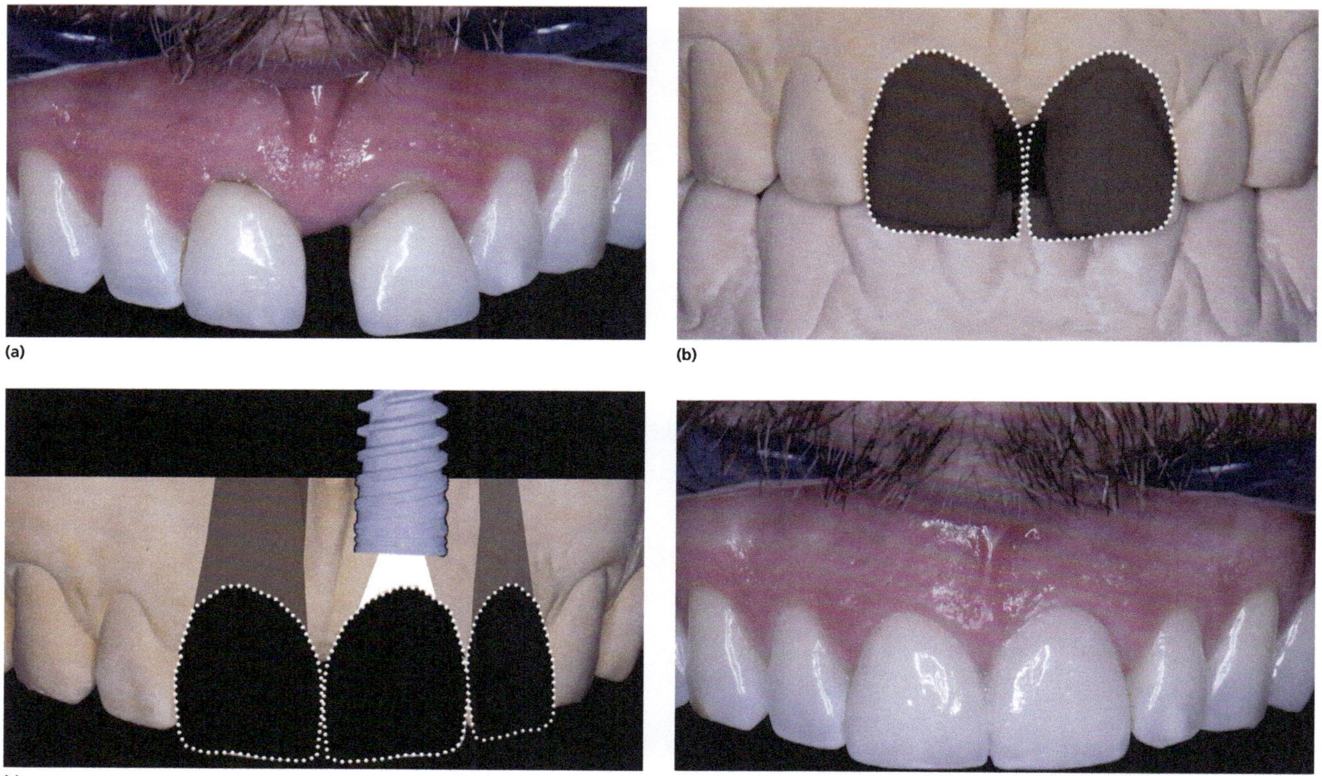

(a) (b) (c) (d)

Figure 1.10 (a) Anterior retracted preoperative image demonstrating a hopeless maxillary left central incisor with a large midline diastema. (b) Esthetic analysis on laboratory study cast; idealized right and left centrals incisors superimposed over the existing sites. (c) Planning for dental implant position with planned tooth proportion changes. (d) Retracted anterior view of definitive results right and left centrals incisors. The patient accepted slightly larger than ideal central incisor restorations in order to avoid having to restore the lateral incisors.

The patient in Figure 1.10 presented for implant consultation to replace a hopeless maxillary left central incisor. The right central incisor had a favorable prognosis. The primary esthetic challenge was a large midline diastema developed following buccal migration of the left incisor secondary to advanced periodontal disease (Figure 1.10a). Prior to treatment, a digital plan was presented to the patient for approval, and to determine if additional treatment of the adjacent teeth would be required to achieve ideal proportions and symmetry (Figure 1.10b and c). The patient accepted slightly larger than ideal central incisor restorations in order to avoid having to restore the lateral incisors (Figure 1.10d).

In cases having a long tapered crown shape and significant interproximal bone and papilla loss, restoration of the teeth adjacent to the implant with veneers or full-coverage restorations may be required in order to move the interproximal contact point apically. This change can achieve a more overall esthetic result, but can result in less than ideal tooth esthetics and squarer proportions. If complex restorative treatments are required to achieve ideal esthetics, it is preferable to advise the patient of this possibility during the treatment planning stage, and have all members of the implant team involved in the decision-making process.

Figure 1.11a–c presents a patient with significant occlusal and esthetic compromise resulting from years of parafunctional occlusal habits combined with chemical erosion and periodontal attachment loss. Performing preoperative direct restorative mock-up procedures can allow these patients to be presented with potential treatment options. In this instance, composite resin was layered and cured onto the incisal aspects without the use of etching or adhesive (Figure 1.11d). Orthodontic wax was used to fill in the open interproximal spaces or "black triangles," creating the illusion that those spaces had been closed (Figure 1.11e and f). This intraoral mock-up was evaluated by the patient, documented with photographs, and duplicated with an alginate impression for the creation of a mock-up cast. The desired final contours were completed with a diagnostic wax-up, allowing predictable replication of contours by the laboratory technician. The definitive porcelain restorations with modified shape and proportions are shown in Figure 1.11g and h.

Inter-arch and vertical space

Inter-arch and vertical space requirements can be one of the most confounding aspects of implant restorative treatment planning, making it imperative to complete a thorough analysis of the inter-arch space in all excursions of the mandible. For single restorations, adequate occlusal thickness for the restorative

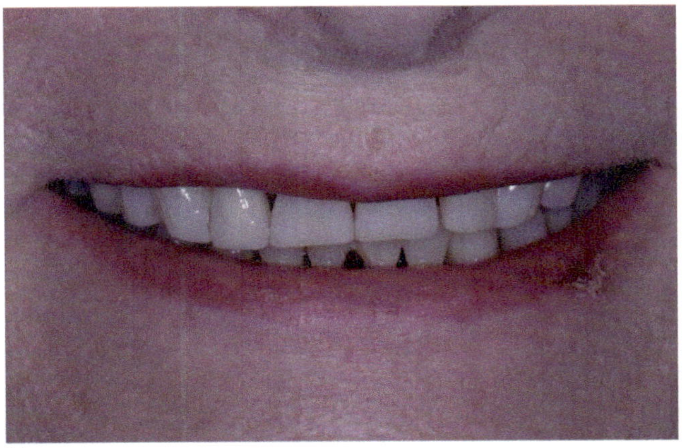
(a)

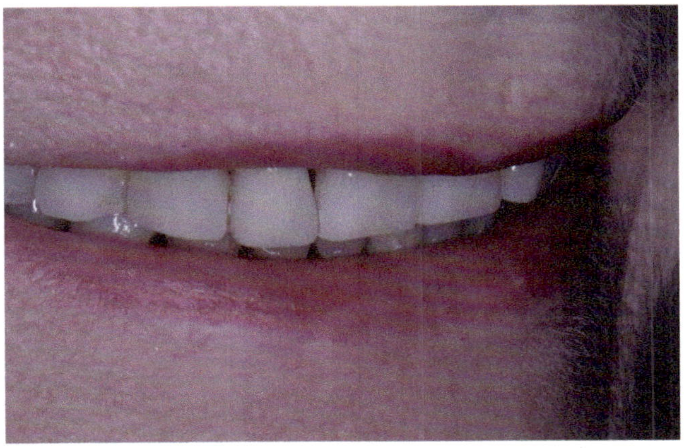
(b)

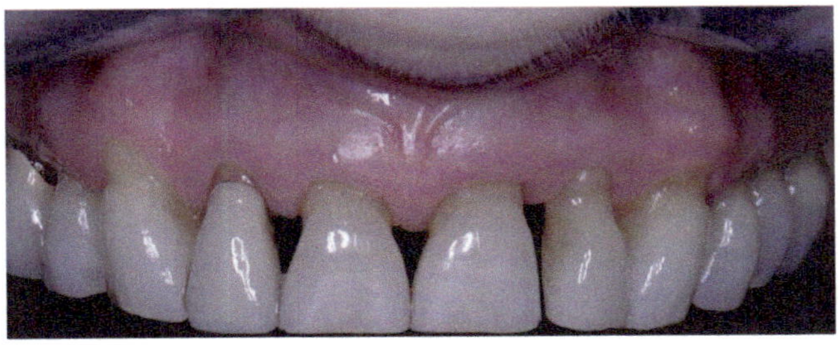
(c)

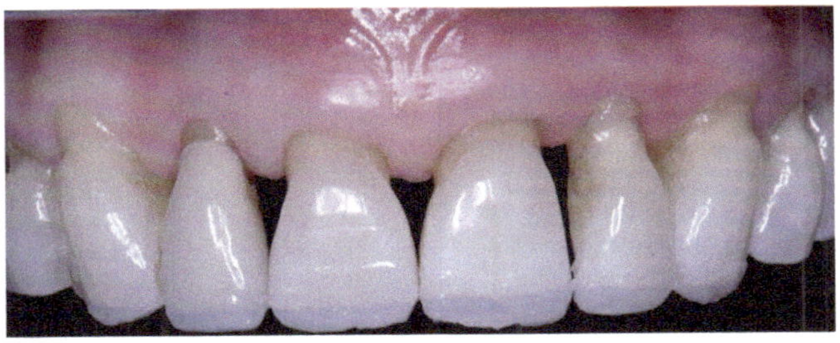
(d)

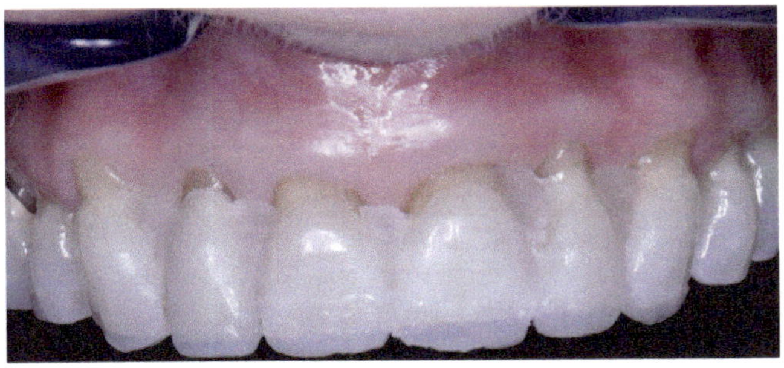
(e)

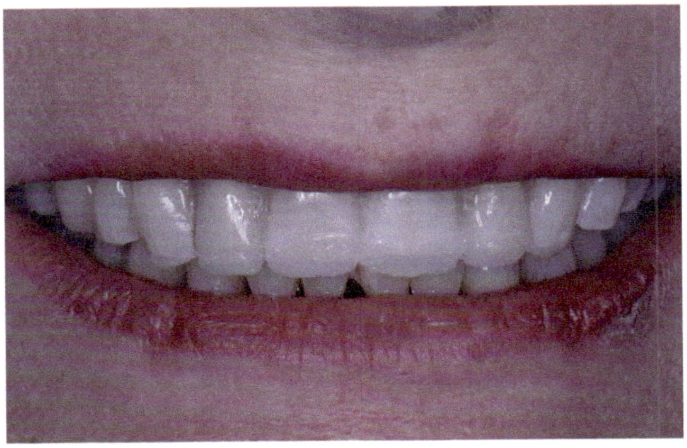
(f)

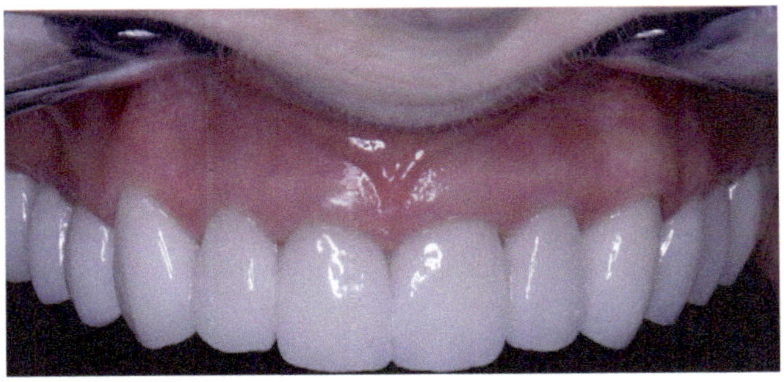
(g)

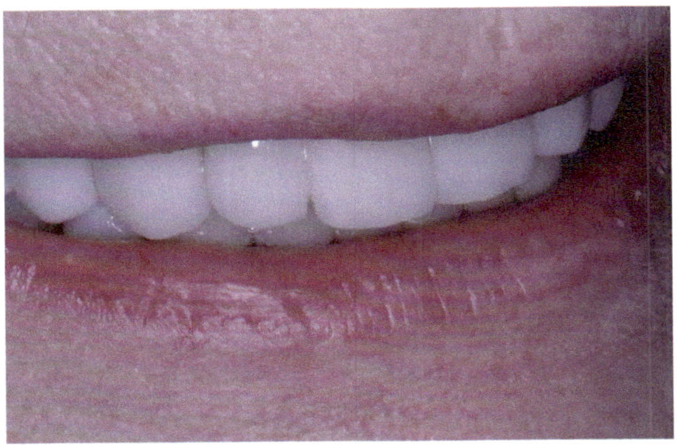
(h)

Figure 1.11 (a) Anterior smile view presents a patient with significant occlusal and esthetic compromise resulting from parafunctional occlusal habits combined with chemical erosion and periodontal recession. (b) Right lateral smile view. (c) Retracted view of the maxillary teeth. (d) Retracted maxillary anterior "mock-up" with rapid freehand addition of composite resin (without bonding agent). (e) Retracted maxillary anterior "mock-up" with white orthodontic wax pressed into gingival embrasures. (f) Anterior smile view of completed rapid "mock-up." (g) Anterior retracted view of completed definitive restorations with modified shape and proportions. (h) Right lateral smile view of completed definitive restorations.

material is mandatory[18] (Figure 1.12a). For zirconium or metal, a minimum of 1.0 mm is required. For lithium disilicate and porcelain-fused-to-metal (PFM) restorations, a minimum of 1.5 mm thickness is required. The cross-sectional areas required for connector zones for splinted multiple unit restorations are 12 mm^2 for short-span zirconia/PFM and 20 mm^2 for longer span zirconia bridges and PFM restorations. Modification of inadequate inter-arch dimension and an abnormal occlusal plane due to extruded opposing teeth can be completed with restorative and/or orthodontic procedures, although the vertical depth of implant placement also must be considered for single restorations. Vertical surgical bone reduction may be needed to achieve adequate prosthetic space for full-arch implant rehabilitations (Figure 1.12b).

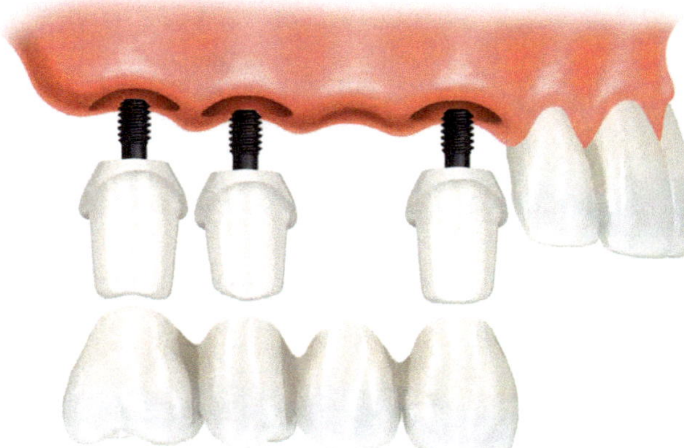

(a)

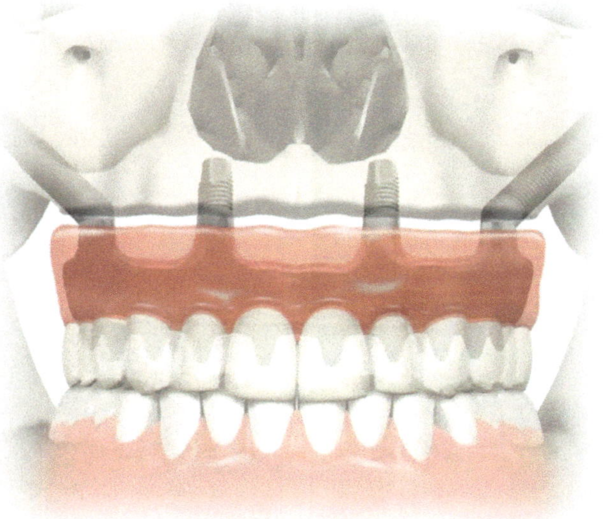

(b)

Figure 1.12 (a, b) Inter-arch and vertical space requirements for prosthesis design need to account for the vertical height of the abutment, major connector, and restorative materials. *Source:* Nobel Biocare. Reproduced with permission of Nobel Biocare, Yorba Linda, CA.

Occlusal stability

Occlusal stability can be improved by idealizing the maxillary anterior cingulum region to provide a stable platform for light centric contacts of implant crowns with the incisal edges of the mandibular anterior teeth. Similarly, recreating simple cusp-to-fossae occlusal contacts in posterior implant restorations should be the goal.

Anterior guidance

Anterior guidance describes the role of the anterior teeth to provide disclusion of the posterior teeth during mandibular movements. The angle of this guidance should be steep enough to achieve posterior disclusion as well as adequate vertical space between the posterior teeth during disclusion. To minimize the effects of potentially damaging forces, the angle of the anterior guidance should be kept to a minimum to reduce lateral and protrusive forces exerted on the anterior teeth.[19] The use of facebow-mounted casts will aid diagnosis, restoration development with the aid of provisionals, and preservation of this critical relationship for use by the laboratory technician.

Phonetics

Natural tooth position and the contours of a fixed or removable prosthesis will influence the quality of speech. Poor tissue profile design with fixed bridges also can lead to difficulty in home-care access and professional maintenance. Poor planning can lead to exaggerated thickness of a removable overdenture or fixed bridge, making it difficult for patients to tolerate the contours and adapt functionally. Improperly designed air space (inadequate pontic design) under a fixed prosthesis (particularly in maxillary arch) can lead to air escape at the tissue level, causing difficulty with pronunciation of silibants.[20] Evaluation of esthetics and phonetics is dynamic, and requires the patient to pronounce "E," "M," "S," "F," and "V" sounds. Having the patient pronounce "E" will exaggerate lip movements and permit easier visualization of the full extent of the esthetic zone. "M" sounds are used to determine the relaxed rest position (vertical dimension of occlusion at rest), as well as the amount of tooth display at rest. In order for "S" sounds (i.e. closest speaking space or vertical speech dimension) to be clear and not "SH-like," the edges of the mandibular anterior incisors should come in "near" contact ("almost" touching) with the lingual of the maxillary incisal edges. Variations can be addressed and corrected as necessary. Finally, for correct pronunciation of "F" and "V" sounds, the incisal edges of the maxillary central incisors ideally need to make contact with the dry–wet line of the lower lip.

Dynamic evaluation of these sounds helps the clinician determine the angulation of the incisal third of the maxillary teeth/implant crowns. The use of provisional restorations can be helpful in facilitating prosthesis design, allowing minor adjustments and a trial period prior to the definitive restoration. Variations expected with each patient can be addressed and corrected. Esthetic zone analysis and the balance of dento-gingival esthetics also require this functional phonic assessment.

The esthetic zone: pink and white esthetic concepts

The esthetic zone is on display during normal speech or animation. Included in the esthetic zone are the "white" esthetics[21] (teeth – presence or absence, symmetry, proportions, etc.) and "pink" esthetics[22] (gingiva – presence or absence, symmetry, color, texture, etc.). White and pink esthetic scores can be helpful for objective assessment as well as in clinical research.[23] However, the overall esthetic outcome is multifactorial and depends on patient expectations and the levels of gingival display. A fundamental challenge in contemporary esthetic implant dentistry is providing a restoration with the proper balance of soft and hard tissue esthetics. Soft tissue contours are critical in high demand cases, and are only predictable with adequate underlying bone support.[24] Bone augmentation, soft tissue augmentation, or a combination are often required in order to provide the foundation for the restoration of esthetic balance (see also Chapters 5, 7, and 8). These augmentation procedures are time-consuming, involve significant financial commitment, and often require the involvement of multiple specialists.

At times, minimally invasive treatment philosophy may dictate a different approach from traditional implant reconstructions. A patient requiring extensive bone augmentation and soft tissue procedures to reconstruct a large alveolar defect may benefit from a less invasive treatment with short, narrow, or angled implant placement (see Chapters 10–12). These techniques can be used with a prosthesis designed with pink porcelain or pink acrylic for replication of the gingival contours.[25] Similarly, a patient with severe periodontal bone loss desiring a full-arch reconstruction may benefit from a less invasive treatment such as a full-arch, screw-retained prosthesis supported by four implants compared with a traditional fixed prosthetic approach involving bilateral bone augmentation and eight or more implants (see "The failing dentition/completely edentulous patient" section and Chapter 12).

A patient who was treated with a minimally invasive approach is demonstrated in Figure 1.13. The patient suffered a traumatic injury to the anterior maxilla. Clinical and periapical radiographic images showed a significant bone and soft tissue defect after loss of the right lateral incisor, canine, and first premolar teeth (Figure 1.13a and b). It was possible to reconstruct this large defect with an implant-supported restoration including a pink esthetic fixed prosthetic with excellent white and pink balance and shade match (Figure 1.13c). The use of a screw-retained prosthesis allowed for periodic removal as needed for prosthesis maintenance and repair.

Placement of the transition line between the prosthetic teeth and soft tissue is an important consideration with the use of pink porcelain or acrylic for replacement of missing soft tissue. Often, the transition line can detract from an otherwise acceptable result. In patients with a low lip line, the vertical or horizontal placement of the transition line is usually not critical. However, all patients should be evaluated for possible maximum display of the prosthesis during an exaggerated smile ("E" sounds). If the transition line is in view, acceptability of the esthetics should be discussed and finalized with the patient. If a horizontal transition line is unacceptable, the implant position may need to be more apical or a labial flange can be used to modify the prosthesis to move the transition line apically with the use of a bar overdenture prosthesis design (see Figure 1.20 and discussion further on). This also requires adequate prosthetic space but allows for adequate hygiene maintenance. The addition of a flange to a fixed prosthesis will result in poor prosthesis contours and limit access for hygiene and professional maintenance, even with the use of a screw-retained prosthesis in these challenging scenarios. Planning and appropriate implant positioning must be determined by the prosthetic plan.

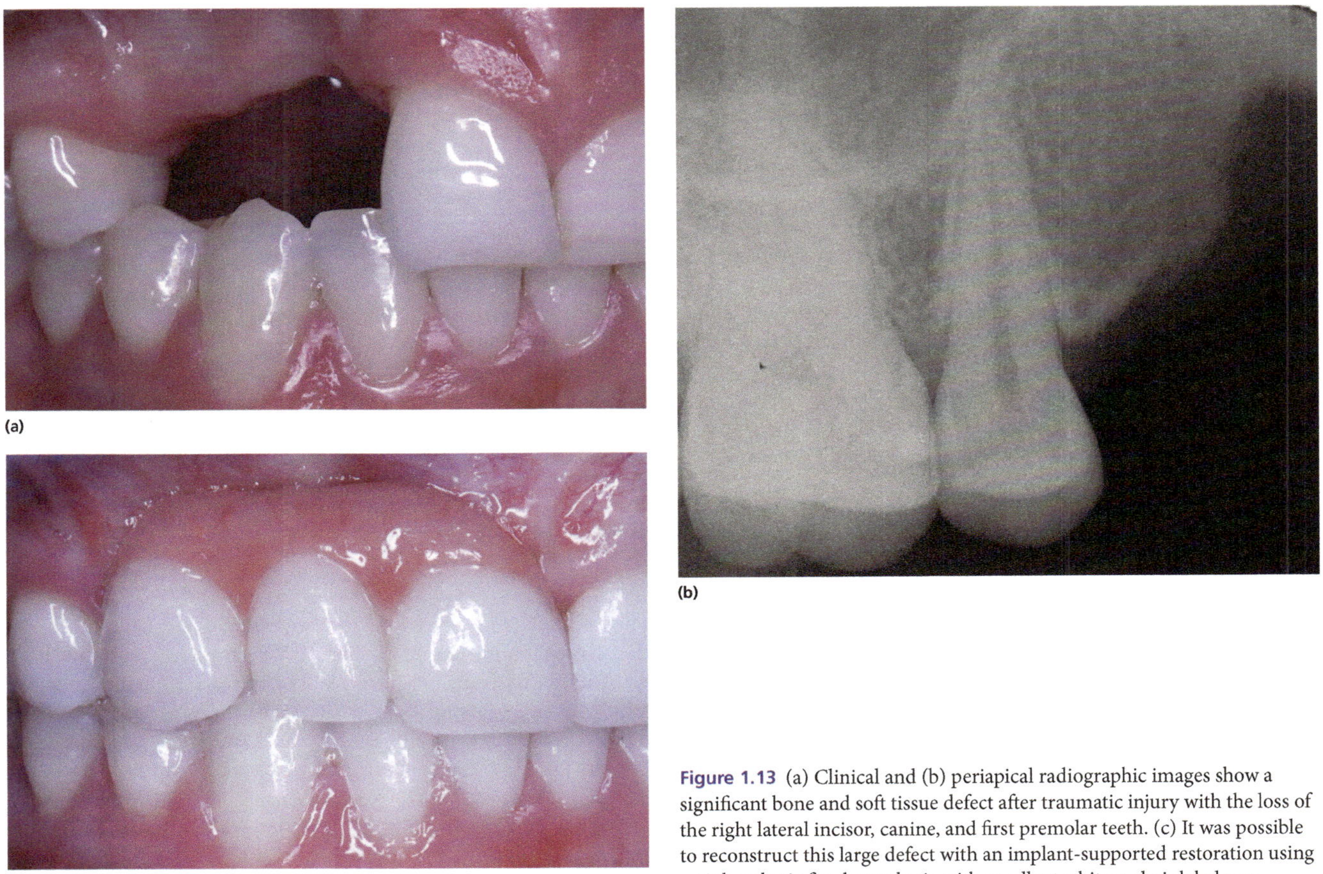

(a) (b) (c)

Figure 1.13 (a) Clinical and (b) periapical radiographic images show a significant bone and soft tissue defect after traumatic injury with the loss of the right lateral incisor, canine, and first premolar teeth. (c) It was possible to reconstruct this large defect with an implant-supported restoration using a pink esthetic fixed prosthetic with excellent white and pink balance.

Planning for ideal implant position

The *interproximal space* between implants and/or teeth is an important consideration for bone and soft tissue stability.[17] Dental implants have no periodontal attachment apparatus with the associated blood supply to help to maintain the interproximal height of bone that is critical for predictable soft tissue levels. Table 1.1 provides a summary of the key dimensions and a classification for tooth and implant spacing and interproximal vertical soft tissue height.[26]

These tissue levels are the result of the bucco-palatal bone width[27] and the vertical and horizontal crestal bone remodeling secondary to the establishment of the biologic width around implants[28] (see Chapter 8, Figure 8.3a and b). For an implant adjacent to a natural tooth, an interproximal distance of 1.0–1.5 mm is required to avoid interproximal bone loss. Between adjacent implants, an interproximal distance of 3.0–3.5 mm must be maintained to prevent or minimize interproximal bone loss.[29] If adjacent implants are placed too close, exaggerated vertical bone loss can result due to merging of the two zones of horizontal crestal remodeling between the implants.[28] Platform-switching and implant design modifications also can help to minimize this remodeling when these crucial interproximal distances cannot be achieved[30] (see further discussion in Chapters 3 and 4).

The ideal *corono-apical position* or depth of placement of the implant prosthetic platform should be 2.0–3.0 mm below the gingival zenith of the proposed implant restoration.[1] The patient shown in Figure 1.14 presented with an esthetically displeasing conventional bonded bridge replacing the maxillary lateral incisors bilaterally. With careful planning for the final level of the free gingival margins of the right and left maxillary lateral incisors, appropriate implant placements were achieved. Figure 1.14b shows an anterior retracted clinical view with superimposed proposed implants in position, with the red lines representing the desired height of the free gingival zeniths. The dotted white lines represent the desired outlines of the new restorations. The provisional crowns are shown in Figure 1.14c after initial soft tissue maturation.

Bucco-lingual implant positioning also is important in maintaining esthetic and functional stability.[31] In the esthetic zone, the buccal plate thickness of natural teeth measures between 0.5 and 2.5 mm at the crest.[32] Preserving this buccal bone or augmentation with hard tissue grafting at implant placement should ensure that a thickness of 2.0 mm or greater is maintained to have predictable and stable hard and soft tissue contours over the facial aspect of the implant.[24] Relationships of the osseous crest and correct bucco-lingual implant placement and trajectory are demonstrated in Figure 1.15. This male patient presented with a chief complaint of a non-restorable, endodontic-treated maxillary left central incisor.

Table 1.1 Salama *et al.* classification of predicted height of interdental papillae

Class	Restorative environment	Proximity limitations (mm)	Vertical soft tissue limitations (mm)
1	Tooth–tooth	1.0	5.0
2	Tooth–pontic	N/A	6.5
3	Pontic–pontic	N/A	6.0
4	Tooth–implant	1.5	4.5
5	Implant–pontic	N/A	5.5
6	Implant–implant	3.1	3.5

Source: Salama H, Salama MA, Garber D, Adar P. The interproximal height of bone: a guide-post to predictable aesthetic strategies and tissue contours in anterior tooth replacement. Pract Periodontics Aesthet Dent. 1998; 10: 1131–1141.[26]

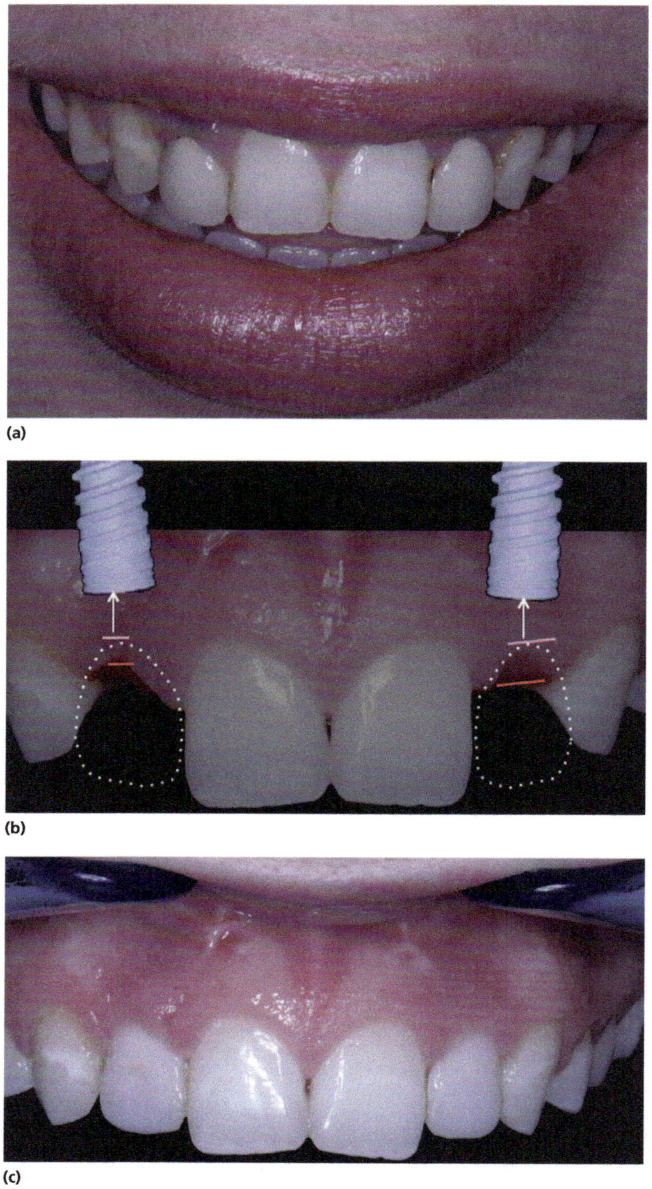

Figure 1.14 (a) Anterior smile view preoperative resin-bonded PFM bridges replacing teeth 7 and 10. (b) Anterior retracted view with superimposed proposed implants 7 and 10 (red lines represent free gingival margins of preoperative restorations; pink lines represent desired height of free-gingival zeniths; dotted white lines represent desired outlines of new restorations 7 and 10). (c) Anterior retracted view of provisional implant crowns 7 and 10 after soft tissue maturation.

(Figure 1.15a) There was significant recurrent decay within the canal preparation (Figure 1.15b). The surrounding soft and hard tissues appeared adequate for a planned implant-supported restoration. The interproximal bony peaks were intact 4.5 mm apical from the desired interproximal contact zones on the mesial and distal (Figure 1.15c). The osseous crest was located 3.0 mm away from the buccal and lingual free gingival margins.

Digital treatment planning included superimposition of the left central incisor mirror image over the edentulous space (Figure 1.15d and e) to evaluate the mesio-distal space requirements.

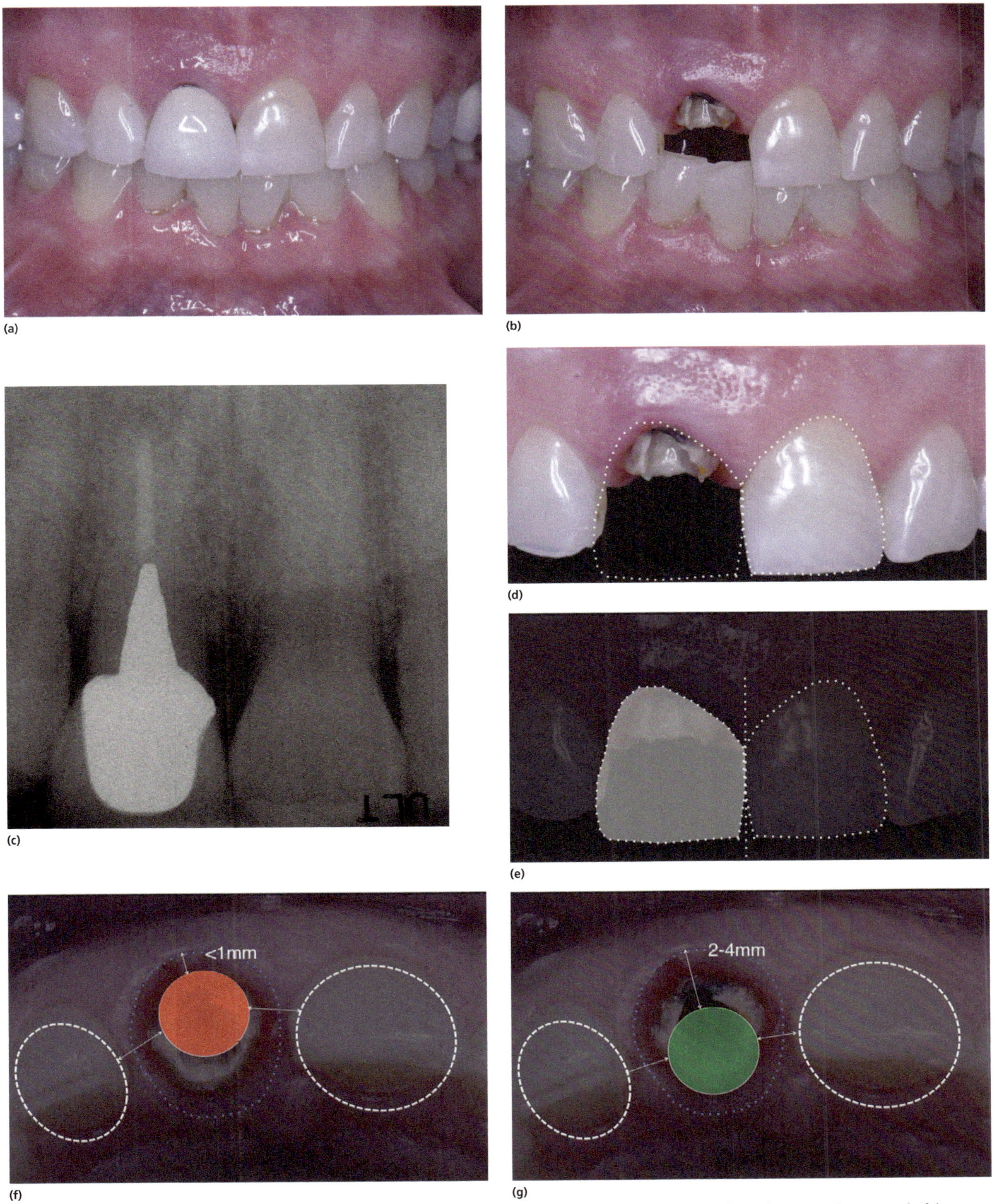

Figure 1.15 (a) Retracted anterior preoperative view of failing maxillary right central incisor. (b) Occlusal view of root fragment after removal of the failing crown. (c) Preoperative periapical radiograph showing intact interproximal bone. (d) Anterior retracted view with superimposed mirror image tracing for tooth shape analysis. (e) Superimposed mirror image tracing for tooth shape analysis with proposed midline and the shaded outline of the proposed restoration. (f) Occlusal view of dangerous bucco-lingual positioning for implant placement in the esthetic zone (too facial). (g) Occlusal view of idealized bucco-lingual positioning for implant planning in the esthetic zone, maintaining at least 2 mm facial gap.

(Continued)

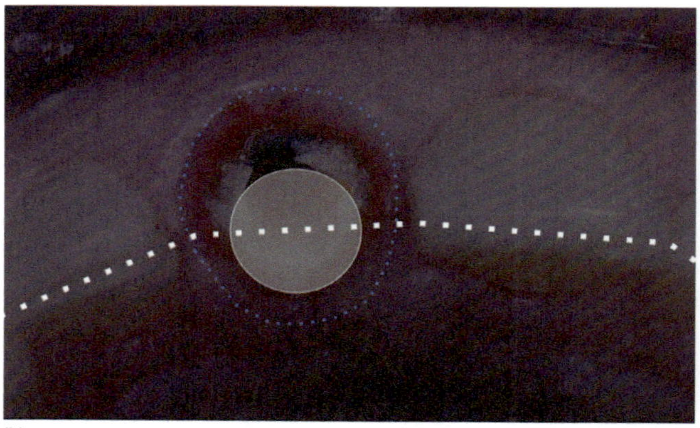

(h)

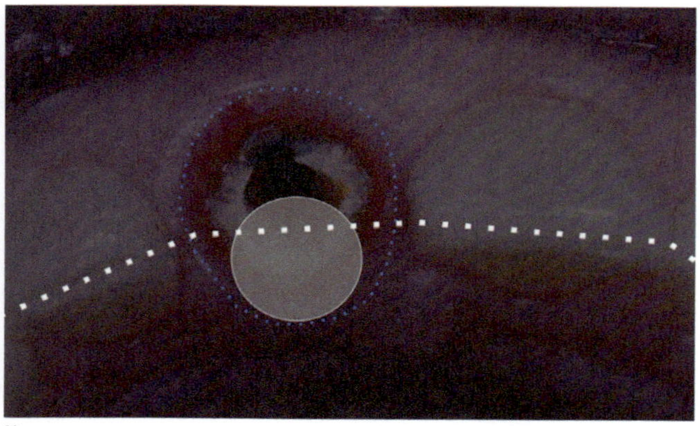

(i)

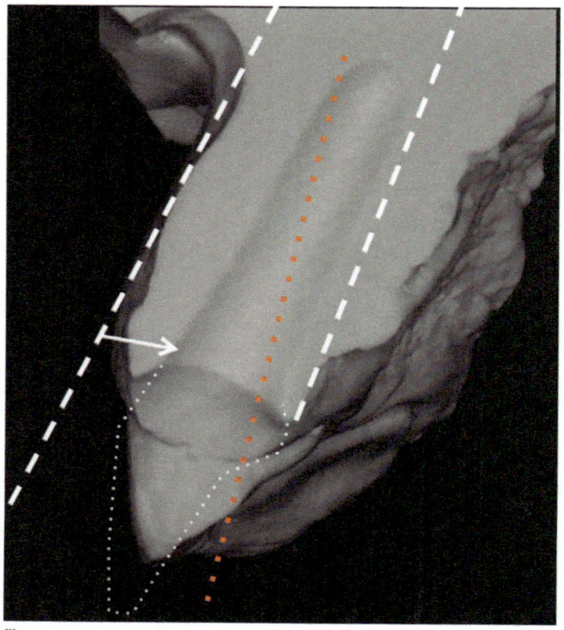

(j)

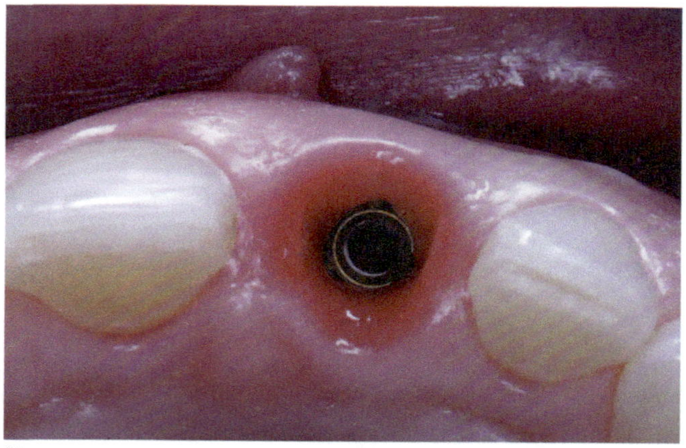

(k)

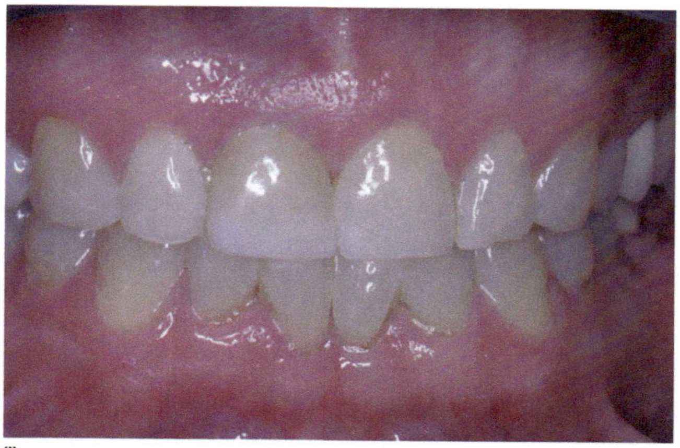

(l)

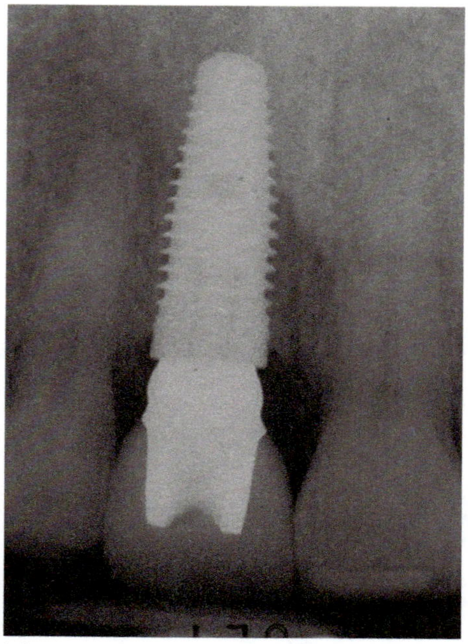

(m)

Figure 1.15 (Continued)
(h) Occlusal view of analysis of bucco-lingual angulation with the access hole location for planned restoration through the incisal edge of the future crown. (i) Occlusal view of analysis of bucco-lingual angulation with the access hole location for planned restoration through the cingulum of future crown. (j) Lateral view of the study cast with a sagittal view representation of (i) showing implant angulation relative to desired restored crown anatomy. The location of the access hole for screw retention is visualized through the cingulum. (k) Occlusal view of the implant and peri-implant soft tissues 4 months post-extraction with an immediate fixed provisional restoration. (l) Anterior retracted view of definitive implant crown at the central incisor. (m) Periapical radiograph of definitive implant restoration.

Correct bucco-lingual positioning of the implant fixture was critical for stable bone and soft tissues and a predictable esthetic result. Ideally, the buccal surface of the implant fixture, when measured at the restorative margin, should be located at least 2.0 mm lingual to the buccal plate contour. If the buccal plate thickness is less than 2.0 mm there is increased risk of soft tissue recession and exposure of the implant abutment. Facial positioning is at risk for horizontal remodeling and recession (Figure 1.15f). A reference line can be made tangent to the buccal bone contours of the adjacent teeth. Implant positioning should be at least 2.0 mm lingual to this reference, and bone augmentation is often necessary (Figure 1.15g).

Bucco-lingual angulation must also be considered in the choice of screw or cement retention for the provisional and definitive restorations. The advantages of screw retention in avoiding peri-implant inflammation and bone loss are well known.[33] In Figure 1.15h, the angulation shown would have resulted in the retention screw emerging at the incisal edge of the restoration (i.e. too far to the buccal). In order to allow adequate restorative material thickness at the incisal edge, a retention screw access opening must be through the cingulum of the restoration, and this dictates that the implant osteotomy be more upright and palatally-positioned (Figure 1.15i). Correct implant positioning with regard to apical trajectory is required in order to achieve optimal positioning of the retention screw for screw-retained implant restorations (Figure 1.15j). This positioning allows an optimal facial bone gap dimension for grafting with immediate implant placement (see Chapters 18 and 19). At 4 months post-extraction, implant placement and immediate provisionalization were undertaken. Figure 1.15k shows the occlusal view of the implant position and peri-implant soft tissues. A periapical radiograph and clinical images demonstrate the definitive implant crown (Figure 1.15l and m).

Implant size selection is dependent on the residual bone volume and desired prosthetic emergence diameter of the tooth to be replaced.[1] Ideally, 3-D imaging should be completed preoperatively to evaluate surgical anatomy of the proposed implant site(s) (see Chapter 2). Implant length should be selected to stay a minimum of 2.0 mm away from the floor of the nose, sinus, and roof of the inferior alveolar canal or from known undercuts. Implant diameter should be selected to maintain the facial and interproximal surrounding bone dimensions as described previously. Often, choosing a slightly narrower diameter implant in favor of maintaining a greater facial and interproximal bone volume can be prudent. Anticipated occlusal loads for a given site also should be taken into consideration, as well as the mechanical risks of using narrow-diameter or short implants versus bone augmentation and the use of standard-diameter/length implants[34,35] (see Chapter 3).

Treatment planning

After review of the diagnostic findings, critical evaluation includes assessment of the patient's anatomy for the presence of any bone or soft tissue defects (see Flowchart 1.1). What are the *patient's expectations,* and are there esthetic zone demands? (See Flowchart 1.2.) Provisional options must be considered with fixed, immediate, or removable appliances and a contingency plan made in the event that a fixed prosthesis is not possible based on the actual surgical outcome. Implications from any *soft tissue transition line* planned for the prosthesis, tooth display, and teeth missing, as well as the patient's age, desires, attrition, and previous dental treatments must be understood (see Flowchart 1.3). Any need to modify incisal edge position of teeth, to employ crown lengthening, and/or to increase vertical dimension of occlusion to enhance esthetics and phonetics must be confirmed. Patients with severe attrition and/or a failing dentition may have exaggerated freeway space or significant dentoalveolar extrusion that will adversely affect the maxillary central incisor position or not allow adequate prosthetic space, requiring occlusal plane changes or treatment with bone reduction and a full arch restoration (see Flowchart 1.4). It is important to assess the skill and experience level of the treatment team to ensure that a minimally invasive treatment approach is indicated and can be completed in a predictable fashion.

The single missing tooth

If a *single tooth* is to be extracted, there must be adequate bone at the buccal plate and interproximal areas to support the buccal soft tissues and interproximal papillae. Esthetic zone demands should be understood (see Flowchart 1.1). With a *soft tissue defect* at a single tooth site, investigation and correction of any underlying bone defect must be addressed whether by bone and soft tissue augmentation as staged procedures (see Chapters 5–8) or with orthodontic supereruption of the adjacent tooth/teeth (see Chapter 20). Slight modification of crown contours and/or the restoration of adjacent teeth may be required to adequately close an existing diastema or compromised embrasure space (Figure 1.9). Use of artificial pink tissue replacement is possible, although often challenging (Figure 1.13).

The female patient in Figure 1.16a and b presented with an implant-supported restoration that had been done after traumatic loss of her maxillary left central incisor. There were significant hard and soft tissue defects present, and the left lateral incisor was rotated to the mesial. There was asymmetry of the maxillary central incisors and a moderately high lip line. No treatment and several treatment options were discussed, including: (i) orthodontic forced eruption of the right central incisor and left lateral incisor to enhance the surrounding tissue, tooth alignment, and rotation; (ii) a conventional fixed bridge supported by the left lateral and right central; (iii) conventional removable partial denture; and/or (iv) prosthetic illusion to minimize the effect of the soft tissue defect with a conventional resin-bonded laminate on the adjacent lateral incisor and alteration of the contours of the replacement crown and left lateral incisor.

Esthetic analysis of two treatment options under consideration can be seen in Figure 1.16c and d, and demonstrates the potential crown contours and gingival level predictions. Treatment option 1 required correction of the gingival recession defect at the left lateral incisor and restorations with contour modifications at the left central and lateral incisors as well as a composite restoration gingivo-mesially at the right central incisor (Figure 1.16c). Treatment option 2 would maintain a longer left lateral incisor to avoid further surgery/orthodontics to correct the gingival recession defect and partially compensate for the slightly longer gingival (apical) margin at the left central incisor (Figure 1.16d). This option would minimize treatment time, the number of procedures, and cost. Owing to the previous extended treatment time (1.5 years at presentation), the patient chose option 2. By slightly altering the facial crown contours and proportions (for the implant crown, facial laminate veneer for the adjacent lateral incisor, and a composite bonding of the right central incisor), the actual size discrepancies were optically minimized by subtle illusions. The treatment resulted in improved symmetry and proportions, as seen in the retracted (Figure 1.16e) and full smile views (Figure 1.16f).

The hopeless tooth

This patient shown in Figure 1.17a–c presented with significant internal root resorption on the right maxillary central incisor.

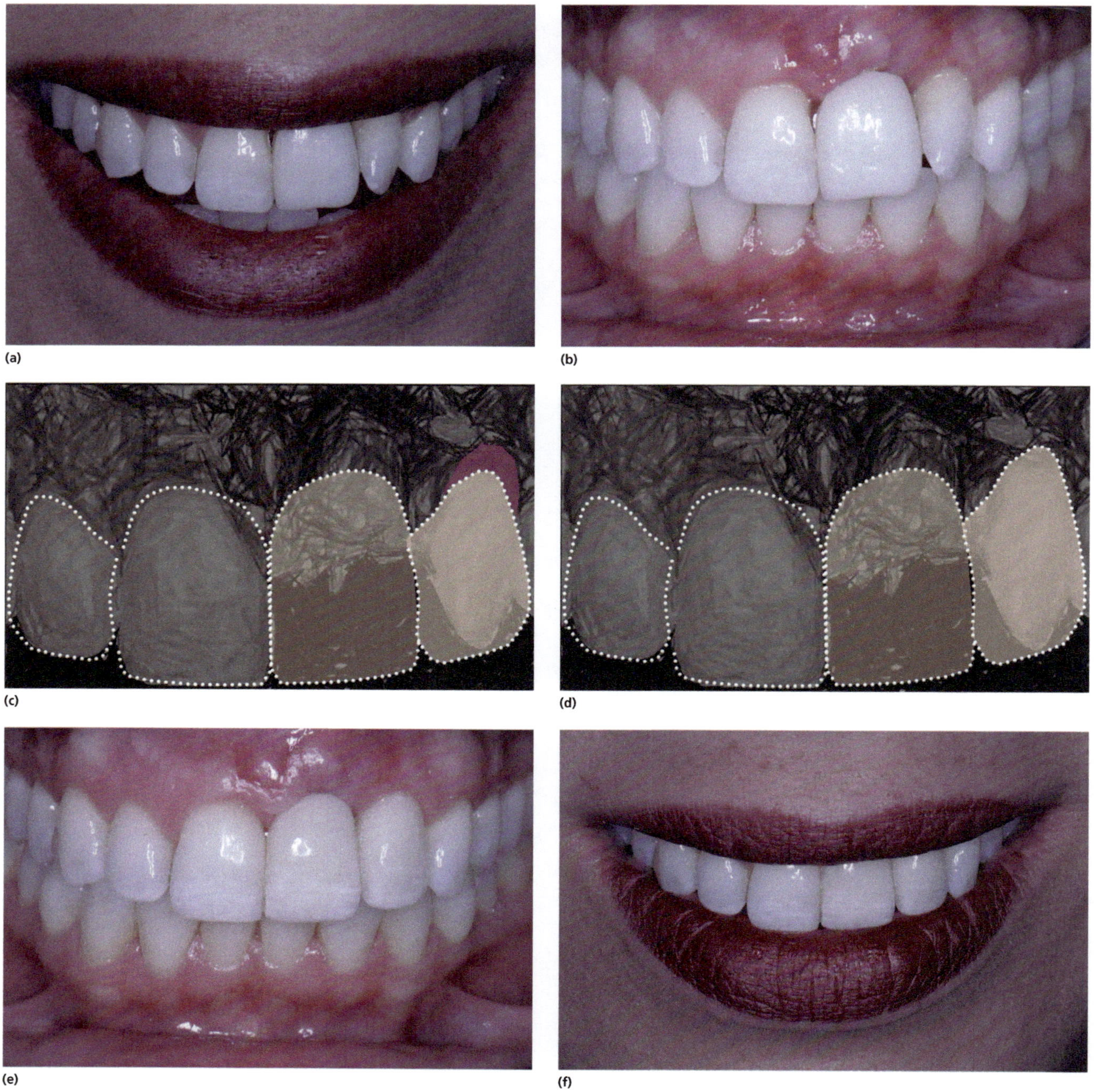

Figure 1.16 (a) Smile view of this female patient after traumatic loss of her maxillary left central incisor. (b) Anterior retracted view of an implant-supported restoration at the maxillary left central incisor, with anterior dental asymmetry and compromised bone and soft tissue levels. (c) Esthetic analysis of treatment option 1 with restoration of gingival recession defect at the left lateral incisor and restorations with proposed contour modifications at the left central and lateral incisors as well as composite gingivo-mesially at the right central incisor. (d) Esthetic analysis of treatment option 2 maintains a longer left lateral incisor to avoid further surgery/orthodontics to correct gingival recession defect. This also partially compensates for the slightly longer gingival (apical) margin at the left central incisor. (e) Anterior retracted view of definitive results after restorations with contour modifications at the left central (implant-supported crown) and lateral incisors (conventional laminate) as well as composite gingivo-mesially at the right central incisor. (f) Anterior smile view of definitive results.

Adequate contours of hard and soft tissues were present for an implant-supported restoration, and consideration was made for a minimally invasive treatment plan (see Flowchart 1.1). Extraction and immediate implant placement for a screw-retained crown included an immediate, non-functional provisional crown with indirect fabrication from a modified study cast (Figure 1.17d). After 4 months healing, Figure 1.17e and f show the frontal and occlusal views. The definitive screw-retained porcelain-fused-to-zirconia restoration displays the emergence contours typical of this anatomic location, and the ideal screw access location can be seen after insertion on the master cast (Figure 1.17g and h). The definitive screw-retained restoration is seen in clinical and periapical

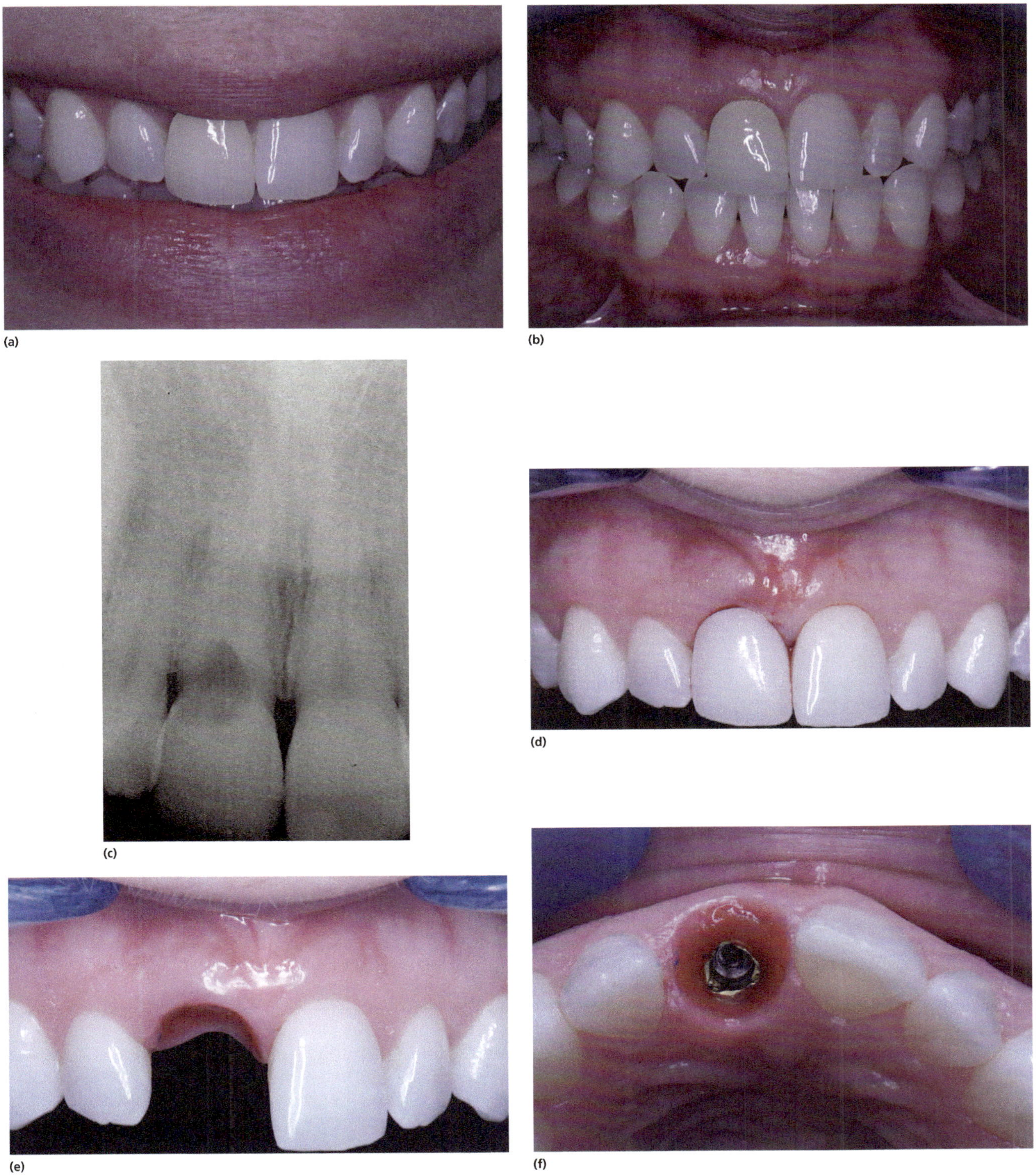

Figure 1.17 (a) Anterior smile view of patient with a failing right maxillary central incisor. (b) Retracted anterior view showing adequate contours of hard and soft tissues present. (c) Periapical radiograph demonstrating a large lesion secondary to internal resorption of the right maxillary central incisor and adequate interproximal bone heights. (d) Extraction and immediate implant reconstruction was completed with placement for screw retention of an immediate non-functional provisional crown. (e) The frontal and (f) occlusal views demonstrate the excellent soft tissue response on removal of the provisional crown 4 months after immediate implant placement with immediate provisional restoration.

(Continued)

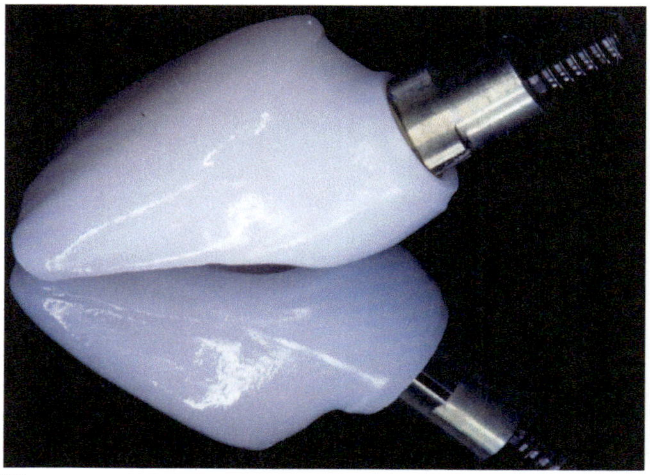

(g)

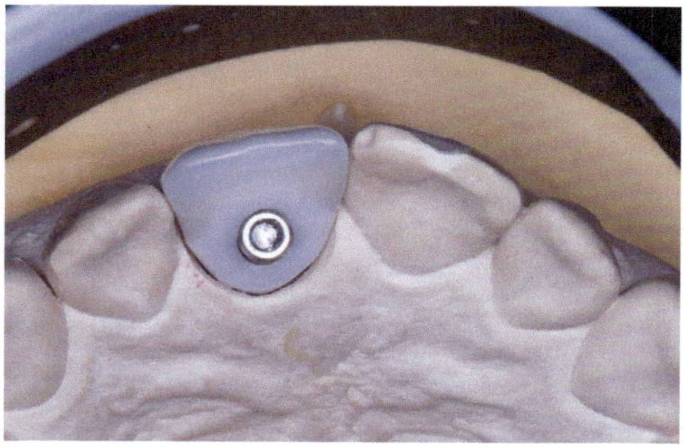

(h)

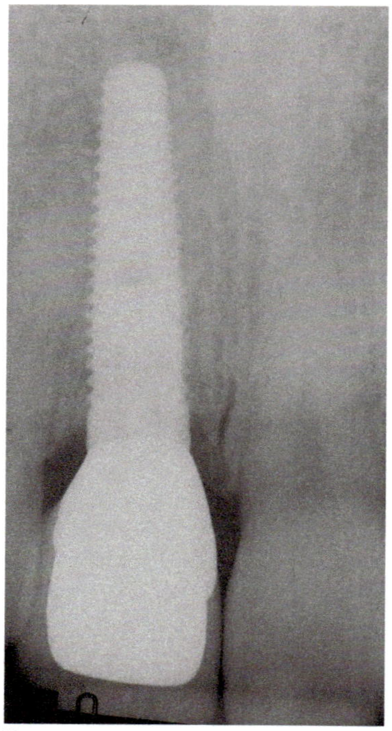

(i)

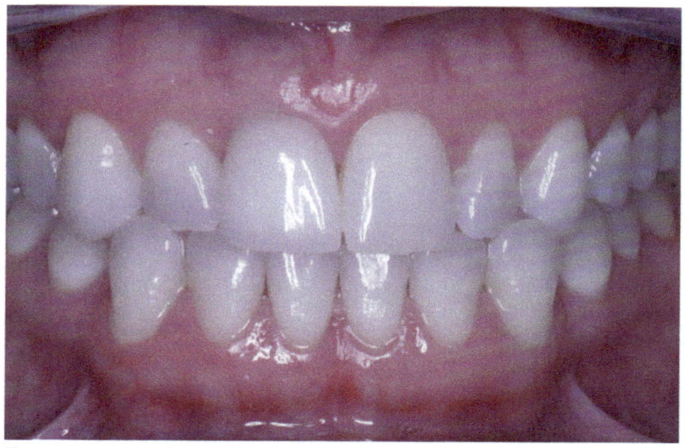

(j)

Figure 1.17 (Continued)
(g) Definitive porcelain-fused-to-zirconia screw-retained crown displays the emergence contours typical of this anatomic location. (h) Definitive screw-retained crown, and the ideal screw access location is shown on the master cast. (i) Periapical radiograph of definitive restoration at the right central incisor shows excellent bone contours and implant positioning with screw retention. (j) A retracted anterior view demonstrates the definitive result with excellent bone and soft tissue contours and implant positioning after immediate implant placement with immediate provisional restoration.

radiographic images to have excellent bone and soft tissue contours after this minimally invasive treatment (Figure 1.17i and j).

Multiple missing teeth

After completion of the diagnostic evaluation of sites with more than one missing tooth, compromises detected with interdental spaces, tooth proportions, and other parameters may require orthodontic treatment, surgical augmentation, and/or prosthetic modifications of adjacent teeth using contour and illusions to improve harmony (see Flowcharts 1.2 and 1.3). Often, staging treatment with initial site augmentation can allow a subsequent minimally invasive approach with guided surgery (see Chapter 9). A comprehensive review of the limitations and predictability of the treatment options should be discussed with the patient.

The patient seen in Figure 1.18a and b presented complaining of an unacceptable implant restoration. Examination revealed implant-supported fixed restorations at the right and left central and right lateral incisors and a restored natural left lateral incisor. There was asymmetry with tooth shape and size discrepancies contributing to an overall displeasing esthetic result. Discussion addressed the esthetic limitations of having adjacent implants in the esthetic zone, and possible treatment options included: (i) restoring the existing adjacent implants with a definitive prosthesis; (ii) submerging one or more implants and converting the affected site(s) to a pontic(s); or (iii) removing and replacing some or all of the implants. Often, in such challenging circumstances, consideration of a diagnostic provisional phase can be helpful in assessing the teeth, soft tissues, and patient expectations (see Chapter 4). The diagnostic provisional restoration used in this patient had improved contours to attempt to correct the esthetic deficiencies and assess the soft tissue and patient responses (Figure 1.18c). The new provisional was designed with the contact points 3.0–3.5 mm crestal to

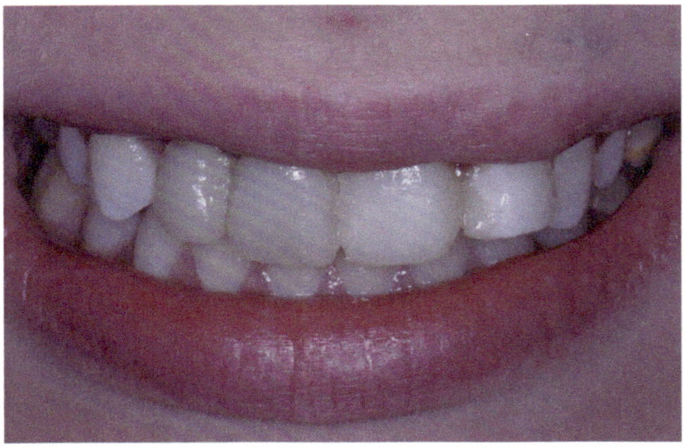
(a)

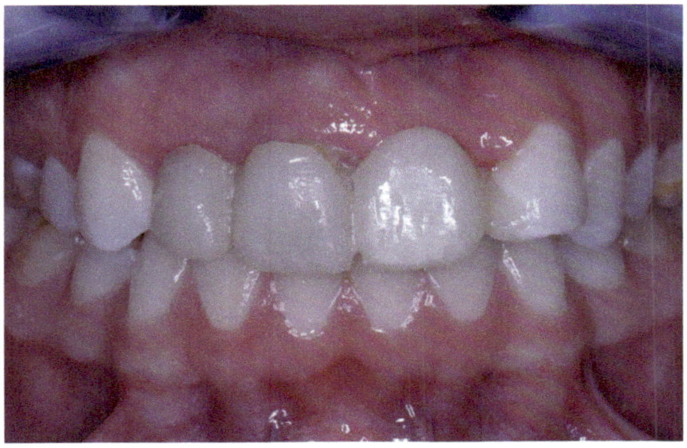
(b)

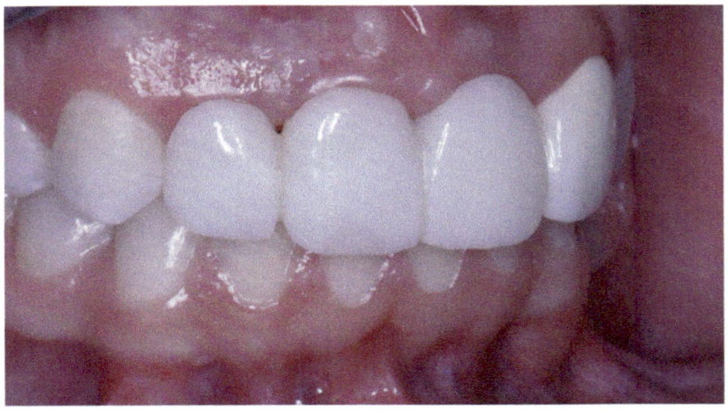
(c)

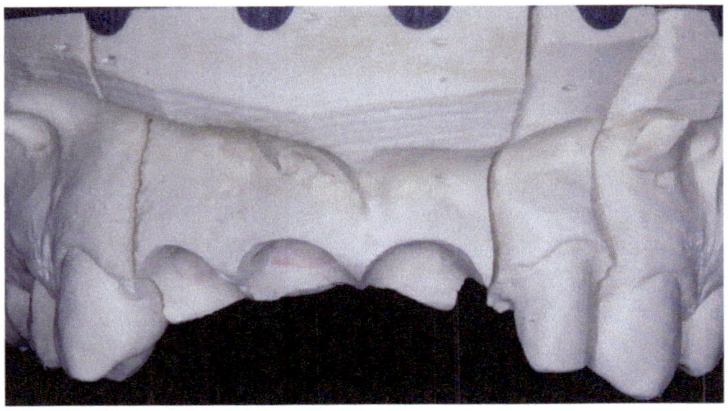
(d)

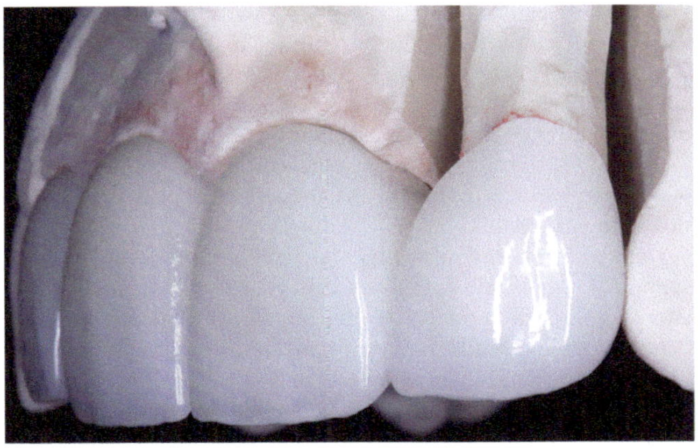
(e)

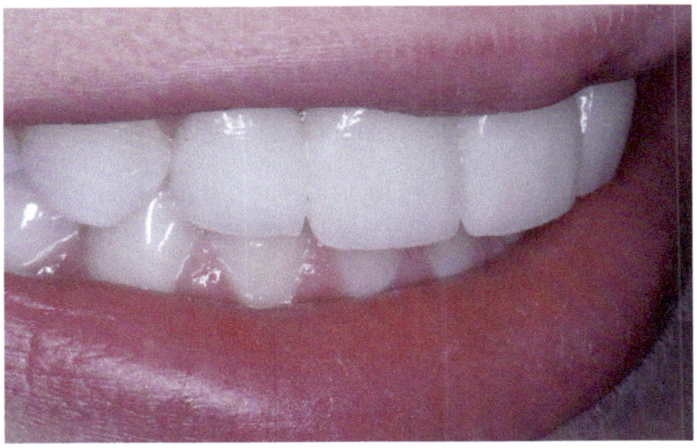
(f)

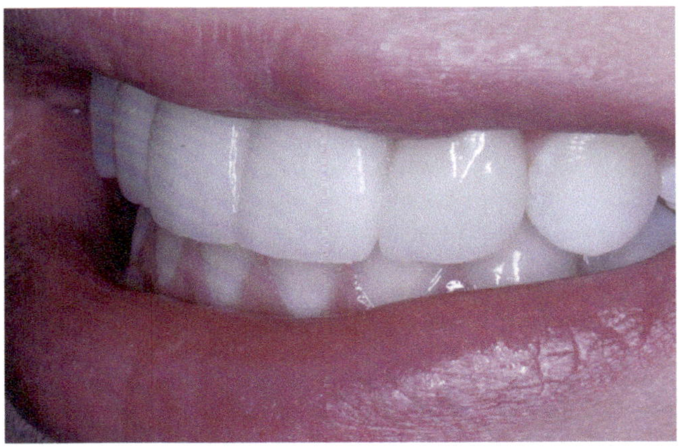
(g)

Figure 1.18 (a) Preoperative smile and (b) retracted view revealed implant-supported fixed restorations at the right lateral and central, and left central incisor locations, with a restored natural left lateral incisor. Apparent tooth shape and size discrepancies and asymmetry were noted, contributing to an overall displeasing esthetic result. (c) Clinical right lateral view of provisional anterior restorations 1 week after placement, designed to correct the esthetic deficiencies, with the contact points 3.0–3.5 mm crestal to the interproximal bone peaks. (d) Anterior and (e) lateral views of customized master cast demonstrating peri-implant tissue profiles on individual implant crowns (right and left central and right lateral incisors) and conventional crown (left lateral incisor). (f, g) Clinical lateral smile views and

(Continued)

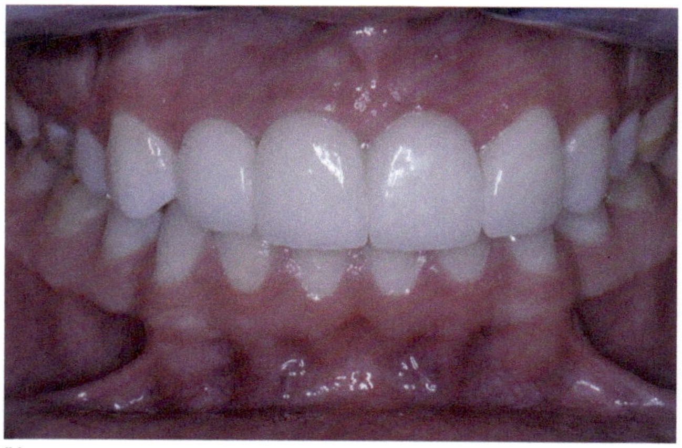

(h)

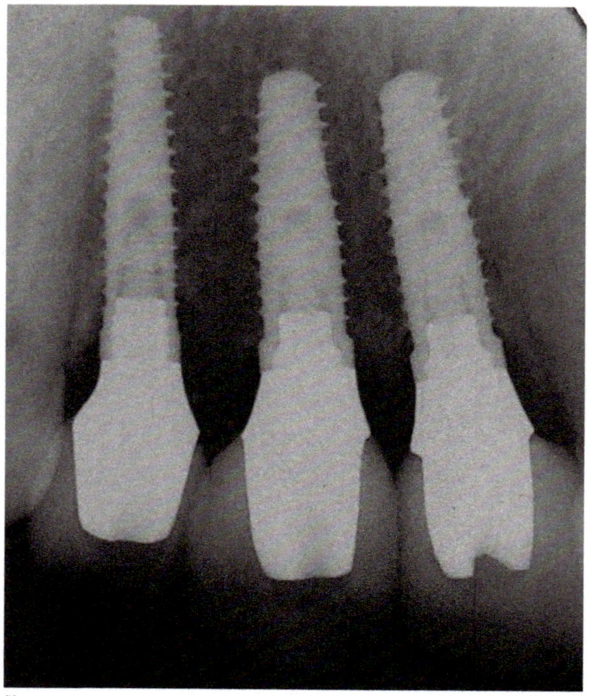

(i)

Figure 1.18 (Continued)
(h) retracted anterior view of the definitive restorations in position with improvement of the white and pink esthetic balance. (i) Periapical radiograph of definitive restoration after insertion.

the interproximal bone peaks. These changes satisfied the patient's chief complaint and allowed the provisional to act as a guide for the final restorative procedures.

During fabrication of the definitive prosthesis, emphasis was placed on transferring the tissue height information to the dental laboratory with custom impression copings and the idealized fixed provisional bridge as the impression transfer. The master cast was modified with custom peri-implant soft tissue emergence profiles at the central and right lateral incisors and a conventional crown at the left lateral incisor (Figure 1.18d and e). Clinical and periapical radiographic images of the definitive restorations are seen in Figure 1.18f–i.

The failing dentition/completely edentulous patient

Treatment considerations for the failing dentition or a fully edentulous patient represent the comprehensive application of prosthetic dentistry principles. Soft tissue display on animation increases the esthetic demand and care in establishing an acceptable prosthesis to the soft tissue transition line (see Flowchart 1.4). The esthetics and phonetics will be determined by the maxillary central incisor positions as the foundation. Minimally invasive treatment options can include implant placement at the time of tooth extraction with two implants placed to support an overdenture after osseointegration is achieved. From a minimally invasive perspective, an immediate implant-supported fixed prosthesis can be ideal. This approach is well-accepted for implant placement at the time of tooth extraction or for fully edentulous patients. The indications for four, six, or more implants are discussed further in Chapters 12 and 21. With adequate primary implant stability, anterior–posterior spread, and adequate prosthetic space, immediate provisional restoration is highly predictable in the mandible. In the maxilla, computed-tomography-guided surgery can be a great asset with planning and completion of the procedure and provisional restoration (see Chapter 9). Alternatively, when planning for fixed full-arch reconstructions, sequential implant placement can be completed in the posterior regions with immediate non-loaded provisional restorations in the premolar esthetic areas. After osseointegration, the posterior segments can be restored with immediate implant and provisional reconstruction of the anterior sites (see Chapter 19). This can allow for continual wear of a fixed prosthesis in the esthetic zone during an extended transition period to an implant-supported, full-arch fixed prosthesis. Figure 1.19a–c show panoramic radiographs of a patient who received sequential immediate implant reconstruction in the maxilla.

Despite the many advantages of fixed restorations, implant-supported removable prostheses can be a viable and less costly alternative. As often required in the maxilla, the flange of an overdenture can be used to hide the transition line. Another advantage is that a removable prosthesis may be utilized with smaller vertical space requirements than a conventional hybrid restoration (cast or milled titanium superstructure processed with acrylic and plastic teeth). As patients age, utilization of a removable bridge (i.e. Marius bridge, spark erosion bar designs, machined-milled designs with plungers, etc.) becomes particularly beneficial, as these prostheses can be designed so as not to move under function but require little force for removal (see Flowchart 1.4). However, the patient should understand the challenges involved in fabricating a removable prosthesis that does not have some degree of movement. Resilient attachments can be designed with a precision metal housing incorporated into the intaglio surface of the denture to help ensure long-term stability and serviceability, and to prevent prosthesis fracture. Figure 1.20a and b demonstrates an implant-supported maxillary precision bar prosthesis secured with plungers in bilateral molar regions.

Vertical space and interarch dimensions require careful consideration as there is typically a need for more prosthetic space with a hybrid design with cantilever components (14 mm) than with

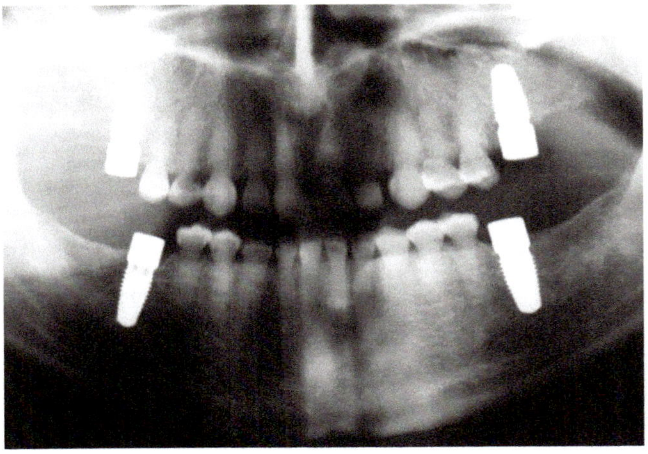

(a)

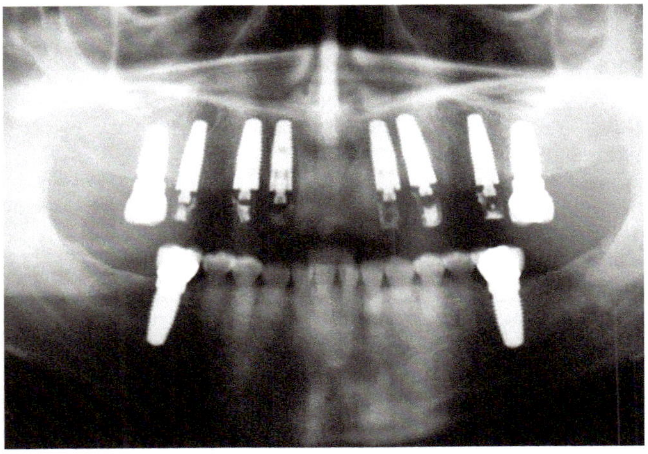

(b)

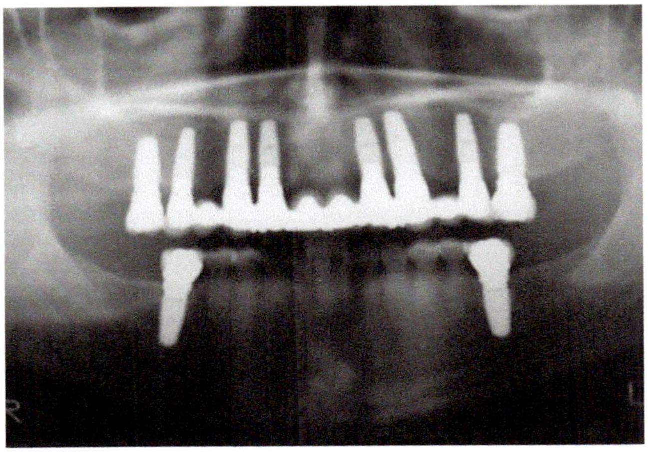

(c)

Figure 1.19 (a–c) Panoramic radiographic series demonstrating sequential implant reconstruction of the maxilla maintaining fixed esthetic provisional restoration through the treatment phases. © Daniel R. Cullum.

a removable bar overdenture or conventional PFM or zirconia bridges. The total height requirements for all implant and prosthetic components must be considered, including the abutment and/or bar, the retentive component and/or bar, the bar superstructure, the denture base acrylic, the pink restorative material, and the teeth (see Flowchart 1.4). All components must be used with due consideration to their material strength, flexion, and wear. For example, a full-arch zirconia appliance in the mandible opposing a complete upper denture can result in wear of maxillary plastic denture teeth, potentially compromising the maxillary smile esthetics over time. Further considerations include reparability and durability. A hybrid restoration with a cast framework is highly reparable

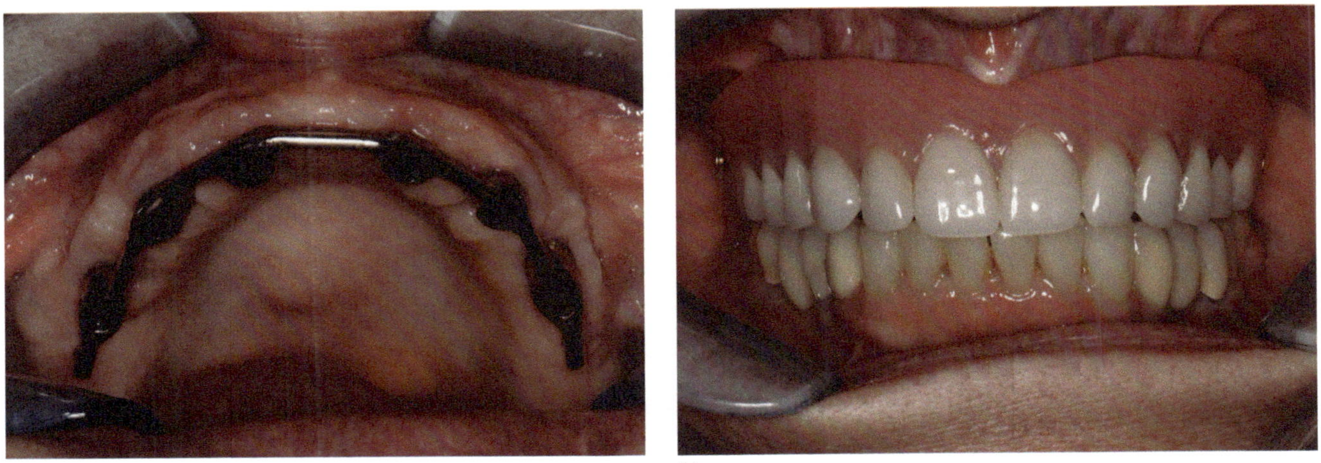

(a) (b)

Figure 1.20 (a, b) Clinical images of an implant-supported maxillary precision bar prosthesis design secured with plungers in the bilateral molar regions. Restoration by Earl Ness DDS MSD. © Daniel R. Cullum.

and can be re-processed with changes in tooth or base dimensions, whereas a PFM or zirconia restoration cannot. Patients with clenching or bruxing habits may benefit from a resilient plastic occlusal surface of a hybrid restoration. Some patients and clinicians prefer the esthetic results of a PFM or zirconia restoration, and patients may require indefinite night guard use with these reconstructions.

Immediate extraction cases, particularly when tooth loss is secondary to severe attrition and/or non-restorable caries, often display loss of vertical dimension over time due to loss of tooth structure and simultaneous dento-alveolar extrusion (Figure 1.21a and b). In these complex cases, simply opening the vertical dimension is insufficient, often resulting in esthetic and functional compromises, including inadequate maxillary incisor display (see Flowchart 1.4). In these cases, the surgical plan must account for required prosthetic space, and bone reduction may be required (Figure 1.21c). After implant insertion, the direct abutment pick-up technique can be used for immediate prosthesis fabrication incorporating a prosthetic design that corrects maxillary incisal edge position (Figure 1.21d–f).

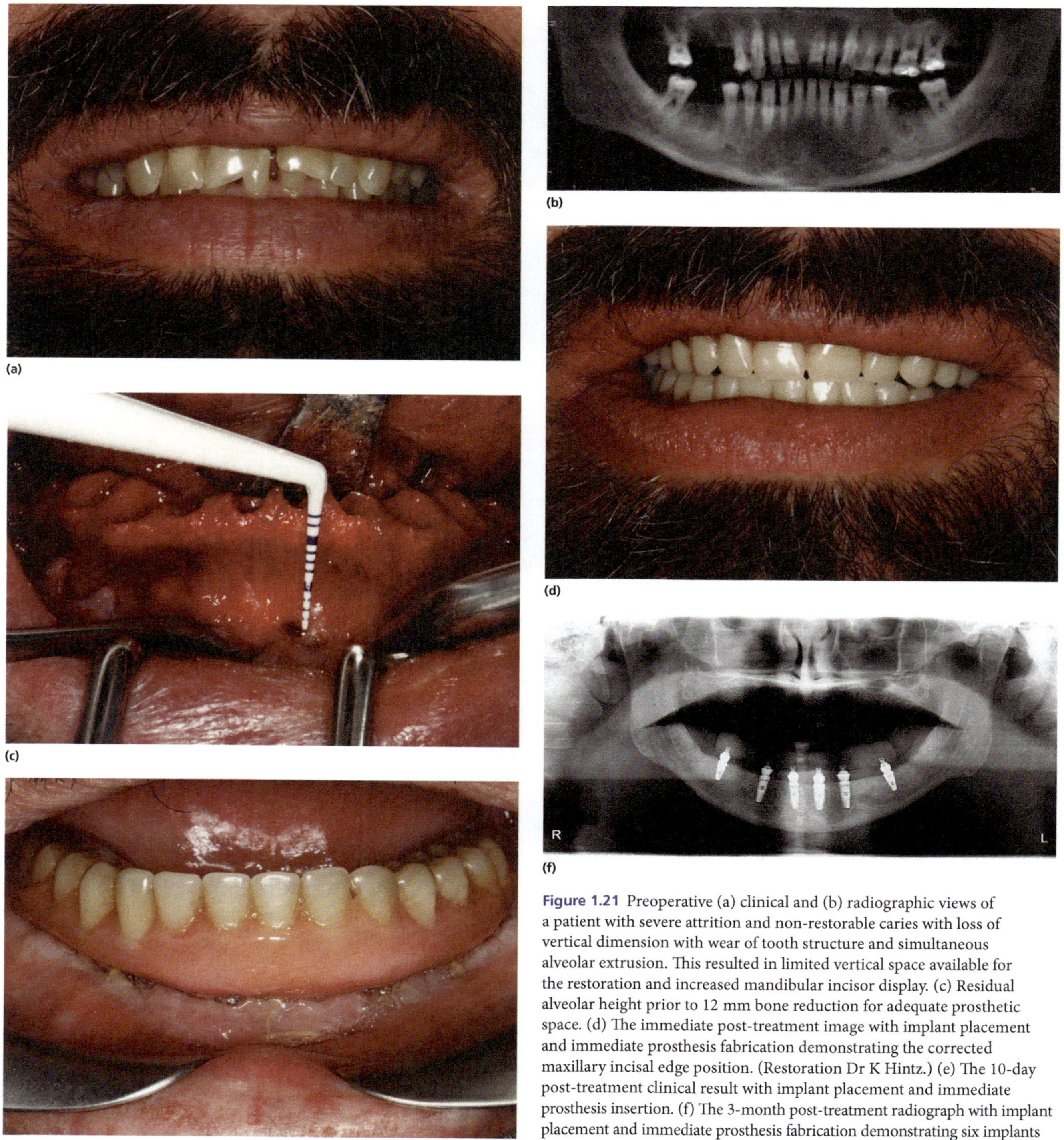

Figure 1.21 Preoperative (a) clinical and (b) radiographic views of a patient with severe attrition and non-restorable caries with loss of vertical dimension with wear of tooth structure and simultaneous alveolar extrusion. This resulted in limited vertical space available for the restoration and increased mandibular incisor display. (c) Residual alveolar height prior to 12 mm bone reduction for adequate prosthetic space. (d) The immediate post-treatment image with implant placement and immediate prosthesis fabrication demonstrating the corrected maxillary incisal edge position. (Restoration Dr K Hintz.) (e) The 10-day post-treatment clinical result with implant placement and immediate prosthesis insertion. (f) The 3-month post-treatment radiograph with implant placement and immediate prosthesis fabrication demonstrating six implants placed for maximum anterior–posterior spread. © Daniel R. Cullum.

The provisional phase can greatly facilitate final prosthesis design and patient satisfaction.

Conclusions

The prosthetic aspects of diagnosis and treatment planning can become more complex if less invasive surgical procedures are anticipated. Clinical evaluation of facial, dento-facial (including the esthetic zone), dento-gingival (gingival architecture, teeth, and occlusion), and phonetic implications must be undertaken. Many diagnostic tools are available, including CBCT imaging, and will help in planning possible therapeutic interventions. Developing an accurate diagnosis is best achieved using a systematic process that is purposeful and meant to gain the patient's full understanding and support. A plan is rarely a singular option, but rather a discussion encompassing multiple possibilities. Application of the concepts of prosthetic camouflage and illusion, white and pink balance, prosthetic space, and prosthesis soft tissue transition lines should be considered. Skill and judgment remain paramount, and minimally invasive approaches require clinicians to be proficient and able to anticipate, prevent, and/or manage potential surgical and prosthetic complications. This chapter has discussed principles for the diagnosis, treatment planning, and prosthetic restoration of commonly encountered clinical situations in the context of employing minimally invasive procedures.

Acknowledgments

A special thank you to Barry Bartee for review and assistance with this chapter.

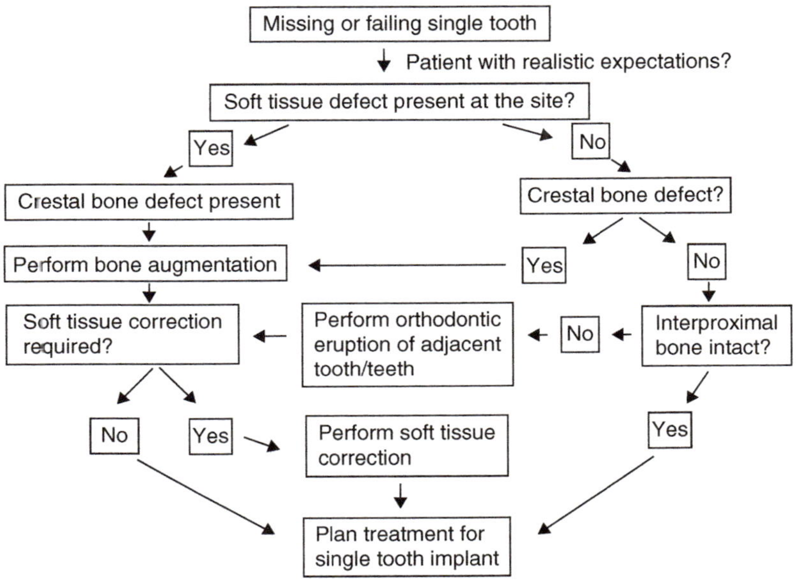

Flowchart 1.1

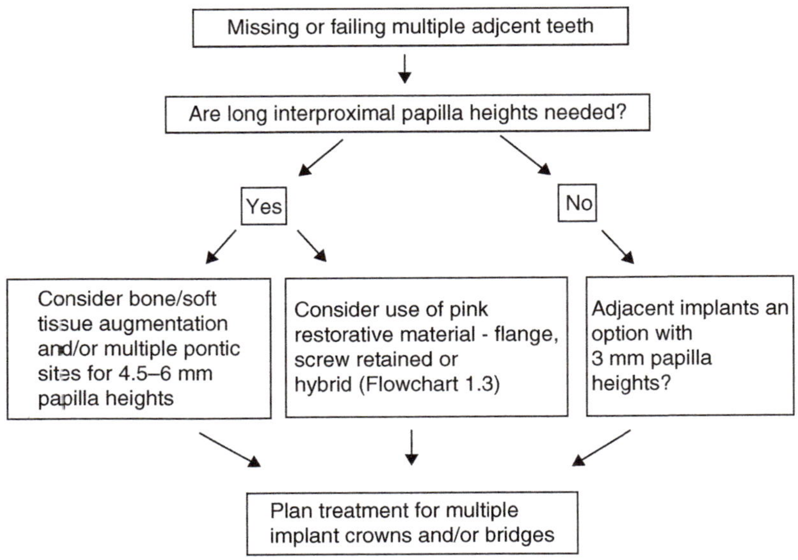

Flowchart 1.2

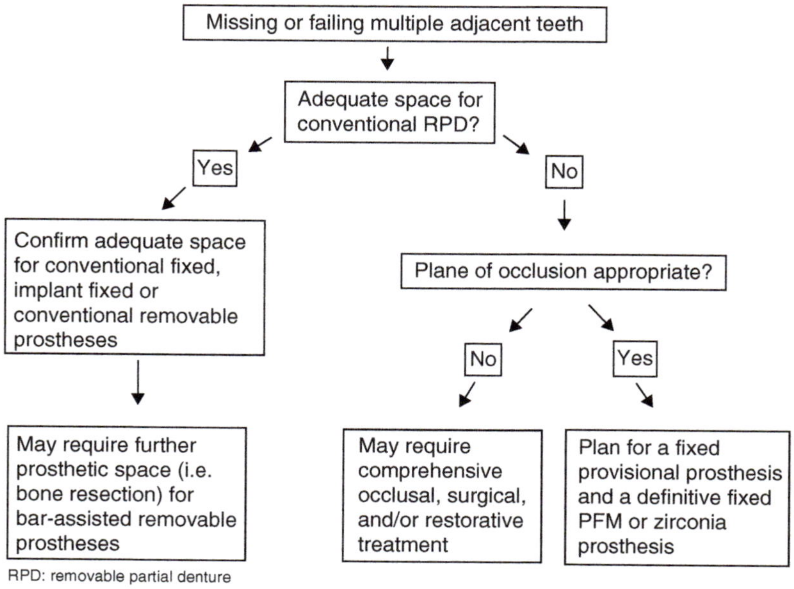

Flowchart 1.3

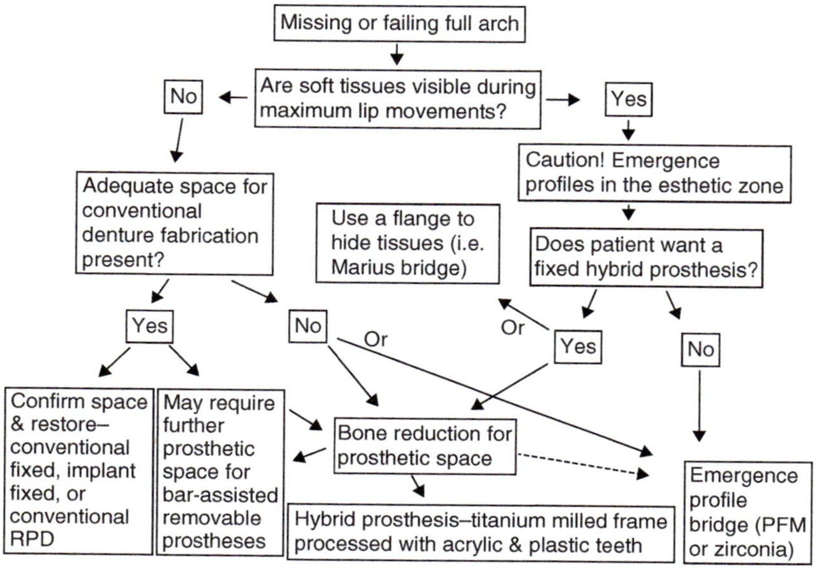

Flowchart 1.4

References

1. Elian N. Dental implants: the biology of esthetic integration. In: Aesthetic Restorative Dentistry: Principles and Practice, Tarnow D, Chu S, Kim J, eds. Mahwah, NJ: Montage Media, 2008, pp. 497–516.
2. Tyndall D, Price J, Tetradis S, et al. American Academy of Oral and Maxillofacial Radiology. Position statement of the American Academy of Oral and Maxillofacial Radiology on selection criteria for the use of radiology in dental implantology with emphasis on cone beam computed tomography. Oral Surg Oral Med Oral Pathol Oral Radiol 2012; 113: 817–826.
3. Rosenfeld A, Mandelaris G, Tardieu P. Prosthetically directed implant placement using computer software to ensure precise placement and predictable prosthetic outcomes. Part 1: diagnostics, imaging, and collaborative accountability. Int J Periodontics Restorative Dent 2006; 26: 215–221.
4. Garber D, Belser U. Restorative driven implant placement with restoration-generated site development. Compend Contin Educ Dent 1995; 16: 796–804.
5. Chiche G, Pinault A. Esthetics of anterior fixed prosthodontics. Chicago, IL: Quintessence Books, 1994.
6. Orentlicher G, Goldsmith D, Abboud M. Computer-guided planning and placement of dental implants. Atlas Oral Maxillofac Surg Clin North Am 2012; 20: 53–79.
7. Goldstein RE. Change Your Smile. Chicago, IL: Quintessence, 1984.
8. Rufenacht C. Fundamentals of Esthetics. Chicago, IL: Quintessence, 1990.
9. Dawson P. Determining the determinants of occlusion. Int J Periodontics Restorative Dent;1983:3: 8–21.
10. Pound E. Applying harmony in selecting and arranging teeth. Dent Clin North Am 1962; 3: 241–258.
11. Vig R, Brundo G. The kinetics of anterior tooth display. J Prosthetic Dent 1978; 39: 502–504.
12. Albino J, Tedesco L, Conny D. Patients' perceptions of dento-facial esthetics: shared concerns in orthodontics and prosthodontics. J Prosthetic Dent 1984; 52: 9–13.
13. Kois J. Predictable single tooth peri-implant esthetics. Five diagnostic keys. Compend Contin Educ Dent 2001; 22: 199–208.
14. Maynard J, Wilson R. Physiologic dimensions of the periodontium significant to the restorative dentist. J Periodontol 1979; 50: 170–174.

15. Kan J, Morimoto T, Rungcharassaeng K. Gingival biotype assessment in the esthetic zone: visual versus direct measurement. Int J Periodontics Restorative Dent 2010; 30: 237–243.
16. Pjetursson B, Thoma, D, Jung R, et al. A systematic review of the survival and complication rates of implant-supported fixed dental prostheses (FDPs) after a mean observation period of at least 5 years. Clin Oral Implants Res 2012; 23: 22–38.
17. Tarnow D, Magner A, Fletcher P. The effect of the distance from the contact point to the crest of bone on the presence or absence of the interproximal dental papilla. J Periodontol 1992; 63: 995–996.
18. Fehmer V, Mühlemann S, Hämmerle CH, Sailer I. Criteria for the selection of restoration materials. Quintessence Int 2014; 45(9): 723–730.
19. Goodacre C, Bernal G, Rungcharassaeng K. Clinical complications in fixed prosthodontics. J Prosthetic Dent 2003; 1: 31–41.
20. Pound E. Let "S" be your guide. J Prosthetic Dent 1977; 38: 482–489.
21. Belser U, Grutter L, Vailati F, et al. Outcome evaluation of early placed maxillary anterior single-tooth implants using objective esthetic criteria: a cross-sectional, retrospective study in 45 patients with a 2- to 4-year follow-up using pink and white esthetic scores. J Periodontol 2009; 80: 140–151.
22. Furhauser R, Florescu D, Benesch T, et al. Evaluation of soft tissue around single-tooth implant crowns: the pink esthetic score. Clin Oral Implants Res 2005; 16: 639–644.
23. Buser D, Chappuis V, Bornstein M, et al. Long-term stability of contour augmentation with early implant placement following single tooth extraction in the esthetic zone: a prospective, cross-sectional study in 41 patients with a 5- to 9-year follow-up. J Periodontol 2013; 84: 1517–1527.
24. Le BT, Borzabadi-Farahani A. Labial bone thickness in area of anterior maxillary implants associated with crestal labial soft tissue thickness. Implant Dent 2012; 21: 406–410.
25. Sumi T, Takeshita K, Takeichi T, et al. Patient-specific gingiva-colored abutments: a case series. Int J Periodontics Restorative Dent 2014; 34: 469–475.
26. Salama H, Salama M, Garber D, Adar P. The interproximal height of bone: a guidepost to esthetic strategies and soft tissue contours in anterior tooth replacement. Pract Periodontics Esthet Dent 1998; 10: 1131–1141.
27. Sigueira S, Pimentel S, Alves R et al. Evaluation of the effects of buccal-palatal bone width on the incidence and height of the interproximal papilla between adjacent implants in esthetic areas. J Periodontol 2013; 84: 170–175.
28. Grunder U, Gracis C, Capelli M. Influence of the 3-D bone-to-implant relationship on esthetics. Int J Periodontics Restorative Dent 2005; 25: 113–119.
29. Tarnow D, Cho S, Wallace S. The effect of inter-implant distance on the height of inter-implant bone crest. J Periodontol 2000; 71: 546–549.
30. Elian N, Bloom M, Dard M, et al. Effect of inter-implant distance (2 and 3 mm) on the height of inter-implant bone crest: a histomorphometric evaluation. J Periodontol 2011; 82: 1749–1756.
31. Chen S, Buser D. Esthetic complications due to implant malpositions: etiology, prevention and treatment. In: Dental Implant Complications: Etiology, Prevention and Treatment, Froum S, ed. Ames, IA: Wiley-Blackwell, 2010, pp. 134–155.
32. Vera C, De Kok I, Reinhold D, et al. Evaluation of buccal alveolar bone dimension of maxillary anterior and premolar teeth: a cone beam computed tomography investigation. Int J Oral Maxillofac Implants 2012; 27: 1514–1519.
33. Wilson, T. The positive relationship between excess cement and peri-implant disease: a prospective clinical endoscopic study. J Periodontol 2009; 80: 1388–1392.
34. Lee E, Gonzalez-Martin O, Fiorellini J. Lingualized flapless implant placement into fresh extracton sockets preserves buccal alveolar bone: a cone beam computed tomography study Int J Periodontics Restorative Dent 2014; 34: 61–68.
35. Renouard R, Nisand D. Impact of implant length and diameter on survival rates. Clin Oral Implants Res 2006; 17(Suppl 2): 35–51.
36. Tawil G, Aboujaoude N, Younan R. Influence of prosthetic parameters on the survival and complication rates of short implants. Int J Oral Maxillofac Implants 2006; 21: 275–282.

CHAPTER 2

Diagnostic Imaging for Patient Evaluation and Minimally Invasive Treatment Planning

Scott D. Ganz
Departments of Restorative Dentistry and Diagnostic Imaging, Rutgers School of Dental Medicine, Newark, NJ, USA
Private Practice, Maxillofacial Prosthodontics and Implant Dentistry, Fort Lee, NJ, USA

Introduction

The continued growth and acceptance of dental implants to replace missing teeth has been dramatic. Dental implant manufacturers have provided clinicians with many innovations by expanding their product lines, improving implant geometry (e.g. thread designs), surface technologies, abutment-to-implant interfaces, and integration with computer-aided design and computer-aided manufacturing (CAD/CAM) of customized prosthetic components.[1] Additionally, there has been a proliferation of biologics, products related to bone and soft tissues and membranes meant to aid in the augmentation of deficient peri-implant hard and soft tissue sites. While most of these innovations relate to the implant after it has been placed, less attention has been focused on the diagnostic phase that takes place prior to a scalpel touching the patient.

During the past 20 years there has in fact been an evolution in diagnostic technology for use with dental implant treatment planning, mainly through the increased use of 3-D imaging modalities. This started with computed tomography (CT), but led to the advent and proliferation of cone beam CT (CBCT) devices. 3-D imaging provides clinicians with an unparalleled appreciation of a patient's individual anatomy. While it is generally understood how important CBCT images are, there are still many misconceptions related to their specific role in assessing a patient's bone for implant placement and the need for associated bone and/or soft tissue grafting procedures. Acquisition of the scan is only the beginning of the diagnostic process.

Cone beam computed tomography data set and software

CT/CBCT scans create a Digital and Imaging Communications in Medicine (DICOM) data set that can be imported into an interactive treatment planning software application, a number of which are available at the present time, including but not limited to, SimPlant® (Dentsply Implant, Waltham, MA), Nobel Clinician® (Nobel BioCare, Gothenberg, Sweden), Invivo5® (Anatomage, San Jose, CA), BlueSky Plan® (BlueSkyBio Grayslake, IL), and coDiagnostix® (Dental Wings GmBH, Chemnitz, Germany). These software applications provide significant new tools to enhance assessment of a patient's anatomy for whatever implant procedure is being planned. They can help to ensure the accuracy of dental implant placement via the fabrication of surgical guides, use of stereolithographic models, and direct links to CAD/CAM technology allowing clinicians to visualize the relationship between the intended implant position(s) and the final prosthetic restoration.[2–5]

There are several basic CT/CBCT radiographic views that are essential for proper treatment planning regardless of the specific software application used. These include axial, coronal, sagittal, cross-sectional, and panoramic views. A computer with appropriate graphics capability is needed to allow display of these interactive 3-D reconstructed views of the intended surgical site. Each of the images needs to be assimilated collectively in order to diagnose every potential implant site, avoid adjacent vital anatomical structures, and plan for ancillary procedures such as grafting procedures, sinus augmentations, ridge-splitting, and tooth extractions.[6] Most commonly, planning mistakes are made when the 3-D tools are not effectively utilized, as many clinicians have inadequate training in the software applications available.

3-D anatomic evaluation

Mandibular alveolar dimensions, undercuts, and the inferior alveolar nerve

The diagnostic process for 3-D planning differs between clinicians depending on training, experience, specific software being utilized, and the type of case presentation. The DICOM data can be visualized with the CBCT device's native software for the initial diagnostic phase. However, clinicians now have the ability to visualize the data in greater detail by importing them into one of many interactive treatment planning software applications with their powerful graphics processors for use on notebook or desktop computers. A 3-D-rendered image can be manipulated, rotated, and magnified for enhanced inspection on the computer screen. In Figure 2.1, the existing anterior teeth, residual roots, and knife-edged alveolar ridge can be seen in relation to the volumetric loss of bone in the posterior mandible. While these images are easy to interpret, they are only one of many views available to aid in the total assessment of the pre-existing anatomy.

Cross-sectional views can be quite revealing, especially for those clinicians who are accustomed to working only with the 2-D information available in panoramic and periapical radiographs (Figure 2.2). It is readily apparent that teeth generally are not surrounded by a large volume of bone, previously described as the "reality of anatomy"[7] (Figure 2.2a). Natural teeth are often buccally situated in the alveolar ridge. There are vital anatomic structures, including vessels and nerves that may be critical to consider prior to implant placement (red arrow, Figure 2.2b). Lingual perforating vessels can cause catastrophic hemorrhagic incidents if damaged during dental implant placement.[8–13] The course of the inferior alveolar nerve can be successfully traced and depicted in

Minimally Invasive Dental Implant Surgery, First Edition. Edited by Daniel R. Cullum and Douglas Deporter.

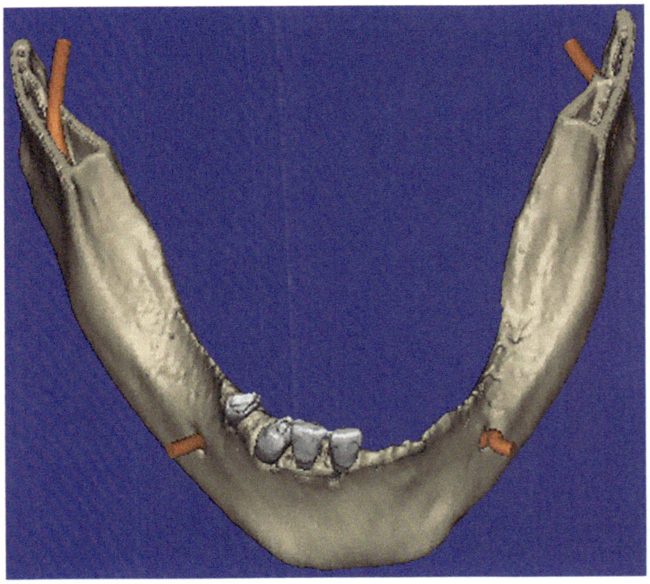

(a)

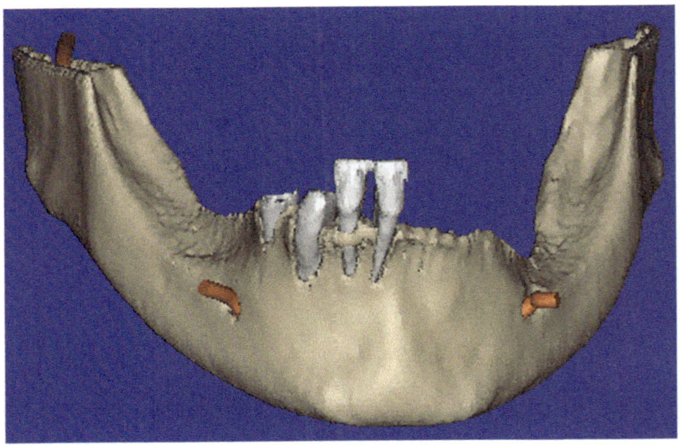

(b)

Figure 2.1 (a, b) A 3-D reconstructed view of the remaining mandibular teeth and knife-edged alveolar ridge seen in relation to the volumetric posterior bone loss.

most software applications from the entrance into the mandible at the lingula to the exit at the mental foramen (seen in orange in Figure 2.3a–c). A knife-edged ridge of the alveolar process can also be clearly visualized. The posterior mandible exhibits a severe lingual undercut (Figure 2.3b and c) that would be undetected with conventional periapical or panoramic radiography, and could result in complications if perforated during implant site preparation.[14,15] Additionally, the posterior mandible can be a donor site for block bone grafting; and if used for this purpose, visualizing the path of the inferior alveolar nerve and its proximity to the buccal cortex is essential to prevent nerve injury and potential paresthesia.[16] The topography of the posterior mandible can be further illustrated by slicing or "clipping" through the 3-D reconstructed image, as seen in Figure 2.3c.

Advances in software capabilities with tools that allow virtual tooth extraction (Figure 2.4a and b) and alteration of image opacity can further aid planning by clinicians.[17] The lateral 3-D reconstructed mandibular view in Figure 2.5a and b was manipulated to alter its opacity, thus making it possible to see the volumetric bone loss and the location of the mental foramen and the entire path of the underlying inferior alveolar nerve. This manipulation with software has been termed "selective transparency."[6,16] The ability to manage the transparencies of individual parts of a patient's anatomy or of simulated implants, abutments, virtual teeth, or optical information imported from desktop computers or intraoral scanners greatly enhances diagnostic accuracy.

The maxillary sinus, ostiomeatal complex, pathology and grafting

The maxilla is an integral part of the skull containing the maxillary teeth, associated sinus and nasal cavities, nerves, and vessels. An axial image of the maxilla reveals the bilateral maxillary sinus cavities,

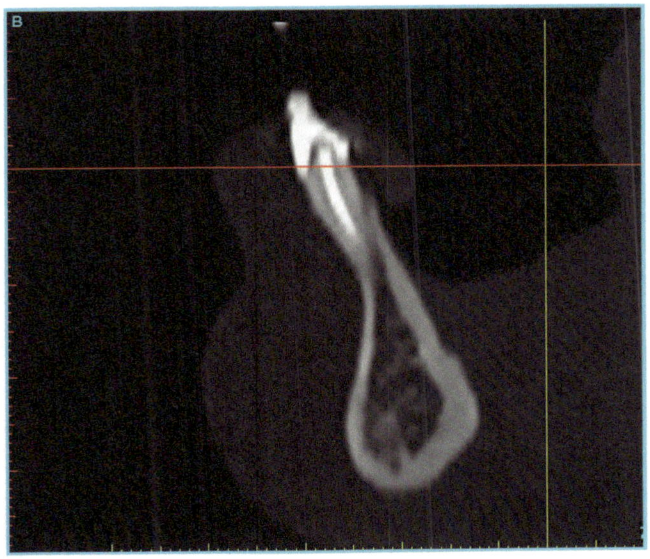

(a)

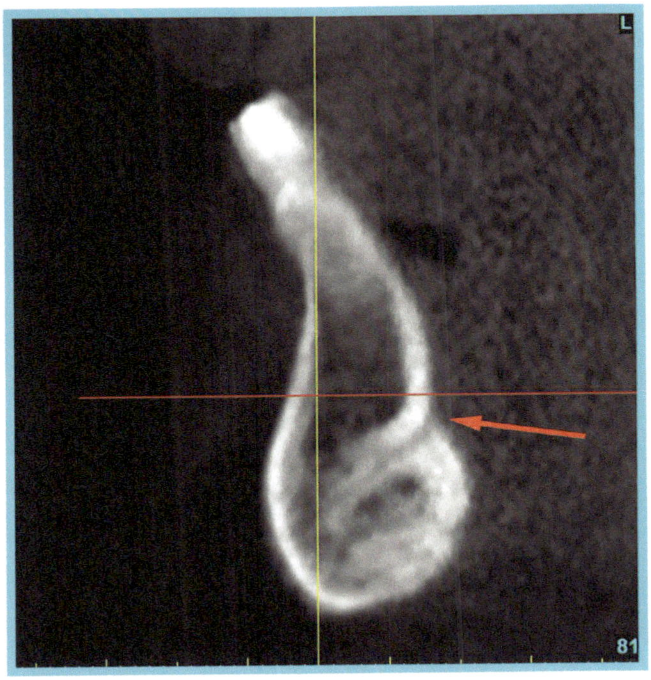

(b)

Figure 2.2 (a) The cross-sectional view of the buccal bone. (b) At the midline of the symphysis, lingual perforating vessels are often found (arrow).

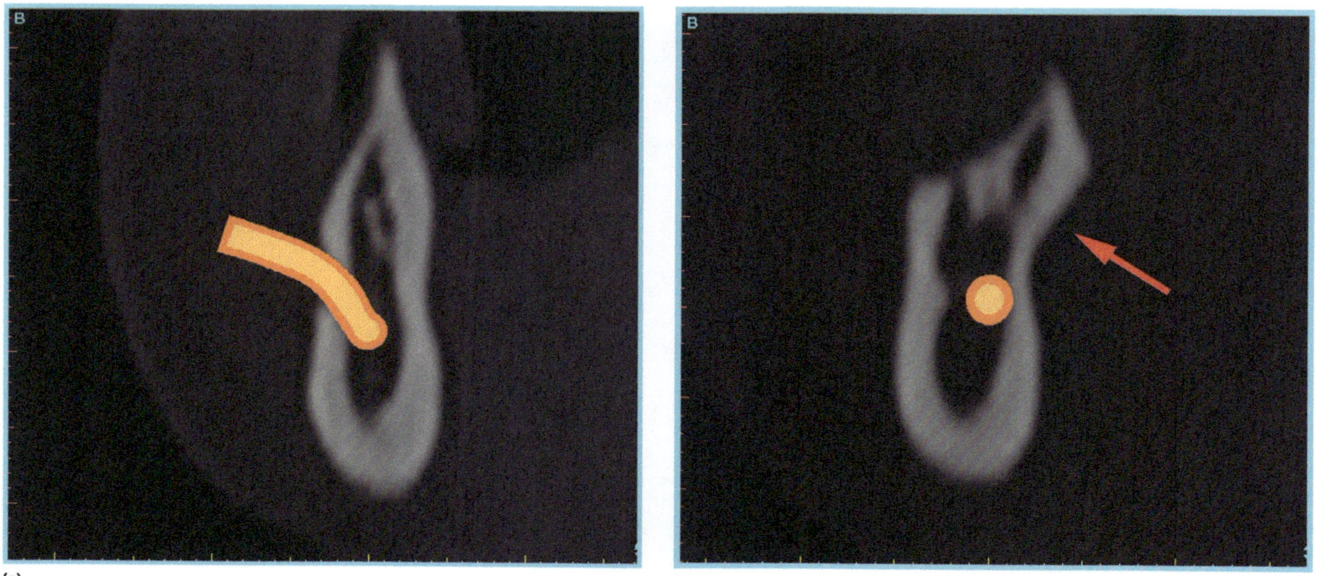

(a) (b)

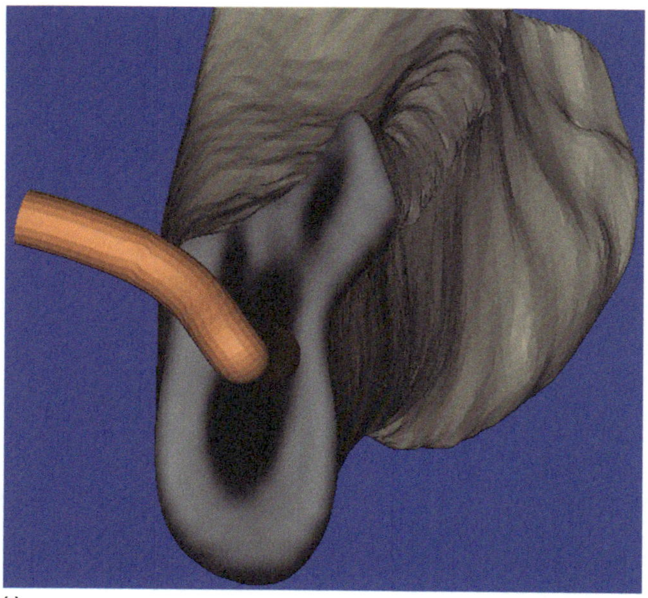

(c)

Figure 2.3 (a) Cross-sectional view of the nerve (orange) exiting the mental foramen. (b) The posterior mandible exhibits a severe lingual undercut (arrow) undetected with conventional periapical or panoramic radiography. (c) The topography of the posterior mandible illustrated by slicing or "clipping" through the 3-D reconstructed image.

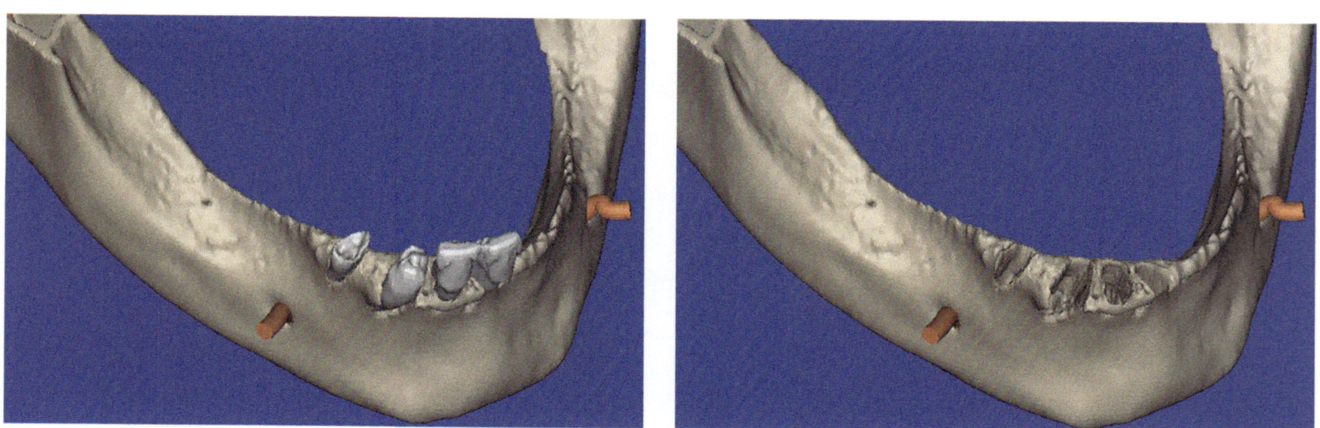

(a) (b)

Figure 2.4 (a, b) Advanced software functionality allows virtual extraction of teeth helping to visualize the residual sockets as an aid in planning.

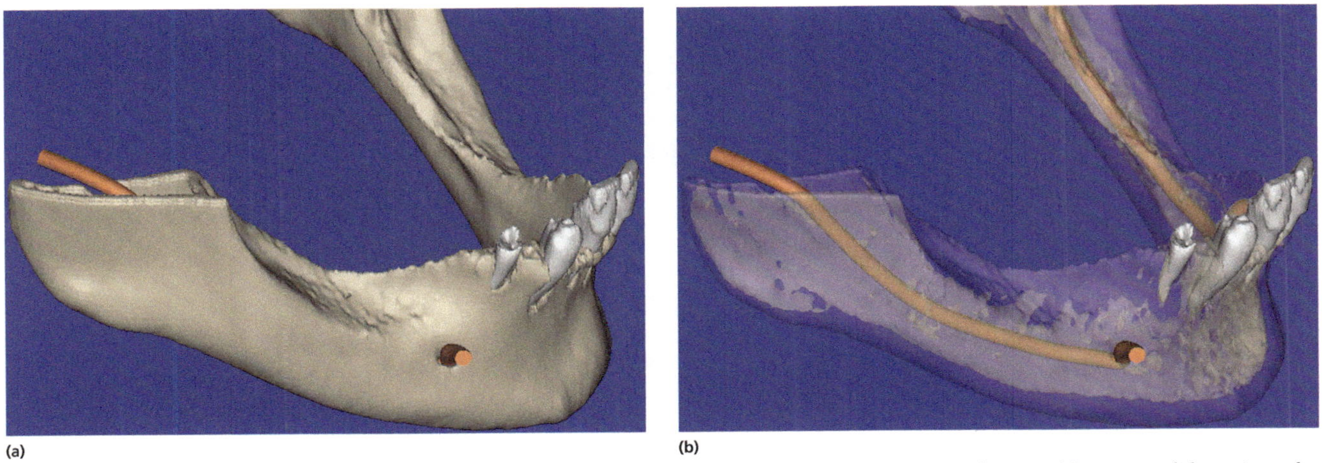

Figure 2.5 The lateral 3-D reconstructed mandibular view (a) was manipulated to alter its opacity to help inspect the mental foramen and the entire path of the underlying inferior alveolar nerve (b).

turbinates, and ethmoid and sphenoid sinuses (Figure 2.6a). Of particular interest in this view is the area of drainage for the frontal, anterior ethmoid, and maxillary sinuses called the ostia, ostiomeatal complex, or ostiomeatal unit. A narrowing or blockage of the ostia can cause sinus inflammation and potential serious complications, and is important to assess when sinus grafting is being considered as part of implant treatment. The coronal images reveal the maxillary sinuses, but also show the right and left endentulous aveoli (Figure 2.6b). Scrolling through the images revealed a clear left sinus but pathology in the right sinus (green arrow, Figures 2.7 and 2.8a).

When considering implant placement in the posterior maxilla, the volume of alveolar ridge and the proximity of the maxillary sinus floor must be assessed. Cross-sectional images allow for an excellent appraisal of the lateral and medial walls of the sinus and crestal bone volume (Figure 2.8a). The thin cortical bone and lack of alveolar ridge height in this example would indicate the need for a significant sinus graft (red arrows). A small polyp can be seen on the lateral wall (green arrow). The maxillary sinus walls are known to house vascular canals, which can often be visualized with CBCT imaging[18–22] (Figure 2.8b, red arrows). Jung et al. examined 250 patients scheduled for implant surgery and found a maxillary arterial endosseous anastomosis in 52.8% of cases.[23] Additionally, measurements were

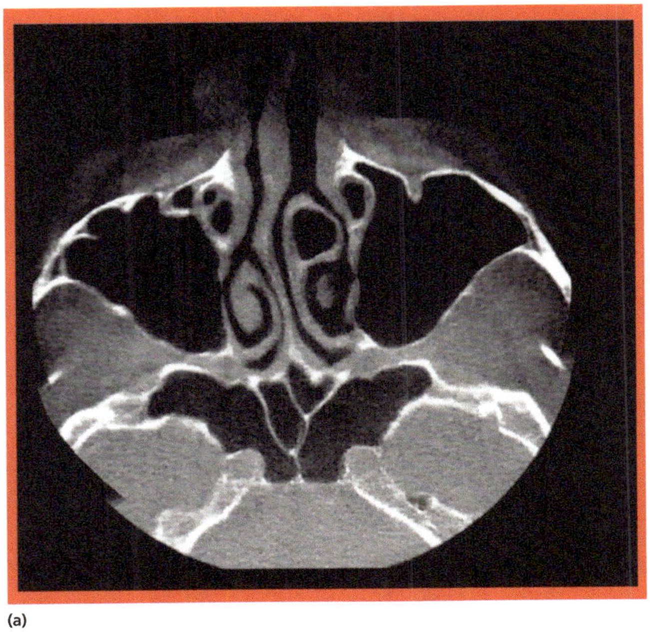

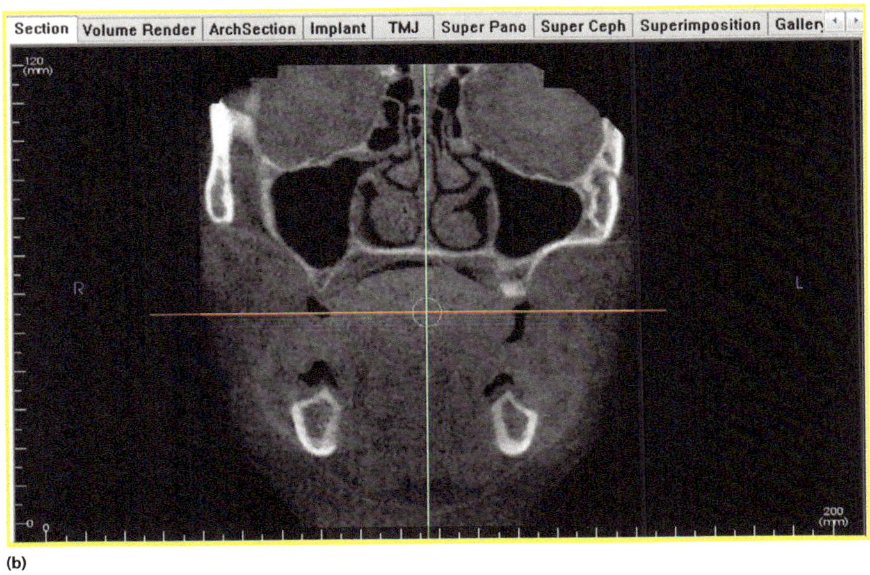

Figure 2.6 (a) An axial image of the maxilla reveals the bilateral maxillary sinus cavities, nasal turbinates, and the ethmoid and sphenoid sinuses. (b) The coronal images reveal the maxillary sinuses and the right and left alveoli.

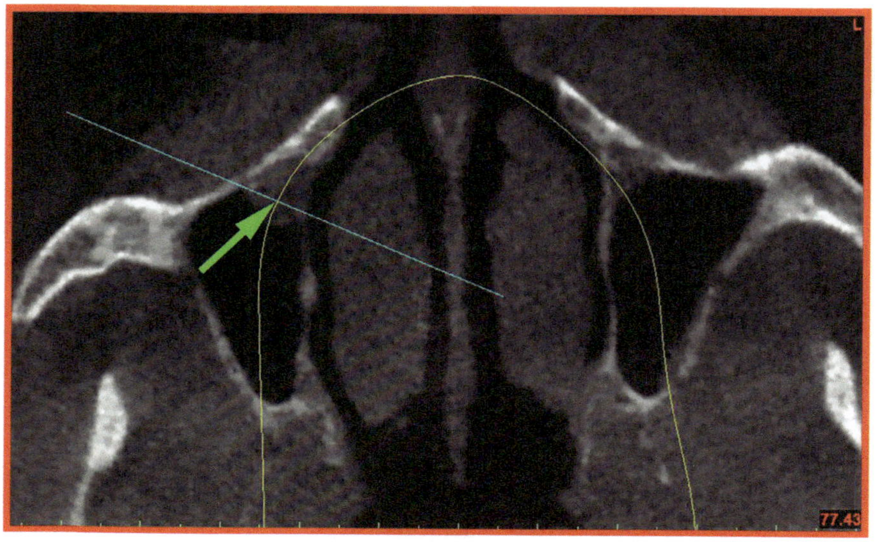

Figure 2.7 The axial slice revealed a normal left sinus, but soft tissue pathology in the right sinus (green arrow).

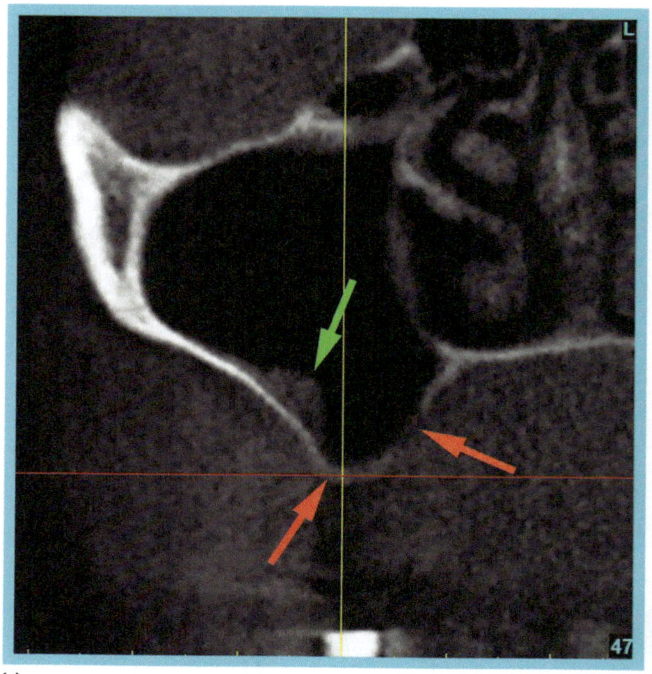

(a)

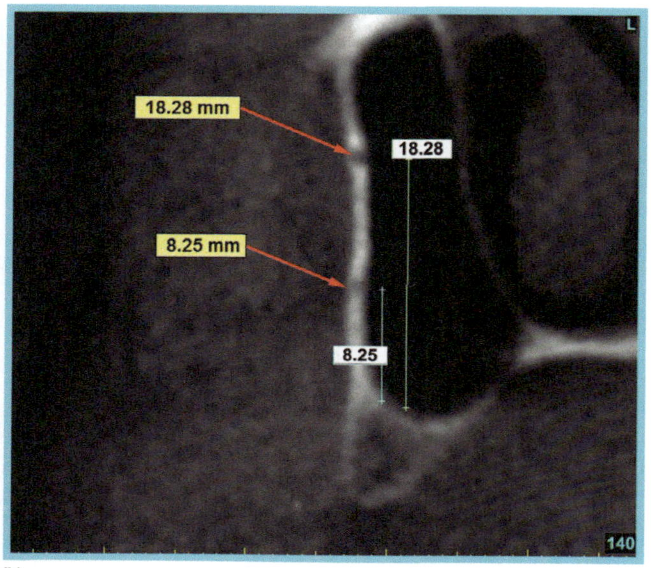

(b)

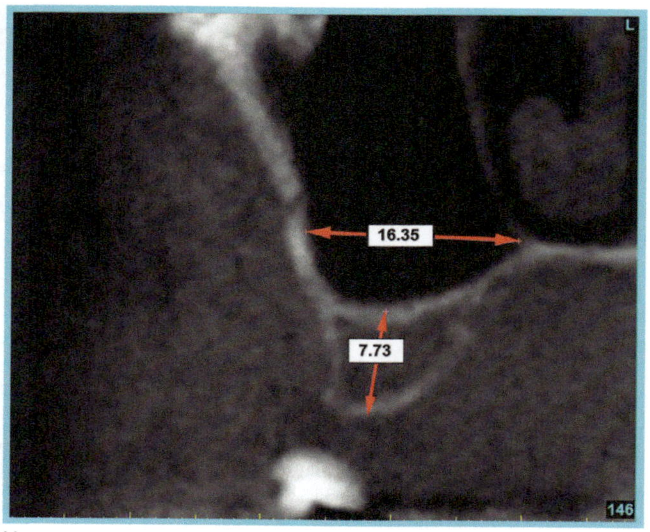

(c)

Figure 2.8 (a) Cross-sectional images allow for an excellent appraisal of the lateral and medial walls of the sinus, the deficient crestal bone (red arrows), and sinus pathology (green arrow). (b) Inspection of the lateral sinus wall with undistorted measurement of distances to intra-osseous vessels seen in the cross-sectional slice. (c) Measurements made from the lateral to medial walls help to estimate bone graft volume needed to prepare the sinus for subsequent dental implant placement.

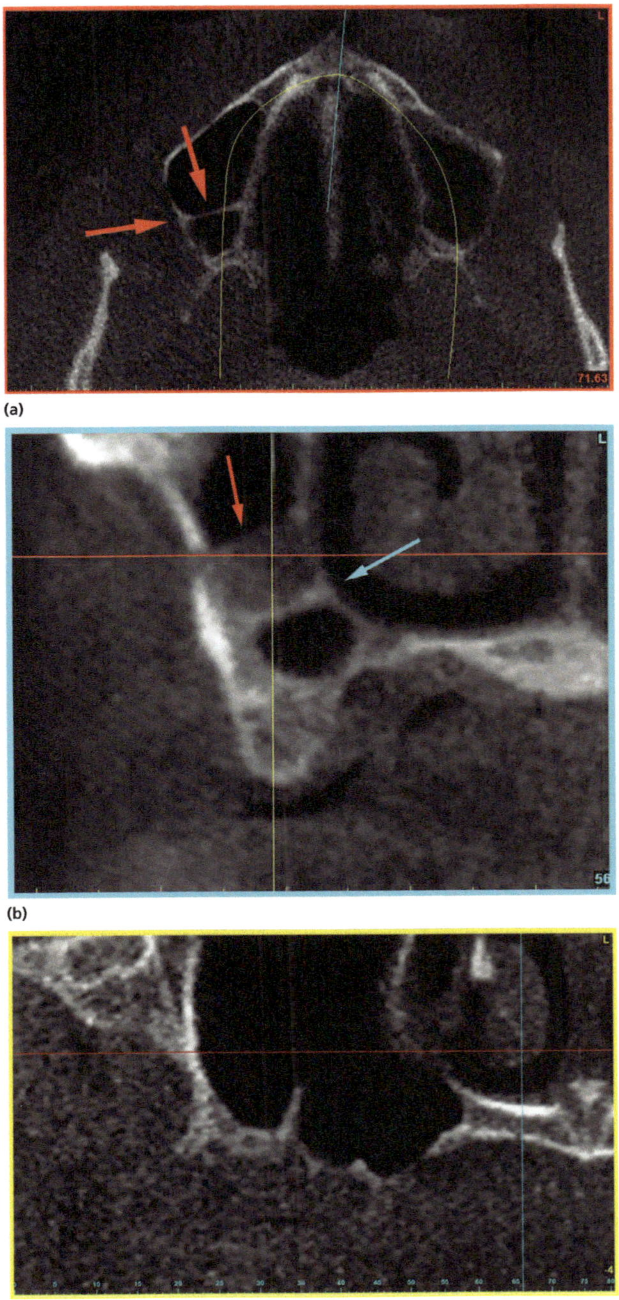

(a)

(b)

(c)

Figure 2.9 (a) The axial image revealing the location and extent of sinus septa (red arrows). (b) Cross-sectional slices are useful in visualizing septa (blue arrow) from the lateral to medial sinus walls and potential pathology within the sinus (red arrow).

made from the floor of the sinus to the vascular canals by tooth position. The mean perpendicular distance was found to be shortest in the first molar region (7.58 ± 3.19 mm) and longest in the first premolar region (9.2 ± 3.22 mm). The mean distance from the alveolar crest to the vascular canal was also found to be shortest when measured in the first molar region (14.79 ± 4.04 mm) and longest in the first premolar region (18.92 ± 4.86 mm). Elian et al. also used CBCT imaging to evaluate the distribution of the maxillary artery in 50 patients undergoing sinus augmentation procedures.[24] In their study the vessel was found in 51.4% of right maxillary sinuses and 54.3% of left maxillary sinuses. The average height from the alveolar crest was found to be 16.4 mm (±3.5 mm). Measurements can be made from the lateral to medial walls to estimate the volume of bone graft materials that will be needed to prepare the sinus for subsequent dental implant placement (Figure 2.8c). It is not unusual to find a width of greater than 18–20 mm. The height and width of the residual alveolar crest also can be determined, and can help clinicians in choosing the appropriate surgical intervention for restoration of the posterior maxilla (e.g. open grafting versus trans-alveolar sinus elevation; see Chapter 15).

Access for lateral window or open sinus augmentation procedures can be complicated by the thickness of the lateral sinus wall, the thickness/thinness of the Schneiderian membrane, and the presence of intra-osseous vessels, sinus pathology, and bony septa.[18–27] The presence of sinus septa can lead to intraoperative complications such as sinus membrane perforation. The use of CBCT imaging can help clinicians to avoid this complication.[8,14,16,22–27] The axial image is particularly useful in revealing the locations and extent of sinus septa, as depicted in Figure 2.9a (red arrows), as are cross-sectional slices (blue arrow, Figure 2.9b). They will also reveal pathology within the sinus (red arrow, Figure 2.9b). Navigating through the coronal slices can pick up even narrow bony projections (Figure 2.9c), helping the clinician to plan the location for surgical intervention. In a review of 150 publications accessed via PubMed and relating to sinus septa and CBCT, Wen et al.[28] found only 10 studies that met their selection criteria. Their conclusion was that "antral septa are one of the most common causes of membrane perforation during sinus augmentation," and they proposed a classification for management of septa during sinus augmentation procedures with three categories – easy (E), moderate (M) and difficult (D) – along with treatment approaches for each category.

The dental literature supports the concept that a thorough understanding of maxillary sinus topography is needed for successful surgical intervention as part of dental implant treatment.[8,16,18–29] The CBCT axial view can alert the clinician to potential pathology that may alter the proposed treatment plan, and/or result in referral for a consultation and review by an oral and maxillofacial radiologist (see left sinus pathology – arrows in Figure 2.10). Pathologies can be seen as unilateral or bilateral lesions, and can be appreciated in a variety of CBCT views (Figure 2.11a and b). While often inconsequential, as in the case of a mucous retention cyst, a differential diagnosis based upon symptomology and clinical presentation is needed prior to any sinus grafting or implant placement.

The preoperative condition of a maxillary sinus can be seen in Figure 2.12a. Utilizing advanced software tools, a prediction of the graft volume required to fill this sinus was simulated and measured (Figure 2.12b). The desired implant receptor site could then be assessed in several views, allowing for an adequate volume of

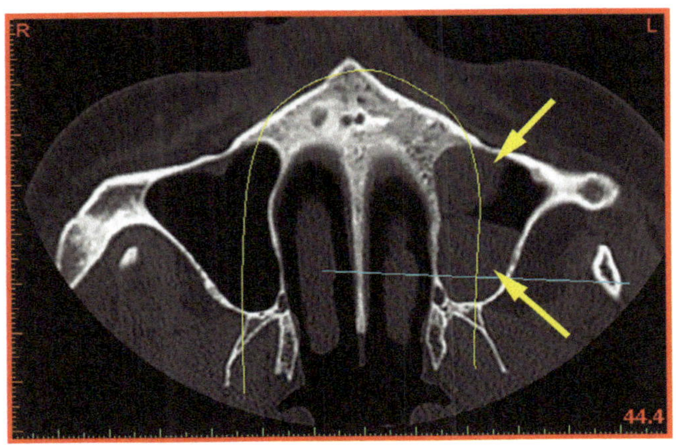

Figure 2.10 Sinus pathology evident in the left axial view (yellow arrows).

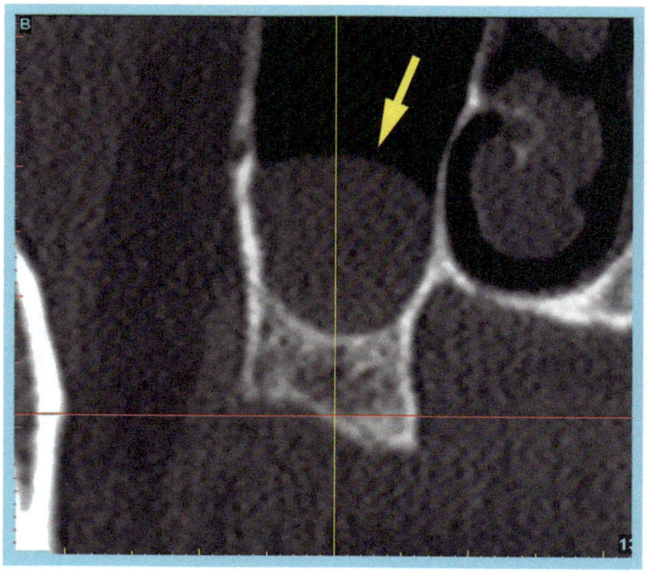

(a)

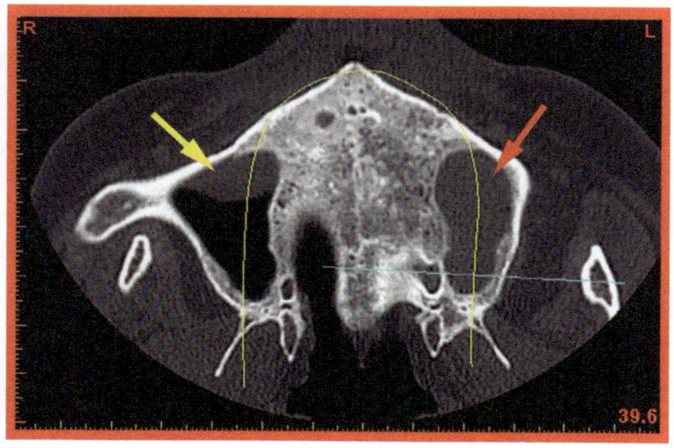

(b)

Figure 2.11 Sinus pathology in the cross-sectional view (a) and axial views (b) depicted by arrows.

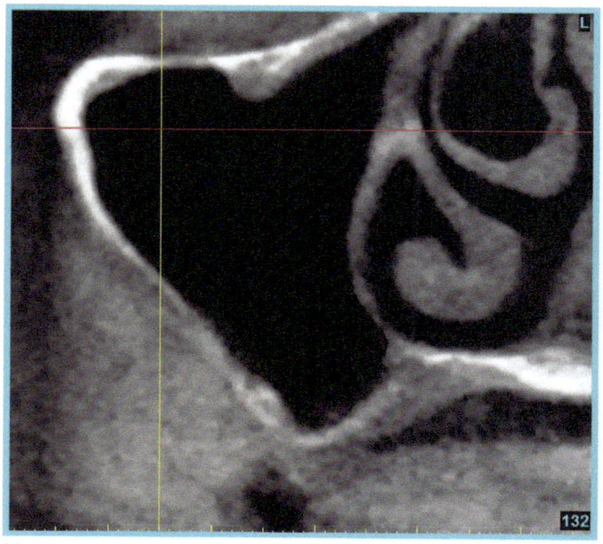

(a)

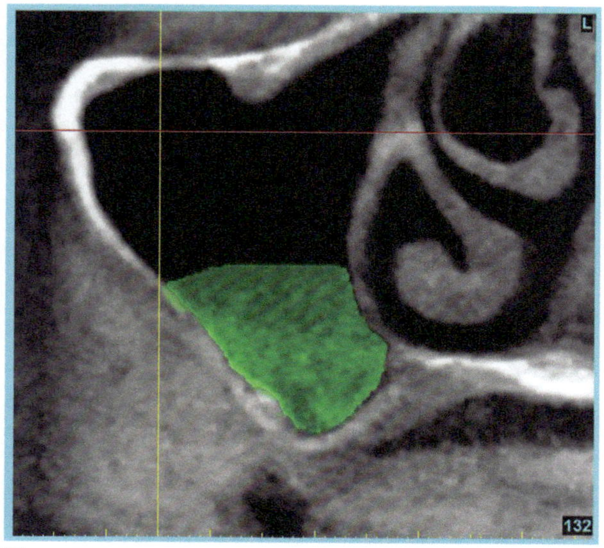

(b)

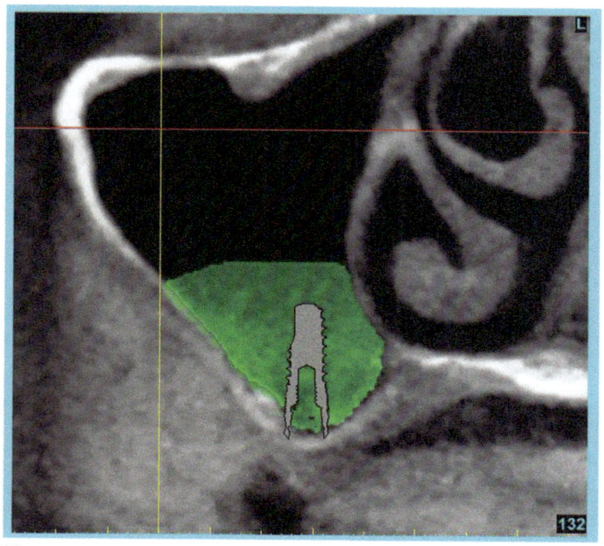

(c)

Figure 2.12 (a) The preoperative condition of a normal maxillary sinus. (b) Advanced software tools can simulate the graft volume required to fill the sinus (green). (c) The simulated implant site assessed in several views allows for an appreciation of the volume of bone needed to surround the body of the implant.

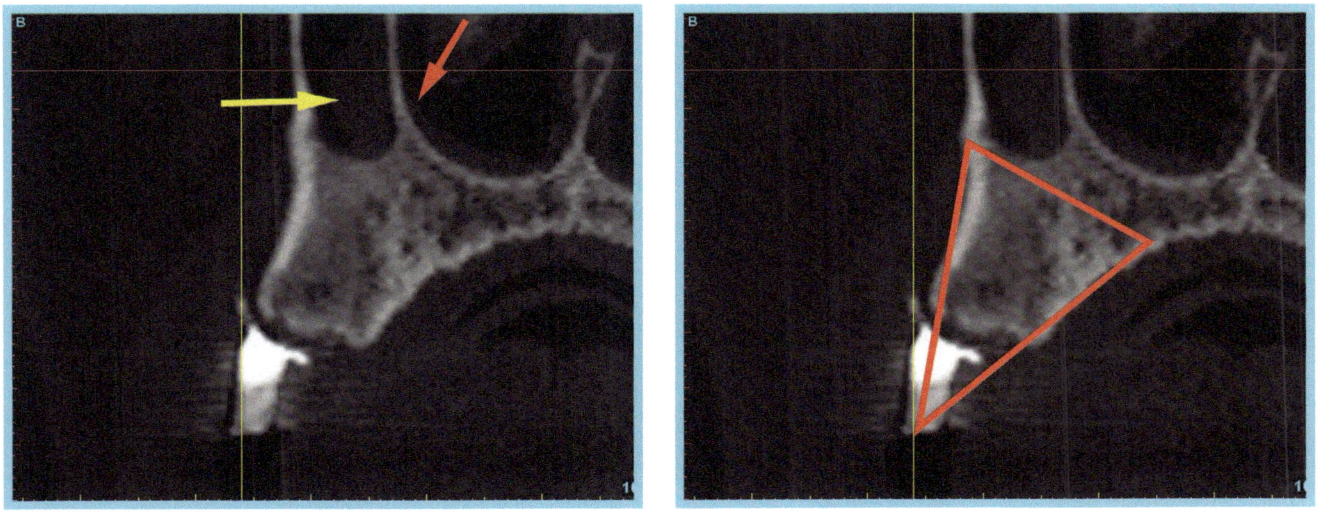

(a) (b)

Figure 2.13 (a) The alveolus is clearly visualized at the junction between the nasal cavity (red arrow) and the anterior extent of the maxillary sinus (yellow arrow). (b) The "triangle of bone" (TOB) concept creates a decision tree for potential implant placement based upon the zone of available bone.

bone to surround the body of the implant in all dimensions (Figure 2.12c). CBCT is therefore an essential imaging modality to help avoid complications related to sinus augmentation procedures and subsequent implant reconstruction.

In the anterior maxilla, cross-sectional images help to define potential implant sites based on available bone.[5–7,17,30–33] In the example in Figure 2.13a, the alveolus can be clearly visualized at the junction between the nasal cavity (red arrow) and the anterior extent of the maxillary sinus (yellow arrow). The "triangle of bone" (TOB) concept as described by the author (Table 2.1) will help in deciding whether implants can be placed in the available bone volume[4–8,17,31,34,35] (Figure 2.13b). The cross-sectional imaging also helps to define the extent of bone loss surrounding adjacent teeth, to estimate the height of the facial cortical plate, and to provide a view of the palatal bone that cannot be appreciated with conventional radiology (Figure 2.14a). The anterior maxilla also houses the incisive canal, an important

Table 2.1 The "triangle of bone" decision tree

- Evaluate the bone (density, thickness of cortical plates)
- Determine if there is enough bone within the TOB to place an implant
- Recognize the presence of a concavity (facial and lingual)
- Determine if bone grafting will be required
  - onlay graft particulate
  - onlay bone block
  - ridge splitting
- Determine width and length of proposed implant
- Determine straight-walled or tapered design implant
- Determine one- or two-piece implant design
- Determine the desired restorative abutment type
  - screw-retained restoration
  - cement-retained restoration
- Determine if soft tissue grafting will be required
- Determine method of implant placement
  - delayed placement
  - one-stage placement with healing collar
  - immediate restoration

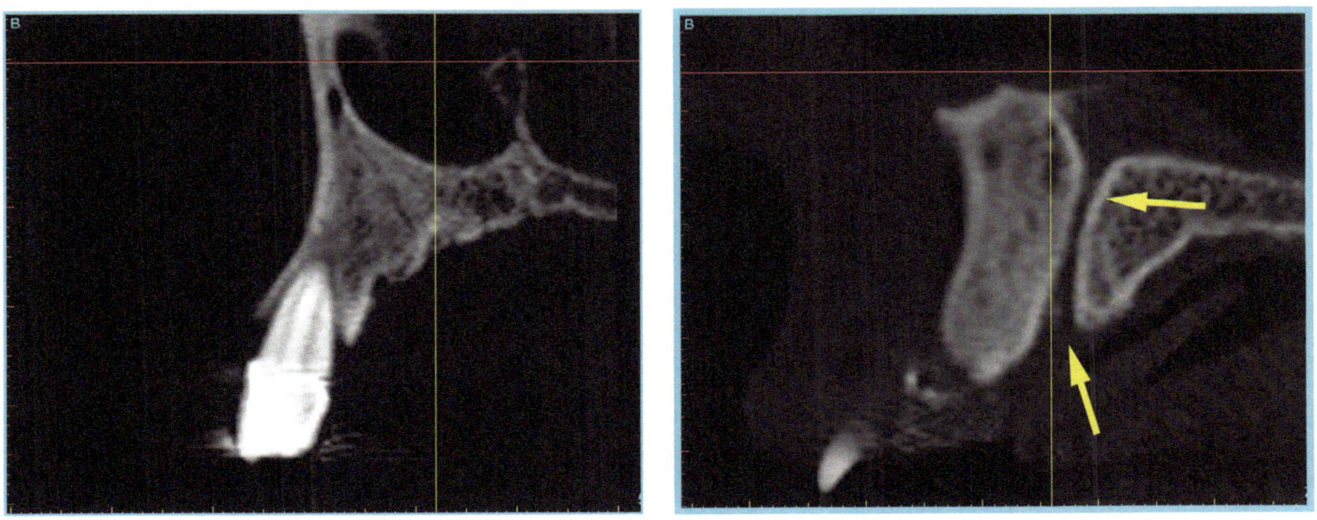

(a) (b)

Figure 2.14 (a) This cross-sectional slice reveals the extent of bone loss surrounding adjacent teeth, the height of the facial cortical plate, and a view of the palatal bone that cannot be appreciated with conventional radiology. (b) The anterior maxilla also houses the incisive canal that varies substantially from patient to patient (yellow arrows).

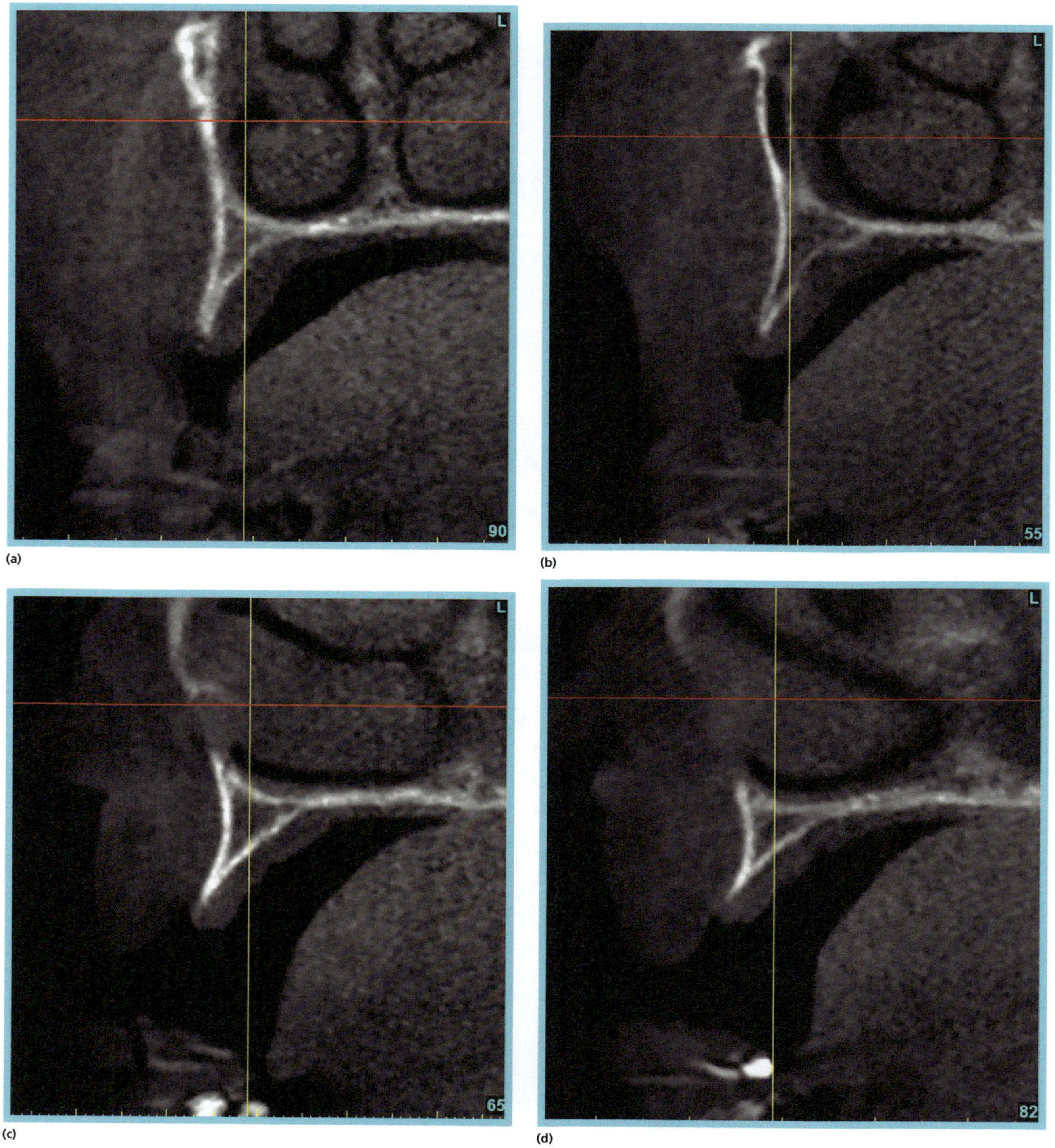

Figure 2.15 (a–d) The anterior maxilla in this case exhibited severe alveolar resorption, making it impossible for dental implant placement without ancillary augmentation procedures to reconstruct the lost volume.

anatomic landmark that varies substantially from patient to patient (Figure 2.14b). Often, the anterior maxilla may exhibit severe alveolar resorption, making it difficult or impossible for dental implant placement without ancillary augmentation procedures to reconstruct the lost volume (Figure 2.15a–d). In these severe cases, CBCT imaging can be useful to evaluate potential autogenous graft donor sites in the ramus or anterior symphysis.[16,17,30]

Clinical applications for diagnostic and restorative driven treatment planning

This section will demonstrate application of CBCT diagnostics for a 44-year-old male patient who presented for consultation regarding a definitive long-term solution to replace his congenitally missing maxillary lateral incisors. The patient's chief complaint was the poor esthetics of the two retained deciduous

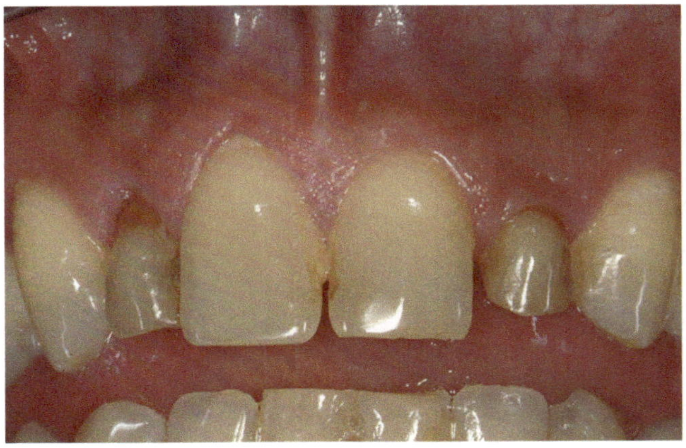

Figure 2.16 Preoperative photograph of the maxillary deciduous lateral incisors.

lateral incisors (Figure 2.16). He did not wish to involve any additional teeth in the restorative plan. Several issues were identified, including poor oral hygiene, mucogingival discrepancies, and asymmetry of shape and varied length of the clinical crowns, mesio–distal inter-tooth distances, and tooth discoloration (Figure 2.17a and b). Periapical radiographs revealed root resorption (Figure 2.18). The roots exhibited little if any bone support, resulting in a completely unfavorable crown/root ratio for conventional prosthodontic treatment. The radiographs appeared to show good bone density and a favorable relationship bilaterally of the adjacent roots of the central incisor and cuspid teeth for potential implant placement. In addition, there appeared to be ample bone height beyond the apices of the natural tooth roots but below the floor of the nose and maxillary sinus (see arrows in Figure 2.18) for site preparation.

Following case presentation, the patient declined conventional prosthetic options and confirmed his desire for dental implants with extraction and immediate provisional restoration if possible. A CBCT scan was completed to fully appreciate the maxillary anatomy. The right lateral incisor periapical radiograph can be seen along with the corresponding cross-sectional CBCT view in Figure 2.19a. The left lateral incisor periapical radiography can be seen with its corresponding cross-sectional CBCT view in Figure 2.19b. The thicknesses of the facial and palatal cortical plates and intermedullary bone density could be easily determined in

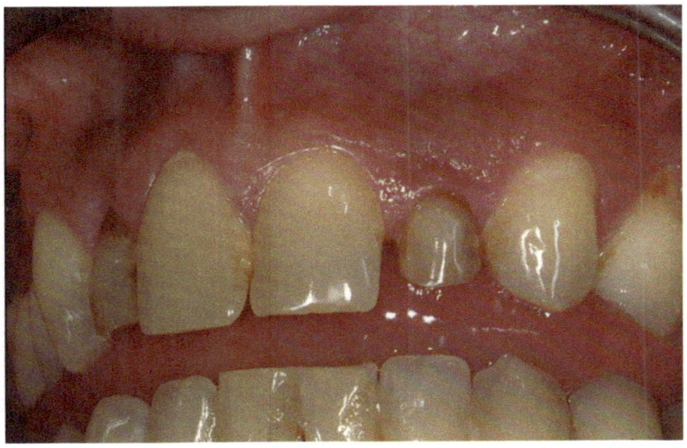

(a)

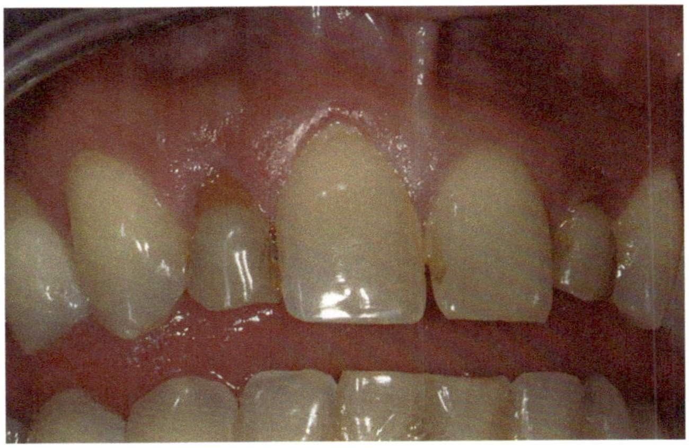

(b)

Figure 2.17 (a) Left side and (b) right side preoperative clinical appearance.

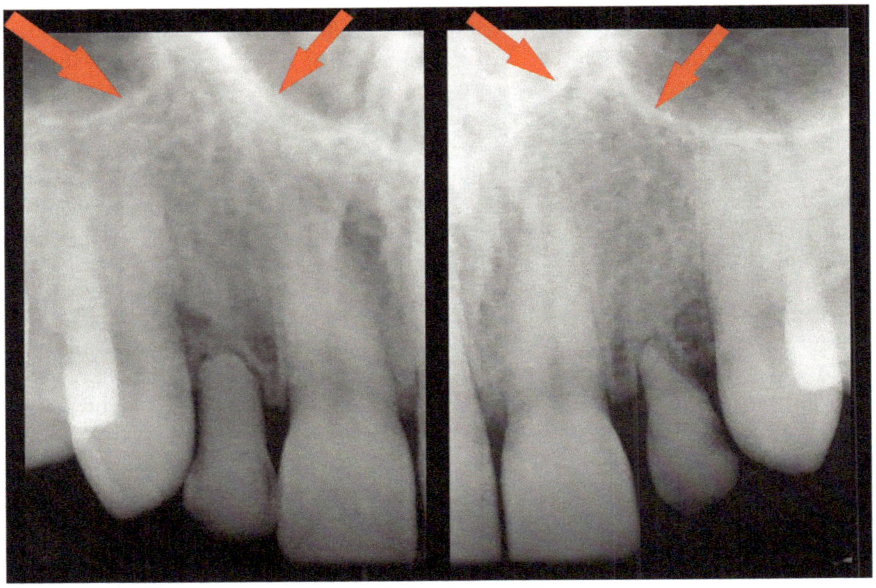

Figure 2.18 Preoperative periapical radiographs demonstrating limited residual roots and excellent apical bone height. Red arrows demonstrate the 2-D inferior position of the nasal (medial) and sinus (lateral) cavities.

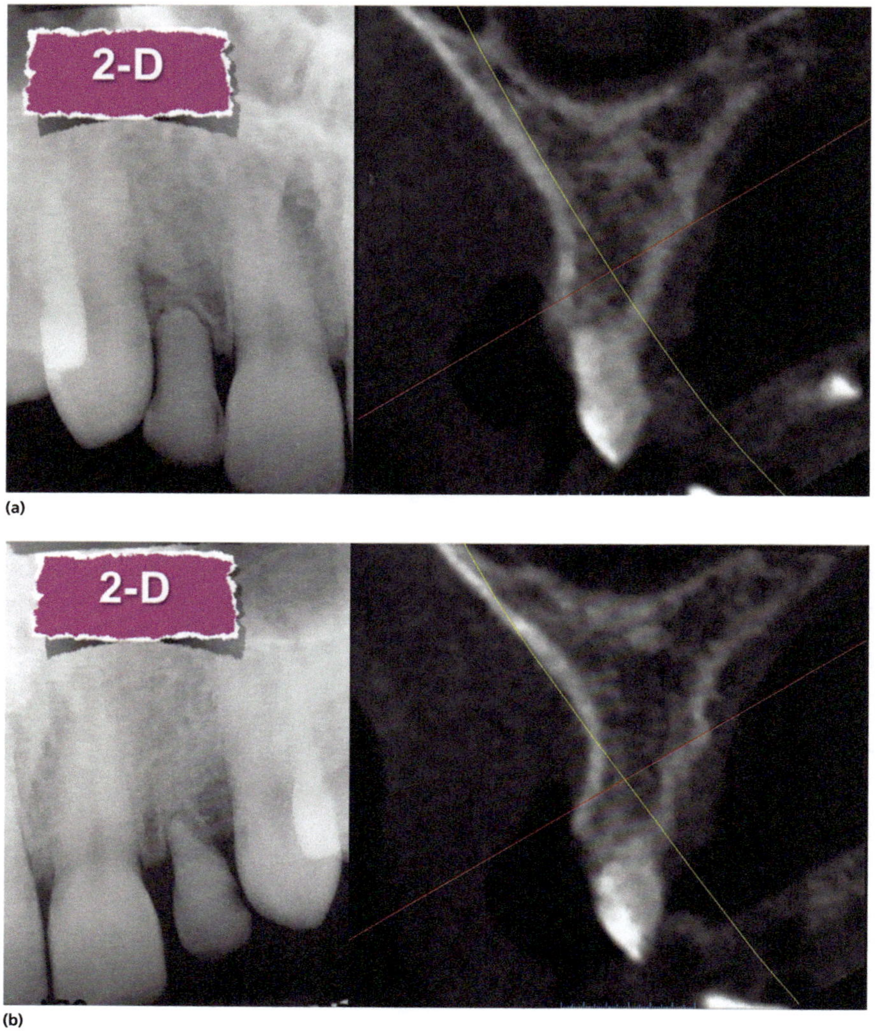

Figure 2.19 Periapical versus cross-sectional CBCT images of (a) right side and (b) left side.

the cross-sectional views, although not appreciated at all in the periapical radiographs. Placing a cotton roll under the lip helped to provide a clear assessment of the facial plate by separating the soft tissue vestibule from bone, a technique previously described as the "lip-lift" technique.[26,36,37]

Axial views helped to visualize the root morphology of adjacent teeth, the location of the incisal canal, and the facial–palatal dimensions of the potential implant sites (Figure 2.20a). The alveolar bone could be assessed apical to the deciduous tooth roots, and the inter-root distances mesio–distally could be measured to determine the diameter of the proposed implant. Using the manufacturer's implant library contained within the software (SimPlant®, Materialise Dental, Dentsply International), simulated implants were placed within the axial slices (Figure 2.20b). This placement was preliminary, as it did not indicate whether the implant could be placed within the existing bone volume along its entire length. In order to determine the actual bone volume, additional views were needed, specifically the cross-sectional images.

The cross-sectional slice was used to determine the "zone" into which the implant could be placed, that is the TOB.[38] The base of this triangle is formed by the widest area of available bone, and is connected to the apex of the triangle at a point that bisects the alveolar ridge approximately 5 mm above the crest (Figure 2.21a). If there is adequate width between the facial and palatal cortical plates, a simulated implant can be positioned to bisect the triangle, thus allowing the implant to be surrounded by the greatest available bone volume and placed within a pyramidal shape from the crest to the apex of the implant (Figure 2.21b). The TOB can be helpful in creating a decision tree to evaluate a potential implant receptor site not only for the placement of an implant, but also as a link to the restorative phase and in deciding if bone or soft tissue grafting will be required for successful outcomes (Table 2.1). The TOB concept will aid the clinician in planning based upon the quality of the bone, thickness of the cortical plates, and identification of any concavity that may be present on the facial or lingual aspect of the alveolus. If there is a concavity, the topography of the bone defect can help decide

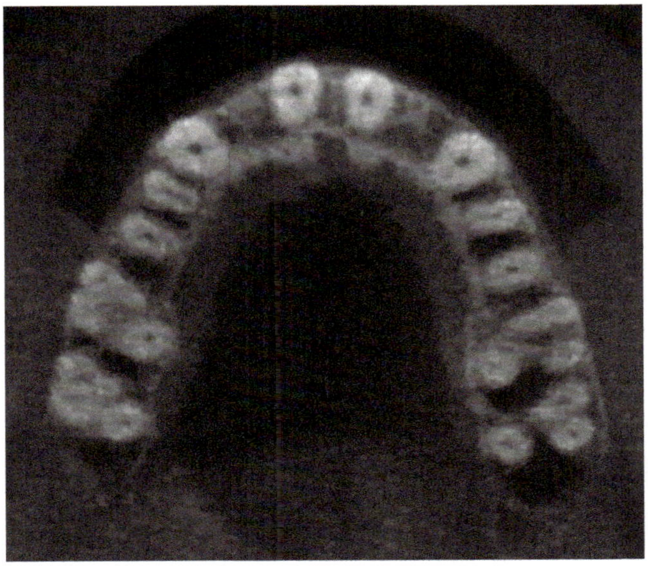

(a)

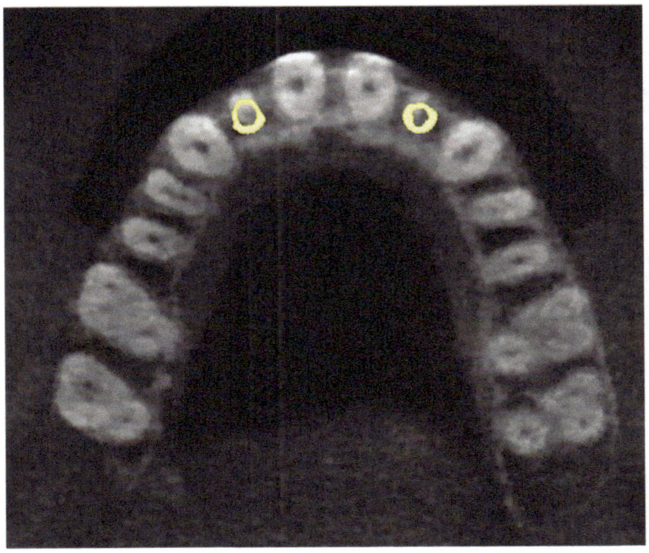

(b)

Figure 2.20 (a) Preoperative axial CBCT view. (b) Preoperative axial view with simulated implant placement (yellow).

what type of grafting would be appropriate, such as particulate, block grafting, or ridge-splitting. The TOB can help in deciding the appropriate length and width of the implant to be placed, and if a straight-walled or tapered implant design should be chosen. As many implant companies offer one-piece implants, the TOB provides important information regarding this type of design as it fits within the surgical and restorative requirements. Implant positioning within the TOB can be a determinant for either screw-retained or cement-retained restorations based upon the apico-coronal angulation in relationship to the envelope of the tooth. If the "lip-lift" technique is utilized, the soft tissue biotype can be assessed to decide if additional soft tissue grafting may be needed. Finally, the TOB can help define the method of placement; that is, delayed placement, one-stage placement with healing collar, or immediate restoration. Implant stability must be confirmed at placement before choosing immediate loading. Variations with interactive treatment planning software should follow the same decision tree as described in Table 2.1. It is recommended that all available views be utilized with the manipulative/simulation tools of the software (Invivo5®, Anatomage, Inc., San Jose, CA) to maximize diagnostic accuracy in positioning the implant properly (Figure 2.22a and b).

Perhaps the most impressive view is the reconstructed 3-D model after all scatter has been removed (Figure 2.23). This preoperative computer-generated model allows inspection with various software tools to enhance the diagnostic process. It is important to note that these images provide an excellent

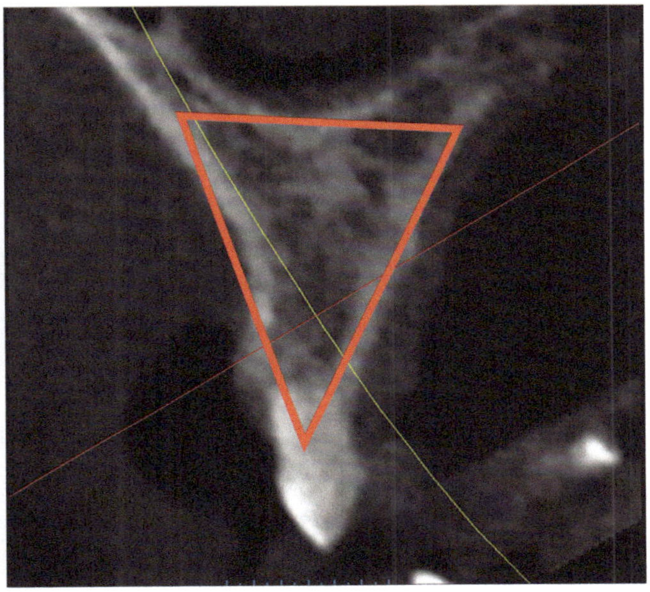

(a)

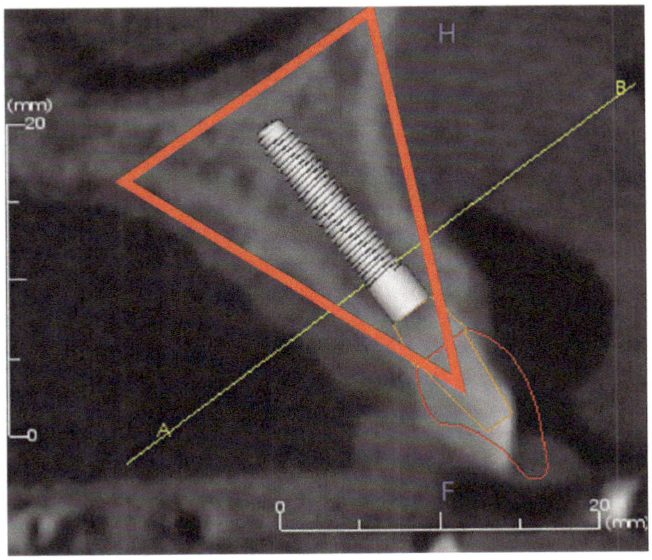

(b)

Figure 2.21 (a) TOB on cross-sectional view. (b) TOB with simulated implant placement.

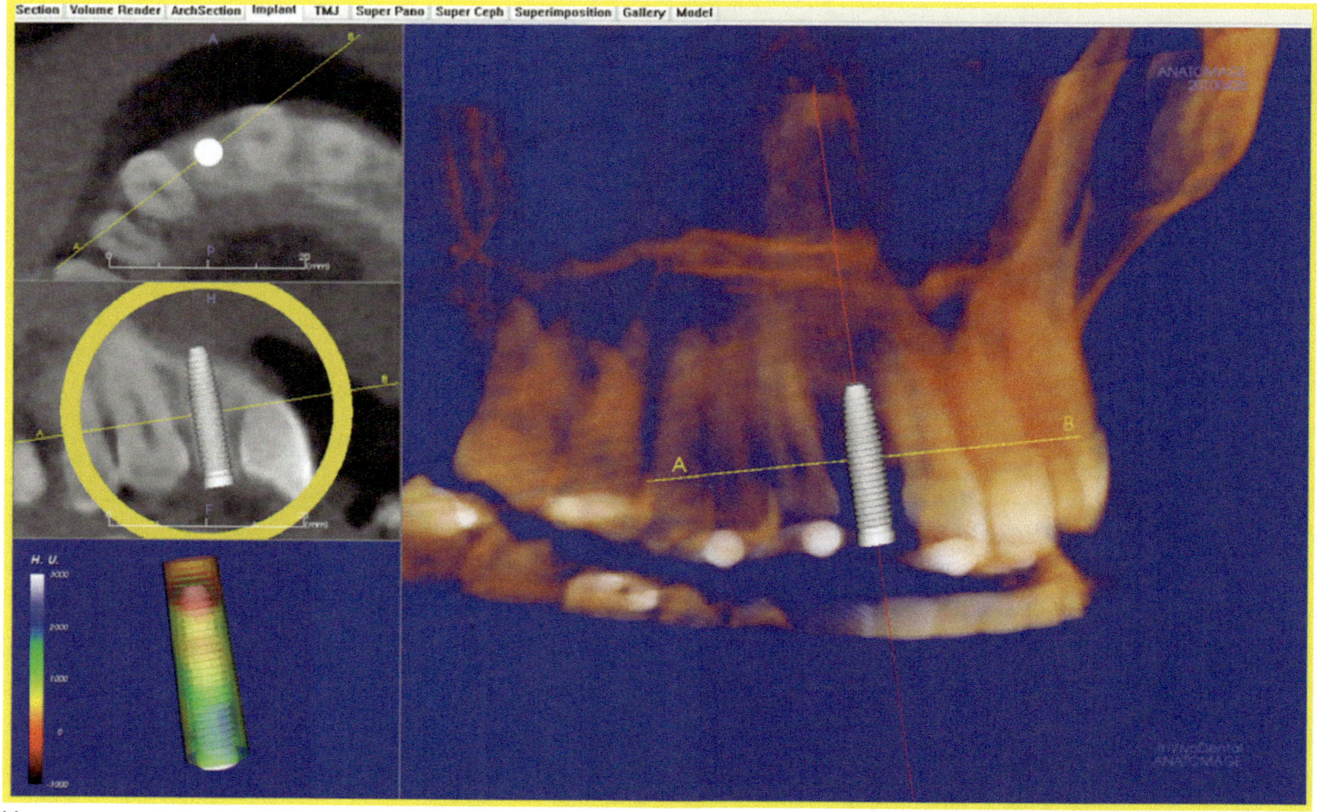

(a)

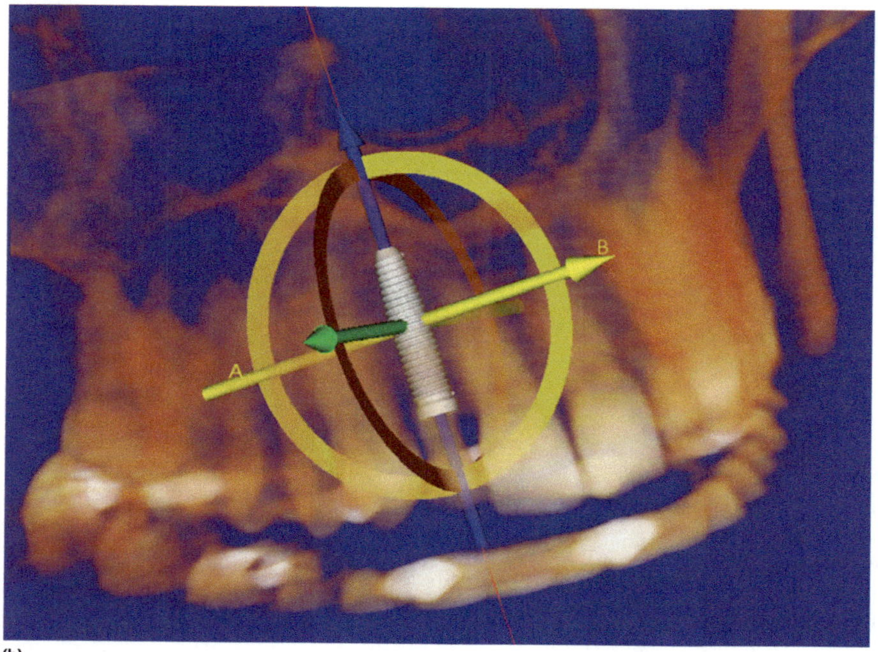

(b)

Figure 2.22 (a, b) Screen shots of interactive treatment planning software application.

foundation for communication between all members of the implant team, including the dental laboratory, and the patient. The initial simulated placement of the implants can be modified within the confines dictated by the adjacent vital anatomy and opposing occlusion. It is advisable to have some type of projection extending from the implant beyond the occlusal table to indicate the trajectory of the implant as it links to the abutment and clinical crown (Figure 2.24a). Using "selective transparency," certain objects can be made to appear opaque or translucent to provide further assistance in the diagnostic phase (Figure 2.24b).[6,16]

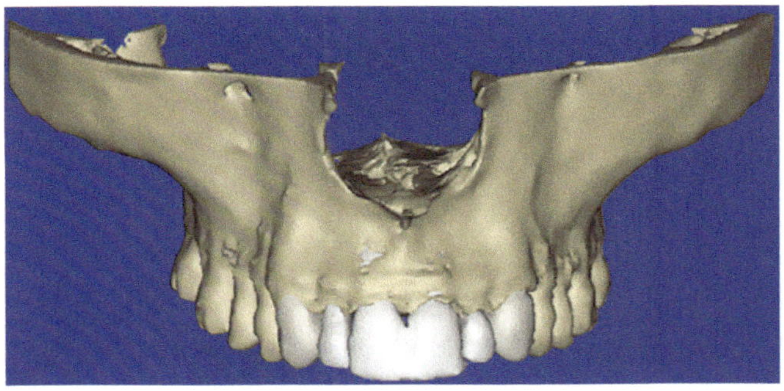

Figure 2.23 The 3-D reconstructed maxillary volume.

The combination of interactive views allows for realistic simulated implant positioning based upon the anatomical and restorative requirements of the case. During this process the appropriate lengths and widths of implants can be determined, as well as choice of straight-walled or tapered implant designs. In order to achieve true restoratively-driven implant reconstruction there must be a complete visualization of the implant within bone, but also the future abutment and crown (Figure 2.25a). The lip can be separated from the facial bone by placing a cotton roll in the vestibule (red line). Without the "lip-lift" technique, the superimposed gray values of the lip would obscure assessment of the thickness of the facial plate and overlying soft tissues. In the example, a "virtual" tooth was created for each of the missing lateral incisor teeth. A projection was then extended from the coronal aspect of the implant through the virtual tooth and about 4–6 mm above the occlusal plane (Figure 2.25b).

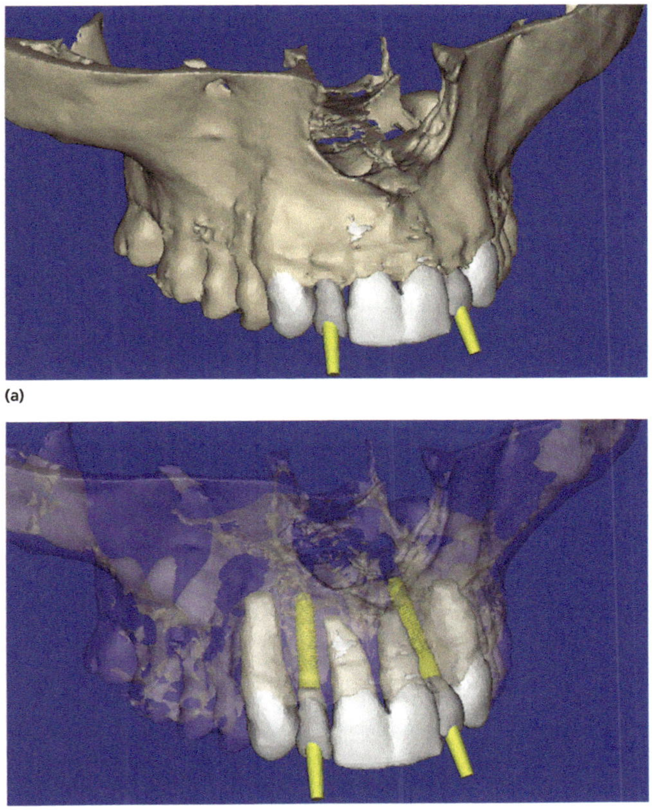

(a)

(b)

Figure 2.24 (a) Using simulated abutment projections (yellow) helps to define the trajectories for the implants.(b) Selected transparency was used to reveal the roots of the adjacent teeth.

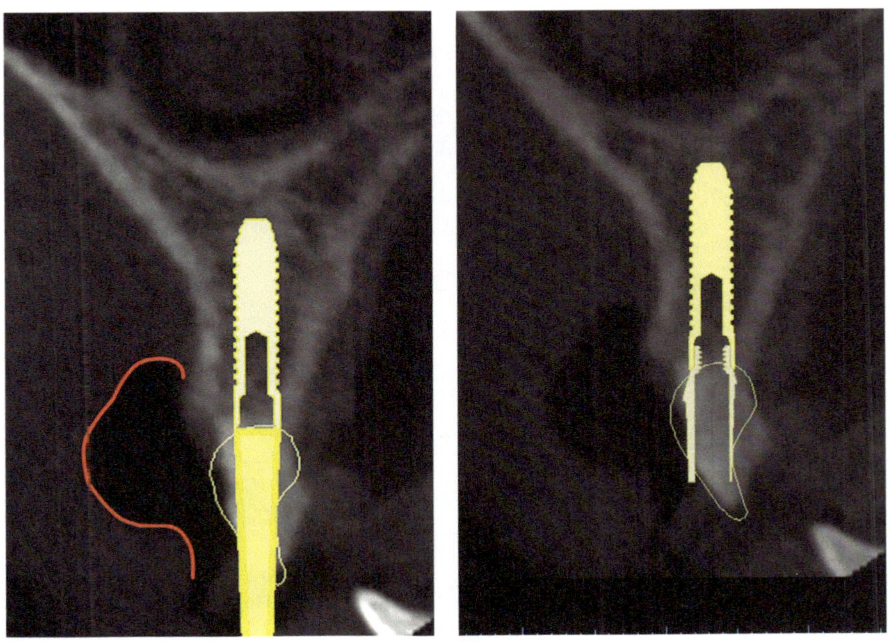

(a)

(b)

Figure 2.25 (a) Cross-sectional CBCT view with abutment projection. The red line indicates positioning of a cotton roll for the "lip lift " technique. (b) Cross-sectional CBCT view with implant and future crown outline.

Screw-retained versus cement-retained positioning concepts

Restorative design decisions should be made during the diagnostic and planning phase of implant treatment. Using the TOB concept, the simulated implant and abutment can be repositioned to accommodate either a cement-retained or screw-retained restoration. When the implant is placed to bisect the TOB, often it will result in a cementable abutment design being needed for the resulting facial–incisal emergence of the restorative projection. The relationship of the implant–abutment complex can be appreciated by slicing through the 3-D model (Figure 2.26). Appropriate abutments can be chosen from the manufacturer's library (Figure 2.27a). The abutment can be visualized through the translucent virtual tooth (Figure 2.27b). For the example shown, a straight abutment was chosen and prepared accordingly to fit within the confines of the restoration. Another option to help in keeping the implant within the greatest volume of bone can be to use an angulated abutment (Figure 2.27c).

When the final restoration is planned to be screw-retained, the implant position must be adjusted to ensure that it remains within the confines of the pre-existing bone volume. Ideally, the screw-access hole required to secure the abutment will emerge from the cingulum aspect of the proposed restoration (Figure 2.28a). In the example, while the implant does emerge on the palatal aspect of the tooth, sectioning through the 3-D reconstructed view shows its apex may perforate the facial cortical plate (Figure 2.28b). The 3-D reconstructed view demonstrates that the desired trajectory through the tooth will result in the potential complication of apical perforation (Figure 2.28c).

To summarize, there are several conclusions that can be drawn for the patient shown in this sample diagnostic exercise: (1) the most favorable implant position, bisecting the TOB, will require a cement-retained restoration; (2) if a screw-retained restoration were to be planned, the implant position would result in apical perforation of the facial cortical plate; (3) if a screw-retained restoration is essential, then either an angulated screw-receiving abutment will be needed or the implant placement will require bone grafting and/or ridge-splitting surgery to accommodate the necessary trajectory; and, (4) immediate placement and

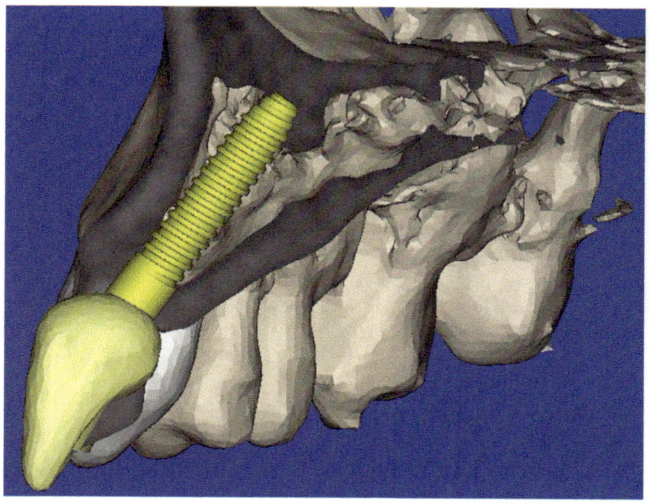

Figure 2.26 Cross-sectional 3-D model including the virtual crown.

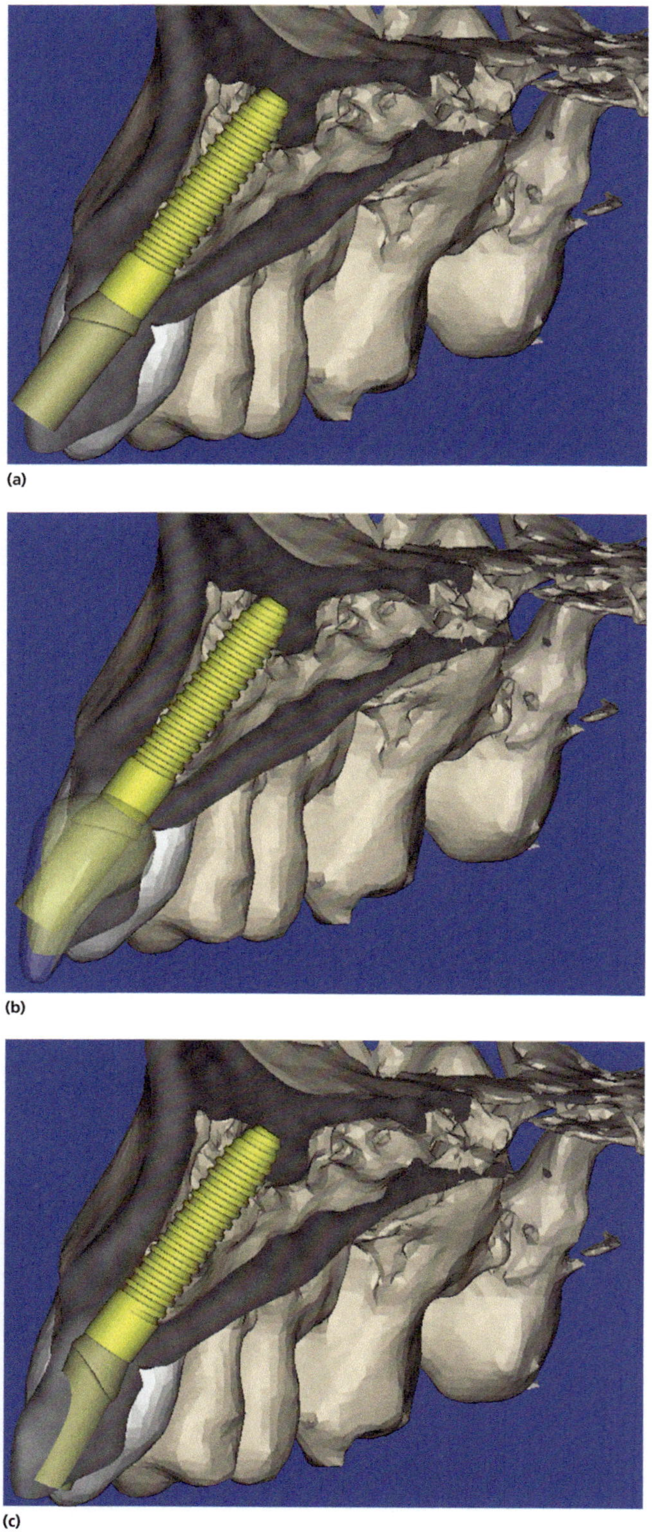

(a)

(b)

(c)

Figure 2.27 (a) Cross-sectional 3-D model of implant and abutment. (b) Cross-sectional image of the 3-D model for the implant, abutment, and virtual crown. (c) 3-D cross-sectional image with an angled abutment within the virtual crown.

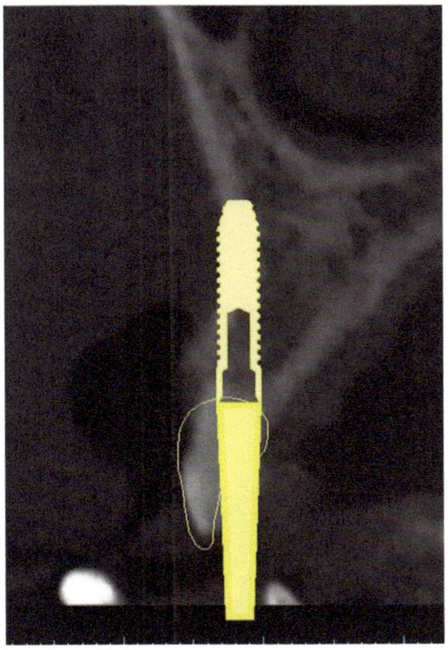

(a)

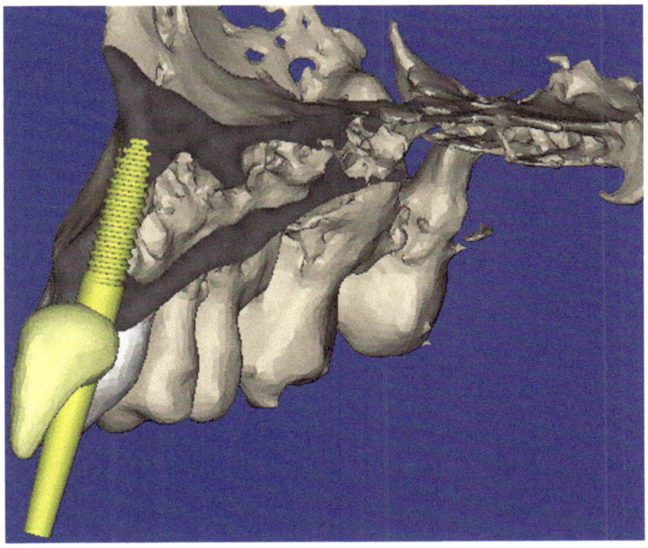

(b)

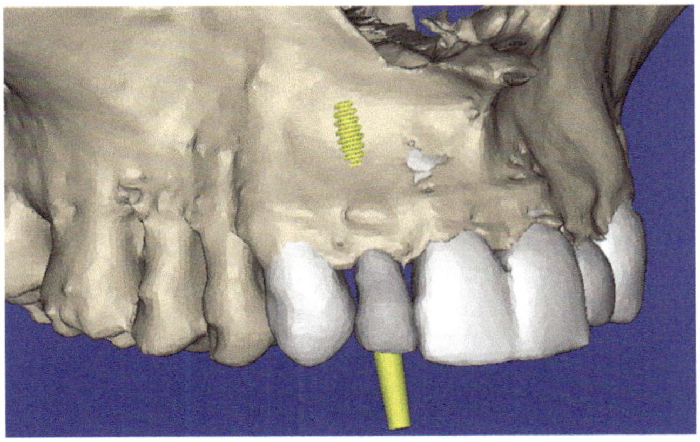

(c)

Figure 2.28 (a) Positioning for a screw-retained crown with screw emergence through the cingulum. (b) Reconstructed view shows positioning for a screw-retained crown may result in apical perforation. (c) 3-D reconstructed view shows screw-retained positioning results in perforation of the facial cortical plate.

provisional restoration is possible owing to the limited root structure of the retained primary teeth and the intact apical bone (see Chapter 19). This allows for a more predictable use of guided surgery for apical drill purchase than in a larger root form defect of a permanent tooth. If the 3-D images are not fully appreciated and implants are placed freehand for a screw-retained treatment plan, apical perforation of the facial plate could result. Therefore, it is advisable to consider the entire implant–abutment–crown complex for each prospective implant site and how this relates to the volume of bone present.[4–8,17,34,35,39–56]

The past several years have seen the evolution of what has been termed "digital dentistry." This all-inclusive term embodies the concepts proposed within this chapter, and has been greatly enhanced by the introduction of intraoral optical scanners and laboratory-based desktop scanning devices. A new set of diagnostic modalities has become available through the merging of these technologies.[57,58] A stone cast can be fabricated first from an intraoral impression (Figure 2.29a). It can then be placed in a desktop optical scanner to convert the physical cast into a digital file. The digital output is formed from the "point cloud" of information generated from the surface scan and turned into an STL (stereolithography or Standard Tessellation Language) file to be used in CAD/CAM fabrication or rapid prototyping. The same information can be obtained using an intraoral scanning device, eliminating the need for a physical impression or cast. The STL file of the stone cast or intraoral image can be visualized with 3-D viewing software or imported directly into the implant planning software (Figure 2.29b). Using tools within the software application, the new STL file can be merged with the CBCT data set and reconstructed into a 3-D model (Figure 2.29c). The red arrow in Figure 2.29c represents the stone cast superimposed onto the 3-D model of the maxilla (yellow arrow).

After the two data sets have been merged, the planning phase can continue. CBCT scans, while delivering lower radiation exposure to patients, were not designed to create images of the natural teeth or occlusal surfaces in high enough resolution. Therefore, the

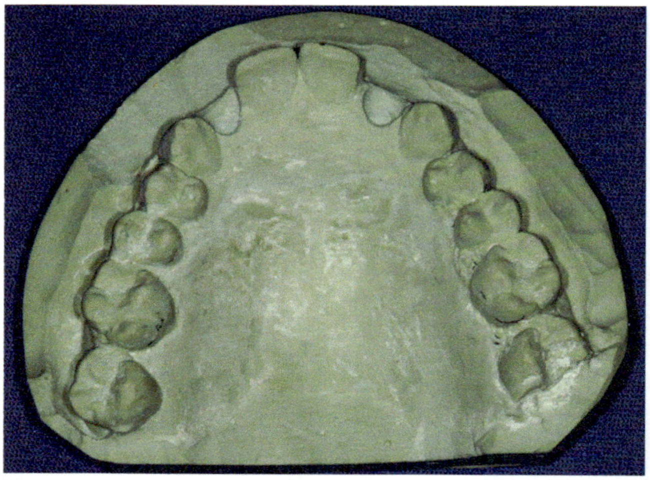
(a)

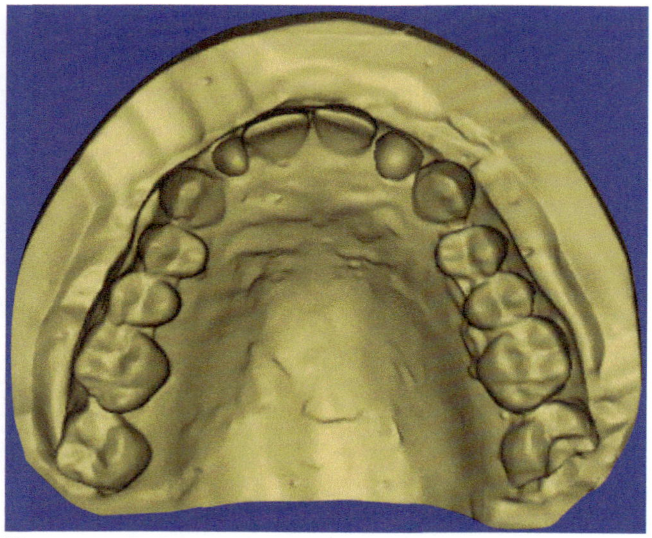
(b)

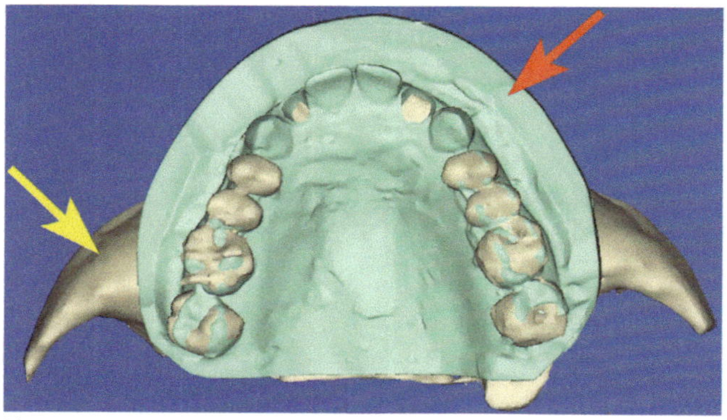
(c)

Figure 2.29 (a) The stone cast with good surface detail. (b) Optical scan of the stone cast. (c) The digital model of stone cast merged with CBCT data.

representation of the occlusal surfaces may not be ideal for the fabrication of a tooth-borne surgical guide, which needs to be closely adapted to the teeth. The lack of surface detail can be overcome by merging the optical scanned data set of the intraoral impression and resultant stone cast, or an intraoral optical impression. After the stone cast is merged with the implant planning file, the digital "virtual" abutment can be seen (Figure 2.30a and b). The smooth contours and surface detail are excellent. It is also possible to visualize the implant and abutment placement in a variety of views for final verification, and to provide the foundation for the fabrication of a tooth-borne surgical template (Figure 2.31a and b). A final plan was established that allowed for a minimally invasive surgical intervention consisting of tooth extractions, placement of two implants, and immediate provisional restorations.

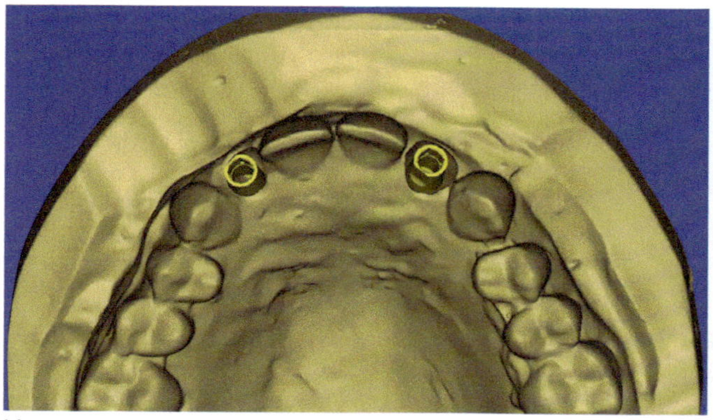
(a)

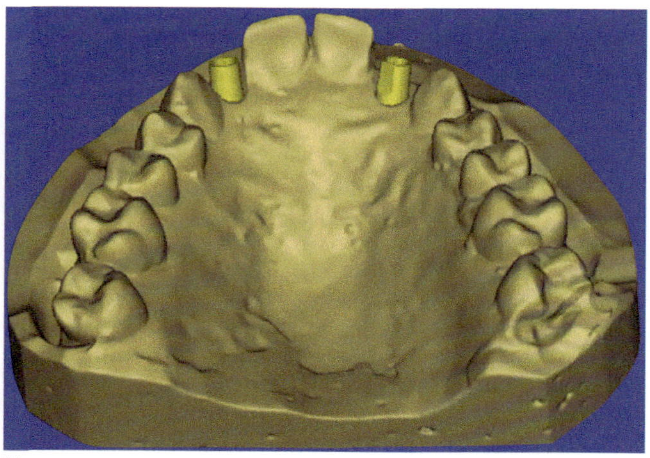
(b)

Figure 2.30 The digital model with (a) digital "virtual" abutments and (b) abutments.

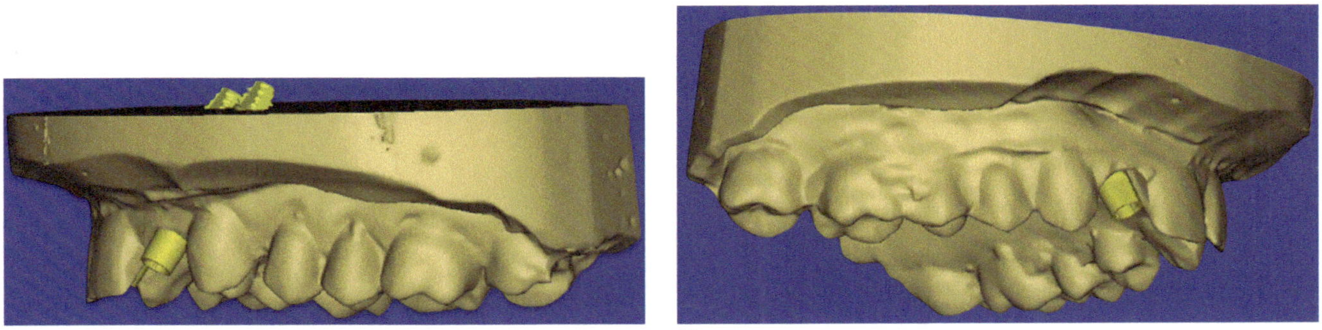

(a) (b)

Figure 2.31 (a) Side view of the digital model with abutments. (b) Digital model with abutments.

Clinical applications: surgical phase

Once the patient had agreed to the proposed treatment plan, the software planning was completed and a surgical guide (template) ordered and fabricated using a stereolithographic process (Materialise® Dental, Dentsply, Inc.). On the day of surgery, the two deciduous teeth were carefully removed using periotomes and a flapless approach used to preserve the surrounding soft tissues. The short residual roots on the extracted teeth can be seen in Figure 2.32. Extraction resulted in minimal residual alveolar defects, optimizing the apical drilling for osteotomy preparation. The tooth-borne surgical guide was seated securely in the patient's mouth (Figure 2.33). Stainless steel guide cylinders can be seen within the surgical template. The single template allowed for the utilization of a sequence of special "guide keys" that corresponded to the diameters of the sequential drills provided by the implant manufacturer. Osteotomies were then prepared for both implants (Figure 2.34). Each implant was placed to the correct depth and positioned to receive a straight abutment for a cement-retained crown (Figure 2.35). The soft tissues were relatively untouched as the unprepared abutment was attached to the left implant (Figure 2.36). All abutment preparation was completed on implant analogs in advance of the surgical intervention (Figure 2.37). In this manner the marginal adaptation of the temporary acrylic restoration could be managed as an "indirect" laboratory procedure prior to insertion. The transitional acrylic restorations were cement-retained (Figure 2.38). Although there is still controversy regarding cement- versus screw-retained prosthetic designs, it is always important to control the cement–abutment interface to prevent late complications related to migration of cement into the sulcus. Note the soft tissue contours on the day of the surgery without

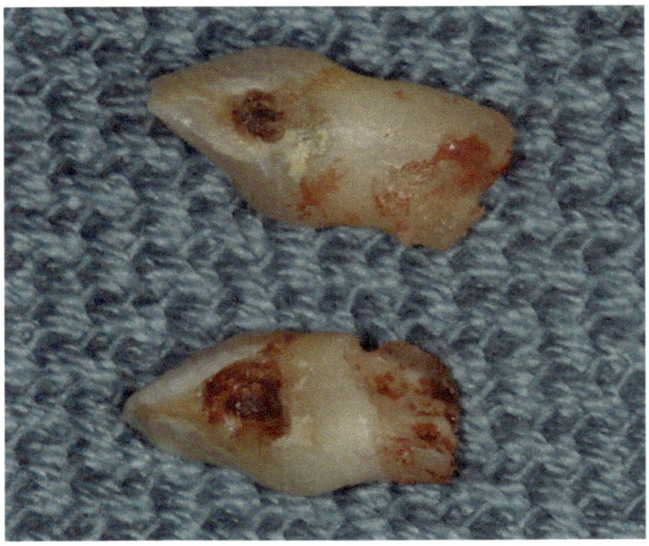

Figure 2.32 Extracted primary teeth confirming short residual root forms per software planning.

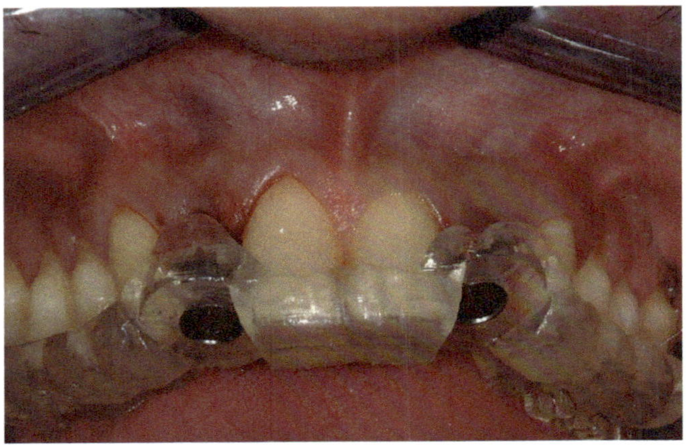

Figure 2.33 The tooth-borne surgical template.

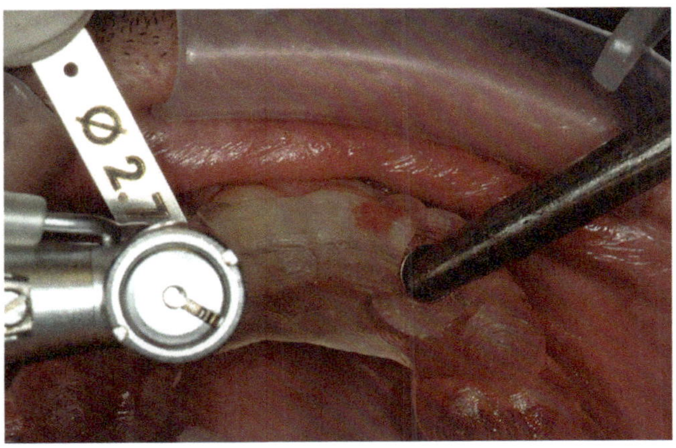

Figure 2.34 Sequential drilling through surgical template with the drill-specific guide key.

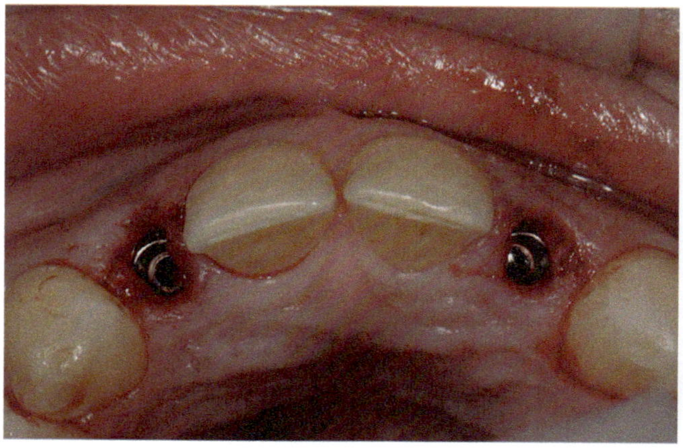

Figure 2.35 Clinical picture after placement of both implants.

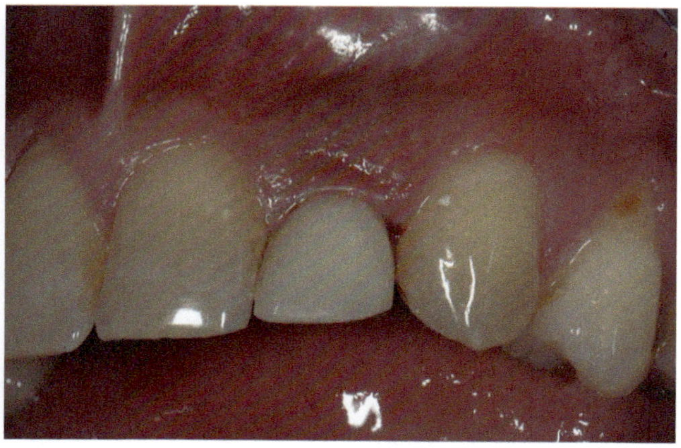

Figure 2.38 Left transitional resin temporary in place.

any sutures being placed. The progress of soft tissue healing was evaluated at 2 weeks and found to be excellent (Figure 2.39a and b). Post-operative periapical radiographs confirmed accurate positioning of the implants (Figure 2.40a and b).

After a healing period of 3 months, an open-tray impression was utilized to transfer the relationship of the implants to the dental laboratory technician for fabrication of the definitive restorations (Figure 2.41). The maturation of the soft tissue and the morphologically contoured temporary restorations helped to create the proper sulcus form and emergence profiles. The ceramo-metal restorations were fabricated on custom abutments, as seen in Figure 2.42a and b. The mature sulcus surrounding the right lateral incisor abutment provided natural-appearing interdental papillae (Figure 2.43). The final restorations blended naturally with the surrounding dentition, and demonstrated excellent soft tissue emergence, sulcus form, and interdental papillae (Figure 2.44a and b). Final periapical radiographs taken at 24 months post-surgery revealed a smooth transition from implant to abutment to the definitive restorations, and confirmed stability of crestal interproximal bone (Figure 2.45).

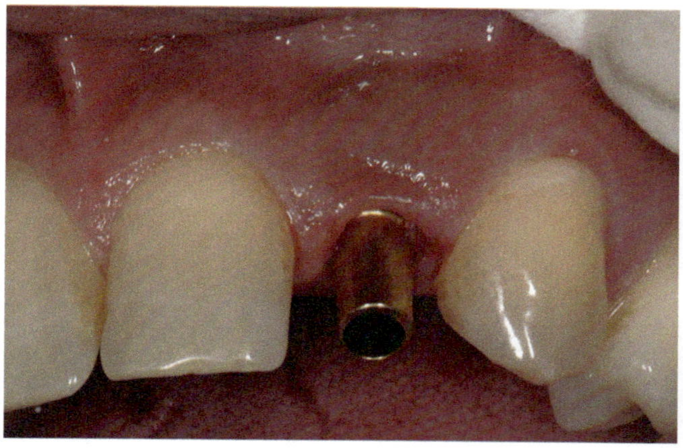

Figure 2.36 Unprepared abutment placed onto the left implant.

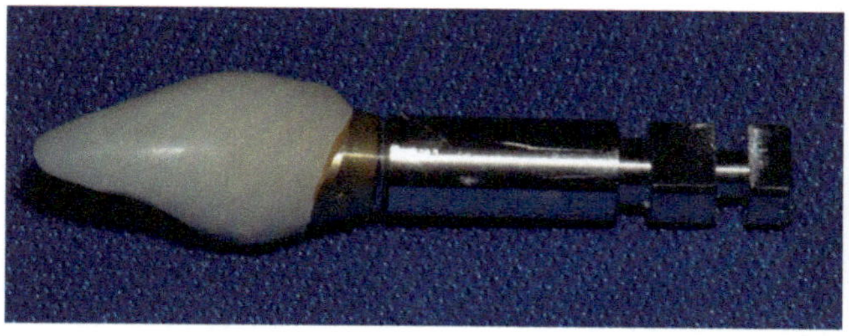

Figure 2.37 Temporary restoration connected to the implant analog.

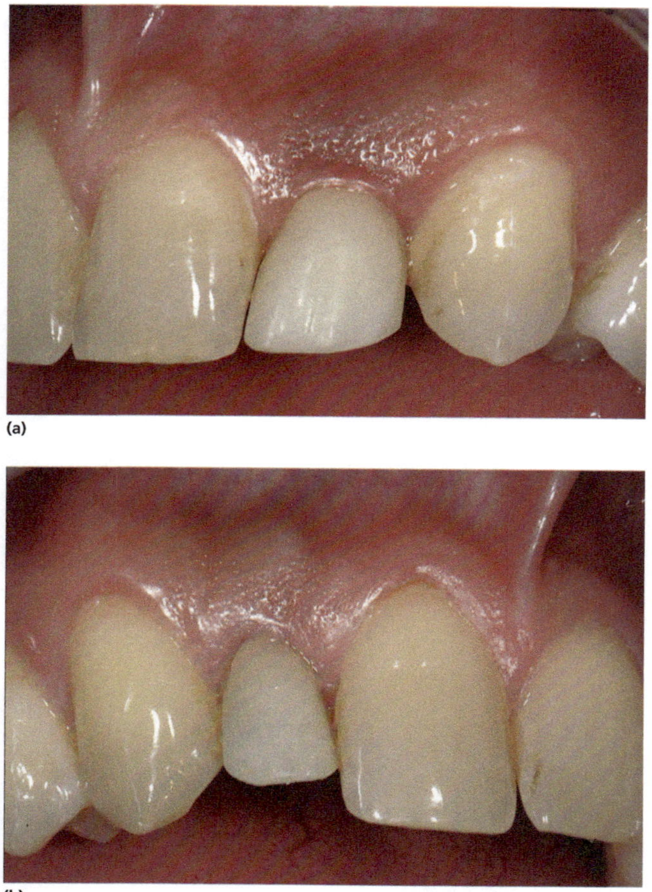

(a)

(b)

Figure 2.39 Clinical appearance at 2 weeks following (a) left implant placement surgery and (b) right implant placement surgery.

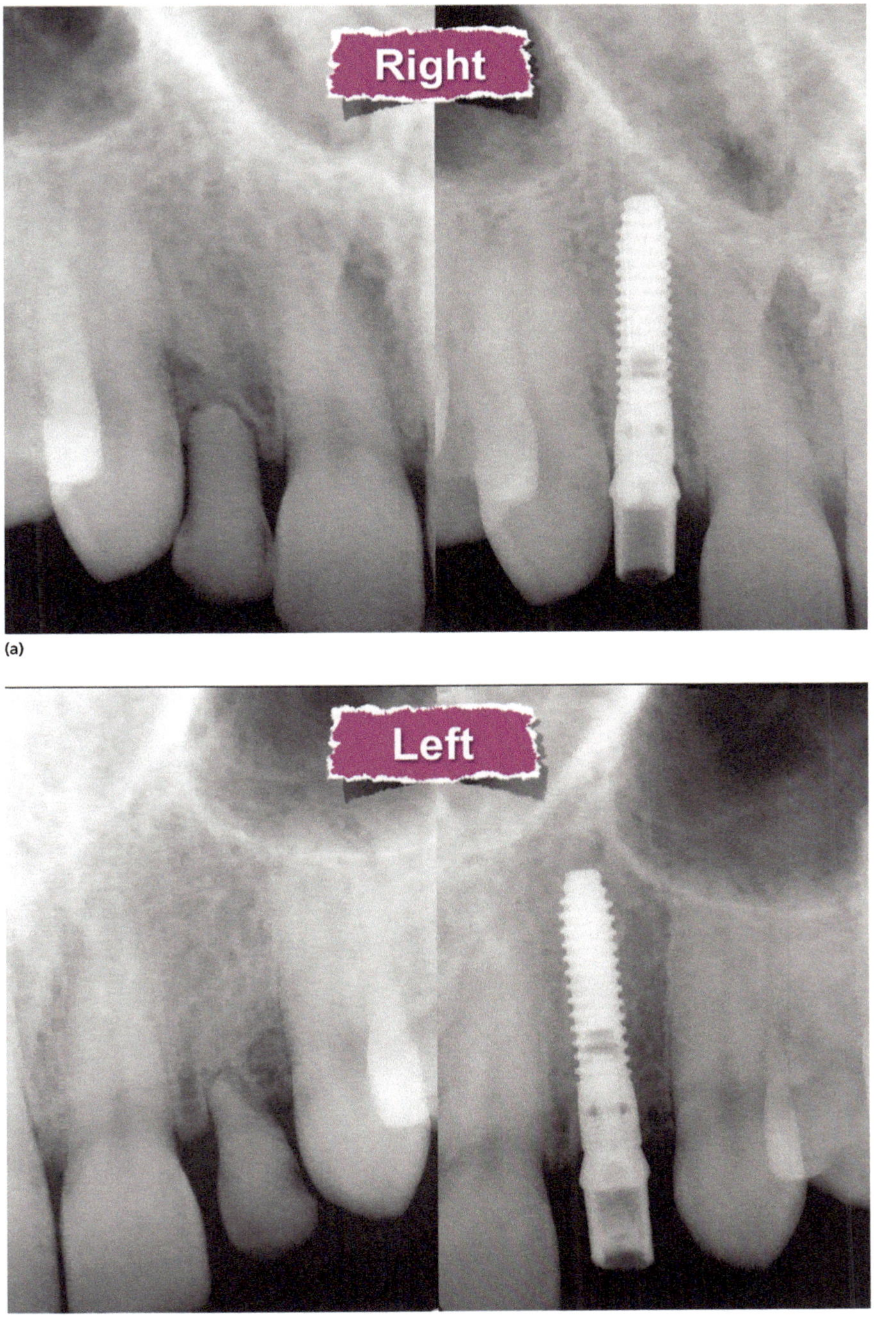

(a)

(b)

Figure 2.40 Preoperative and post-operative radiographs of the (a) right and (b) left lateral incisor implant.

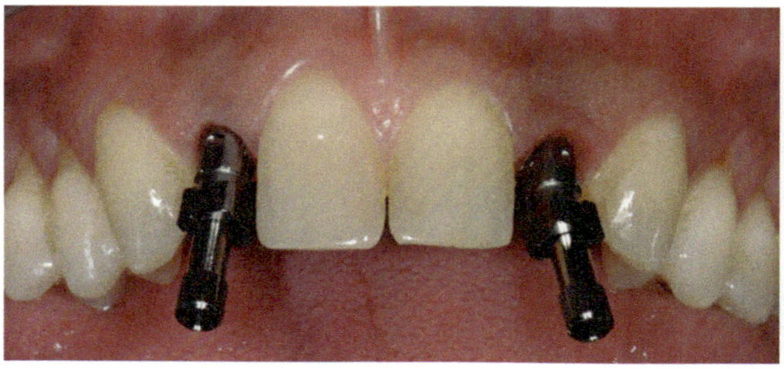

Figure 2.41 Open-tray fixture-level impression transfer copings in position.

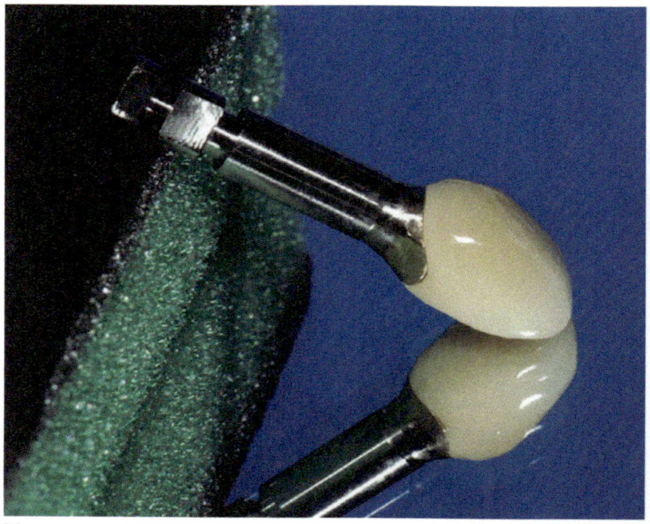

(a)

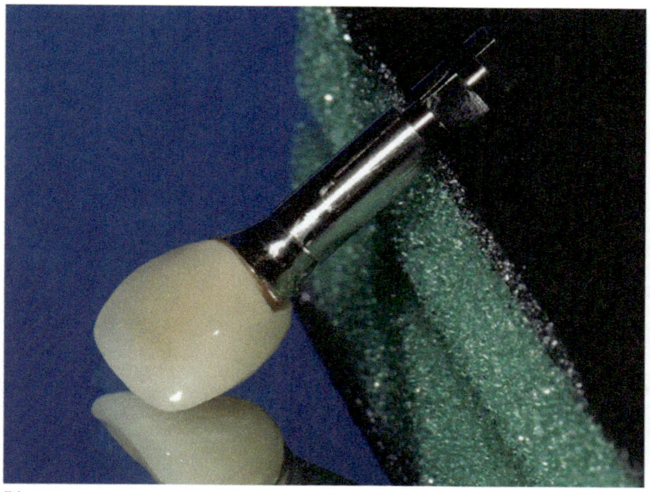

(b)

Figure 2.42 (a, b) Ceramo-metal restorations on the implant analogs.

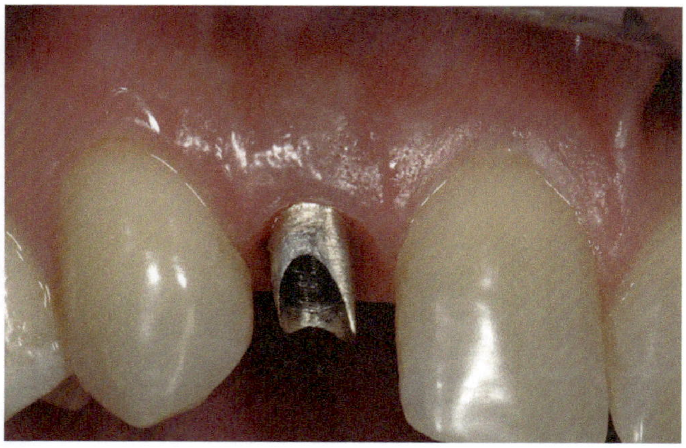

Figure 2.43 Custom post for the right implant with a good soft tissue profile.

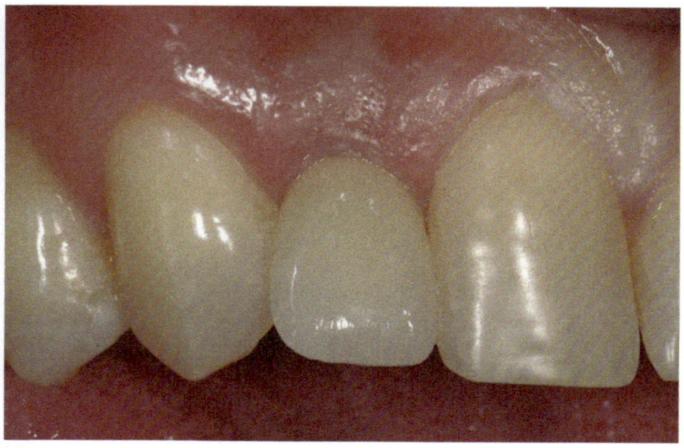

(a)

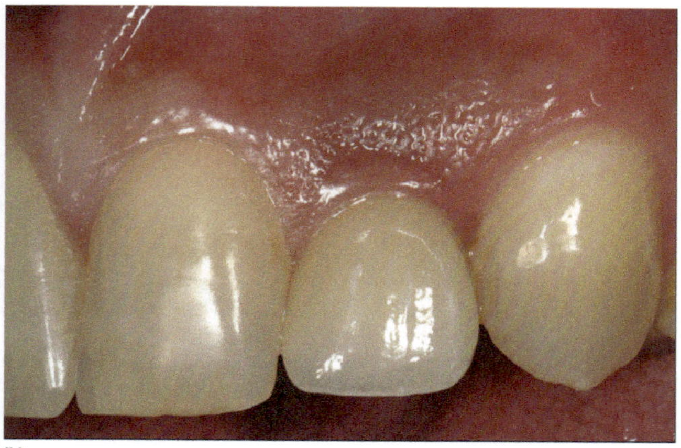

(b)

Figure 2.44 Final ceramo-metal restoration on the (a) right and (b) left lateral incisor.

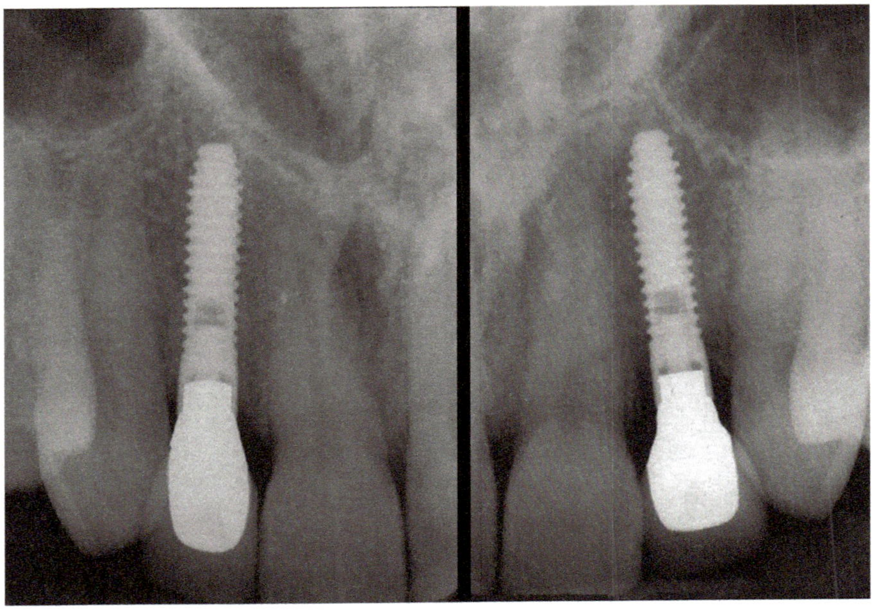

Figure 2.45 Final periapical radiographs taken at 24 months post-surgery for the right and left lateral incisor implant restorations.

Conclusions

Implant dentistry has become one of the most predictable treatment modalities that clinicians can offer to patients who are missing or will be losing teeth. Improvements in implant design, ancillary biologics, and prosthetic interfaces have helped enormously, but less attention has been directed toward the diagnostic phase of implant treatment, which also has evolved considerably. The use of computer-based technology, such as CBCT, provides further improvements in surgical accuracy and restorative outcomes. The purpose of this chapter was to review concepts as to the state-of-the-art technology available to clinicians in case diagnosis and planning. A step-by-step process was used to illustrate the diagnostic, surgical, and restorative phases necessary to execute a minimally invasive surgical intervention consisting of tooth extractions, immediate placement of two implants, and immediate provisional restoration. In addition, CBCT technology offers an excellent means of communication between all members of the dental implant team. The use of images in case presentations can provide one of the best educational tools to inform patients of their treatment options. Standardized protocols need to be developed to aid clinicians in understanding how best to utilize 3-D CBCT images for implant planning with greater accuracy, and execute the plan from within the interactive treatment planning software, using either a freehand surgical approach or with a CT-derived template for surgical guidance (see Chapter 9). The adoption and utilization of CT-based technology will only improve as the industry provides updated tools to integrate and merge the CBCT scan to the implant planning phase, template fabrication, surgical intervention, and CAD/CAM fabrication of abutments and restorations. Merging these technologies with intraoral scanning, and/or optical scanning of physical impressions or stone casts, will be refined, improving accuracy of the diagnostic, surgical, and restorative phases of dental implant reconstruction.

References

1. Ganz SD. Dental implantology: an evolving treatment modality. Compend Contin Educ Dent 2013; 34: 628–629.
2. Orentlicher G, Goldsmith D, Abboud M. Computer-guided planning and placement of dental implants. Atlas Oral Maxillofac Surg Clin North Am 2012; 20: 53–79.
3. Orentlicher G, Abboud M. Guided surgery for implant therapy. Oral Maxillofac Surg Clin North Am 2011; 23: 239–256.
4. Ganz SD. Use of stereolithographic models as diagnostic and restorative aids for predictable immediate loading of implants. Pract Proced Aesthet Dent 2003; 15: 763–771.
5. Ganz SD. Techniques for the use of CT imaging for the fabrication of surgical guides. Atlas Oral Maxillofac Surg Clin North Am 2006; 14: 75–97.
6. Ganz SD. Cone beam computed tomography-assisted treatment planning concepts. Dent Clin North Am 2011; 55: 515–536.
7. Ganz SD. The reality of anatomy and the triangle of bone. Inside Dent 2006; 2(5): 72–77.
8. Ganz SD. Implant complications associated with two- and three dimensional diagnostic imaging technologies. In: Dental Implant Complications – Etiology, Prevention, and Treatment, FroumSJ, ed. Chichester: Wiley-Blackwell, 2010, pp. 71–99.
9. Hofschneider U, Tepper G, Gahleitner A, Ulm C. Assessment of the blood supply to the mental region for reduction of bleeding complications during implant surgery in the interforaminal region. Int J Oral Maxillofac Implants 1999; 14: 379–383.
10. Leong DJ, Chan HL, Yeh CY, et al. Risk of lingual plate perforation during implant placement in the posterior mandible: a human cadaver study. Implant Dent 2011; 20: 360–363.
11. Longoni S, Sartori M, Braun M, et al. Lingual vascular canals of the mandible: the risk of bleeding complications during implant procedures. Implant Dent 2007; 16: 131–138.
12. Mardinger O, Manor Y, Mijiritsky E, Hirshberg A. Lingual perimandibular vessels associated with life-threatening bleeding: an anatomic study. Int J Oral Maxillofac Implants 2007; 22: 127–131.
13. Tepper G, Hofschneider UB, Gahleitner A, Ulm C. Computed tomographic diagnosis and localization of bone canals in the mandibular interforaminal region for prevention of bleeding complications during implant surgery. Int J Oral Maxillofac Implants 2001; 16: 68–72.
14. Lin MH, Mau LP, Cochran DL, et al. Risk assessment of inferior alveolar nerve injury for immediate implant placement in the posterior mandible: a virtual implant placement study. J Dent 2014; 42: 263–270.
15. Chan HL, Benavides E, Yeh CY, et al. Risk assessment of lingual plate perforation in posterior mandibular region: a virtual implant placement study using cone-beam computed tomography. J Periodontol 2011; 82: 129–135.

16. Ganz SD. Utilization of three-dimensional imaging technology to enhance maxillofacial surgical applications In: Peterson's Principles of Oral and Maxillofacial Surgery, MiloroM, GhaliGE, LarsenP, WaiteP, eds. Shelton, CT: People's Medical House, 2012, pp. 179–200.
17. Ganz SD. Defining new paradigms for assessment of implant receptor sites. The use of CT/CBCT and interactive virtual treatment planning for congenitally missing lateral incisors. Compend Contin Educ Dent 2008; 29: 256–267.
18. Solar P, Geyerhofer U, Traxler H, et al. Blood supply to the maxillary sinus relevant to sinus floor elevation procedures. Clin Oral Implants Res 1999; 10: 34–44.
19. Van den Bergh JP, ten Bruggenkate CM, Disch FJ, Tuinzing DB. Anatomical aspects of sinus floor elevations. Clin Oral Implants Res 2000; 11: 256–265.
20. Anamali S, Avila-Ortiz G, Elangovan S, et al. Prevalence of the posterior superior alveolar canal in cone beam computed tomography scans. Clin Oral Implants Res 2015; 26(1): e8–e12.
21. Chan HL, Misch K, Wang HL. Dental imaging in implant treatment planning. Implant Dent 2010; 19: 288–298.
22. Ella B, Sédarat C, Noble Rda C, et al. Vascular connections of the lateral wall of the sinus: surgical effect in sinus augmentation. Int J Oral Maxillofac Implants 2008; 23: 1047–1052.
23. Jung J, Yim JH, Kwon YD, et al. A radiographic study of the position and prevalence of the maxillary arterial endosseous anastomosis using cone beam computed tomography. Int J Oral Maxillofac Implants 2011; 26: 1273–1278.
24. Elian N, Wallace S, Cho SC, et al. Distribution of the maxillary artery as it relates to sinus floor augmentation. Int J Oral Maxillofac Implants 2005; 20(5): 784–787.
25. Angelopoulos C, Aghaloo T. Imaging technology in implant diagnosis. Dent Clin North Am 2011; 55: 141–158.
26. Benavides E, Rios HF, Ganz SD, et al. Use of cone beam computed tomography in implant dentistry: The International Congress of Oral Implantologists consensus report. Implant Dent 2012; 21: 78–86.
27. Mardinger O, Abba M, Hirshberg A, Schwartz-Arad D. Prevalence, diameter and course of the maxillary intraosseous vascular canal with relation to sinus augmentation procedure: a radiographic study. Int J Oral Maxillofac Surg 2007; 36: 735–738.
28. Wen SC, Chan HL, Wang HL. Classification and management of antral septa for maxillary sinus augmentation. Int J Periodontics Restorative Dent 2013; 33: 509–517.
29. Tyndall DA, Price JB, Tetradis S, et al. American Academy of Oral and Maxillofacial Radiology. Position statement of the American Academy of Oral and Maxillofacial Radiology on selection criteria for the use of radiology in dental implantology with emphasis on cone beam computed tomography. Oral Surg Oral Med Oral Pathol Oral Radiol 2012; 113: 817–826.
30. Elian N, Ehrlich B, Jalbout Z, et al. A restoratively driven ridge categorization, as determined by incorporating ideal restorative positions on radiographic templates utilizing computed tomography scan analysis. Clin Implant Dent Relat Res 2009; 11: 272–278.
31. Ganz SD. Focus on: CBCT technology. Dent Today 2012; 31(5): 17.
32. Rosenfeld AL, Mandelaris GA, Tardieu PB. Prosthetically directed implant placement using computer software to ensure precise placement and predictable prosthetic outcomes. Part 1: diagnostics, imaging, and collaborative accountability. Int J Periodontics Restorative Dent 2006; 26: 215–221.
33. Rosenfeld AL, Mandelaris GA, Tardieu PB. Prosthetically directed implant placement using computer software to ensure precise placement and predictable prosthetic outcomes. Part 2: rapid-prototype medical modeling and stereolithographic drilling guides requiring bone exposure. Int J Periodontics Restorative Dent 2006; 26: 347–353.
34. Ganz SD. The triangle of bone – a formula for successful implant placement and restoration. Implant Soc 1995; 5(5): 2–6.
35. Ganz SD. Presurgical planning with CT-derived fabrication of surgical guides. J Oral Maxillofac Surg 2005; 63(Suppl 2): 59–71.
36. Ganz SD. Use of CT diagnostics, stereolithography and CT derived templates to enhance dental implant placement and immediate load protocols. Presented at the 27th Annual Convention of the American Association of Dental Maxillofacial Radiographic Technicians, Phoenix, AZ, 2005.
37. Ganz SD. CT/CBCT diagnosis and treatment planning concepts for bone grafting applications. In: Implant Site Development, SonickM, HwangD, SaadounAP, eds. Chichester: Wiley-Blackwell, 2012, pp. 101–120.
38. Ganz SD. Using interactive technology: "in the zone with the triangle of bone". Dent Implantol Update 2008; 19(5): 33–38.
39. Abboud M, Kobren LB, Orentlicher G. Implant complications: biomechanical and esthetic considerations – a prosthodontist's perspective. Compend Contin Educ Dent 2013; 34(Spec No. 7): 20–24.
40. Arisan V, Karabuda ZC, Ozdemir T. Accuracy of two stereolithographic guide systems for computer-aided implant placement: a computed tomography-based clinical comparative study. J Periodontol 2010; 81: 43–51.
41. Azari A, Nikzad S. Flapless implant surgery: review of the literature and report of 2 cases with computer-guided surgical approach. J Oral Maxillofac Surg 2008; 66: 1015–1021.
42. Cassetta M, Stefanelli LV, Giansanti M, Calasso S. Accuracy of implant placement with a stereolithographic surgical template. Int J Oral Maxillofac Implants 2012; 27: 655–663.
43. Chaar MS, Att W, Strub JR. Prosthetic outcome of cement-retained implant-supported fixed dental restorations: a systematic review. J Oral Rehabil 2011; 38: 697–711.
44. D'haese J, Van De Velde T, Komiyama A, et al. Accuracy and complications using computer-designed stereolithographic surgical guides for oral rehabilitation by means of dental implants: a review of the literature. Clin Implant Dent Relat Res 2012; 14: 321–335.
45. Da Rocha PV, Freitas MA, de Morais Alves da Cunha T. Influence of screw access on the retention of cement-retained implant prostheses. J Prosthetic Dent 2013; 109: 264–268.
46. De Brandão ML, Vettore MV, Vidigal Júnior GM. Peri-implant bone loss in cement- and screw-retained prostheses: systematic review and meta-analysis. J Clin Periodontol 2013; 40: 287–295.
47. Katsoulis J, Pazera P, Mericske-Stern R. Prosthetically driven, computer-guided implant planning for the edentulous maxilla: a model study. Clin Implant Dent Relat Res 2009; 11: 238–245.
48. Lee A, Okayasu K, Wang HL. Screw- versus cement-retained implant restorations: current concepts. Implant Dent 2010; 19: 8–15.
49. Koop R, Vercruyssen M, Vermeulen K, Quirynen M. Tolerance within the sleeve inserts of different surgical guides for guided implant surgery. Clin Oral Implants Res 2013; 24: 630–634.
50. Ozan O, Turkyilmaz I, Ersoy AE, et al. Clinical accuracy of 3 different types of computed tomography-derived stereolithographic surgical guides in implant placement. J Oral Maxillofac Surg 2009; 67: 394–401.
51. Shadid R, Sadaqa N. A comparison between screw- and cement-retained implant prostheses. A literature review. J Oral Implantol 2012; 38: 298–307.
52. Michalakis KX, Hirayama H, Garefis PD. Cement-retained versus screw-retained implant restorations: a critical review. Int J Oral Maxillofac Implants 2003; 18: 719–728.
53. Noelken R, Donati M, Fiorellini J, et al. Soft and hard tissue alterations around implants placed in an alveolar ridge with a sloped configuration. Clin Oral Implants Res 2014; 25: 3–9.
54. Sammartino G, Della Valle A, Marenzi G, et al. Stereolithography in oral implantology: a comparison of surgical guides. Implant Dent 2004; 13: 133–139.
55. Valente F, Schiroli G, Sbrenna A. Accuracy of computer-aided oral implant surgery: a clinical and radiographic study. Int J Oral Maxillofac Implants 2009; 24: 234–242.
56. Vandeweghe S, Cosyn J, Thevissen E, et al. A 1-year prospective study on Co-Axis implants immediately loaded with a full ceramic crown. Clin Implant Dent Relat Res 2012; 14(Suppl 1): e126–e138.
57. Lee CY, Ganz SD, Wong N, Suzuki JB. Use of cone beam computed tomography and a laser intraoral scanner in virtual dental implant surgery: part 1. Implant Dent 2012; 21: 265–271.
58. Wouters V, Mollemans W, Schutyser F. Calibrated segmentation of CBCT and CT images for digitization of dental prostheses. Int J Comput Assist Radiol Surg 2011; 6: 609–616.

CHAPTER 3

Risk Assessment and Avoiding Complications

David Dara Yarmand,[1] Douglas Deporter,[2] & Daniel R. Cullum[3]
[1]Private Practice, OMS, Toronto, ON, Canada
[2]Discipline of Periodontics, Faculty of Dentistry, University of Toronto, Toronto, ON, Canada
[3]Private Practice, Coeur d'Alene, ID; Loma Linda University Department of OMS, Loma Linda, CA; UCLA Department of OMS, Los Angeles, CA, USA

Introduction

As with all surgical procedures, there are risks associated with the placement of dental implants, and whole books have been written on this topic.[1] By reducing the invasiveness of implant procedures and reducing the overall number of surgeries, these risks can be minimized. Additionally, the clinician's level of training and experience will play a significant role in avoiding complications and achieving successful treatment outcomes. However, the greatest potential for reducing risks and complications can be achieved by careful preoperative assessment of the patient's health and expectations, appropriate clinical and radiographic examinations, and 3-D computer-assisted planning (see Chapters 2 and 9).

Risks associated with patient health and habits

There appear to be few absolute medical contraindications for dental implant treatment.[2] They include recent myocardial infarction or stroke, a recent joint or valvular prosthesis, a state of immunosuppression, active treatment for malignancy including recent head and neck radiotherapy, drug and/or alcohol abuse, psychiatric illness, and intravenous bisphosphonate treatment. However, patients who have been long-term users of oral bisphosphonate drugs (e.g. Fosamax®, Merck, Whitehouse, NJ, or Actonel®, Proctor & Gamble, Cincinnati, OH) or RANK-L inhibitors (Prolia®, Amgen Inc, Thousand Oaks, CA) for the management of osteoporosis or steroid-induced osteopenia also can be considered at increased risk for implant complications, specifically implant loss or osteonecrosis.[3–5] Anti-resorptive medications (including bisphosphonates and RANK-L inhibitors) function primarily by interfering with the activity of osteoclasts, and in so doing increase bone density while decreasing bone vascularity. However, the pathophysiology of the resulting disease has not been fully established, and there is still great controversy as to the mechanism of medication-related osteonecrosis of the jaw[6] (MRONJ, formerly known as bisphosphonate-related osteonecrosis of the jaw). MRONJ is notoriously difficult to resolve in jaw sites affected by intravenous bisphosphonate usage, and may require long-term antibiotic use or in some instances extensive resective jaw surgery.

Yip et al.[7] presented retrospective data on implant failure in women taking oral bisphosphonates (January 1997 to December 2004) prior to their being identified as a risk factor for MRONJ and implant failures. Over 1100 implants had been placed in 337 women aged 40 years and older, with implant failures in 114 women. The main study variable was oral bisphosphonate use at the time of implant treatment, while covariates included patient age at treatment, year of implant placement, smoking status, implant location, implant surface type, as well as implant diameter and length. After adjusting for all covariates, women who had been using oral bisphosphonates were 2.7 times more likely to have had an implant failure. Oral bisphosphonate with combined use of corticosteroids[6] or other co-morbidities may adversely affect implant outcomes without the occurrence of osteonecrosis.

The American Association of Oral and Maxillofacial Surgeons' position paper on bisphosphonate-related osteonecrosis of the jaws in 2009 recommended discontinuation of oral bisphosphonates 3 months prior to and 3 months after dentoalveolar surgery.[5] However, there is currently limited evidence substantiating such a recommendation. The 2014 American Association of Oral and Maxillofacial Surgeons' guidelines suggest a "drug holiday" only with patients at higher risk of developing MRONJ, such as patients using anti-resorptive medication for 4 years or longer and/or with other co-morbidities, such as glucocorticoid use, diabetes, and smoking.[6] The current drug holiday strategy is to have a drug-free period 2 months prior and 2 months after any invasive dental procedures. However, these guidelines still cannot be supported or refuted because of the limited data available, leaving the decision to the clinician's judgment.

The general consensus for management of patients with diabetes mellitus is that there should be no contraindication to having implant treatment if the diabetes is well-controlled, with hemoglobin A_{1C} levels below 7[8] and a stable periodontal condition. Patients with diabetes are at increased risk of developing periodontitis;[9] however, successful periodontal treatment does lead to improved glycemic control in diabetics.[10] Elimination of co-morbidities, such as poor oral hygiene and smoking, and the use of an appropriate antibiotic regimen with surgery will be important to successful implant treatment outcomes.[11,12] Taking a careful patient medical history to discover previous oral surgical treatments and their outcomes can be helpful.[13] Other medical conditions that might affect outcomes with dental implants, such as Sjögren's syndrome, Parkinson's disease, Crohn's disease, and organ transplantation have not been adequately studied to formulate recommendations.[14]

Minimally Invasive Dental Implant Surgery, First Edition. Edited by Daniel R. Cullum and Douglas Deporter.

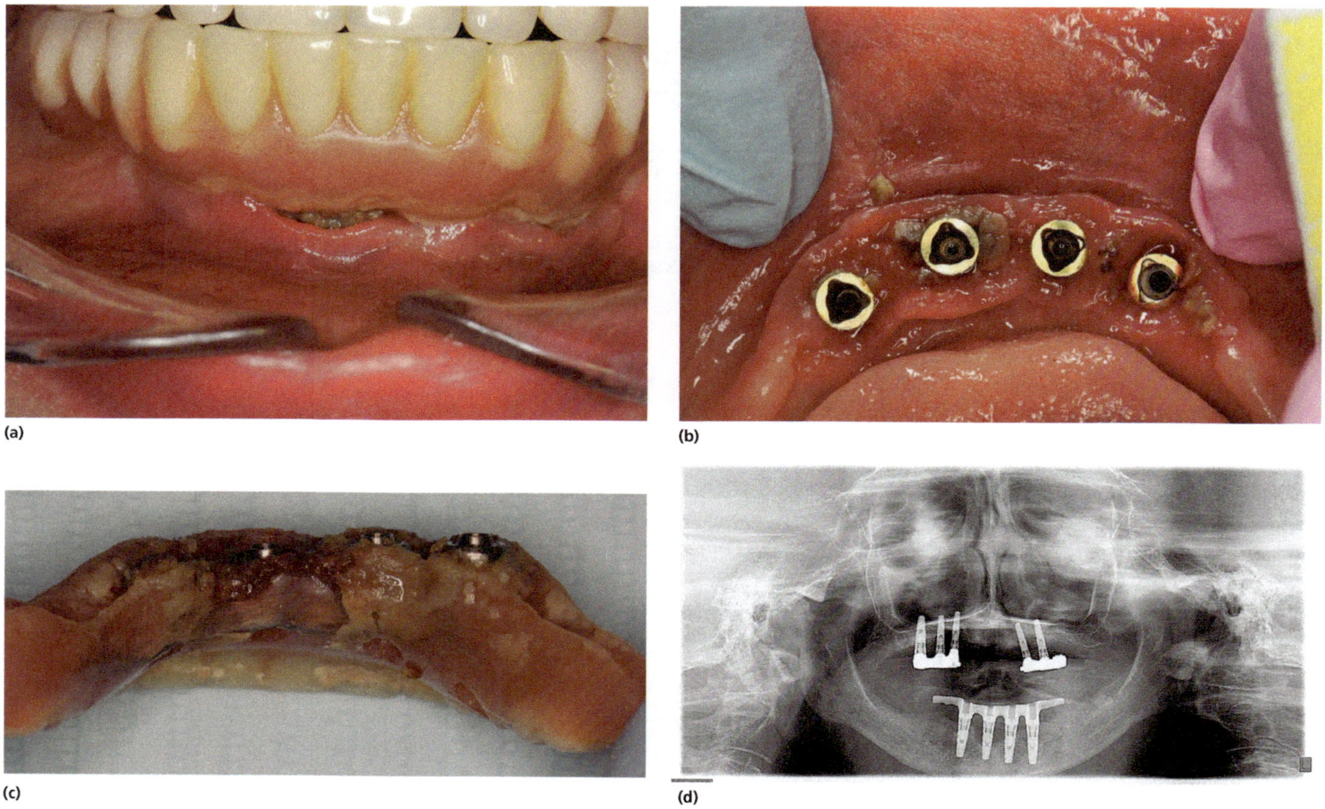

Figure 3.1 (a) Clinical view of a fixed implant-supported prosthesis showing accumulation of food debris as well as plaque and calculus under the denture due to a poor prosthetic design (case provided by Dr David Chvartszaid, Toronto, ON). (b) Occlusal view of the implants and soft tissue. The tissue appears inflamed due to chronic irritation. (c) The intaglio surface is irregular with a poor, unhygienic prosthetic design making it difficult to clean. (d) Radiograph showing the resulting crestal bone loss that has affected most notably the second implant from the right.

Patients who have poor oral hygiene habits and/or accessibility challenges with adequate hygiene due to poor prosthesis design, will most likely show greater peri-implant bone loss and risk of peri-implantitis than those with good hygiene and prostheses designed for cleansiblity[15,16] (Figure 3.1). Patients who smoke cigarettes are at higher risk for implant complications and failure, especially in posterior maxilla,[17] regardless of implant type and surface texture.[18] Along with the existing subantral bone height, smoking is considered a major risk factor following maxillary sinus augmentation,[19] especially with simultaneous dental implant placement. Lin et al.[20] reported that implant failure in smokers who had sinus grafting with simultaneous implant placement was as high as 40%. Patients are often categorized into groups as per their smoking history, and many clinicians consider patients who smoke 10 or fewer cigarettes per day not to be at elevated risk. Others, however, have reported that even this level of smoking can be detrimental;[21] so, the best approach may be to assume that smokers are always at greater risk than non-smokers and to make this fact clear to patients who smoke and are unable to stop. Smoking also increases peri-implant crestal bone loss after onset of implant function,[22–24] and this may become increasingly important in the future given that many clinicians have moved to using short dental implants. Short implants are currently defined as those having designed intrabony lengths of ≤8 mm[25] (see also Chapter 10). While there are no existing data on the relative importance of crestal bone loss for short versus long dental implants, biomechanically, any loss of crestal bone from a short implant may have greater impact than with longer implants. The occurrence of peri-implant crestal bone loss often is due to peri-implantitis, and smoking predisposes to this as well,[26] especially in the maxilla. Smokers also have a higher prevalence of periodontitis,[27] which if not adequately treated may provide a source of microbial pathogens for the initiation of peri-implantitis.[28,29] There is a greater risk of peri-implantitis in smoking patients with concurrent or even a past history of treated periodontitis.[30–32] Patients who are susceptible to periodontitis have a higher risk of developing peri-implantitis if periodontal pocket depths of ≥5 mm remain after active periodontal therapy.[32] It is possible for aggressive pathogens to transfer from periodontally affected teeth to adjacent implants,[29] although different key pathogens may be involved in periodontitis versus peri-implantitis.[33] Patients with a history of treated periodontal disease will require regular and thorough periodontal maintenance care for long-term success with dental implants.[34]

Another patient habit suggested to be a risk for implant treatment is bruxism; however, the effect of bruxism on progressive bone loss and subsequent implant failure is inconclusive. In two recent review papers,[35,36] the authors concluded that while bruxism may predispose implant prostheses to mechanical complications, there is less evidence to suggest that the habit leads to implant failure. Little data exist on the relationship between bruxism and implant length, particularly short implant length. Tawil et al.[37] reported data primarily from the posterior mandible with machine-turned, threaded implants in lengths of ≤10 mm and found no relationship between bruxism and peri-implant crestal bone loss. One implant fracture occurred after an extended functional period in one patient with severe bruxism, likely due to metal fatigue. No mention was made of whether or not this patient had been using a night guard. An example of a fractured implant is shown in Figure 3.2. Practitioners often provide their implant patients having known bruxing habits with protective night guards. This is certainly not contraindicated, as such an appliance will help to protect implant crowns from excessive wear and tear and fracture of implant components, assuming adequate patient compliance. Further considerations for bruxing patients include whether the patient has a single implant-supported restoration or multiple units and whether or not "cross-arch" stabilization was employed. The load-bearing ability of a single-unit restoration with a "protected occlusion" provided by support of contiguous natural teeth is at less risk compared with, for example, a posterior free-end restoration or an anterior implant-supported restoration without protrusive guidance. Questions still remain about the role of inflammation and crestal bone loss in the presence of excessive occlusal forces. Prosthetic challenges abound in these situations and are discussed further under prosthetic risk factors below.

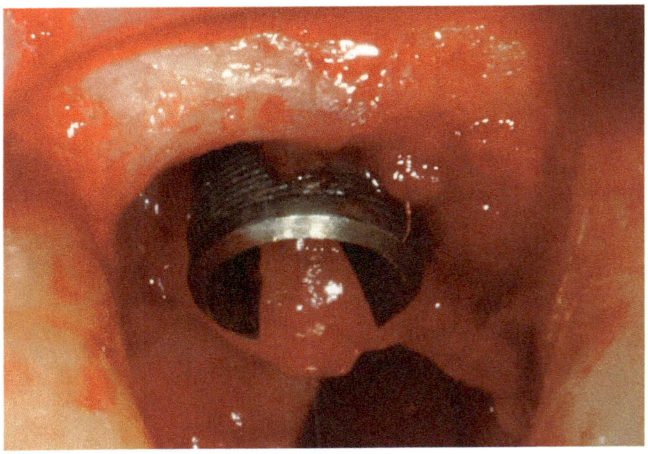

(a)

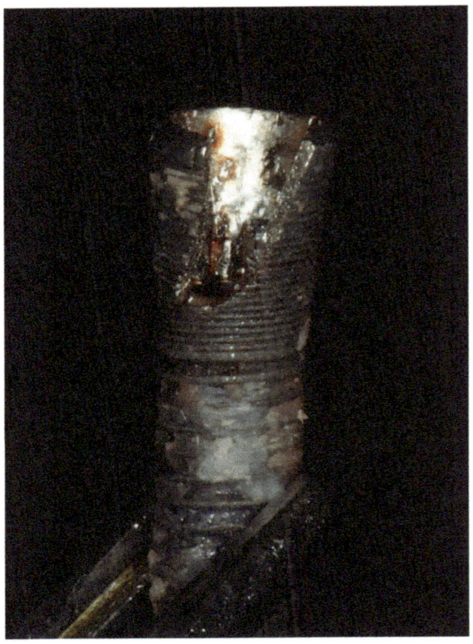

(b)

Figure 3.2 (a) The implant shown fractured on the palatal aspect resulting in peri-implant inflammation and bone loss. (b) View of the fractured implant after removal.

Anatomic risk factors

The greatest loss in alveolar ridge dimension following tooth extraction without socket preservation (see Chapter 5) is in bucco-lingual/palatal bone width, and is accentuated mid-buccally.[38] This eventuality can prevent or complicate placement of a dental implant. Flap elevation at the time of implant surgery can compromise blood supply to buccal bone, with further vertical bone loss during the early healing phase. If buccal bone thickness after implant osteotomy site preparation is <2 mm, it has been recommended that augmentation grafting is essential to prevent unwanted buccal bone loss,[39,40] exposure of the buccal implant surface, associated gingival recession, and even peri-implantitis. In esthetic areas, the surgeon must ensure that there is an adequate facial bone volume after healing, as late soft tissue recession can result in esthetic compromise (Figure 3.3). Therefore, the majority of implants will require buccal bone augmentation, since buccal bone thickness impacts on the thickness of overlying soft tissues[41] (see also Chapter 8). Sites with reduced interproximal bone height also impact negatively on treatment outcomes since optimal gingival papilla reformation requires that the distance from the peak of interproximal bone to the contact point of the implant crown and adjacent tooth or of two adjacent implant crowns be <5 mm.[42,43]

Local bone density may also be a risk factor if the site is primarily cancellous in nature, or if the patient presents with osteoporosis or osteopenia undiagnosed or in treatment with anti-resorptive medications as discussed previously. Surgical management of these sites can be enhanced by using slightly undersized osteotomies,[44] avoiding implants that require countersinking,[45,46] and using moderately rough-surfaced implants[47] and/or implants that are tapered and/or self-tapping for increased initial implant stability as compensation for the compromised bone density. Advantage also may be gained by using increased diameter implants if this is feasible within the existing alveolar ridge housing.

Inadequate width and thickness of peri-implant keratinized gingival tissue is considered by some clinicians to be a risk to implant outcomes, and soft tissue grafting procedures may be employed for augmentation (see Chapter 8), including those sites with a thin gingival biotype. Sites with limited or absent peri-implant keratinized soft tissue will often display soft tissue mobility, which can be uncomfortable for the patient and predispose the area to traumatic injury and resorption of underlying crestal bone. Peri-implant attached keratinized tissue requires adequate bone volume support and should be at least 2 mm in both apico-coronal width[48] and overall thickness[49] to avoid the risk of buccal bone loss, soft tissue recession, and exposure of

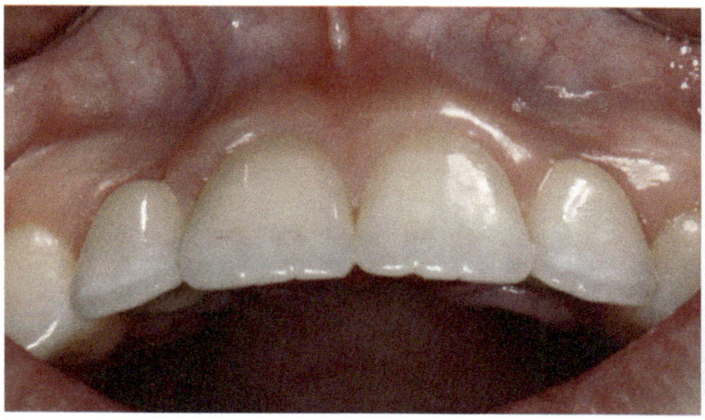

(a)

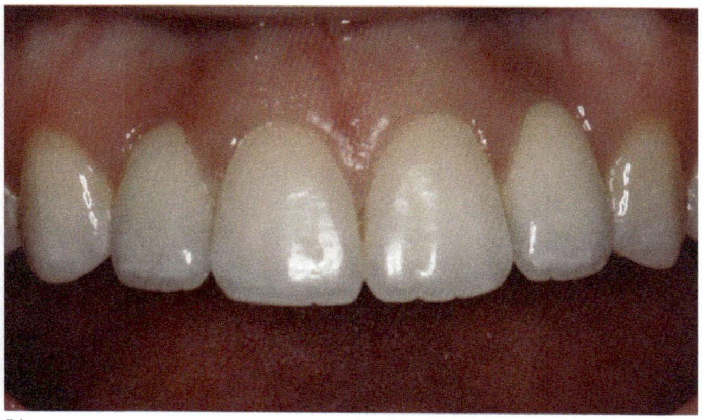

(b)

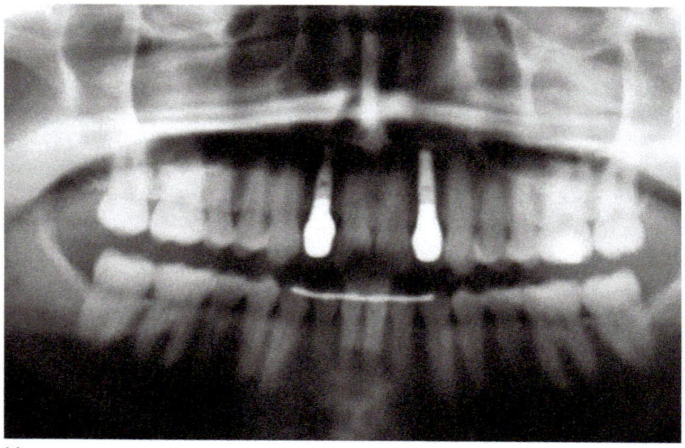

(c)

Figure 3.3 (a) Occlusal view showing inadequate bone and soft tissue volume at the facial aspect of implants at the lateral incisor positions resulting in a compromised esthetic result and thin soft tissue. (b) A facial view of the sites shows a thin soft tissue biotype with recession and tissue color compromise, which did not present until 2 years after restoration. Late findings of bone remodeling and soft tissue volume changes can result from inadequate initial facial bone thickness (<2 mm). (c) The corresponding panoramic radiograph demonstrates good implant positioning and maintenance of the interproximal bone heights. © Daniel R. Cullum.

buccal implant surface (Figure 3.4). If rough implant surfaces become exposed, there may be an increased risk of further bone loss because of bacterial colonization and establishment of peri-implantitis. In one study[50] in which implants with plasma-sprayed hydroxyapatite surfaces were used, implant failures in sites with <2 mm keratinized soft tissue width were 10 times higher (29.5% failure) than where ≥2 mm of keratinized tissue existed (2.9% failure). Once the rough hydroxyapatite surfaces became denuded of bone and contaminated with bacterial plaque, progressive bone loss occurred. Similar results were found with rough-surfaced titanium plasma-sprayed implants.[51,52] While moderately rough implant surfaces, such as particle-blasted and/or acid-etched surfaces, under healthy conditions may have less crestal bone loss than machined-surface implants,[53] surface exposure following resorption of thin buccal bone can lead to peri-implantitis.[54]

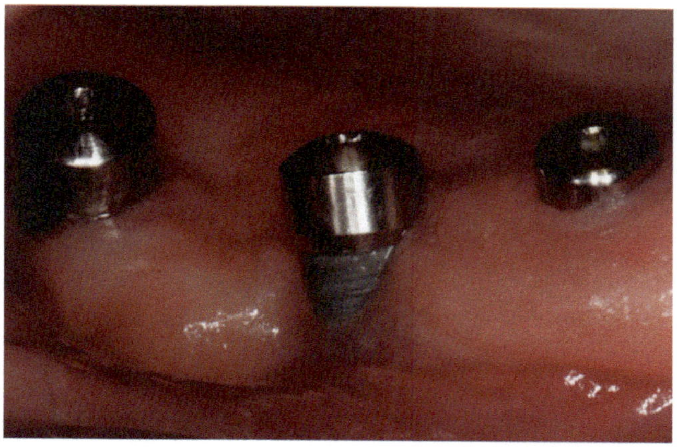

Figure 3.4 Tissue recession exposing implant threads. The tissue quality is of a thin biotype with visible buccal bone loss compared with the thick keratinized tissue and bone support associated with the two adjacent implants. © Daniel R. Cullum.

Peri-implant mucositis is a bacteria-related, soft tissue inflammation around implants not unlike gingivitis around teeth,[55,56] and smoking increases the risk of this condition.[57] Peri-implant mucositis is independent of implant type, and its key parameter is bleeding upon gentle probing (Figure 3.5). Its incidence is far greater than peri-implantitis,[58] and it should always be addressed with debridement and improved patient homecare, although it may take longer to resolve than gingivitis since it is associated with a greater host inflammatory reaction.[59] Other mucosal disorders, such as lichen planus, do not appear to be a contraindication for implant treatment,[60] although more thorough investigation of possible untoward outcomes is needed. Patients with oral lichen planus do appear to be at greater risk to peri-implant mucositis; but as with all mucositis lesions, these patients should be managed with debridement and good homecare.

Peri-implantitis is a progressive lesion, and is becoming a common challenge in implant dentistry (Figure 3.6). Data published in 2012 showed the occurrence of this problem to range from 2% to 44% of implants under assessment.[61] Experimental work in dogs[62] has shown that, once plaque contamination of moderately rough implant surfaces is established using the ligature model,

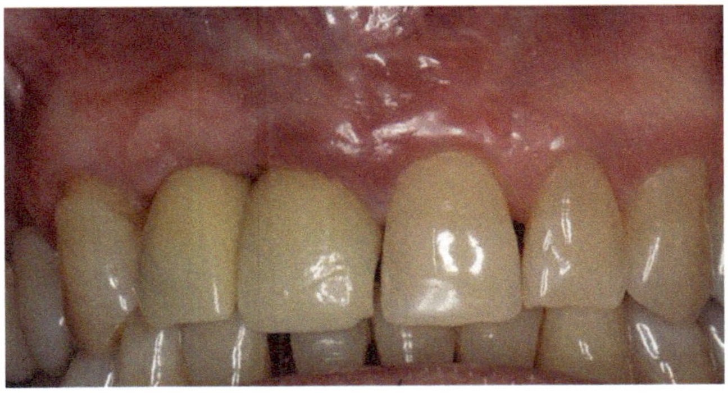

(a)

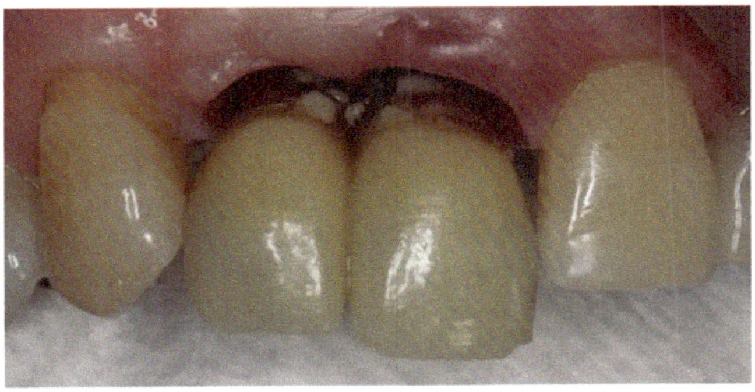

(b)

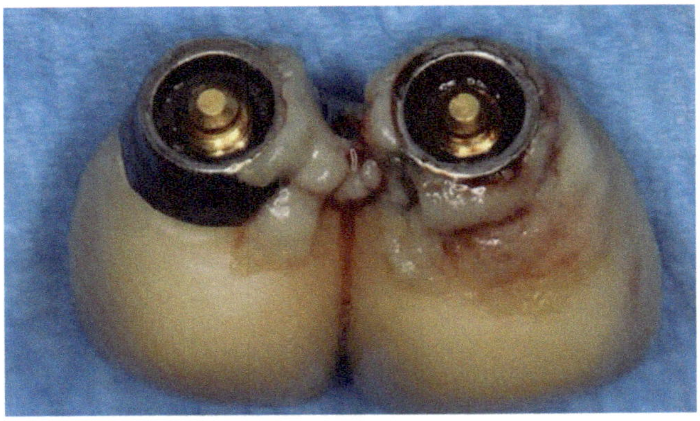

(c)

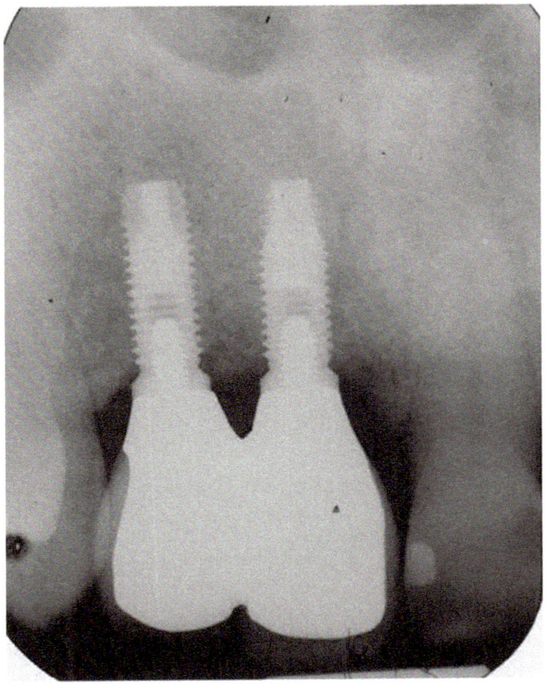

(d)

Figure 3.5 Clinical example of peri-implant mucositis. (a) The soft tissue is inflamed with a slight mucoid discharge. (b) As the prosthesis was being removed, heavy subgingival deposits were seen; and, (c) were found to be extensive following prosthesis removal. (d) No peri-implant bone loss was detected in this radiograph taken at the time. (case provided by Dr David Chvartszaid, Toronto, ON).

significantly greater spontaneous progression of peri-implant bone loss will occur with moderately rough surfaces compared with machined surfaces after ligature removal. Exposed implant surfaces meant to remain buried in bone can become a problem depending on many factors, including patient homecare, smoking, presence of periodontal disease, history of treated periodontal disease, type of periodontal disease, and regularity and quality of professional periodontal maintenance care. One recent study suggested that patients who had previously been treated for aggressive periodontal disease were at 14 times greater risk of developing peri-implantitis than periodontally healthy subjects.[63] Others have suggested that it is the quality of periodontal maintenance care rather than the use of moderately rough-surfaced implants or a history of treated periodontal disease that affects peri-implantitis risk.[34,64,65] Periodontally compromised patients with at least one residual periodontal pocket of depth ≥6 mm were more likely to develop peri-implantitis than similar patients without such residual periodontal pockets.[66] If such pockets cannot be eliminated, the patient should be placed on a more frequent recall program for scaling and root planing, perhaps in conjunction with subgingival medications like Arrestin® (OraPharm Inc., Horsham, PA), a topical preparation of minocycline. Strong consideration also should be given to removing the refractory offending tooth/teeth and or implant.

The history of an extraction site must be considered when planning implant treatment.[67] The clinician must ensure that all root fragments and periapical pathology have been eliminated. Periapical residual infections can contaminate a bone graft (Figure 3.7) or an implant whether placed immediately or in delayed fashion by retrograde tracking leading to an implant periapical lesion and eventual failure.[68–70] Immediate implant placement in an acutely infected socket should not be performed unless the contaminated site can be meticulously debrided and cleared of any residual pathology, and even then caution must be exercised. In addition to the implant site itself, adjacent teeth can also factor into the survival of an implant.[70] Even in the absence of any clinical or radiographic signs, an asymptomatic endodontically treated tooth can lead to failure of adjacent implants.[71] The implications of this can be troubling, and establishing guidelines can pose a challenge as it would not seem reasonable to recommend extraction of all endodontically treated teeth proximating an implant.

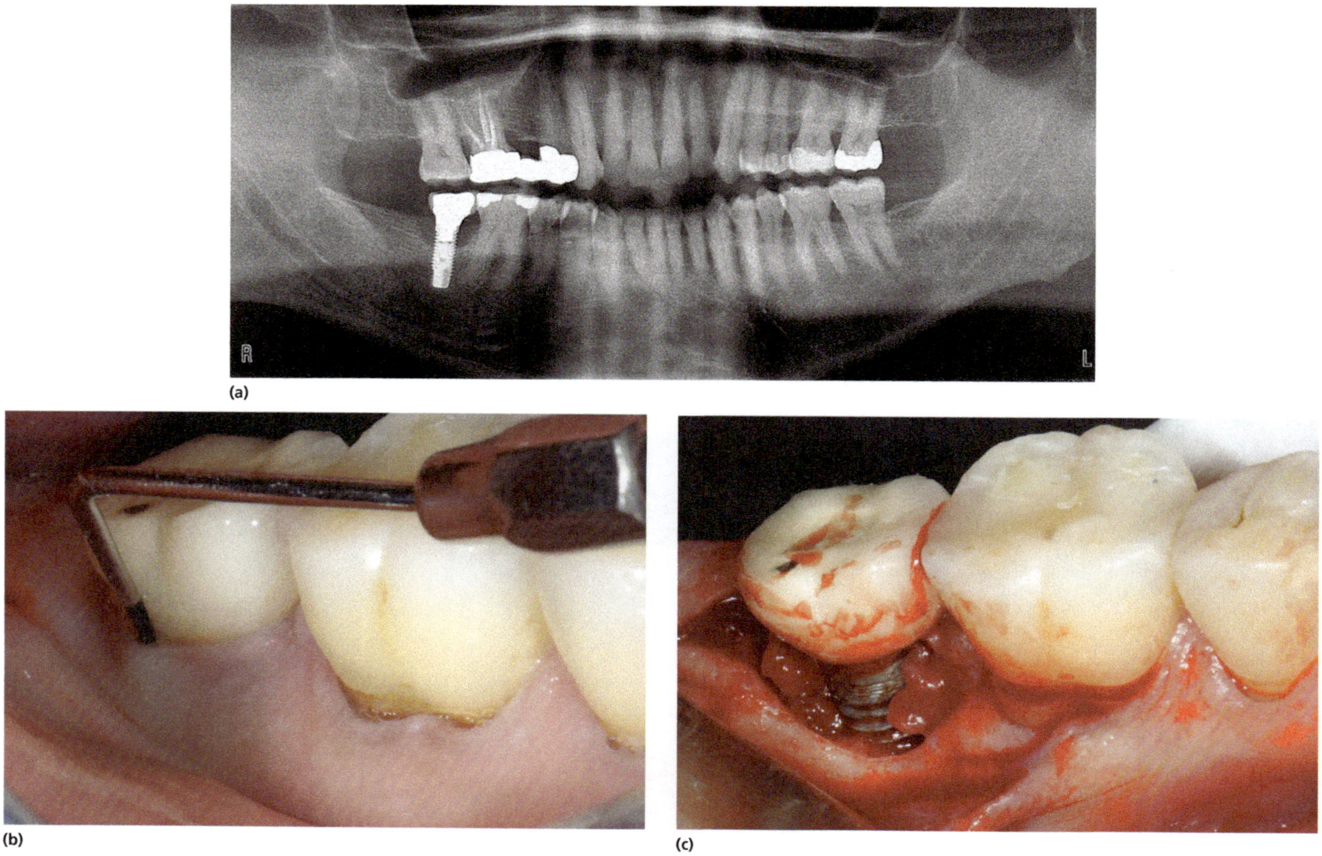

Figure 3.6 (a) A panoramic radiograph showing bone loss around the implant in the mandibular right second molar site. (b) Probing depths in excess of 10 mm were found at the buccal and lingual surfaces of the implant crown. Delayed bleeding and purulent discharge also were noted. (c) A flap was reflected showing the denuded implant surface as well as the bony trough and granulation tissue resulting from the inflammatory response.

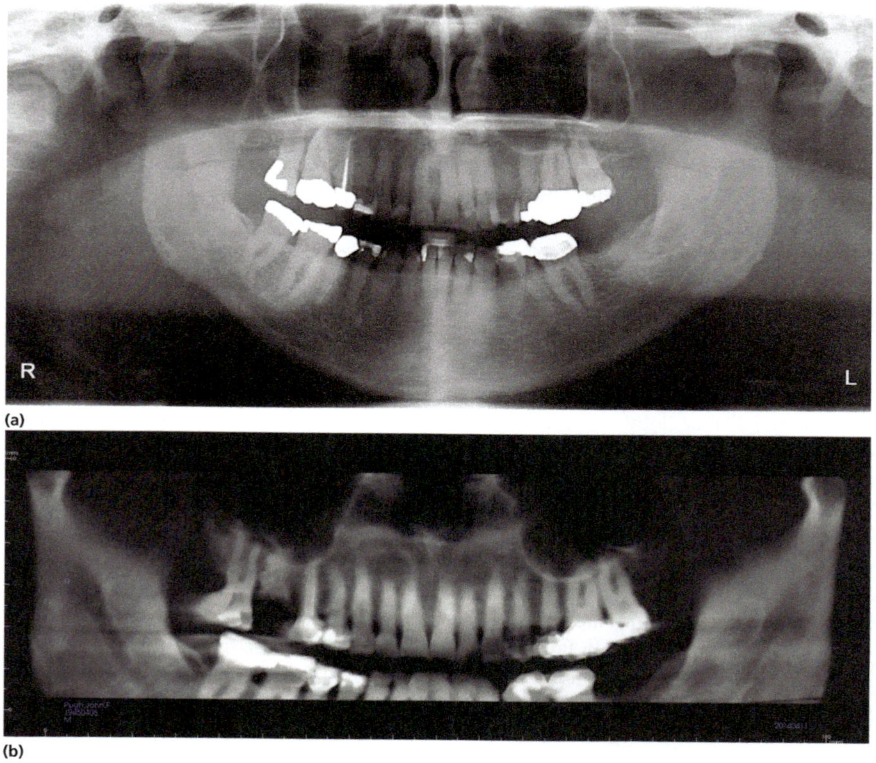

Figure 3.7 (a) A preoperative radiograph shows tooth #3, which was removed and site preservation grafting completed. (b) At the 6-month follow-up visit, a periapical radiolucency was seen at tooth #2 and is directly communicating with the adjacent bone graft. The graft was subsequently compromised.

(Continued)

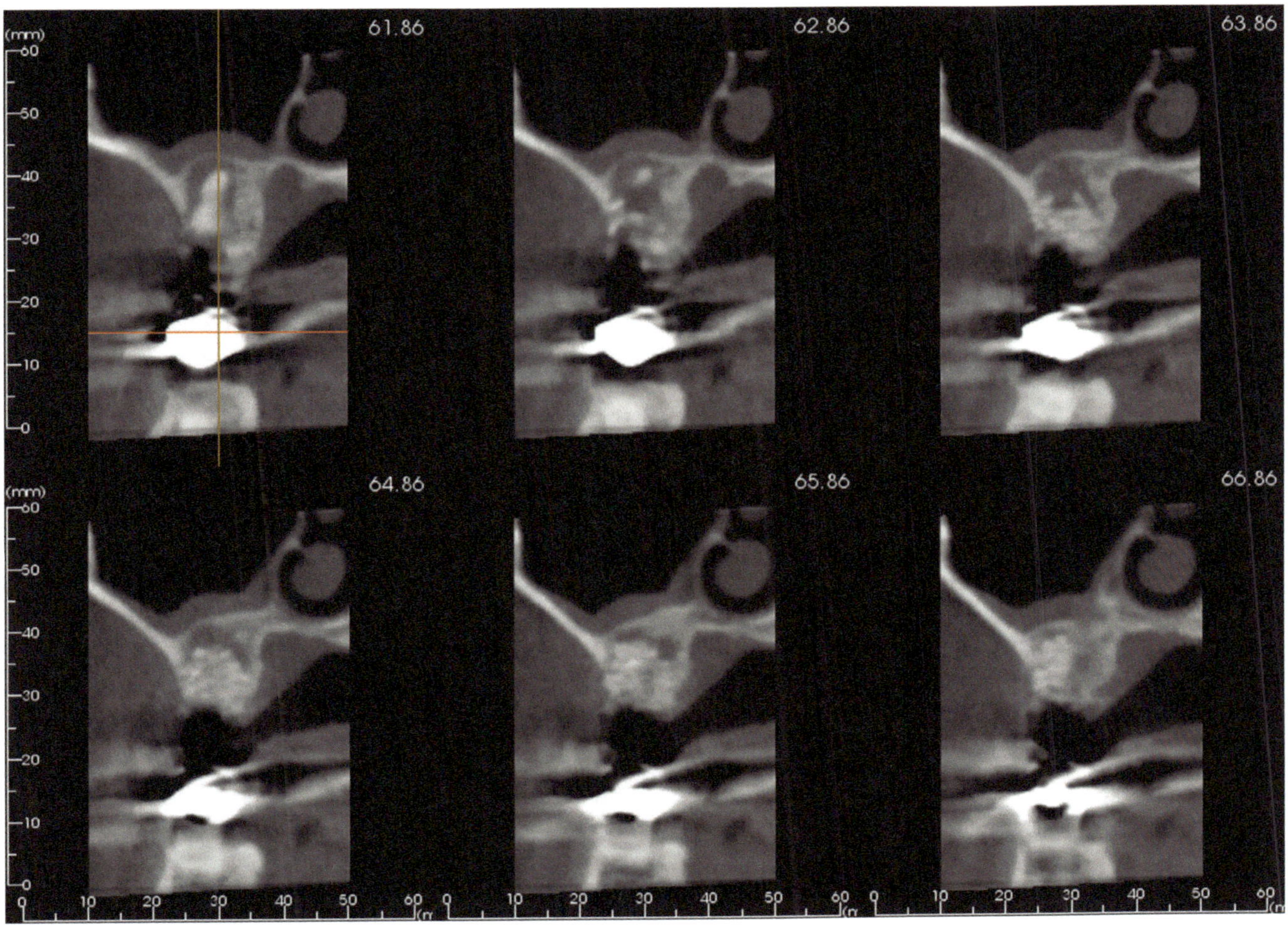

(c)

Figure 3.7 (Continued)
(c) Cross-sectional CBCT views show contamination and infection of the grafted site originating from tooth #2. © Daniel R. Cullum.

Prosthetic risk factors

The final prosthetic outcome with an implant restoration is at risk to a variety of factors. The treatment plan developed must be based on multiple diagnostic esthetic and anatomic factors as incorporated into a "restorative driven" plan (see Chapters 1 and 2). These principles include 3-D implant position, implant proximity to contiguous teeth and/or implants, implant diameter, emergence profile, and mode of retention (see Chapter 8, Figure 8.3). Regarding positioning in the bucco-lingual/palatal dimension, if an implant is positioned or angled too far buccally, it is likely that the buccal bone will be too thin to support overlying soft tissues. This will likely result in gingival recession, a longer than desired clinical crown, or even exposure of the implant surface[72,73] (Figure 3.8a and b; see Chapter 8, Figure 8.3d) Conversely, if an implant is positioned too far lingually/palatally, it may be necessary to use a custom provisional restoration for emergence profile development (see Chapter 4) and to avoid a ridge-lap crown design and the associated poor access for daily homecare. Also, in the latter situation, the implant crown may impinge upon the tongue space and become an irritation or affect speech.

An intended implant site also must have sufficient bone width in the mesio-distal dimension or there is the risk of damaging adjacent tooth roots. If there remains insufficient interproximal bone between an implant and a tooth or between two implants, then vertical bone loss may occur and the bone height may be inadequate to allow for an acceptable gingival papilla to reform. Implant site preparation should preserve at least 1.5 mm of bone between an implant and the adjacent teeth[74] or >3 mm between two adjacent implants.[75] This mesio-distal positioning is independent from the bucco-palatal positioning, as shown in Figure 3.3, where facial bone loss has occurred; however, adequate interproximal support has remained because of proper mesio-distal implant positioning[73] (see Chapter 8, Figure 8.3c and d).

A tendency for loss in height of the inter-implant bone peak will occur as inter-implant distance decreases below 3 mm,[76,77] although this bone loss can be modified using platform switching (see later). Implants placed >3 mm apart showed a mean loss in height of the interproximal bone peak of 0.45 mm, while those with ≤3 mm distance showed a loss of 1.04 mm.[78] In situations where the inter-implant distance is suboptimal (i.e. <3 mm), the lateral bone losses (1.4 mm) of the two adjacent implants could join, resulting in a significant reduction in the height of the inter-implant bone peak (Figure 3.9) impacting support for adequate soft tissue papilla reformation.[78]

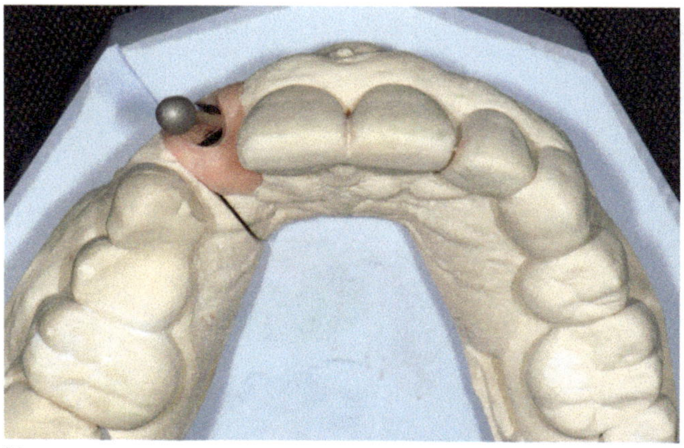

(a)

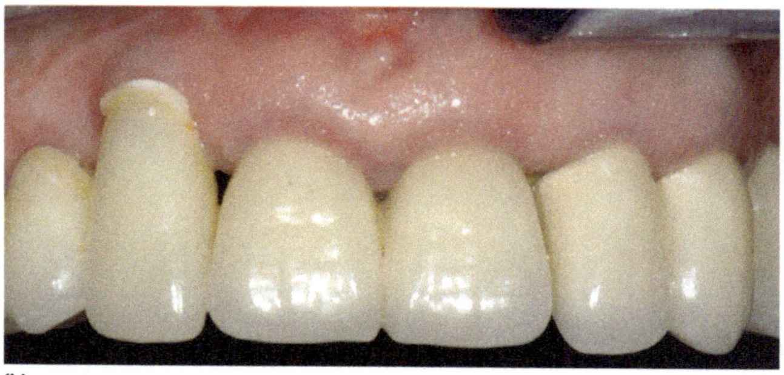

(b)

Figure 3.8 (a) The stone model for an implant at site #7 shows the positioning and excessive facial angulation of the fixture. (b) Clinically, this resulted in an apical gingival margin position and an unesthetic and overly long clinical crown.

While placing adjacent implants ≥3 mm apart reduces the risk of inter-implant bone loss,[77] it does not ensure the maintenance or reformation of an interproximal papilla. Tarnow et al.[78] reported that with two adjacent implants the mean papilla height from the interproximal bone crest was 3.4 mm with a range of 1–7 mm. Sigueira et al.[79] found that satisfactory inter-implant papillae (Jemt types "2" or "3"[80]) formed primarily when the distance from the interproximal bone peak to the contact point between the two implant crowns was ≤5 mm. Papilla formation did not seem to be related to gingival biotype.

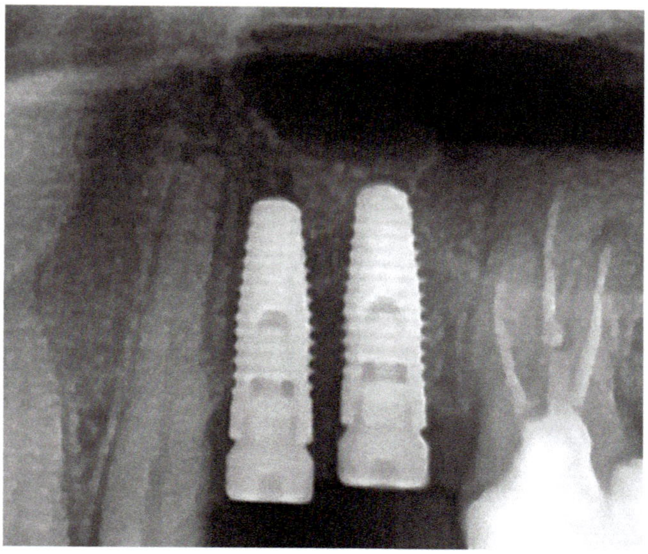

Figure 3.9 A radiograph of two adjacent implants violating the desired 3 mm inter-implant distance. Significant bone loss between the failing implants can be seen, and they were subsequently removed.

The means of retention for a fixed prosthesis (i.e. cement or screw retained) can contribute significant risk for both provisional and definitive restorations. In situations where the patient has a high scalloped/triangular tooth form or with deeply placed implants, it is important that screw-retained prostheses be used since it will be extremely difficult to ensure that no cement flash has been left behind. However, in the case of anterior implants, the facial angulation must be well behind the incisal edge to allow for the screw access to exit in the cingulum (see Chapters 1, 2, and 4). Cement fragments can be difficult if not impossible to see on radiographs, and if left behind will almost certainly initiate an inflammatory reaction that can lead to peri-implantitis and eventual implant failure[81] (Figure 3.10).

Advances in implant design with two-piece implant systems include "platform switching" of the implant abutment interface and broad application of a tapered internal connection (Figure 3.11). The principle of platform switching, which uses a prosthetic abutment smaller in diameter than the implant itself, allows for a medial or inward horizontal repositioning of the implant–abutment interface ("microgap").[82] This design feature can be created in an implant body by the manufacturer or achieved by the clinician by using a compatible abutment of lesser diameter than the implant platform. The effect of platform switching is to create a horizontal component for the total linear length required for biologic width formation,[83,84] thereby reducing both lateral and vertical bone loss adjacent to the implant platform and allowing the biologic width to be located more coronally,[85] an obvious advantage in the esthetic zone. Platform switching may also lower the effect of occlusal loading and stress concentration at the cervical bone–implant interface.[86] Generally, the increased biologic width accommodation created about the circumference of an implant by platform switching is around 0.35 to 0.5 mm, which can result in significantly less radiographically detectable interproximal crestal bone loss[84,87,88] and better soft tissue support.[89]

Following a study in minipigs in which implants with diameter-reduced prosthetic abutments were separated by either 2 mm or 3 mm, Elian et al.[90] observed similar levels of inter-implant crestal bone loss in both groups. They concluded that "platform switching" may allow clinicians to place adjacent implants closer than 3 mm without losing interproximal bone height, or in the case of an implant adjacent to a tooth without damaging the attachment apparatus of the tooth. Similar conclusions were drawn from a human clinical study when measuring the effects of platform switching on implants adjacent to teeth.[91] Platform switching is not intended as a replacement for accurate and precise implant placement. It merely allows for slightly increased flexibility in tighter spaces (see also Chapter 18). Alternatively, a narrow-diameter implant (≤3.5 mm) may be considered, assuming that precautions have been taken to ensure that the implant will not be subjected to excessive occlusal force and that sufficient soft tissue thickness exists to provide for the development of an acceptable emergence profile for the implant crown (see also Chapter 11).

Soft tissue enhancements were observed with platform switching using moderately rough-surfaced implants placed in the dog mandible.[92] The authors found that the connective tissue component of biologic width was located more coronally and occupied the microgap region, when compared with non-platform-switched

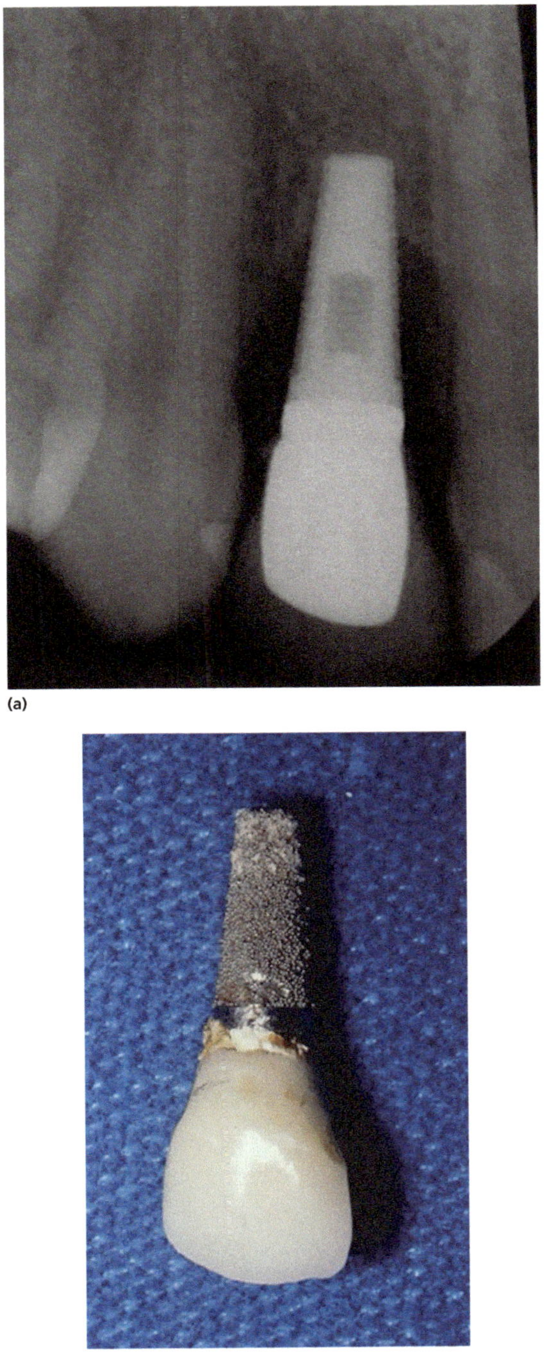

(a)

(b)

Figure 3.10 (a) A periapical radiograph showed extensive peri-implant crestal bone loss. (b) After implant removal, cement was visible on the buccal aspect.

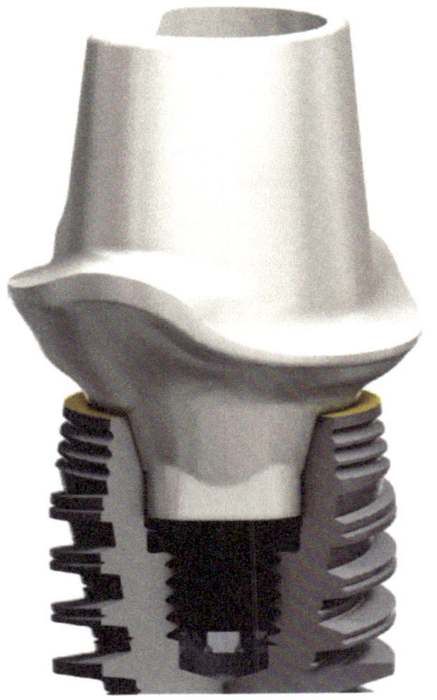

Figure 3.11 An implant design showing both platform switching and a tapered internal connection. *Source:* Nobel Biocare. Reproduced with permission of Nobel Biocare.

implants. It is yet to be documented that this shift in biologic width will translate into better papilla formation between implants and result in long-term esthetic stability.

The concept of "one abutment, one time"[93] is based on the notion that eliminating abutment changes and placing a final abutment at the time of implant placement can avoid disruption of the soft tissue apparatus and minimize crestal bone loss. In fact, it has been shown that frequent removal and replacement of healing caps (five times or more in a 6-month period) can lead to apical migration of the connective tissue zone.[94] However, changing from a healing abutment to a permanent abutment as a single event does not result in a change in the dimension and quality of the transmucosal attachment.[95]

Development of an acceptable prosthetic emergence profile for any implant can be challenging. In addition to optimal implant positioning bucco-lingually/palatally and mesio-distally, the implant's position apico-coronally in relation to adjacent teeth is crucial. Ideally, the implant platform should be positioned at least 2–3 mm apical to the future soft tissue margin of the implant crown,[96] so that the emergence profile can be developed within the confines of the peri-implant biologic width or what is referred to as "running room."[97] The minimal inter-occlusal space required would depend on the final restoration. A cement-retained single restoration would need at least 7 mm of clearance from the implant platform to the opposing dentition, while a screw-retained "one piece" UCLA-type crown can be placed in as little as 4.5–5 mm of inter-occlusal space.[98] With palatal positioning, the implant may need to be placed 1 mm deeper to add additional "running room."[99] In all situations, the use of a fixed provisional prosthesis will assist in developing the optimal emergence profile possible (see Chapter 4). Figure 3.12a shows a compromised inter-occlusal distance secondary to overextrusion of the opposing dentition and high riding crest. Implants were placed and custom healing caps were made to develop optimal emergence profiles (Figures 3.12b and c). Orthodontics and temporary anchorage devices (see Chapter 20) were used to intrude the opposing dentition and increase inter-occlusal space (Figure 3.12d and e). The final position of opposing teeth after orthodontic intrusion can be seen on the panoramic radiograph in Figure 3.12f showing adequate space for fixed restoration.

Occlusal design schemes for implant restorations have generally followed from concepts governing the natural dentition, as mandibular movements are generally the same for patients with

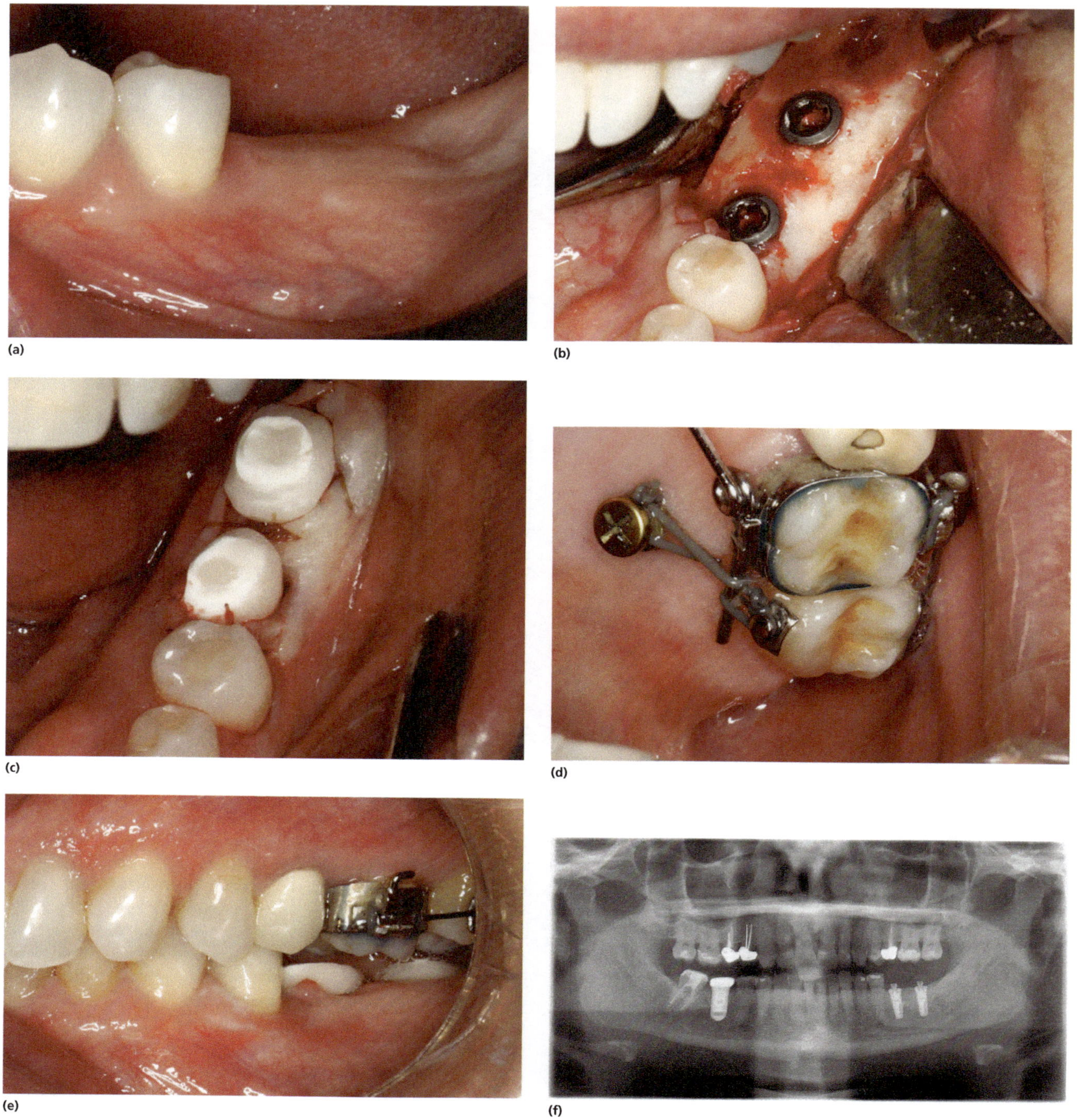

Figure 3.12 (a) Compromised inter-occlusal distance secondary to extrusion of the opposing dentition and a high-riding crest. (b) Implants were placed. (c) Custom healing caps were made after integration with uncovering, to develop optimal emergence profiles. (d, e) The opposing dentition was orthodontically impacted with the use of a temporary anchorage device to increase the available inter-occlusal space. (Orthodontic treatment by Dr J. Hintz.) (f) Panoramic radiograph showing the final position of the opposing teeth after orthodontic intrusion, confirming adequate space for crown placement. © Daniel R. Cullum.

natural teeth versus those with implants.[100] Implants are essentially ankylosed to the surrounding bone and lack proprioception and shock-absorbing capabilities. The load-sharing ability, adaptation to occlusal forces, and "mechano-perception" are significantly reduced with dental implants, necessitating different occlusal considerations for implants as opposed to natural teeth. It is important to note, however, that there is currently no evidence-based, universally accepted, implant-specific concept of occlusion.[101]

As with restorations on natural teeth, implant overloading can contribute to both prosthetic and biologic complications. Cantilevered restorations, parafunction, and premature contacts all can have detrimental effects on the implant-prosthetic complex,[102–104] although the impact of all these factors is controversial as previously discussed. Concepts of occlusion, including "balanced occlusion," "group function," and "mutually protected occlusion," must be followed when planning for an implant-supported prosthesis.[105] Occlusal plan modifications with an implant-protected occlusion include occlusal load sharing, reduced occlusal table and anatomic changes, and elimination of direct occlusal contacts on implants with poor biomechanics such as reduced crown-to-root ratio or off-axis loading.[106,107] Other basic principles of occlusion apply with dental implants. Principles such as (1) anterior guidance, (2) bilateral stability and wide freedom in centric occlusion, (3) even distribution of contacts and forces, (4) eliminating interferences, and (5) balanced and even lateral excursive movements need to be observed.[101]

In the mixed implant–natural tooth dentition, premature occlusal contacts must be avoided on an implant restoration, and instead be distributed over the natural teeth.[108] Compression of natural teeth during function should not allow untoward loading on the implants. Similarly, anterior teeth have greater lateral and apical movements compared with implants during eccentric excursion, and it has been suggested that the anterior guidance of implant-supported prostheses should be as shallow as possible to reduce the potential load from lateral shear forces.[109] Overall, the prosthetic goal should be to reduce cantilever length, to eliminate excursive contacts with loading within the implant diameter, to narrow the bucco-lingual dimension of the prosthesis, and to reduce the angle of disclusion and cusp inclination.

Surgical risks

There are a number of surgical risks that may be encountered in the placement of dental implants. Some of these risks can be reduced or eliminated by using the minimally invasive techniques described in this book. However, unexpected complications can and will occur, and the implant surgeon must have sufficient training and experience to anticipate and manage complications appropriately.[110] Careful planning in advance of the procedure is required as it will prepare the surgeon to manage the unexpected more effectively under duress, should complications arise.[111] Surgical risks range from damage to the mandibular neurovascular bundle to life-threatening hemorrhage.[112] Appropriate preoperative radiographs are an important first step, but some would argue that cone beam computer-assisted tomography (CBCT) scans should be part of the diagnostic protocol (see Chapter 2). CBCT becomes particularly crucial in areas of questionable anatomy, such as the position of the neurovascular bundle or the shape and dimensions of the maxillary sinus. It is also invaluable in determining the pre-existing volume of bone that is present. Choosing short implants (see Chapter 10) along with infiltration anesthesia rather than a mandibular nerve block[113] may reduce complications associated with posterior mandibular implant placement.

The majority of surgical and implant procedures are accomplished using mucoperiosteal flap elevation to allow direct observation of the surgical site. Because of the morbidity associated with large flap elevations and the early post-surgical compromise of blood supply to buccal bone, some clinicians have promoted the use of flapless implant surgical procedures.[114] This alternative, however, is for the very experienced, often with the aid of computer-assisted treatment planning and computer-generated surgical guides (see Chapter 9) since the risk of intraoperative complications is higher.[115] Less experienced surgeons should utilize more open procedures for adequate visualization and predictability. For example, with tooth extraction where access is inadequate for complete debridement of apical pathology, a traditional crestal mucoperiosteal flap may be employed. If the crestal buccal plate is intact, a semi-lunar vestibular incision may be employed for access as a less invasive approach (see Chapter 21, Figure 21.1).

Severe hemorrhage during dental implant surgery is rare, but there is the risk of penetrating the lingual cortical plate of bone and lacerating an artery, producing a life-threatening sublingual hematoma and airway obstruction. This complication has been most commonly reported in the anterior mandible since the floor of the mouth is occupied by branches of the submental, sublingual, and mylohyoid arteries.[116,117] Severe hemorrhage also may occur if the arterial supply to the maxillary sinus is severed during manipulation of the lateral wall of the sinus to permit sinus access for direct sinus grafting.[118,119] This is relatively rare, since this artery (an anastomosis of the posterior superior alveolar and infraorbital arteries) follows an intrabony course and is normally located well above the maxillary alveolar ridge (see Chapter 2, Figure 2.8b).[120] It has been estimated that in about 20% of open sinus grafting procedures this artery will be encountered,[121] making it prudent to consider use of a piezosurgical device rather than surgical burs to prepare the access window in the lateral sinus wall (see Chapter 13). Arterial damage is less likely to result from an indirect sinus elevation using osteotomes or other crestal techniques (see Chapter 15), but at least one case of a severe hemorrhage requiring hospitalization following this procedure has been reported.[122]

Infection following dental implant placement is rare with correct protocol including preoperative rinsing with chlorhexidine and a loading dose of antibiotic.[112,123] Infection of the maxillary sinus can be a serious complication of open sinus grafting[124–126] and usually requires removal of the graft material or endoscopic sinus surgery to open a non-patent ostium. Infection rarely results following the indirect sinus elevation procedure, which gains access to the sinus space through crestal bone. Preoperative clinical evaluation with a careful history and imaging (see Chapter 2) are important to rule out pre-existing dental pathology or sinus disease that could compromise the outcome (Figure 3.13). Smoking increases the risk of sinus infection following open sinus grafting,[127] making smoking cessation highly desirable for the patient. Testori et al.[128] have published a list of 19 recommendations meant to reduce the risk of sinus infection. Some of these include careful selection of patients with healthy sinuses, preoperative computed tomography scans, antibiotic prophylaxis, and preop chlorhexidine mouth rinsing.

A comprehensive review of possible risks associated with open sinus grafting was also published by Wallace,[129] the most common being tears in the Scheiderian membrane, which can often be challenging to repair. Less risk for tears is associated with the indirect or crestal sinus elevation originally presented by Summers.[130,131] If careful case selection is undertaken, implant outcomes with both sinus approaches are similar if not slightly better with the indirect approach.[132]

There has been the occasional report of dental implants being displaced into the sinus cavity, either at the time of implant placement or subsequently during initial site healing[133,134] (Figure 3.14). The situation may arise following either open window or trans-crestal sinus floor elevation. Risk factors appear to be increased with the use of cylindrical rather than tapered implants, narrower diameter implants, and inadequate initial implant stability.[135] Compromise of implant stability can result from an overlying removable prosthesis, over-instrumentation, or lateral thermal damage

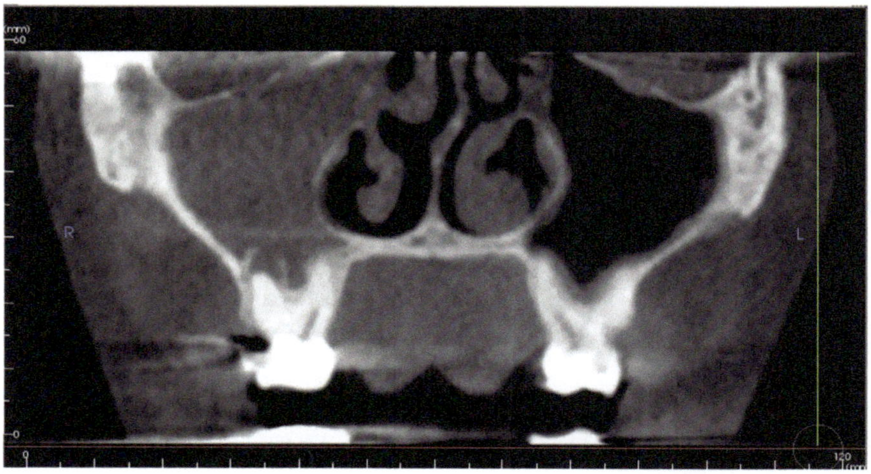

Figure 3.13 An axial CBCT image of a maxillary sinus with complete opacification of the right sinus secondary to a dental abcess and chronic sinusitis.

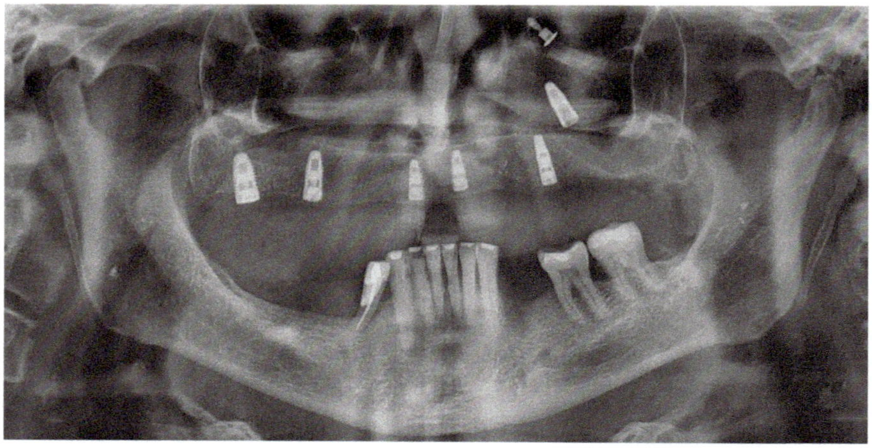

Figure 3.14 A panoramic radiograph showing an implant displaced into the maxillary sinus. Further apically, the cover screw is also visible.

at osteotomy preparation leading to loss of primary stability and implant micromovements. These complications may be the result of inadequate implant site development and limited surgical training or experience.[110]

Other risks associated with placement of dental implants include damage to adjacent teeth, fracture of the mandible, or the remote possibility of an allergic reaction to titanium. Soehardi et al.[136] surveyed 198 hospital-based oral and maxillofacial surgeons regarding the occurrence of mandibular fractures in patients under their care for implant treatment. The incidence of fracture was estimated to be 0.05% of approximately 475,000 implants placed between 1980 and 2007. It was determined that mandibles with ≤10 mm in the symphysis region were at greatest risk and that penetration of the inferior border was to be avoided. Almost half of the fractures occurred as a late complication and seemed to be linked to loss of peri-implant crestal bone. If an implant in the anterior mandible of ≤10 mm height had bone loss affecting >50% of implant length, removal was recommended due to the increased risk of fracture. This is especially notable since 48% of the fractures resulted in serious complications such as osteomyelitis and non-union. Cases of suspected allergy have been reported in the orthopedic and cardiovascular literature, although there is a lack of data regarding the incidence and prevalence of allergies with dental implants.[137]

With orthopedic implants, "fretting corrosion" can occur with wear and loading of two opposing metal surfaces, resulting in release of metal particles and a foreign-body reaction by macrophages. Similar "corrosion" seems unlikely with dental implants, but is conceivable at a much reduced level at the implant abutment interface. In a recent review article,[138] titanium allergy has been suspected in some instances of dental implant failure, leading the authors to suggest that this complication may have been under-reported. Preez et al.[139] published a case of a patient who developed a severe soft tissue reaction to a dental implant, and Egusa et al.[140] reported a patient who developed facial eczema following treatment with an implant-retained overdenture. In both of these suspected allergic reactions, removal of the implants led to apparent resolution of the soft tissue abnormalities.

Conclusions

There are few medical contraindications to the placement of dental implants provided that adequate preoperative planning has been undertaken and that the clinician has the necessary skills and training to understand and manage any inherent risks. Medical history and co-morbidities play an important role, and special consideration must be given to patients who have been on long-term anti-resorptive medications, such as oral bisphosphonates and RANK-L inhibitors. Patient habits, including poor oral hygiene and smoking, can lead to poor treatment outcomes, including implant failure. Patients with current or even a past history of treated moderate to severe periodontitis will be at elevated risk to develop implant infection and mid- to long-term failure. Placement of dental implants in the esthetic zone (i.e. the maxillary anterior) comes with significant risks of esthetic failure and patient dissatisfaction so that the inexperienced clinician should consider referral of such patients to more experienced colleagues for optimal treatment outcomes. Also, clinicians inexperienced in management of complications such as sinus infection or major hemorrhage are best advised to limit implant surgery to straight-forward implant protocols commensurate with their experience and employ open exposure techniques rather than minimally invasive approaches.

References

1. Froum S. Dental Implant Complications: Etiology, Prevention, and Treatment. Ames, IA: Wiley-Blackwell, 2012.
2. Hwang D, Wang H-L. Medical contraindications to implant therapy: part I: absolute contraindications. Implant Dent 2006; 15: 353–360.
3. Wang H-L, Weber D, McCauley L. Effect of long-term oral bisphosphonates on implant wound healing: literature and a case report. J Periodontol 2007; 78: 584–594.
4. Marx R, Cillo J, Ulloa J. Oral bisphosphonate-induced osteonecrosis: prediction of risk factors using serum CTX testing, prevention, and treatment. J Oral Maxillofac Surg 2007; 65: 2397–2410.
5. Advisory Task Force on Bisphosphonate-Related Ostenonecrosis of the Jaws, American Association of Oral and Maxillofacial Surgeons. American Association of Oral and Maxillofacial Surgeons position paper on bisphosphonate-related osteonecrosis of the jaws. J Oral Maxillofac Surg 2007; 65: 369–376.
6. Ruggiero SL, Dodson TB, Fantasia J, et al. American Association of Oral and Maxillofacial Surgeons position paper on medication-related osteonecrosis of the jaws – 2014 update. J Oral Maxillofac Surg 2014; 72: 1938–1956.
7. Yip J, Borrell L, Cho S-C, et al. Association between oral bisphosphonate use and dental implant failure among middle-aged women. J Clin Periodontol 2012; 39: 408–414.
8. Droumaguet C, Balkau, B, Simon D, et al. Use of HbA1C in predicting progression to diabetes in French men and women. Data from an epidemiological study on the insulin resistance syndrome (DESIR). Diabetes Care 2006; 29: 1619–1625.
9. Mealey B, Oates T. Diabetes mellitus and periodontal diseases. J Periodontol 2006; 77: 1289–1303.
10. Teeuw W, Gerdes V, Loos B. Effect of periodontal treatment on glycemic control of diabetic patients. Diabetes Care 2010; 33: 421–427.
11. Javed F, Romanos G. Impact of diabetes mellitus and glycemic control on the osseointegration of dental implants: a systematic literature review. J Periodontol 2009; 80: 1719–1730.
12. Marchand F, Raskin A, Dionnes-Hornes A, et al. Dental implants and diabetes: conditions for success. Diabetes Metab 2012; 38: 14–19.
13. Michaeli E, Weinberg I, Nahlieli O. Dental implants in the diabetic patient: systemic and rehabilitative considerations. Quintessence Int 2009; 40: 639–645.
14. Bornstein M, Cionca N, Mombelli A. Systemic conditions and treatments as risks for implant therapy. Int J Oral Maxillofac Implants 2009; 24(Suppl): 12–27.
15. Lindquist L, Carlsson G, Jemt T. A prospective 15-year follow-up of mandibular fixed prostheses supported by osseointegrated implants. Clin Oral Implants Res 1996; 7: 329–336.
16. Sereno G, Strom C. Peri-implantitis in partially edentulous patients: association with inadequate plaque control. Clin Oral Implants Res 2009; 20: 169–174.
17. Bain C, Moy P. The association between the failure of dental implants and cigarette smoking. Int J Oral Maxillofac Implants 1993; 8: 609–615.
18. Noorwali O, Alremthi H, Deporter D. The influence of smoking on moderately rough-surfaced dental implants: a literature review. J Implant Adv Clin Dent 2011; 3(5): 51–59.
19. Testori T, Weinstein R, Taschieri S, et al. Risk factor analysis following maxillary sinus augmentation: a retrospective multicenter study. Int J Oral Maxillofac Implants 2012; 27: 1170–1176.
20. Lin T, Chen L, Cha J, et al. The effect of cigarette smoking and native bone height on dental implants placed immediately in sinuses grafted by hydraulic condensation. Int J Periodontics Restorative Dent 2012; 32: 255–261.
21. Karoussis I, Muller S, Salvi G, et al. Association between periodontal and peri-implant conditions: a 10-year prospective study. Clin Oral Implant Res 2004; 15: 1–7.
22. Lindquist L, Carlsson G, Jemt T. Association between marginal bone loss around osseointegrated mandibular implants and smoking habits. J Dent Res 1997; 76: 1667–1674.
23. Penarrocha M, Palomar M, Sanchis J, et al. Radiologic study of marginal bone loss and its relationship to smoking, implant location and morphology. Int J Oral Maxillofac Implants 2004; 19: 861–867.
24. Wennstrom J, Zurdo J, Karlsson S, et al. Bone level change at implant-supported fixed partial dentures with and without cantilever extension after 5 years in function. J Clin Periodontol 2004; 31: 1077–1083.
25. Renouard R, Nisand D. Impact of implant length and diameter on survival rates. Clin Oral Implants Res 2006; 17(Suppl 2): 35–51.
26. Haas R, Haimbock W, Mailath G, et al. The relationship of smoking on peri-implant tissue: a retrospective study. J Prosthetic Dent 1996; 76: 592–596.
27. Tomar S, Asma S. Smoking-attributable periodontitis in the United States: findings from NHANES. J Periodontol 2000; 71: 743–751.
28. Gouvoussis J, Sindhusake D, Yeung S. Cross-infection from periodontitis sites to failing implant sites in the same mouth. Int J Oral Maxillofac Implants 1997; 12: 666–673.
29. Aoki M, Takanashi K, Matsukubo T, et al. Transmission of periodontopathic bacteria from natural teeth to implants. Clin Implant Dent Rel Res 2012; 14: 406–411.
30. Renvert S, Persson G. Periodontitis as a potential risk factor for peri-implantitis. J Clin Periodontol 2009; 36(Suppl 10): 9–14.
31. Mombelli A, Muller N, Cionca N. The epidemiology of peri-implantitis. Clin Oral Implants Res 2012; 23(Suppl 6): 67–76.
32. Pjetursson B, Helbing C, Weber H, et al. Peri-implantitis susceptibility as it relates to periodontal therapy and supportive care. Clin Oral Implants Res 2012; 23: 888–894.
33. Koyanagi T, Sakamoto M, Takeuchi Y, et al. Comprehensive microbiological findings in peri-implantitis and periodontitis. J Clin Periodontol 2013; 40: 218–226.
34. Quirynen M, Abarca M, van Assche N, et al. Impact of supportive periodontal therapy and implant surface roughness on implant outcome in patients with a history of periodontitis. J Clin Periodontol 2007; 34: 805–815.
35. Salvi G, Bragger U. Mechanical and technical risks in implant therapy. Int J Oral Maxillofac Implants 2009; 24(Suppl): 69–85.
36. Manfredini D, Poggio C, Lobbezoo F. Is bruxism a risk factor for dental implants? A systematic review of the literature. Clin Implant Dent Relat Res 2014; 16: 460–469.
37. Tawil G, Aboujaoude N, Younan R. Influence of prosthetic parameters on the survival and complication rates of short implants. Int J Oral Maxillofac Implants 2006; 21: 275–282.
38. Covani U, Ricci M, Bozzolo G, et al. Analysis of the pattern of alveolar ridge remodeling following single tooth extraction. Clin Oral Implants Res 2011; 22: 820–825.
39. Spray J, Black C, Morris H, Ochi S. The influence of bone thickness on facial marginal bone response: stage 1 placement through stage 2 uncovering. Ann Periodontol 2000; 5: 119–128.
40. Qahash M, Susin C, Polimeni G, et al. Bone healing dynamics at buccal peri-implant sites. Clin Oral Implants Res 2008; 19: 166–172.
41. Le B, Borzabadi-Farahani A. Labial bone thickness in area of anterior maxillary implants associated with crestal labial soft tissue thickness. Implant Dent 2012; 21: 406–410.
42. Choquet V, Hermans M, Adriaenssens P, et al. Clinical and radiographic evaluation of the papilla level adjacent to single-tooth dental implants. A retrospective study in the maxillary anterior region. J Periodontol 2001; 72: 1364–1371.
43. Tarnow D, Elian N, Fletcher P, et al. Vertical distance from the crest of bone to the height of the interproximal papilla between adjacent implants. J Periodontol 2003; 74: 1785–1788.
44. Blanco J, Alvarez E, Munoz F, et al. Influence on early osseointegration of dental implants installed with two different drilling protocols: a histomorphometric study in rabbit. Clin Oral Implant Res 2010; 22: 92–99.
45. Degidi M, Daprile G, Piattelli A, Carinci F. Evaluation of factors influencing resonance frequency analysis values, at insertion surgery, of implants placed in sinus-augmented and non-grafted sites. Clin Implant Dent Relat Res 2007; 9: 144–149.
46. Vidyasagar L, Salms G, Apse P, Teibe U. The influence of site preparation (countersinking) on initial dental implant stability. An *in vitro* study using resonance frequency analysis. Stomatologija, Baltic Dent Maxillofac J 2004; 6: 14–16.
47. Albrektsson T, Wennerberg A. Oral implant surfaces: part I – review focusing on topographic and chemical properties of different surfaces and *in vivo* responses to them. Int J Prosthodont 2004; 17: 536–43.
48. Bouri A, Bissada N, Al-Zahrani M, et al. Width of keratinized gingiva and the health status of the supporting tissues around dental implants. Int J Oral Maxillofac Implants 2008; 23: 323–326.

49. Linkevicius T, Apse P, Grybauskas S, et al. The influence of soft tissue thickness on crestal bone changes around implants: a 1-year prospective controlled clinical trial. Int J Oral Maxillofac Implants 2009; 24: 712–719.
50. Block M, Gardiner D, Kent J, et al. Hydroxyapatite-coated cylindrical implants in the posterior mandible: 10-year observations. Int J Oral Maxillofac Implants 1996; 11: 626–633.
51. Haas R, Mensdorff-Pouilly N, Mailath G, Watzek G. Survival of 1,920 IMZ implants followed for up to 100 months. Int J Oral Maxillofac Implants 1996; 11: 581–588.
52. Astrand P, Engquist B, Anzen B, et al. A three-year follow-up report of a comparative study of ITI Dental Implants® and Branemark System Implants® in the treatment of the partially edentulous maxilla. Clin Implant Dent Rel Res 2004; 6: 130–141.
53. Zechner W, Trinki N, Watzek G., et al. Radiologic follow-up of peri-implant bone loss around machine-surfaced and rough-surfaced interforaminal implants in the mandible functionally loaded for 3 to 7 years. Int J Oral Maxillofac Implants 2004; 19: 216–221.
54. Ostman P-O, Hellman M, Albrektsson T, Sennerby L. Direct loading of Nobel Direct® and Nobel Perfect® one-piece implants: a 1-year prospective clinical and radiographic study. Clin Oral Implants Res 2007; 18: 409–418.
55. Lang N, Bosshardt D, Lulic M. Do mucositis lesions around implants differ from gingivitis lesions around teeth? J Clin Periodontol 2011; 38(Suppl 11): 182–187.
56. Task Force on Peri-implantitis. Peri-implant mucositis and peri-implantitis: a current understanding of their diagnoses and clinical implications. J Periodontol 2013; 84: 436–443.
57. Karbach J, Callaway A, Kwon Y-D, et al. Comparison of five parameters as risk factors for peri-implant mucositis. Int J Oral Maxillofac Implants 2009; 24: 491–496.
58. Zeza B, Pilloni A. Peri-implant mucositis treatments in humans: a systematic review. Ann Stomatol (Roma) 2012; 3(3–4): 83–89.
59. Salvi G, Aglietta M, Eick S, et al. Reversibility of experimental peri-implant mucositis compared with experimental gingivitis in humans. Clin Oral Implants Res 2012; 23: 182–190.
60. Hernandez G, Lopez-Pintor R, Arriba L, et al. Implant treatment in patients with oral lichen planus; a prospective-controlled study. Clin Oral Implants Res 2012; 23: 726–732.
61. Huynh-Ba G. Peri-implantitis: "tsunami" or marginal problem? Int J Oral Maxillofac Implants 2013; 28: 334–337.
62. Berglundh T, Gotfredsen K, Zitzmann N, et al. Spontaneous progression of ligature induced peri-implantitis at implants with different surface roughness: an experimental study in dogs. Clin Oral Implants Res 2007; 18: 655–661.
63. Swierkot K, Lottholz P, Flores-de-Jacoby L, et al. Mucositis, peri-implantitis, implant success, and survival of implants in patients with treated aggressive periodontititis: 3- to 16-year results of a prospective long-term cohort study. J Periodontol 2012; 83: 1213–1225.
64. Roos-Jansaker A-M, Lindahl C, Renvert S. Nine- to fourteen-year follow-up of implant treatment. Part II: presence of peri-implant lesions. J Clin Periodontol 2006; 33: 290–295.
65. Costa F, Takenaka-Martinez S, Cota L, et al. Peri-implant disease in subjects with and without preventive maintenance: a 5-year follow-up. J Clin Periodontol 2012; 39: 173–181.
66. Cho-Yan Lee J, Mattheos N, Nixon K, et al. Residual periodontal pockets are a risk indicator for peri-implantitis in patients treated for periodontitis. Clin Oral Implants Res 2012; 23: 325–333.
67. Park S, Sorenson W, Wang H. Management and prevention of retrograde peri-implant infection from retained root tips: two case reports. Int J Periodontics Restorative Dent 2004; 24: 422–433.
68. Sussman H, Moss S. Localized osteomyelitis secondary to endodontic implant pathosis: a case report. J Periodontol 1993; 64: 306–310.
69. Jalbout Z, Tarnow D. The implant periapical lesion: four case reports and review of the literature. Pract Proced Aesthet Dent 2001; 13: 107–112.
70. Shaffer M, Juruaz D, Haggerty P. The effect of periradicular endodontic pathosis on the apical region of adjacent implants. Oral Surg Oral Med Oral Path Oral Radiol Endod 1998; 86: 578–581.
71. Brisman D, Brisman A, Moses M. Implant failures associated with asymptomatic endodontically treated teeth. J Am Dent Assoc 2001; 132: 191–195.
72. Chen S, Buser D. Esthetic complications due to implant malpositions: etiology, prevention and treatment. In: Dental Implant Complications: Etiology, Prevention and Treatment, FroumS, ed. Ames, IA: Wiley-Blackwell, 2010, pp. 134–155.
73. Grunder U, Gracis S, Capelli M. Influence of the 3-D bone to implant relationship on esthetics. Int J Periodontics Restorative Dent 2005; 25: 113–119.
74. Salama H, Salama M, Garber D, Adar P. The interproximal height of bone: a guidepost to esthetic strategies and soft tissue contours in anterior tooth replacement. Pract Periodontics Aesthet Dent 1998; 10: 1131–1141.
75. Tarnow D, Cho S, Wallace S. The effect of inter-implant distance on the height of inter-implant bone crest. J Periodontol 2000; 71: 546–549.
76. Kois J. Predictable single tooth peri-implant esthetics: five diagnostic keys. Compend Contin Educ Dent 2001; 22: 199–208.
77. Kupershmidt I, Levin L, Schwartz-Arad D. Inter-implant bone height changes in anterior maxillary immediate and non-immediate adjacent dental implants. J Periodontol 2007; 78: 991–996.
78. Tarnow D, Elian N, Fletcher P, et al. Vertical distance from the crest of bone to the height of the interproximal papilla between adjacent implants. J Periodontol 2003; 74: 1785–1788.
79. Sigueira S, Pimentel S, Alves R, et al. Evaluation of the effects of buccal–palatal bone width on the incidence and height of the interproximal papilla between adjacent implants in esthetic areas. J Periodontol 2013; 84: 170–175.
80. Jemt T. Regeneration of gingival papillae after single-implant treatment. Int J Periodontics Restorative Dent 1997; 17: 326–333.
81. Wilson T. The positive relationship between excess cement and peri-implant disease: a prospective clinical endoscopic study. J Periodontol 2009; 80: 1388–1392.
82. Scarano A, Assenza B, Piattelli M, et al. Inter-implant distance and crestal bone resorption: a histologic study in the canine mandible. Clin Implant Dent Relat Res 2004; 6: 150–156.
83. Lazzara R, Porter S. Platform switching: a new concept in implant dentistry for controlling post-restorative crestal bone levels. Int J Periodontics Restorative Dent 2006; 26: 9–17.
84. Vela-Nebot X, Rodríguez-Ciurana X, Rodado-Alonso C, Segalà-Torres M. Benefits of an implant platform modification technique to reduce crestal bone resorption. Implant Dent 2006; 15: 313–320.
85. Rodriguez-Ciurana X, Vela-Nebot X, Segala-Torres M, et al. The effect of inter-implant distance on the height of the inter-implant bone crest when using platform-switched implants. Int J Periodontics Restorative Dent 2009; 29: 141–151.
86. Maeda Y, Miura J, Taki I, Sogo M. Biomechanical analysis on platform switching: is there any biomechanical rationale? Clin Oral Implants Res 2007; 18: 581–584.
87. Puchades-Roman L, Palmer R, Palmer P, et al. A clinical, radiographic and microbiologic comparison of Astra Tech and Branemark single tooth implants. Clin Implant Dent Relat Res 2000; 2: 78–84.
88. Cappiello M, Luongo R, Di Lorio D, et al. Evaluation of peri-implant bone loss around platform-switched implants. Int J Periodontics Restorative Dent 2008; 28: 347–355.
89. Gardner D. Platform-switching as a means to achieving implant esthetics. N Y State Dent J 2005; 71: 34–37.
90. Elian N, Bloom M, Dard M, et al. Effect of inter-implant distance (2 and 3 mm) on the height of inter-implant bone crest: a histomorphometric evaluation. J Periodontol 2011; 82: 1749–1756.
91. Vela X, Mendez V, Rodriguez X, et al. Crestal bone changes on platform-switched implants and adjacent teeth when the tooth-implant distance is less than 1.5 mm. Int J Periodontics Restorative Dent 2012; 32: 149–155.
92. Cochran D, Mau LP, Higginbottom F, et al. Soft and hard tissue histologic dimensions around dental implants in the canine restored with smaller-diameter abutments: a paradigm shift in peri-implant biology. Int J Oral Maxillofac Implants 2013; 28: 494–502.
93. Canullo L, Bignozzi I, Cocchetto R, et al. Immediate positioning of a definitive abutment versus repeated abutment replacements in post-extractive implants: 3-year follow-up of a randomized multi-centre clinical trial. Eur J Oral Implantol 2010; 3: 285–296.
94. Abrahamsson I, Berglundh T, Lindhe J. The mucosal barrier following abutment dis/reconnection. An experimental study in dogs. J Clin Periodontol 1997; 24: 568–572.
95. Abrahamsson I, Berglundh T, Sekino S, Lindhe J. Tissue reactions to abutment shift: an experimental study in dogs. Clin Implant Dent Relat Res 2003; 5: 82–88.
96. Buser D, Martin W, Belser U. Optimizing esthetics for implant restorations in the anterior maxilla: anatomic and surgical considerations. Int J Oral Maxillofac Implants 2004; 19(Suppl): 43–61.
97. Cavallaro J, Greenstein G. Prosthodontic complications related to non-optimal dental implant placement. In: Dental Implant Complications: Etiology, Prevention and Treatment, FroumS, ed. Ames, IA: Wiley-Blackwell, 2010, pp. 156–171.
98. Priest G. Soft tissue development with provisional and definitive implant restorations. In: Implant Site Development, SonickM, HwangD, eds. Ames, IA: Wiley-Blackwell, 2012, pp. 398–418.
99. Gartner J, Mushimoto K, Weber H, Nishimura I. Effect of osseointegrated implants on the coordination of masticatory muscles: a pilot study. J Prosthetic Dent 2000; 84: 185–193.
100. Kim Y, Oh T, Misch C, Wang H. Occlusal considerations in implant therapy: clinical guidelines with biomechanical rationale. Clin Oral Implants Res 2005; 16: 26–35.

101. Duyck J, Van Oosterwyck J, De Cooman M, et al. Magnitude and distribution of occlusal forces on oral implants supporting fixed prostheses: an *in vivo* study. Clin Oral Implants Res 2000; 11: 465–475.
102. Naert I, Quirynen M, Van Steenberghe D, Darius P. A study of 589 consecutive implants supporting complete fixed prosthesis. Part II: prosthetic aspects. J Prosthetic Dent 1992; 68: 949–956.
103. Miyata T, Kobyashi Y, Araki H, et al. The influence of controlled occlusal overload on peri-implant tissue. Part 3: a histological study in monkeys. Int J Oral Maxillofac Implants 2000; 15: 425–431.
104. Hobo S, Ichida E, Garcia L. Ideal occlusion. In: Osseointegration and Occlusal Rehabilitation. Quintessence Publishing Company, 1989, pp. 315–328.
105. Misch C, Bidez M. Implant-protected occlusion: a biomechanical rationale. Compend Contin Educ Dent 1994; 14: 1330–1334.
106. Misch C, Bidez M. Implant-protected occlusion. Int J Dent Symp 1994; 2: 32–37.
107. Sekine H, Komiyama Y, Hotta, H, Yoshida K. Mobility characteristics and tactile sensitivity of osseointegrated fixture-supporting systems. In: Tissue Integration in Oral Maxillofacial Reconstruction, van SteenbergheD, ed. Amsterdam: Elsevier, 1986, pp. 326–332.
108. Weinberg L, Kruger B. A comparison of implant/prosthesis loading with four clinical variables. Int J Prosthodont 1995; 8: 421–433.
109. Chen Y, Kuan C, Wang Y. Implant occlusion: biomechanical considerations for implant-supported prostheses. J Dent Sci 2008; 3: 65–74.
110. Wheeler S, Bollinger,C. Complications or substandard care? Risks of inadequate implant training. J Calif Dent Assoc 2009; 37: 647–651.
111. Renouard F, Charrier J-G. The Search for the Weakest Link. An Introduction to the Human Factors. Chatillon: Ewen Editions, 2012.
112. Misch C, Wang H-L. Implant surgery complications: etiology and treatment. Implant Dent 2008; 17: 159–168.
113. Heller A, Shankland W. Alternative to inferior alveolar nerve block anesthesia when placing mandibular dental implants posterior to the mental foramen. J Oral Implantol 2001; 27: 127–133.
114. Parmigiani-Izquierdo J, Sanchez-Perez A, Cabana-Munoz M. A pilot study of post-operative pain felt after two implant surgery techniques: a randomized blinded prospective clinical study. Int J Oral Maxillofac Implants 2013; 28: 1305–1310.
115. Wilson T. Complications associated with flapless surgery. In: Dental Implant Complications: Etiology, Prevention and Treatment, FroumS, ed. Ames, IA:, Wiley-Blackwell, 2012, pp. 341–354.
116. Kalpidis C, Setayesh R. Hemorrhaging associated with endosseous implant placement in the anterior mandible: a review of the literature. J Periodontol 2004; 75: 631–645.
117. Rosano G, Taschieri S, Gaudy J, et al. Anatomic assessment of the anterior mandible and relative hemorrhage risk in implant dentistry: a cadaveric study. Clin Oral Implants Res 2009; 20: 791–795.
118. Lee C. Brisk, prolonged pulsatile hemorrhage during the sinus graft procedure: a case report with discussion on intra-operative hemostatic management. Implant Dent 2010; 19: 189–195.
119. Hong Y-H, Mun S-K. A case of massive maxillary sinus bleeding after dental implant. Int J Oral Maxillofac Surg 2011; 40: 758–760.
120. Rosano G, Taschieri S, Gaudy J-F, et al. Maxillary sinus vascular anatomy and its relation to sinus lift surgery. Clin Oral Implants Res 2011; 22: 711–715.
121. Elian N, Wallace S, Cho S-C, et al. Distribution of the maxillary artery as it relates to sinus floor augmentation. Int J Oral Maxillofac Implants 2005; 20: 784–787.
122. Jensen S, Eriksen J, Schiodt M. Severe bleeding after sinus floor elevation using the transcrestal technique: a case report. Eur J Oral Implantol 2012; 5: 287–291.
123. Cardemil C, Ristevski Z, Alsen B, Dahlin C. Influence of different operatory setups on implant survival rate: a retrospective clinical study. Clin Implant Dent Relat Res 2009; 11: 288–291.
124. Schwartz-Arad D, Herzberg R, Dolev E. The prevalence of surgical complications of the sinus graft procedure and their impact on implant survival. J Periodontol 2004; 75: 511–516.
125. Sohn D-S, Lee J-K, Shin H-I, et al. Fungal infection as a complication of sinus bone grafting and implants: a case report. Oral Surg Oral Med Oral Pathol Oral Radiol Endod 2009; 107: 375–380.
126. Urban I, Nagursky H, Church C, Lozada J. Incidence, diagnosis, and treatment of sinus graft infection after sinus floor elevation: a clinical study. Int J Oral Maxillofac Implants 2012; 27: 449–457.
127. Barone A, Santini S, Sbordone L, et al. A clinical study of the outcomes and complications associated with maxillary sinus augmentation. Int J Oral Maxillofac Implants 2006; 21: 81–85.
128. Testori T, Drago L, Wallace S, et al. Prevention and treatment of post-operative infections after sinus elevation surgery: clinical consensus and recommendations. Int J Dent 2012; 2012: 365809.
129. Wallace S. Complications in lateral window sinus elevation surgery. In: Dental Implant Complications: Etiology, Prevention and Treatment, FroumS, ed. Ames, IA: Wiley-Blackwell, 2011, pp. 284–309.
130. Summers R. The ostotome technique: part 3 – less invasive methods of elevating the sinus floor. Compend Contin Dent Educ 1994; 15: 698–708.
131. Rosen P. Complications with the bone-added osteotome sinus floor elevtion: etiology, prevention and treatment. In: Dental Implant Complications: Etiology, Prevention and Treatment, FroumS, ed. Ames, IA: Wiley-Blackwell, 2011, pp. 310–324.
132. Del Fabbro M, Wallace S, Testori T. Long-term implant survival in the grafted maxillary sinus. A systematic review. Int J Periodontics Restorative Dent 2013; 33: 773–783.
133. Flanagan D. A method to retrieve a displaced dental implant from the maxillary sinus. J Oral Implantol 2009; 35(2): 70–74.
134. Chen L, Cha J. Dental implant migration into two different maxillary sinus cavities. J Implant Adv Clin Dent 2012; 4(4): 21–25.
135. Moreno-Galindo P, Padial-Molina M, Avila G, et al. Complications associated with implant migration into the maxillary sinus cavity. Clin Oral Implants Res 2012; 23: 1152–1160.
136. Soehardi A, Meijer G, Manders R, Stoelinga P. An inventory of mandibular fractures associated with implants in atrophic edentulous mandibles: a survey of Dutch oral and maxillofacial surgeons. Int J Oral Maxillofac Implants 2011; 26: 1087–1093.
137. Schuh A, Lill C, Honle W, Effenberger H. Prevalence of allergic reactions to implant materials in total hip and knee arthroplasty. Zentralbl Chir 2008; 133: 292–296 (in German).
138. Siddiqi A, Payne A, DeSilva R, Duncan W. Titanium allergy: could it affect dental implant integration? Clin Oral Implants Res 2011; 22: 673–680.
139. Preez L, Butow K, Swart T. Implant failure due to titanium hypersensitivity/allergy? Report of a case. SADJ 2007; 62: 24–25
140. Egusa H, Ko N, Shimazu T, Yatani H. Suspected association of an allergic reaction with titanium dental implants: a clinical report. J Prosthetic Dent 2008; 100: 344–347.

CHAPTER 4

The Provisional Restoration: A Diagnostic, Functional, and Esthetic Template

Aldo Leopardi[1] & Daniel R. Cullum[2]

[1]Private Practice, Prosthodontist, Greenwood Village, CO, USA

[2]Private Practice, Coeur d'Alene, ID; Loma Linda University Department of OMS, Loma Linda, CA; UCLA Department of OMS, Los Angeles, CA, USA

Introduction

In the contemporary practice of implant dentistry, patients have come to expect good esthetic outcomes with implant-supported fixed restorations, especially in the esthetic zone. With adequate bone and soft tissue quality and quantity, normal levels of interproximal bone on contiguous teeth and correct 3-D positioning, this esthetic expectation is generally achievable with single implant-supported restorations. However, it is far more challenging and less predictable with facial implant positioning, bone and/or soft tissue deficiencies, when two or more adjacent implants are placed, and with narrow-diameter implants used to treat sites with reduced bone volume. Customized soft tissue manipulation with a transitional prosthesis can be completed after implant site healing and osseointegration.[1] This process can create favorable soft tissue and abutment contours at the gingival zenith, root eminence and interproximal regions for optimal esthetics and function for the final restoration. While there are little data from well-controlled clinical studies, many accomplished clinicians employ these techniques routinely for significant improvement with patient esthetics and function. An additional benefit of the fixed provisional process is further time for soft tissue maturation prior to final restoration without the duress of a removable appliance. The tissue manipulation process can require multiple visits and increased treatment time, needing the full support and cooperation of the patient. This is one of the highest art forms of clinical restorative dentistry to achieve the utmost esthetic and functional result for the patient. This chapter will review relevant literature on this topic, discuss components and techniques, as well as clinical application with treated cases.

Bone and soft tissue considerations

In order to achieve optimal soft tissue contours with dental implant restorations, ideal bone volume, soft tissue support, and 3-D implant placement are crucial[2–4] (see Chapters 1 and 3). Attention to the known critical distances between an implant and an adjacent tooth or between adjacent implants is also required.[5,6] Further, facial bone thickness must remain >1.8 to 2 mm or be augmented in order to minimize crestal resorption[7] and support adequate thickness of the overlying soft tissues.[8] Immediate implant placement into a fresh extraction socket with normal bone anatomy can result in stable and acceptable soft tissue profiles[9,10] if managed with current strategies (see Chapters 18 and 19). If the extraction socket walls are compromised, and/or the patient has high esthetic demand, a thin tissue biotype, or other findings indicating a complex risk assessment, then delayed implant placement may be more appropriate. Socket grafting with or without buccal bone or connective tissue augmentation at the time of tooth extraction may be a more predictable treatment option in these situations[11,12] (see also Chapters 5 and 8). Whether the surgeon uses an immediate or a delayed protocol, the healed implant site requires good bone support proximally and a mimimal 2 mm thickness on the buccal to ensure long-term implant success[3,8,13] and stable soft tissue levels.[14] The gingival biotype or phenotype of the patient can be described as thin or thick, scalloped or flat, with the thick and flat tissue phenotype being the more common[3,15] (Figure 4.1a; see also Chapter 8). Thin peri-implant gingiva is often associated with narrow, long teeth and scalloped bone/tissue architecture, which can result in greater facial crestal bone resorption and soft tissue recession[16,17] (see Figure 4.1b). Sites with thin gingival biotype often need augmentation with bone and/or soft tissue grafting, to create a gingival thickness adequate to accommodate the biologic width within and the emergence profile of the implant crown and its long-term stability[8,10] (see also Chapter 8).

For single-tooth dental implant sites, a horizontal distance of ≥1.5 mm between the implant and the adjacent tooth roots is required for interproximal bone stability. The interproximal bone height is dependent on the attachment level and periodontal bone support of the adjacent teeth.[18–20] When the interproximal bone height is acceptable and the gingival biotype is thick, satisfactory papilla regeneration is likely.[21] Second-stage uncovering procedures at single-tooth implant sites showed faster reformation of papillae with provisional crowns compared with stock healing caps.[1] However, after 2 years in function the control sites treated with healing abutments showed similar outcomes. A long-term study of denuded human papillae on natural teeth required an extended time of up to 3 years to regenerate papilla height to a mean of 4.3 mm.[21] Application of these concepts to implant therapy would imply that adequate

Minimally Invasive Dental Implant Surgery, First Edition. Edited by Daniel R. Cullum and Douglas Deporter.

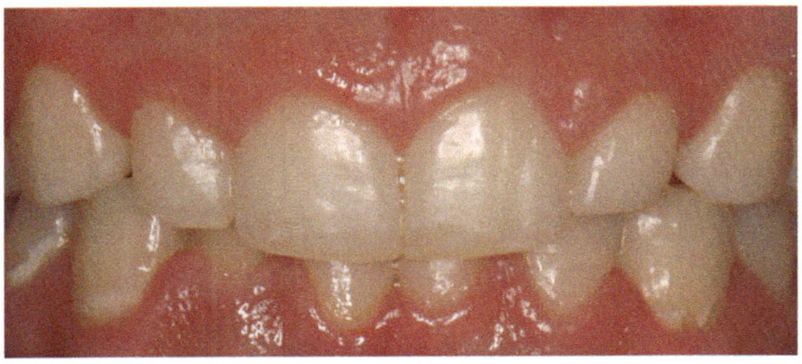

(a)

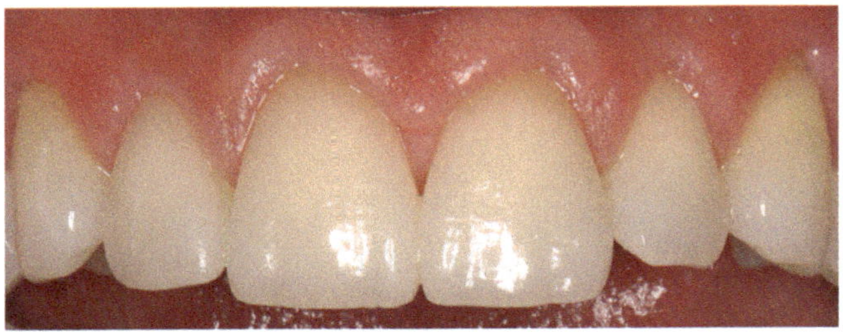

(b)

Figure 4.1 (a) Low scalloped, thick gingival biotype with shorter clinical crowns and papilla heights. (b) High scalloped, thin gingival biotype with more triangular tooth forms are at greater risk of bone and soft tissue recession. © Aldo Leopardi.

prosthetic space be left for papilla ingrowth. Practically, to leave the embrasure open and/or to delay the final restoration for this time period for maturation would be unacceptable for most patients and clinicians.

If the interproximal bone height is compromised on the adjacent tooth, satisfactory papilla maintenance or regeneration between tooth and implant is unlikely.[22] However, the situation can be manipulated so that the distance from the interproximal bone height of the tooth is no more than 4.5 mm apical to the contact point between the tooth and implant crowns.[14] Alternatively, the treatment plan and implant positioning can be altered with use of a pontic, which may maintain a taller soft tissue papilla[5,6,23] (Table 4.1; see Chapter 1). Using a fixed provisional restoration allows the clinician to develop different crown contours in an attempt to optimize papillary and facial gingival contours. A restoration with a square-shaped crown form will fill the embrasure space with restorative material and prevent the anticipated soft tissue regeneration when there is adequate adjacent interproximal bone.

Table 4.1 The interproximal height of bone and soft tissue considerations

Proximity limitations	Restorative environment (mm)	Vertical soft tissue limitations (mm)
Tooth–tooth	1	5
Tooth–pontic	N/A	6.5
Tooth–implant	1.5	4.5
Implant–pontic	N/A	5.5
Implant–implant	3	3.5
Pontic–pontic	N/A	6

After Salama H, Salama M, Garber D, and Adar P, Journal of Practical Periodontics.[23]

Biologic width

"Biologic width" around the neck of a dental implant constitutes a mucosal seal needed to protect the underlying bone. Its minimal overall thickness is approximately 3 mm including 1 mm of sulcus depth, 1 mm of epithelial attachment, and 1 mm of connective tissue between the periosteal covering of bone and the epithelial attachment.[24,25] The connective tissue component of the peri-implant biologic width will have circumferentially oriented collagen fibers, except perhaps with laser-ablated implant collar and/or abutment surfaces, where some oriented fibrous connective tissue attachment to implant surface seems possible (see Chapter 6). If the soft tissues overlying an implant are too thin to accommodate biologic width requirements, peri-implant crestal bone will be resorbed to allow reformation of the requisite soft tissue thickness.[16,26] The result may be metal translucency at the abutment margin or unwanted exposure of the implant surface with an unsatisfactory esthetic outcome. Thick soft tissue over an implant provides greater opportunity to develop a pleasing emergence profile and gingival zenith. However, deep peri-implant sulci may create a serious risk if cement-retained implant crowns are planned since subgingival cement remnants may be impossible to detect. Retained cement will almost certainly initiate an inflammatory response that will lead to crestal bone loss with treatment compromise or failure.[27–29]

With two-piece implant systems, the implant–abutment interface ("microgap") is generally initially positioned at the level of the alveolar crest, and biologic width will be established in relation to this interface. With two-piece implants placed in dogs, regardless of whether submerged or non-submerged healing was used, the most coronal bone-to-implant contact was about 2 mm apical to the microgap.[30] This loss in crestal bone was driven by the need for the connective tissue and epithelial components of biologic width to separate crestal bone from the microgap with its bacterial deposits and micromovements under function.[31–33] While it has been reported that repeated removal and replacement of abutments onto an implant may have deleterious effects on crestal bone because of disruptions of the soft tissue seal,[34] further studies and significant clinical experience are at conflict with this concept.[35,36] Challenges with the concept of "one abutment, one time" include limited restorative options (primarily cement-retained), residual excess cement,[37] and limited soft tissue manipulation capabilities with suboptimal emergence profiles.

Adjacent implants

When adjacent implants are placed, the horizontal distance between the two implants influences the stability of the inter-implant crestal bone. A tendency for loss in height of the inter-implant bone peak will occur as inter-implant distance decreases below 3 mm.[38,39] Clinical data for implants with >3 mm inter-implant dimension showed a mean loss in height of the interproximal bone peak of 0.45 mm, while those with ≤3 mm inter-implant bone showed a mean loss in height of 1.04 mm.[6] Histological data from animal experiments using two-piece, moderately rough implants showed that vertical crestal inter-implant bone loss decreased from 1.98 mm for a 2 mm inter-implant distance to 0.23 mm for a 5 mm inter-implant distance.[39] A horizontal or lateral component has also been shown for this inter-implant bone loss in addition to the more commonly discussed vertical component[6,40,41] (see Figure 8.3a and b).

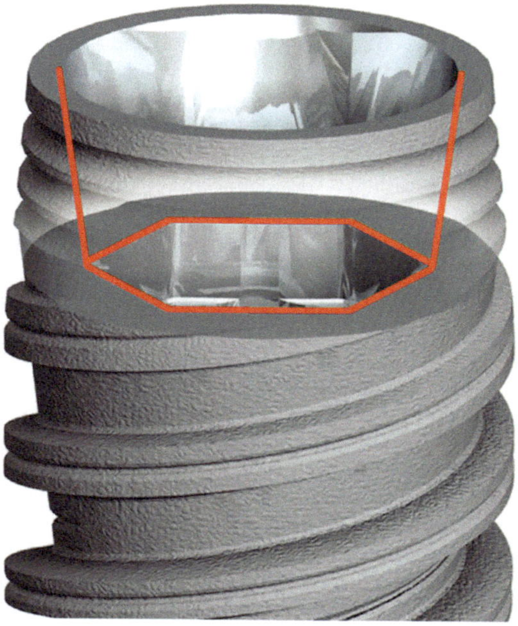

Figure 4.2 The use of an internal tapered connection reduces the dimension of the microgap and abutment micromotion under function. *Source:* Nobel Biocare. Reproduced with permission of Nobel Biocare.

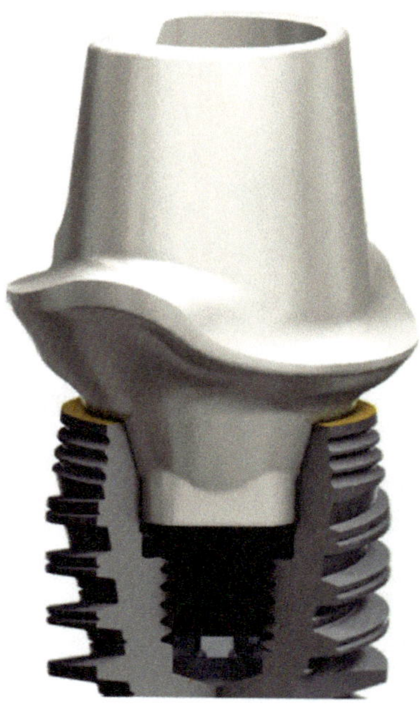

Figure 4.3 Platform switching moves the implant–abutment interface (microgap) medially to reduce the vertical height requirement of the biologic width. *Source:* Nobel Biocare. Reproduced with permission of Nobel Biocare.

Following re-entry of two-piece minimally rough implants and establishment of biologic width, investigators noted approximately 1.4 mm of horizontal marginal bone loss in relation to each of the two approximating implant surfaces.[6] In situations where the inter-implant distance was suboptimal (i.e. <3 mm), the lateral bone losses of the two adjacent implants could fuse, resulting in a significant reduction in the height of the inter-implant bone peak meant to support the soft tissue papilla.[6] Placing adjacent implants ≥3 mm apart reduces the risk of this unwanted inter-implant bone loss; however, it does not ensure the maintenance or reformation of an interproximal papilla. Tarnow et al.[40] reported that the mean height of papilla from the interproximal bone crest was 3.4 mm with a range of 1 mm to 7 mm (2 mm: 16.9%; 3 mm: 35.3%; or 4 mm: 37.5%). Advances in implant design with two-piece implant systems such as "platform switching" of the implant abutment interface and broad application of internal Morse taper connections (Figure 4.2) may improve this situation by maintaining interproximal bone, thereby increasing papillary volume and height.

"Platform switching or shifting"

The principle of platform switching utilizes a prosthetic abutment smaller in diameter than the implant itself, which allows for a medial or inward horizontal repositioning of the implant—abutment interface (microgap)[42] (Figure 4.3). This design feature can be created in an implant body by the manufacturer or achieved by the clinician using a compatible abutment of lesser diameter than the implant platform. The effect of platform switching is to create a horizontal component for the total linear length required for biologic width formation.[42,43] The effect will be to reduce both lateral and vertical bone loss adjacent to the implant neck and allow the biologic width to be located more coronally,[44] an obvious advantage in the esthetic zone. Platform switching also may lower the effect of occlusal loading and stress concentration at the cervical bone–implant interface.[45]

Generally, a horizontal component of 0.35–0.5 mm of biologic width is created about the circumference of an implant by "platform switching." Studies indicate this design feature results in less interproximal crestal bone loss on radiographic evaluation[43,46,47] and better soft tissue support.[48] Cochran et al.[49] found that the connective tissue component of biologic width was located more coronal with platform-switched implants compared with non-platform-switched implants in the dog mandible. Similar findings with less interproximal bone loss were reported in animal[50] and human studies,[51] using a significant platform-switching and steep Morse taper implant design. Elian et al.[52] concluded that platform switching may allow clinicians to place adjacent implants closer to each other than 3 mm without losing interproximal bone height. Also, this design can help avoid damaging the attachment apparatus when an implant is placed adjacent to a tooth. Similar conclusions were drawn from a human clinical study for the implant-to-tooth scenario.[53] Whether platform shifting results in long-term stability with better papilla formation between implants requires further investigation.[54]

Implant design features that maintain stable crestal bone and soft tissue, including macro design, surface treatment, tapered internal connections (Figure 4.2) and platform switching (Figure 4.3), are all exciting concepts that appear to have a positive influence on long-term esthetic and functional outcomes, but further research and discussion are necessary.[54]

Provisional restoration

Provisional restorations are of significant benefit in creating natural-looking final implant restorations with acceptable and stable soft tissue profiles.[55–59] A removable provisional prosthesis often is prepared as an economic compromise in the esthetic zone. This can be an adequate "space-filling" appliance for temporary esthetics over the months of implant integration for the majority of patients who are not candidates for immediate provisional restoration. An Essix® design is somewhat less esthetic and less durable than a removable partial denture. However, it is less expensive and useful for patients with a significant overbite to avoid occlusal displacement of an appliance and traumatic injury to the underlying surgical site.[58] During the immediate post-implant healing interval, the removable appliance should have no direct contact on the healing tissues or implant healing abutment. Use of a removable appliance for ovate pontic site development has limited application at implant sites.[60] Tooth-borne provisionals are also an excellent consideration if the adjacent teeth are involved in the restorative process. When implants are being used to replace two or more contiguous teeth, a fixed provisional prosthesis supported by natural teeth or transitional implants are the methods of choice to avoid denture pressure at the intaglio surface and micromotion on healing implant sites.[56–58]

After implant integration and soft tissue healing, fabrication of an implant-supported, screw-retained fixed provisional crown can be completed. The advantages of this technique are significant for site development, offering excellent control and precision in guiding the final soft tissue contours with a prototype restoration.[56,60] Subgingival contours of fixed provisional restorations can be used to shape and optimize peri-implant gingival tissues, particularly those on the facial aspect.[60–64] Provisional restoration can promote development of improved papillary and marginal gingiva tissue contours, in particular with reduced-diameter implants (see also Chapter 11). Development of an esthetically pleasing emergence profile for an implant crown requires understanding of the limitations of peri-implant bone and soft tissue parameters, including gingival biotype, biologic width, implant-to-tooth and implant-to-implant critical distances, platform switching, and contact point-to-proximal bone crest critical distances.

Further advantages of fixed provisional restorations include:

1 The surgeon and restorative team can observe the soft tissue profile developing with the provisional and make appropriate changes to the prosthesis if need be.
2 The surgeon can see the impact of implant positioning and design features on the restorative treatment sequence, allowing them to confirm or modify future treatment choices.
3 The patient can sign off on the esthetic outcome before the final restoration.
4 The provisional facilitates communication with the laboratory technician.
5 The final restoration can easily be inserted into the established soft tissue profile developed by the provisional.

Provisional abutments

Direct and indirect provisional fabrication techniques have been advocated.[56] The patient evaluation must include assessment of overbite, overjet, and the occlusal plane. The deep bite patient can pose significant challenges to avoiding direct occlusal contact on excursive movements of the mandible with function and parafunction. This requires an adequate thickness of restorative material and strength of the abutment to withstand the time interval of the provisional phase. Manufacturers have produced numerous designs and materials. Challenges with "plastic" provisional abutments include longevity and fracture at the abutment–restorative material interface.

Screw retention greatly simplifies the restorative process by avoiding cement displacement on placement and subsequent modifications of the provisional. Modified techniques with cement-retained restorations include fabrication of a custom abutment with the margin at or above the gingival level, and venting of the crown via duplication of the abutment to "pre-cement" the crown and remove any excess prior to placement in the patient's mouth (Figure 4.4). These applications and indications for cement-retained provisional restorations should be reserved for those rare instances when implant placement is not acceptable for screw retention (see Chapter 19).

Many philosophical discussions can be made about the concepts and clinical applications of plastic, ceramic, titanium, zirconia, or other abutments for provisionalization. For immediate provisional restoration, plastic abutments using a "direct" screw-retained pick-up technique are demonstrated in Chapter 19. The advantages of resiliency[65] and simple modification in the surgical setting outweigh the potential for material delamination, fracture, and fatigue. For application at a healed site, as presented in this chapter, an "indirect" screw-retained provisional titanium abutment with laboratory fabrication is the recommended technique for optimal emergence profile development. The provisional abutment must allow for repeated recontouring and reshaping, sometimes over an extended time interval to allow adequate soft tissue maturation. Perhaps future developments in the digital world will produce fabrication or milling of multiple abutments with incremental sizes and/or shape modifications in a cost-effective way. Additionally, compensation for eccentric or palatal positioning cannot be completed without customization as a secondary prosthetic process. There is not currently any system that allows immediate custom final abutment fabrication with broad clinical application.

Provisional fabrication and impression techniques

Case study 4.1

This case study (Figure 4.5) demonstrates the custom anterior impression and post technique for the fabrication of an indirect screw-retained provisional restoration. A temporary abutment was used with this provisional after initial impression and preparation. The process required repeated adjustments to the intaglio surface, with a minimum of 6 weeks needed to develop the tissue profiles.

A closed tray impression was completed with pre-impression patient images and confirmatory periapical radiographs (Figure 4.5a–d). Fabrication of the master soft tissue cast was completed (Figure 4.5e), and a combination peak acrylic and titanium base provisional abutment used (Figure 4.5f). The provisional abutment was seated on the model with removal of soft tissue (Figure 4.5g) to produce the desired emergence profile in wax. Abutment preparation was completed with blocking out of undercuts using wax (Figure 4.5h). A pretreatment laboratory vacuform template was constructed (Figure 4.5i) from a diagnostic work-up master cast (not shown here), and separating medium (petroleum jelly) was

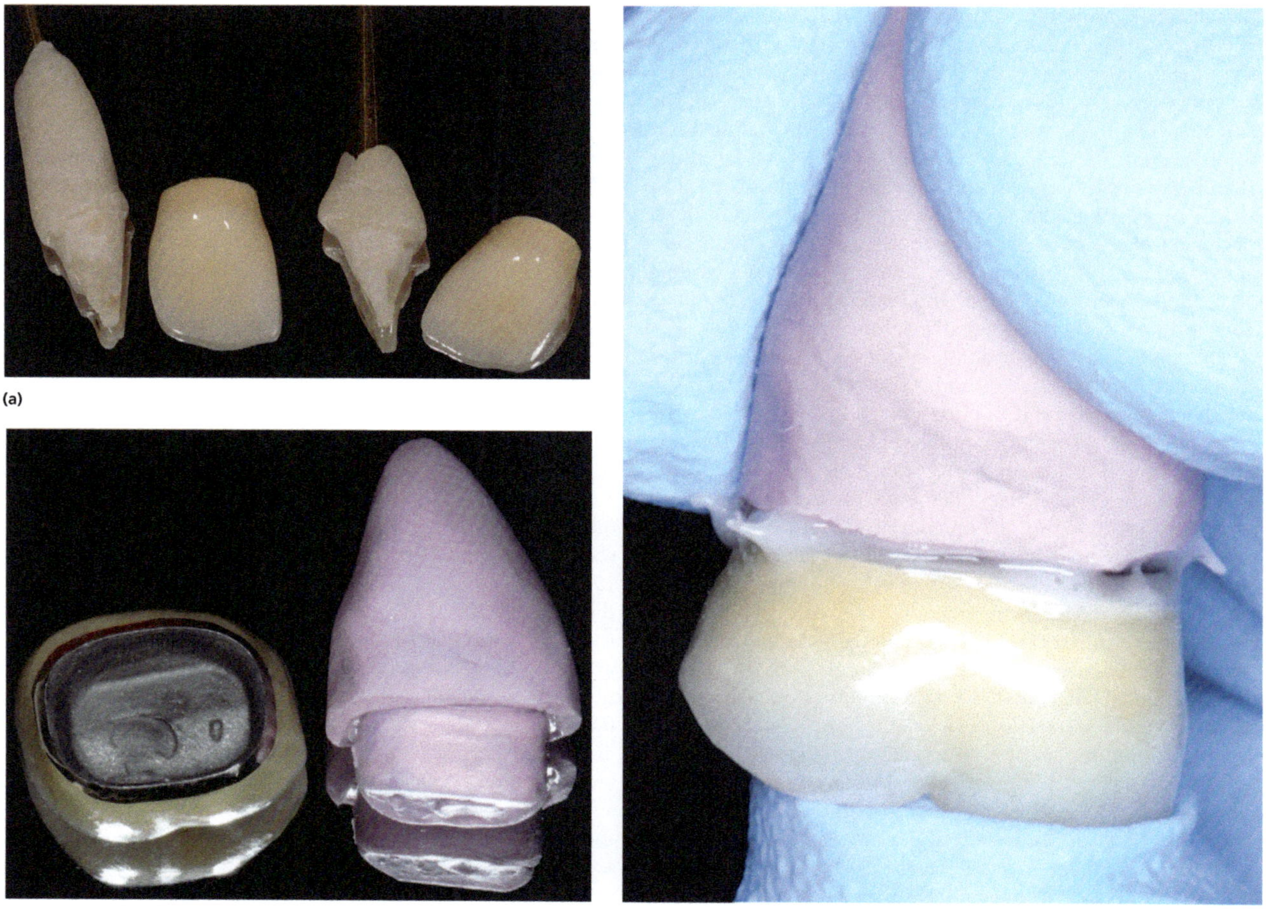

(a)

(b)

(c)

Figure 4.4 (a–c) Fabrication of a secondary "die" or abutment can be used as a technique with cemented crowns to seat and extrude excess cement for complete removal prior to seating in the patient. © Aldo Leopardi.

placed on the cast followed by indirect acrylic of matched shade (Figure 4.5j). The provisional restorations were trimmed and polished to the desired contours for maxillary lateral incisors (Figure 4.5k), and the screw-retained temporary abutments seated on the cast (Figure 4.5l). The patient can be seen on clinical and radiographic images after 3 weeks with provisional restorations in place in Figure 4.5m–o. These titanium–polymer combination abutments were for short-term use of up to 6–8 weeks.

The next series of images (Figure 4.6) for the same patient demonstrate construction of titanium-based, screw-retained provisional restorations for the maxillary first premolar teeth. These were needed to serve as longer term provisionals; that is, good for about 6–12 months. Temporary titanium cylinders are recommended where modification of the emergence profile is needed. However, the use of prefabricated, contoured titanium abutments is also an option where subgingval emergence modification is not necessary. The decision can be made after impression-taking by evaluation of the patient and master cast with and without the soft tissue mask. Fabrication of the master soft tissue cast can be completed with removal of soft tissue and placement of a titanium provisional or stock abutment. Figure 4.6a–d demonstrates use of a stock precontoured titanium abutment. The desired emergence profile was produced in wax (reverse) with block-out of the undercuts and use of a vacuform template constructed in the laboratory from a diagnostic work-up master cast (not shown here). Separating medium (petroleum jelly) was placed on the cast, followed by application of a metal primer and bonding agent and use of resin tint modifier opaque to blockout the metal base. (Figure 4.6e and f). The desired provisional resin was placed (Triad®, Dentsply), light cured (Figure 4.6g), and then removed and trimmed to the appropriate contours (Figure 4.6h and i). The abutments and crowns were cleansed and delivered to the patient. Blanching of tissue typically occurs with insertion, but should resolve within 5–10 min. The screw-retained provisional can be seen in position after 3 weeks in Figure 4.6j. The patient should be reassessed after 2 weeks to determine if further adjustments to the intaglio surface are needed. The process requires a minimum 6 weeks to develop the desired tissue profiles.

Fabrication of custom impression posts for the maxillary right and left lateral incisors in this case study is demonstrated in Figure 4.7a–f. Capturing the intaglio information of the

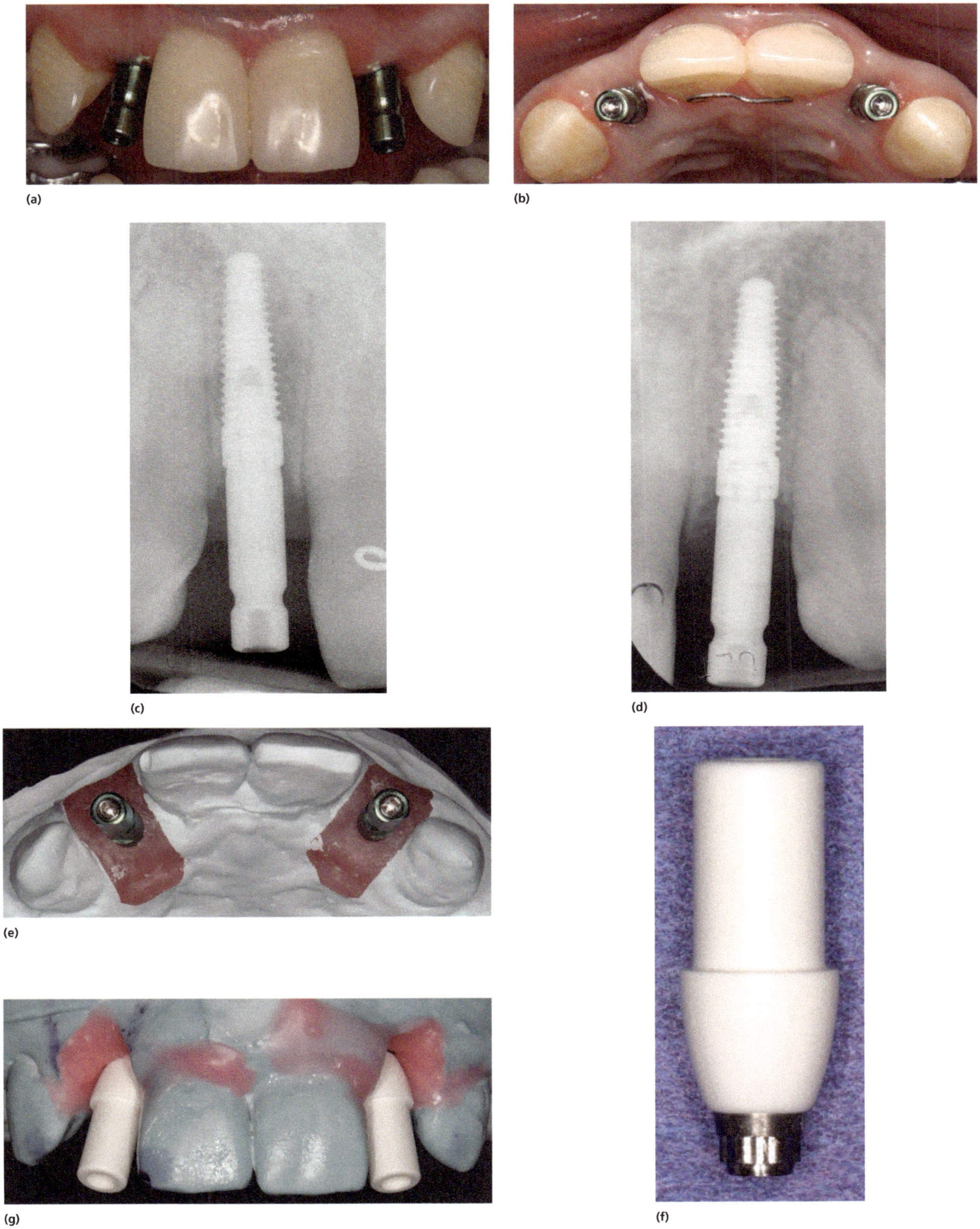

Figure 4.5 (a, b) Healed implant sites with impression copings in place. The implants demonstrate excellent palatal positioning and angulation appropriate for screw retention. (c, d) The corresponding radiographs confirmed complete impression coping seating. (e) A closed-tray impression was used to fabricate the master cast with simulated soft tissue at the implant sites. (f) A combination PEEK polymer and titanium base provisional abutments were used. (g) Provisional abutments were seated onto the working model with removal of simulated soft tissue to produce the desired emergence profile in wax.

(Continued)

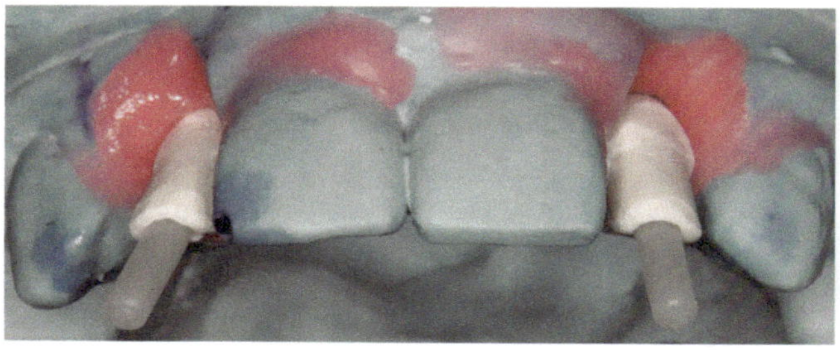

(h)

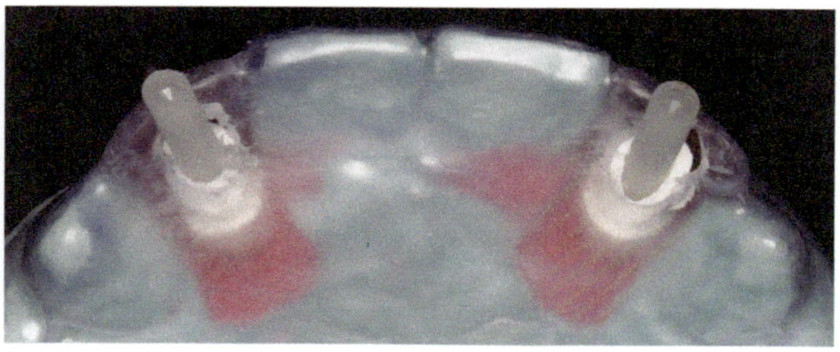

(i)

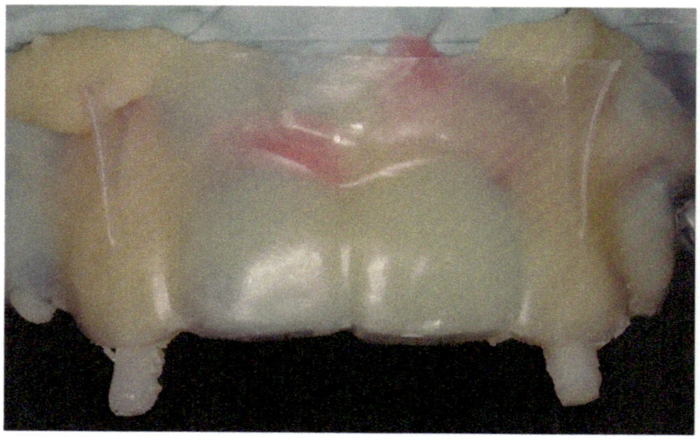

(j)

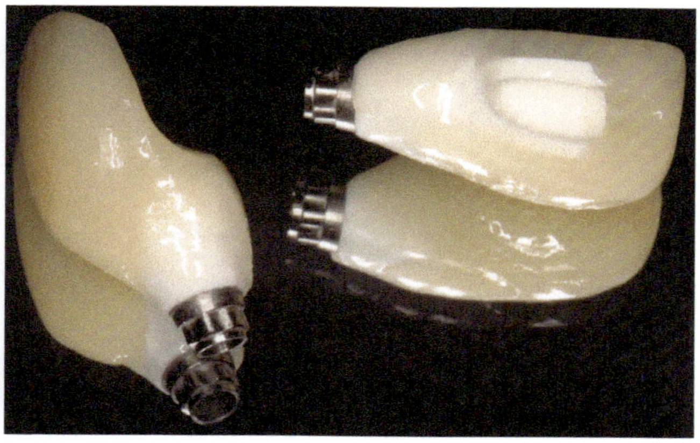

(k)

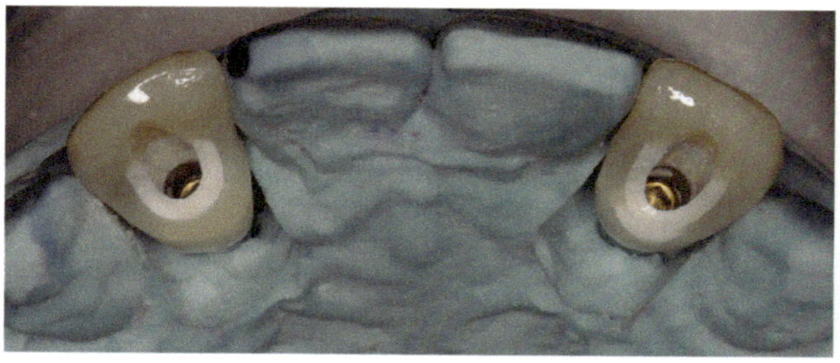

(l)

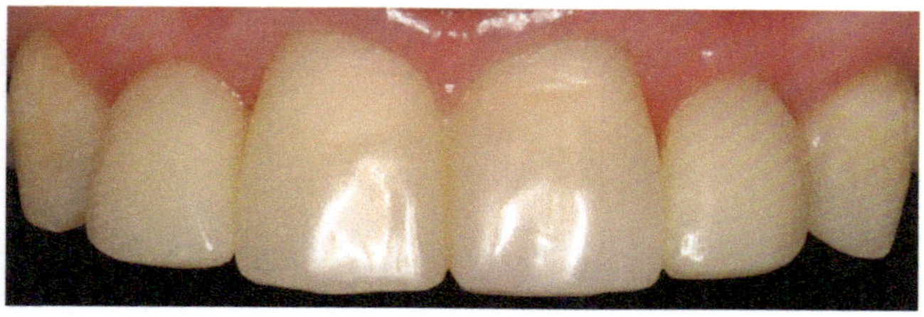

(m)

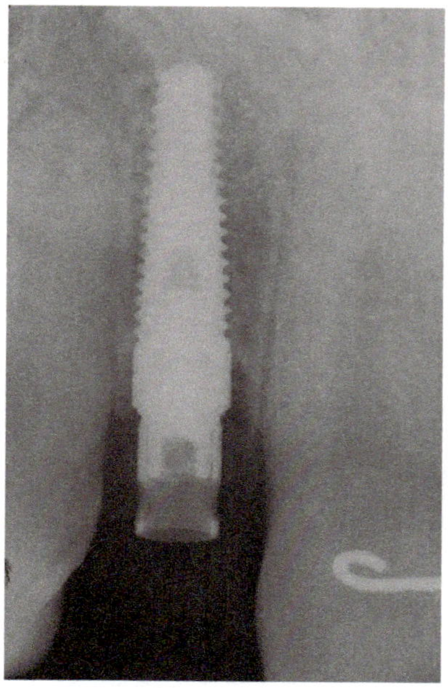

(n)

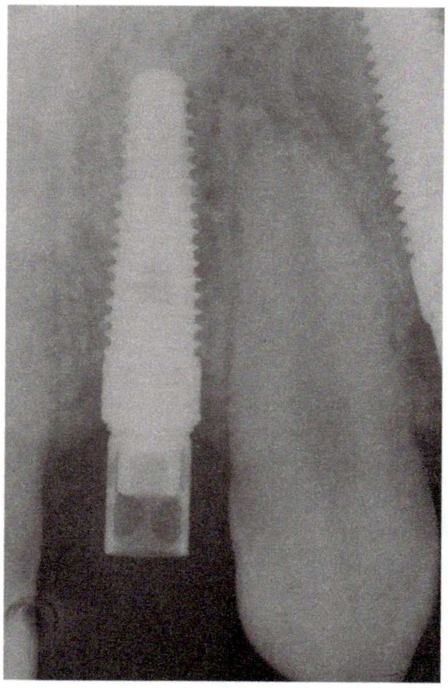

(o)

Figure 4.5 (Continued)
(h) Initial abutment preparation was completed and the undercuts on the master cast blocked out with wax. (i) A vacuform template was constructed in the laboratory from a diagnostic work-up master cast. (j) Separating medium (petroleum jelly) was placed on the master cast. An indirect technique was used by filling of the vacuform template with light-cured provisional material (Triad, Dentsply) of matched shade followed by delivery to the master cast.
(k) After curing, the provisional screw-retained restorations were removed from the cast and trimmed and polished to the desired contours for the maxillary lateral incisors. (l) Provisional screw-retained restorations were seated onto the cast. (m–o) These clinical and radiographic images demonstrate the soft tissue contours with provisional restorations in place for 3 weeks. © Aldo Leopardi.

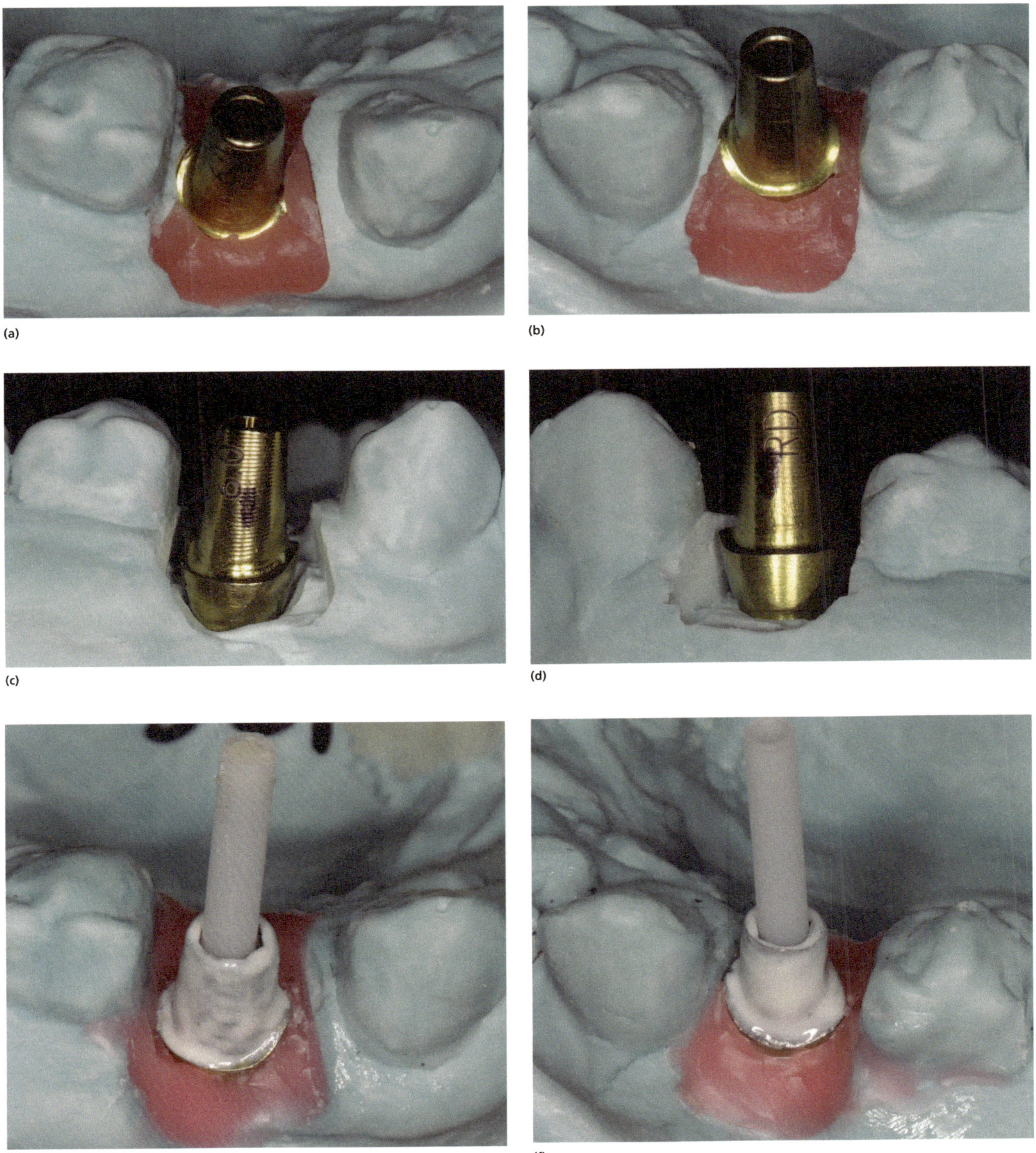

Figure 4.6 (a–d) After fabrication of the master soft tissue cast was completed, screw-retained, stock precontoured titanium abutments were placed and the case evaluated with the soft tissue mask in place and after its removal. (e, f) The desired emergence profile was produced in wax (reverse) with block-out of undercuts. The abutments were prepared with application of metal primer and bonding agent, use of resin tint opaque modifier to block out the metal and a separating medium placed on the cast. *(Continued)*

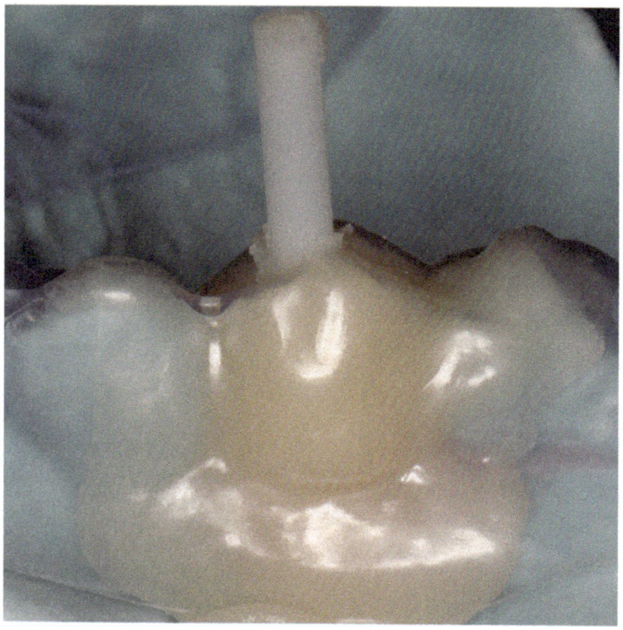

(g)

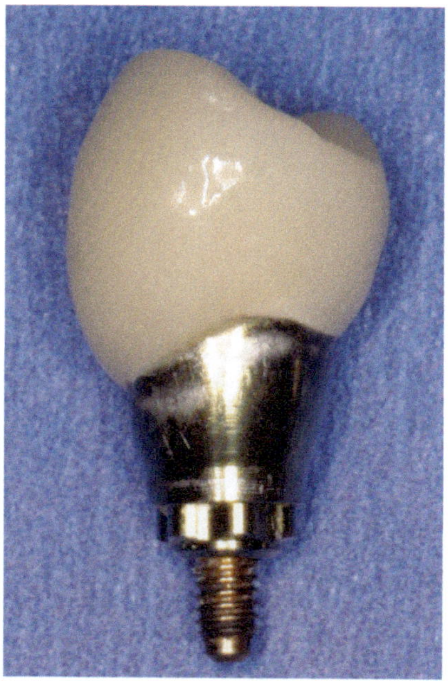

(h)

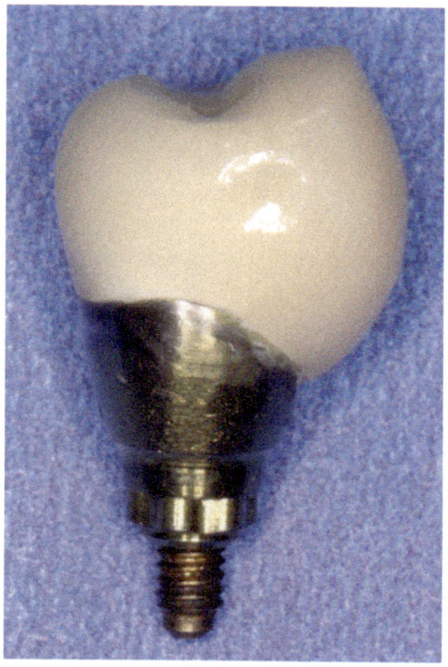

(i)

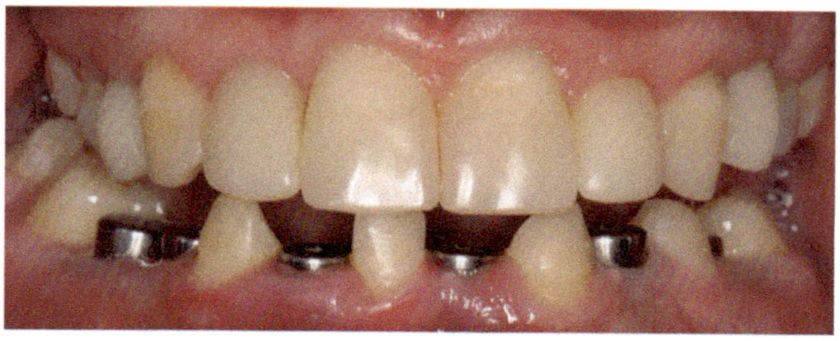

(j)

Figure 4.6 (Continued)
(g) A vacuform template was filled with the desired provisional resin (Triad, Dentsply) and cured. (h, i) The provisional restorations were removed from the master cast, trimmed to appropriate contours, and polished. (j) The restorations were cleansed and delivered to the patient. Typically, blanching of the soft tissue occurs with insertion; this should resolve within several minutes. The screw-retained provisional restoration can be seen in position after 3 weeks. © Aldo Leopardi.

prototype provisional restorations was completed after contour modifications and tissue maturation. The prototypes were placed back onto the cast (Figure 4.7a), and a medium-body vinyl polysiloxane impression material injected to record the soft tissue profiles (Figure 4.7b). The prototypes were removed from the cast (Figure 4.7c), and open-tray impression posts inserted with a light-cured or chemical-cured resin placed into the gap (GC pattern resin – chemical cured, GC pattern resin™ LS, GC America) (Figure 4.7d). After adequate time for curing, the custom impression copings were removed and trimmed (Figure 4.7e). The custom posts now were ready to deliver to the patient for the master impression appointment (Figure 4.7f). Fabrication of the screw-retained final restorations included customization of precontoured stock zirconia abutments (Figure 4.7g). Restorations and periapical radiographs can be seen in Figure 4.7h–j 3 weeks after insertion. Pretreatment and long-term follow-up images for the patient with an excellent esthetic and stable clinical result are presented in Figure 4.7k and l.

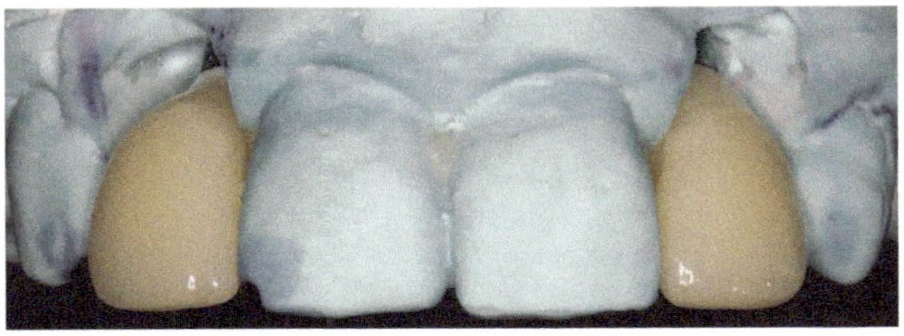

(a)

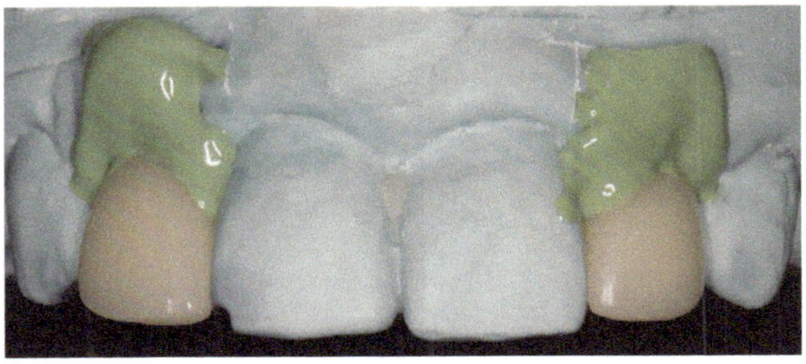

(b)

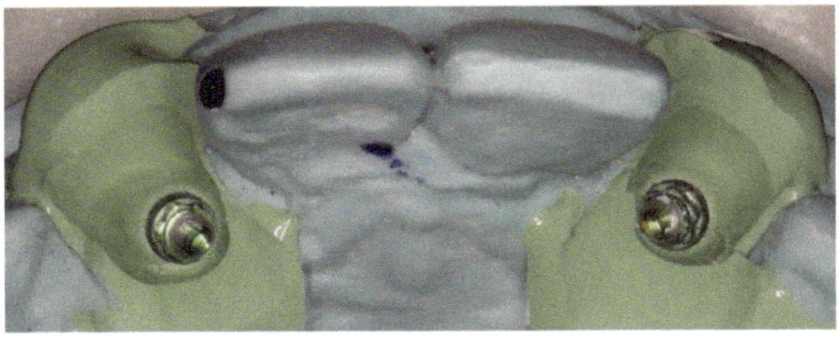

(c)

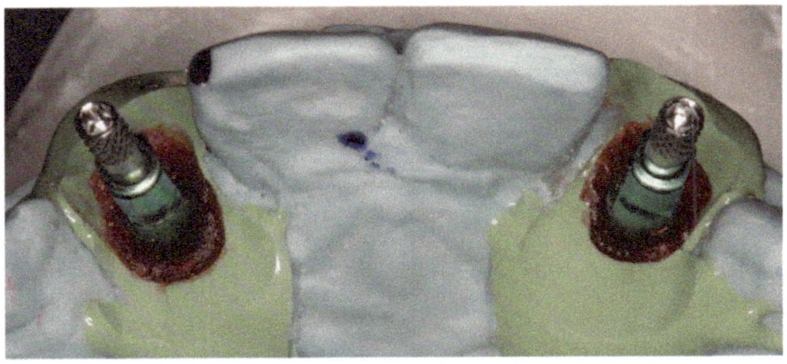

(d)

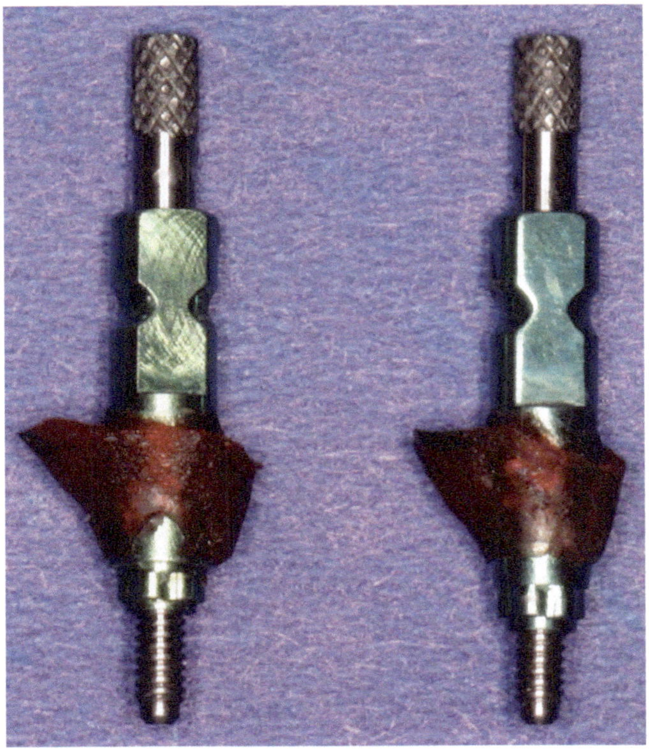

(e)

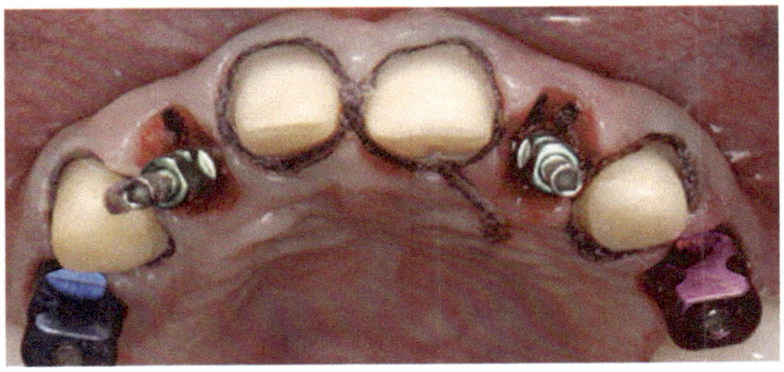

(f)

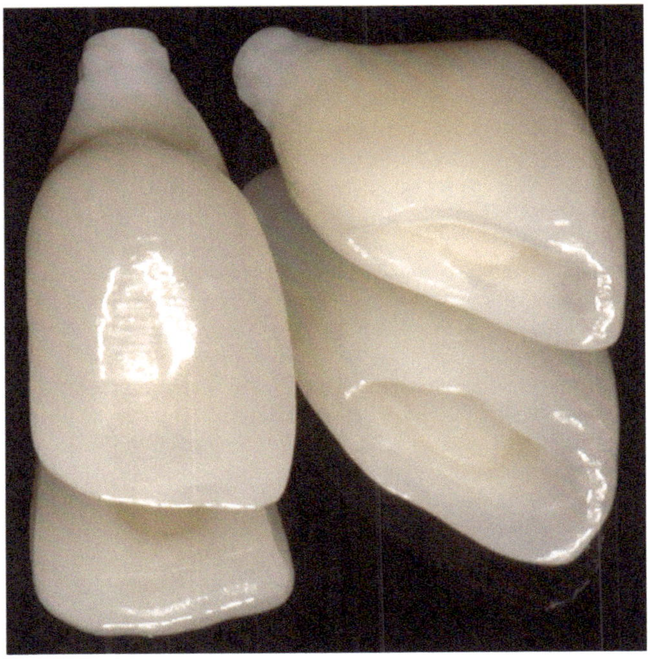

(g)

Figure 4.7 (a) Custom impression posts for case study 4.1 maxillary right and left lateral incisors are shown here. The prototypes were placed back onto the cast. (b) A medium-body vinyl polysiloxane impression material was injected onto the cast to record the soft tissue profile. (c) The prototypes were removed from the cast. (d) Open-tray impression posts were placed using a light-cured or chemical-cured resin (GC pattern resin™ LS, GC America). (e) After adequate time for curing, the custom impression copings were removed and trimmed. (f) Posts now were ready to deliver to the patient during the master impression appointment. (g) Fabrication of the screw-retained final restorations included customization of precontoured stock zirconia abutments. *(Continued)*

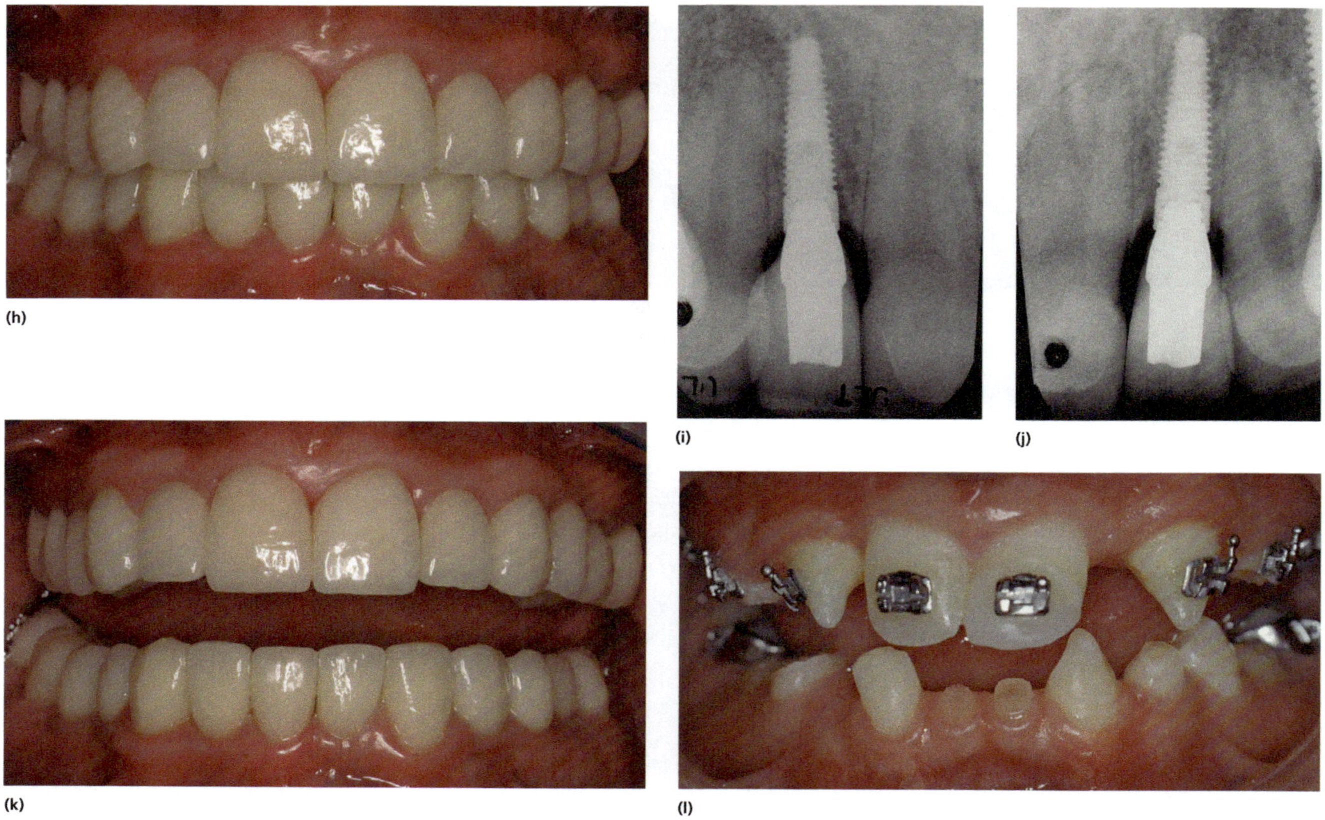

Figure 4.7 (Continued)
(h–j) Shown here are the inserted restorations and periapical radiographs 3 weeks after insertion. (k, l) Definitive restoration and pretreatment images for the patient can be seen confirming an excellent esthetic and stable clinical result. © Aldo Leopardi.

Tissue manipulation and sculpting

Case study 4.2

Figure 4.8 shows how to manipulate soft tissues with a prototype provisional restoration. The most significant changes to tissue profiles will occur around the last 1.5 mm of the intaglio area prior to emergence through the gingiva. With the addition of provisional materials to the sub-emergence contour, the tissue will move apically. Alternatively, if material is removed from the intaglio area, the tissue can move coronally. This patient lost tooth #9 after failed endodontic and restorative treatments, while teeth #8 and #10 had been treated 4 years previously with porcelain veneers. Six months after extraction and grafting of the left maxillary central incisor, excellent tissue contours and volume can be seen in Figure 4.8a. A surgical guide was used for staged implant placement. The patient wore a removable partial denture for interim esthetics. Uncovering and placement of a healing abutment were completed after adequate time for integration. After a minimum 8 weeks for soft tissue healing (Figure 4.8b), an impression coping was inserted (Figure 4.8c) and the casting and fabrication of a composite fused to titanium screw-retained prototype was completed (as described in case study 4.1). The prototype provisional restoration was delivered to the patient. It is necessary to allow an additional 2 weeks for tissue maturation (Figure 4.8d) prior to modifying the prototype. The facial gingival margin in this case was 1.5 mm coronal to the contralateral tooth. The anticipated effect of contour change on the gingival profile is demonstrated in Figure 4.8e and f with the planned addition of facial contour using a triangular pad of flowable, light-cured composite resin (or acrylic with the brush technique). By adding restorative material to the mid-facial intaglio area (last 1.5 mm) with trimming and polishing, the tissue was displaced coronally to achieve the desired soft tissue profile. Figure 4.8g shows the clinical presentation after provisional modification and revision of the veneers of the adjacent teeth (provisional veneers) after two more weeks for tissue maturation. The custom impression post technique (as described above) was used to fabricate the definitive restorations (Figure 4.8h and i). Clinical "try-in" was completed to confirm and modify the definitive restorations. The clinical and radiographic images 3 weeks after delivery of the definitive restorations are shown in Figure 4.8j–l, and included a screw-retained porcelain fused to zirconium implant crown at the maxillary left central incisor and revised porcelain laminate veneers at the adjacent teeth.

Case study 4.3

The patient seen in Figure 4.9 presented with congenitally missing maxillary lateral incisor teeth. The permanent maxillary canine teeth had already been moved to the lateral incisor positions and the deciduous canines had been left in the canine positions. The

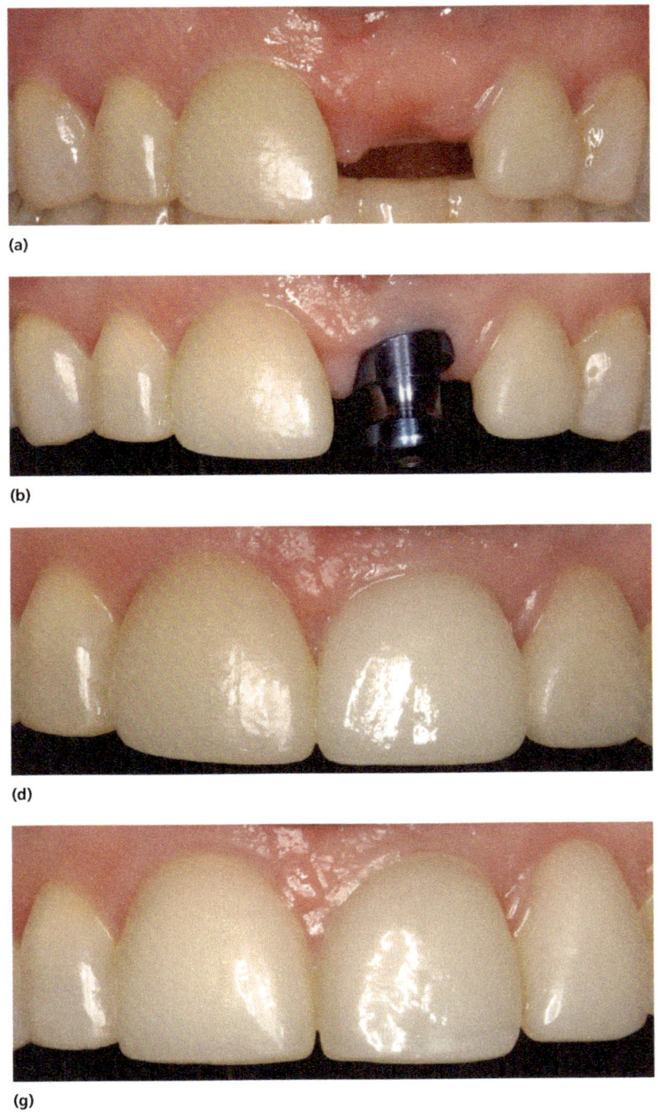

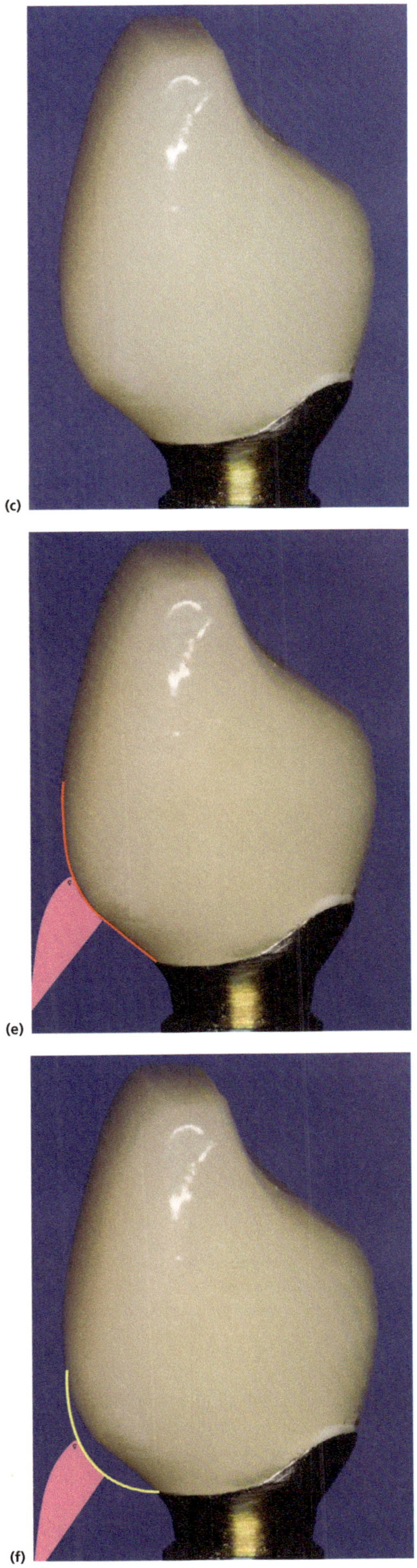

Figure 4.8 (a) Excellent tissue contours and volume can be seen at the maxillary left central incisor site 6 months after extraction and site preservation grafting. (b) After the minimum 8 weeks of soft tissue healing, a closed-tray impression coping was inserted and the impression completed. (c) A titanium (Triad fused to titanium) screw-retained prototype was fabricated as described in case study 4.1. (d) The prototype provisional restoration was delivered to the patient. After 2 weeks of soft tissue maturation, the facial gingival margin is approximately 1.5 mm coronal to that of the contralateral tooth. (e, f) The anticipated effect of contour change on the gingival profile is demonstrated here with the addition of facial contour using a triangular pad of flowable light-cured composite resin. By adding restorative material to the mid-facial intaglio area (last 1.5 mm), the tissue was displaced coronally to achieve the desired soft tissue profile. (g) The clinical presentation after provisional modification and two more weeks for tissue maturation. Temporary veneers also were placed on the adjacent teeth.

(Continued)

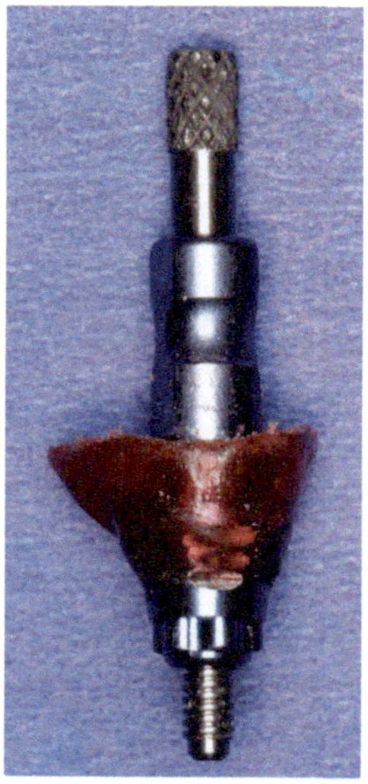

(h)

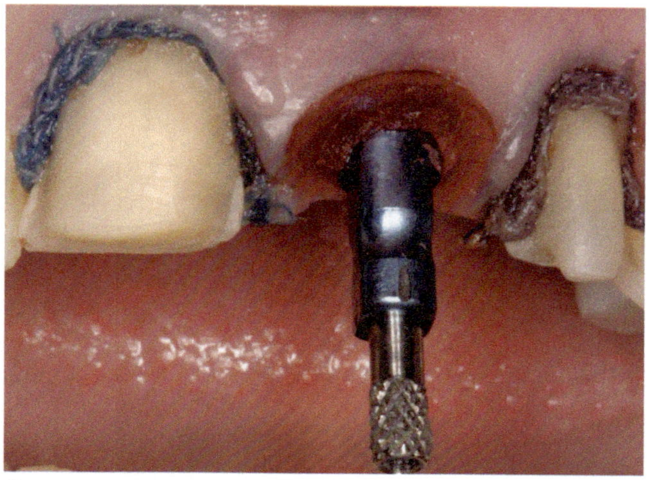

(i)

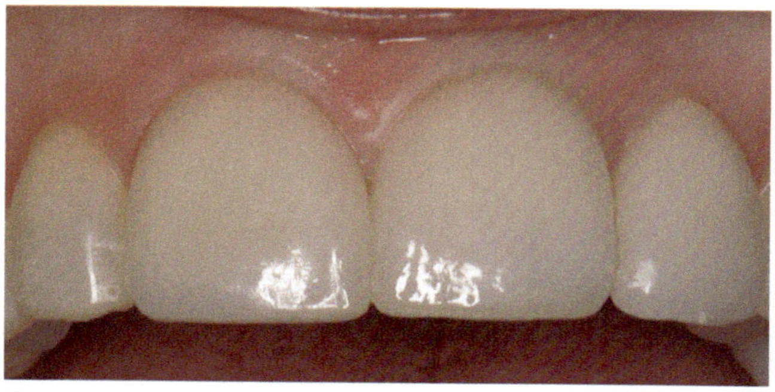

(j)

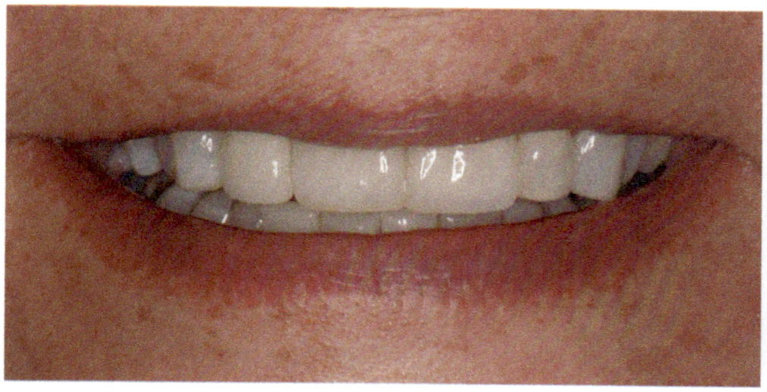

(l)

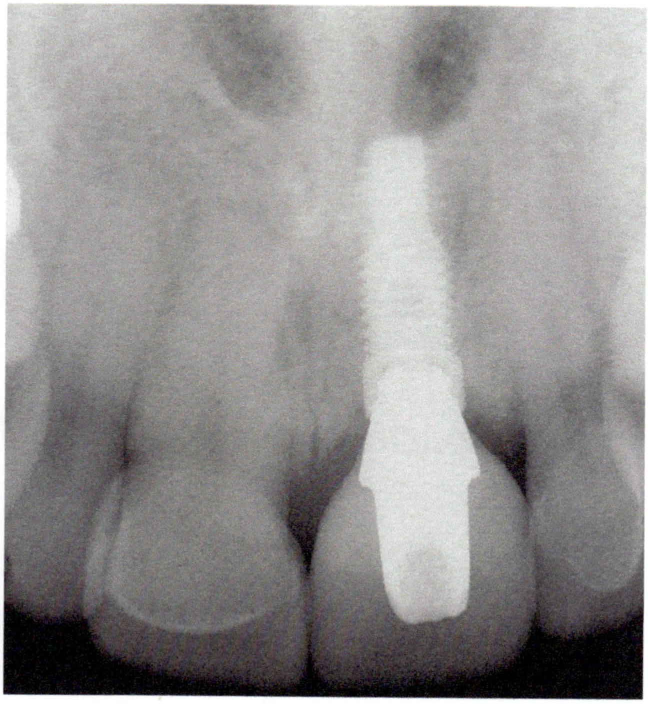

(k)

Figure 4.8 (Continued)
(h, i) The custom impression post technique was used to fabricate the definitive restorations. Clinical "try-in" was completed to confirm the final contours. (j–l) The clinical and radiographic images 3 weeks after delivery of the definitive restorations, which included a screw-retained porcelain fused to zirconium implant crown at the maxillary left central incisor and revised porcelain laminate veneers at the adjacent teeth. © Aldo Leopardi.

patient's treatment plan included adult orthodontics, removal of the deciduous canines, and moving the canines back to their normal positions. After completion of orthodontic movements, placement of 3.0 mm diameter implants was completed at the lateral incisor sites using a minimally invasive, guided procedure. The initial patient presentation is documented in Figure 4.9a and b. The patient accepted the proposed treatment and can be seen in Figure 4.9c after orthodontic treatment was completed with a surgical guide in position. Implants were placed single stage with a guided minimally invasive approach.

After 4 months healing, palatal implant positioning can be seen with excellent facial tissue volume (Figure 4.9d). Using the open-tray technique (Figure 4.9e), the impression was completed after radiographic confirmation of the abutment seatings (Figure 4.9f

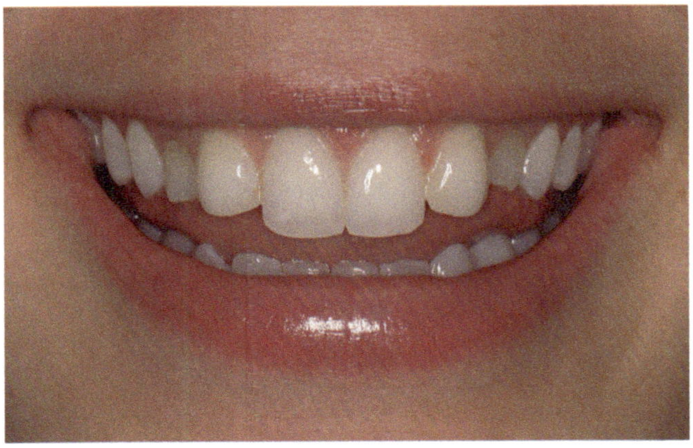
(a)

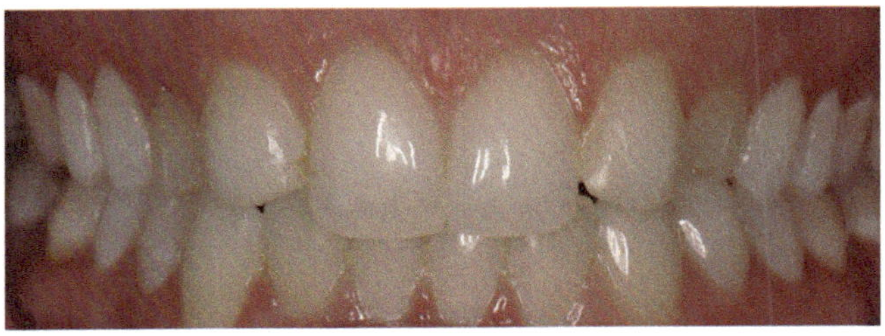
(b)

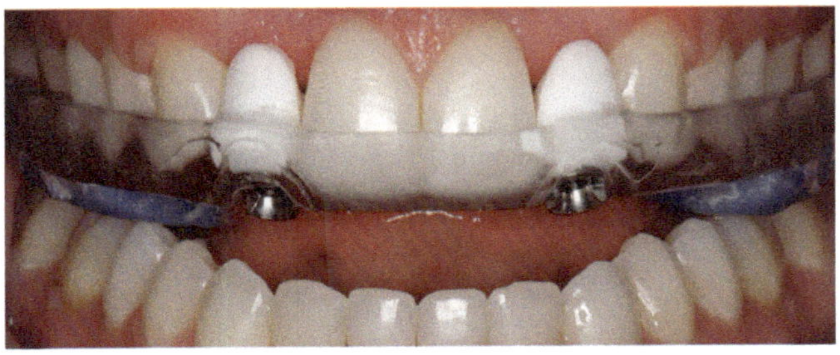
(c)

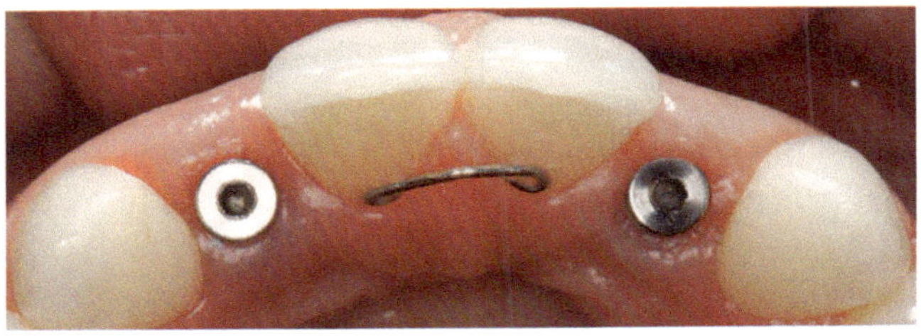
(d)

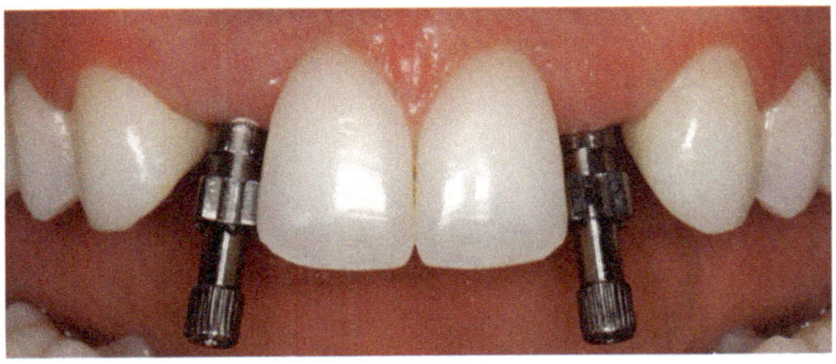
(e)

Figure 4.9 (a) The patient presented with retained primary canines and permanent canines that had been moved into the lateral incisor positions. (b) The patient elected to proceed with adult orthodontics, removal of deciduous canines, and movement of the canines back to normal canine positions. (c) The patient is seen here after orthodontic treatment in preparation for implant placement with a surgical guide in position. Implants were placed using a single-stage protocol with a guided minimally invasive approach. (d) After 4 months healing, palatal implant positioning can be seen with excellent facial tissue volume. (e–g) Open-tray impression technique was used following radiographic confirmation of abutment seating.

(Continued)

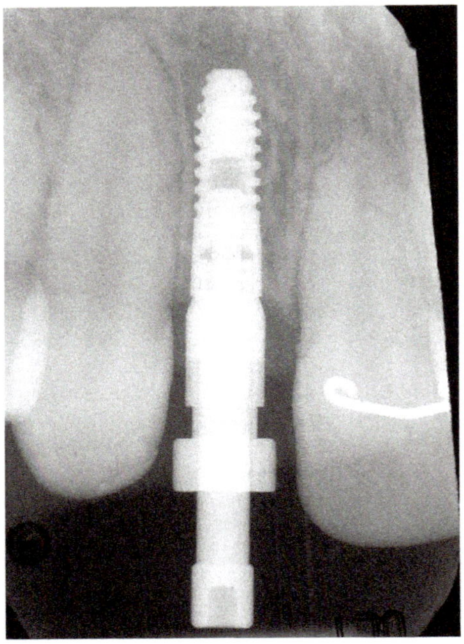
(f)

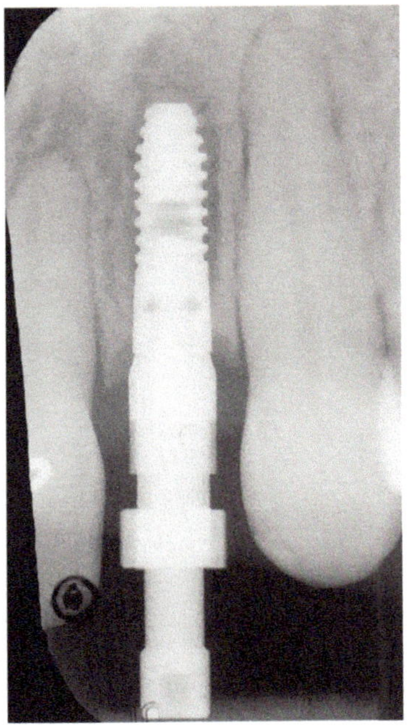
(g)

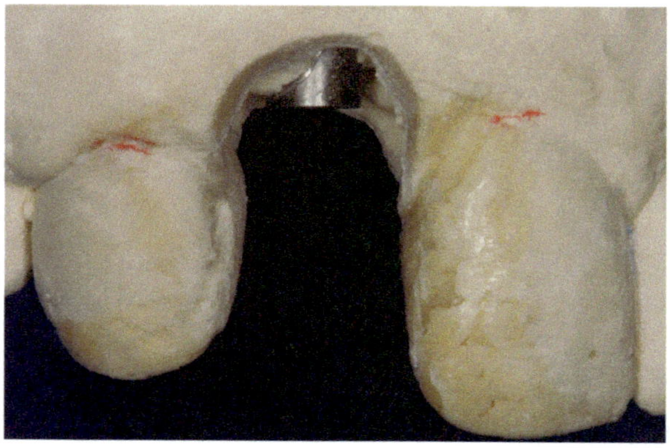

(h)

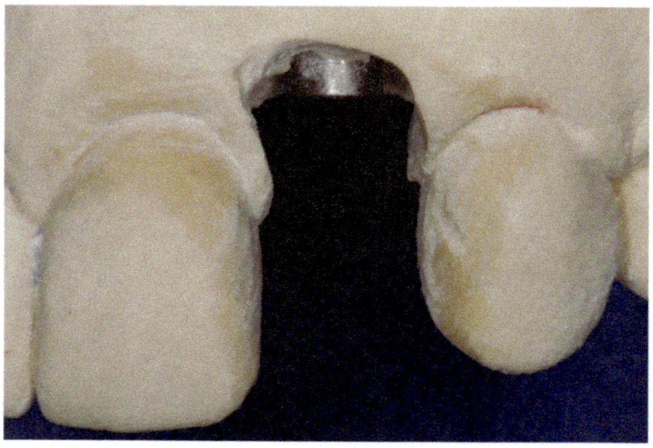

(i)

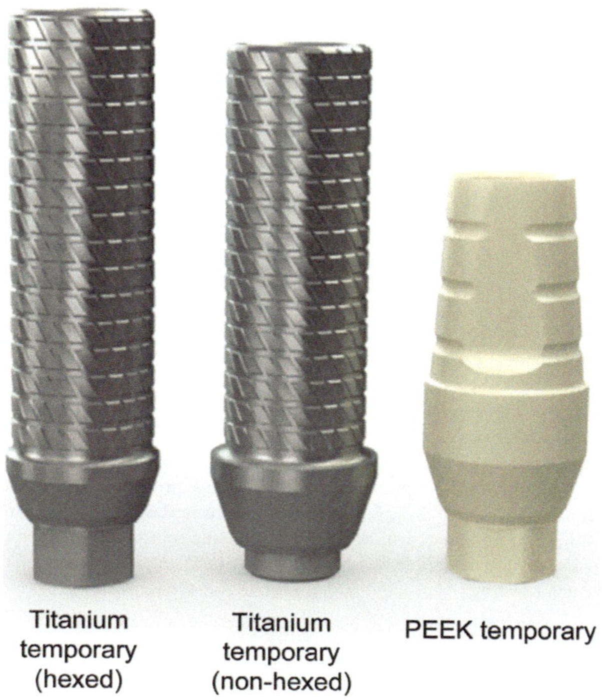

(j)

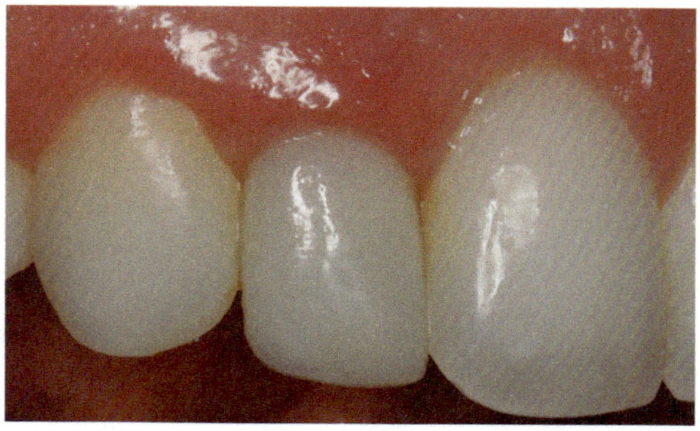

(k)

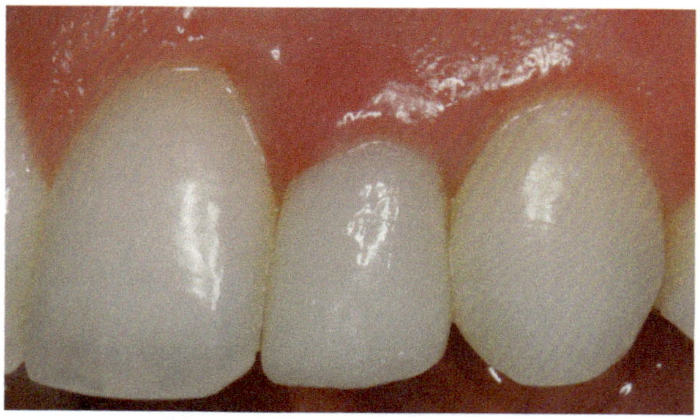

(l)

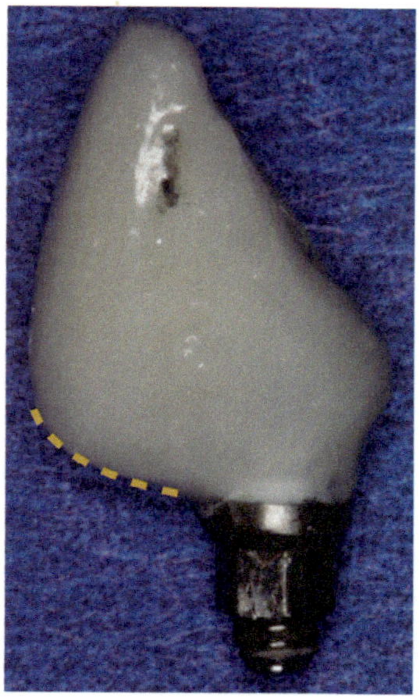

(m)

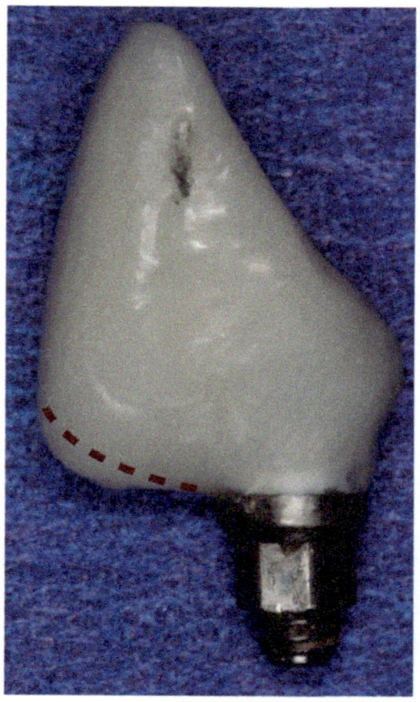

(n)

Figure 4.9 (Continued)
(h, i) The implant-level impression was used to prepare the working cast (as described previously). Implants had been placed well in the buccal–palatal dimension for screw-retained restorations. However, the placements were slightly shallow (2 mm apical to the future mid-facial free gingival margins), as can be seen here on the working model. (j) This figure displays the available 3.0 mm diameter provisional abutments: titanium engaging (hex index), titanium non-engaging, and PEEK polymer engaging (BioHorizons, Birmingham, AL). The provisional restorations in this case were fabricated using the 3.0 mm diameter engaging titanium abutments. *Source:* BioHorizons, Inc. Reproduced with permission of BioHorizons, Inc. (k, l) The soft tissue contours of the provisional restorations of the maxillary lateral incisors can be seen here 1 week following insertion. (m, n) The prototype provisional abutment used for this left maxillary lateral incisor required addition of contour to the mid-facial area (i.e. the last 1.5 mm of the emergence profile). © 4.9a–i, k–n, Aldo Leopardi.

and g). The implant-level impression was used for fabrication of the working cast (as described previously). The implants had been placed well in the buccal–palatal dimension for screw-retained restorations, but the placements were slightly shallow (2 mm apical to the future mid-facial free gingival margins) as visualized on the working model (Figure 4.9h and i). Figure 4.9j displays the available 3.0 mm diameter provisional abutments: titanium engaging (hex index), titanium non-engaging, and PEEK polymer (engaging). Provisional restorations were fabricated using the 3.0 mm diameter engaging titanium abutment. One week after insertion the soft tissue contours of the provisional restorations of the maxillary lateral incisors can be seen in Figure 4.9k and l. The prototype provisional abutment at the left maxillary lateral incisor required addition of contour to the mid-facial area (Figure 4.9k and l); that is, the last 1.5 mm of the emergence profile (Figure 4.9m and n).

After 4 weeks, the mid-facial tissue profile was progressing well; however, the prototypes were impinging on the interproximal papillae (Figure 4.10a and b). A radiograph of the right central incisor also showed less than 4.5 mm distance between height of interproximal bone and contact area with the provisional crown form (Figure 4.10c). The provisional restorations were placed on the cast (Figure 4.10d and e) and the contact areas opened up to within 5 mm of the interproximal bone height and finished (Figure 4.10f and g). The restorations were reinserted (Figure 4.10h and i) and, as a result, the papillae reformed after 6 weeks (Figure 4.10j and k). The soft tissue profile development was completed by 12 weeks and is documented with restorations in place (Figure 4.10l and m) and after removal (Figure 4.10n–p) showing excellent gingival architecture and health. At this point, the custom post-impression technique (Figure 4.10q) was used (as discussed previously). During bisque bake try-in, minor adjustments with resin were made to close inadequate interproximal contacts and improve interproximal emergence profile on the definitive restoration (provisional prototype, Figure 4.10r, and modified bisque bake, Figure 4.10s). The modifications were completed with the technician, and the crowns finished and delivered. The esthetic result can be seen in retracted views in Figure 4.10t and u. Pretreatment and post-treatment full-smile views demonstrate the significant esthetic improvement produced by appropriate treatment planning and careful application of the provisional restorative phase (Figure 4.10v and w).

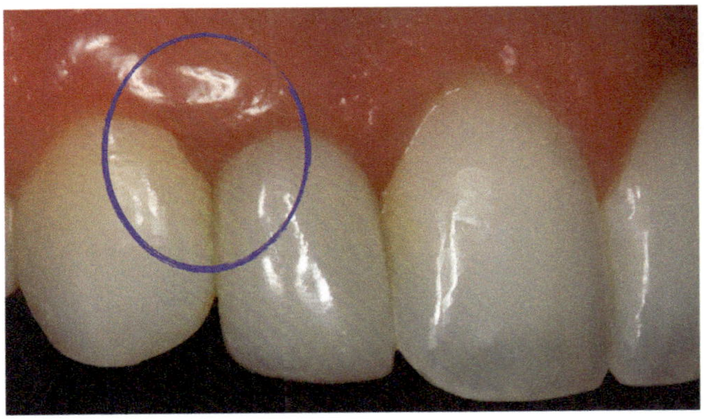

(a)

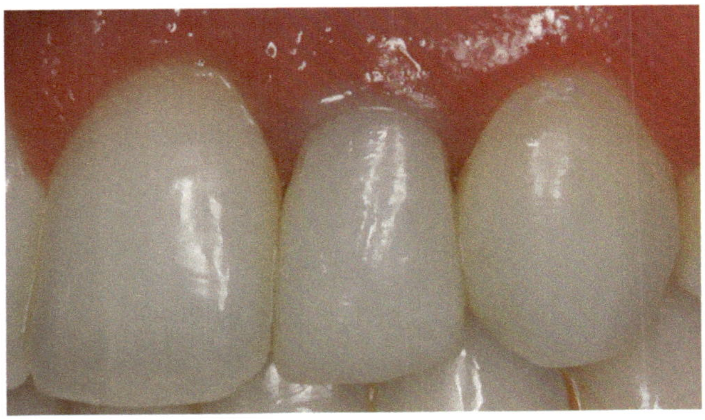

(b)

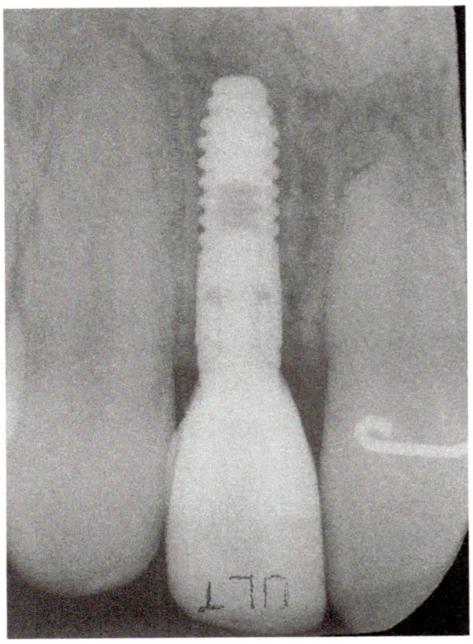

(c)

Figure 4.10 (a, b) After 4 weeks, mid-facial contour can be seen to have shaped well. However, the prototypes are impinging on the interproximal papillae. (c) A radiograph of the right lateral incisor showed less than a 4.5 mm distance between the height of interproximal bone and the contact area of the provisional crown form.

(Continued)

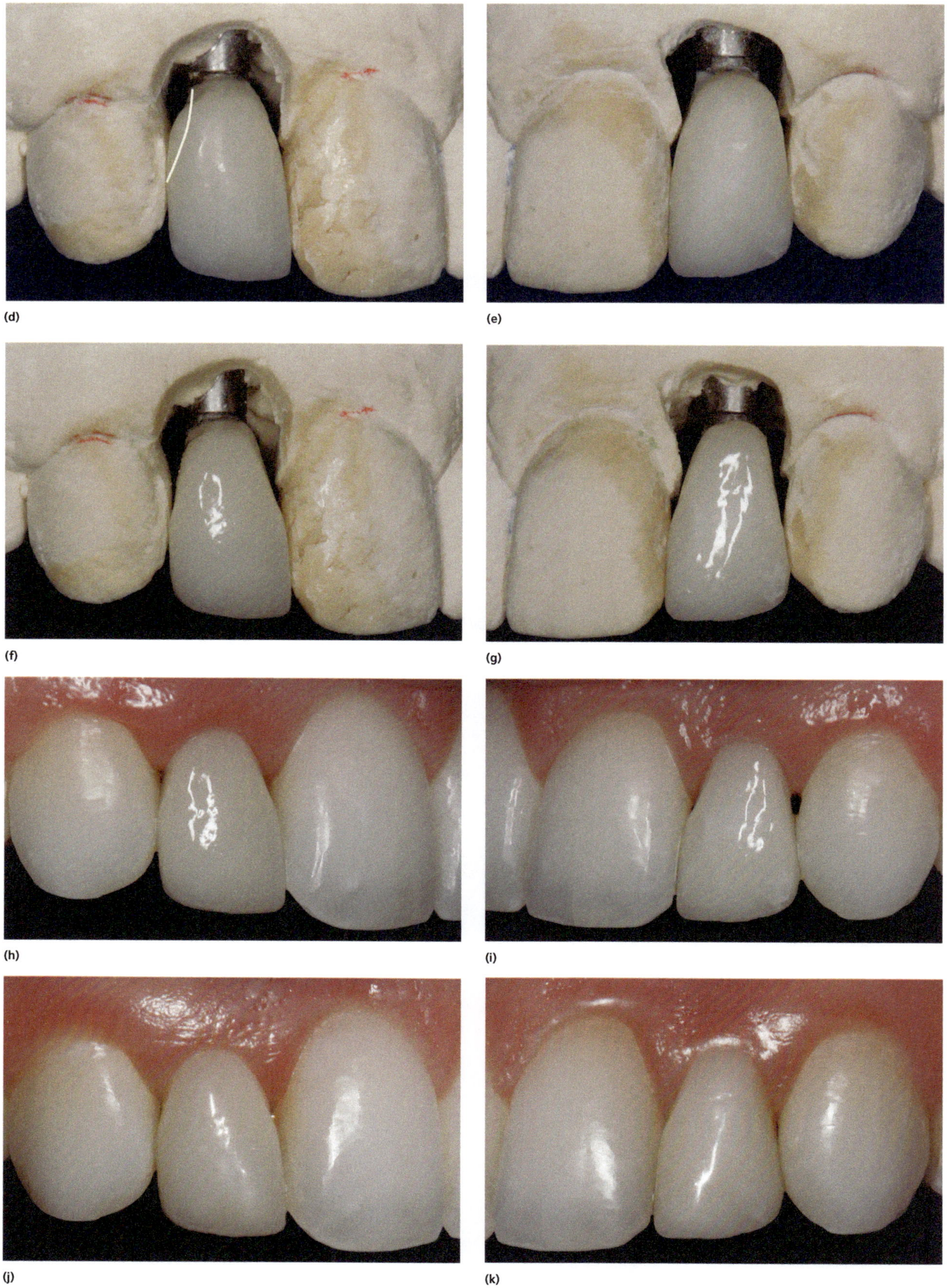

Figure 4.10 (Continued)
(d, e) The provisional restorations are shown here after placement onto the cast. The line indicates the areas of contour change needed. (f, g) Contact areas were opened up to a point within 5 mm from the interproximal bone height and finished. (h, i) The restorations are shown here after re-insertion (day of). (j, k) The clinical change 6 weeks after the contour adjustments, and with the papillae reformed.

(Continued)

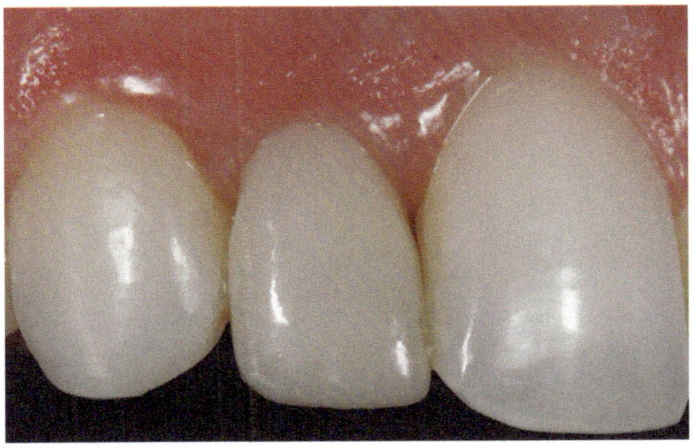

(l)

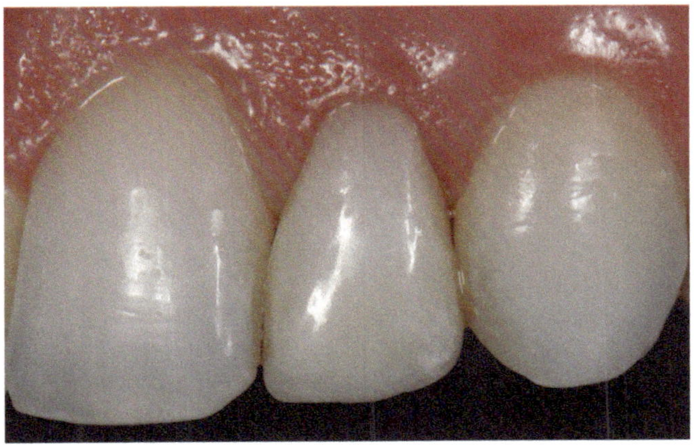

(m)

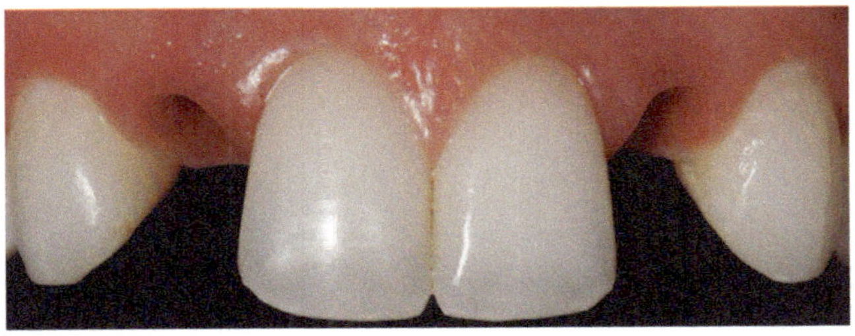

(n)

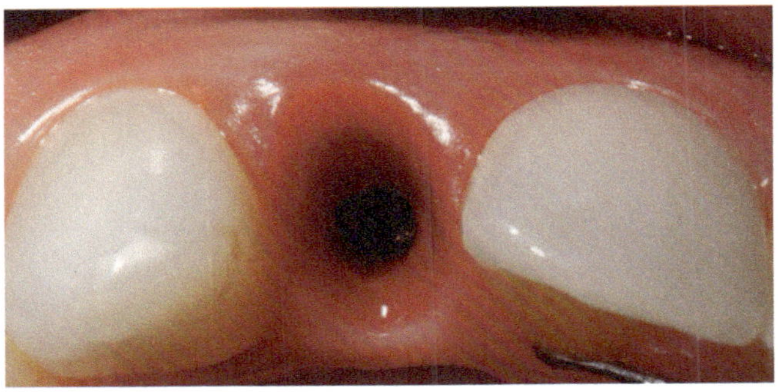

(o)

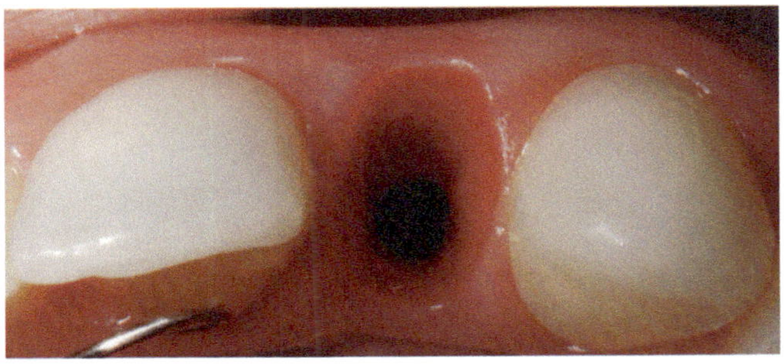

(p)

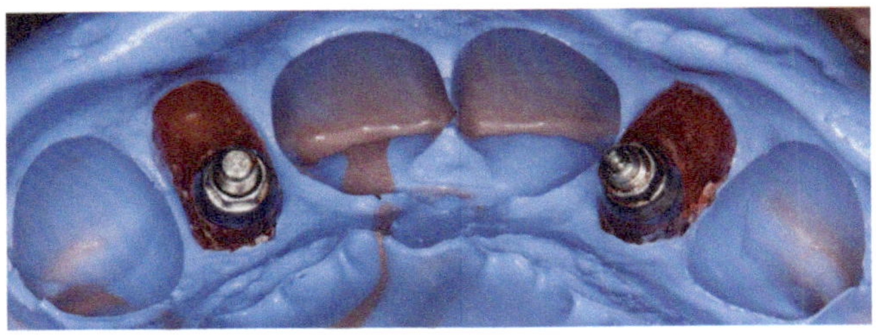

(q)

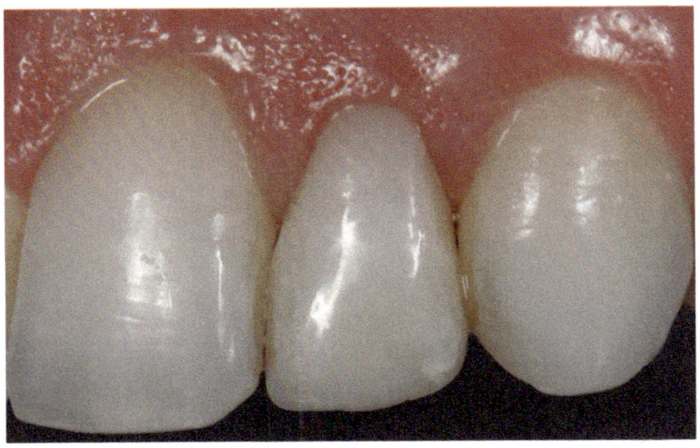

(r)

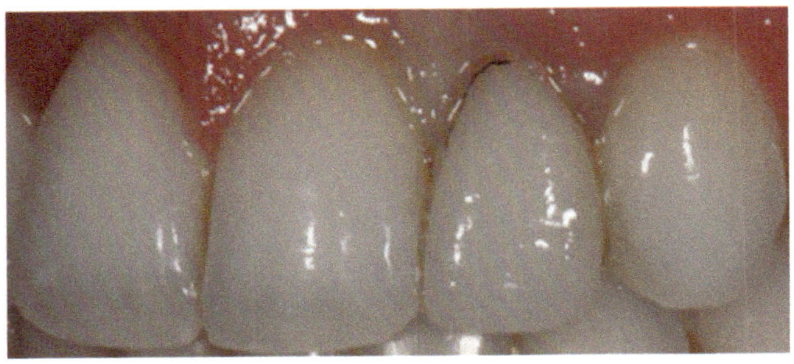

(s)

Figure 4.10 *(Continued)*
(l, m) The soft tissue profile development was completed at 12 weeks, and is documented here with restorations in place. (n–p) The soft tissue contours and thickness can be visualized after provisional removal showing excellent gingival architecture and health. (q) The custom post-impression technique was performed as discussed previously. (r, s) During bisque bake try-in, minor adjustments with resin were made to close the open interproximal contacts and improve the interproximal emergence profile of the definitive restoration – provisional prototype (r) and modified bisque bake (s).

(Continued)

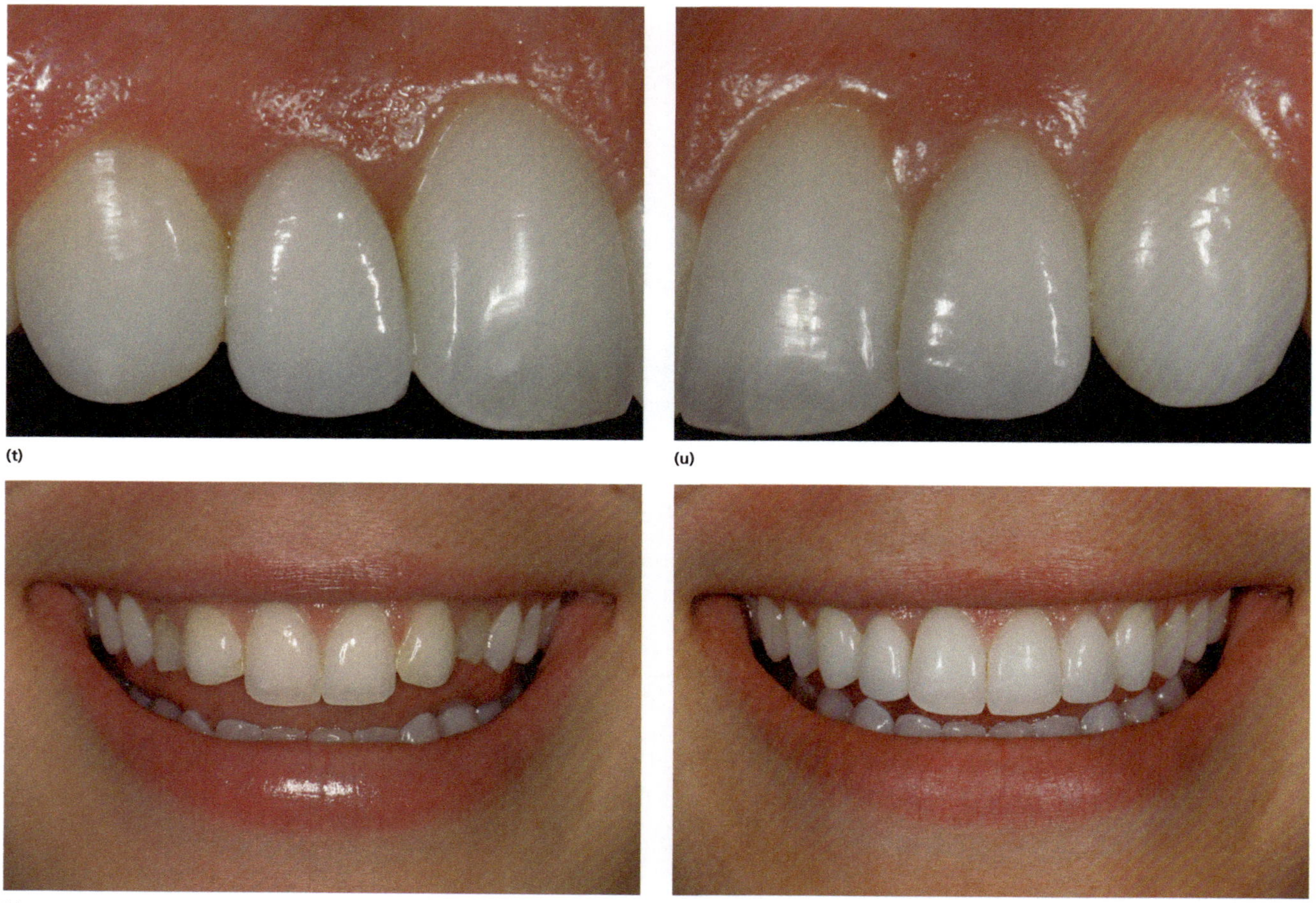

(t) (u) (v) (w)

Figure 4.10 (Continued)
(t, u) The modifications were completed with the technician, and the crowns finished and delivered with the esthetic result shown in these retracted views. (v, w) Pretreatment and restoration full-smile views demonstrated significant esthetic improvement produced by using appropriate treatment planning and application of carefully prepared provisional restorations. © Aldo Leopardi.

Conclusions

The use of provisional restorations offers patients and clinicians the ability to improve overall esthetic and functional treatment outcomes. The approach provides fixed interim restorations and helps to develop facial emergence profile/tissue contours with appropriate interproximal embrasures and to determine if additional soft tissue augmentation procedures are indicated for further esthetic improvements. It also assists in the construction of accurate custom implant platform-level impression posts to capture the emergence profile created by the provisional restoration and facilitates the creation of an accurate master cast to aid selection and design of the appropriate abutment. Provisional restorations also aid with comprehensive treatment planning, allowing visualization of interim esthetics, time for tissue maturation, and to determine if any additional esthetic and/or functional tooth-borne treatment needs are required.

References

1. Jemt T. Restoring the gingival contour by means of provisional resin crowns after single-implant treatment. Int J Periodontics Restorative Dent 1999; 19: 21–29.
2. Saadoum A, Touati B. Soft tissue recession around implants: is it still unavoidable – Part I. Pract Proced Aesthet Dent 2007; 19: 55–62.
3. Kois J. Predictable single tooth peri-implant esthetics. Five diagnostic keys. Compend Contin Educ Dent 2001; 22: 199–208.
4. Lee E, Gonzalez-Martin O, Fiorellini J. Lingualized flapless implant placement into fresh extraction sockets preserves buccal alveolar bone: a cone beam computed tomography study. Int J Periodontics Restorative Dent 2014; 34: 61–68.
5. Tarnow D, Magner A, Fletcher P. The effect of the distance from the contact point to the crest of bone on the presence or absence of the interproximal dental papilla. J Periodontol 1992; 63: 995–996.
6. Tarnow D, Cho S, Wallace S. The effect of inter-implant distance on the height of inter-implant bone crest. J Periodontol 2000; 71: 546–549.
7. Spray J, Black C, Morris H, Ochi S. The influence of bone thickness on facial marginal bone response: stage 1 placement through stage 2 uncovering. Ann Periodontol 2000; 5: 119–128.
8. Le B, Borzabadi-Farahani A. Labial bone thickness in the area of anterior maxillary implants associated with crestal labial soft tissue thickness. Implant Dent 2012; 21: 406–410.
9. Kan J, Rungcharassaeng K. Immediate placement and provisionalization of maxillary anterior single implants: a surgical and prosthodontic rationale. Pract Proced Aesthet Dent 2000; 12: 817–824.
10. Kan J, Rungcharassaeng K, Lozada J, Zimmerman G. Facial gingival tissue stability following immediate placement and provisionalization of maxillary anterior single implants: a 2- to 8-year follow-up. Int J Oral Maxillofac Implants 2011; 26: 179–187.
11. Bartee B, Lignelli J. Guided tissue regeneration in implant dentistry: techniques for management of localized bone defects. In: Oral and Maxillofacial Surgery, vol. 1, 2nd ed., FonsecaR, BarberH, MathesonJ, eds. St. Louis, MO: Saunders Elsevier, 2009, pp. 428–457.

12. Iasella J, Greenwell H, Miller R, et al. Ridge preservation with freeze-dried bone allograft and a collagen membrane compared to extraction alone for implant site development: a clinical and histologic study in humans. J Periodontol 2003; 74: 990–999.
13. Qahash M, Susin C, Polimeni G, et al. Bone healing dynamics at buccal peri-implant sites. Clin Oral Implants Res 2008; 19: 166–172.
14. Choquet V, Hermans M, Adriaenssens P, et al. Clinical and radiographic evaluation of papilla level adjacent to single-tooth dental implants. A retrospective study of the maxillary anterior region. J Periodontol 2001; 72: 1364–1371.
15. De Rouck T, Eghbali R, Collys K, et al. The gingival biotype revisited: transparency of the periodontal probe through the gingival margin as a method to discriminate thin from thick gingiva. J Clin Periodontol 2009; 36: 428–433.
16. Linkevicius T, Apse P, Grybauskas S, et al. The influence of soft tissue thickness on crestal bone changes around implants: a 1-year prospective controlled clinical trial. Int J Oral Maxillofac Implants 2009; 24: 712–719.
17. Fu J, Yeh H, Tatarakis N, et al. Tissue biotype and its relation to the underlying bone morphology. J Periodontol 2010; 81: 569–574.
18. Esposito M, Ekestubbe A, Grondahl K. Radiological evaluation of marginal bone loss at tooth surfaces facing single Brånemark implants. Clin Oral Implants Res 1993; 4: 151–157.
19. Choquet V, Hermans M, Adriaenssens P, et al. Clinical and radiographic evaluation of the papilla level adjacent to single-tooth dental implants. A retrospective study in the maxillary anterior region. J Periodontol 2001; 72: 1364–1371.
20. Schropp L, Flemming I, Kostopoulos L, Wenzel A. Inter-proximal papilla levels following early versus delayed placement of single-tooth implants: a controlled clinical trial. Int J Oral Maxillofac Implants 2005; 20: 753–761.
21. Van der Veldon U. Regeneration of the interdental soft tissues following denudation procedures. J Clin Periodontol 1982; 9: 455–459.
22. Romeo E, Lops D, Rossi A, et al. Surgical and prosthetic management of interproximal region with single-implant restorations: 1-year prospective study. J Periodontol 2008; 79: 1048–1055.
23. Salama H, Salama M, Garber D, Adar P. The interproximal height of bone: a guidepost to esthetic strategies and soft tissue contours in anterior tooth replacement. J Pract Periodontics Aesthet Dent 1998; 10: 1131–1141.
24. Abrahamsson I, Berglundh T, Wennstrom J, Lindhe J. The peri-implant hard and soft tissues at different implant systems: a comparative study in the dog. Clin Oral Implants Res 1996; 7: 212–219.
25. Baumann G, Rapley J, Hallmon W, Mills M. The peri-implant sulcus. Int J Oral Maxillofac Implants 1993; 8: 273–280.
26. Berglundh T, Lindhe J. Dimension of the peri-implant mucosa. Biological width revisited. J Clin Periodontol 1996; 23: 971–973.
27. Task Force on Peri-implantitis. Peri-implant mucositis and peri-implantitis: a current understanding of their diagnoses and clinical implications. J Periodontol 2013; 84: 436–443.
28. Wilson T. The positive relationship between cement excess and peri-implant disease: a prospective clinical endoscopic study. J Periodontol 2009; 80: 1388–1392.
29. Linkevicius T, Puisys A, Vindasiute E, et al. Does residual cement around implant-supported restorations cause peri-implant disease? A retrospective case analysis. Clin Oral Implants Res 2013; 24: 1179–1184.
30. Hermann J, Cochran D, Nummikoski P, Buser D. Crestal bone changes around titanium implants. A radiographic evaluation of unloaded non-submerged and submerged implants in the canine mandible. J Periodontol 1997; 68: 1117–1130.
31. Ericsson I, Persson L, Berglundh T, et al. Different types of inflammatory reactions in peri-implant soft tissues. J Clin Periodontol 1995; 22: 255–261.
32. Broggini N, McManus L, Hermann J, et al. Persistent acute inflammation at the implant–abutment interface. J Dent Res 2003; 82: 232–237.
33. Hermann J, Schoolfield J, Schenk R, et al. Influence of the size of the micro-gap on crestal bone changes around titanium implants. A histometric evaluation of unloaded non-submerged implants in the canine mandible. J Periodontol 2001; 72: 1372–1383.
34. Abrahamsson I. The mucosal barrier following abutment dis-reconnection. An experimental study in dogs. J Clin Periodontol 1997; 24: 568–572.
35. Abrahamsson I, Berglundh T, Sekino S, Lindhe J. Tissue reactions to abutment shift: an experimental study in dogs. Clin Implant Dent Relat Res 2003; 5: 82–88.
36. Piñeyro A, Tucker LM. One abutment–one time: the negative effect of uncontrolled abutment margin depths and excess cement-a case report. Compend Contin Educ Dent 2013; 34: 680–684.
37. Sailer I, Mühlemann S, Zwahlen M, et al. Cemented and screw-retained implant reconstructions: a systematic review of the survival and complication rates. Clin Oral Implants Res. 2012; 23(Suppl 6): 163–201.
38. Kupershmidt I, Levin L, Schwartz-Arad D. Inter-implant bone height changes in anterior maxillary immediate and non-immediate adjacent dental implants. J Periodontol 2007; 78: 991–996.
39. Scarano A, Assenza B, Piattelli M, et al. Inter-implant distance and crestal bone resorption: a histologic study in the canine mandible. Clin Implant Dent Relat Res 2004; 6: 150-156.
40. Tarnow D, Elian N, Fletcher P, et al. Vertical distance from the crest of bone to the height of the interproximal papilla between adjacent implants. J Periodontol 2003; 74: 1785–1788.
41. Grunder U, Gracis S, Capelli M. Influence of the 3-D bone to implant relationship on esthetics. Int J Periodontics Restorative Dent 2005; 25: 113–119.
42. Lazzara R, Porter S. Platform switching: a new concept in implant dentistry for controlling post-restorative crestal bone levels. Int J Periodontics Restorative Dent 2006; 26: 9–17.
43. Vela-Nebot X, Rodríguez-Ciurana X, Rodado-Alonso C, Segalà-Torres M. Benefits of an implant platform modification technique to reduce crestal bone resorption. Implant Dent 2006; 15: 313–320.
44. Rodriguez-Ciurana X, Vela-Nebot X, Segala-Torres M, et al. The effect of inter-implant distance on the height of the inter-implant bone crest when using platform-switched implants. Int J Periodontics Restorative Dent 2009; 29: 141–151.
45. Maeda Y, Miura J, Taki I, Sogo M. Biomechanical analysis on platform switching: is there any biomechanical rationale? Clin Oral Implants Res 2007; 18: 581–584.
46. Puchades-Roman L, Palmer R, Palmer P, et al. A clinical, radiographic and microbiologic comparison of Astra Tech and Brånemark single tooth implants. Clin Implant Dent Relat Res 2000; 2: 78–84.
47. Cappiello M, Luongo R, Di Lorio D, et al. Evaluation of peri-implant bone loss around platform-switched implants. Int J Periodontics Restorative Dent 2008; 28: 347–355.
48. Gardner D. Platform switching as a means to achieving implant esthetics. N Y State Dent J 2005; 71: 34–37.
49. Cochran D, Mau LP, Higginbottom F, et al. Soft and hard tissue histologic dimensions around dental implants in the canine restored with smaller-diameter abutments: a paradigm shift in peri-implant biology. Int J Oral Maxillofac Implants 2013; 28: 494–502.
50. Novaes A, Barros R, Muglia V, Borges G. Influence of inter-implant distances and placement depth on papilla formation and crestal resorption: a clinical and radiographic study in dogs. J Oral Implantol 2009; 35(1): 18–27.
51. Veis A, Parissis N, Tsirlis A, et al. Evaluation of peri-implant marginal bone loss using modified abutment connections at various crestal level placements. Int J Periodontics Restorative Dent 2010; 30: 609–617.
52. Elian N, Bloom M, Dard M, et al. Effect of inter-implant distance (2 and 3 mm) on the height of inter-implant bone crest: a histomorphometric evaluation. J Periodontol 2011; 82: 1749–1756.
53. Vela X, Mendez V, Rodriguez X, et al. Crestal bone changes on platform-switched implants and adjacent teeth when the tooth–implant distance is less than 1.5 mm. Int J Periodontics Dent 2012; 32: 149–155.
54. Rodriguez A, Rosenstiel S. Esthetic considerations related to bone and soft tissue maintenance and development around dental implants: report of the Committee on Research in Fixed Prosthodontics of the American Academy of Fixed Prosthodontics. J Prosthetic Dent 2012; 108: 259–267.
55. Chee W, Donovan T. Use of provisional restorations to enhance soft tissue contours for implant restorations. Compend Contin Educ Dent 1998; 19: 481–489.
56. Santosa R. Provisional restoration options in implant dentistry. Aust Dent J 2007; 52: 234–242.
57. Cho S-C, Shetty S, Froum S, et al. Fixed and removable provisional options for patients undergoing implant treatment. Compend Contin Educ Dent 2007; 28: 604–609.
58. Moskowitz E, Sheridan J, Celenza F, et al. Essix appliances. Provisional anterior prosthesis for pre and post implant patients. N Y State Dent J 1997; 63: 32–35.
59. Kan J, Rungcharassaeng K, Kois JC. Removable ovate pontic for peri-implant architecture preservation during immediate implant placement. Pract Proced Aesthet Dent 2001;13: 711–715.
60. Priest G. Soft tissue development with provisional and definitive implant restorations. In: Implant Site Development, SonickM, HwangD, eds. Hoboken, NJ: John Wiley and Sons, Inc., 2012, pp. 398–418.
61. Biggs W. Placement of a custom implant provisional restoration at the second-stage surgery for improved gingival management: a clinical report. J Prosthetic Dent 1996; 75: 231–233.
62. Higginbottom F, Belser U, Jones J, Keith S. Prosthetic management of implants in the esthetic zone. Int J Oral Maxillfac Implants 2004; 19(Suppl): 62–72.
63. Macintosh D, Sutherland M. Method for developing an optimal emergence profile using heat-polymerized provisional restorations for single-tooth implant-supported restorations. J Prosthetic Dent 2004; 91: 289–292.
64. Saadoun A, Sebbab P. Immediate implant placement and temporization: literature review and case studies. Compend Contin Educ Dent 2004; 25: 277–298.
65. Gracis S, Nicholls J, Chalupnik J, Yuodelis R. Shock-absorbing behavior of five restorative materials used on implants. Int J Prosthodont 1991; 4: 282–291.

SECTION II

Technology and Surgery

CHAPTER 5

Extraction Site Management for Ridge Preservation and Implant Site Development

Barry Bartee[1] **& Daniel R. Cullum**[2]

[1]Osteogenics Biomedical, Inc., Lubbock, TX, USA

[2]Private Practice, Coeur d'Alene, ID; Loma Linda University Department of OMS, Loma Linda, CA; UCLA Department of OMS, Los Angeles, CA, USA

Introduction

The treatment complications of alveolar bone loss seen after tooth extraction are well known.[1,2] In sites where dental implants are planned, even slight changes in alveolar ridge contours may affect the ability of the implant team to deliver a satisfactory implant restoration. Loss of bone may require placement of shorter or smaller diameter implants, and/or necessitate complex surgical[3–5] and/or prosthodontic interventions to achieve the desired result.[6–8] While bone loss at healed extraction sockets can be partially regenerated by augmentation grafting, a less invasive and more predictable approach may be to employ grafting procedures to preserve ridge anatomy during initial site healing. This chapter will discuss the rationale and sample techniques for this treatment concept. In particular, flapless grafting with "modified" Bio-Col® and the use of "open barrier" techniques without primary wound closure, using high-density (i.e. non-porous) polytetrafluoroethylene (hd-PTFE) membranes will be reviewed and discussed.

Rationale for alveolar ridge preservation

The current definition of esthetic success in implant dentistry includes a natural appearance for peri-implant soft tissues. While challenging to achieve, the ideal implant restoration should include soft tissues that have the correct proportion of keratinized gingiva and alveolar mucosa, minimal disruption of the position of the mucogingival junction, and minimal soft tissue scarring.[9–13] The level of the gingival margin should be symmetrical with respect to the contralateral tooth, and soft tissues should exhibit natural color, contour, texture, and tone, including the interdental papillae being proportional with respect to adjacent and contralateral teeth. Thickness of soft tissues should be adequate to render the underlying implant and restorative margins inconspicuous. All of these soft tissue requirements are dependent on a foundation of adequate bone volume, contour, and density, not only to achieve primary implant stability, but also to provide a framework for support of soft tissues surrounding the implant.[14–16] A direct correlation of soft tissue thickness to underlying bone anatomy/thickness has recently been advanced.[17]

When tooth loss occurs, the surrounding hard and soft tissues heal with very different kinetics. Competition occurs between the rapidly proliferating soft tissue cells and the more slowly developing bone-derived cells to fill any existing defects. In the typical extraction site, the apical two-thirds of the socket is quickly repaired with appositional bone growth from the socket walls, while the coronal one-third is filled with fibrous scar tissue. Clinically, this pattern of secondary wound healing and contraction results in a convex crestal alveolar ridge anatomy. Significant remodeling of alveolar crest and buccal cortical plate then occurs during the next 2–3 months, resulting in further loss of bone and soft tissue volume. The extent of alveolar remodeling is affected by a myriad of anatomic, cellular, biochemical, environmental, and biomechanical factors that vary greatly among individual patients. The clinical challenge is that changes experienced for an individual patient are difficult to predict. However, controlled studies of socket healing in relatively intact sockets indicate that as much as 2–4 mm loss in alveolar ridge bucco-lingual width and 1–3 mm loss in height can occur in the first 6 months.[18–21] Ultimately, as much as 40–50% of alveolar width and 20–30% of height can be irreversibly lost in the first year following extraction.[22] Over time, atrophy ultimately results in the thin, knife-edge ridge or total loss of the alveolus down to basal bone. Fortunately, most of these effects of tooth loss can be prevented in the short term and reduced significantly over longer periods by ridge preservation grafting and a minimally invasive surgical approach.

Frequently, patients presenting for dental implants have severely compromised alveolar ridge anatomy as a result of root fracture, endodontic treatment failure, facial trauma, or chronic destructive periodontitis. Many times the affected teeth have already been removed without consideration for the ultimate treatment plan, resulting in larger defects than would otherwise have occurred. Our goal is to have a healed site with contour preservation, avoiding hard and/or soft tissue defects that increase the challenge of reconstruction without compromised esthetics and long-term stability.

The biology of extraction socket healing

To develop effective clinical strategies to reduce the extent of alveolar ridge resorption post-extraction, it is helpful to review the process of normal extraction socket healing. While it is recognized that the minimally traumatic extraction technique helps to minimize ridge resorption, a certain amount of tissue trauma is unavoidable. With the initial incision and soft tissue flap reflection, there is disruption of the dento-gingival attachment and periosteum, while luxation of the tooth root can cause microfractures of the alveolar walls, which can stimulate bone remodeling.[23] The forces needed for tooth removal (rotation, shear, tension, and compression) cause further damage to surrounding bone by disrupting its microcirculation.[24]

Minimally Invasive Dental Implant Surgery, First Edition. Edited by Daniel R. Cullum and Douglas Deporter.

Following tooth removal, blood from the damaged vessels and bone enters the socket, and platelets are activated to aggregate and seal ruptured vessels. As platelet degranulation occurs, growth factors are released locally. A loose network of fibrin forms, entrapping blood cells and platelets into an organized clot. An inflammatory phase ensues, first dominated by polymorphonuclear neutrophils and later by macrophages needed for initial cellular debridement of the wound.[25] At the coronal aspect of the socket, the initial fibrin clot begins to retract below the soft tissue due to further platelet activity and cross-linking of fibrin. The resulting void is then subject to contamination with saliva, bacteria, and oral debris, all of which can interfere with optimal wound healing. Clot lysis ensues within 48 h by the action of plasmin, a fibrinolytic enzyme. By the fourth day, enzymes from oral bacteria have further degraded the clot, and regenerating epithelium from the oral mucosa begins to grow over the clot surface.[26] The combination of clot retraction, lysis, and epithelial migration results in incomplete bone regeneration in the upper one-third of the socket.[27]

In the apical two-thirds of the socket, the blood clot is simultaneously degraded enzymatically and replaced by a highly vascular, amorphous granulation tissue rich in fibroblasts and new capillaries. By the eighth day, this granulation tissue becomes invaded by new blood vessels from the socket walls. At 14 days, the granulation tissue begins to be replaced by a collagen-rich, organized provisional connective tissue matrix. Revascularization and maturation of the provisional matrix progresses in an apical to coronal direction and from the lateral aspects of the socket towards the center. By 21 days approximately two-thirds of the socket has become filled with provisional matrix and immature, poorly mineralized, woven bone. Mineralization of the provisional connective tissue matrix begins at the apex and periphery of the socket, progressing centrally and coronally, partially filling the socket with immature bone by 6 weeks. At this point, the woven bone begins to remodel into organized and highly mineralized lamellar bone.[28]

In addition to cellular and molecular events, there are biomechanically induced changes in the surrounding tissues of the healing socket. With tooth loss, mechanical stimulation of surrounding bone is significantly reduced. Fibers of the periodontal ligament, typically involved in force transfer between teeth and bone, no longer exist. There are vascular changes on several fronts. Incisions have been made, flaps reflected, and vessels torn with loss of the periodontal vascular plexus. All of these changes affect the microcirculation of buccal cortical bone, leading to its rapid loss. Indeed, the greatest loss of alveolar bone volume occurs on the buccal aspect,[29] often resulting in a concavity and esthetic compromise for later implant placement.

Guided bone regeneration applied to extraction sites

The use of occlusive barriers to guide bone regeneration was first shown by Dahlin et al.[30] These investigators used occlusive barriers to cover critical-size surgically created bone defects in rat mandible. Defects covered with a barrier filled with bone, while those not covered with a barrier showed ingrowth of fibrous scar tissue only. Following this work, guided-tissue-regeneration membranes were introduced in clinical dentistry for the management of periodontal defects, but were soon being tested in covering extraction sockets. In early reports, extraction sockets were essentially treated as large periodontal defects by debridement, isolation with membrane, and primary soft tissue closure. Results indicated that the concept was valid, with experimental sites demonstrating near-complete bone regeneration in sockets with immediate implant placement.[31] A reduction in ridge resorption was also noted when compared with controls.[18,19,32] However, the macroporous nature of early barrier materials, especially those made from expanded (i.e. porous) PTFE, made them unsuitable for routine use in extraction site grafting because of the need to achieve and maintain primary soft tissue closure for the duration of healing. If these barriers became exposed, infection ensued, and the results were at best similar to those for controls.

There are several problems with the need for primary flap closure using guided-tissue-regeneration membranes in socket preservation grafting. The flap manipulation needed to achieve primary closure is time-consuming, requires vertical releasing incisions, and compromises the periosteal blood supply. All of these procedures increase surgical trauma and patient morbidity. Mobilizing a flap to create a coronally advanced, tension-free primary closure also impacts soft tissue architecture. The mucobuccal fold is reduced and the position of the mucogingival junction is raised coronally with reduced keratinized tissue and associated unfavorable esthetics in the final rehabilitation. An additional disadvantage can be the need for a second surgery to remove a non-resorbable barrier like porous PTFE, a titanium mesh, or tenting screws. This can add further invasiveness and time. While collagen-based barrier membranes do not require later removal, they also are most often used with complete flap closure and its attendant untoward effects. These challenges led to the development of materials and procedures for open grafting techniques to manage extraction defects such as a collagen matrix in the Bio-Col technique[33] or the hd-PTFE membrane approach developed by Bartee.[34]

Minimally invasive surgical protocol

The patient is prepared following a standard surgical protocol including oral chlorhexidine rinses bid (3 days preoperatively) and antibiotic (amoxicillin 2G or similar antimicrobial spectrum coverage). Standard surgical instrumentation can be supplemented with various "Proximator®" designs (H&H Company, Ontario, CA) (Figure 5.1). After completion of local anesthesia, an atraumatic surgical technique is necessary to minimize bone and soft tissue injury with tooth removal. Crush and tear injuries along with increasing the dimensions of any bony defects will impair the vascular supply, increase inflammatory response, and compromise healing. Development of gentle surgical skills with experience and judgment can significantly enhance treatment outcomes. Often, the residual tooth or root fragment is compromised by caries, endodontic treatment, or fracture, adding to the challenge of atraumatic removal. Proper force application reduces surgical injury. A "flapless" approach utilizes incision of the crestal fibers around the residual root, followed with development of an alveolar–periodontal ligament space purchase. This is developed in a circular rotational application of force following the curvature of the root–alveolar interface. Traditional "periotomes" fulfill this function poorly owing to their flat functional surfaces. The radius of curvature of the Proximator-style of instrument is a significant advantage to reduce trauma and increase surgical efficiency (Figure 5.1a and b).

Working the Proximator along the palatal aspect from the mesial to distal interproximal areas progressively mobilizes the root. A finger rest with the dominant hand and palpation of the labial aspect of the extraction site with the non-dominant hand gives the surgeon a continuous tactile sense of reduced compliance or root ankylosis to avoid buccal plate fracture. Care must be taken to avoid direct elevation forces on thin buccal bone and control application of force on the palatal root surface, so as to avoid sudden root

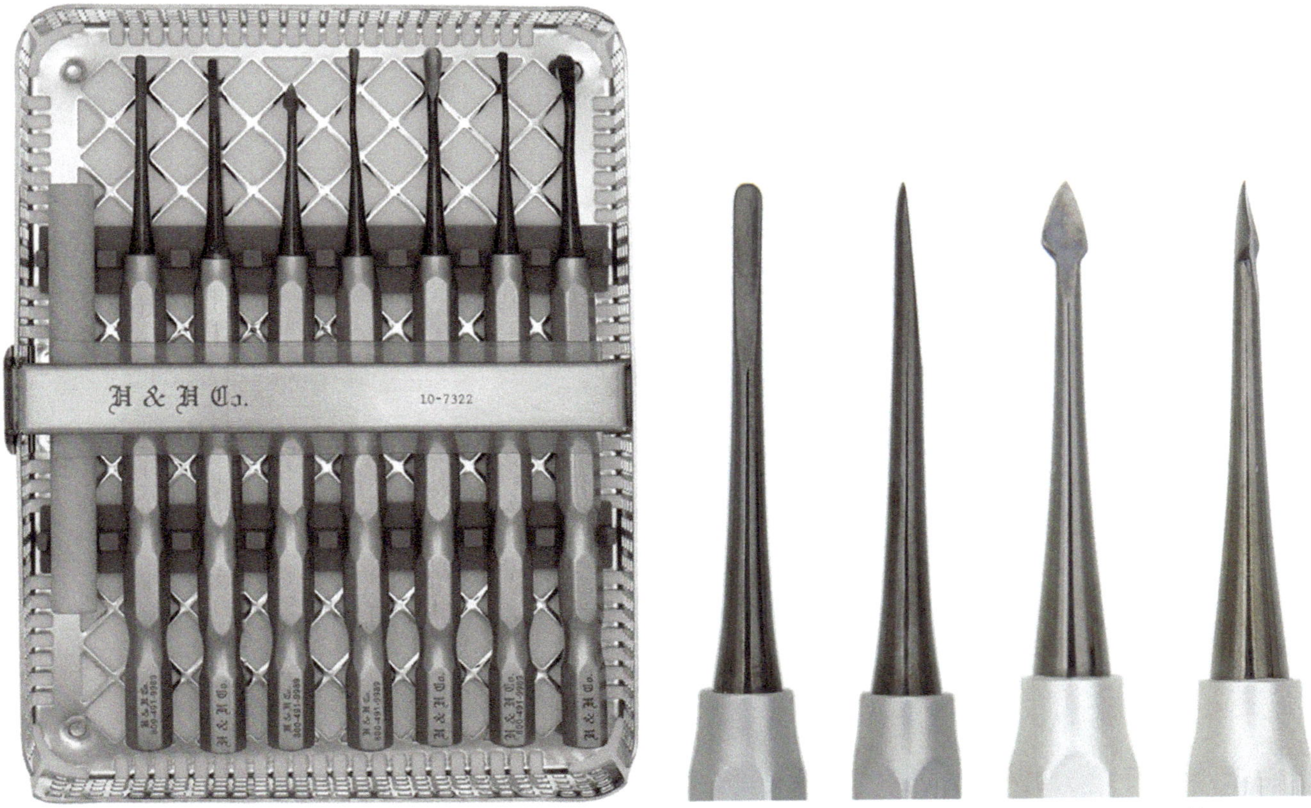

(a) (b) (c) (d) (e)

Figure 5.1 (a) "Proximator" instrument kit with specialized shapes for atraumatic root extraction (H&H Company, Ontario CA). (b–e) The radius of curvature of the Proximator-style of instrument is a significant advantage to reduce trauma and increase surgical efficiency. Instruments with a rounded and "spear" shaped tips are the most helpful in management of challenging root removal. *Source* (a): H&H Company, Ontario, CA, USA. Reproduced with permission of H&H Company.

displacement to the buccal and fracture an intact buccal plate. Use of instruments with rounded and "spear"-shaped tips can be most helpful in management of challenging root removal (Figure 5.1a and b). Sectioning the tooth root may be necessary with inadequate mobilization or ankylosis. Ultrasonic bone surgery also offers an enhanced extraction protocol with ankylotic root fragments or thin buccal bone (see Chapter 13).

After root delivery, site assessment is completed with direct probing of bone and soft tissue dimensions. This is critical as there is no direct observation with a flapless approach. Findings of a relative bony defect or an intact interproximal height of bone and labial plate determine the site preservation approach to be used. Sockets that are intact with 2–4 mm of soft tissue thickness on the labial and 3–5 mm at the interproximal regions and small labial defects (less than one-third of the buccal plate mesio-distal dimension) offer adequate healing potential for the "modified" Bio-Col approach. Sites with a defect greater than one-third of the facial plate width or a defect extending into the interproximal bone may result in reduced site dimensions after healing and require a more aggressive grafting approach with an hd-PTFE open-barrier technique or a traditional guided bone regeneration approach with open flap exposure and primary closure by labial flap advancement or pedicle flap closure.

Aggressive debridement of the extraction site is necessary with sharp double-ended curettes to ensure complete removal of periodontal remnants and granulations. This requires a systematic and sequential progression around the complete bone margins. Cleansing with povidine iodine 2% solution can be helpful in cases of gross bacterial contamination of the site with chronic infection or root fracture and possible anaerobic bacterial contamination. Repeated irrigation with sterile saline should be used to cleanse and debride the wound to achieve a healthy bleeding bone surface. Removal of granulation tissue can be assisted with sharp rongeurs, including those with a compact tip design (Figure 5.2a and b). Additional instruments for graft placement are seen in Figure 5.2c.

The "modified" Bio-Col technique for ridge preservation

The Bio-Col technique is a minimally invasive approach for socket preservation.[33] Its advantage lies in a flapless approach, thus preserving periosteum and blood supply to thin residual crestal lamellar bone and soft tissue. Following tooth removal using a minimally traumatic protocol, evaluation of the extraction socket will determine if the Bio-Col technique is indicated. Appropriate sites are those with optimal healing potential; that is, minimal soft tissue disturbance and minimal to no damage to the buccal and lingual/palatal cortical plates. Larger defects or vertical defects extending into the interproximal region(s) are better managed with an open- or closed-barrier technique as discussed later. If the Bio-Col technique is selected, the debrided extraction socket is gently packed with a mineralized, particulate graft material such as bovine xenograft (e.g. Bio-Oss®, Geistlich, Princeton, NJ) which acts as an

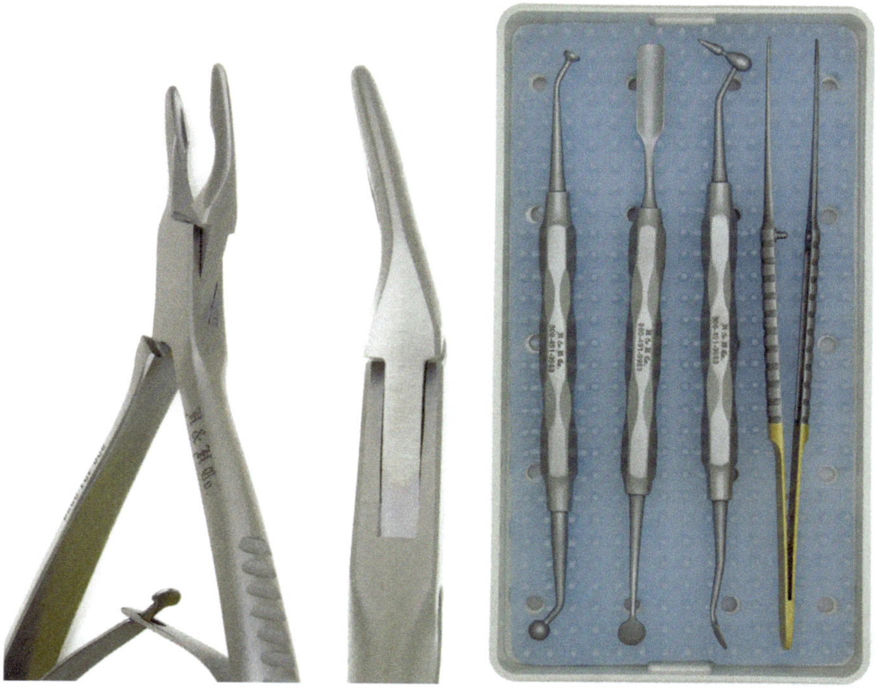

(a) (b) (c)

Figure 5.2 (a–c) Instruments to facilitate access for minimally invasive grafting include mini-rongeurs and specialized instrument kit for preparing and placing the graft materials. *Source:* H&H Company, Ontario, CA, USA. Reproduced with permission of H&H Company.

osteo-conductive scaffold that will support new bone formation and minimize loss in bucco-lingual/palatal alveolar ridge dimension. The graft particles are then covered with a layer of an absorbable collagen sponge (e.g. Ora-Plug®, Salvin Dental, Charlotte, NC) secured with a figure-of-eight fixation suture. Cyanoacrylate (e.g. PeriAcryl®, GluStitch Inc., Delta, BC, Canada) is then flowed over the exposed surface to protect the collagen from salivary enzyme degradation, mechanical trauma, and/or micromotion during initial healing. This technique is particularly applicable for extraction sites with single-rooted teeth where the progression of secondary intention wound healing from the periphery can quickly coalesce for wound closure. Because of the greater dimensions of molars, fibrin deposition and granulation from the wound periphery will take longer; and for larger defects, consideration of the hd-PTFE open-barrier technique can be helpful.

Suggested clinical modifications of the Bio-Col technique include using other graft materials (e.g. mineralized allograft or alloplastic material) in order to achieve different wound healing kinetics, or using autologous venous blood to saturate graft particles and the collagen plug prior to their placement. These steps have been suggested to improve healing by incorporating native growth factors from platelet degranulation. Alternatively, commercially available growth factor such as recombinant human platelet-derived growth factor (rhPDGF – GEM 21S®, Osteohealth Inc., Shirley, NY) can be used in an "off-label" application (see Chapter 7). Additionally, protection of the collagen from any contact with saliva or mechanical trauma during surgery or the early healing period is important. The salivary enzymes quickly begin degradation of the collagen and can result in early exposure of the graft material. A light-cured periodontal dressing (Barricaid™, Dentsply-Caulk, Milford, DE) can be placed over the wound to protect the collagen layer, and this is especially helpful at larger multirooted tooth defects. While these additions to the original Bio-Col technique can add significantly to treatment outcomes, they have yet to be clearly documented in controlled clinical studies.

A "modified" Bio-Col technique is demonstrated for a non-restorable left mandibular first molar in Figure 5.3a. The tooth was removed carefully with an atraumatic approach using root sectioning and Proximators for maximum site preservation and minimal hard and soft tissue damage (Figure 5.1). The site was assessed with a periodontal probe to have intact bone margins, and soft tissue granulations were excised with a micro-rongeur (Figure 5.2). Particulate graft material was saturated in autologous venous blood (Figure 5.3b) and packed into the defect up to the surrounding bone margins. A collagen plug was sectioned (Figure 5.3d) and saturated with autologous venous blood or here with rhPDGF (GEM 21S®, Osteohealth, Shirley, NY). The sectioned collagen plug was placed as a single layer and stabilized with a "figure of eight" chromic gut fixation suture (Figure 5.3d). Light-cured periodontal dressing was placed over the exposed wound site and onto the adjacent teeth to protect the collagen. The patient continued on chlorhexidine oral rinse for 10–14 days and oral antibiotics for 5 days. The patient was seen at 10 days post-op for removal of the periodontal dressing, at which time grafted sites typically demonstrate fibrin deposition with minimal inflammation. The dressing can be replaced for an additional 10 days of wound protection (if any graft granules are visible) or the patient may transition to a removable appliance without soft tissue contact for esthetic management. A second post-operative visit is completed at 3 weeks, as seen in Figure 14.3e, and typically shows complete granulation and maturing epithelium. Radiographic images demonstrate the bone dimensions preoperatively at the failing tooth and grafted site after 6 months' healing (Figure 5.3f and g), after which an implant was placed. At surgery, significant buccal bone volume was demonstrated with flap exposure prior to apical positioning (Figure 5.3h).

Application of the Bio-Col technique in the esthetic zone is demonstrated at a failing maxillary right central incisor with a buccal fistula (Figure 5.4a). Atraumatic removal of the fractured root was followed by site assessment, aggressive site debridement, excision of the fistula,

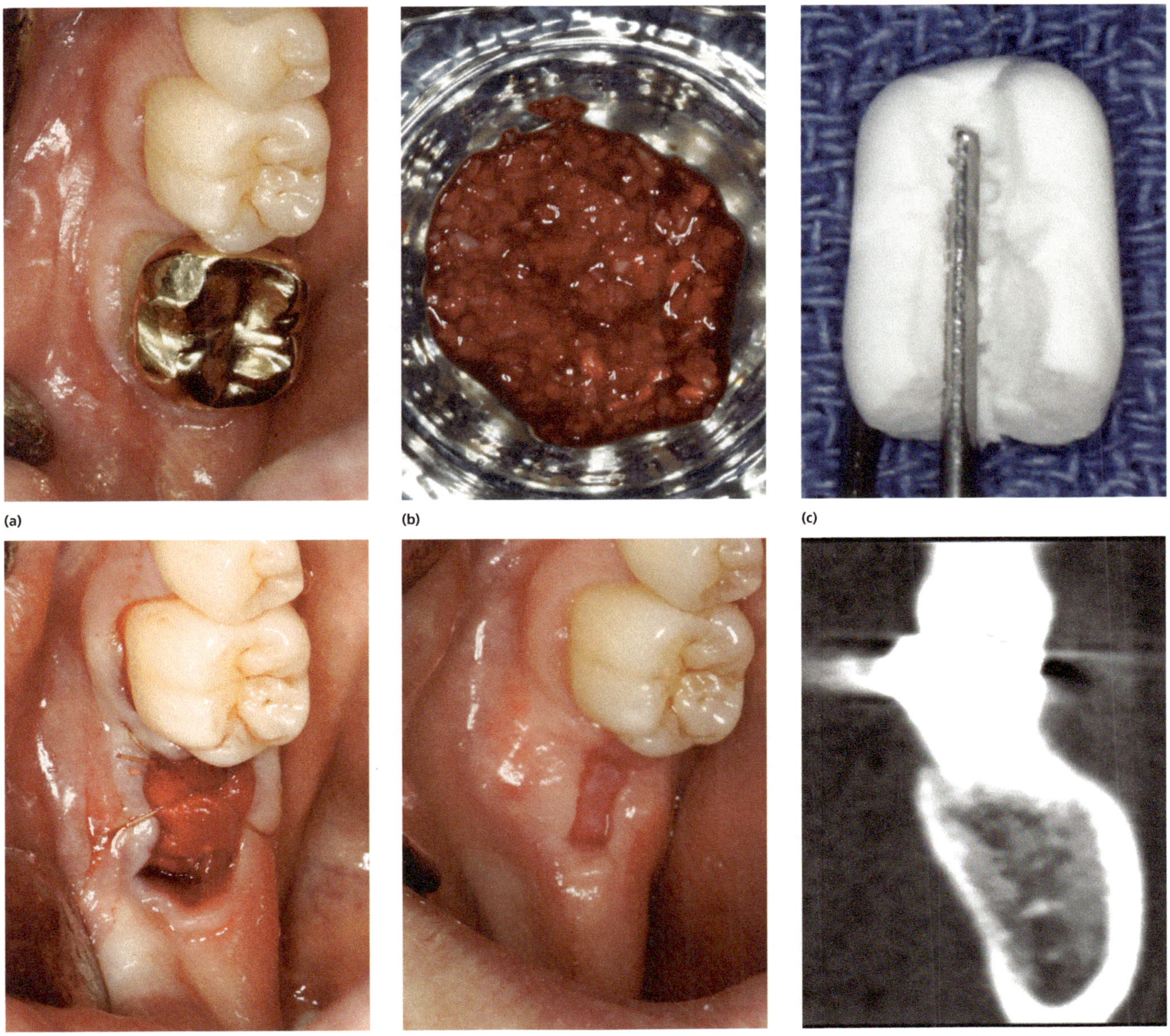

(a) (b) (c) (d) (e) (f)

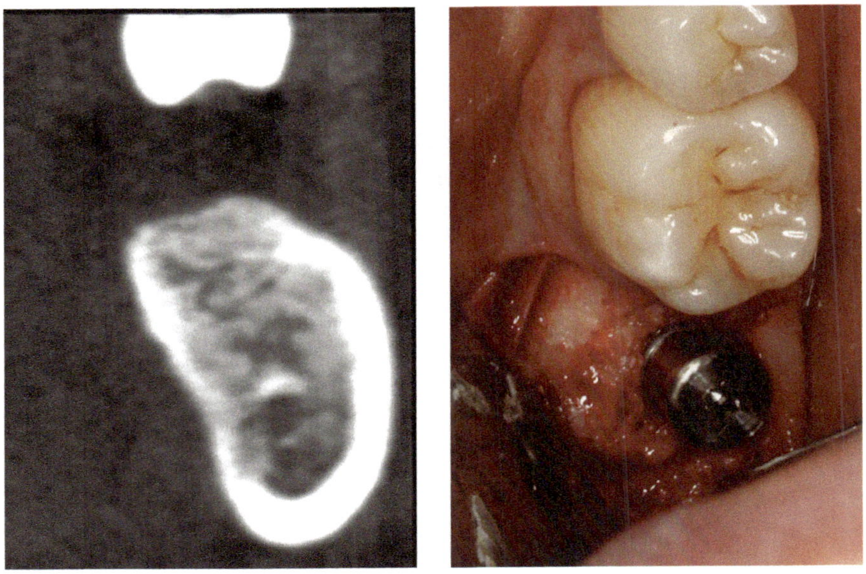

(g) (h)

Figure 5.3 The modified Bio-Col® technique is demonstrated at a non-restorable mandibular first molar region. (a) Failing mandibular right first molar occlusal view. (b) Particulate xenograft saturated in venous autologous blood (Equimatrix®, Osteohealth, Shirley, NY). (c) Sectioned collagen plug (Ora-Plug®, Salvin Dental, Charlotte, NC). (d) Extraction site following minimally invasive surgery after particulate grafting and placement of a sectioned collagen plug saturated in rhPDGF (GEM 21S®, Osteohealth, Shirley, NY) and a figure-of-eight chromic suture (4-0). (e) Healing site after 3 weeks demonstrating maturing epithelium. (f) Open exposure of the grafted site after 6 months' healing and implant placement (5 mm diameter) demonstrating buccal bone volume. (g) Pretreatment cone beam computed tomography (CBCT) cross-sectional radiographic view of the failing molar site. (h) CBCT cross-sectional radiographic view of the grafted edentulous site after 6 months' healing, immediately prior to implant placement. © Daniel R. Cullum.

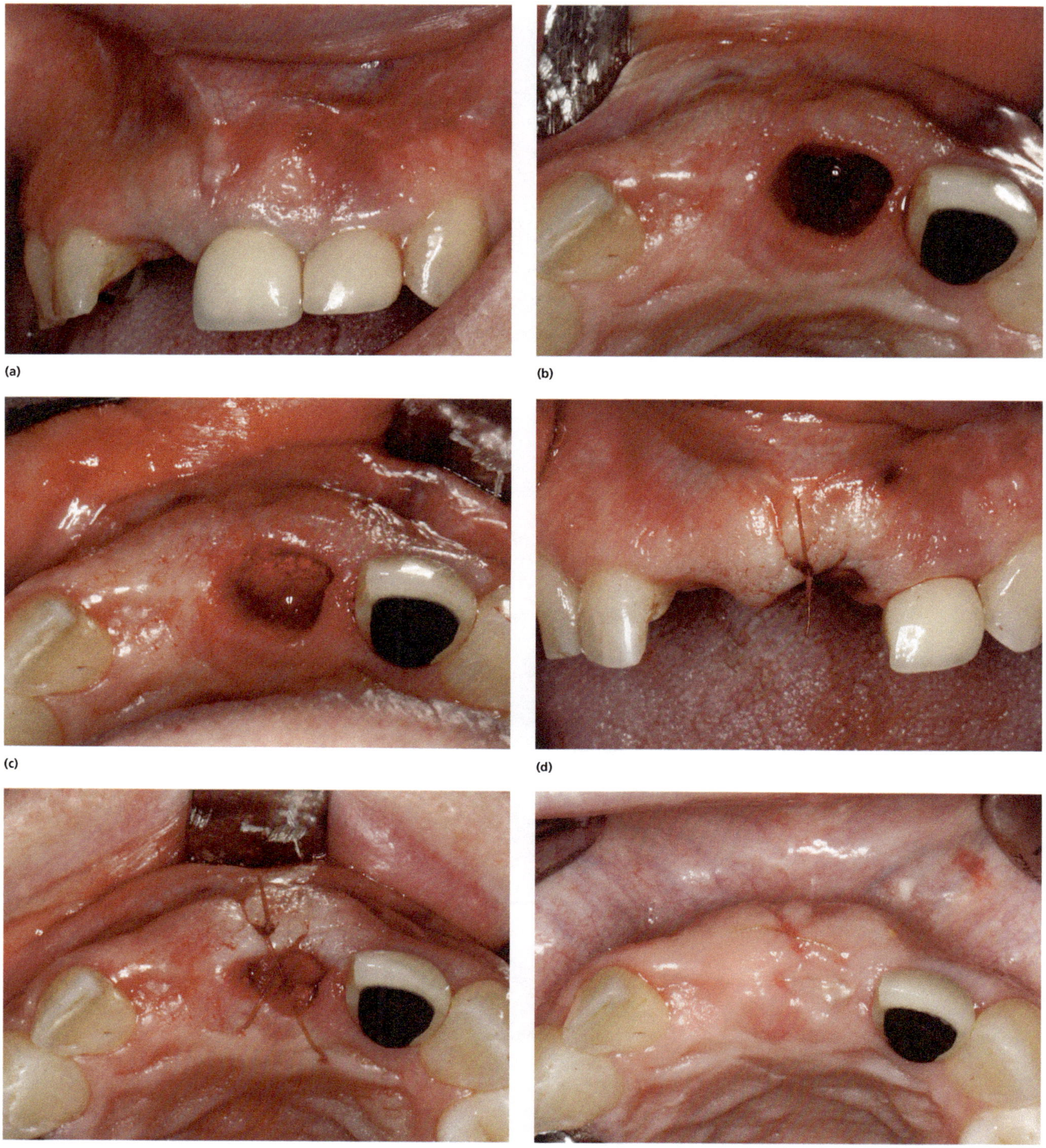

(a) (b) (c) (d) (e) (f)

Figure 5.4 (a) Failing maxillary right central incisor with a buccal fistula. (b) Atraumatic removal of the fractured root and socket debridement is completed. (c) The residual defect is grafted with mineralized allograft up to the surrounding bone margins. (d) Facial and (e) occlusal views showing the sectioned collagen plug saturated in rhPDGF (GEM 21S®, Osteohealth, Shirley, NY) after being placed in the crestal soft tissue defect and secured with a figure-of-eight 4-0 chromic suture. (f) Occlusal view after 10 days' healing.

(Continued)

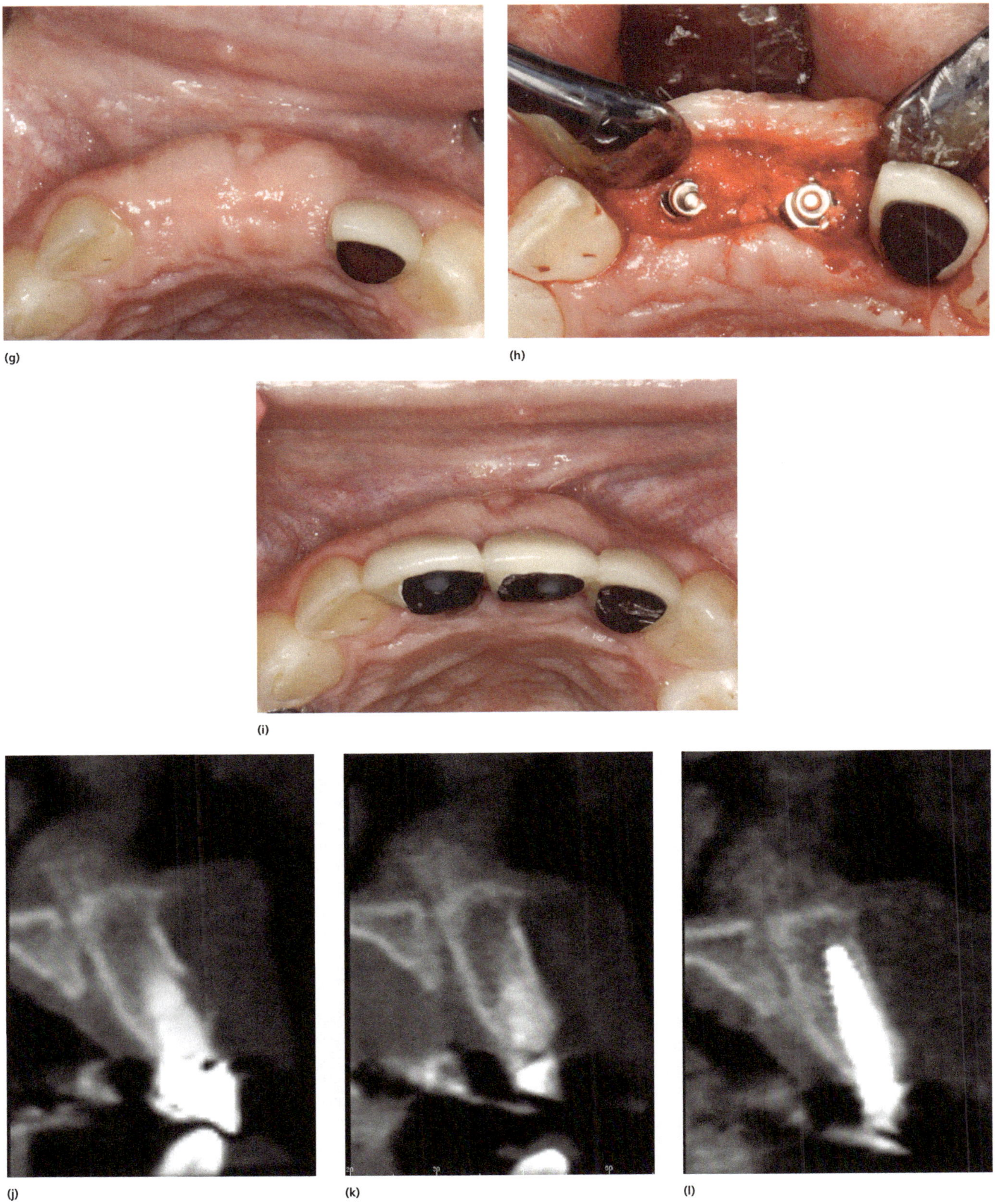

Figure 5.4 (Continued)
(g) Occlusal view after 4 months' healing. (h) Occlusal view of implant placement demonstrating buccal bone volume after modified Bio-Col® technique. (i) Final buccal dimensions can be visualized after restoration. (j–l) CBCT cross-sectional radiographs of the site demonstrate bone dimensions preoperative, 4 months post-operative, and after restoration. © Daniel R. Cullum.

and grafting of the defect as described previously (Figure 5.4b and c). The extraction site defect was filled with a 3 mm thick horizontal sectioned portion of collagen plug, which was saturated in rhPDGF ("off-label" application of GEM 21S®, Osteohealth, Shirley, NY) and secured with a figure-of-eight chromic gut suture (Figure 5.4d and e). Early wound healing can be seen at 10 days in Figure 5.4f. Ridge preservation and healing with adequate bone volume can be seen after 4 months (Figure 5.4g). Implant placement is completed with limited flap exposure demonstrating buccal bone volume maintenance (Figure 5.4h). Final buccal dimensions and volume can be visualized after restoration (Figure 5.4i). CBCT cross-sectional radiographs of the site demonstrate the bone dimensions preoperative, 4 months postoperative, and after restoration (Figure 5.4j–l).

Protection of the exposed collagen in the immediate postoperative period is a critical factor in achieving success with this technique. While some mechanical protection is given from a non-impinging Essix® retainer (Raintree Essix Inc., Metairie, LA), many clinicians have noted findings on follow-up of totally exposed graft material with apparent complete resorption of the collagen. While this will typically close by secondary intention, some graft particles are lost and alveolar volume of the graft is reduced. The judicious use of a cyanoacrylate surface layer or the physical protection of periodontal dressing (Barricaid®, Dentsply-Caulk, Milford, DE) are paramount to the predictability of this technique.

Open-barrier techniques

Larger extraction defects, such as those of a single molar tooth, multiple tooth defects, or defects that include substantial loss of buccal or lingual/palatal cortical plate, may not be appropriate for the Bio-Col technique. While the original porous PTFE membranes can work well with these types of defects, primary soft tissue closure is a major technical challenge, and bacterial cell penetration with resulting infection can occur with exposure to the oral environment. This limitation led to the development of a second-generation PTFE barrier membrane[34,35] formed from hd-PTFE (Figure 5.5). Hd-PTFE is impervious to bacteria, and if properly adapted over the grafted socket has a very low incidence of infection. Animal studies confirmed the efficacy of hd-PTFE as a guided tissue regeneration material, and US Food and Drug Administration clearance was granted in 1994. Techniques for use of these hd-PTFE barriers can be very effective and relatively inexpensive for a variety of clinical applications, as will now be described.[36]

The Cytoplast® (hd-PTFE) ridge preservation technique

Evidence of the efficacy of hd-PTFE used in socket preservation grafting without primary closure was shown in a recent comparative, clinical, and histologic study.[37] In sockets grafted with mineralized bone allograft and covered with hd-PTFE, vertical bone loss at 4 months post-extraction was −0.25 mm while horizontal loss was −0.30 mm. This compared favorably with sockets grafted with mineralized bone allograft and covered with acellular human dermis (−1.10 mm vertical and −0.44 mm horizontal loss). Histomorphometric analysis revealed a vital bone percentage of 47.4% for hd-PTFE and 41.8% for the human dermis membrane group. In a retrospective, non-randomized human study reporting on 276 treated sockets, predictable bone regeneration was found with no reported cases of infection associated with the exposed hd-PTFE membranes.[38] Dental implant success rates in bone regenerated with the hd-PTFE technique for a case series with 5-year results showed 98% survival of 99 implants placed into the regenerated bone.[39]

Results of another published series of 420 treated cases using hd-PTFE with and without lyophilized mineralized bone allograft indicated preservation of bone, preservation of the position of the mucogingival junction, and formation of adequate keratinized tissue,[40] as was earlier reported by Barber et al.[41] The technique is indicated for any extraction site where ridge preservation is desired, and can also be employed in conjunction with immediate implant placement. Normally, a particulate graft material is used under the membrane, although Barboza et al.[40] have shown that the graft may in fact not be needed, at least if sufficient buccal cortical bone remains to support the membrane. If additional soft tissue augmentation is desired in thin gingival biotype cases, the technique may be modified by adding a layer of collagen membrane or autogenous connective tissue under the hd-PTFE layer.

Contraindications include existing cigarette smoking, uncontrolled chronic periodontal disease, or acute infection with swelling and drainage. Chronic periodontal and/or periapical infections are relative contraindications, but may not present increased risk provided that preoperative antibiotics are prescribed along with aggressive site debridement.

The patient shown in Figure 5.6 was a 43-year-old female with a recent history of discomfort and swelling affecting the maxillary left cuspid tooth. The tooth showed class I mobility and 5 mm of buccal gingival recession with marginal inflammation (Figure 5.6a). The radiograph in Figure 5.6b suggested external root resorption; as a

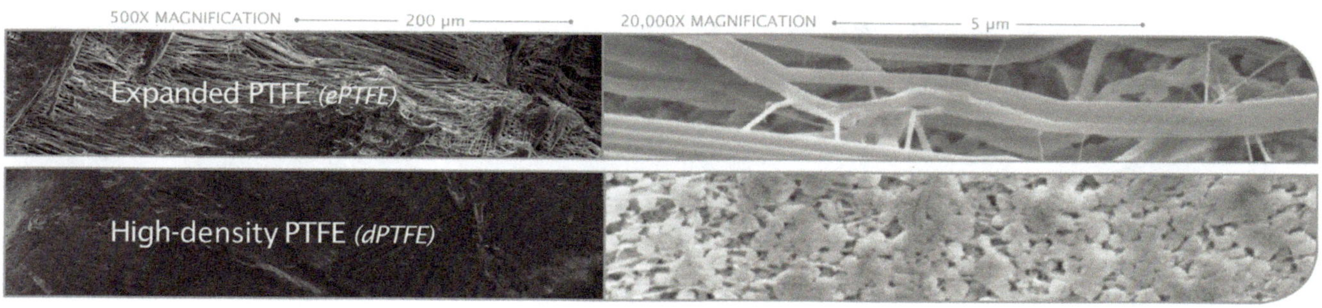

Figure 5.5 Scanning electron microscopic comparison of expanded PTFE (ePTFE) and hd-PTFE. At 500×, the "node and fibril" structure typical of ePTFE can be seen, whereas the surface of hd-PTFE appears more dense without distinct fibrils. At 20,000×, individual ePTFE fibrils are shown, demonstrating a highly porous structure. At 20,000× the submicrometer pore size of hd-PTFE can be appreciated. *Source:* Implant Site Development and Extraction Site Grafting Technical Manual. Osteogenics Clinical Education, 2012. Reproduced with permission of Dr Barry Bartee, Osteogenics Biomedical, Inc. Lubbock, TX, USA.

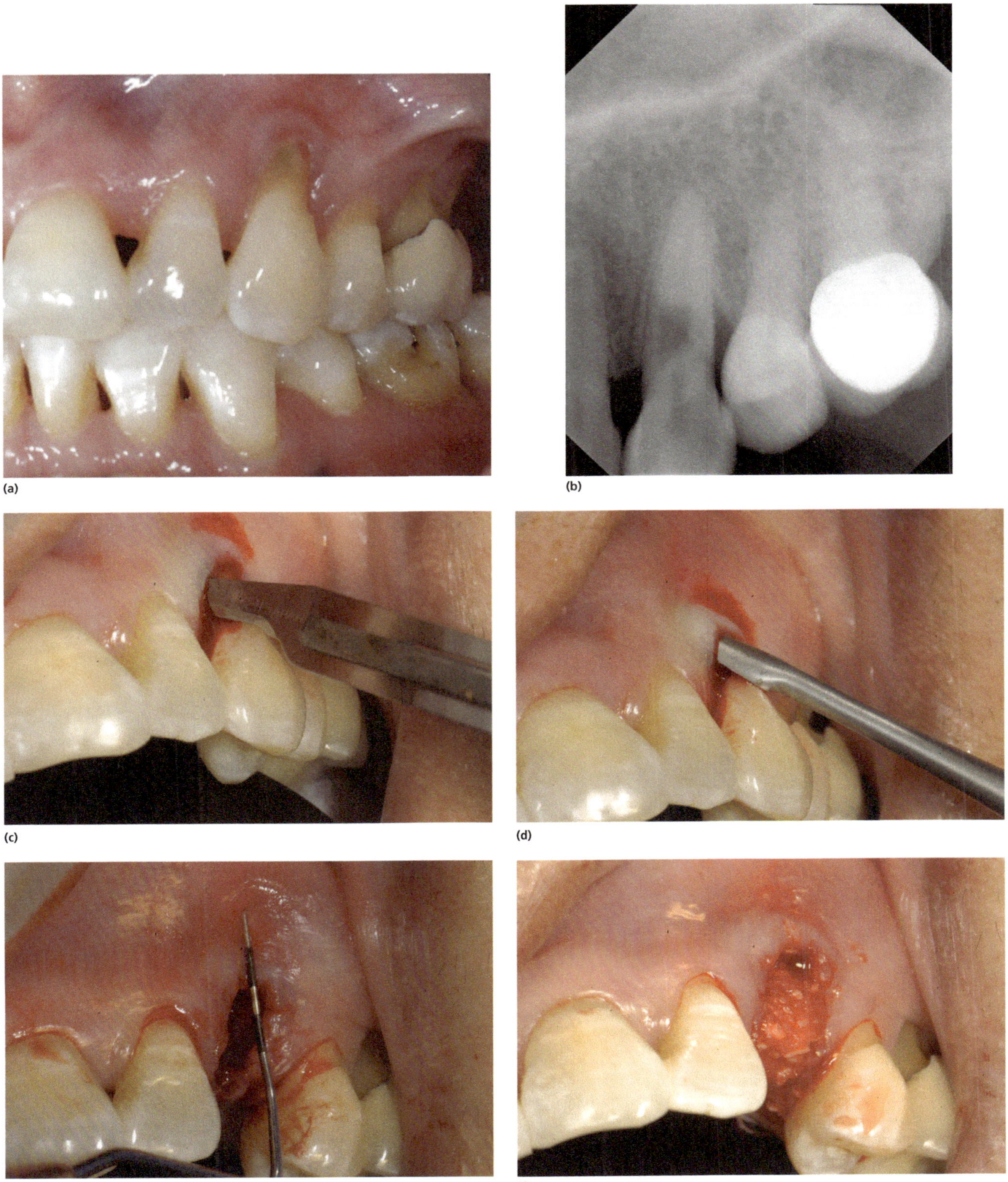

Figure 5.6 (a) Clinical photograph of the symptomatic maxillary left cuspid tooth. (b)Periapical radiograph showed external root resorption. (c) A circumferential intra-sulcular incision was made to free the marginal soft tissues. (d) A micro-periosteal elevator was used in initial flap elevation to start to create a soft tissue pouch into which to insert the barrier material. (e) The buccal bone level was found to be 6 mm apical to the buccal soft tissue margin likely as a result of the external root resorptive activity. (f) A combination of particulate mineralized and demineralized allograft materials was used to graft the socket. *(Continued)*

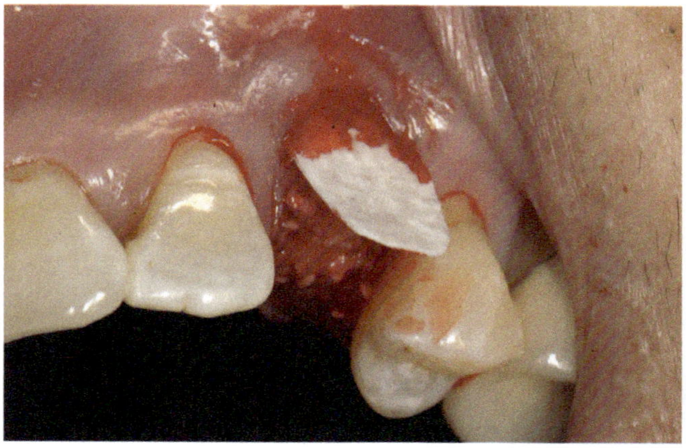

(g)

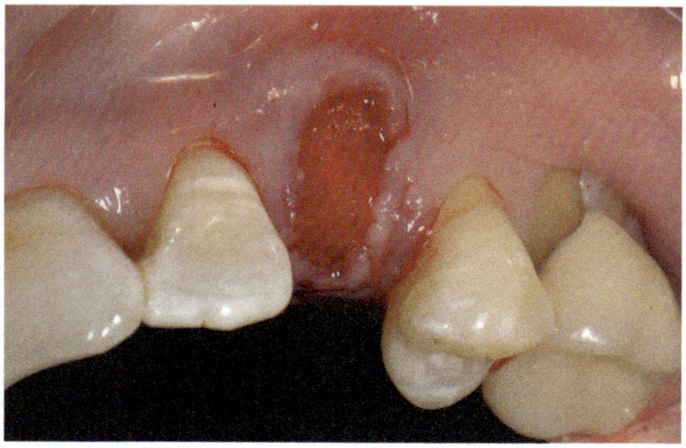

(h)

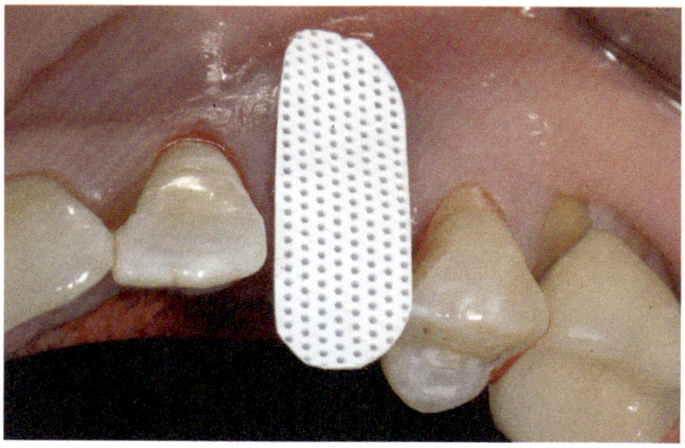

(i)

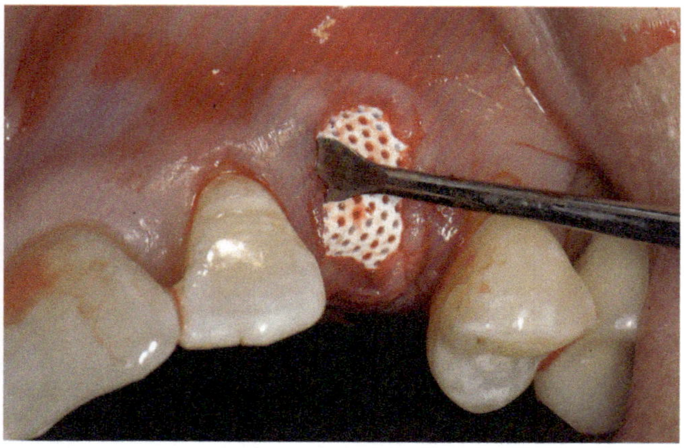

(j)

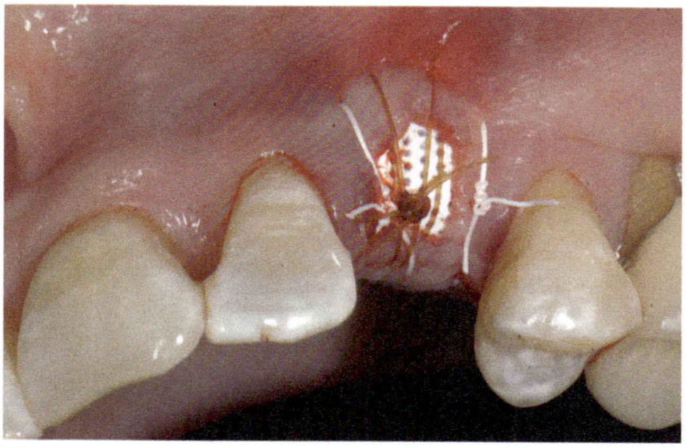

(k)

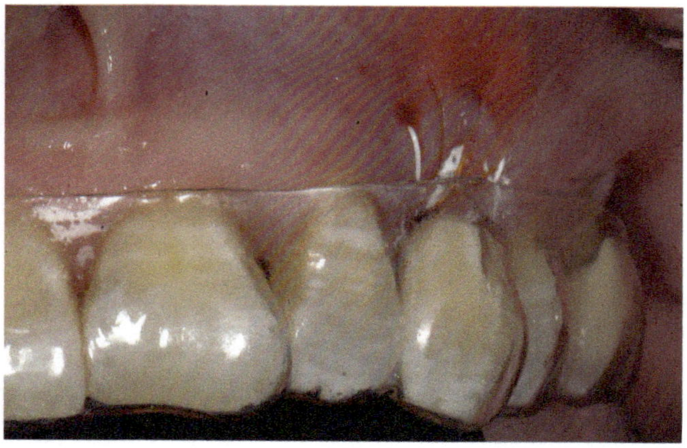

(l)

Figure 5.6 (Continued)
(g) A collagen membrane was prepared to provide a first layer of protection for the grafted socket. (h) The collagen membrane was inserted onto the surrounding bone margins on the buccal, palatal, and interproximal regions. (i) The hd-PTFE barrier was trimmed to create rounded edges and with adequate length to cover the socket and rest on 3–4 mm of the peripheral bone. (j) The hd-PTFE barrier was carefully inserted to avoid bent edges and underlying dead space. (k) Sutures were used to stabilize the barrier. (l) The inserted Essix® retainer used for temporization.

result, endodontic treatment of the tooth was contraindicated. In such cases, an intrasulcular incision with a 15-C blade is preferred for access. If severe caries is present, and appears to extend subcrestally, flap reflection to gain improved visualization may be needed (Figure 5.6c). Otherwise, a minimally invasive technique should be the priority in order to preserve blood supply to thin buccal cortical bone and interdental papillae. However, flap reflection should be adequate to expose sufficient bone (3–4 mm) buccally and linguo-palatally to receive and support the membrane within a subperiosteal pocket (Figure 5.6d). The use of periotomes, Proximators, careful surgical sectioning of teeth, and gentle luxation and extraction forces is recommended. Following extraction, the external root resorption lesion was apparent and the buccal bone level demonstrated 6 mm of bone loss (Figure 5.6e). All soft tissues within the socket, including remnants of periodontal ligament, were removed with sharp curettes. Special care should be taken to remove any pathogenic soft tissues at the apices of failed endodontic treated teeth, as this tissue may harbor persistent pathogenic bacteria and lead to later problems.[42] There should be adequate bleeding noted from the socket walls. Otherwise, decortication of socket walls can be done with a #2 round surgical bur to assure a source of mesenchymal cells and provide for more rapid revascularization. Following debridement, particulate graft material (30% demineralized, freeze-dried allograft and 70% mineralized, freeze-dried allograft) was gently packed into the socket with a small curette, taking care to distribute the material evenly throughout the socket and any associated defects (Figure 5.6f). Overpacking of the socket with graft is contraindicated as this can impede early ingrowth of blood vessels.

A double-membrane technique was employed by first using a resorbable collagen membrane to cover the graft materials (Cytoplast® RTM Type I collagen, Osteogenics Biomedical Inc.). This membrane was trimmed to rest on 3–4 mm of buccal and palatal bone and on the interdental bone crests as well (Figure 5.6g and h). An hd-PTFE membrane (Cytoplast TXT-200®, Osteogenics Biomedical Inc.) was trimmed with scissors to fit the site and placed over the collagen membrane and into the prepared buccal and palatal subperiosteal pouches. This membrane was carefully trimmed so as to fit precisely over the socket and associated bone defect, extending 3.0–4.0 mm onto bone beyond the socket margins for support (Figure 5.6i and j). The corners of the membrane should be gently rounded and smooth. Sutures were used to stabilize the membrane and eliminate dead space under the barrier (Figure 5.6k).

Management of the interdental tissue will vary depending on the clinical situation. In posterior sites, and where access and visualization of the entire socket is required, the papillae are divided midcrestally and the membrane placed to lie on the interdental crestal bone. However, the membrane must be trimmed so as to stay at least 1.0 mm away from the adjacent tooth roots. In the esthetic zone, where the gingival biotype is thin, rather than incising and elevating the interdental papillae, they should be left intact and simply undermined to create space for membrane placement. When properly placed, the membrane should lie passively across the socket and under the flap margins (Figure 5.6k). It should be smooth without wrinkles or folds that could potentially allow bacterial migration beneath it. If necessary, the membrane can be stretched slightly over a gloved fingertip or curved over an instrument handle to help achieve the required shape for a passive fit before final membrane insertion. Any stray bone graft particles between membrane and flap are removed. Care should also be taken not to puncture the membrane during trimming, placement, and suturing so as to avoid potential for bacterial leakage through the membrane. If two pieces of membrane are being used, as in the case of multiple adjacent extraction sites, care should be taken to avoid overlapping the membrane segments, particularly in an area where they might become exposed to the oral environment. Such an overlap can provide ready access to bacterial migration under the membrane. In these situations, either a single larger membrane should be used or the two membranes placed independently with complete soft tissue coverage between their contiguous exposed edges.

Monofilament PTFE suture is recommended for wound closure (Figure 5.6k). Good, tension-free adaptation of the flap to the membrane and elimination of dead space are required. A "figure-of-eight" suture technique may be used in single sockets or, alternatively, two interdental interrupted sutures can be placed across the interdental papillae combined with a horizontal mattress suture placed across the mid portion of the socket. Covering the wound site with light-cured periodontal dressing can aid in wound protection. A temporary prosthesis, if present, should be carefully trimmed to avoid placing pressure from the pontic onto the surgical site. Even soft liners or tissue conditioners should not be in direct contact with the grafted site during the first 3 weeks, and the occlusion should be carefully adjusted to prevent micromotion of the temporary prosthesis during function. In the case being demonstrated, an Essix A+® removable retainer (Raintree Essix Inc., Metairie, LA) was used for temporization (Figure 5.6l).

The patient was seen for follow-up at 1 week to confirm adequate oral hygiene. She was instructed in the local application of chlorhexidine rinse to the exposed membrane using a Q-tip. The PTFE sutures, which cause minimal inflammatory response, can be left in place for 10–14 days or even longer. Suture removal in this case was at 2 weeks, and the membrane inspected to ensure complication-free healing. Gentle pressure applied to the exposed membrane with an instrument handle or Q-tip should reveal a solid, non-compressible and non-tender graft site. The membrane was removed non-surgically after 3–4 weeks of site healing by grasping it with tweezers and tugging gently (Figure 5.7a).

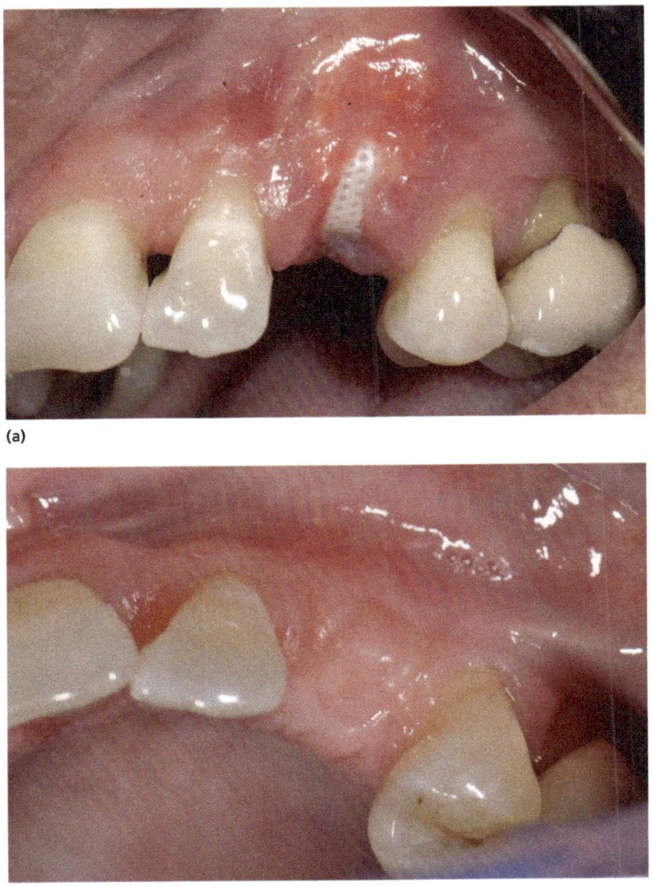
(a)
(b)

Figure 5.7 (a) The site at 3 weeks of healing immediately before non-surgical removal of the barrier. (b) At 6 weeks the site has healed well with good ridge width retention and formation of abundant keratinized tissue.

Normally, by 21–28 days of site healing, there will be a dense, vascular connective tissue matrix in the socket, and early osteogenesis will be occurring in its apical two-thirds.[43,44] Larger defects, or those missing one or more socket walls, may require additional time before membrane removal, but it is not necessary to leave the membrane longer than 6–8 weeks. The membrane is removed by grasping the exposed surface with cotton forceps and gently tugging it from the tissue bed. Topical anesthetic may be applied in advance if desired for membrane removal. A glistening, well-vascularized, well-consolidated graft should be observed at that time. If loose graft particles are observed, they can be removed with sterile irrigation. Once the barrier is gone, the epithelium of adjacent gingival tissues will migrate across the osteoid matrix during the following 7–10 days. By 6 weeks, a thick, keratinizing gingiva will have formed over the grafted socket, and the natural soft tissue architecture, including the interdental papillae, will have been preserved (Figure 5.7b).

Complications, such as soft tissue dehiscence seen as flap retraction, are rare but can occur. Cases with pre-existing infection and/or total loss of buccal or palatal plate are at increased risk for this complication. The risk may be reduced with careful flap dissection, meticulous tissue handling, and precise suturing. Using a double-barrier technique can also be of benefit where minimal buccal bone remains. If dehiscence and further membrane exposure occur, the exposed area should be kept clean and free of plaque using chlorhexidine and a Q-tip. Care should be taken during cleaning to prevent disruption of the membrane for at least 3 weeks, at which time the membrane can be removed as per usual protocol, and further healing should proceed as normal. The most common reason for dehiscence and flap retraction is vascular compromise of the soft tissues. This may occur due to over-tightening of sutures or stretching of the flap beyond the capability of its small arteries and capillaries to supply blood to the flap margins. Tension-free suturing should be the goal. Periosteal-releasing incisions and split-thickness dissection can be used to aid in this objective. If used, vertical relieving incisions should be made at least 8–10 mm away from the membrane, or the width of one to two teeth away from the defect margins. With the use of prophylactic antibiotics, antiseptic rinses, and precise technique, post-operative infection is rare. The presence of purulent drainage, bad taste, or foul odor in the post-operative period indicates infection of the graft. A simple method to evaluate the health of the tissue under the membrane is to gently touch the exposed membrane with a dental mirror handle or Q-tip. The membrane and underlying tissue should be firm, with no exudate or fluid movement noted when gentle pressure is applied. If infection is suspected under the membrane, it should immediately be removed. Failure of the graft may or may not occur with minor infection depending on the time of membrane removal.

In the case being demonstrated, 4 months' site healing was allowed. At that time the soft (Figure 5.8a and b) and hard tissues (Figure 5.8c) were deemed to have healed adequately. Comparing the soft tissue levels, it was apparent that at least 5 mm of buccal vertical keratinized tissue gain was achieved in the area of the previous recession. In the 4-month radiograph, approximately 4 mm of vertical bone gain at the buccal plate defect had occurred. A small, minimally invasive "u"-shaped flap was raised over the intended implant site, leaving the adjacent papillae intact (Figure 5.8d). The exposed bone was found to be adequate to maintain at least 2 mm of buccal bone thickness following osteotomy site preparation, and the bone was type III.[45] A threaded 4 mm × 13 mm implant (Tapered, Screw-Vent®, Zimmer Dental, Carlsbad, CA) was placed, and the small buccal flap apically repositioned to maximize keratinized tissue (Figure 5.8e). After 4 months' site healing, the implant was deemed ready for restoration, with good bone healing demonstrated on the radiograph (Figure 5.8f). The buccal soft tissue profile appeared satisfactory (Figure 5.8g). An implant-level impression was made, and a custom zirconia abutment was fabricated (Figure 5.8h). The implant was progressively loaded starting with a custom acrylic crown, and then finally restored with an all-ceramic crown. The implant restoration can be seen after 16 months (Figure 5.8i) on a periapical radiograph (Figure 5.8j) and CBCT scan of the site (Figure 5.8k), confirming adequate retention of buccal cortical bone along the full implant length.

A second case demonstrates a molar site preservation in a 50-year-old male patient (Figure 5.9a). The mandibular right second molar was deemed hopeless due to a vertical root fracture and ensuing periapical infection. The first molar had been removed without site preservation 3 months earlier (Figure 5.9a and b), resulting in an alveolar ridge deficiency. The past dental history included a bruxing habit that had resulted in other cracked teeth requiring endodontic treatment and full crowns. A panoramic radiograph (Figure 5.9b) revealed a large periapical radiolucency affecting the second molar, while the preoperative CBCT scan (Figure 5.9c) confirmed a large bone defect with vertical loss of buccal plate in the first molar extraction site.

The patient was premedicated with amoxicillin (loading dose 1 h before procedure). Under local anesthesia and conscious sedation, the second molar was extracted and its socket debrided of all soft tissue. The cortical socket walls were still present (Figure 5.9d), and a vertical root fracture was confirmed on the extracted tooth. The poorly healed socket of the first molar also was debrided of all remaining soft tissues. After copious saline irrigation, both socket defects were filled with a combination of 70% mineralized, freeze-dried allograft and 30% demineralized, freeze-dried allograft (Figure 5.9e). An hd-PTFE barrier was trimmed to fit over the augmented defects, overlapping the adjacent bone margins by 2–3 mm (Figure 5.9f). The soft tissue flap was trimmed to remove any inflamed granulation tissue, and then sutured with PTFE suture (Figure 5.9g). No attempt was made to obtain primary closure, leaving the hd-PTFE barrier exposed over the crest. After 3 weeks of site healing, the sutures and barrier were removed using only topical anesthetic.

At 6 months post-extraction, a new CBCT scan was performed (Figure 5.10a). Regeneration of the buccal contour and ridge height in the first molar site was evident (Figure 5.10b). Bone formation in the second molar site also appeared satisfactory (Figure 5.10c). There was good soft tissue healing with adequate thickness and keratinization (Figure 5.10d). At the time of implant placement, a mid-crestal incision was used, and after flap reflection good bone healing was seen, permitting the placement of wider diameter threaded dental implants (Tapered, Screw-Vent®, Zimmer Dental, Carlsbad, CA). A 4.7 mm × 11 mm implant was used in the first molar location, while a 4.7 mm × 10 mm implant was placed in the second molar site, both without complications. Bone quality was good (type II of Lekholm and Zarb[45]) (Figure 5.10e–g). A bone biopsy was taken during osteotomy preparation at the first molar site. Histological examination of this biopsy revealed the vital bone percentage to be 86% with 13% residual allograft (Figure 5.10h). The implants were loaded progressively by placing an acrylic fixed prosthesis after initial site healing. This temporary prosthesis was allowed to function for 6 months before being replaced by the final porcelain-to-metal fixed implant-supported bridge (Figure 5.10i and j).

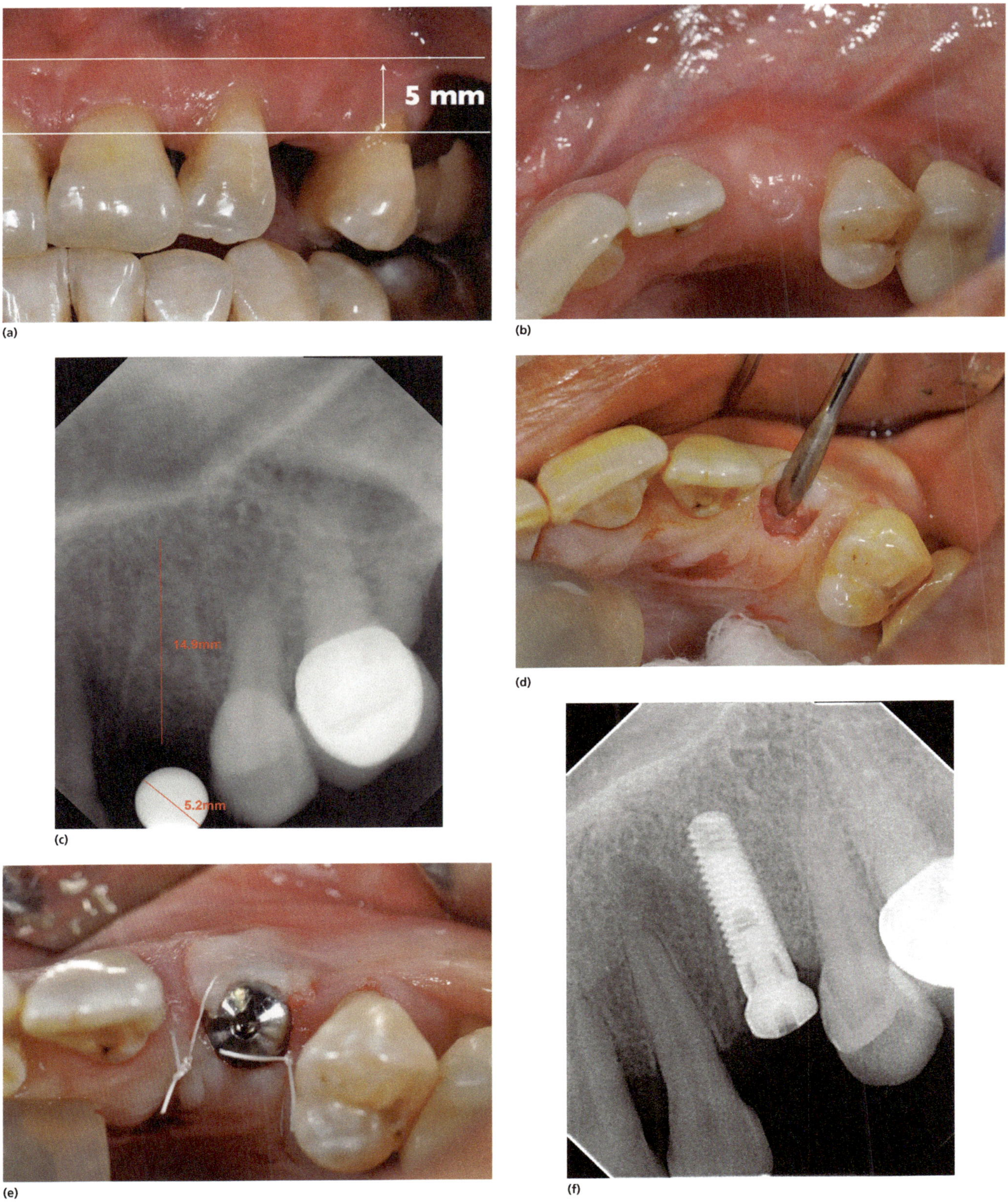

Figure 5.8 (a) Four-month post-ridge preservation soft tissue profiles. Compare with the pretreatment defect Figure 5.6a and e. (b) Soft tissue profile after 4 months' healing. (c) Four-month bone healing is shown in this radiograph. (d) Minimally invasive implant site preparation with a small, u-shaped flap elevation preserving the adjacent papillae. (e) The implant placed and soft tissue sutured. The flap was repositioned apically to retain and further thicken the keratinized tissue. (f) A radiograph of the implant after 4 months' site healing.

(Continued)

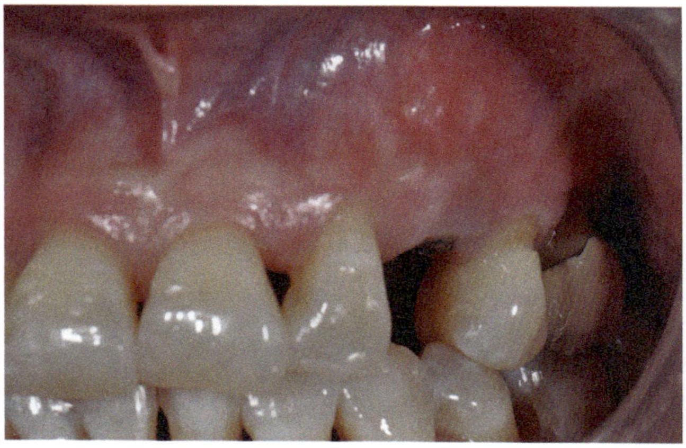

(g)

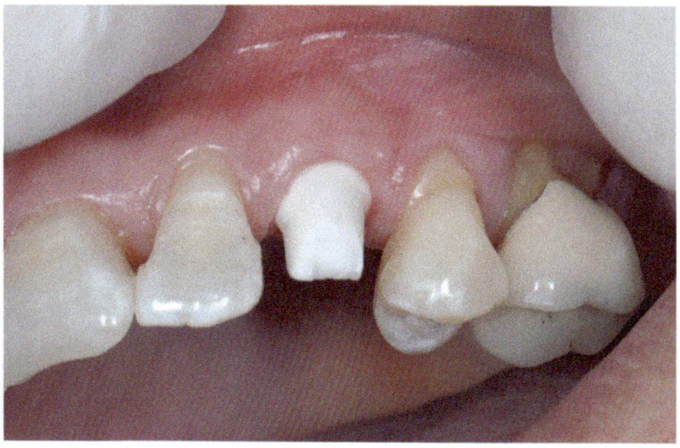

(h)

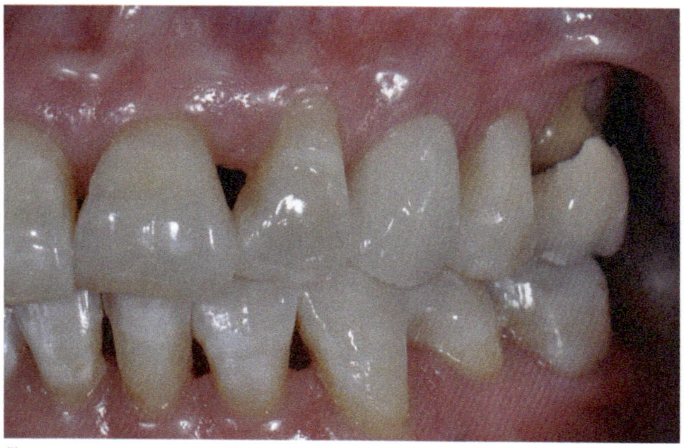

(i)

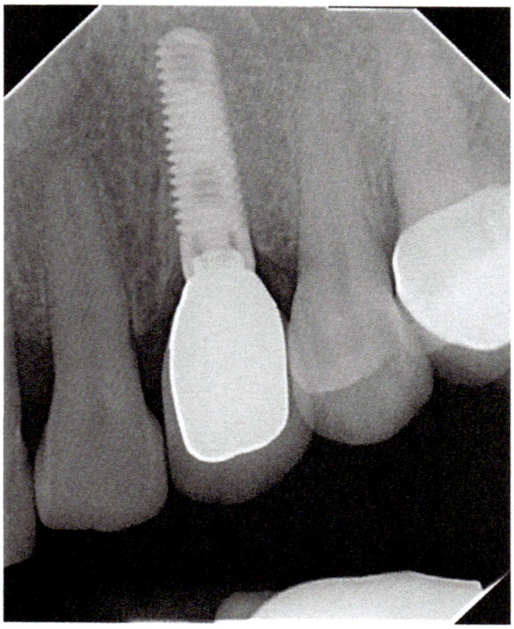

(j)

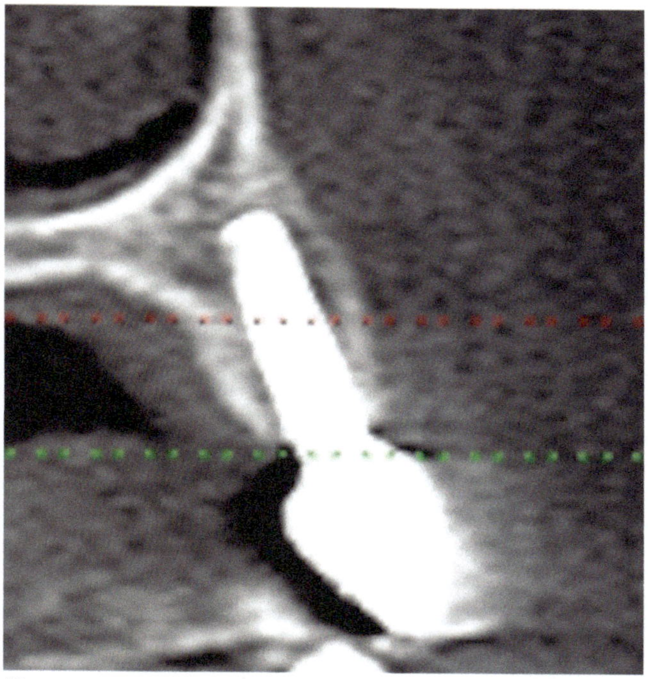

(k)

Figure 5.8 (Continued)
(g) The buccal soft tissues 4 months following implant placement. (h) The implant restoration included a custom zirconia abutment. (i) Post-restoration clinical view after 16 months. (j) A post-restoration radiograph taken after 16 months of clinical function. (k) A CBCT scan at 16 months reveals adequate retention of buccal cortical bone for the whole implant length.

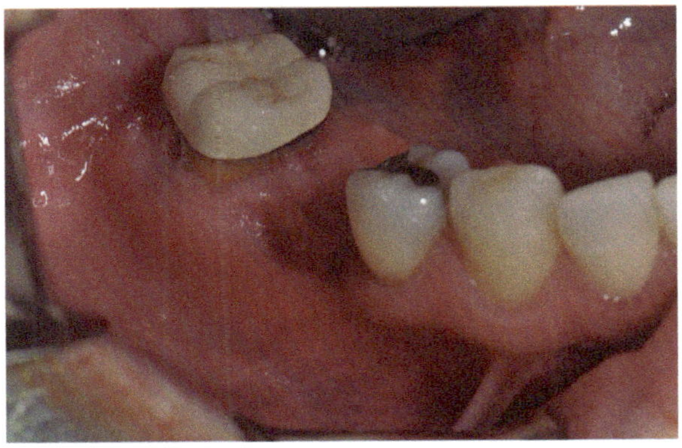

(a)

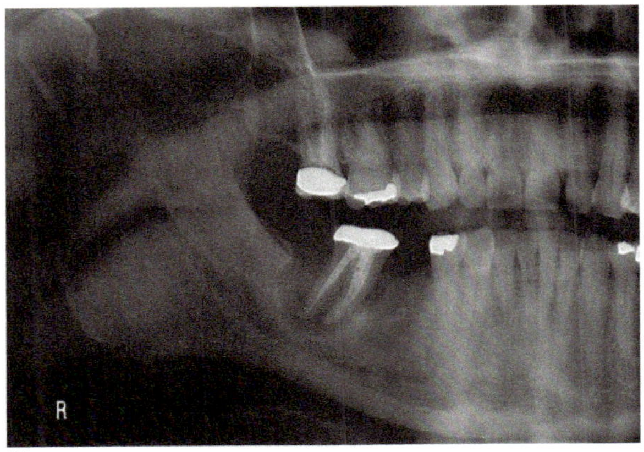

(b)

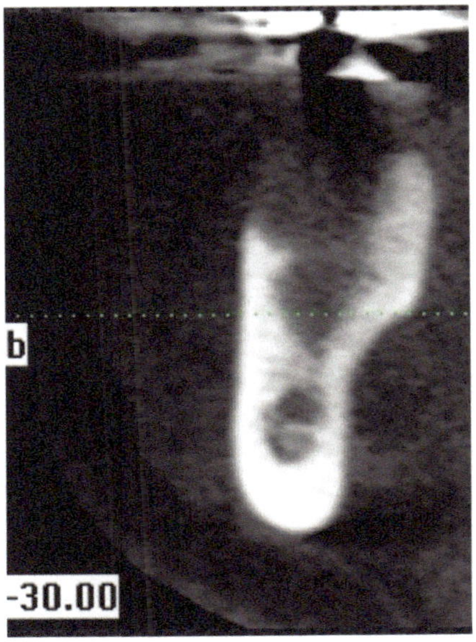

(c)

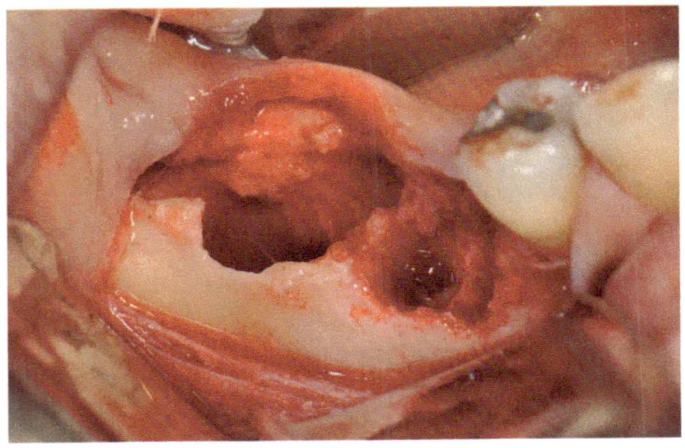

(d)

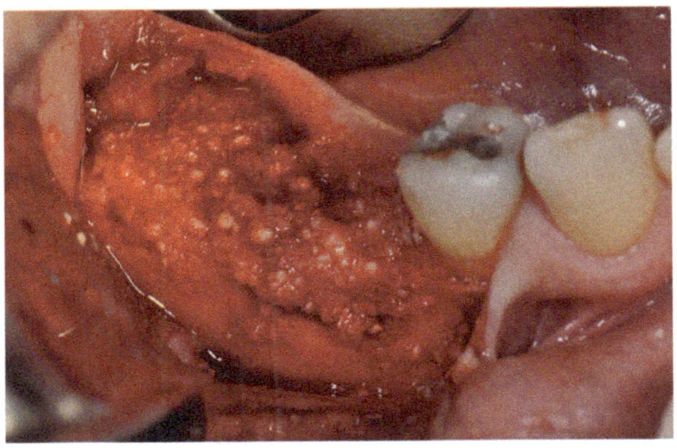

(e)

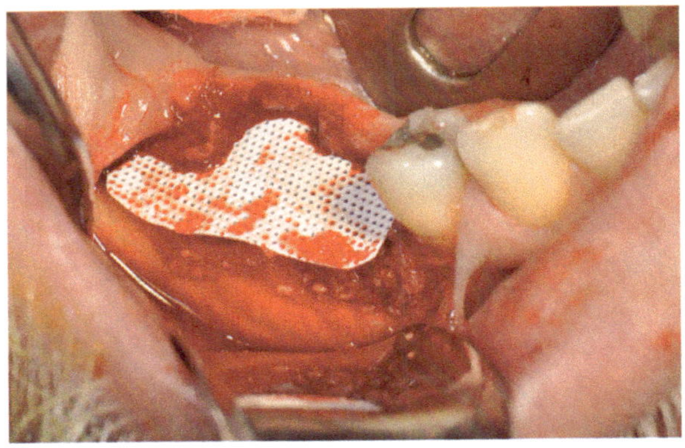

(f)

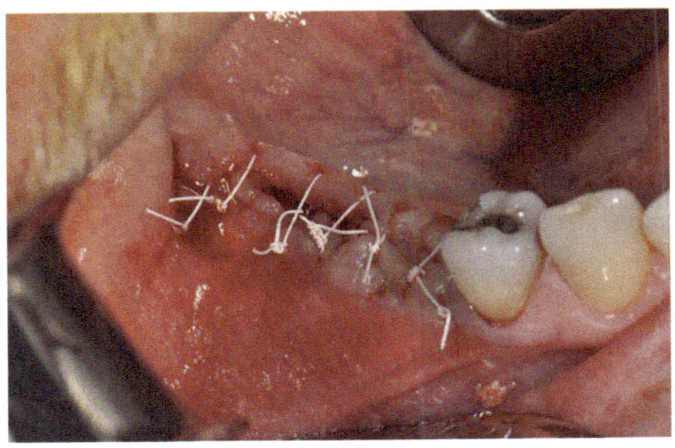

(g)

Figure 5.9 (a) The healing tissue profile in the previously extracted first molar site which had not been preserved with grafting appears abnormal with likely loss of buccal bone, later confirmed with a computed tomography scan (see (c)). (b) The mandibular right second molar was deemed hopeless and showed extensive bone loss secondary to a root fracture. Evidence of recent extraction of the first molar can be seen. (c) The preop computed tomography scan shows extensive bone loss in the previously extracted mandibular first molar site. (d) The socket walls at the second molar site were largely intact, while following debridement the first molar site shows inadequate bone healing. (e) The debrided sockets were filled with a combination freeze-dried allograft that had both a mineralized and demineralized portion. (f) The graft material was covered with an hd-PTFE barrier. (g) The soft tissues were sutured with no effort being made to gain complete flap closure.

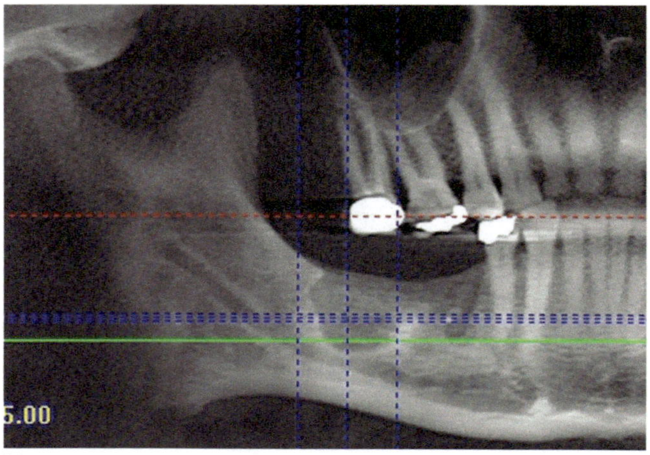

(a)

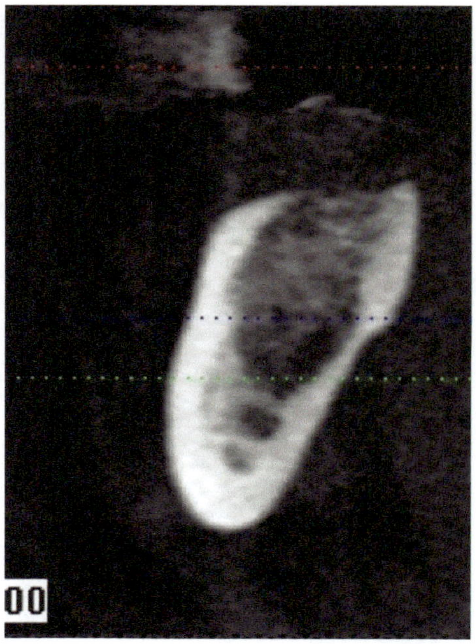

(b)

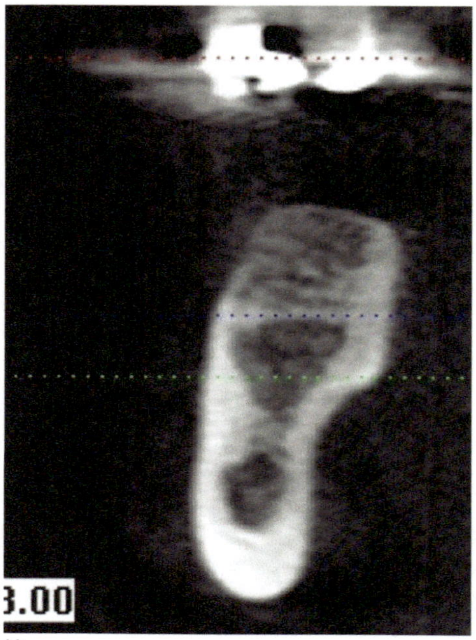

(c)

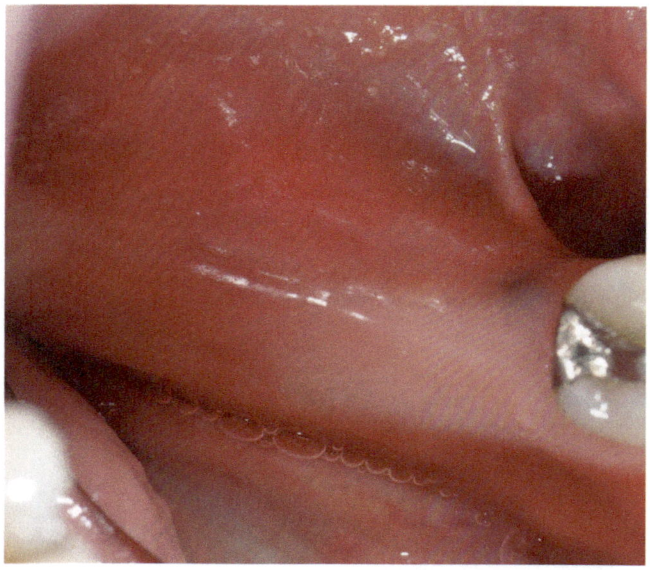

(d)

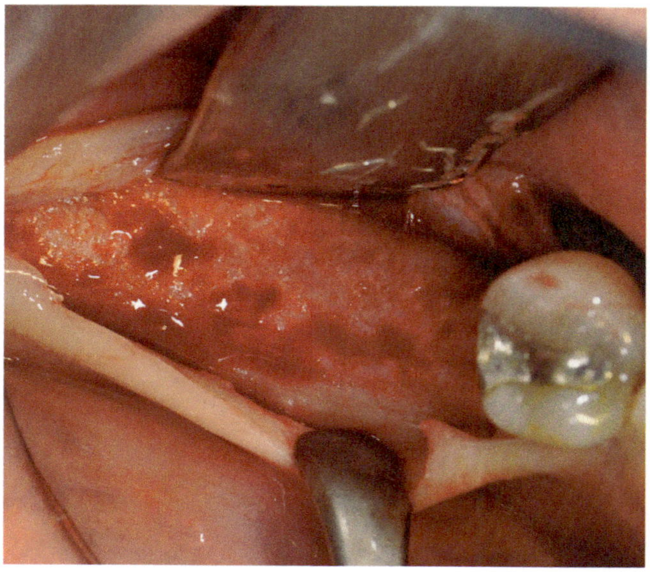

(e)

Figure 5.10 (a) A 6-month post-extraction CBCT scan showed good healing at the second molar site and regeneration of buccal plate and lost vertical height at the first molar site. (b) Cross-sectional image of right mandibular second molar. (c) Cross-sectional image of right mandibular first molar. (d) Complete soft tissue healing can be seen 6 months after extraction and socket preservation grafting. (e) A wide, flat, healed bony ridge is seen after 6 months' healing and flap reflection. (f) Two 4.8 mm diameter threaded implants were placed. (g) The soft tissue were sutured following single-stage implant placement. (h) The histological findings following 6 months of healing at the grafted first molar site. (i) A clinical photograph of the completed implant-borne prosthesis. (j) The baseline post-treatment radiograph.

(Continued)

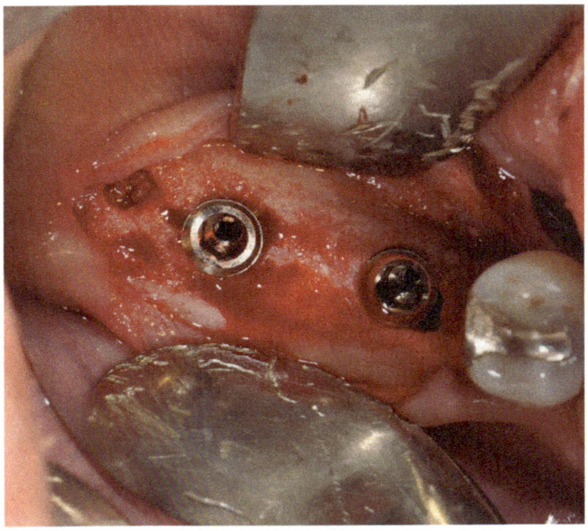
(f)

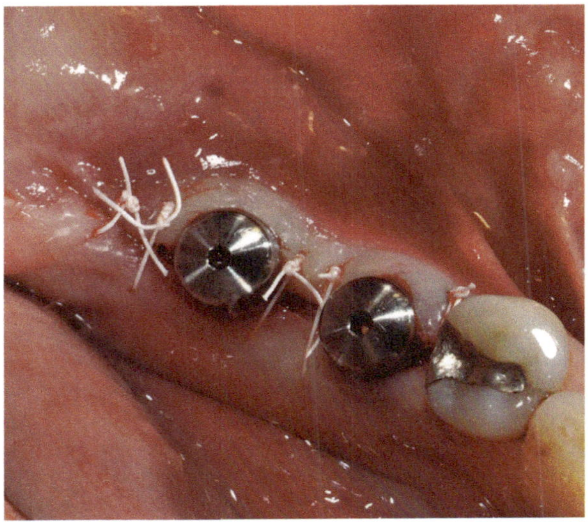
(g)

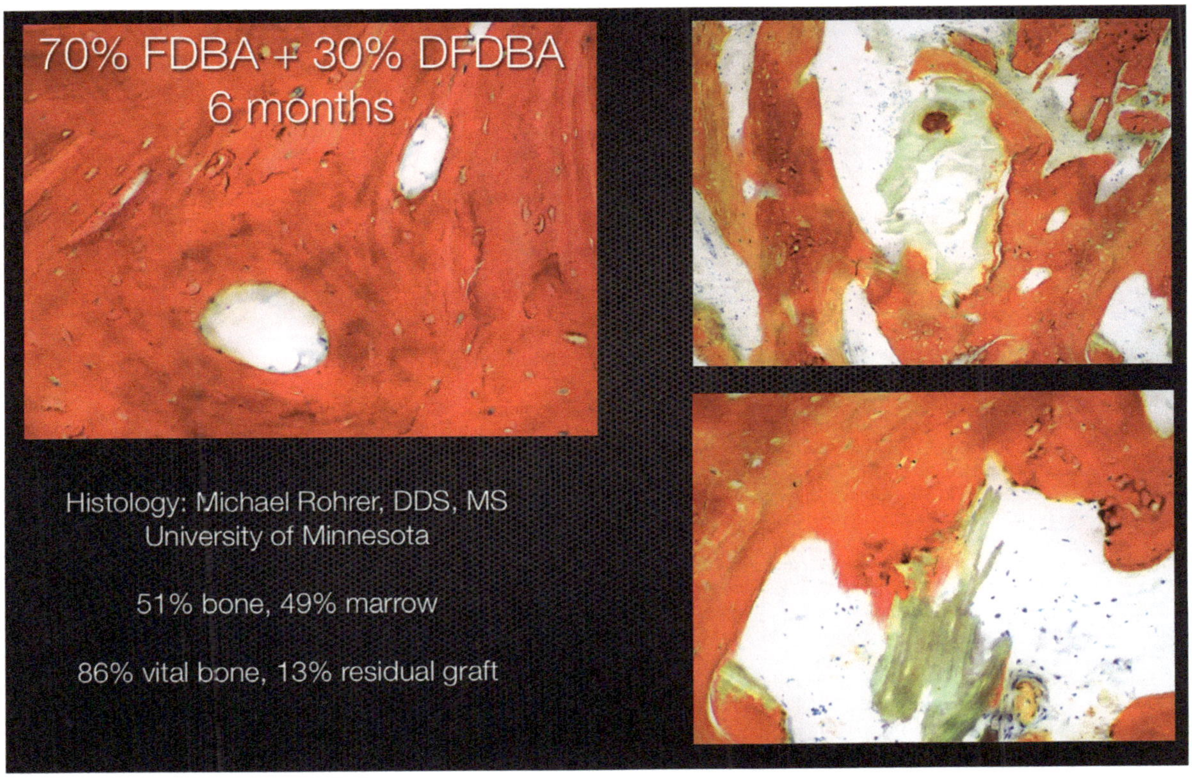

(h)

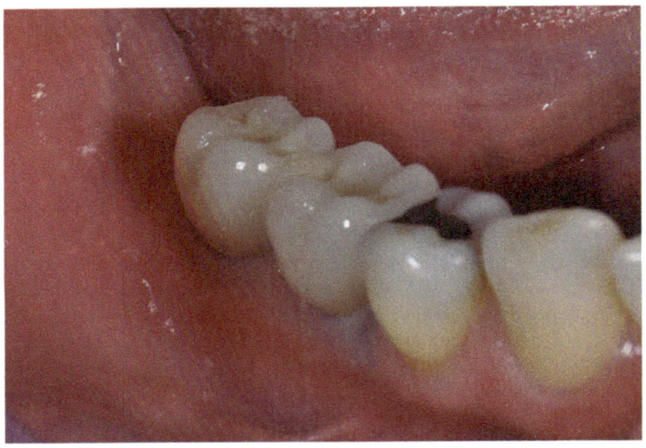
(i)

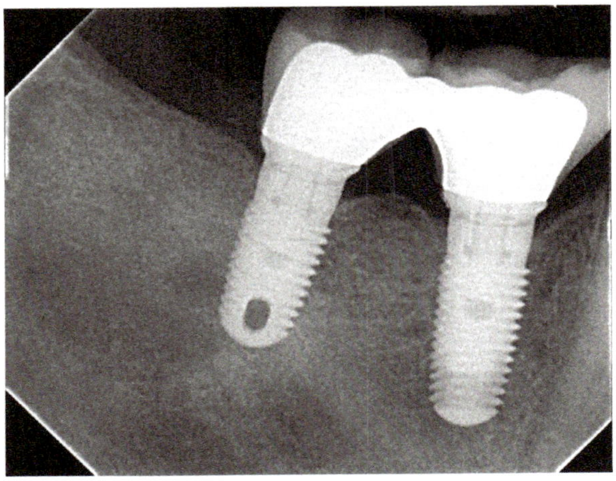
(j)

Figure 5.10 (Continued)

Conclusions

Extraction site ridge preservation techniques have become an essential part of contemporary dental implant practice. Our efforts to replace hopeless teeth with esthetic and functional restorations are greatly enhanced with the application of minimally invasive extraction and secondary closure techniques. The Bio-Col technique and modifications thereof offer a minimally invasive grafting option for management of residual extraction socket defects using a flapless approach to preserve periosteal vascular supply. For larger extraction sites or for those that have suffered extensive loss of buccal and/or lingual/palatal cortical plates, guided tissue regeneration using a mineralized particulate graft with hd-PTFE ridge preservation technique is an "inexpensive workhorse" with broad application. These "open-barrier" regeneration techniques provide the secondary benefits of preserving soft tissue and vestibular morphology, and even of enhancing width of keratinized gingiva. Clinical experience with these techniques in daily patient care has proven to be predictable, practical, and enjoyable.

References

1. Atwood D. Reduction of residual ridges. A major oral disease entity. J Prosthetic Dent 1971; 26: 266– 279.
2. Atwood D. Bone loss of the edentulous alveolar ridges. J Periodontol 1979; 50: 11–21.
3. Rocchietta I, Fontana F, Simion M. Clinical outcomes of vertical bone augmentation to enable dental implant placement: a systematic review. J Clin Periodontol 2008; 35: 203–215.
4. Pereira M, de Freitas P, da Rosa T, Xavier C. Understanding distraction osteogenesis on the maxillary complex: a literature review. J Oral Maxillofac Surg 2007; 65: 2518–2523.
5. Esposito M, Grusovin M, Rees J, et al. Effectiveness of sinus lift procedures for dental implant rehabilitation: a Cochrane systematic review. Eur J Oral Implantol 2010; 3: 7–26.
6. Coachman C, Salama M, Garber D, et al. Prosthetic gingival reconstruction in a fixed partial restoration. Part 1: introduction to artificial gingiva as an alternative therapy. Int J Periodontics Restorative Dent 2009; 29 :471–477.
7. Coachman C, Salama M, Garber D, et al. Prosthetic gingival reconstruction in fixed partial restorations. Part 3: laboratory procedures and maintenance. Int J Periodontics Restorative Dent 2010; 30: 19–29.
8. Salama M, Coachman C, Garber D, et al. Prosthetic gingival reconstruction in the fixed partial restoration. Part 2: diagnosis and treatment planning. Int J Periodontics Restorative Dent 2009; 29: 573–581.
9. Sclar AG. Strategies for management of single tooth extraction sites in aesthetic implant therapy. J Oral Maxillofac Surg 2004; 62(Suppl 2): 90–105.
10. Fürhauser R, Florescu D, Benesch T, et al. Evaluation of soft tissue around single-tooth implant crowns: the pink esthetic score. Clin Oral Implants Res 2005; 16: 639–644.
11. Lai H, Zhang Z, Wang F, et al. Evaluation of soft tissue alteration around implant-supported single-tooth restoration in the anterior maxilla: the pink esthetic score. Clin Oral Implants Res 2008; 19: 560–564.
12. Belser U, Grütter L, Vailati F, et al. Outcome evaluation of early placed maxillary anterior single-tooth implants using objective esthetic criteria: a cross-sectional, retrospective study in 45 patients with a 2- to 4-year follow-up using pink and white esthetic scores. J Periodontol 2009; 80: 140–151.
13. Cho H, Lee J, Um H, Chang B. Esthetic evaluation of maxillary single-tooth implants in the esthetic zone. J Periodont Implant Sci 2010; 40: 188–193.
14. Grunder U, Gracis S, Capelli M. Influence of the 3-D bone-to-implant relationship on esthetics. Int J Periodontics Restorative Dent 2005; 25: 113–119.
15. Kan J, Rungcharassaeng K, Lozada J, Zimmerman G. Facial gingival tissue stability following immediate placement and provisionalization of maxillary anterior single implants: a 2- to 8-year follow-up. Int J Oral Maxillofac Implants 2011; 26: 179–187
16. Lee A, Fu J, Wang H. Soft tissue biotype affects implant success. Implant Dent 2011; 20: e38–e47.
17. Le B, Borzabadi-Farahani A. Labial bone thickness in areas of maxillary anterior implants associated with crestal labial soft tissue thickness. Implant Dent 2012; 21: 406–410.
18. Lekovic V, Kenney E, Weinlaender M, et al. A bone regenerative approach to alveolar ridge maintenance following tooth extraction. Report of 10 cases. J Periodontol 1997; 68: 563–570.
19. Lekovic V, Camargo P, Klokkevold P, et al. Preservation of alveolar bone in extraction sockets using bioabsorbable membranes. J Periodontol 1998; 69: 1044–1049.
20. Iasella J, Greenwell H, Miller R, et al. Ridge preservation with freeze-dried bone allograft and a collagen membrane compared to extraction alone for implant site development: a clinical and histologic study in humans. J Periodontol 2003; 74: 990–999.
21. Van der Weijden F, Dell'Acqua F, Slot D. Alveolar bone dimensional changes of post-extraction sockets in humans. J Clin Periodontol 2011; 36: 1048–1058.
22. Schropp L, Wenzel A, Kostopoulos L, Karring T. Bone healing and soft tissue contour changes following single-tooth extraction: a clinical and radiographic 12-month prospective study. Int J Periodontics Restorative Dent 2003; 23: 313–323.
23. Verna C, Dalstra M, Lee T, et al. Micro-cracks in the alveolar bone following orthodontic tooth movement: a morphological and morphometric study. Eur J Orthod 2004; 26: 459–467.
24. Novaes A, Macedo G, Suaid F, et al. Histologic evaluation of the buccal and lingual cortical bone plates in anterior dog teeth: possible influence on implant dentistry. J Periodontol 2011; 82: 872–877.
25. NanciA, ed. Repair and regeneration of oral tissues. In: Ten Cate's Oral Histology: Development, Structure, and Function. St. Louis, MO: Mosby Elsevier, 2008, pp. 388–389.
26. Cawson R, Odell E. Cawson's Essentials of Oral Pathology and Oral Medicine, 8th ed. Philadelphia, PA: Churchill Livingstone Elsevier, 2008, p. 114.
27. Amler M. The sequence of tissue regeneration in human extraction wounds. Oral Surg Oral Med Oral Pathol 1969; 27: 309–318.
28. Araújo M, Lindhe J. Dimensional ridge alterations following tooth extraction. An experimental study in the dog. J Clin Periodontol 2005; 32: 212–218.
29. Covani U, Ricci M, Bozzolo G, et al. Analysis of the pattern of alveolar ridge remodeling following single tooth extraction. Clin Oral Implants Res 2011; 22: 820–825.
30. Dahlin C, Linde A, Gottlow J, Nyman S. Healing of bone defects by guided tissue regeneration. Plast Reconstr Surg 1988; 81: 672–676.
31. Warrer L, Gotfredsen K, Hjørting-Hansen E, Karring T. Guided tissue regeneration ensures osseointegration of dental implants placed into extraction sockets. An experimental study in monkeys. Clin Oral Implants Res 1991; 2: 166–171.
32. Nemcovsky C, Serfaty V. Alveolar ridge preservation following tooth extraction of maxillary anterior teeth. Report on 23 consecutive cases. J Periodontol 1996; 67: 390–395.
33. Sclar AT. The Bio-Col technique. In: Soft Tissue and Esthetic Considerations in Implant Therapy. Chicago, IL: Quintessence, 2003, pp. 75–104.
34. Bartee B. The use of high density polytetrafluoroethylene to treat osseous defects: clinical reports. Implant Dent 1995; 4: 21–26.
35. Bartee B, Carr J. Evaluation of a high-density polytetrafluoroethylene membrane as a barrier to facilitate guided bone regeneration in the rat mandible. J Oral Implantol 1995; 21: 88–95.
36. Bartee B, Lignelli J. Guided tissue regeneration in implant dentistry: techniques for management of localized bone defects. In: Oral and Maxillofacial Surgery, vol. 1, 2nd ed, FonsecaR, BarberH, MathesonJ, eds. St. Louis, MO: Saunders Elsevier, 2009: 428–457.
37. Fotek P, Neiva R, Wang H. Comparison of dermal matrix and polytetrafluoroethylene membrane for socket bone augmentation: A clinical and histologic study. J Periodontol 2009; 80: 776–785.
38. Hoffmann O, Bartee B, Beaumont C, et al. Alveolar bone preservation in extraction sockets using non-resorbable dPTFE membranes: a retrospective non-randomized study. J Periodontol 2008; 79: 1355–1369.
39. Zafiropoulos G, Deli G, Bartee B, Hoffmann O. Single-tooth implant placement and loading in fresh and regenerated extraction sockets. Five-year results: a case series using two different implant designs. J Periodontol 2010; 81: 604–615.
40. Barboza E, Stutz B, Ferreira V, Carvalho W. Guided bone regeneration using non-expanded polytetrafluoroethylene membranes in preparation for dental implant placements: A report of 420 cases. Implant Dent 2010; 19: 2–7.
41. Barber HD, Lignelli J, Smith B, Bartee B. Using a dense PTFE membrane without primary closure to achieve bone and tissue regeneration. J Oral Maxillofac Surg 2007; 65: 748–752.
42. Nelson S, Thomas G. Bacterial persistence in dentoalveolar bone following extraction: a microbiological study and implications for dental implant treatment. Clin Implant Dent Relat Res 2010; 12: 306–314.
43. Cardaropoli G, Araújo M, Lindhe J. Dynamics of bone tissue formation in tooth extraction sites. An experimental study in dogs. J Clin Periodontol 2003; 30: 809–818.
44. Cardaropoli G, Araújo M, Hayacibara R, et al. Healing of extraction sockets and surgically produced – augmented and non-augmented – defects in the alveolar ridge. An experimental study in the dog. J Clin Periodontol 2005; 32: 435–440.
45. Lekholm U, Zarb G. Patient selection and preparation. In: Tissue-Integrated Protheses: Osseointegration in Clinical Dentistry, BrånemarkPI, ZarbG, AlbrektssonT, eds. Chicago, IL: Quintessence, 1985, pp. 199–208.

CHAPTER 6

Engineering Biologic Width and Tissue Levels with Implant and Abutment Surface Preparation

Myron Nevins,[1] Cary A. Shapoff,[2] Khalid Al Hezaimi,[3] & David M. Kim[1]
[1]Division of Periodontology, Department of Oral Medicine, Infection and Immunity, Harvard School of Dental Medicine, Boston, MA, USA
[2]Private Practice, Fairfield, CT, USA
[3]Research Chair for Growth Factors and Bone Regeneration, King Saud University, Riyadh, Saudi Arabia

Introduction

In the natural dentition, gingival collagen fibers attach directly via cementum to the tooth root surface by means of Sharpey's fibers,[1] with the junctional epithelium (JE) immediately occlusal to these fibers adhering to the tooth via hemi-desmosomes. Goldman described the Sharpey's fiber attachment to cementum as the physiologic factor preventing apical downgrowth of epithelium in the healthy periodontium.[2] In contrast, with the majority of dental implant devices, gingival connective tissue fibers generally do not attach to implant surfaces, but merely encircle the implant periphery as a fibrous tissue capsule.[3–5] However, implant collar surfaces treated by laser ablation have a surface topography allowing for a more tooth-like gingival attachment, and the information on this design concept will be discussed in this chapter.

The mucosal barrier surrounding dental implants is referred to as the peri-implant "biologic width," a term borrowed from the natural dentition.[6] This biologic seal exists around dental implants generally at the level of the implant to abutment interface ("microgap") with two-piece implants. It consists of epithelial and connective tissue components. The thickness of connective tissue has been shown to be approximately 1.5 mm,[7] which, as stated, takes the form of a fibrous capsule with collagen fibers oriented circumferentially. If this thickness is less than 1.5 mm, crestal bone loss will occur until the minimal thickness is established. This was shown by Berglundh and Lindhe[8] in a dog study in which the investigators thinned the connective tissue portion on the inside aspect of peri-implant flaps at the time of abutment connection and studied the healing response microscopically. Wound healing of the area consistently demonstrated bone loss to accommodate for the re-establishment of the required connective tissue thickness. Since connective tissue fibers do not insert directly into the implant surface, a true seal cannot be formed; as a consequence, peri-implant soft tissues display inflammatory cell infiltrates more or less universally.[9]

The laser-ablated surface

Laser treatment of implant surfaces is termed "laser ablation," and this can be used to create precise circumferential microgrooves in the transgingival neck and/or abutment segments of dental implants by metal vaporization, localized melting, and rapid resolidification. This type of implant surface microgeometry has been shown to have directional effects on the orientation of bone cells, fibroblasts, and epithelial cells, both *in vitro* and *in vivo*. For example, Ricci and coworkers[10–12] reported that cultured fibroblasts grown on microgrooved polystyrene surfaces vapor-deposited with titanium oxide became oriented or channeled ("contact guidance") in the direction of the grooves. In comparison, the same cells grown on non-grooved surfaces showed a random growth pattern. Fibroblast orientation by grooved substrates also determines the pattern of collagen synthesis by these cells in culture.[13] Groove widths and depths of 6–12 μm appeared to channel cells most efficiently.[11] Specifically, 12 μm grooves appeared the most hospitable to bone cells while inhibiting fibrous tissue growth relative to bone cell growth, whereas 8 μm grooves promoted horizontal orientation of fibroblasts while also inhibiting their migration across the grooves, in effect acting as a fibroblast migration barrier.

Weiner et al.[14] used a dog model to examine the responses of crestal bone, soft connective tissue, and epithelium to laser microtextured collars used on particle-blasted, threaded dental implants. Overall collar length was 2 mm, and was prepared with three different surface zones. The deepest zone of 0.8 mm width received computer-controlled, laser-ablated microgrooves of 12 μm width and 10 ± 3 μm depth. The middle zone of 0.7 mm width received microgrooves of 8 μm width and 4 ± 1 μm depth, while the uppermost 0.5 mm of collar had a machine-turned (i.e. relatively smooth or planar) surface. Control implants had collars that were fully machine-turned. Histometric data were prepared for unloaded implants as well as for those loaded for 3 or 6 months. Unloaded test implants that had healed in a submerged condition for 3 months showed either bone or soft tissue elements on the microgrooves depending on the characteristics of the host tissue in contact with the implant surface. The machined collar surfaces of unloaded control implants showed only soft tissues. For loaded test implants, epithelial tissue was in contact primarily with the machine-turned coronal 0.5 mm of collar. The laser-created microgrooves showed soft connective tissue attachment more coronally and bone attachment more apically. The machine-turned collars (MTCs) of loaded control implants showed mostly soft tissue contact and greater crestal bone saucerization than did test implants. Somewhat similar findings were published by Shin and Han[15] using the same implant designs, but with immediate implantation into dog extraction sockets followed by 3 months' healing before animal termination.

Minimally Invasive Dental Implant Surgery, First Edition. Edited by Daniel R. Cullum and Douglas Deporter.

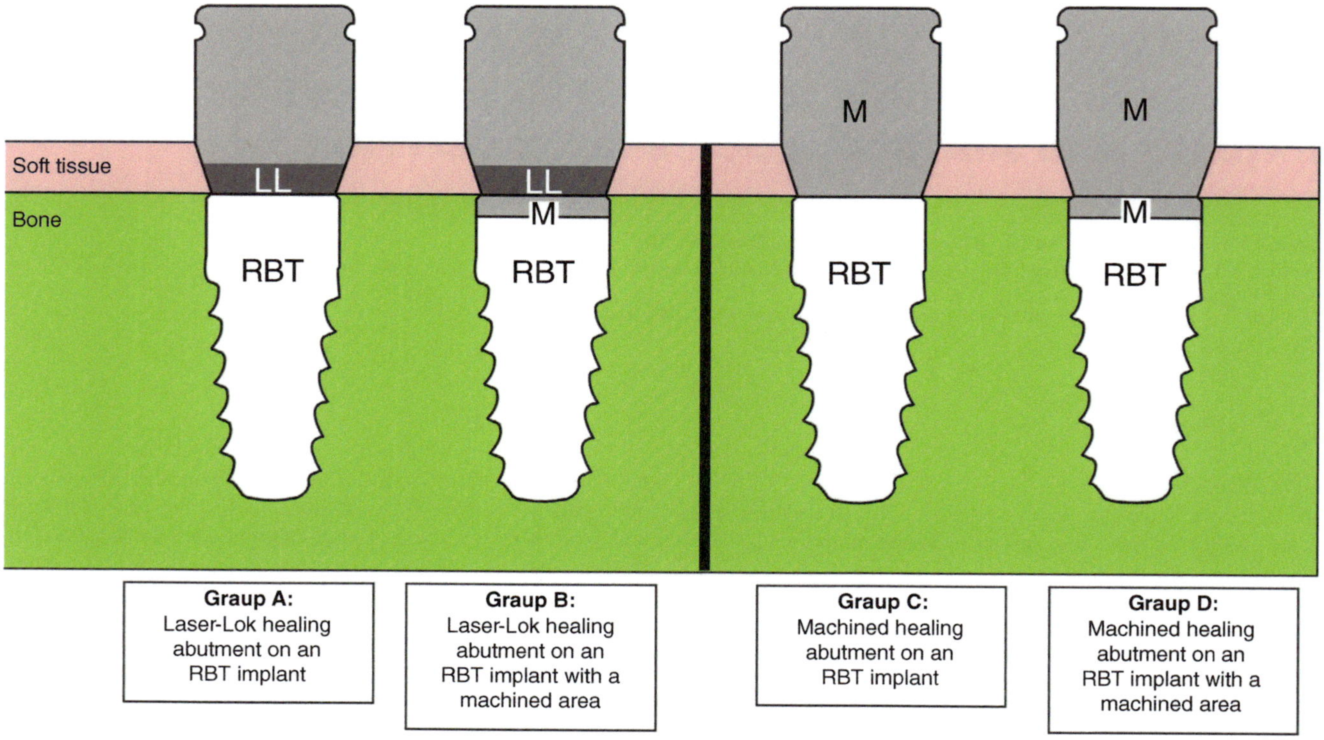

Figure 6.1 The four cohorts. LL: Laser-Lok® (BioHorizons, Birmingham, AL); RBT: resorbable blast texturing; M: machined surface.

However, substantial resorption of buccal bone occurred as the extraction socket walls remodeled, thus reducing the benefit of the laser microgrooves on buccal compared with lingual surfaces.

Nevins et al.[16] also used a dog model to study healing in relation to 8 μm wide laser-ablated microgrooves created on implant abutments rather than on implant collars. All implants were threaded with particle-blasted surfaces, and four implant–abutment combinations were studied (Figure 6.1). Group A consisted of implants that were fully particle-blasted; that is, had no MTC segment. Their abutments had an apical (i.e. immediately coronal to the implant-abutment microgap) 0.7 mm wide zone of laser microgrooves. Group B implants had a 0.3 mm wide MTC and their abutments were identical to group A. Group C implants had fully particle-blasted surfaces and fully machine-turned abutments, while group D implants had a 0.3 mm MTC and fully machine-turned abutments.

Every effort was made to place the implant prosthetic platforms level with the osseous crest (Figure 6.2) in order to allow later accurate histologic assessment of remodeled crestal bone levels. All abutments were installed at the time of implant placement surgery, and 3 months healing was allowed before animal termination. Abutment types were assigned randomly to each implant (Figure 6.3).

Histologic, high-resolution micro-computed tomography (CT), and scanning electron microscopy (SEM) observations of groups A and B demonstrated bone and soft connective tissue attachments (Figures 6.4, 6.5, 6.6, and 6.7), with the latter showing

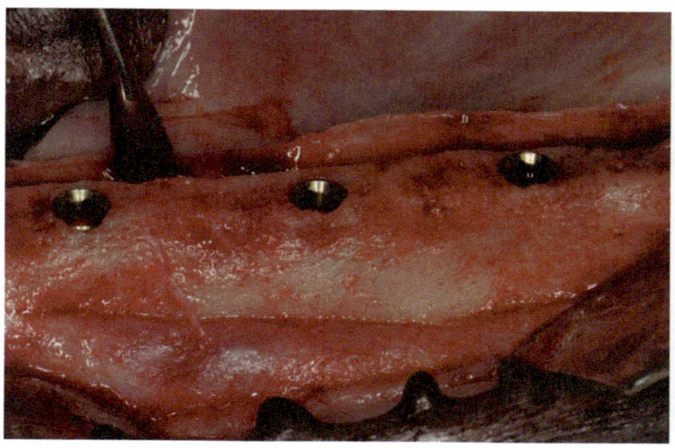

Figure 6.2 Implant platforms were placed as level as possible with the osseous crest to allow for accurate histologic assessment of crestal bone levels.

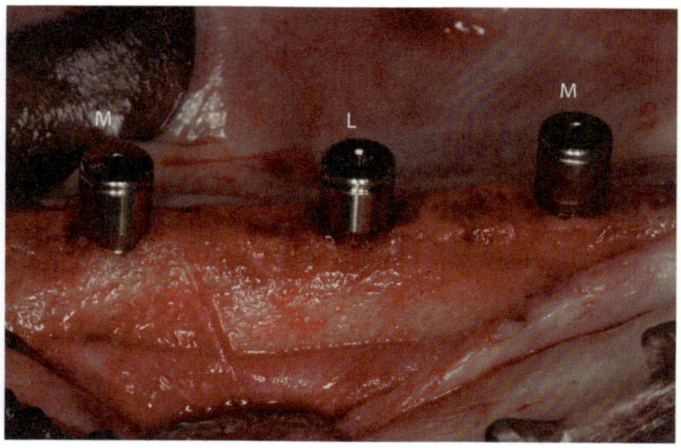

Figure 6.3 LL microgrooved healing abutment (L) and standard machined-surface healing abutments (M) were placed on the implants at the time of implant placement.

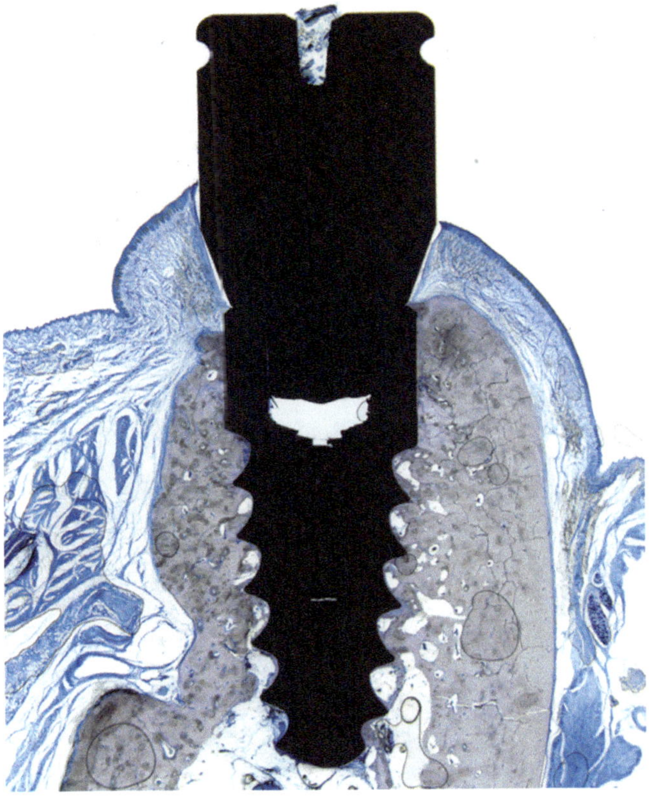

Figure 6.4 Bucco-lingual light microscopic section of a group A specimen demonstrating osseointegration and crestal bone levels.

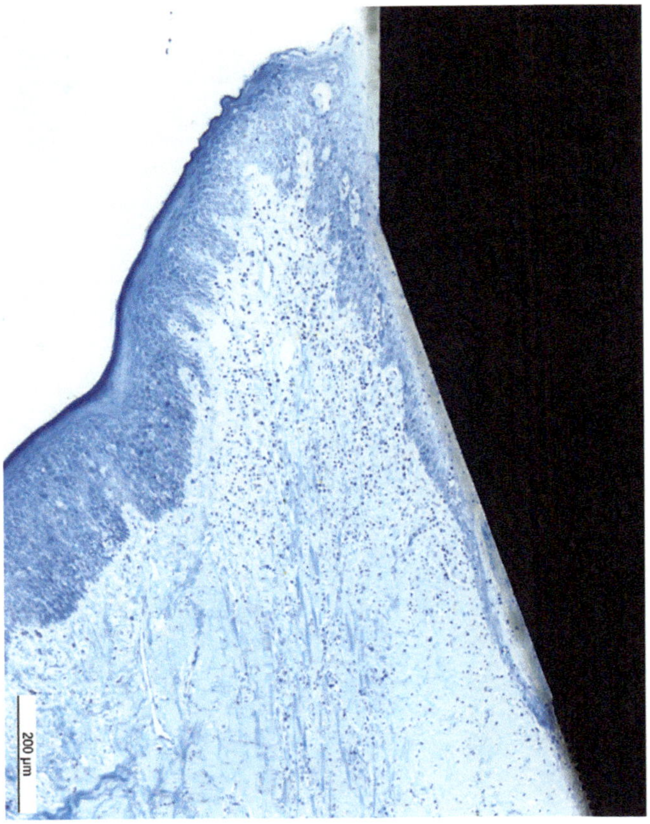

Figure 6.5 At group A sites, the JE ended at the coronal-most LL grooved area. Apical to the JE, healthy connective tissue fibers attached perpendicularly to the laser-ablated channels.

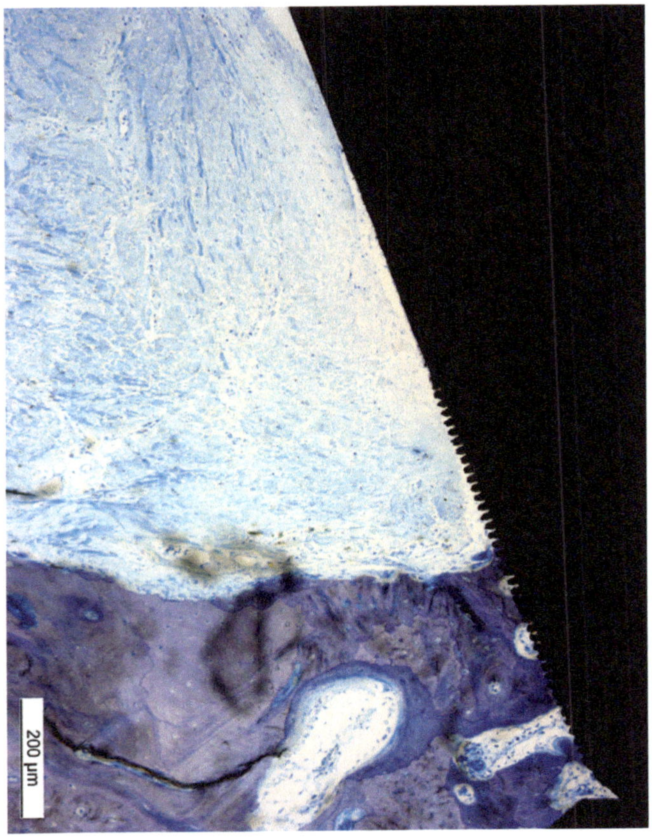

Figure 6.6 In this group A specimen, regenerated bone was attached to the LL abutment surface and the IAJ microgap was eliminated.

perpendicularly oriented fibers in relation to the microgrooves on test abutments. Apical migration of JE was inhibited and crestal bone resorption prevented by the laser-treated zone on the abutments. In group A, there was even bone growth into the microgap and onto the abutment microgrooves in some specimens (Figure 6.6). Micro-CT examination corroborated the histologic findings. SEM examination demonstrated dense connective tissue networks attached to laser microgrooves (Figure 6.7). A more or less similar outcome was seen

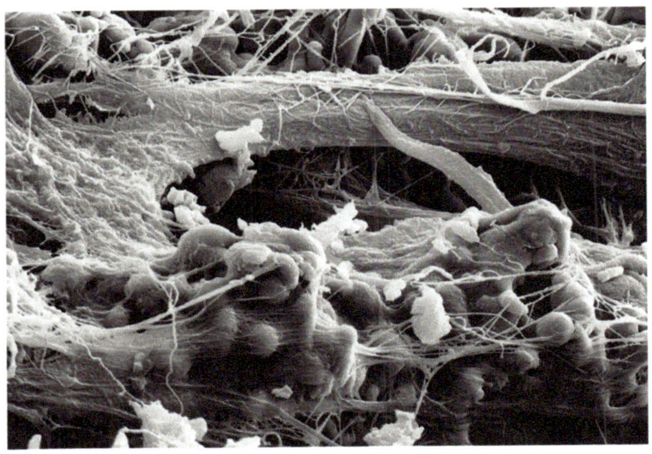

Figure 6.7 Intense fibroblastic cellular activity and dense networks of connective tissue fibers occurred on the LL microgrooved areas of abutments in all group A specimens.

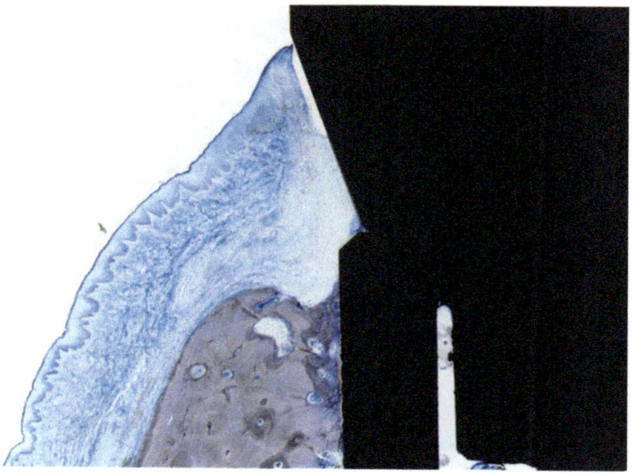

Figure 6.8 A light microscopic section of a group B specimen demonstrating native and new bone (darker stain) on the implant surface. This probably is the result of the correction of drilling disparity, but it is evidenced that the supracrestal connective tissue fiber has prohibited apical migration of epithelium, allowing the bone to respond in an aseptic environment.

with group B specimens. The abutment microgrooved zones showed oriented connective tissue attachment, inhibition of JE migration, and limited crestal bone loss (Figures 6.8 and 6.9).

In group C (fully particle-blasted implants with fully machine-turned abutments), the formation of a long JE along the abutment and particle-blasted collar segments prevented oriented connective tissue attachment (Figure 6.10). A similar outcome was seen in group D (0.3 mm MTC and fully machine-turned abutment) with the addition of some crestal bone loss adjacent to the MTC (Figure 6.11) In

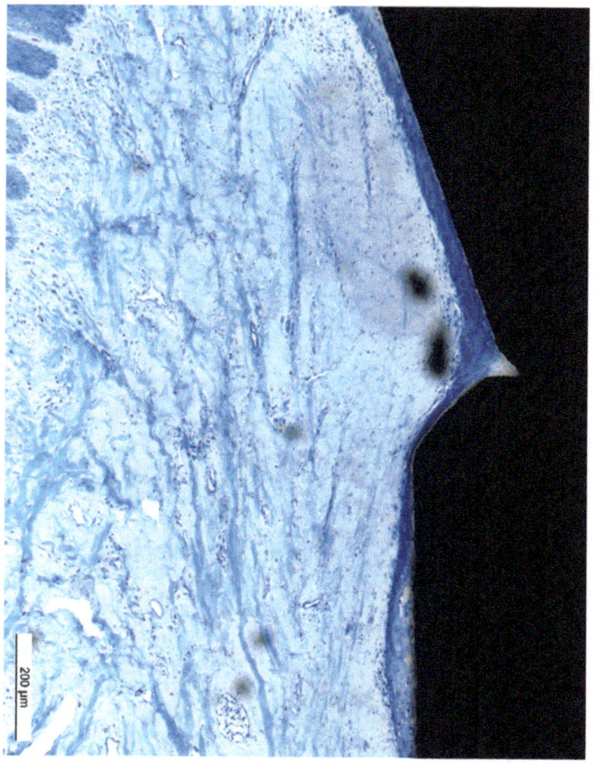

Figure 6.10 A group C specimen with a long JE seen along the abutment and implant MTC surfaces, preventing connective tissue fibers from forming the protective barrier seen in groups A and B.

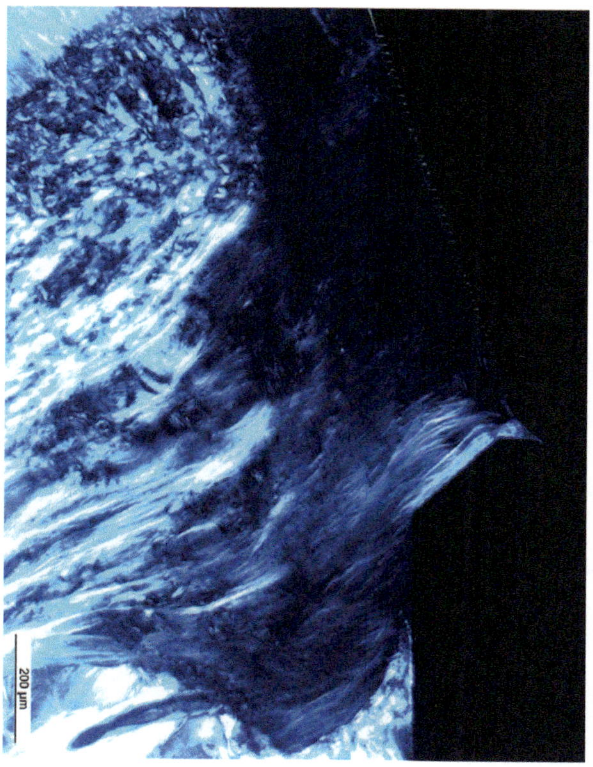

Figure 6.9 A polarized light microscopic view of a group B specimen demonstrating perpendicularly oriented connective tissue fibers against the entire surface of the LL microgrooved area.

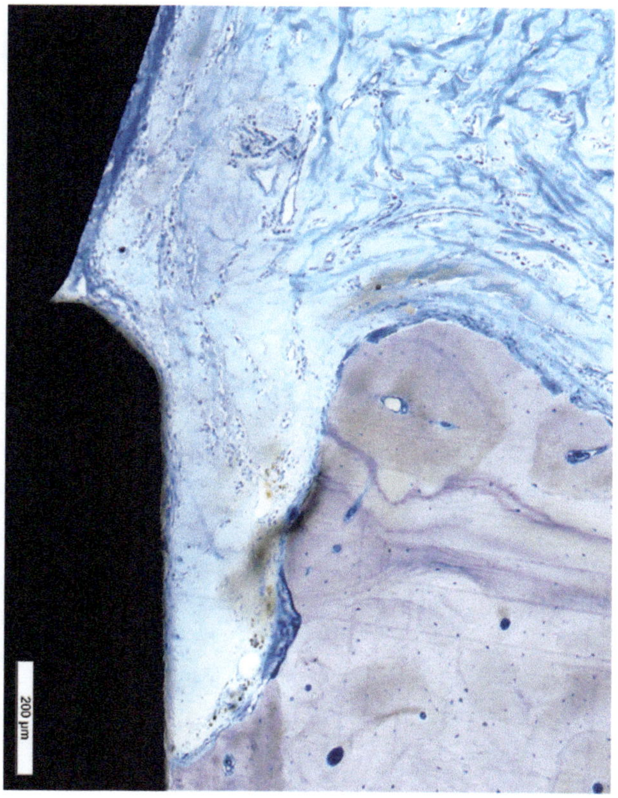

Figure 6.11 A group D high-power specimen demonstrated apical JE migration, resulting in significant crestal bone resorption.

both groups C and D, micrograps were never protected by bone or connective tissue attachment, making them more likely to be contaminated with microbial plaque.[17]

Human histologic evidence of a connective tissue attachment to a dental implant

The first human proof-of-principle study with implants having laser-ablated surfaces on their collar segments was done using the LL dental implant device by Nevins et al.[18] (Figure 6.12). The study was designed to investigate the possibility of achieving a physical connective tissue attachment to laser-created microgrooves on the implant collar segment. Four patients were selected to receive enough implants so that one implant per patient could be harvested for examination, while the remaining implants would allow for an implant-supported restoration. Implants had collars with three distinct surface treatments. The most apical 0.8 mm of collar (i.e. at the level of implant–abutment connection) had laser-created microgrooves of 12 μm width and 12 μm depth. An intermediate 0.7 mm collar zone had microgrooves of 8 μm width and 6 μm depth, while the most coronal 0.5 mm zone of collar had a machine-turned surface finish (Figure 6.12). Healing abutments were delivered at the time of initial implant placement. Every effort was made at that time to ensure that the 0.7 mm zone meant to develop soft tissue attachment was supracrestal both mesially and distally. The patients were monitored at 1, 2, 3, 4, 8, 12, and 24 weeks after surgery to ensure adequate supragingival plaque removal and, if need be, given repeated oral hygiene instruction. At 6 months, the four designated implants were harvested *en bloc* together with the adjacent soft and hard tissues so as to preserve the soft tissue attachment. The specimens were then prepared for examination using light microscopy, SEM, and micro-CT.

The implants were osseointegrated with histologic evidence of direct bone contact (Figures 6.13 and 6.14). There was a connective tissue attachment to the LL microgrooves with no signs of inflammation. Peri-implant soft tissues consisted of a dense, collagenous lamina propria covered with a stratified, squamous, keratinizing epithelium that was continuous with a para-keratinized sulcular epithelium that lined the lateral surface of the peri-implant sulcus (Figure 6.14). Between the apical termination of JE and alveolar bone crest, connective tissue was directly apposed onto implant surface (Figure 6.15). Polarized light microscopy of this area confirmed functionally oriented

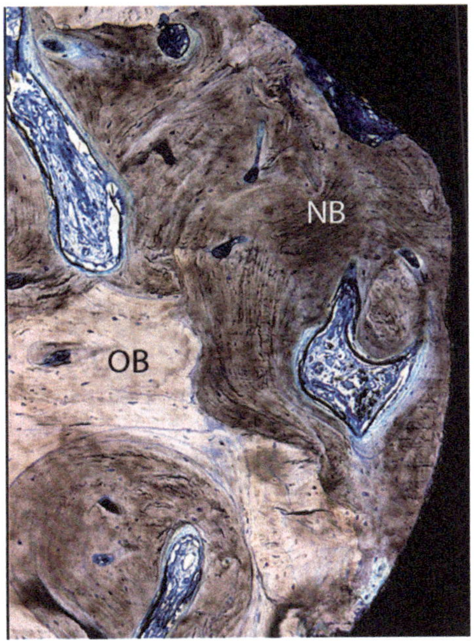

Figure 6.13 A ground section showing intimate osseointegration of this implant. Note the intense remodeling activity in the area of newly formed bone (NB). OB: local old bone.

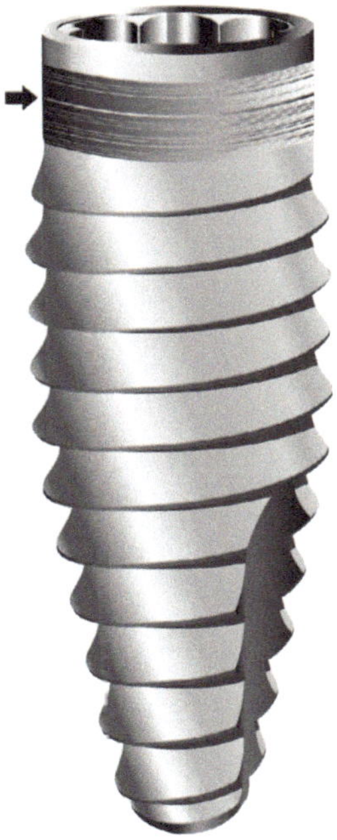

Figure 6.12 The LL collar of a dental implant. The most coronal zone of 0.5 mm has a machine-turned surface. The black arrow distinguishes the upper laser-ablated zone, which consists of 8 μm microgrooves that are 6 μm deep, from the lower laser-ablated zone, which consist of 12 μm microgrooves that are 12 μm deep.

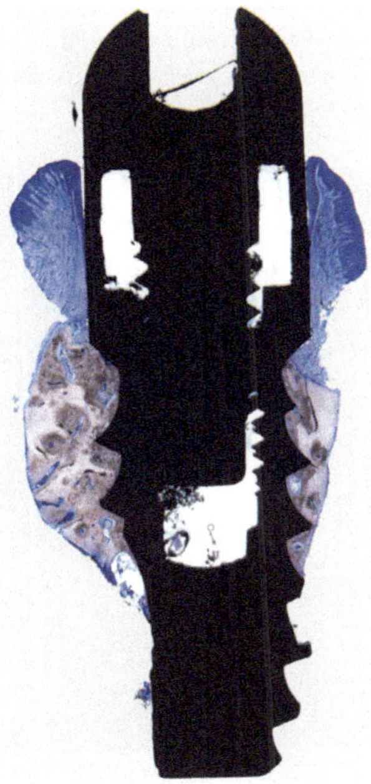

Figure 6.14 A ground section of specimen stained with toluidine blue–Azure II.

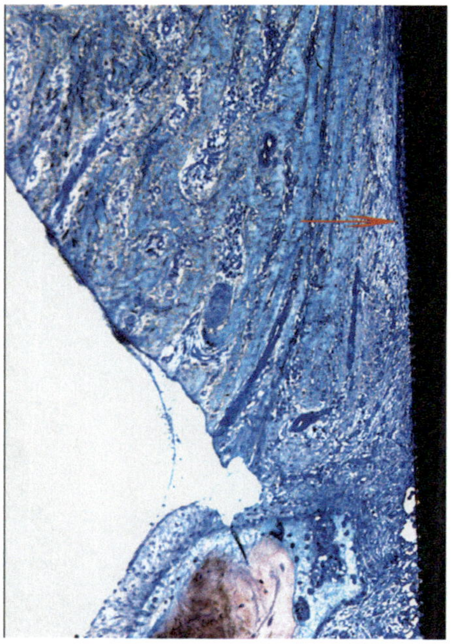

Figure 6.15 Higher magnification of Figure 6.14 identifies the apical extent of the JE (red arrow). There is a connective tissue attachment to the laser microchannel surface that extends to the point of bone attachment.

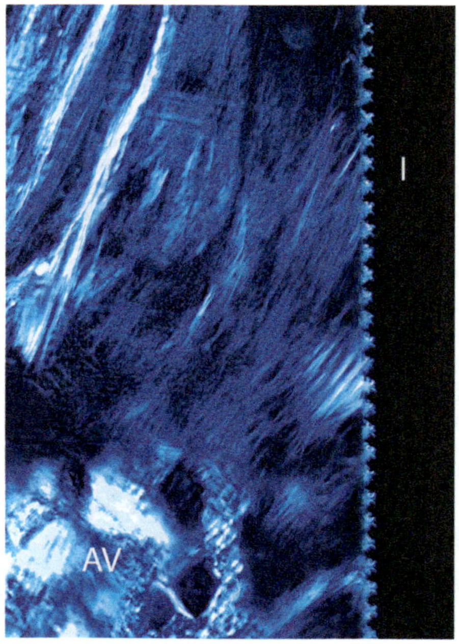

Figure 6.16 View of the connective tissue in contact with the laser microgrooves (Figure 6.14 at higher magnification and with polarized light). Note the functional orientation of the collagen fibers toward the implant surface. I: implant; AV: alveolar bone crest.

collagen fibers extending toward the surface microgrooves (Figure 6.16), while SEM of a corresponding area of the specimen confirmed the presence of physically attached collagen fibers (Figures 6.17 and 6.18). It appeared that the connective tissue attachment was instrumental in inhibiting apical migration of the epithelium, thus preserving crestal bone.

A follow-up human proof-of-principle study[19] examined the effect of providing laser-ablated microgrooves on implant abutment surfaces (Figure 6.19). Two patients requiring multiple implants to restore their missing dentition completed informed consent to receive an extra implant that could be removed without affecting their treatment. Implants were placed as level to the osseous crest as possible, and healing abutments with laser-ablated microgrooves added immediately. Flaps were closed tension free. At 10 weeks, one implant from each patient was removed *en bloc* together with adjacent soft and hard tissues, and the removal sites reconstructed to restore natural ridge contour. Histologic examination demonstrated normal peri-abutment soft tissues without evidence of inflammatory cell infiltrate at the implant-to-abutment junction (IAJ) at low magnification (Figures 6.20, 6.21, 6.22, 6.23, 6.24, and 6.25). Excellent bone-to-implant contact was noted with no evidence of crestal bone loss (Figure 6.20). At higher magnification, dense connective tissue was in intimate contact with the abutment surface microgrooves. Healthy connective tissue extended apically into the IAJ with no signs of the inflammatory

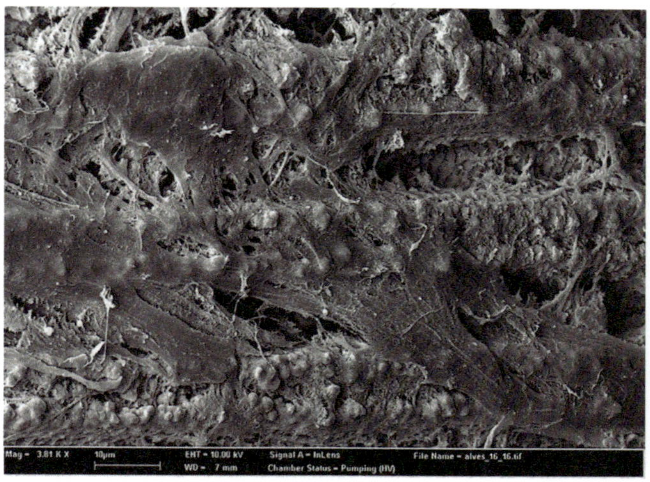

Figure 6.17 SEM image showing collagen fibers attached to the rough implant surface (original magnification ×3810).

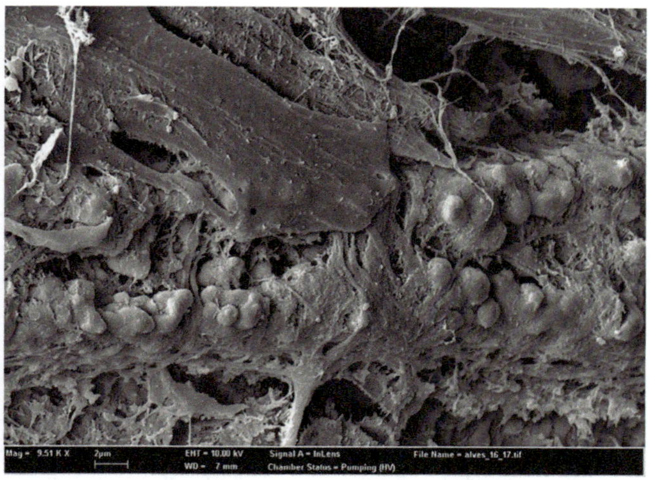

Figure 6.18 Higher magnification of area shown in Figure 6.17 (original magnification ×9510).

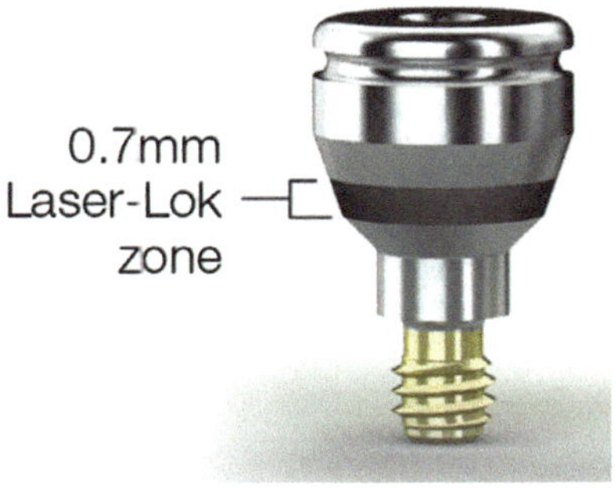

Figure 6.19 Healing abutment with a 0.7 mm LL microgrooved zone.

cell infiltrates frequently described at this junction.[9] Equally important, there was no evidence of epithelial migration along the surface of the abutment (Figures 6.20, 6.21, 6.22, 6.24, and 6.25).

Polarized light imagery of mesial and distal surfaces revealed dense, obliquely oriented connective tissue fibers attaching directly to the LL grooved abutment surfaces (Figure 6.25). In addition, connective tissue had interposed itself directly into the region of the IAJ, effectively eliminating microgap-propagated inflammatory problems.

Another LL healing abutment study was performed by Geurs et al.[20] In two patients, laser-ablated healing abutments along with their surrounding soft tissues were biopsied after 6 weeks of healing. Once again, collagen fibers were attached and oriented perpendicular to the microgrooved surface.

Pecora et al.[21] provided prospective, controlled clinical data for a group of 15 patients and 20 pairs of LL and control implants. Both implant models were tapered, threaded, and particle-blasted. The test implant was the implant device used by Nevins et al.,[18] while the control implant had a 2 mm collar that was fully machine-turned (MTCs). During 37 months of clinical monitoring, the test LL implants showed significantly less pocket probing depth than controls, while at

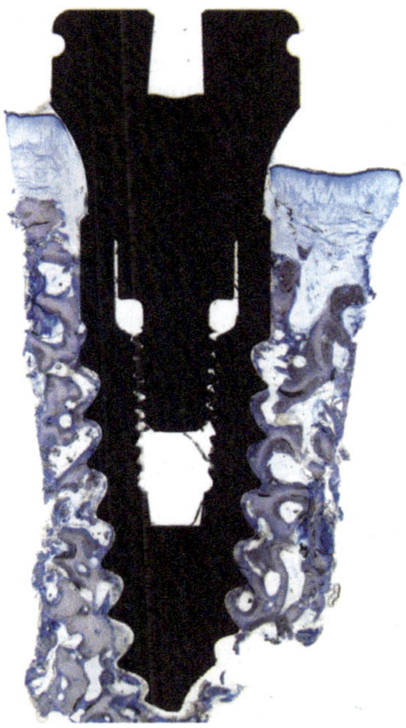

Figure 6.20 At low magnification, peri-abutment soft tissues are healthy with no inflammatory cell infiltrate at the IAJ. A long JE is absent, and excellent bone-to-implant contact is noted at all implant threads.

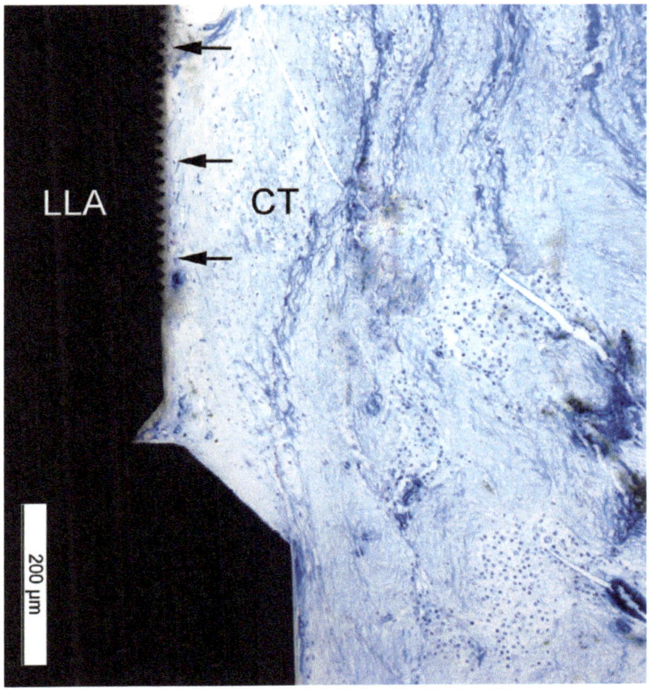

Figure 6.21 At higher magnification, direct contact (arrows) is seen between the abutment microchannels and adjacent connective tissue. Evidence of a long JE is absent. LLA: LL abutment; CT: connective tissue.

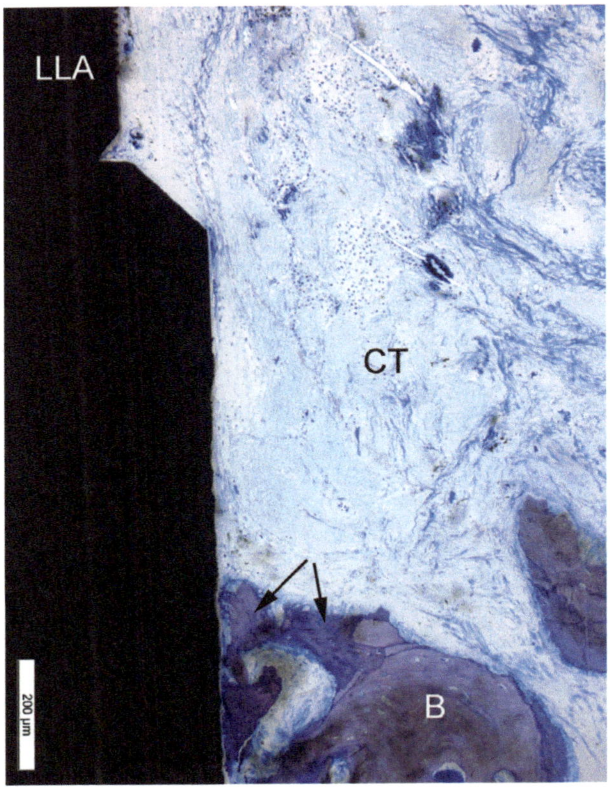

Figure 6.22 Crestal bone can be seen in close contact with the implant collar surface, with no evidence of bone loss apparent, and even new bone formation (arrows). LLA: LL abutment; CT: connective tissue; B: bone.

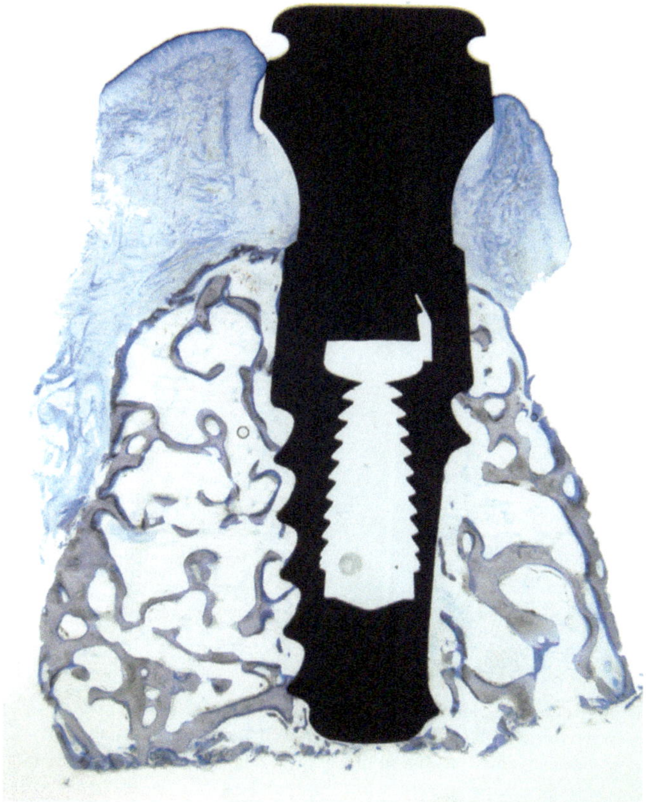

Figure 6.23 Low power view of an *en bloc* specimen to show healthy connective tissue against all borders of the abutment surface. No evidence is seen of crestal bone loss on either side of the implant collar.

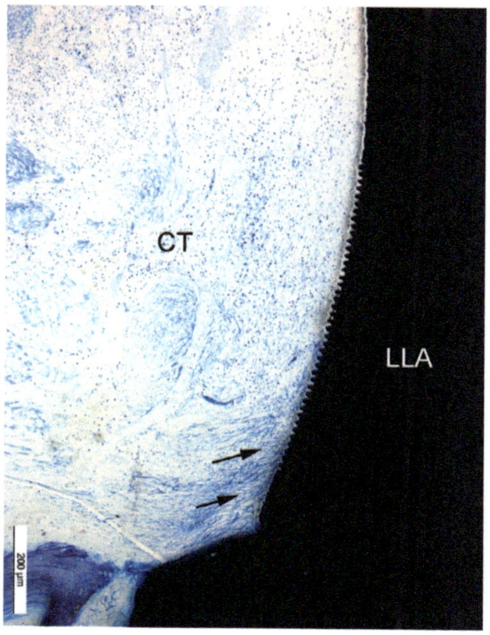

Figure 6.24 At higher power, dense connective tissue (arrows) is seen in intimate contact with the abutment microgrooved surface. LLA: LL abutment; CT: connective tissue.

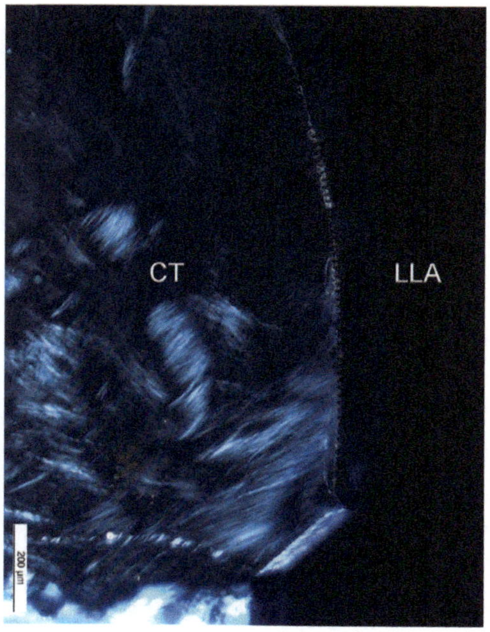

Figure 6.25 Polarized light image to demonstrate dense, obliquely oriented connective tissue fibers inserting directly into the laser microchannel abutment surface. LLA: LL abutment; CT: connective tissue.

7 months and later they also showed less crestal bone loss (0.59 mm versus 1.94 mm) in radiographs. Similar results were presented by Botos et al.[22] who placed LL as test and Nobel Select® (NS; Nobel Biocare, Gothenburg, Sweden) as control, the latter implants having fully machined collars. Fifteen edentulous patients each received two of each implant type in the interforaminal region of mandible. One of each type was loaded immediately by supporting ball-retained overdentures, while the remaining two implants in each patient acted as non-loaded controls. Pocket probing depths and crestal bone loss for loaded LL implants were both significantly less than for controls at 6 and 12 months (e.g. 0.72 mm versus 1.13 mm bone loss at 12 months). Bone loss was also less for non-loaded LL implants.

The radiographic data for bone loss with LL implants presented by Pecora et al.[21] and Botos et al.[22] were similar to earlier non-controlled retrospective data from a long-term study presented by Shapoff et al.[23] This study was conducted in a single private office on 41 consecutively treated patients (mean age, 62 years) who received 60 LL dental implants between February 2005 and January 2007. Using the submerged healing technique, 37 implants were placed in the maxilla and 13 were placed in the mandible. Thirty-nine (78%) of the 50 implants were placed in the anterior regions, and the remaining 11 implants (22%) were placed in molar sites. At re-entry after a mean healing time of 4.8 months, laser-treated abutments were connected to the healed implants.

Post-operative radiographs were taken after re-entry, after final restoration, and at 1, 2, and 3 years of function. These digital radiographs were imported into Photoshop CS3 with Analysis Toolkit for analysis. Mesial and distal crestal perpendicular bone lengths were standardized with known mid-axis implant lengths. Crestal bone lengths were then averaged per implant, and the mean bone level changes computed. There was one implant failure as a result of an endodontic abscess of an adjacent tooth, making a total of 49 implants available for radiographic analysis. Crestal bone levels were expressed in

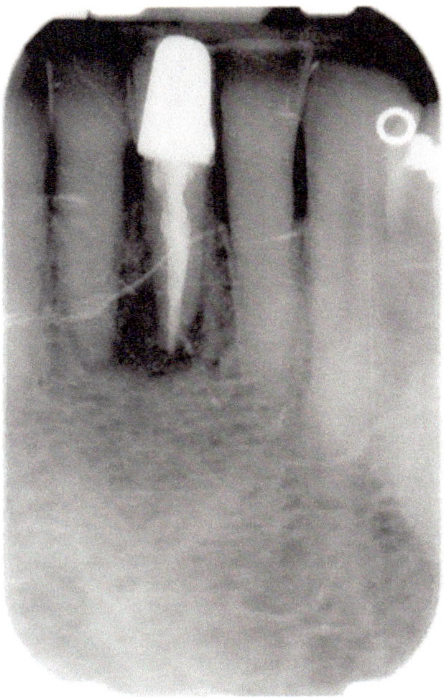

(a)

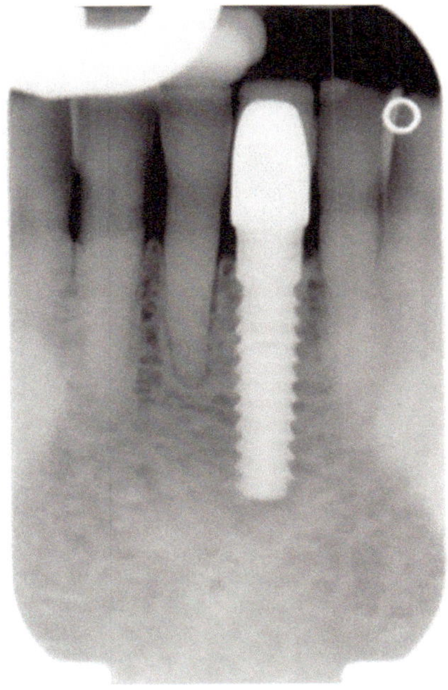

(b)

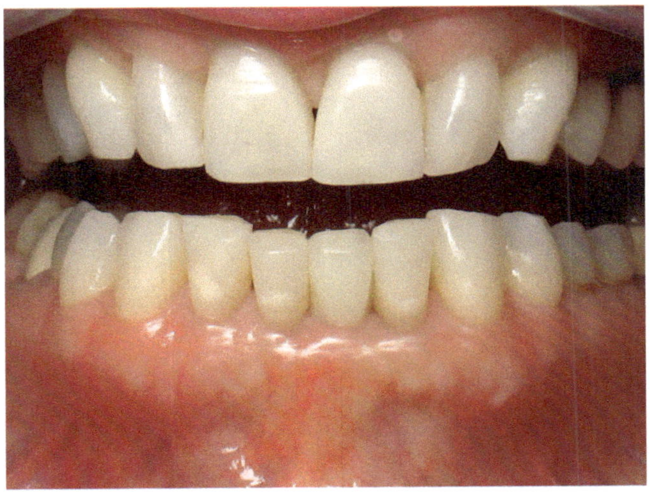

(c)

Figure 6.26 (a) Initial radiograph of a defect around the mandibular left central incisor. The site showed complete loss of the facial plate, and the implant was placed using a staged protocol with bone graft and resorbable barrier membrane. (b) Two-year radiograph of restored case demonstrating stable crestal bone level. (c) Two-year clinical picture of (b).

millimeters from the top of the implant platform to the first bone-to-implant contact. Forty-one of the original 49 implants had post-restoration radiographs after 2 years (Figure 6.26), while 30 implants had radiographs after 3 years (Figure 6.27a–e). A small number of implants were followed radiographically for even longer periods of time (Figure 6.27f). The mean crestal bone level change after 2 years was −0.44 ± 0.10 mm, while the mean change after 3 years was −0.46 ± 0.12 mm. No statistically significant differences in the mean bone loss could be detected between years 2 and 3 ($p > 0.05$). In addition, data from implants placed in edentulous sites, previously grafted sites, or as immediate implants did not show statistically significant differences. The minimal bone loss seen with laser microchannel abutment surfaces may be partially due to minimization of crestal bone stress. Alexander et al.[24] used finite element analyses to compare stresses predicted following axial and side loading for implants with laser-treated versus MTCs. The LL treated collars were predicted to exhibit significantly lower peak stress on crestal bone (22.6 MPa for laser versus 91.9 MPa for machine-turned).

Clinical application of a LL 3.5 mm platform implant (BioHorizons, Birmingham, AL) can be seen with three-year follow-up findings for a 21-year-old female patient with restoration of a congenitally missing maxillary lateral incisor (Figure 6.28). This patient demonstrated crestal/interproximal bone stability on periapical radiograph and clinical soft tissue health and esthetics.

An example of an immediate extraction and implant placement for a maxillary right central incisor can be seen on the radiograph in Figure 6.29a for a 78-year-old female after 2 years of implant function (4.5 mm platform LL tapered internal implant; Biohorizons, Birmingham, AL) (Figure 6.29a). A clinical photograph of the 2-year result is presented in Figure 6.29b.

A final case demonstration is seen in Figure 6.30a with radiographic findings at 10 years after placement of a prototype LL microchannel 1 mm collar implant. Crestal bone levels can be seen within 0.5 mm of the top of the collar. Clinical photographic images of the restoration after 8 years demonstrate maintenance of gingival papilla height and facial contour (Figure 6.30b).

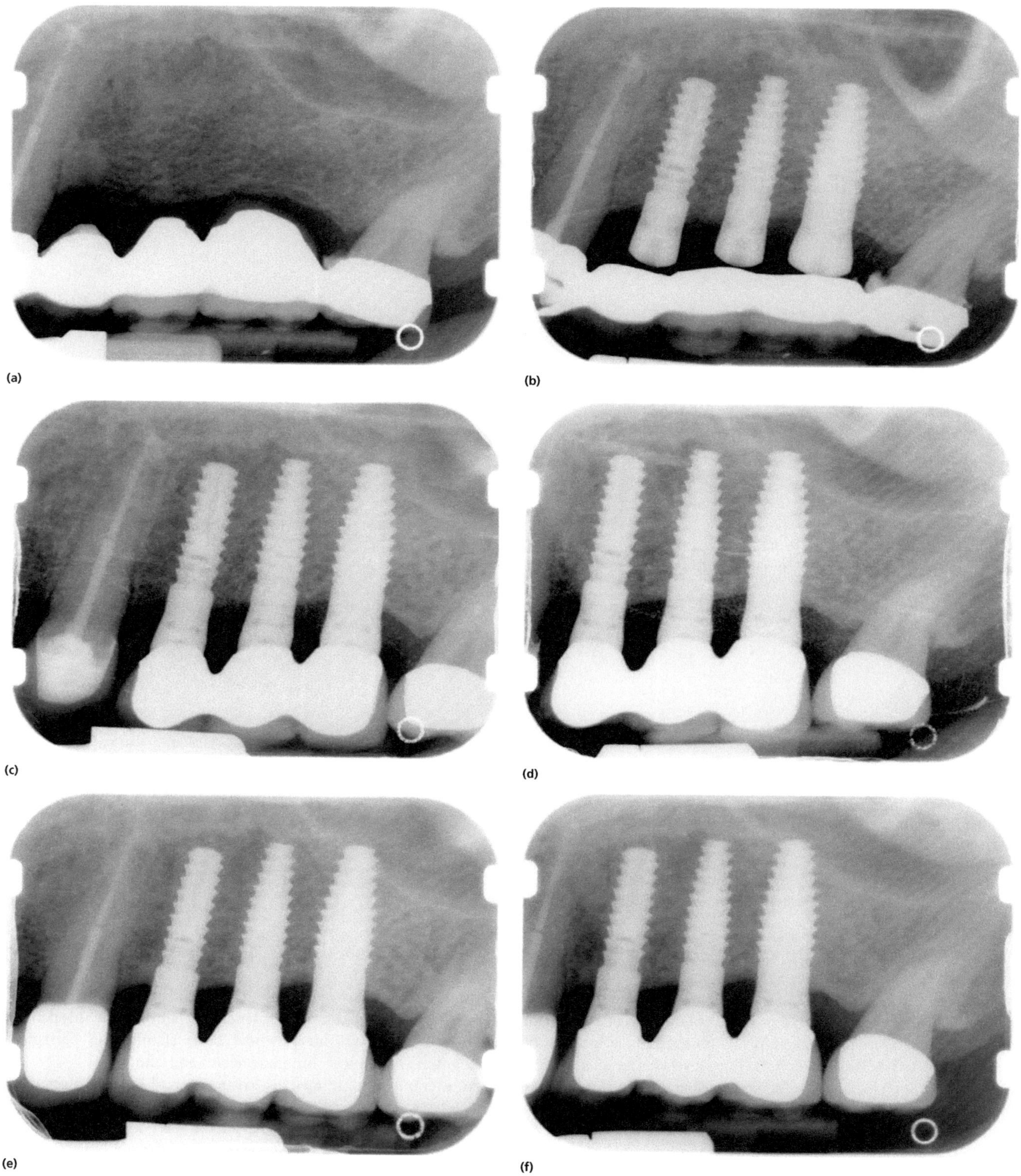

Figure 6.27 (a–c) A patient with a failed fixed partial denture in the maxillary left posterior region. A CT scan revealed a ridge width of 4–5 mm, requiring a ridge-splitting technique at the time of implant placement: (a) initial radiograph; (b) digital radiograph of the implants placed; (c) after 1 year in function. (d–f) Long-term post-restoration follow-up digital radiographs demonstrate crestal bone stability at (d) 2 years, (e) 3 years, and (f) 4 years.

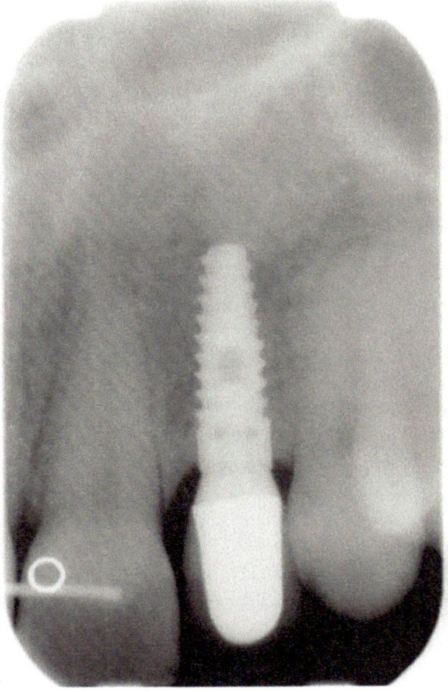
(a)

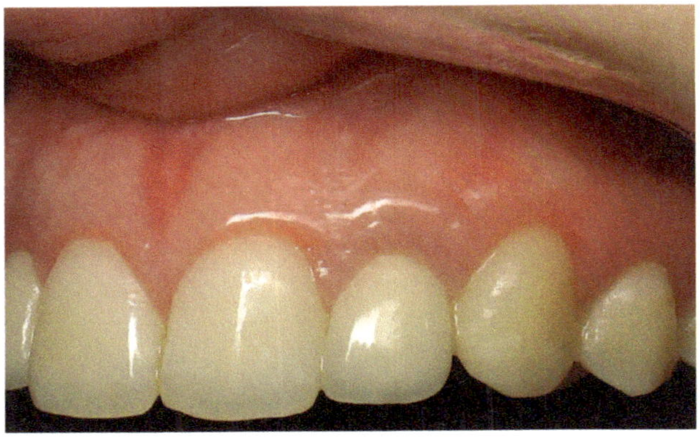
(b)

Figure 6.28 (a) Radiograph at 3 years of a LL 3.5 mm platform implant (BioHorizons, Birmingham, AL) placed in a narrow ridge of a congenitally missing left maxillary lateral incisor in this 21-year-old female. (b) Clinical photograph of restored maxillary lateral incisor. Note crestal bone level at coronal aspect of LL microchannel collar.

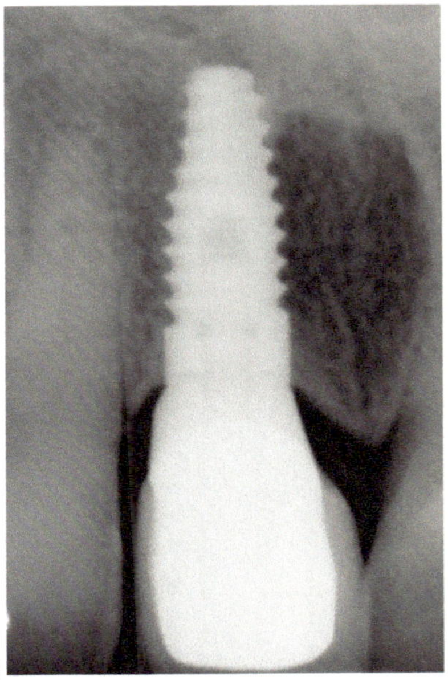
(a)

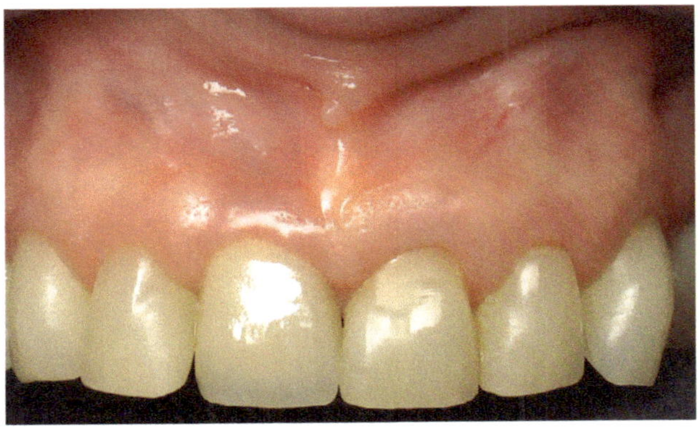
(b)

Figure 6.29 (a) Radiograph at 2 years following immediate extraction and implant placement of the maxillary right central incisor with a 4.5 mm platform LL tapered internal implant (BioHorizons, Birmingham, AL). (b) Clinical photograph of 2-year result in 78-year-old female.

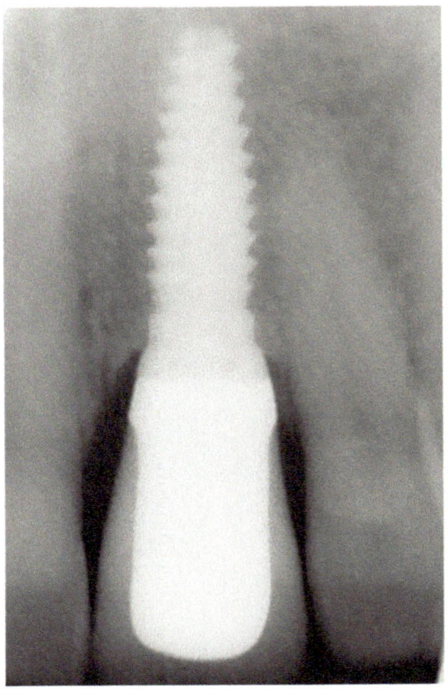
(a)

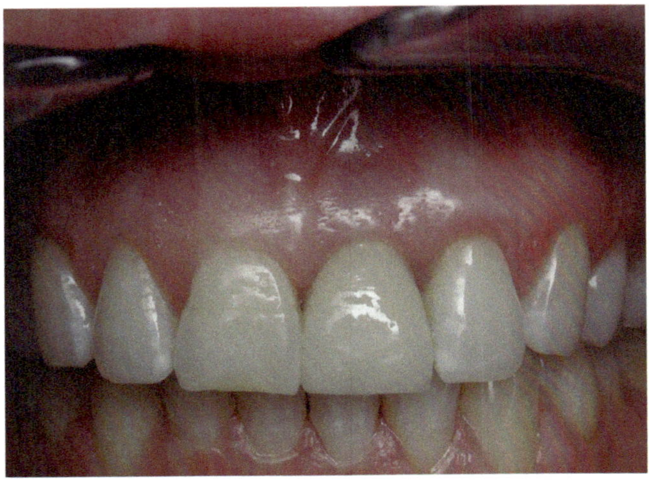
(b)

Figure 6.30 (a) Radiograph at 10 years utilizing prototype LL microtextured 1 mm collar implant. Note crestal bone levels within 0.5 mm of top of collar. (b) Clinical photograph of restored implant at 8 years with maintenance of gingival papilla height and facial contour.

Conclusions

Surface microgrooves of a defined size range can be created on implant collar and abutment surfaces by laser ablation, and result in a true peri-implant oriented soft connective tissue attachment much like that seen on the cementum layer of a natural tooth root surface. This type of soft tissue attachment to the implant collar appears to limit crestal bone loss and reduce the likelihood of soft tissue inflammation, assuming good patient home care. The question remains, however, whether these beneficial effects can be maintained over time with repeated perturbations of the soft tissue attachment during function and maintenance care. This key question begs long-term clinical study.

References

1. Nanci A. Periodontium. In: Ten Cate's Oral Histology. Development, Structure and Function. St. Louis, MO: Mosby Elsevier, 2013, pp. 205–232.
2. Goldman H. The behavior of transseptal fibers in periodontal disease. J Dent Res 1957; 36: 249–254.
3. Listgarten M, Lang N, Schroeder H, Schroeder A. Periodontal tissues and their counterparts around endosseous implants. Clin Oral Implants Res 1991; 2: 1–19.
4. Berglundh T, Lindhe J, Ericsson I, et al. Different types of inflammatory in peri-implant soft tissues. J Clin Periodontol 1995; 22: 255–261.
5. Schierano G, Ramieri G, Cortese M, et al. Organization of the connective tissue barrier around long-term loaded implant abutments in man. Clin Oral Implants Res 2002; 13: 460–464.
6. Gargiulo A, Wentz M, Orban B. Dimensions of the dentogingival junction in humans. J Periodontol 1969; 32: 261–267.
7. Abrahamsson I, Berglundh T, Wennstrom J, Lindhe J. The peri-implant hard and soft tissues at different implant systems. A comparative study in the dog. Clin Oral Implants Res 1996; 7: 212–219.
8. Berglundh T, Lindhe J. Dimension of the peri-implant mucosa. Biological width revisited. J Clin Periodontol 1996; 23: 971–973.
9. Ericsson I, Persson L, Berglundh T, et al. Different types of inflammatory reactions in peri-implant soft tissues. J Clin Periodontol 1995; 22: 255–261.
10. Ricci J, Charvet J, Frenkel S, et al. Bone response to laser micro-textured surfaces. In: Bone Engineering, DaviesJE, ed. Toronto: EM Squared, 2000, pp. 282–294.
11. Ricci J, Grew J, Alexander H. Connective tissue responses to defined biomaterial surfaces. I. Growth of rat fibroblast and bone marrow cell colonies on micro-grooved substrates. J Biomed Mater Res A 2008; 85: 313–325.
12. Grew J, Ricci J, Alexander H. Connective tissue responses to defined biomaterial surfaces. II. Behavior of rat and mouse fibroblasts cultured on micro-grooved substrates. J Biomed Mater Res A 2008; 85: 326–335.
13. Glass-Brudzinski J, Perizollo D, Brunette D. Effects of substratum surface topography on the organization of cells and collagen fibers in collagen gel cultures. J Biomed Mater Res 2002; 61: 608–618.
14. Weiner S, Simon J, Ehrenberg D, et al. The effects of laser micro-textured collars upon crestal bone levels of dental implants. Implant Dent 2008; 17: 217–228.
15. Shin S, Han D. Influence of micro-grooved collar implants on tissue healing. Clin Oral Implants Res 2010; 21: 804—814.
16. Nevins M, Kim M, Jun S, Guze K. Histologic evidence of connective tissue attachment to laser micro-grooved abutments. A canine study. Int J Periodontics Restorative Dent 2010; 30: 245–255.
17. Broggini N, McManus L, Hermann J, et al. Persistent acute inflammation at the implant-abutment interface. J Dent Res 2003; 82: 232–237.
18. Nevins M, Nevins M, Camelo M, et al. Human histologic evidence of a connective tissue attachment to a dental implant. Int J Periodontics Restorative Dent 2008; 28: 111–121.
19. Nevins M, Camelo M, Nevins ML, et al. Connective tissue attachment to laser-micro-grooved abutments: a human histological case report. Int J Periodontics Restorative Dent 2012; 32: 385–392.
20. Geurs N, Vassilopoulos P, Reddy M. Histologic evidence of connective tissue integration on laser micro-grooved abutments in humans. Clin Adv Periodontics 2011; 1: 29–33.
21. Pecora G, Ceccarelli R, Bonelli M, et al. Clinical evaluation of laser micro-texturing for soft tissue and bone attachment to dental implants. Implant Dent 2009; 18: 57–66.
22. Botos S, Yousef H, Zweig B, et al. The effects of laser micro-texturing on the dental implant collar on crestal bone levels and peri-implant health. Int J Maxillofac Implants 2011; 26: 492–498.
23. Shapoff C, Lahey B, Wasserlauf P, Kim D. Radiographic analysis of crestal bone levels around Laser-Lok® collar dental implants. Int J Periodontics Restorative Dent 2010; 30: 129–137.
24. Alexander H, Ricci J, Hrico J. A mechanical basis for bone retention around dental implants. J Biomed Mater Res B Appl Biomater 2009; 88: 306–311.

CHAPTER 7

Recombinant Human Bone Morphogenetic Protein-2 or Recombinant Human Platelet-Derived Growth Factor BB in Extraction Site Preservation and Bone Augmentation

Craig M. Misch,[1,2] Marc L. Nevins,[3] & Jason A. Boch[4,5]
[1]Oral & Maxillofacial Surgery and Prosthodontics, Sarasota, FL, USA
[2]Department of Implant Dentistry, New York University, New York, NY, USA
[3]Boston Periodontics & Dental Implants, Boston, MA, USA
[4]Harvard School of Dental Medicine, Department of Oral Medicine, Infection, and Immunity, Boston, MA, USA
[5]Private Practice, Wayland, MA, USA

Introduction

Successful dental implant treatment requires that there be adequate alveolar ridge height and width to enable placement of an implant(s) of appropriate design and dimensions. This often requires repair and/or augmentation grafting of existing bone defects using autogenous bone collected via secondary invasive surgical procedures. Tissue engineering with growth factors has emerged as a promising alternative source of material for these purposes.[1] Tissue engineering promotes the interaction of native, or in some instances undifferentiated, osteoprogenitor cells[2] with scaffolding matrices impregnated with genetically engineered growth factors such as bone morphogenetic proteins (BMPs) or platelet-derived growth factors (PDGFs).[2–6] These two cytokines have been extensively studied. For example, intraoral clinical applications of recombinant human BMP-2 (rhBMP-2) have included extraction socket preservation and repair,[7,8] sinus augmentation grafting,[9,10] and alveolar ridge augmentation.[11,12]

BMPs are naturally occurring osteoinductive proteins found in bone, while recombinant human PDGF-BB (rhPDGF-BB) enhances wound healing by stimulating committed osteogenic and other cellular functions required for regeneration of tissues, including chemotaxis, mitogenesis, cell proliferation, and angiogenesis.[2] BMPs were first reported by Urist,[13] who found that bone matrix demineralized with acid released substances that could produce heterotopic bone formation in non-bone sites such as dermis or muscle. This quickly led to the idea that demineralized bone allografts might be beneficial as a graft for intraoral purposes.[14,15] However, while this material did under ideal circumstances lead to bone formation in bone defects or following sinus grafting, it was not effective in regenerating lost periodontal ligament and cementum, making it far from the ideal periodontal grafting material. On the other hand, in animals and humans, rhPDGF-BB can promote regeneration of all three periodontal tissues (bone, periodontal ligament, and cementum). Early studies applied rhPDGF-BB in canine and non-human primate models of periodontal disease, either alone or in combination with insulin-like growth factor-1 (IGF-1). Later, a multicenter prospective randomized human clinical trial utilized the combination of rhPDGF-BB and IGF-1 to treat intrabony periodontal angular and furcation defects.[16] Changes in linear bone height and measurements of osseous defect fill at re-entry were statistically significant, with furcation defects responding most favorably (2.8 mm horizontal osseous fill). The ability of rhPDGF-BB combined with demineralized freeze-dried bone allograft (DFDBA) to achieve periodontal regeneration also has been demonstrated in humans.[17,18] The investigators used retrieved histological specimens and observed regeneration with new bone, periodontal ligament, and cementum at and coronal to notches created in both periodontal intrabony and furcation defects.

A logical concern with surgical delivery of growth factors is their duration of action since they are typically given as a single bolus dose. The period of stimulation by BMP-2 can be extended by using DFDBA as carrier since further BMPs present in carefully prepared DFDBA will be released and have a delayed effect as allograft particles are resorbed.[2] Likewise, when rhPDGF-BB is administered during periodontal surgery, there can be a prolonged effect with increased bone turnover for up to 6 weeks.[19] This prolonged effect occurred despite the reported 4.2 hr half-life and more than 96% clearance by 4 days in a dog model of naturally-occurring periodontal disease.[20] These longer lasting biologic effects may be the result of neo-vascularization induced by rhPDGF-BB-mediated production of vascular endothelial growth factor during wound healing, in addition to its mitogenic and chemotactic effects on mesenchymal cells.[6,21]

Fiorellini et al.[7] conducted a randomized human, multicenter study evaluating two concentrations of rhBMP-2 (0.75 m/mL, 1.5 mg/mL) in the repair of extraction socket buccal wall defects at future dental implant sites. An absorbable collagen sponge (ACS) was utilized as the carrier for BMP molecules. The sockets were filled with an rhBMP-2–ACS combination, and primary soft tissue closure obtained. At 4 months, patients treated with the higher concentration of rhBMP-2 had significantly greater bone augmentation. Comparison of cross-sectional computed tomography (CT) scan images taken immediately post-extraction and 4 months later showed an average bone width gain of 3.53 mm at the crest. Nevertheless, 14% (3/18) of the grafted sockets required additional bone augmentation at the time of later dental implant placement, perhaps because collagen rather than DFDBA had been used as

Minimally Invasive Dental Implant Surgery, First Edition. Edited by Daniel R. Cullum and Douglas Deporter.

carrier. The 1.5 mg/mL concentration became the dose used by Medtronic (Memphis, TN, USA) to produce Infuse®, a commercially available rhBMP-2 product approved for human clinical use.

The efficacy of rhPDGF-BB was initially established in a large randomized controlled prospective clinical study combining it with a passive synthetic scaffold of beta-tricalcium phosphate to regenerate periodontal defects.[22,23] Since then, clinicians have sought to utilize the tissue engineering benefits of rhPDGF-BB, in an "off-label" application, by combining it with other commonly used bone replacement graft materials, including DFDBA or mineralized freeze-dried bone allograft (FDBA) to form growth factor-enhanced matrices for periodontal regeneration as well as for dental implant site development.[1,24,25] Clinical studies using rhPDGF-BB have consisted of case reports or case series, and provided both histologic and clinical evidence. In a case series, rhPDGF-BB was combined with FDBA to treat periodontal bone defects, and clinical re-entry showed complete defect fill with bone.[18] Allograft scaffolds also have been used successfully to deliver rhPDGF-BB for extraction socket ridge preservation and for localized ridge augmentation procedures.[25,26] Xenografts, too, have been proposed as a carrier vehicle for rhPDGF-BB, and preclinical studies support their use for periodontal and ridge augmentation procedures.[27,28] Another preclinical canine study, and later two human case reports, investigated the use of a deproteinized, cancellous bovine block infused with rhPDGF-BB to achieve vertical ridge augmentation.[29,30] Results indicated that sites using this combination without a barrier membrane demonstrated greater bone formation and superior replacement of graft material with host bone compared with xenograft block alone. Similar results were obtained using an equine bone block combined with rhPDGF-BB.[31] Although data were limited, the investigators suggested that a barrier might not be needed with these combinations of materials, or even be a disadvantage by excluding periosteal progenitor cells, which are easily stimulated by PDGF-BB.[2]

Recombinant human bone morphogenetic protein-2 for extraction socket defects

The horizontal and vertical loss of alveolar bone following tooth extraction is well documented.[32,33] Horizontal alveolar bone loss occurs shortly after tooth removal and can approach 50% of ridge width within the first year.[34] This outcome can have a significant impact on the ability to place dental implants optimally, if at all, especially in the esthetic zone.[35] Immediate dental implant placement into an extraction socket does not prevent this resorptive bone remodeling process,[36] and is contraindicated when significant buccal bone defects exist.[37] In anterior sites, immediate implant placement also may result in unfavorable buccal soft tissue recession, leading to esthetic flaws that are difficult if not impossible to resolve.[38] These problems can often be avoided with extraction site preservation grafting and/or repair. While there is generalized agreement that socket preservation techniques are beneficial in minimizing post-extraction bone loss (see also Chapter 5), there is no consensus on the ideal graft material and technique.[39] Conventional augmentation with bone grafting for future implant placement have employed various particulate graft materials with or without protective barrier membranes[40] (see also Chapter 14). When socket walls are intact, an osteoconductive graft material such as a mineralized xenograft[41,42] with or without a protective barrier may often suffice. However, when one or more socket walls are missing, the healing environment for bone fill is somewhat compromised.[43] Elian et al.[44] classified extraction sockets according to morphology of the buccal cortex. Type 1 sockets were those with all walls intact, including the buccal, while type 2 sockets were those with up to 50% of buccal cortex missing, and type 3 sockets those with 50% or more missing. Type 2 and 3 sockets are often encountered following removal of teeth with long-standing endodontic infections, root fractures or trauma, and with teeth having prominent, facially positioned roots. These defects with loss of buccal bone often require autogenous bone or osteoinductive and/or mitogenic graft materials. While DFDBAs may contain low levels of BMPs if properly sourced and processed,[45,46] rhBMP-2 provides a more concentrated and reliable source of BMPs.

In a recent case series report, Misch[8] evaluated rhBMP-2/ACS (Infuse; Medtronic, Memphis, TN) for the repair of Elian type 3 bone defects (>50% buccal bone loss) following removal of maxillary central incisors. The as-received rhBMP-2/ACS (Infuse) was mixed with a small amount of mineralized bone allograft; the latter was meant to act as a bulking agent to reduce graft compression by the replaced soft tissue flap,[47,48] and to compensate for the fact that primary soft tissue closure was not always achievable. CT scans were used to evaluate alveolar buccal bone repair. Implant placement was possible in all grafted sites after 4–6 months' healing without the need for further bone augmentation. A comparison of pre- and post-operative CT scans showed only slight post-treatment loss (1.07 mm) in alveolar bucco-palatal width at the crest. Lack of primary soft tissue closure over the graft nor the lack of protective barrier materials did not appear to have complicated or compromised treatment outcomes. The regenerated bone was assessed clinically as primarily cancellous in nature.

Recombinant human bone morphogenetic protein-2–absorbable collagen sponge socket repair technique

As indicated, since osteoconductive bone substitutes such as xenografts on their own may be efficacious in preserving sockets with all walls intact, use of growth factors like rhBMP-2–ACS is reserved for sites where significant alveolar defects exist. Using rhBMP-2–ACS graft on its own may suffice in single extraction sockets. However, in larger surgical sites involving more than a single socket, especially those with loss of interdental as well as buccal bone, the repositioned flap can compress the ACS and compromise outcomes. In these situations, methods to support the flap and protect the graft should be employed, such as by adding a mineralized allograft as bulking agent, or by protecting the graft with titanium mesh. Although the presence of chronic periapical infection does not appear to compromise outcomes, acute infection would contraindicate immediate post-extraction site grafting.

Extensive flap elevation for the procedure is discouraged in order to minimize disruption of blood supply to bone via periosteal vessels.[49] If needed for access to remove chronically infected apical tissue, a remote incision can be made in the mucosa or at the mucogingival junction over the root apex, leaving the marginal tissues and their blood supply intact. Periapical radiographs with adjunctive "bone sounding" may be sufficient to diagnose pathology and evaluate surrounding bone. However, preoperative cone beam CT (CBCT) may be beneficial, especially in the esthetic zone to help to evaluate tooth position and presence or absence of buccal bone. CBCT may not, however, show thin buccal bone reliably, and may overestimate buccal fenestrations and dehiscences.[50]

Patients are typically administered a loading dose of antibiotic (amoxicillin or clindamycin), a corticosteroid (dexamethasone), and 0.12% chlorhexidine rinse. Following tooth removal and thorough socket debridement, the bony socket walls are evaluated to determine the extent of the defect. If indicated, an XXS Infuse bone graft kit (Medtronic, Memphis, TN, USA) is used, and includes a

1/2″ × 2″ collagen sponge and 0.7 mL of rhBMP-2 (1.5 mg/ml). Fifteen minutes before use, the rhBMP-2 is applied to the sponge so as to saturate it. Thereafter, the collagen sponge is cut into smaller pieces with scissors, and if appropriate mixed with a mineralized allograft or xenograft material (25–50% by volume) for a beneficial bulking effect. The graft should be placed into the extraction socket in increments and gently compressed to fill the socket to the level of the interdental alveolar bone margins of the contiguous teeth. A piece of collagen sponge alone without added rhBMP-2 can then be used to cover the graft, and is secured using PTFE, polypropylene, or chromic gut interrupted sutures in a crisscross pattern over the socket.

Provisional tooth replacement can be accomplished with a bonded temporary bridge, an Essix® retainer, or possibly an acrylic removable partial denture. However, the provisional prosthesis should not place any pressure onto the grafted site. The patient should continue the prescribed antibiotic (amoxicillin or clindamycin) for a week, and rinse with 0.12% chlorhexidine twice daily. A short-term tapering dose of corticosteroid therapy also can be prescribed for 2 days, and the grafted site is allowed to heal for 4–6 months prior to dental implant placement. Waiting longer will produce a denser bone quality, although in softer bone undersizing the osteotomy and/or using hand osteotomes for site development can be employed to ensure optimal initial implant stability.

A sample case is shown in Figures 7.1, 7.2, and 7.3. Figure 7.1 shows the pretreatment status for a failed maxillary left central

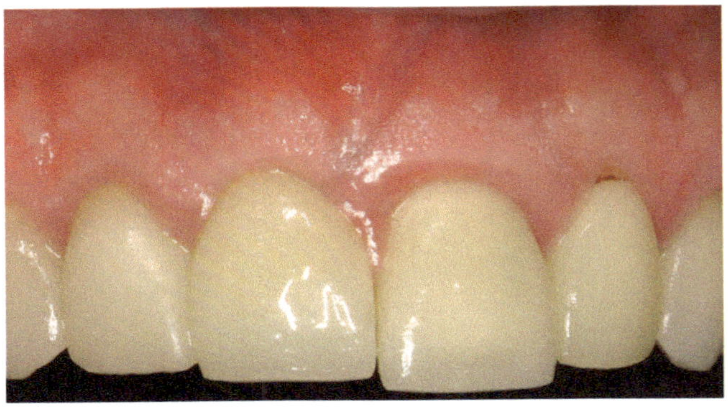

(a)

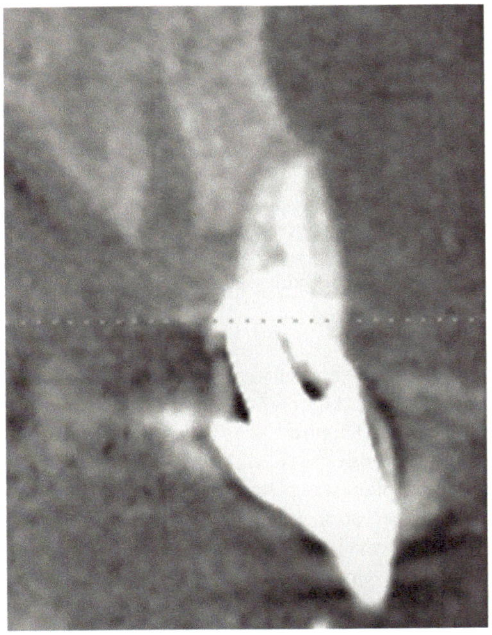

(b)

Figure 7.1 (a) Preoperative view of the failed maxillary left central incisor. (b) CT scan image reveals a lack of facial bone and root fracture with palatal bone loss. *Source:* Misch CM. The use of recombinant human bone morphogenetic protein-2 for the repair of extraction socket defects: a technical modification and case series report. Int J Oral Maxillofac Implants 2010; 25: 1246–1252.[8] Reproduced with permission of Quintessence Publishing Co., Inc.

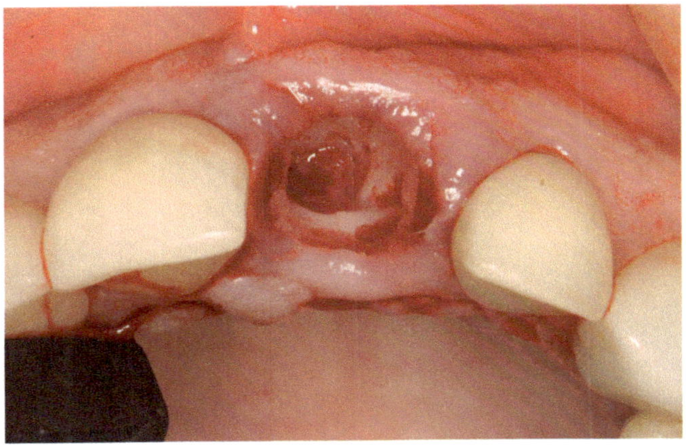

(a)

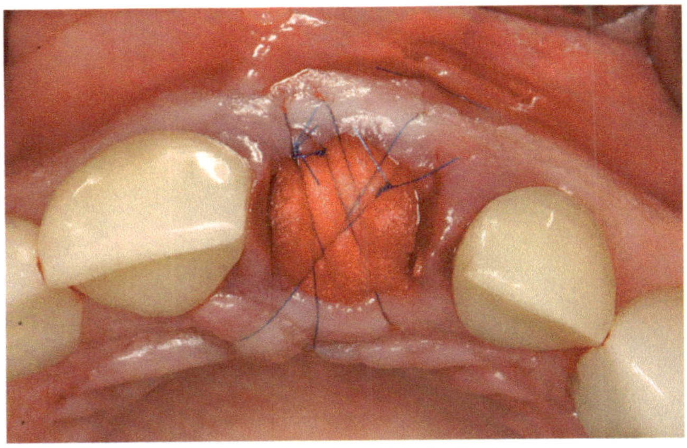

(b)

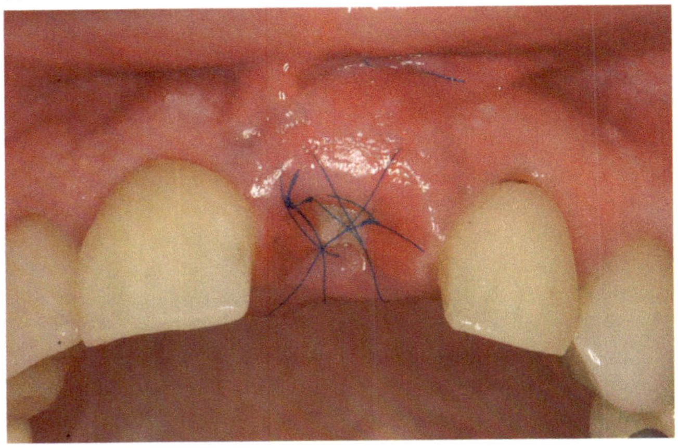

(c)

Figure 7.2 (a) An occlusal view of the extraction socket and bone defect. (b) The socket was grafted with rhBMP-2–ACS and secured with cross-sutures. (c) Healing at 1 week following the extraction and grafting. *Source:* Misch CM. The use of recombinant human bone morphogenetic protein-2 for the repair of extraction socket defects: a technical modification and case series report. Int J Oral Maxillofac Implants 2010; 25: 1246–1252.[8] Reproduced with permission of Quintessence Publishing Co., Inc.

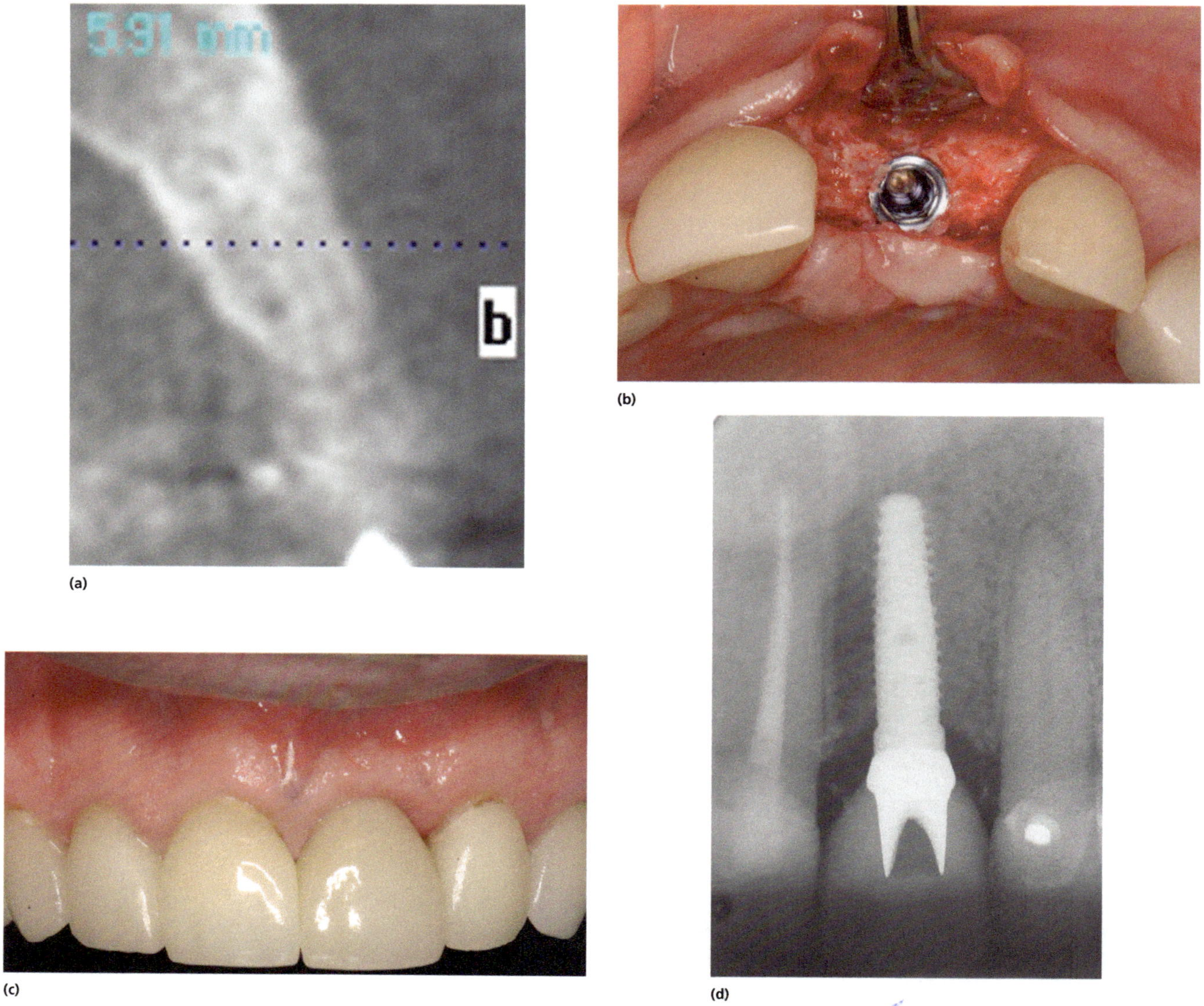

Figure 7.3 (a) Cross-sectional CT scan image of the healed graft site at 5 months. (b) An occlusal view of the implant. Note the regeneration of the buccal and palatal bone. (c) Final cement-retained implant crown. (d) Periapical radiograph of the restored implant reveals favorable integration. (a, b) *Source:* Misch CM. The use of recombinant human bone morphogenetic protein-2 for the repair of extraction socket defects: a technical modification and case series report. Int J Oral Maxillofac Implants 2010; 25: 1246–1252.[8] Reproduced with permission of Quintessence Publishing Co., Inc.

incisor. The CT scan image indicated a lack of buccal bone and a root fracture associated with a palatal bone defect as well. Following tooth extraction and socket debridement (Figure 7.2a), the socket was grafted with rhBMP-2–ACS secured with cross-sutures (Figure 7.2b). Healing at the 1 week post-op is shown in Figure 7.2c. A cross-sectional CT image taken after 5 months' site healing showed a successful outcome (Figure 7.3a). Implant placement was done thereafter, at which time good regeneration of buccal bone was confirmed (Figure 7.3b). Following site healing, the implant was restored with a single, cement-retained crown (Figure 7.3c and d).

A second case is shown in Figures 7.4 and 7.5. The maxillary right central incisor failed due to endodontic complications (Figure 7.4a). A cross-sectional CT image revealed a lack of buccal bone (Figure 7.4b). A flap was not raised, but after socket debridement a periodontal probe indicated the extent of buccal bone loss (Figure 7.4c). The socket was grafted with rhBMP-2–ACS as described previously (Figure 7.4d), and showed straightforward healing after 1 week (Figure 7.4e). The grafted site appeared successful in the 4-month cross-sectional CT scan (Figure 7.5a), at which time an implant was placed (Figure 7.5b–d).

When site preservation is not completed at the time of tooth extraction, and especially following a significantly traumatic extraction or with extensive periodontal bone loss, a significant defect can result. Horizontal and/or vertical ridge augmentation grafting may be needed later to develop sufficient bone volume to permit dental implant placement. There are a number of procedures available for this augmentation, including onlay block grafting with autogenous, allogeneic, or xenogeneic materials, ridge-splitting (using various approaches, including piezoelectric bone surgery), guided bone regeneration (GBR), and distraction osteogenesis. When large osseous defects are encountered, autogenous grafts have

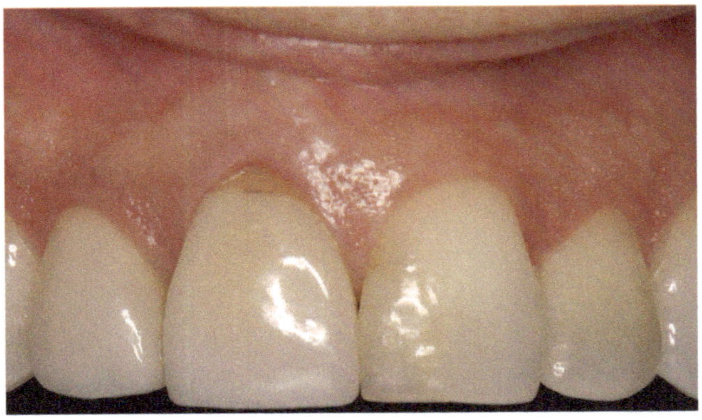

(a)

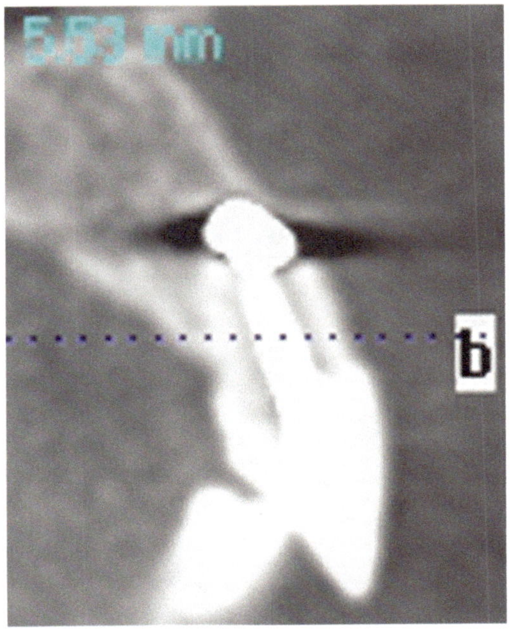

(b)

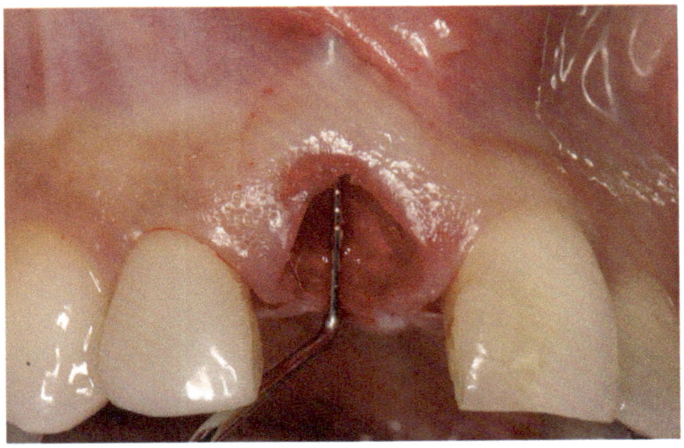

(c)

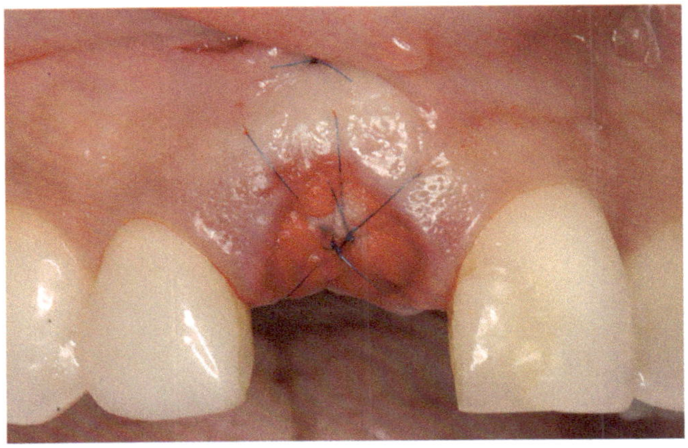

(d)

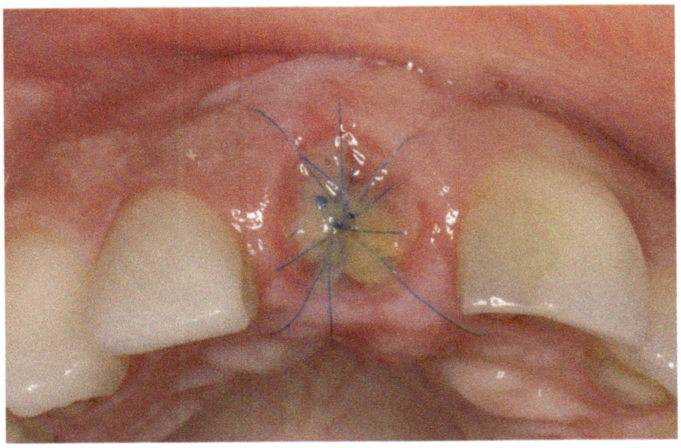

(e)

Figure 7.4 (a) Preoperative view of the failed maxillary right central incisor. (b) Cross-sectional CT scan image reveals a lack of facial bone over the endodontic treated failed incisor. (c) A probe was used to evaluate the buccal bone defect. (d) The socket was grafted with rhBMP-2–ACS and secured with cross-sutures. (e) Healing at 1 week following the extraction and grafting. *Source:* Misch CM. The use of recombinant human bone morphogenetic protein-2 for the repair of extraction socket defects: a technical modification and case series report. Int J Oral Maxillofac Implants 2010; 25: 1246–1252.[8] Reproduced with permission of Quintessence Publishing Co., Inc.

been used alone or in combination with bone substitutes.[51,52] The osteogenic properties of autogenous bone offer significant advantages in these situations. For large onlay augmentation procedures, autogenous extraoral (e.g. femur, tibia) block bone grafts may be needed, often with the overlying protection of a titanium mesh. For smaller defects, intraorally harvested cortical blocks (e.g. chin, ramus) or particulate autograft material protected with titanium mesh or barrier membranes may be considered.[52,53] In both scenarios, however, use of rhBMP-2–ACS is currently under investigation as a replacement.[11,12] However, it should be noted that while the use of Infuse for socket preservation has been approved by the US Food and Drug Administration, at the time of publication of this book its use for augmentation of healed ridge defects is still considered an off-label application.

Although ACS has been found to be a good carrier for rhBMP-2, as already stressed, it is not cross-linked, and, as a consequence, has poor space maintenance properties in resisting compression from repositioned flaps. The sponge is comprised of type 1 bovine collagen and undergoes resorption over a 4–12-week period.[54] In spinal fusion surgery, rhBMP-2–ACS has been sequestered in implantable titanium cages to resist compressive forces from the surrounding tissues. In oral applications, titanium mesh or polyethylene

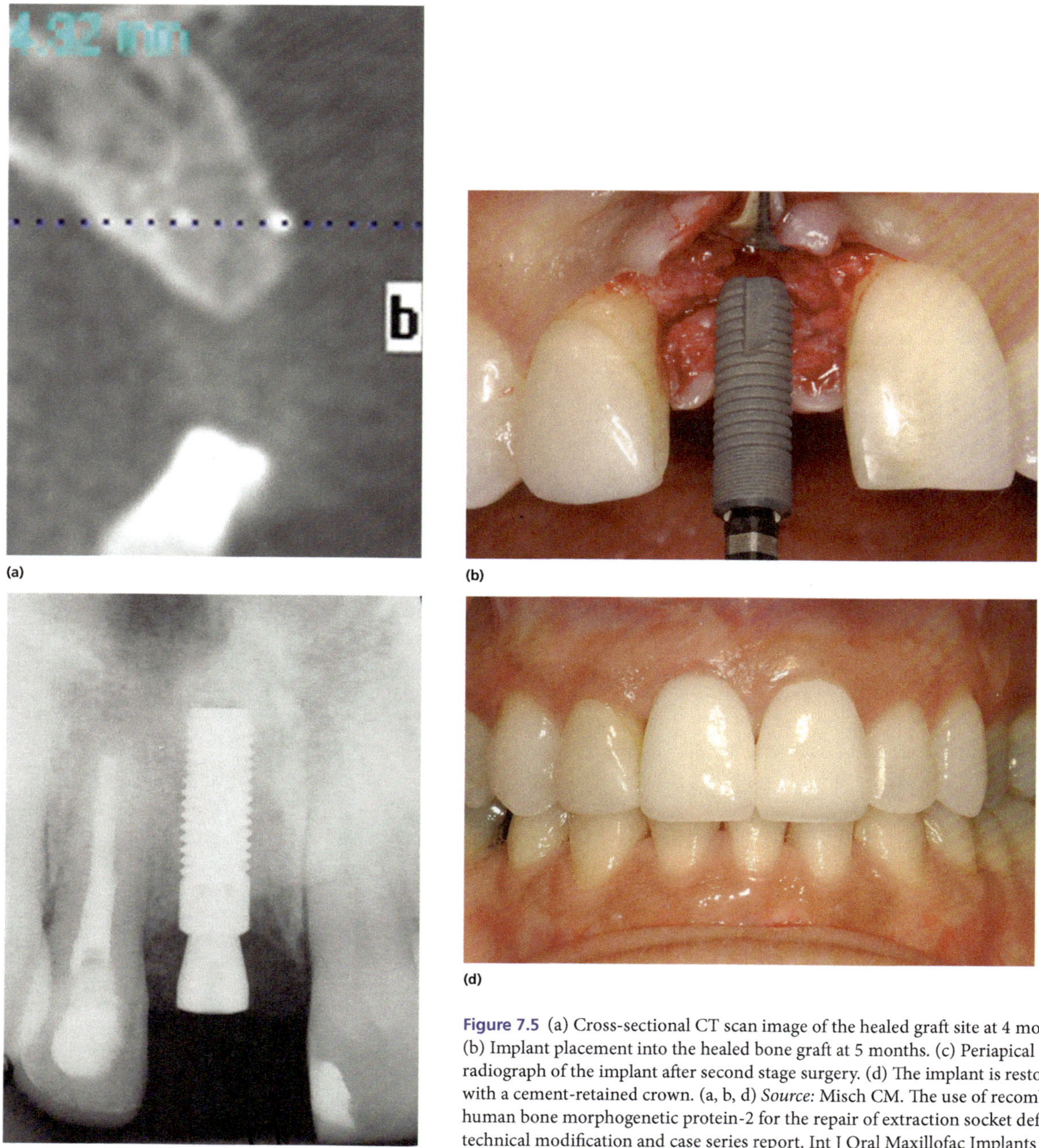

Figure 7.5 (a) Cross-sectional CT scan image of the healed graft site at 4 months. (b) Implant placement into the healed bone graft at 5 months. (c) Periapical radiograph of the implant after second stage surgery. (d) The implant is restored with a cement-retained crown. (a, b, d) *Source:* Misch CM. The use of recombinant human bone morphogenetic protein-2 for the repair of extraction socket defects: a technical modification and case series report. Int J Oral Maxillofac Implants 2010; 25: 1246–1252.[8] Reproduced with permission of Quintessence Publishing Co., Inc.

mesh have been proposed to protect rhBMP-2-ACS.[55] Mesh thickness should be adequate to resist flexing and micromovements during healing, but thin enough to trim and mold to the desired ridge shape. A 0.2 mm thick mesh appears to fulfill these requirements.[12] The ideal mesh design and pore size have not been determined, but one study suggests a macromesh may be preferable to a micromesh design in order to permit passage of nutrients from the soft tissue flap and rapid revascularization.[56] Although titanium mesh is biocompatible and structurally favorable, its disadvantage is the need to remove it at a later time.

The use of titanium mesh for bone augmentation should not be confused with the concept of GBR which uses a cellular occlusive barrier membrane to impede soft tissue penetration and allow slower growing bone cells to repopulate osseous defects without interference from overlying gingival fibroblasts.[57] On the other hand, titanium mesh is not cellular occlusive, and principally acts as a protective support to maintain space and facilitate osteogenesis. Covering rhBMP-2-ACS grafts with an occlusive barrier membrane does not seem to provide any advantage, and may even be biologically counterproductive as it impedes revascularization from the soft tissue flap.[56,58–60] Existing human trials using rhBMP-2-ACS for bone augmentation did not employ GBR occlusive barrier membranes.[7,9–11] When rhBMP-2-ACS is used for augmentation of healed extraction site defects, thorough preparation of the osseous recipient site is needed to expose endosteal and bone marrow cells upon which the BMP will have its effect. All soft tissue remnants must be removed and the cortex of the recipient site perforated in multiple sites with a bur to allow access to marrow. Primary tension-free closure of soft tissue flaps over the grafted site is recommended to prevent wound dehiscence and early exposure of mesh. Although late mesh exposures are fairly well tolerated,[61,62] early mesh exposure can be detrimental to success.[11] RhBMP-2–ACS in combination with titanium mesh can be used for the augmentation of horizontal, vertical, or combined 3-D ridge deficiencies. A preoperative CT scan is needed to assess ridge morphology and extent of jaw atrophy. Study casts can be used to plan for the amount of graft and size of titanium mesh required. A diagnostic wax-up of the planned reconstruction can even be used to preform the mesh into the desired shape prior to surgery.[63] Stereolithographic models produced from a CT scan may also be used for this purpose.[52]

The patient should receive a preoperative loading dose of antibiotic (amoxicillin or clindamycin), corticosteroid (dexamethasone), and a 0.12% chlorhexidine rinse. The use of corticosteroids will reduce but not eliminate post-operative swelling. Nevertheless, with the larger doses of rhBMP-2 typically needed for ridge augmentation cases, patients should be warned of the possibility of significant post-operative edema. The rhBMP-2–ACS graft is prepared just prior to surgery to allow adequate time for protein binding to the sponge. The appropriate total dosage of rhBMP-2 is determined by the defect size and volume of the planned augmentation. A useful guideline is to plan for approximately 1.5 mg of rhBMP-2 for each two-tooth span.[11] The collagen sponges included in the Infuse bone graft kit should be evenly saturated with reconstituted rhBMP-2 (1.5 mg/mL) liquid. A minimum of 15 min is required for binding of the growth factor to the collagen carrier before it is placed into the surgical site. The collagen sponge is then cut into smaller pieces with scissors, and mixed with particulate mineralized bone allograft (20–50% by volume) as a bulking agent.

Following local anesthesia, a crestal incision is typically made to extend well beyond the graft margins. Remote vertical releasing incisions are made as needed, and a broad-based mucoperiosteal flap developed to expose the ridge deficiency and identify local anatomy. A 0.2 mm thick mesh is trimmed with scissors to cover the desired area of augmentation. The mesh is formed into a U-shape over the ridge area and molded to the bone with a periosteal elevator. The formed mesh is then removed and overextended margins trimmed, with care taken to remove any sharp edges or unsupported metal struts. All soft tissue remnants are removed from bone and the cortex of the ridge generously perforated to produce bleeding using a small round carbide bur. Pilot holes for mesh fixation screws also can be prepared at this time. The concave portion of the mesh is then packed with the rhBMP-2–ACS and particulate allograft combination, and then the mesh with graft is reinserted over the ridge and compressed into place. A minimum of two monocortical fixation screws (4.0 mm length) should be placed buccally to secure the mesh. Additional palatal or lingual fixation screws are inserted if flexure of the mesh or micromovement is a concern. A scalpel blade is used to incise the periosteum along the base of the buccal flap to obtain release for its advancement over the grafted site. Lingual flap release can be accomplished in the posterior mandible by dissecting to the mylohyoid ridge and stretching the thin periosteum with a gloved finger. Flap margins are then advanced over the mesh and approximated without tension. Flaps are closed primarily with PTFE, polyethylene, or polyglactin 910 mattress and/or interrupted sutures.

The patient should continue with an antibiotic for the first week and rinse twice daily using 0.12% chlorhexidine solution. The healing soft tissues over the grafted site will often appear erythematous from the BMP-enhanced vascular response. Ideally, temporary esthetic tooth replacement should be accomplished with a fixed provisional prosthesis or removable Essix appliance. If, however, a soft tissue borne prosthesis is planned, it should not be worn until the incision is completely healed, typically at least 2 weeks, and the patient should follow a soft diet for at least 2 months, following which relining with tissue conditioner may be needed for continued cosmetic use and light function.

The grafted site will need to heal for at least 6 months, although longer healing times may produce better bone quality. A further CT scan is recommended prior to implant placement surgery in order to evaluate site healing and bone density, and to select the appropriate size implant(s). If done after 5–6 months' graft site healing, the CT scan may reveal a density less than native bone, especially in the mandible. At the time of implant surgery, a flap design similar to that used previously is needed to facilitate mesh removal. Fixation screws are removed, and an edge of the mesh freed and held with a hemostat to permit its careful sharp dissection from the overlying soft tissues. Fibrous tissue typically will have encapsulated the mesh, and this tissue must be reflected from underlying bone to expose the true extent of ridge augmentation. Implant osteotomies are prepared according to the manufacturer's drilling protocol, but in sites where width augmentation was developed, care is needed to ensure that implant drills do not deviate into the softer regenerated bone. A side-cutting Lindemann bur may be useful to allow preferential preparation of the osteotomy along its denser side of native bone. The density of bone regenerated by rhBMP-2 varies, but is often average to soft (type III[64]), making it prudent to consider a submerged implant healing protocol.

A sample case is shown in Figures 7.6, 7.7, 7.8, 7.9, and 7.10. The patient suffered from hypodentia (Figure 7.6a) and wished to have replacement of the missing maxillary cuspid teeth with dental implant-supported crowns (Figure 7.6b and c). The preoperative CT scans showed knife-edge thin alveolar ridges (Figure 7.6d and e). A large, full-thickness mucoperiosteal flap was elevated to expose both cuspid sites (Figure 7.7a), and a composite graft of rhBMP-2–ACS, FDBA, and autogenous platelet-rich plasma prepared (Figure 7.7b). When ready, this graft combination was placed into each defect site and covered with trimmed titanium mesh secured with monocortical fixation screws (Figure 7.7c and d). After site healing, the meshes were removed and implant osteotomies prepared (Figure 7.8a–c).

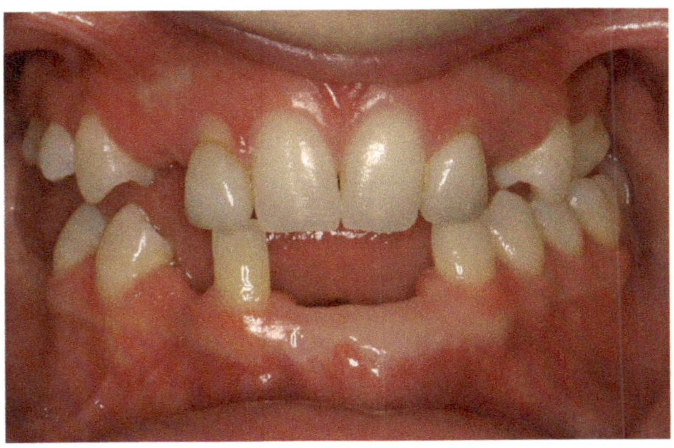

(a)

Figure 7.6 (a) Preoperative view of patient with hypodontia.

(Continued)

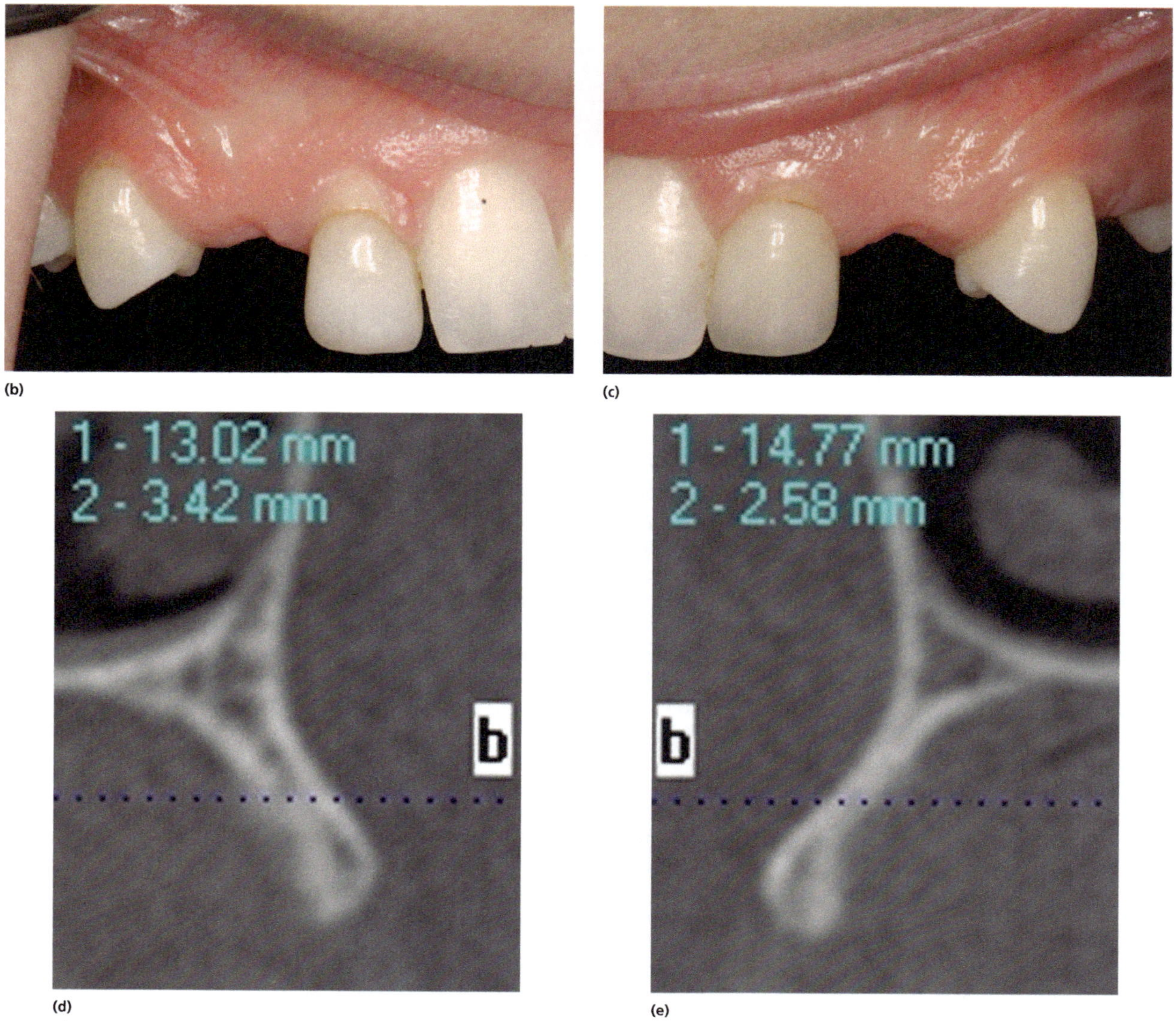

Figure 7.6 (Continued)
(b) Missing maxillary right cuspid #6. (c) Missing maxillary left cuspid #11. (d) CT scan image of the maxillary right cuspid site. (e) CT scan image of the maxillary left cuspid site.

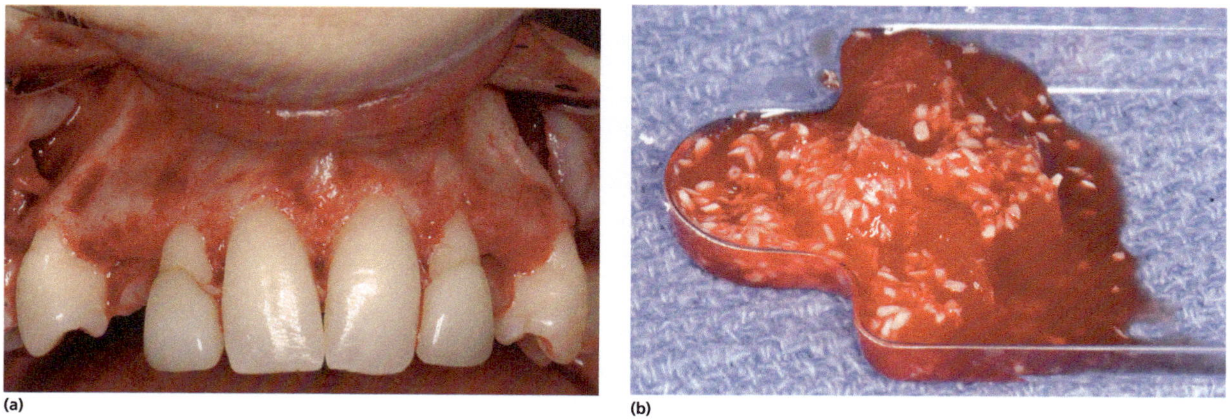

Figure 7.7 (a) Mucoperiosteal flap is elevated to expose the maxillary ridges. (b) A composite graft mixture of rhBMP-2–ACS plus mineralized allograft plus platelet-rich plasma.

(*Continued*)

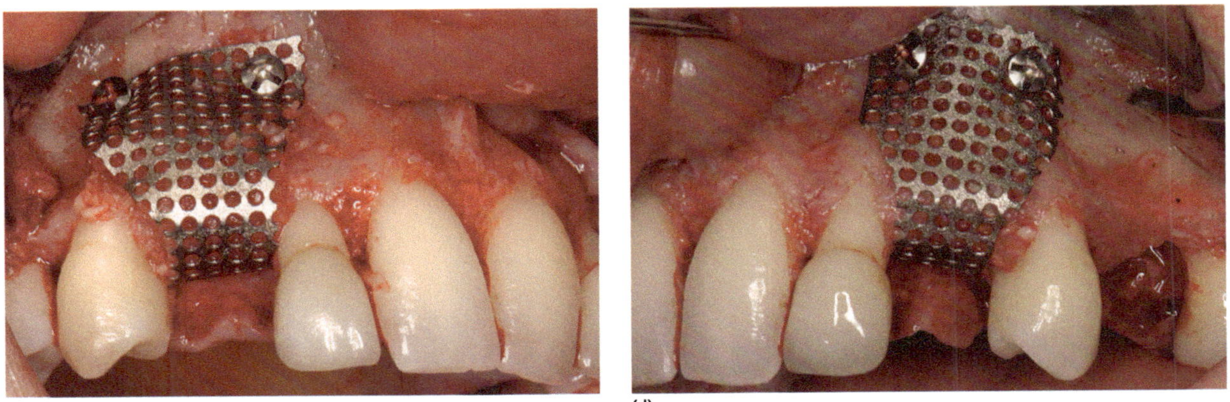

(c) (d)

Figure 7.7 (Continued)
(c) The maxillary right ridge is augmented with the composite graft supported by titanium mesh. (d) The maxillary left ridge is augmented with the composite graft supported by titanium mesh.

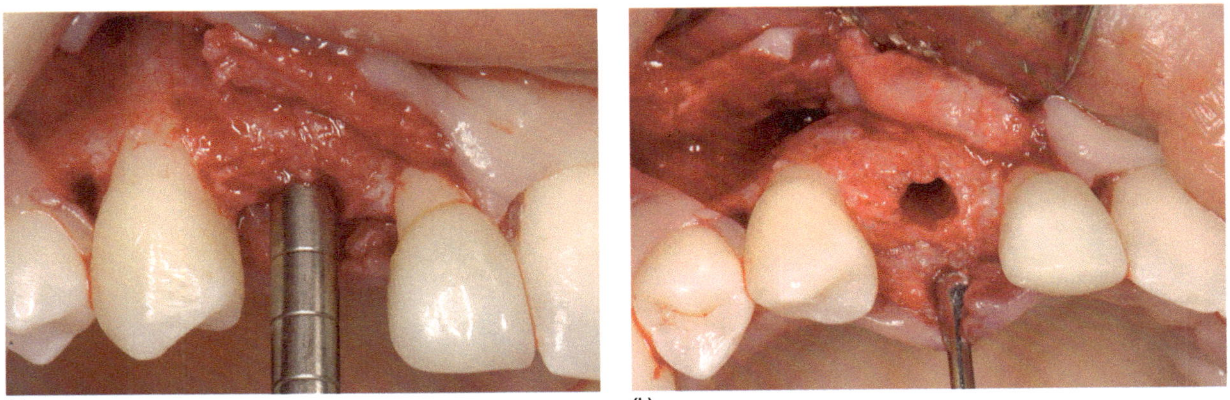

(a) (b)

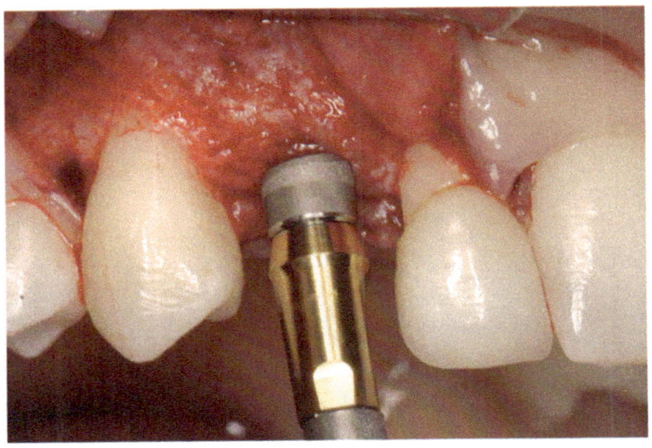

(c)

Figure 7.8 (a) The regenerated bone is D3 quality, so the implant osteotomy is prepared with osteotomes. (b) An occlusal view of the reconstructed ridge and the implant osteotomy. (c) The tapered implant is inserted for submerged healing.

Bone quality was type III, making it necessary to use hand osteotomes for implant site development. When the mesh was removed from the left cuspid defect, there was a pseudoperiosteal soft tissue underlying it and covering the regenerated bone surface (Figure 7.9). The final implant restorations for the patient are shown in Figure 7.10.

A final case shows a patient requiring the use of titanium mesh with rhBMP-2–ACS to restore a resorbed mandibular bone defect. The patient initially had a large bone cyst requiring enucleation (Figure 7.11a). After cyst removal and site healing, a cross-sectional CT scan revealed complete loss of buccal bone (Figure 7.11b), which was confirmed clinically at the time of flap reflection (Figure 7.11c). A composite graft of rhBMP-2–ACS and FDBA was prepared and packed into the concavity of a shaped and trimmed titanium mesh (Figure 7.11d). The mesh was subsequently placed over the defect and secured with monocortical fixation screws (Figure 7.11e). After 6 months' healing, the mesh was removed and three implants placed. At that time, substantial increase in ridge width was demonstrated (Figure 7.11f and g).

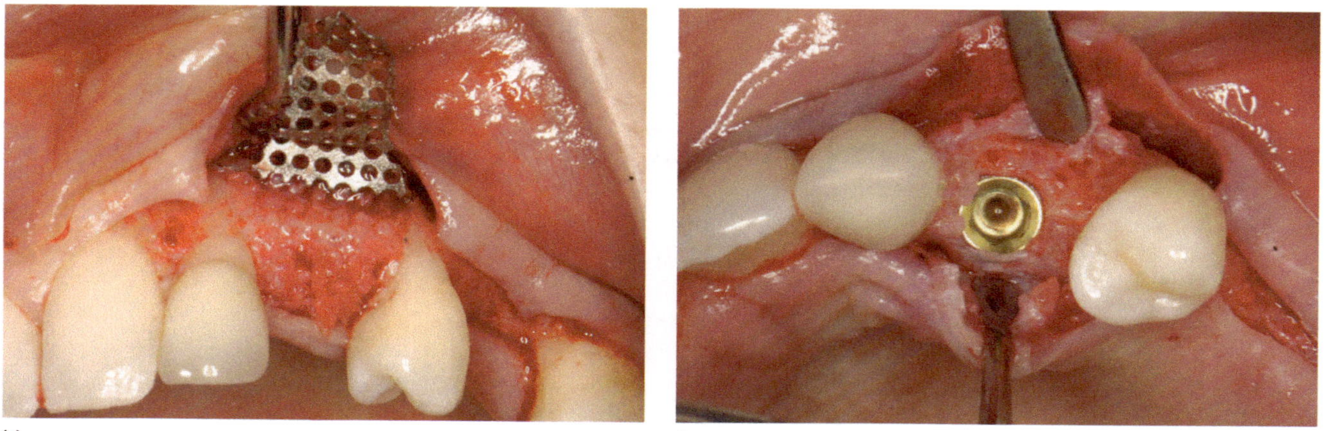

(a) (b)

Figure 7.9 (a) Removal of the titanium mesh reveals a "pseudoperiosteum" over the maxillary left reconstructed ridge. (b) An occlusal view of the implant in the maxillary left ridge.

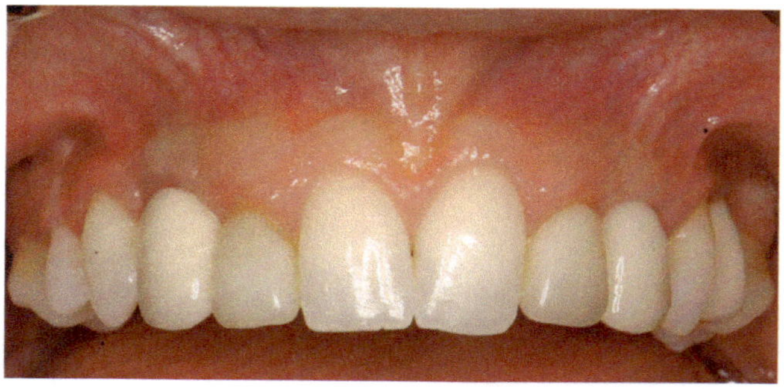

Figure 7.10 The healed implants are restored with single crowns.

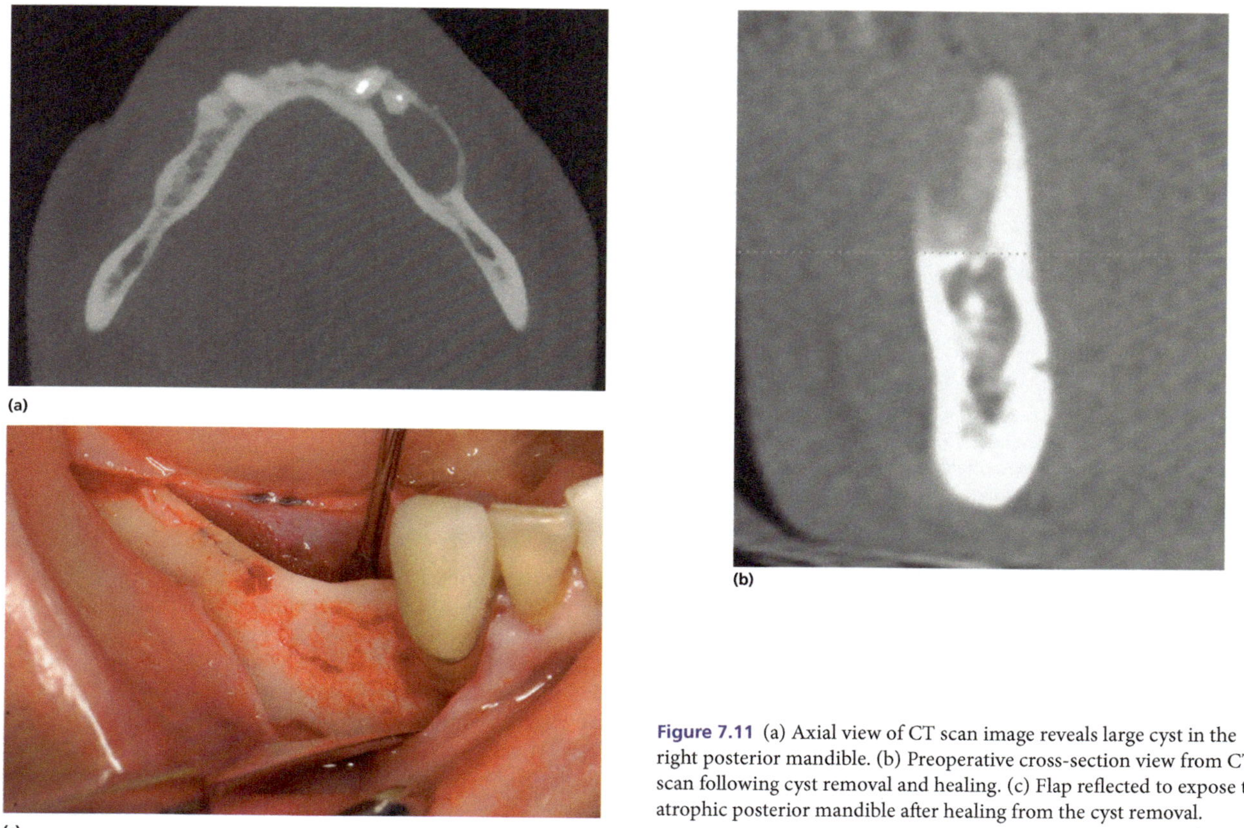

(a) (b) (c)

Figure 7.11 (a) Axial view of CT scan image reveals large cyst in the right posterior mandible. (b) Preoperative cross-section view from CT scan following cyst removal and healing. (c) Flap reflected to expose the atrophic posterior mandible after healing from the cyst removal.

(Continued)

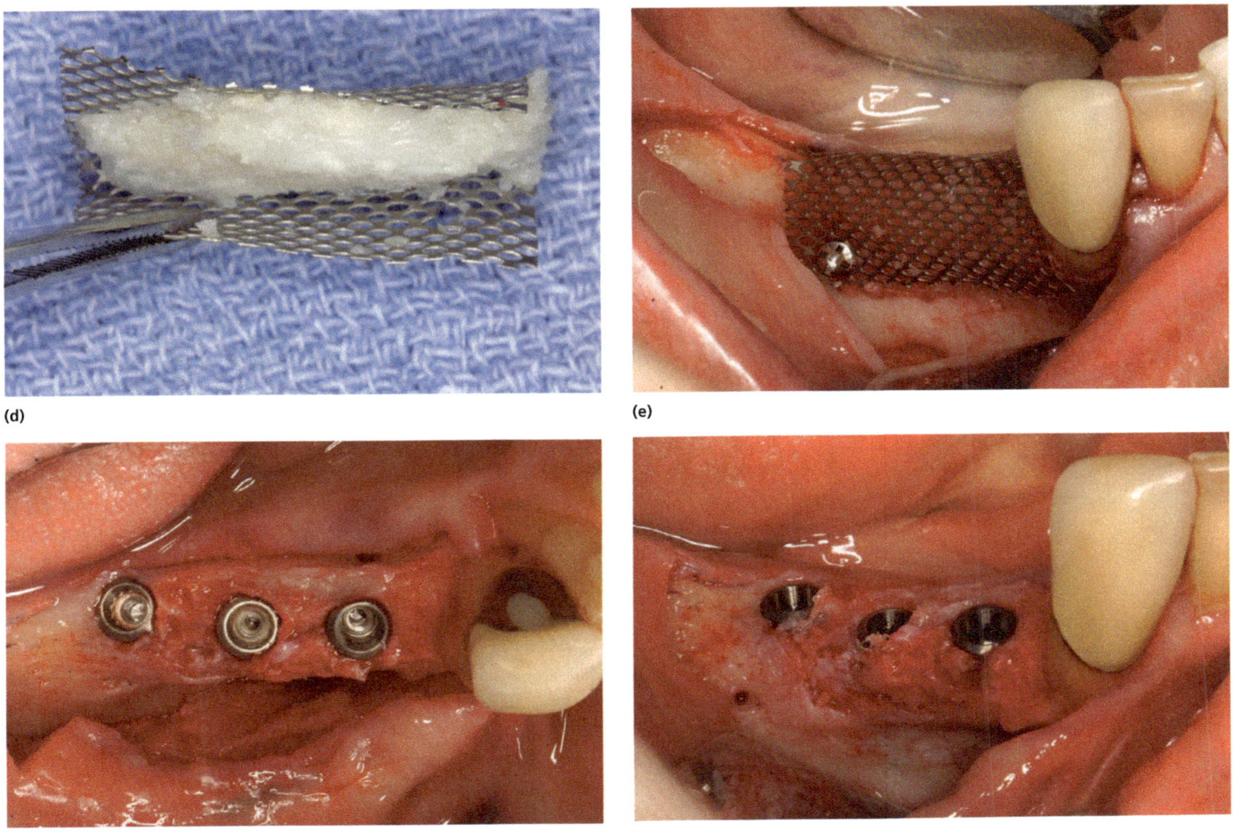

(d) (e) (f) (g)

Figure 7.11 (Continued)
(d) The rhBMP-2–ACS mixed with allograft is packed into the concave area of the titanium mesh. (e) The titanium mesh and graft is secured over the atrophic ridge with monocortical fixation screws. (f) After 6 months' healing, the mesh was removed and three 4.0 mm diameter implants were inserted. (g) A lateral view of the reconstructed site and implant placement in the right posterior mandible. *Source:* Misch CM. Bone augmentation of the atrophic posterior mandible for dental implants using rhBMP-2 and titanium mesh: clinical technique and early results. Int J Periodontics Restorative Dent 2011; 31; 581–589.[12] Reproduced with permission of Quintessence Publishing Co., Inc.

Recombinant human platelet-derived growth factor BB for extraction socket defects

A clinical study by McAllister et al.[65] compared tooth sockets grafted with rhPDGF-BB in combination with either synthetic tricalcium phosphate or xenogeneic mineralized bovine bone/collagen substitute (MCBS) (Bio-Oss Collagen®, Osteohealth, Shirley, NY; 90% bovine bone mineral and 10% porcine collagen). Both treatments were effective methods of socket preservation, but histologic examination showed increased replacement of graft particles and greater vital bone in the coronal portion of sockets grafted with the rhPDGF-BB–MCBS combination as an "off-label" application. Around the same time, Nevins et al.[66] used MCBS as a carrier for rhPDGF-BB to treat buccal plate extraction-site defects, and obtained histologic evidence of robust new bone formation throughout the sockets at 4 months with signs of resorption and replacement of the MCBS at this early timepoint. In a follow-up study in 2011, Nevins et al.[67] compared extraction socket buccal wall defect bone regeneration using MCBS alone or enhanced with either rhPDGF-BB or enamel matrix derivative (EMD). Results indicated more favorable ridge morphology and a trend toward more new bone with rhPDGF-BB-infused MCBS, compared with MCBS alone, MCBS with EMD, or EMD with bone ceramic. The following case examples demonstrate "off-label" clinical applications of rhPDGF-BB in GBR procedures.

Case 7.1

This case presents clinical photographs before treatment and at the 5-month re-entry for an rhPDGF-BB–MCBS-treated case (Figure 7.12). Before grafting, there was a 10 mm vertical buccal plate defect. The socket was thoroughly debrided and packed with the graft combo. After 5 months' healing, the site was re-entered to allow placement of a single dental implant. At that time, it appeared that the defect had completely resolved, and that the grafting had achieved substantial improvement in ridge height and width.

Case 7.2

This second case using rhPDGF-BB shows its application in managing advanced bone loss interproximally between a mandibular right first and second molar. The periodontal pocket depth distally on the first molar was 12 mm, and the radiograph (Figure 7.13a) demonstrated angular bone loss to the apices of the first molar and to 80% on the mesial of the second molar. The prognosis was designated hopeless for the first molar and guarded for the second molar. The first molar was extracted atraumatically after sectioning of the two roots without raising a flap, and the socket debrided. The affected root surface of the second molar site was treated with LANAP® (laser-assisted new attachment procedure protocol[68]), which included laser ablation followed by scaling and root planing

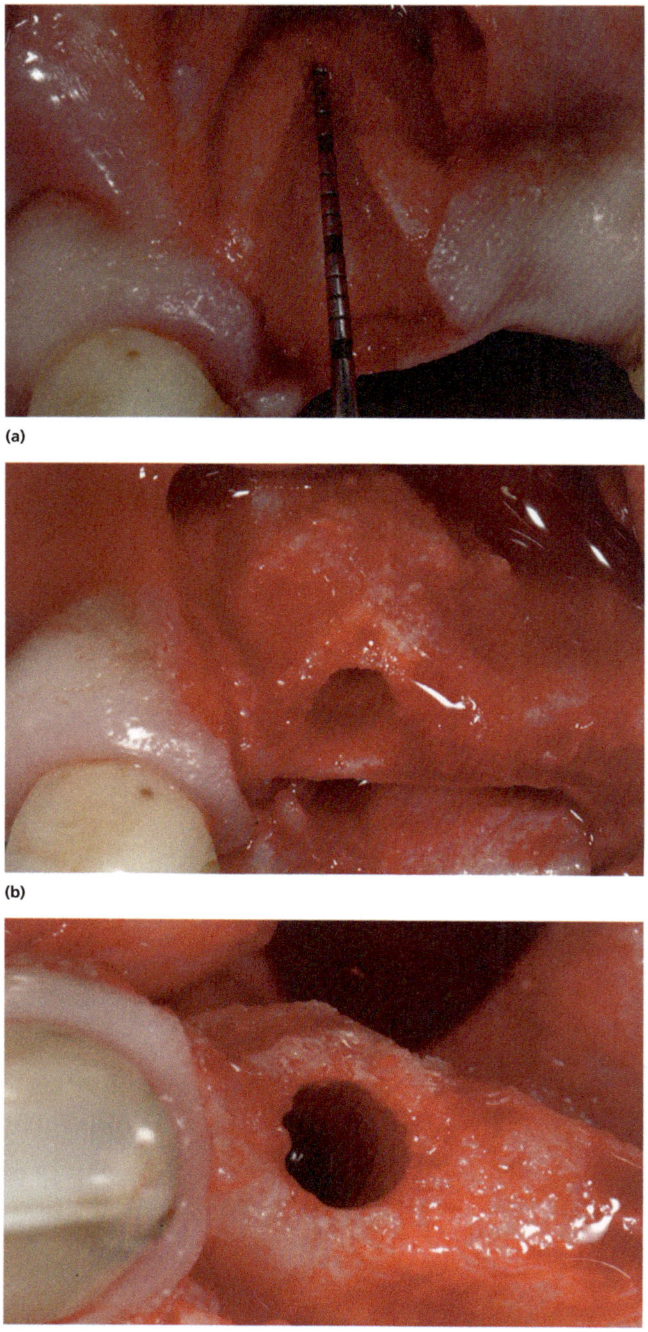

(a) (b) (c)

Figure 7.12 (a) This extraction socket defect has 10 mm loss of buccal plate. It was grafted with a combination of rhPDGF-BB and MCBS (no membrane), and the buccal flap advanced for primary closure. (b, c) The re-entry at 5 months demonstrated robust bone formation, which was confirmed via histologic evaluation. Reprinted with permission of Quintessence Publishing Co., Inc.

with piezo-ultrasonic instrumentation. Finally, the site was grafted with rhPDGF-BB-enhanced DFDBA (a potential source of BMP), and covered with a collagen membrane (Bio-Gide®, Osteohealth Co.) stabilized with medical-grade cyanoacrylate. The 5-week post-operative radiograph (Figure 7.13b) is a preview of the bone healing later demonstrated in the 3.5-month CBCT scan (Figure 7.13c). Surgical re-entry at 8 months demonstrated good bone fill and little evidence of the graft particulate (Figure 7.13d), allowing for implant placement (Figure 7.13e). The prognosis of the second molar also was upgraded following the treatment. The site can be seen on the 3-year periapical radiograph in Figure 7.13f.

Case 7.3

This next case presents the challenge of regenerating bone for future implant placement in a site with significant post-extraction maxillary ridge resorption associated with an ill-fitting removable partial denture (RPD) (Figure 7.14a). A CBCT scan done with an intraoral barium-containing stent fabricated via a diagnostic wax-up was used to establish an accurate diagnosis and treatment intervention (Figure 7.14b–d). A staged approach was chosen and undertaken using growth factors rather than autogenous block grafting. A scaffold was constructed by combining a tenting screw, DFDBA soaked in rhPDGF-BB, and a protective resorbable collagen membrane. This resulted in adequate bone volume (Figure 7.14e) for the later placement of two dental implants (Figure 7.14f).

Case 7.4

This final case presents the treatment sequence for transitioning from a failing maxillary central incisor to a successful implant-supported crown. Multiple treatment options have been proposed for this common dilemma, including immediate implant placement with or without immediate provisional restoration (see Chapter 19), or extraction site preservation (see also Chapter 5) and delayed implant placement. The latter approach was taken for this patient. The preop clinical photograph revealed a thin tissue biotype with recession at the existing crown margin and a high frenum attachment (Figure 7.15a). A CBCT scan (Figure 7.15b) was diagnostically important for decision-making as it indicated a thin labial plate of bone and a buccally angled root. Flapless surgery was used coronally in order to preserve gingival architecture, while a horizontal incision at the mucogingival junction combined with frenectomy allowed access for grafting of the buccal bone undercut (Figure 7.15c–f). The site was grafted with rh-PDGF-BB infused freeze-dried bone allograft protected by a Bio-Gide membrane. The buccal incision was sutured, and medical-grade cyanoacrylate applied occlusally over the exposed membrane surface. An Essix appliance (Figure 7.15g) was used for initial tooth replacement to prevent pressure from a removable partial denture appliance. At the time of later implant placement (Figure 7.15h), a connective tissue graft was placed buccally (Figure 7.15i–k) to augment the thickness of attached tissue and promote long-term stability of marginal tissue.[69–71] The implant site was allowed to heal for 4 months prior to the restorative phase of treatment (Figure 7.15l and m).

This final case employed a minimally invasive approach for extraction socket grafting in the esthetic zone, and while there are cases where this completely flapless approach is appropriate, other situations may require greater surgical access. The benefits of flapless surgery include less soft tissue disturbance, reduced healing time, and less discomfort. However, this type of minimally invasive surgery presents unique challenges for clinicians. There must be adequate visualization for surgical access to debride the defect completely and access to place and stabilize soft and hard tissue graft materials. In addition, it is important to be able to ascertain whether there are unexpected dehiscence or fenestration defects buccally or palato-lingually.

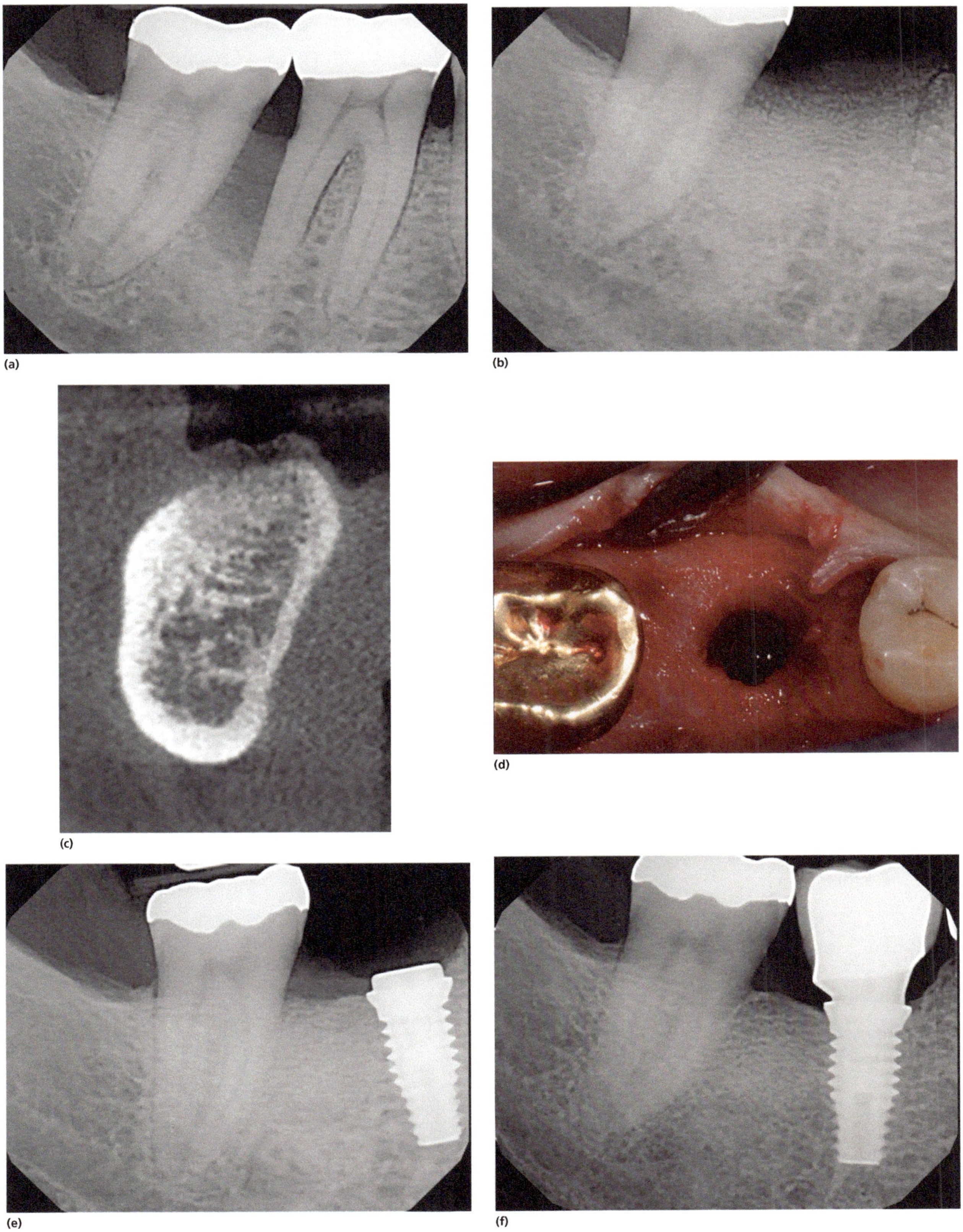

Figure 7.13 (a) This radiograph demonstrates advanced vertical bone loss to the apices of the first molar and to 80% for the second molar, which had hopeless and guarded prognoses respectively. (b) The first molar extraction site was grafted with rhPDGF-BB-enhanced freeze-dried bone allograft covered by a collagen membrane. The growth-factor-enhanced healing resulted in early bone formation and graft biomaterial integration, as evidenced by this 5-week post-operative radiograph. (c) The 3.5-month CBCT scan revealed extensive bone regeneration. (d) The surgical re-entry at 8 months demonstrated the degree of bone fill and little evidence of the graft particulate. (e) The bone fill on the mesial of the second molar allows for ideal implant placement. (f) The 3-year follow-up periapical radiograph.

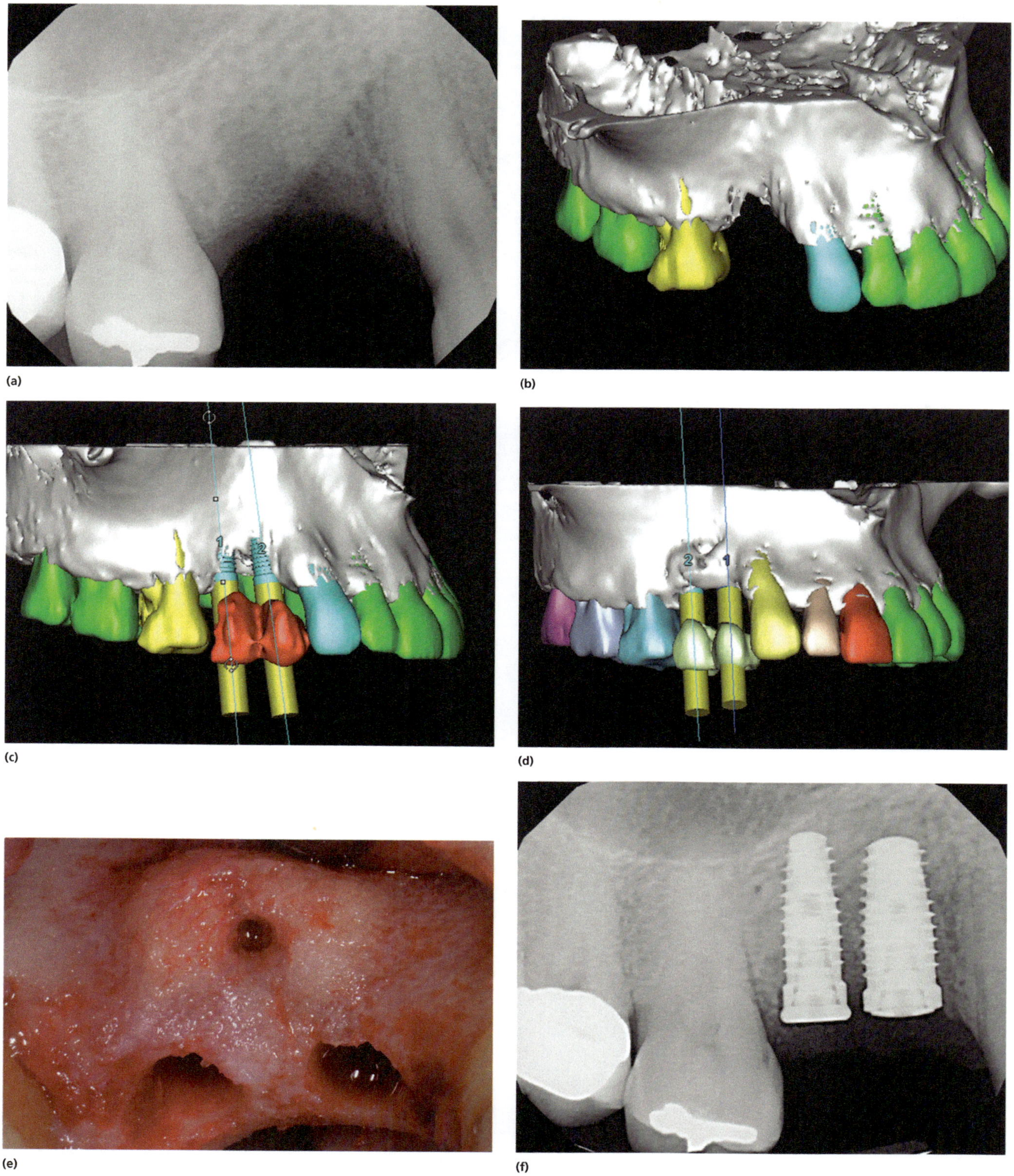

Figure 7.14 (a, b) Note the significant bone loss post-extraction from pressure due to an ill-fitting removable partial denture. (c) A pretreatment CBCT scan using a barium stent fabricated via a diagnostic wax-up allowed an accurate diagnosis and treatment plan. (d) A scaffold system combining a tenting screw, freeze-dried bone allograft (soaked in rhPDGF-BB), and a resorbable membrane were used successfully to regenerate the ridge, as evidenced in the 5-month post-grafting CT scan. (e) Re-entry demonstrated adequate bone for implant placement (Figure 7.3d) and allowed for implant placements. (f) Post-placement radiograph of the implants.

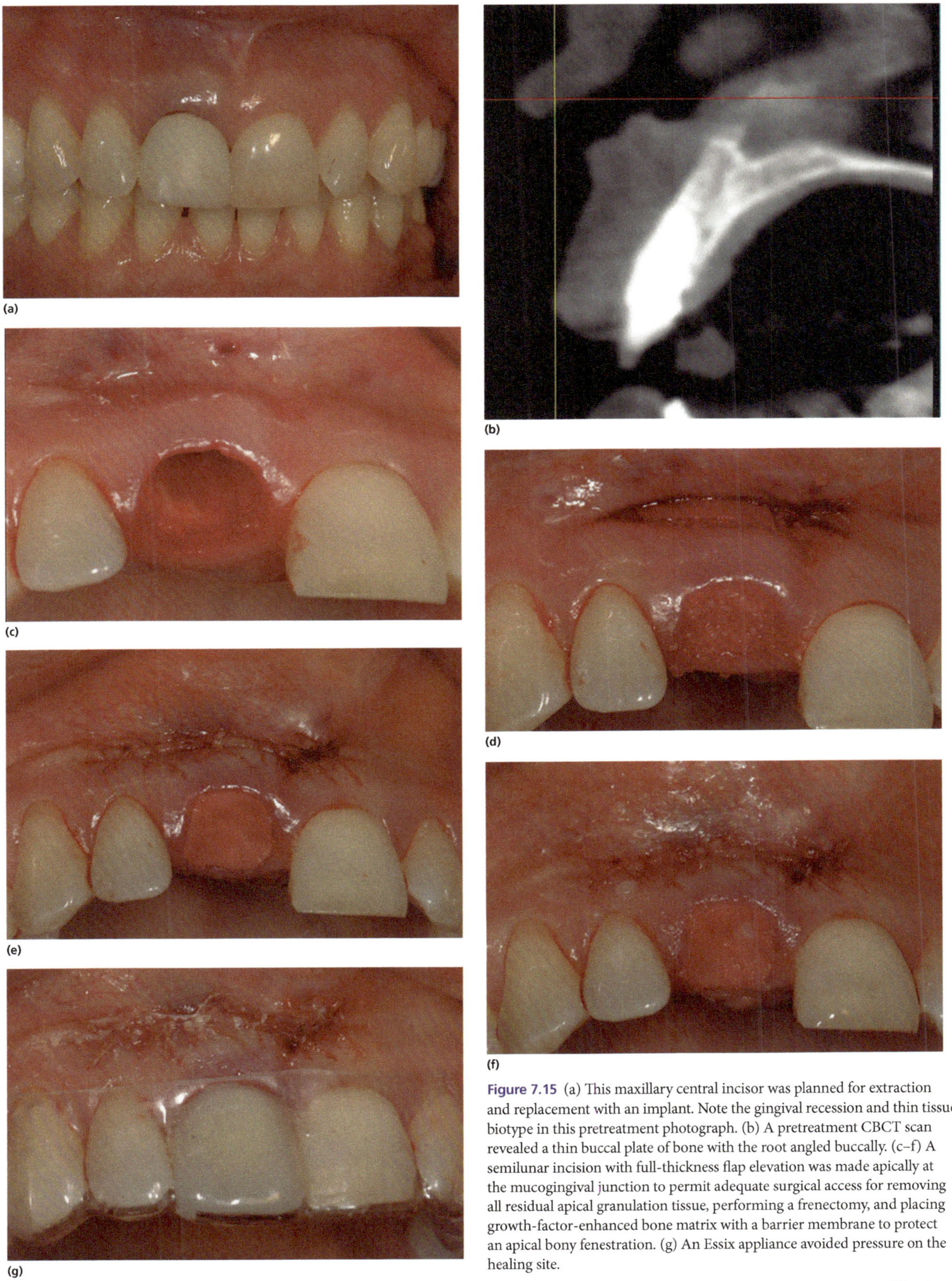

Figure 7.15 (a) This maxillary central incisor was planned for extraction and replacement with an implant. Note the gingival recession and thin tissue biotype in this pretreatment photograph. (b) A pretreatment CBCT scan revealed a thin buccal plate of bone with the root angled buccally. (c–f) A semilunar incision with full-thickness flap elevation was made apically at the mucogingival junction to permit adequate surgical access for removing all residual apical granulation tissue, performing a frenectomy, and placing growth-factor-enhanced bone matrix with a barrier membrane to protect an apical bony fenestration. (g) An Essix appliance avoided pressure on the healing site.

(Continued)

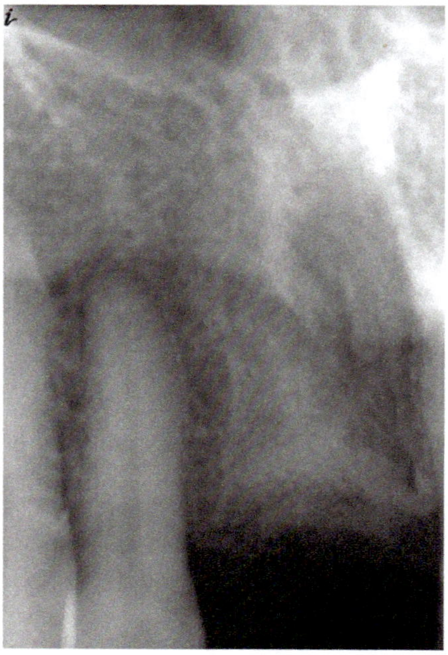

(h)

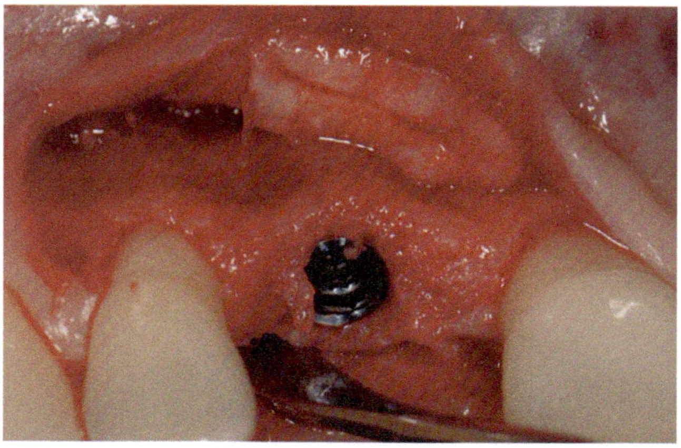

(i)

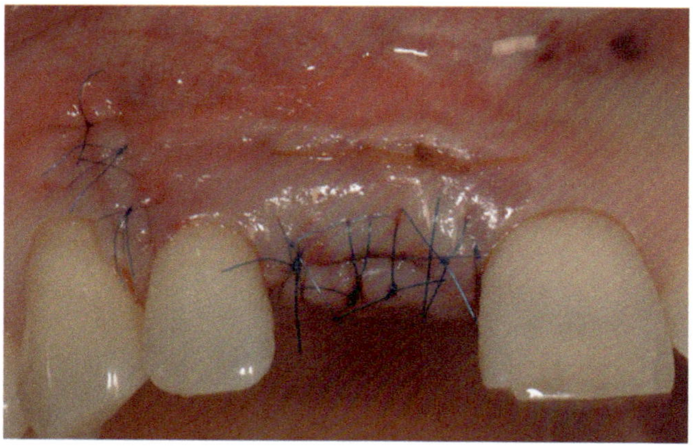

(j)

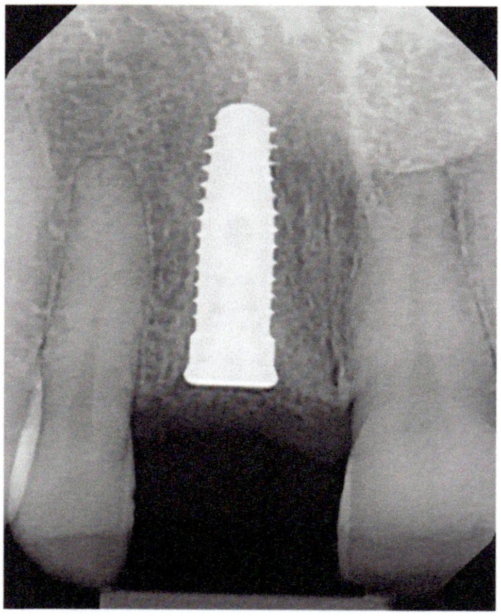

(k)

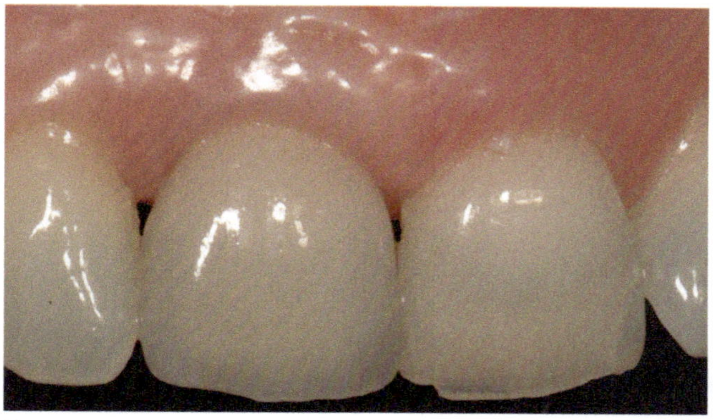

(l)

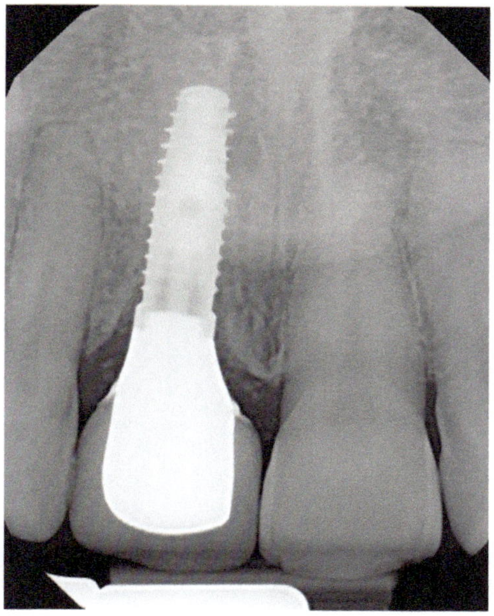

(m)

Figure 7.15 (Continued)
(h) The periapical radiograph 3 months post-extraction. (i–k) Re-entry surgery after 5 months' healing allowed implant placement and connective tissue grafting. (l, m) The final restoration met the patient's functional and esthetic needs.

Discussion

Using rhBMP-2 or rhPDGF-BB can reduce the invasiveness of alveolar bone grafting procedures needed for extraction site preservation or augmentation of healed and resorbed extraction sites by eliminating the need for autogenous bone grafts. However, one limitation is that the bone regenerated may take longer to develop adequate density for dental implant placement.[8,9,59] After 4 months healing, the bone present is still primarily woven, so that use of hand osteotomes and/or undersizing of the osteotomy may be necessary to achieve adequate initial implant stability. Following sinus grafting with rhBMP-2, Boyne et al.[9] reported significantly less radiographic bone density at 4 months than seen at autogenous bone-grafted sites. By 6 months, however, more similar bone density was seen in the two patient groups. A longer healing period of at least six to perhaps nine months also appears to be beneficial when using rhBMP-2 for onlay ridge augmentation.[10,11] However, healing of soft tissues over rhBMP-2 or rh-PDGF-BB grafted sites appears to be accelerated,[8,72] which may be related to the fact that these factors are pleiotropic and play roles in growth and differentiation. They have been found to be chemotactic for endothelial cells, and can also stimulate angiogenesis through the production of vascular endothelial growth factor A by osteoblasts.[73,74] This enhanced vascular response also may explain the erythema often seen in the overlying healing soft tissues, and perhaps even why achieving primary soft tissue closure, at least at sites where titanium mesh was not required, is not as crucial as is the situation with autogenous block grafts or GBR-type procedures using membranes. Compromise in these latter situations also is related to the fact that extensive flap elevation is necessary to place block grafts and to achieve adequate cortical bone support for barrier membranes used in GBR techniques. In contrast, the minimal flap elevation needed in many sites managed with rhBMP-2 or rh-PDGF-BB grafting results in far less disturbance of periosteal blood vessels, the principle source of nourishment of buccal bone.

Conclusions

There is good evidence to support the use of rh-BMP-2 or rhPDGF-BB with various scaffold carriers to reconstruct damaged or previously healed and resorbed extraction site defects; however, many of these applications are "off label." Addition of these growth factors stimulates robust new bone growth compared with osteoconductive graft materials on their own. The wounds require longer healing intervals than sites grafted with autogenous bone do. To the extent that rh-BMP-2 or rhPDGF-BB can reduce or eliminate the need for autogenous bone grafts of either intraoral or extraoral origin, their use will significantly reduce the level of invasiveness for procedures to augment larger immediate or healed extraction site bone defects. These growth factors also may have special application for high systemic risk patients, complex defects, and those with high esthetic demands.

References

1. Kaigler D, Cirelli J, Giannobile W. Growth factor delivery for oral and periodontal tissue engineering. Expert Opin Drug Deliv 2006; 3: 647–662.
2. Boyan B, Ranly D, Schwartz Z. Use of growth factors to modify osteoinductivity of demineralized bone allografts: lessons for tissue engineering of bone. Dent Clinics North Am 2006; 50(2): 217–228.
3. Reddi AH. Role of morphogenetic proteins in skeletal tissue engineering and regeneration. Nat Biotechnol 1998; 16: 247–252.
4. Wozney J, Rosen V, Celeste A. Novel regulators of bone formation: molecular clones and activities. Science 1988; 242: 1528–1534.
5. Hollinger J, Hart C, Hirsch S, et al. Recombinant human platelet-derived growth factor: biology and clinical applications. J Bone Joint Surg Am 2008; 90(Suppl 1): 48–54.
6. Cooke J, Sarment D, Whitesman L, et al. Effect of platelet-derived growth factor on mediators of periodontal wound repair. Tissue Eng 2006; 12: 1441–1450.
7. Fiorellini JP, Howell TH, Cochran D, et al. Randomized study evaluating recombinant human bone morphogenetic protein-2 for extraction socket augmentation. J Periodontol 2005; 76: 605–613.
8. Misch CM. The use of recombinant human bone morphogenetic protein-2 for the repair of extraction socket defects: a technical modification and case series report. Int J Oral Maxillofac Implants 2010; 25: 1246–1252.
9. Boyne PJ, Lilly LC, Marx RE, et al. De novo bone induction by recombinant human bone morphogenetic protein-2 (rhBMP-2) in maxillary sinus floor augmentation. J Oral Maxillofac Surg 2005; 63: 1693–707.
10. Triplett R, Nevins M, Marx R, et al. Pivotal, randomized, parallel evaluation of recombinant human bone morphogenetic protein-2/absorbable collagen sponge and autogenous bone graft for maxillary sinus floor augmentation. J Oral Maxillofac Surg 2009; 67: 1947–1960.
11. Marx R, Armentano L, Olavarria A, Samaniego J. RhBMP-2/ACS grafts versus autogenous cancellous marrow grafts in large vertical defects of the maxilla: an unsponsored randomized open-label clinical trial. Oral Craniofac Tissue Eng 2011; 1: 33–41.
12. Misch CM. Bone augmentation of the atrophic posterior mandible for dental implants using rhBMP-2 and titanium mesh: clinical technique and early results. Int J Periodontics Restorative Dent 2011; 31: 581–589.
13. Urist MR. Bone: formation by autoinduction. Science 1965; 115: 893–899.
14. Rummelhart J, Mellonig J, Gray J, Towley H. A comparison of freeze-dried bone allograft and demineralized freeze-dried bone allograft in human periodontal osseous defects. J Periodontol 1989; 60: 655–663.
15. Schwartz Z, Goldstein M, Raviv E, et al. Clinical evaluation of demineralized bone allograft in a hyaluronic acid carrier for sinus lift augmentation in humans: a computed tomography and histomorphometric study. Clin Oral Implant Res 2007; 18(2): 204–211.
16. Howell T, Fiorellini J, Paquette D, et al. A phase I/II clinical trial to evaluate a combination of recombinant human platelet-derived growth factor-BB and recombinant human insulin-like growth factor-I in patients with periodontal disease. J Periodontol 1997; 68: 1186–1193.
17. Camelo M, Nevins M, Schenk R, et al. Periodontal regeneration in human class II furcations using purified recombinant human platelet-derived growth factor-BB (rhPDGF-BB) with bone allograft. Int J Periodontics Restorative Dent 2003; 23: 213–225.
18. Nevins M, Hanratty J, Lynch S. Clinical results using recombinant human platelet-derived growth factor and mineralized freeze-dried bone allograft in periodontal defects. Int J Periodontics Restorative Dent 2007; 27: 421–427.
19. Sarment D, Cooke J, Miller S, et al. Effect of rhPDGF-BB on bone turnover during periodontal repair. J Clin Periodontol 2006; 33: 135–140.
20. Lynch S, de Castilla G, Williams R, et al. The effects of short-term application of a combination of platelet-derived and insulin-like growth factors on periodontal wound healing. J Periodontol 1991; 62: 458–467.
21. Homsi J, Daud AI. Spectrum of activity and mechanism of action of VEGF/PDGF inhibitors. Cancer Control 2007; 14: 285–294.
22. Nevins M, Giannobile W, McGuire M, et al. Platelet-derived growth factor stimulates bone fill and rate of attachment level gain: results of a large multicenter randomized controlled trial. J Periodontol 2005; 76: 2205–2215.
23. Nevins M, Kao R, McGuire M, et al. PDGF promotes periodontal regeneration in localized osseous defects: 36-month extension results from a randomized, controlled, double-masked clinical trial. J Periodontol 2013;84(4): 456–464.
24. Lynch S, Wisner-Lynch L, Nevins M, Nevins ML. A new era in periodontal and peri-implant regeneration: use of growth-factor enhanced matrices incorporating rhPDGF. Compend Contin Educ Dent 2006; 27: 672–678.
25. Nevins ML, Reynolds MA. Tissue engineering with recombinant human platelet-derived growth factor BB for implant site development. Compend Contin Educ Dent 2011; 32: 20–27.
26. Nevins ML, Camelo M, Nevins M, et al. Minimally invasive alveolar ridge augmentation procedure (tunneling technique) using rhPDGF-BB in combination with three matrices: a case series. Int J Periodontics Restorative Dent 2009; 29: 371–383.
27. Stephan E, Jiang D, Lynch S, et al. Anorganic bovine bone supports osteoblastic cell attachment and proliferation. J Periodontol 1999; 70: 364–369.
28. Nevins M, Nevins ML, Karimbux N, et al. The combination of purified recombinant human platelet-derived growth factor-BB and equine particulate bone graft for periodontal regeneration. J Periodontol 2012; 83: 565–573.
29. Simion M, Rocchietta I, Kim D, et al. Vertical ridge augmentation by means of deproteinized bovine bone block and recombinant human platelet-derived growth factor-BB: a histologic study in a dog model. Int J Periodontics Restorative Dent 2006; 26: 415–423.

30. Simion M, Rocchietta I, Dellavia C. Three-dimensional ridge augmentation with xenograft and recombinant human platelet-derived growth factor-BB in humans: report of two cases. Int J Periodontics Restorative Dent 2007; 27: 109–115.
31. Simion M, Nevins M, Rocchietta I, et al. Vertical ridge augmentation using an equine block infused with recombinant human platelet-derived growth factor-BB: a histologic study in a canine model. Int J Periodontics Restorative Dent 2009; 29: 245–255.
32. Carlsson G, Bergman B, Hedegård B. Changes in contour of the maxillary alveolar process under immediate dentures. A longitudinal clinical and x-ray cephalometric study covering 5 years. Acta Odontol Scand 1967; 25: 45–75.
33. Pietrokovski J, Massler M. Alveolar ridge resorption following tooth extraction. J Prosthetic Dent 1967; 17: 21–27.
34. Schropp L, Wenzel A, Kostopoulos L, Karring T. Bone healing and soft tissue contour changes following single-tooth extraction: a clinical and radiographic 12-month prospective study. Int J Periodontics Restorative Dent 2003; 23: 313–323.
35. Grunder, U, Gracis S, Capelli M. Influence of the 3-D bone-to-implant relationship on esthetics. Int J Periodontics Restorative Dent 2005; 25: 113–119.
36. Covani U, Bortolaia C, Barone A, Sbordone L. Bucco-lingual crestal bone changes after immediate and delayed implant placement. J Periodontol 2004; 75: 1605–1612.
37. Miyamoto Y, Obama T. Dental cone beam computed tomography analyses of post-operative labial bone thickness in maxillary anterior implants: comparing immediate and delayed implant placement. Int J Periodontics Restorative Dent 2011; 31: 215–225.
38. Kan JY, Rungcharassaeng K, Sclar A, Lozada JL. Effects of the facial osseous defect morphology on gingival dynamics after immediate tooth replacement and guided bone regeneration: 1-year results. J Oral Maxillofac Surg 2007; 65(Suppl 1): 13–19.
39. Wang H-L, Kiyonobu K, Neiva RF. Socket augmentation: rationale and technique. Implant Dent 2004; 13: 286–296.
40. Aghaloo TL, Moy PK. Which hard tissue augmentation techniques are the most successful in furnishing bony support for implant placement? Int J Oral Maxillofac Implants 2007; 22(Suppl): 49–70.
41. Nevins M, Carmelo M, De Paoli S, et al. A study of the fate of the buccal wall of extraction sockets of teeth with prominent roots. Int J Periodontics Restorative Dent 2006; 26: 19–29.
42. Brugmani I, Caiazzo A. Efficacy evaluation of a new buccal bone plate preservation technique. A pilot study. Int J Periodontics Restorative Dent 2011; 31: 67–73.
43. Wang HL, Boyapati L. "PASS" principles for predictable bone regeneration. Implant Dent 2006; 15: 8–17.
44. Elian N, Cho S, Froum S, et al. A simplified socket classification and repair technique. Pract Proced Aesthet Dent 2007; 19: 99–104.
45. Schwartz Z, Somers A, Mellonig JT, et al. Ability of commercial demineralized freeze-dried bone allograft to induce new bone formation is dependent on donor age but not gender. J Periodontol 1998; 69: 470–478.
46. Blum B, Moseley J, Miller L, et al. Measurement of bone morphogenetic proteins and other growth factors in demineralized bone matrix. Orthopedics 2004; 27: S161–S165.
47. Barnes B, Boden S, Louis-Ugbo J, et al. Lower dose of rhBMP-2 achieves spine fusion when combined with an osteoconductive bulking agent in non-human primates. Spine 2005; 30: 1127–1133.
48. Kraiwattanapong C, Boden S, Louis-Ugbo J, et al. Comparison of Healos/bone marrow to INFUSE (rhBMP-2/ACS) with a collagen-ceramic sponge bulking agent as graft substitutes for lumbar spine fusion. Spine 2005; 30: 1001–1007.
49. Berglundh T, Lindhe J, Jonsson K, Ericsson I. The topography of vascular systems in the periodontal and peri-implant tissues in the dog. J Clin Periodontol 1994; 21: 189–193.
50. Patcas R, Muller L, Ullrich O, Peltomaki T. Accuracy of cone-beam computed tomography at different resolutions assessed on the bony covering of the mandibular anterior teeth. Am J Orthod Dentofacial Orthoped 2012; 141: 41–50.
51. Simion M, Fontana F, Rasperini G, Maiorana C. Vertical ridge augmentation by expanded-polytetrafluoroethylene membrane and a combination of intraoral autogenous bone graft and deproteinized anorganic bovine bone (Bio Oss®). Clin Oral Implants Res 2007; 18: 620–629.
52. Misch CM. Chapter 24. Autogenous bone grafting for dental implants. In: Oral and Maxillofacial Surgery, vol. 1, 2nd ed., FonsecaRJ, TurveryTA, MarcianiRD, eds. Philadelphia, PA: W.B. Saunders Co., 2008, pp. 344–370.
53. Misch CM. Comparison of intraoral donor sites for onlay grafting prior to implant placement. Int J Oral Maxillofac Implants 1997; 12: 767–776.
54. McKay W, Peckham S, Marotta J. The Science of RhBMP-2. St. Louis, MO: Quality Medical Publishing, 2006, pp. 88–116.
55. Spagnoli DB, Marx RE. Dental implants and the use of rhBMP-2. Oral Maxillofac Surg Clin North Am 2011; 23: 347–361.
56. Gutta R, Baker RA, Bartolucci AA, Louis PJ. Barrier membranes used for ridge augmentation: is there an optimal pore size? J Oral Maxillofac Surg 2009; 67: 1218–1225.
57. Dahlin C, Linde A, Gottlow J, Nyman S. Healing of bone defects by guided tissue regeneration. Plastic Reconstr Surg 1988; 81: 672–676.
58. Jovanovic S, Hunt D, Bernard G, et al. Bone reconstruction following implantation of rhBMP-2 and guided bone regeneration in canine alveolar ridge defects. Clin Oral Implants Res 2007; 18: 224–230.
59. Wozney J, Wikesjo UM. RhBMP-2: biology and applications in oral and maxillofacial surgery and periodontics. In: Tissue engineering, 2nd ed., LynchSE, MarxRE, NevinsM, Wisner-LynchLA, eds. Chicago, IL: Quintessence, 2008, pp. 159–177.
60. Schopper C, Moser D, Spassova E, et al. Bone regeneration using a naturally grown HA/TCP carrier loaded with rhBMP-2 is independent of barrier membrane effects. J Biomed Mater Res A 2008; 85: 954–963.
61. Proussaefs P, Lozada J, Kleinman A, et al. The use of titanium mesh in conjunction with autogenous bone graft and inorganic bovine bone mineral (Bio-Oss) for localized alveolar ridge augmentation: a human study. Int J Periodontics Restorative Dent 2003; 23: 185–195.
62. Louis P, Gutta R, Said-Al-Naief N, Bartolucci A. Reconstruction of the maxilla and mandible with particulate bone graft and titanium mesh for implant placement. J Oral Maxillofac Surg 2008; 66: 235–245.
63. Boyne P. Osseous Reconstruction of the Maxilla and the Mandible: Surgical Techniques Using Titanium Mesh and Bone Mineral. Chicago, IL: Quintessence, 1997, pp. 1–100.
64. Lekholm U, Zarb G. Patient selection. In: Tissue-Integrated Prostheses: Osseointegration in Clinical Dentistry, BrånemarkP-I, AlbrektssonT, ZarbG, eds. 1985. Chicago, IL: Quintessence.
65. McAllister B, Haghighat K, Prasad H, Rohrer M. Histologic evaluation of recombinant human platelet-derived growth factor-BB after use in extraction socket defects: a case series. Int J Periodontics Restorative Dent 2010; 30: 365–373.
66. Nevins ML, Camelo M, Schupbach P, et al. Human histologic evaluation of mineralized collagen bone substitute and recombinant platelet-derived growth factor-BB to create bone for implant placement in extraction socket defects at 4 and 6 months: a case series. Int J Periodontics Restorative Dent 2009; 29: 129–139.
67. Nevins ML, Camelo M, Schupbach P, et al. Human buccal plate extraction socket regeneration with recombinant human platelet-derived growth factor BB or enamel matrix derivative. Int J Periodontics Restorative Dent 2011; 31: 481–492.
68. Belal M, Watanabe H, Ichinose S, Ishikawa I. Effect of Er-YAG laser combined with rh-PDGF-BB on attachment of cultured fibroblasts to periodontally involved root surfaces. J Periodontol 2007; 78: 1329–1341.
69. Fu J, Lee A, Wang H. Influence of tissue biotype on implant esthetics. Int J Oral Maxillofac Implants 2011; 26: 499–508.
70. Grunder U. Placing implants at the time of tooth extraction with and without soft tissue augmentation after a healing period of 6 months: report of 24 consecutive cases. Int J Periodontics Restorative Dent 2011; 31: 9–17.
71. Linkevicius T, Apse P, Grybauskas S, Puisys A. The influence of soft tissue thickness on crestal bone changes around implants: a 1-year prospective controlled clinical trial. Int J Oral Maxillofac Implants 2009; 24: 712–719.
72. Govender S, Csimma C, Genant H, et al. Recombinant human bone morphogenetic protein-2 for treatment of open tibial fractures: a prospective, controlled, randomized study of four hundred and fifty patients. J Bone Joint Surg Am 2002; 84: 2123–2134.
73. Deckers M, van Bezooijen R, van der Horst G, et alS. Bone morphogenetic proteins stimulate angiogenesis through osteoblast-derived vascular endothelial growth factor A. Endocrinology 2002; 143: 1545–1553.
74. Li G, Cui Y, McILmurray L, et al. RhBMP-2, rhVEGF165, rhPTN and thrombin-related peptide, TP508 induced chemotaxis of human osteoblasts and microvascular endothelial cells. J Orthop Res 2005; 23: 680–685.

CHAPTER 8

Periodontal and Peri-Implant Soft Tissue Surgery

Giles Horrocks,[1] Christine Cole,[2] & Daniel R. Cullum[3]
[1,2]Private Practice, Periodontics, Boulder, CO, USA
[3]Private Practice, Coeur d'Alene, ID; Loma Linda University Department of OMS, Loma Linda, CA; UCLA Department of OMS, Los Angeles, CA, USA

Introduction

Periodontal plastic surgery is often necessary for the management of both hard and soft tissue defects around teeth and implants, demanding both skill and innovation from the surgeon. By incorporating literature-based mucogingival surgical procedures with adequate bone volume parameters, an esthetic and stable restoration can be achieved. Further, by refining these techniques and minimizing trauma, the surgical approach can become minimally invasive. Ultimately, the goal should be to limit the number of procedures, duration of treatment, potential morbidity, and/or cost. A key factor in minimally invasive surgical technique is to avoid vascular compromise by eliminating open flap exposure where possible, being selective in the use of vertical releasing incisions,[1] utilizing supraperiosteal tunneling techniques,[2] and repositioning and rotating soft tissue flaps to maintain a vascularized pedicle of tissue at the defect site.[3–5] Additional considerations include combining procedures, minimizing donor site morbidity with minimally invasive harvesting techniques, or using commercially available allografts, xenografts, or biologics. The choice of soft tissue autograft, allograft, or xenograft will be dependent on the existing defect size, the surgeon's preference, and the requirements of the specific augmentation. Esthetic demands may require a combination of techniques to achieve the desired outcome. For minimally invasive surgery, case selection, treatment planning, and surgical technique are more demanding than for staged and/or open procedures. This chapter will present clinical applications of open and closed techniques to advance patient treatment with minimally invasive surgical principles.

Anatomic considerations

Oral soft tissue morphology

The role of oral soft tissues is to maintain a physical barrier to protect teeth and implant sites from invasion by bacteria and/or injury from their by-products. Oral soft tissue morphology also plays an important role in esthetics and long-term soft tissue health.[6–8] Relevant soft tissue types include alveolar mucosa and gingiva, which have rich anastomoses of arterioles and capillaries that facilitate faster healing compared for example with skin in response to injury.[9]

Alveolar mucosa is a loose areolar connective tissue that is non-keratinized and less fibrous, but more vascular than attached gingiva. It is less effective in maintaining health around both teeth and dental implants. Because of its mobility, alveolar mucosa is often unable to withstand the trauma of mastication and daily maintenance. Additionally, oral hygiene procedures can be painful without the support of keratinized tissue, thereby limiting a patient's motivation for appropriate daily maintenance.[10] In contrast, attached gingiva is keratinized and has a thick lamina propria containing dense collagen fibers in closely packed bundles that are firmly attached to the periosteum of underlining bone.[9] It can withstand the compressive and shear forces of mastication and oral hygiene efforts. It has been shown that increasing attached keratinized tissue width around implants to at least 2 mm can reduce the immunologic response to bacterial biofilm[8] and result in less radiographic bone loss and improved indices of soft tissue health.[7]

The gingival biotypes of oral soft tissues in the natural dentition have been described as thin and thick.[11] Kan et al.[12] suggested that periodontal probe visibility through the gingival tissue is a simple way to distinguish a thin from a thick gingival biotype. The thin gingival biotype has a thickness of ≤ 1.5 mm, and commonly results in recession with natural teeth following the onset of an inflammatory process,[13] traumatic tooth brushing, orthodontic tooth movements, or as a result of an underlying root prominence and bony dehiscence. Thin biotype is often associated with a triangular tooth form, thin alveolar bone, and root prominence. This results in the alveolar crestal bone level being at a greater distance from the gingival margin, increasing the risk of soft tissue recession and/or alveolar bone volume loss following tooth extraction. Additionally, the triangular tooth shape leaves an open embrasure space, exacerbating any papillary volume loss. The generally accepted definition of a thick gingival biotype is one with a gingival thickness of >2 mm,[11] and typically is associated with a square tooth form. Thick tissue biotype is also moderately correlated to thicker bone when evaluated by cone beam computed tomography (CBCT).[14] In a review of literature, Hwang and Wang reported a high association between soft tissue flap thickness and complete root coverage with soft tissue grafting for natural teeth.[15] Thick keratinized tissue has also been shown to be of benefit in protecting the periodontium when restorative margins are present.[6] These observations suggest that a thicker tissue biotype might be significant in influencing esthetic treatment outcomes with implants.

The dento-gingival versus implant–gingival complex

The gingival complex of the natural dentition presents as a true soft tissue attachment.[9] The junctional epithelium surrounds the perimeter of the tooth as an epithelial-lined sleeve providing a seal from

Minimally Invasive Dental Implant Surgery, First Edition. Edited by Daniel R. Cullum and Douglas Deporter.

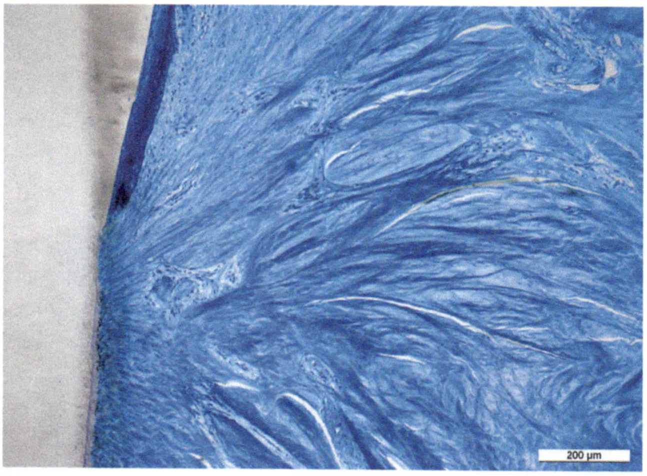

(a)

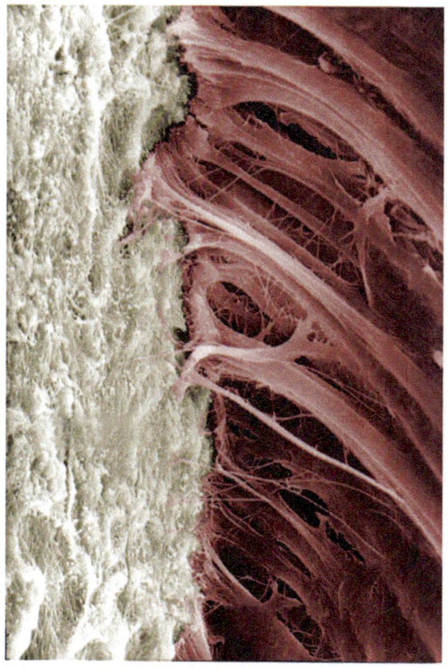

(b)

Figure 8.1 (a) Periodontal attachment–junctional epithelium supported by strong dentogingival fibers. (b) Numerous collagenous fibrils are bundled into one fiber and each fiber is firmly anchored to the mineralized cementum. Courtesy of Dr Peter Schupbach. Nobel Biocare. Reproduced with permission of Nobel Biocare.

the oral environment. It is supported by the underlying lamina propria, which emerges from the alveolar bone and comprises dense collagenous Sharpey's fibers that insert perpendicularly to the root surface into the cementum (Figure 8.1). These components in essence comprise the "biologic width" around natural teeth. Natural teeth also have an extensive vascular complex within the periodontal ligament, which complements that of the surrounding bone.

In contrast to teeth, the implant gingival complex offers a less robust attachment mechanism comprised of connective tissue without true collagen fiber attachment to the implant surface.[16] The junctional epithelium is supported by a lamina propria, but this lacks a perpendicular connective tissue orientation and surface attachment. The usual implant gingival complex is much like an "O"-ring with parallel, circularly oriented collagen fibers (Figure 8.2). The protective seal around an implant is provided by adhesion of the junctional epithelium via hemidesmosomes at the transgingival implant surface. One exception may be a proprietary implant design that uses laser microgrooves created on its neck region and/or prosthetic abutments to promote formation of a more tooth-like soft tissue attachment (see Chapter 6). Nevins and coworkers have shown human[17,18] and animal[19] histologic results confirming a direct attachment of perpendicularly oriented connective tissue fibers to this type of implant surface. The physical barrier created has been suggested to inhibit migration of epithelium and help protect against crestal bone resorption. The periodontal ligament vascular plexis, however, is still absent at the peri-implant soft tissues. For this reason, it has been suggested that peri-implant gingiva may be more susceptible to injury or infection, and can display a stronger inflammatory response than seen in gingiva around natural teeth.[16] Furthermore, animal studies have shown a more rapid progression of peri-implant mucositis to peri-implantitis compared with the progression of gingivitis to periodontitis.[20,21]

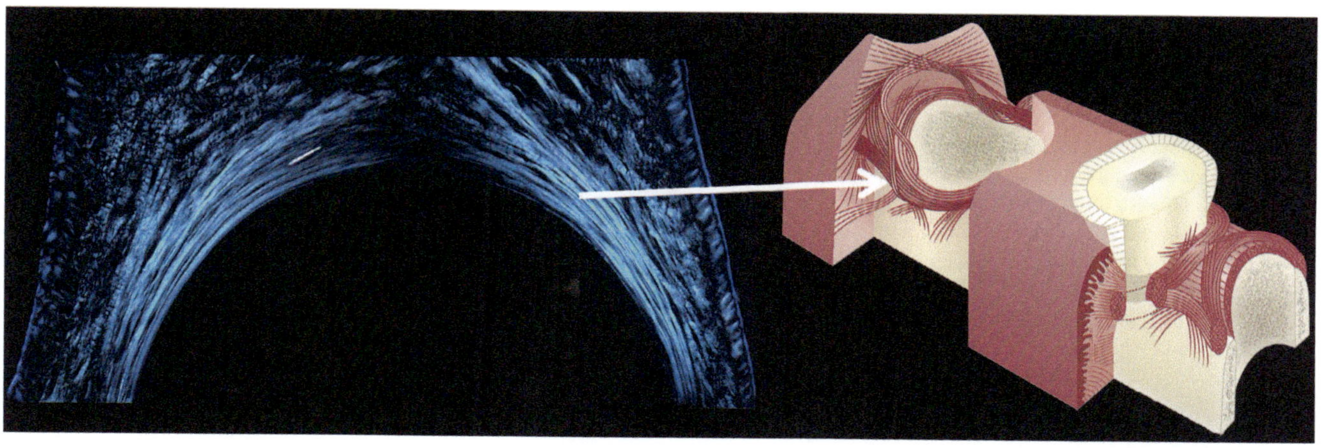

Figure 8.2 "O-ring" stability at the implant–gingival complex is provided by circular fibers as seen on polarized light microscopy, arranged around an implant abutment in an "O-ring" configuration. Courtesy of Dr Peter Schupbach. Nobel Biocare. Reproduced with permission of Nobel Biocare.

Causes of peri-implant inflammation are various and include a foreign body reaction to even small amounts of retained peri-implant crown cement deposits, bacterial plaque accumulation, especially at exposed rough surface implants, and/or implant component mobility and bacterial accumulation at the "microgap" (implant–abutment junction).[22–26]

Quality and quantity of soft tissue and bone support

Bone volume is a key factor in its response to crestal bone loss due to inflammation. While some teeth develop periodontal pocketing and vertical bone defects, others manifest horizontal bone loss and soft tissue recession.[27] The wider the alveolus surrounding a tooth, the more apt the site is to develop a vertical intrabony defect with the onset of inflammatory periodontal disease. However, with narrower alveoli and thin buccal bone, buccal and/or lingual cortical walls can be breached, and bone loss will present in a more horizontal pattern with soft tissue recession. Conceptually, marginal bone remodeling around implants is similar to that of teeth with establishment of the biologic width in relation to the microgap[28] (Figure 8.3). If an alveolus is broad bucco-lingually, the marginal bone may remodel to form a circumferential three-wall bone defect, and the soft tissue height will remain unchanged (Figure 8.3a and c). However, if the cortical bone is thinner than 2 mm, marginal bone remodeling may breach the buccal and lingual plates with bone loss and often manifest clinically as soft tissue recession (Figure 8.3b and d). In the esthetic zone, soft tissue recession and crestal resorption about implants likely will occur if the underlying facial bone is <2 mm in thickness.[29,30]

Many studies have shown the relationship of bone levels and papilla fill,[32,33] but the role of thick soft tissue as a protective barrier against facial and crestal bone loss around implants has recently been presented. Linkevicius et al.[30] observed in a human study 1.45 mm of crestal bone loss with implants placed in sites with thin overlying soft tissues (≤2.5 mm), while sites with thicker soft tissues had a mean of only 0.26 mm of crestal loss. Other studies have shown that the underlying bone volume correlates to the overlying

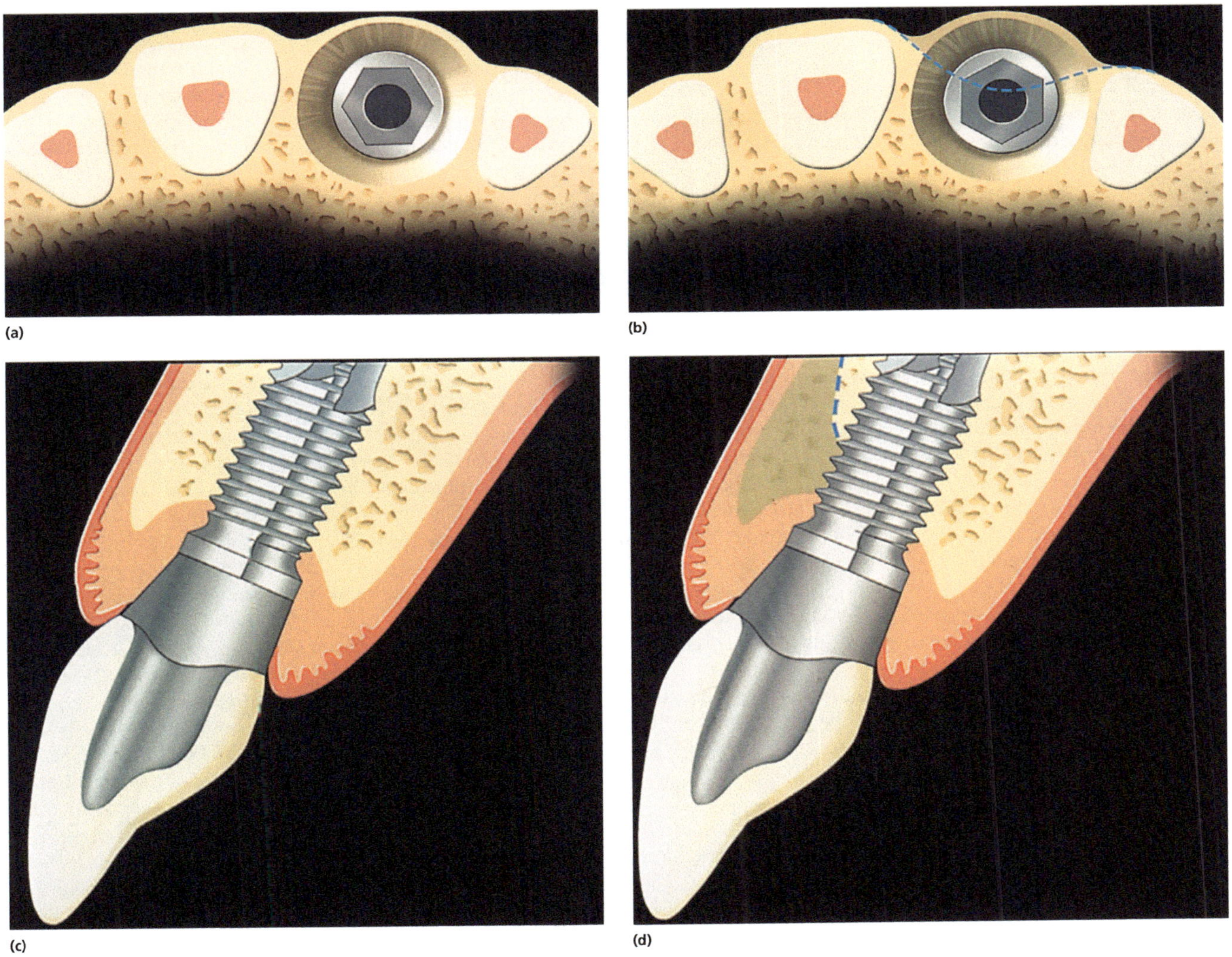

Figure 8.3 (a, c) Peri-implant bone remodeling and crestal bone volume.[28] Good thickness of bone on the buccal side of implant is necessary to support the gingival margin following bone remodeling for establishment of the biologic width. (b, d) Inadequate buccal bone thickness on an implant can result in vertical bone loss and recession of the gingival margin following remodeling needed for biologic width. Grunder et al. 2005.[28] Reproduced with permission of Quintessence Publishing Co., Inc.

tissue thickness. In a retrospective study on anterior implants, Le suggested that thicker facial bone is highly associated with the presence of thicker overlying soft tissue.[31] Whether this reflects the need for thicker soft tissues to maintain the facial bone or the reverse is still unclear. The absence of adequate peri-implant keratinized gingiva may result in higher plaque accumulation and gingival inflammation because of the patient's unwillingness or inability to maintain good homecare.[34,35] In a study of immediate single-tooth implant restorations, patients with thin mucosa often had greater tissue recession, while patients with thick keratinized mucosa tended to maintain more favorable implant papilla height.[36]

Thus, a reasonably wide and thick band of keratinized tissue is recommended to ensure implant treatment success, particularly in the esthetic zone. A 5 mm width of keratinized tissue is recommended around natural teeth for long-term restorative success, with 2 mm of sulcus depth and 3 mm of attached tissue.[6] Without a minimum of 2 mm width[7] and similar thickness,[30] there may be insufficient keratinized tissue about an implant to ensure optimal esthetics, patient comfort, and resistance to the trauma of brushing.[37] A thin peri-implant soft tissue biotype will more likely be subject to crestal bone loss and other complications, especially if there is any deficiency of underlying bone volume.

Surgical considerations

Periodontal plastic surgical procedures, including minimally invasive modifications thereof, require careful preoperative assessment of the dentition. Evaluation of the overall periodontal and restorative status of dentate and edentulous areas, smile assessment, and facial esthetics are crucial to development of a treatment plan (see Chapter 1). Classifications of recession defects in the tooth environment help to predict surgical outcomes, and also guide the surgeon in the choice of flap design. Utilizing the Miller classification for tooth gingival recession defects[38] can help in the implant environment because it predicts outcomes based on the surrounding blood supply and underlying bone support. Also, its consideration of vertical interproximal bone heights framing the recession defect will aid in predicting the potential vertical soft tissue correction. For example, in a Miller class III tooth recession defect, in addition to root exposure beyond the mucogingival junction there is also horizontal interproximal bone loss, and only partial root coverage can be expected regardless of the type of surgical intervention utilized.

The objectives of periodontal plastic surgery in the natural dentition are:

1. To create an adequate width and thickness of attached keratinized gingiva, especially when restorative margins will be covered by gingiva.
2. To correct gingival recessions using root coverage techniques.
3. To relieve the pull of frenum and muscle attachments on the gingival margin.
4. To correct deformities of edentulous ridges.
5. To deepen a shallow vestibule.
6. To assist in orthodontic therapy, by uncovering impacted teeth and ensuring appropriate gingiva is positioned onto the facial surface.

Osseointegrated dental implants, as already noted, lack a periodontal ligament vascular complex; as a result, soft tissue grafting, including that for management of implant recession defects, requires complete soft tissue coverage of graft materials irrespective of the size of defect or the material used. In contrast, in the tooth environment, smaller defects can be treated with minimal surgical intervention and autogenous tissue can be left exposed.[39] Biologic width in the natural dentition occurs above the residual alveolar crest and is comprised of the connective tissue and epithelial attachment that separates the oral environment from bone. However, dental implant biologic width generally forms apically to the implant–abutment junction ("microgap").[40] When facial bone thickness is less than 2 mm, remodeling will result in crestal bone loss[29] and the result will be either soft tissue recession or deeper soft tissue pocket formation than seen with natural teeth. In an effort to eliminate the risk of recession, maintaining or augmenting the site to develop the thickest bone and soft tissue possible seems prudent.

The objectives of peri-implant gingival plastic surgery are to:

1. enhance the width and thickness of existing tissues;
2. ensure that there is sufficient soft tissue to allow good emergence profile development for implant crowns;
3. mask underlying restorative materials;
4. avoid soft tissue recession;
5. offer sufficient tissue resistance to mastication and daily homecare; and
6. facilitate wound closure and healing.[41]

Accurate assessment of the periodontal attachment levels of teeth adjacent to a site intended for extraction or augmentation is critical in predicting final soft tissue and bone levels following tooth loss and implant placement. With attachment loss on adjacent teeth, papilla reformation will be compromised. The vertical anticipated papilla position can be predicted in various implant restorative scenarios; that is, between two adjacent teeth, between an implant and tooth, between two adjacent implants, and at adjacent pontic sites.[33] To increase the predictability of an esthetic outcome the clinician must include these known tissue dimensions in the restorative plan (see Chapters 1 and 4). In most instances, placing two implants adjacent to each other in the esthetic zone will lead to soft tissue contour compromise, particularly in the central/lateral incisor locations. Shorter papilla fill can be expected between adjacent implants (especially with triangular crown form), with a lack of symmetry of the contralateral teeth. The only location in the high esthetic demand case where two adjacent implants may be esthetically acceptable is typically in the central incisor positions. The midline and central/lateral papillae will be shorter, but there will be bilateral symmetry of the shorter distal papillae, thus maintaining relative gingival esthetics. Future application of "platform-switching" designs and narrow implants may alter these planning guidelines, if early experience can be further documented.

The surgical-restorative team should begin with determining the desired final prosthetic outcome and esthetic predictability, and then determine the surgical management for an implant-retained prosthesis or a tooth- or tissue-borne prosthesis. Patients with high esthetic demands and unfavorable bone and/or soft tissue volume may best be managed by tooth-borne fixed prostheses. Alternatively, there will be cases such as the low smile-line patient where function and access for optimal daily home care will outweigh esthetic concerns, allowing adjacent implants to be used successfully. Communicating the limitations of implant soft tissue contours to the patient in advance is an important factor in the success or failure of the treatment. Operator experience is critical in the esthetic zone, and further challenged by the technical demands of minimally invasive soft tissue procedures. In more difficult cases, it may be prudent to consider referral to a more experienced clinician.

While soft tissue augmentation procedures may have limited effect on overall implant survival, they can have a significant role in esthetic success. The use of screw-retained restorations is helpful to avoid the potential for subgingival cement displacement and subsequent inflammatory changes and bone loss. Several implant design features may help to reduce unwanted soft tissue recession. "Platform switching" is an implant design feature using a smaller diameter abutment than the coronal implant platform. The microgap and associated bacteria are moved approximately 0.5 mm to the medial away from the bone crest, helping to reduce inflammatory crestal bone resorption.[42,43] Additionally, with platform switching, the thickness of the overlying soft tissue can be enhanced as the restorative abutment emergence begins narrower at the implant connection. Avoiding rough implant surfaces, especially on the coronal aspect near the microgap (at the trans-gingival portion), or intentionally modifying the surface are considerations. Use of laser microgrooves on the neck region and/or abutment may form a more tooth-like soft tissue attachment of perpendicularly oriented connective tissue fibers to this surface and has been suggested to inhibit migration of epithelium and help protect against crestal bone resorption.[18,19] A further design consideration is the use of a Morse taper internal implant–abutment connection to reduce both the micromotion associated with parallel-walled connections and reduce the size of the microgap.[44]

Flap design principles

In designing a flap for peri-implant soft tissue surgery, consideration must be given to blood supply, surgical handling, achieving tension-free closure, and anticipating the potential effects of post-operative edema. Important factors to be considered for the long-term success of free mucosal and connective tissue grafts include primary fixation without mobility, revascularization, and revitalization from the receptor site. Intimate contact with a highly vascular receptor site is especially critical to the success of free grafts. To be minimally invasive, peri-implant plastic surgical procedures must follow known mucogingival surgical principles, and be completed atraumatically. Crestal flap designs are most commonly used, while tunnel and pedicle designs have shown increasing applications.

The *crestally initiated flap* allows buccal or palatal soft tissues to be manipulated as full-thickness (mucoperiosteal), split-thickness (mucosal-full-thickness connective tissue), superficial layer split-thickness (mucosal-limited connective tissue), or a combination of these flap designs. The crestal incision position can be varied from a mid-crestal to the palatal aspect to increase the ultimate vertical height of buccal keratinized tissue and volume of the flap. Designs also can include maintaining the continuity of the periosteum and palatal connective tissue with the buccal flap in order to extend the flap length, allowing for enhanced volume with primary closure. A buccal incision should follow an envelope design with release at adjacent teeth, marginal release at the mucogingival junction, or maintenance of a trapezoidal shape with vertical releases to optimize vascular supply and promote graft containment. A buccal flap design often requires a periosteal releasing incision at the base of the flap for passive flap advancement and tension-free closure. Application with vertical releasing incisions can reduce the extent of horizontal exposure and enhance coronal positioning, but may reduce vascular supply especially if combined with an apical periosteal releasing incision. If the flap release is not passive (periosteal and muscle release is insufficient) or the flap thickness is compromised by being too thin, wound dehiscence and flap retraction can occur compromising the surgical result.

The traditional *split-thickness flap*[45] design allows for periosteal preservation with maintenance of vascular supply both to the underlying alveolar bone and exposed periosteum for revascularization when used with open soft tissue grafting procedures. The dissection is completed along the supraperiosteal plane by direct incision. The *superficial-layer split-thickness flap*[46] varies from the traditional split-thickness dissection in that the scalpel blade follows the contours of the outer buccal flap rather than the alveolar contour, and may gain adequate mobilization without periosteal release. This dissection allows for maximum flap release and mobility for tension-free closure, and may reduce post-operative bleeding and edema as the muscle layer is not disturbed. It can be very useful in periodontal plastic surgical procedures, allowing placement of a large volume of soft tissue graft without compromising primary closure. Care is needed, however, to keep a reasonable amount of connective tissue within the superficial layer of the flap in order to maintain adequate vascularity and avoid flap perforation.

The *tunnel flap* approach can be supraperiosteal alone, subperiosteal alone, or a combination of both. Originally, the supraperiosteal tunnel flap was designed with a sulcular incison extending to the mucogingival junction for use with connective tissue grafting for root coverage in recession defects.[47] Limited tunnel space is developed and vertical releasing incisions are required to allow graft placement. With the *modified tunnel technique,*[48] a full-thickness dissection to the level of the mucogingival junction is completed and then extended beyond the mucogingival junction in a supraperiosteal fashion. This modification can allow for greater flap mobilization without muscle fiber adhesion, giving greater access for soft tissue augmentation through the initial sulcular incision.

When *bone augmentation* is needed at a future implant site, it is important first to assess the quality and quantity of soft tissues at the recipient site. A thick, broad, passive flap with overlying keratinized gingiva is necessary to withstand the trauma of a large bone augmentation procedure, to maintain vascular supply, and to avoid wound dehiscence. Ensuring a wide zone of keratinized tissue also will help to provide adequate blood supply and the flap strength needed to withstand the forces created by edema and wound contraction. Soft tissue grafting with a xenograft or autograft is sometimes needed as a separate procedure prior to reconstructive bone grafting surgery. Alternatively, simultaneous hard and soft tissue grafting may be possible if adequate overlying flap coverage can be achieved.

Socket preservation grafting at the time of tooth extraction has become a routine procedure to minimize the resulting alveolar ridge resorption (see Chapters 5). Teeth with existing recession and/or a thin gingival biotype also may require soft tissue augmentation at the time of tooth extraction. In cases with a thin scalloped gingival contour, connective tissue grafting at the time of extraction may be necessary to preserve and enhance gingival dimensions. Connective tissue can be placed over the extraction socket and/or into a facial split-thickness tunnel to augment soft tissue volume over the underlying grafted site and prevent shrinkage and recession at the gingival margin. In the thin biotype with a high scalloped gingival architecture, an autograft is more predictable and esthetic than an allograft. When used over socket graft materials, connective tissue can be left exposed at the epithelial margins provided that the grafted tissue obtains vascular supply from the buccal and palatal/lingual supraperiosteal dissection. The connective tissue graft must be supported by bone and secured without mobility. This approach avoids the need for flap advancement to gain primary closure, avoiding distortion of the mucogingival junction. At smaller flapless extraction sites (lateral or most central incisors) a full-thickness gingival tissue "plug" may be grafted into the defect. It must be intimately approximated to the surrounding dental col for adequate vascular supply for regeneration.

Pedicle flap designs maintain their own vascular supply and can offer a more favorable prognosis than free grafts. Development and mobilization of these flaps requires adequate pedicle dimensions and blood supply to maintain flap vitality. Full-thickness designs can be used, but leave a significant defect at the donor site. Split-thickness design flaps are most commonly developed with epithelium and connective tissue or connective tissue and periosteum, maintaining residual coverage over the donor site. The flaps can be repositioned apically, laterally, coronally, or folded back over the pedicle to obtain soft tissue coverage or increased volume at the recipient site. Connective tissue can be grafted more predictably when secured by an overlying flap, especially in situations with a compromised periosteal bed as with an exposed root or implant surface or residual bony defect. The simplest approach is to use the apical positioned flap, which can be completed with a full-thickness or split-thickness dissection as discussed previously. The technical difficulty of these flaps increases from coronal and lateral repositioning to more complex palatal partial thickness designs.

Surgical techniques

Open recipient site preparation

Classic open recipient site preparation for soft tissue grafting generally employs vertical releasing incisions at the buccal line angles on either side of the surgical site. A split-thickness dissection avoiding flap dehiscence is extended beyond the mucogingival junction into the vestibular area. The periosteal bed must be free of muscle attachments and of adequate size to accommodate the intended graft. This will allow a blood supply for the graft from the underlying periosteum with open placement and a bilaminar blood supply with coronal or lateral repositioning to cover the graft, ensuring its survival. The dissection is extended to remove any vestibular mobility and allow the flap to be easily repositioned to the cementoenamel junction or sutured to the vestibule. If the adjacent teeth also require soft tissue grafting, any root convexity beyond the alveolar housing should be reduced and the root surfaces properly prepared. Careful root planing and surface demineralization with an agent such as saturated citric acid should be completed before the grafting.

Soft tissue grafts and open flap techniques

The use of autogenous tissues for soft tissue augmentation around dental implants is well described.[49] The implant surgeon should develop good skills with these techniques in an open flap environment prior to undertaking minimally invasive applications. While the *free gingival graft* has had the longest history and is technically less demanding, donor site morbidity can be significant as it is left with an exposed connective tissue wound base for secondary intention healing. Nevertheless, onlay grafting using full-thickness gingival grafts does have several applications in peri-implant plastic surgery, and can be used either before or during implant placement. For example, it may be needed at edentulous sites that have minimal keratinized tissue, very thin soft tissues, or require a

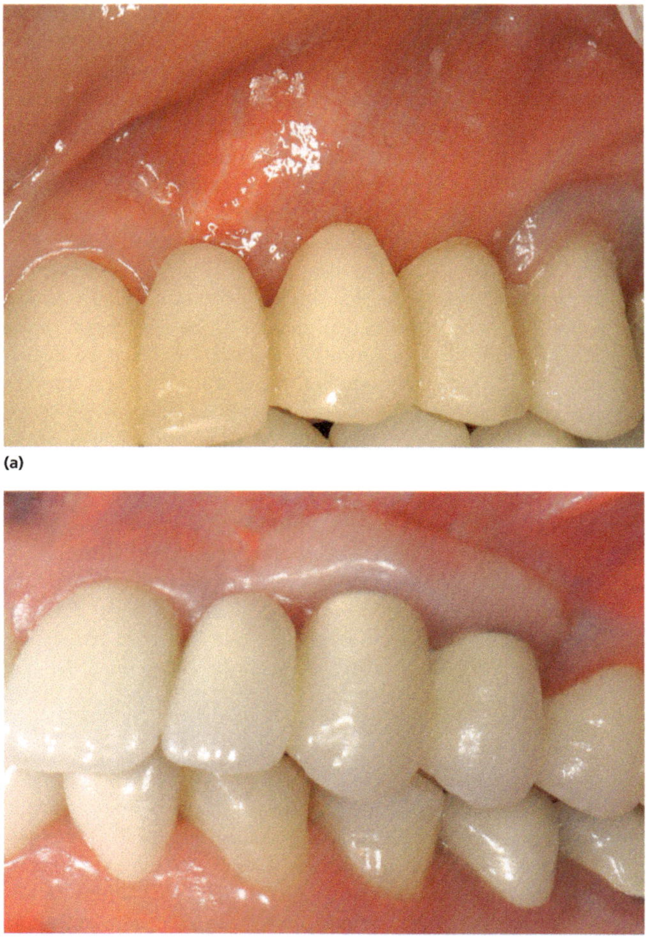

(a)

(b)

Figure 8.4 (a) The clinical presentation of the left maxilla with loss of the facial gingiva at the lateral incisor, canine, and first premolar sites after guided bone regeneration and labial flap advancement for primary wound closure. (b) The implant-supported restorations year after a free gingival graft was placed at the maxillary left canine and first premolar sites providing vestibular extension, frenum release, and an increase in the thickness and width of attached gingiva.

vestibular extension.[50] Figure 8.4a illustrates a case in which lost keratinized tissue needed to be replaced with a free gingival graft prior to implant placement at the maxillary left canine and first premolar sites. Figure 8.4b illustrates the 1-year result after restoration. An anterior cantilever pontic was used to replace the lateral incisor and was supported by implants at the canine and premolar sites.

Connective tissue grafts are more commonly used in periodontal and peri-implant grafting as they offer better color and texture results and have less donor site morbidity. Donor sites that can have suitable amounts of connective tissue include the palate, the tuberosity region, and occasionally other alveolar edentulous areas. The most common area from which to harvest connective tissue is the palate as it has the largest amount of connective tissue and is the most accessible. Palatal harvest of subepithelial connective tissue can be completed from the distal of the canine (avoiding sites with rugae) to the mid first molar region. The connective tissue layer is thinner anterior to the canine than in more posterior regions and is complicated by the nasopalatine foramen with its vascular and neural occupants.

The single incision technique for the collection of connective tissue grafts can be completed with a horizontal incision made 3–5 mm from the free gingival margin of remaining teeth.[51] A partial-thickness dissection is then made to release a palatal epithelial–connective tissue flap that has adequate thickness to minimize the risk of dehiscence (Figure 8.5a). The dissection extends vertically into the palatal vault, ensuring that an adequate thickness of connective tissue and periosteum remains attached to bone for later collection as the connective tissue graft. After ensuring adequate extension of the flap for access to the underlying tissue, the connective tissue and periosteum can be elevated (Figure 8.5c) and harvested with a combination of sharp and blunt dissection (Figure 8.5d). Any adipose tissue that remains attached on the undersurface of the graft is removed, and the graft is maintained in a moist environment until it can be transplanted to the recipient site.

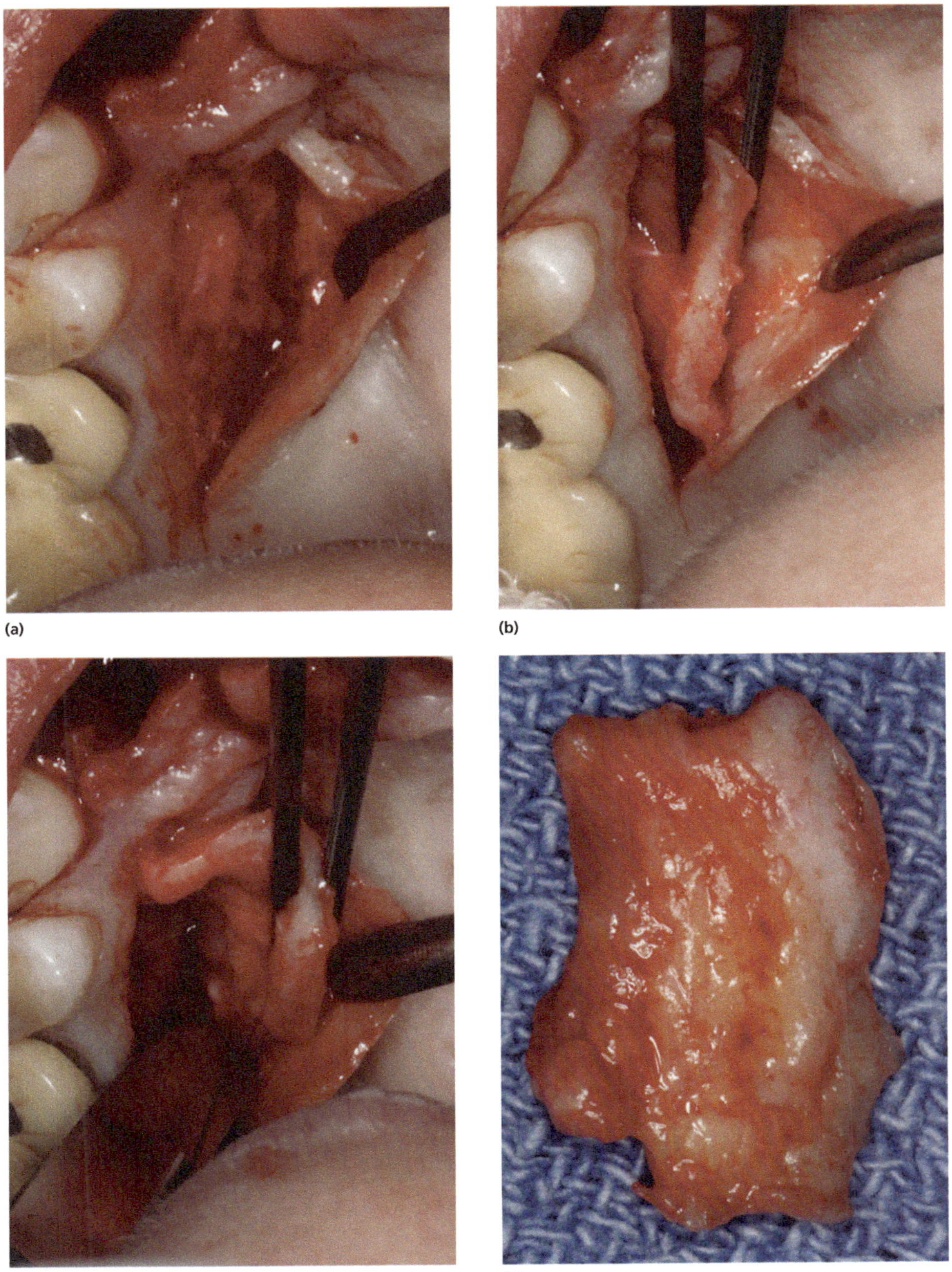

(a) (b) (c) (d)

Figure 8.5 (a) A palatal connective tissue harvest was completed using a curvilinear incision (mid-palatal of the first molar to the distal aspect of central incisor) at a minimum distance of 3 mm from the palatal gingival margin; dissection was done parallel to the palatal surface deep to the vault to gain maximum tissue harvest. Adequate thickness of the overlying epithelial flap is necessary to preserve blood supply and vitality during the donor site healing interval. (b) After ensuring adequate dimensions of the graft, the incision is completed through the remaining connective tissue and the periosteum elevated. (c, d) After the final dissection and capture of the free graft have been completed, the tissue is "defatted" and stored in a saline-soaked gauze. © Daniel R. Cullum.

The use of the *maxillary tuberosity* or other edentulous areas with hyperplastic connective tissue can provide small to even large amounts of connective tissue for augmentation at single- or multiple-tooth/implant sites. The advantage is a significant reduction of donor site morbidity. Using oblique or semilunar incisions can maximize the linear dimensions of the harvested tissue and/or allow shaping it to fit the recipient site (Figure 8.6). Tuberosity access can be more difficult and require specialized instruments, and in some patients the site may have inadequate tissue volume.

Soft tissue grafting with free gingiva, connective tissue or a full-thickness tissue harvest can be used as an autologous barrier in socket preservation grafting.[52] For the patient shown in Figure 8.7, following extraction, debridement, decortication, and hard tissue socket grafting (Figure 8.7a), the defect was covered with a connective graft harvested from the palate (Figure 8.7b). Supraperiosteal

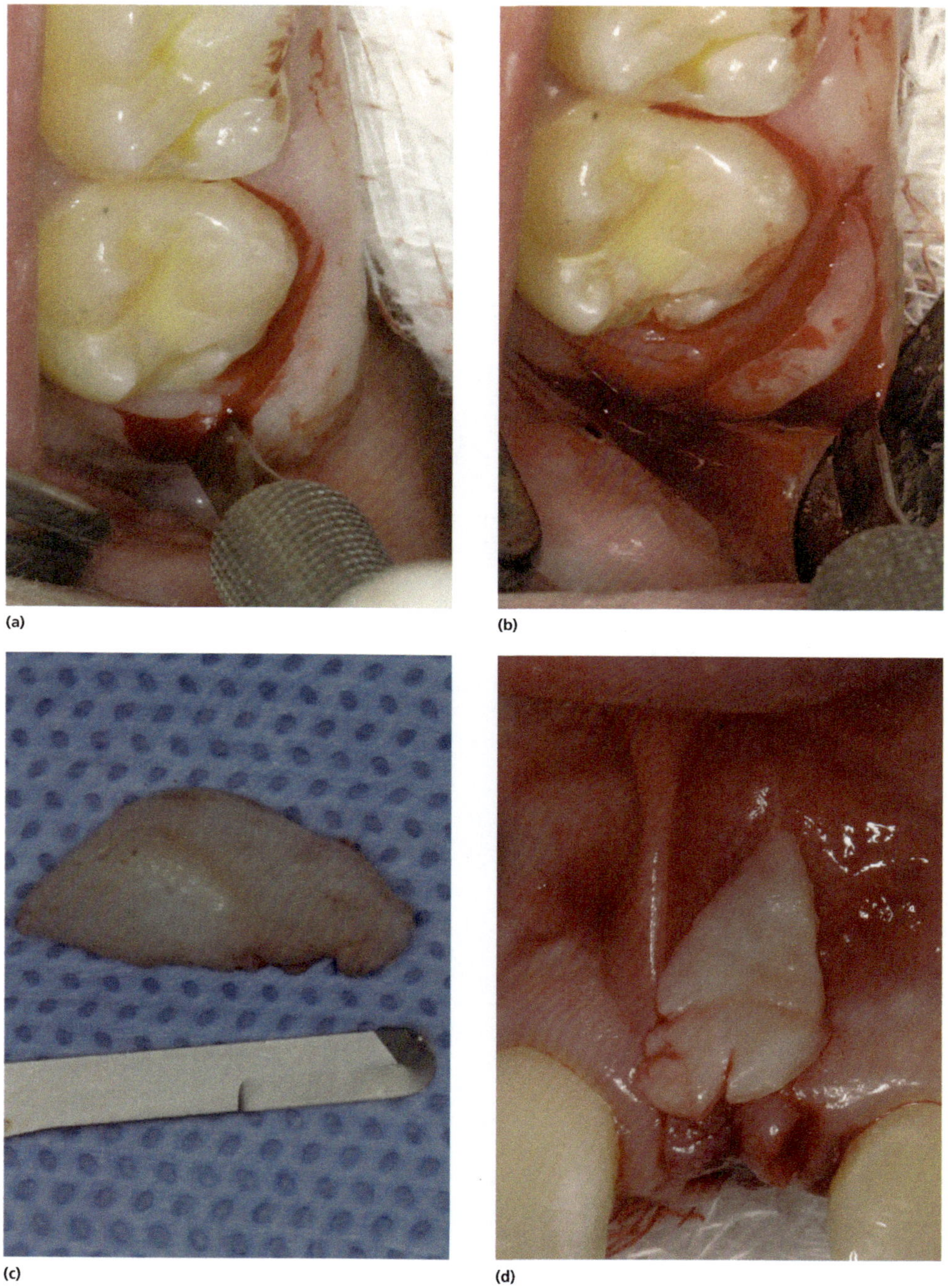

Figure 8.6 (a) A tuberosity connective tissue harvest using an oblique and/or semilunar incision completed from the disto-buccal aspect of the tuberosity to the palatal aspect of the second molar. (b) Joining the oblique incisions can maximize the linear dimensions of the harvested tissue and in designing the graft to fit the recipient site. (c) The harvested tuberosity connective tissue graft. (d) The trimmed connective tissue graft simulating positioning on the buccal soft tissue prior to insertion into the recipient tunnel. © Daniel R. Cullum.

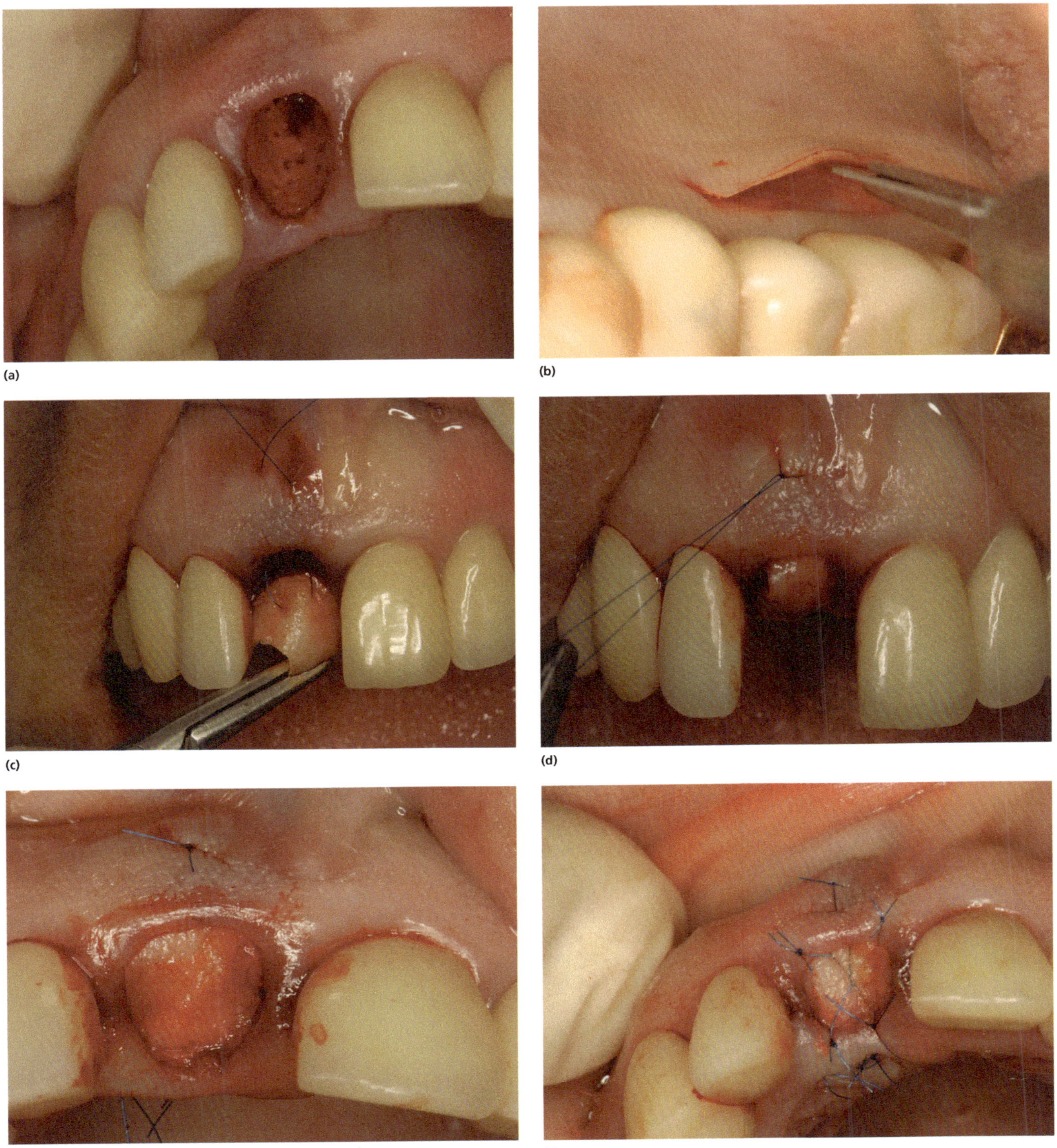

(a) (b) (c) (d) (e) (f)

Figure 8.7 (a) The immediate post-extraction condition of a maxillary right central incisor site after decortication in preparation for socket grafting. (b) A palatal connective tissue donor site demonstrating the mucosal–connective tissue plane of dissection (prior to elevation and harvest of the connective tissue). (c) A buccal supraperiosteal pouch has been prepared. The connective tissue is engaged with a monofilament horizontal mattress suture. (d and e) The connective tissue is pulled into the buccal pouch, then the lingual and sutured. (f) The post-operative view of the connective tissue graft forming a biologic plug at the time of socket grafting of the maxillary right central incisor.

(Continued)

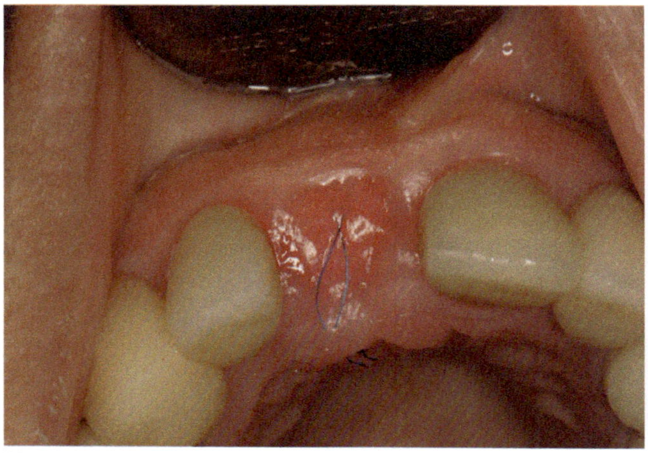
(g)

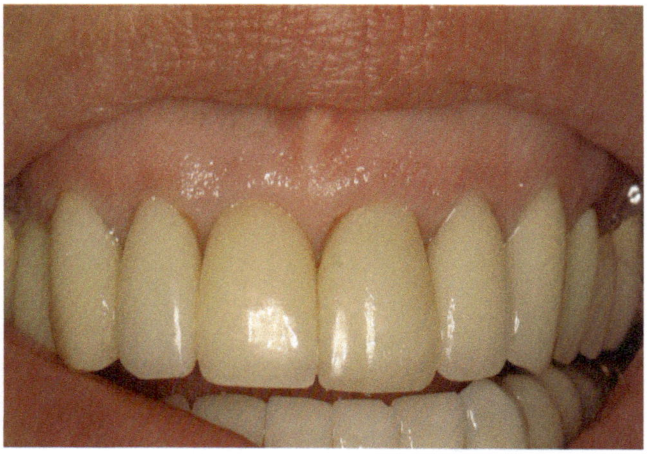
(h)

Figure 8.7 (Continued)
(g) One month healing of a socket bone graft where a connective tissue graft was utilized for socket closure and maintenance of the buccal soft tissue contour. (h) The final restoration of the maxillary right central incisor implant with esthetic gingival contours.

incisions of approximately 3 mm depth were completed under the buccal and palatal flap margins to provide bone support for the connective tissue graft. The graft was secured under the flap margins with facial and palatal pocket horizontal mattress 6-0 monofilament sutures (Figure 8.7c–f). If the harvested tissue is intended to include an epithelial component, care must be taken to ensure that submerged portions of graft are free of epithelium. Figure 8.7g illustrates the grafted site after 4 weeks' healing. The final restoration of the right maxillary central incisor displays excellent hard and soft tissue contours (Figure 8.7h).

In the case shown in Figure 8.8, onlay soft tissue grafting was used for vestibular extension prior to bone grafting and implant reconstruction. The patient had presented with multiple failing mini-implants, and was in need of remedial treatment (Figure 8.8a and b). Findings included difficulty wearing a maxillary prosthesis, reduced vestibular height, bilateral tuberosity hyperplasia, and alveolar irregularities. Additional findings included "combination syndrome"[53] with anterior maxillary bone loss and extrusion of the remaining mandibular anterior teeth. The mini-implants were removed along with extraction of the lower teeth (Figure 8.8c). Connective tissue grafts were taken from the bilateral tuberosity regions (Figure 8.8d and e) as part of a pre-prosthetic tuberosity reduction to reduce the descending plane of occlusion (see Chapter 1). The harvested tissue was shaped to fit the recipient site and positioned as planned for placement (Figure 8.8f and g). Vestibular extension and removal of multiple frenae were completed by surgical incision at the mucogingival junction (Figure 8.8h and i). The incision was continued at a supraperiosteal level into the vestibule bilaterally (Figure 8.8j and k). Vestibular fixation was completed with the coronal flap margin sutured to the vestibular muscle/periosteal base. The connective tissue graft taken from the tuberosity region was trimmed to fit, placed into the wound site, and secured with a slowly resorbing suture (Figure 8.8l). The patient can be seen after 4 weeks' healing in Figure 8.8m. Four-month postoperative healing is demonstrated in Figure 8.8n and o, confirming significant vestibular extension and improved soft tissue contours for future bone grafting/guided surgery reconstruction.

Porcine dermal matrix xenograft (Mucograft®, Geistlich Pharma, Wolhusen, Switzerland) often can be used to avoid the need for autogenous tissue harvesting and permit larger areas to be treated in one intervention. This material can be effective in establishing an increased zone of keratinized tissue and an increase in the depth of the vestibule, but requires some existing keratinized tissue as a source for creeping epithelialization. It also can be used at secondary implant uncovering to treat minimal attached tissue, a significant hyperplastic frenum, and/or to improve limited vestibular depth. In the example in Figure 8.9a, a split-thickness dissection with vestibular extension was completed. Porcine dermal matrix (Figure 8.9b) was saturated in recombinant human platelet-derived growth factor (rhPDGF) to enhance wound healing ("off-label" use of GEM 21S®, Osteohealth, Shirley, NY) and sutured to the wound margins with 5-0 polyglycolic acid resorbable sutures (Figure 8.9c). The flap was apically positioned, and the immediate post-operative result can be seen in Figure 8.9d prior to wound protection with light-cured periodontal dressing (Barricaid®, Dentsply Caulk, York, PA). Early wound healing at 8 weeks (Figure 8.9e) and 6 months following restoration can be seen in Figure 8.9f and g and on panoramic radiographic examination (Figure 8.9h).

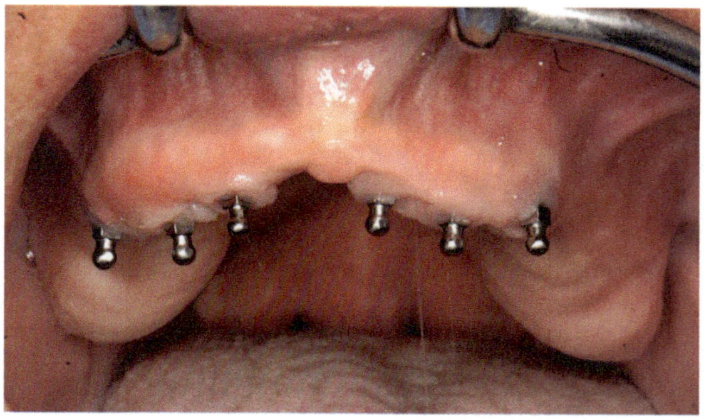
(a)

Figure 8.8 (a, b) Preoperative views of an edentulous maxilla with a failing mini-implant reconstruction and severe anterior bone loss and posterior soft tissue tuberosity hyperplasia.

(Continued)

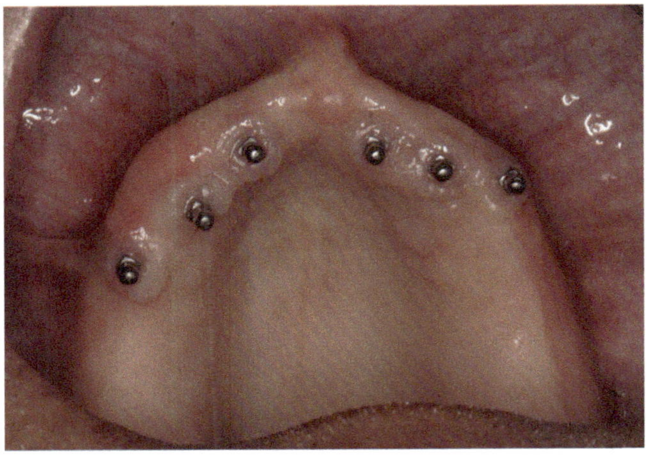

(b)

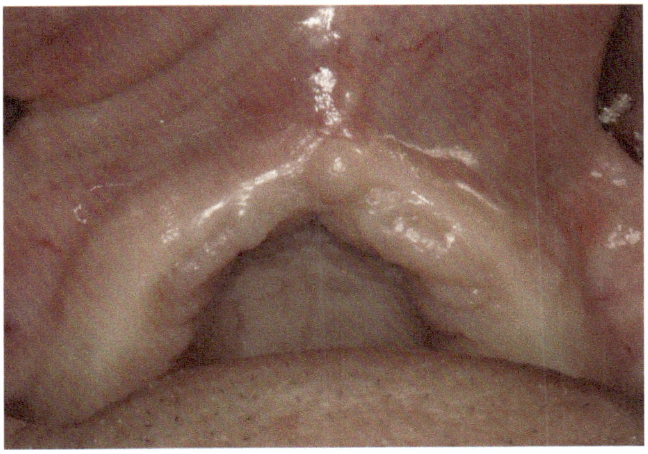

(c)

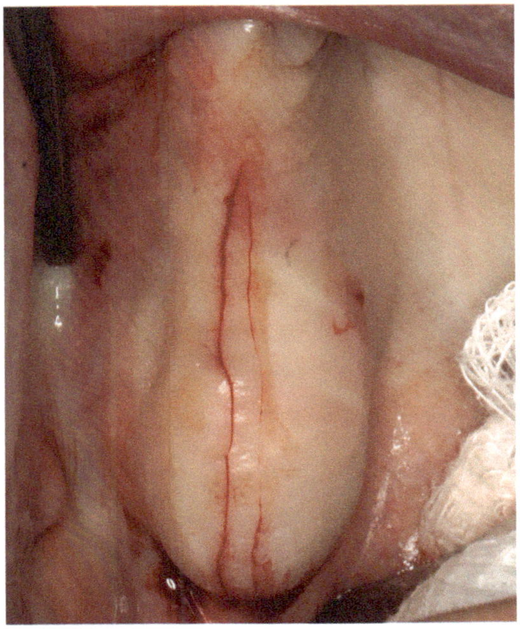

(d)

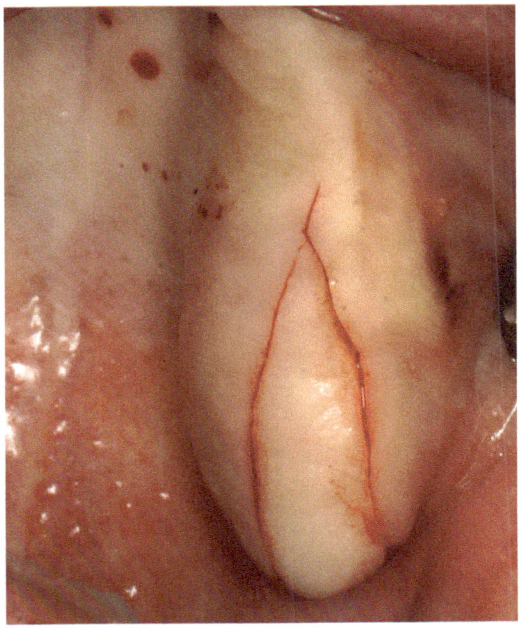

(e)

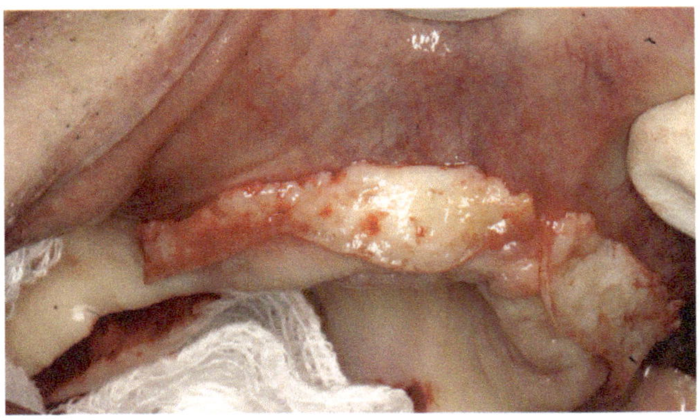

(f)

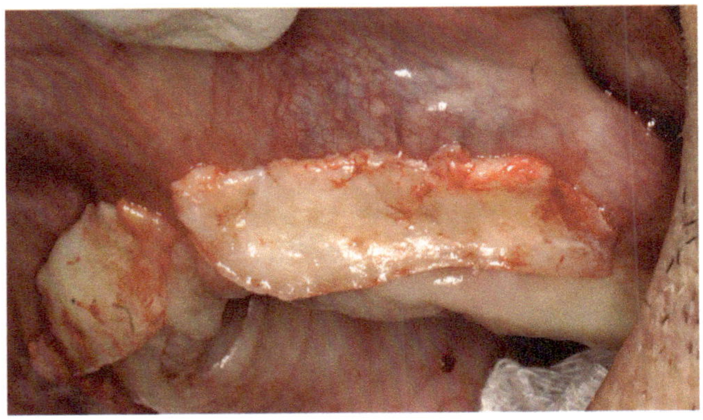

(g)

Figure 8.8 (Continued)
(c) Preoperative view of the atrophic edentulous maxilla after mini-implant removal. (d, e) The incision design for bilateral maxillary tuberosity connective tissue harvest/volume reduction. (f, g) The harvested connective tissue prior to recipient site development and graft placement.

(Continued)

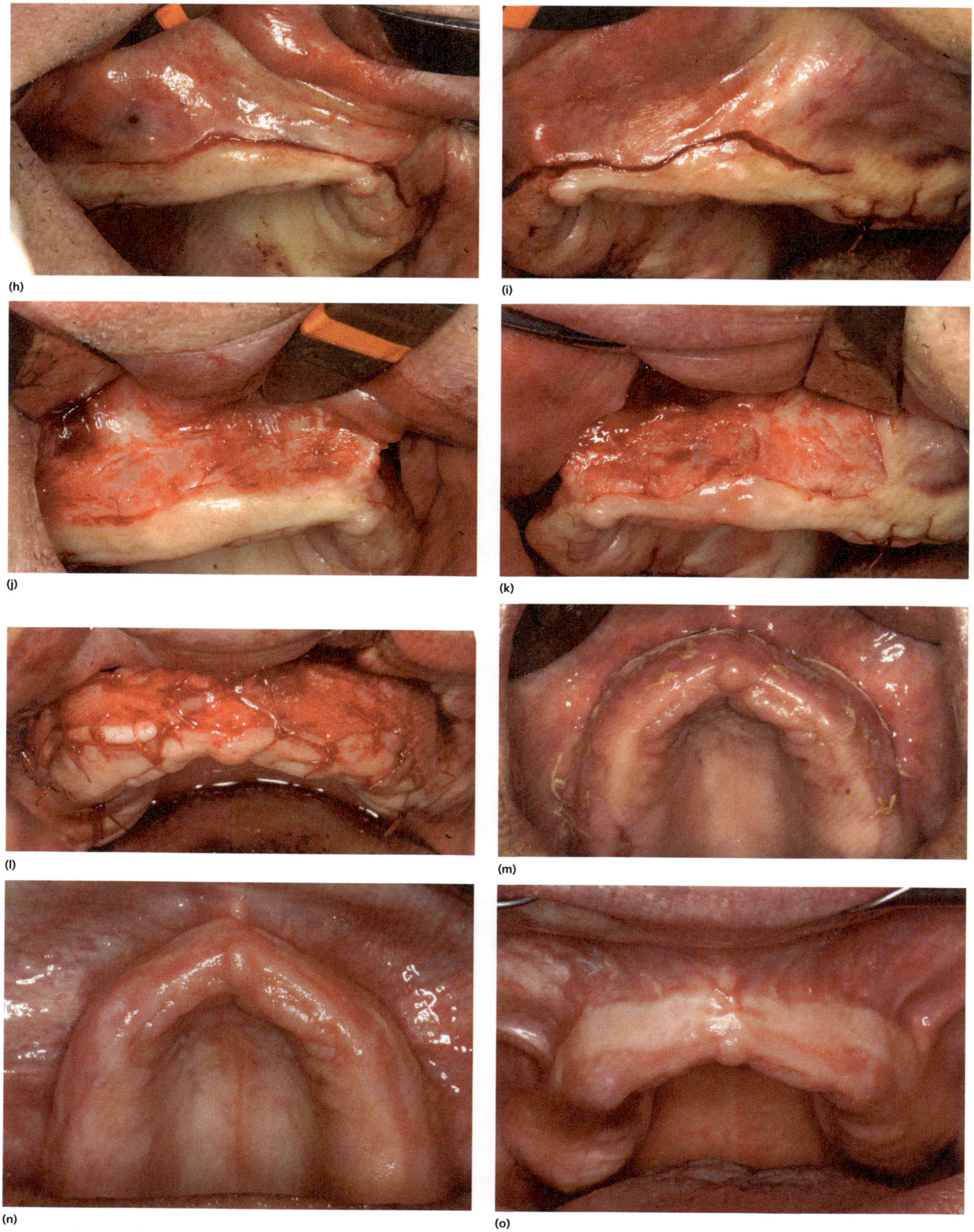

Figure 8.8 (Continued)
(h, i) An incision has been made at the mucogingival junction for a split-thickness dissection. (j, k) The split-thickness dissection has been completed uniformly into the bilateral vestibule and extended to the depth required to remove any muscle pull or instability with lip or cheek mobilization. (l) The crestal tissue was secured to the periosteum at the base of the wound for "vestibular fixation" and the connective tissue grafts were sutured in place with 4-0 Vicryl® (Ethicon, Summerville, NJ). (m) The post-operative image at 4 weeks. (n, o) The soft tissue healing prior to maxillary reconstruction with implants. © Daniel R. Cullum.

A patient who presented with an esthetically compromised implant reconstruction replacing the upper right lateral incisor and canine teeth was managed with a superficial-layer split-thickness flap as demonstrated in Figure 8.10. The challenges of implant position, tooth form, tissue asymmetry, and inadequate bone and soft tissue thicknesses are apparent on clinical and radiographic examination, with recession and translucency of the restorative abutments through the soft tissues (Figure 8.10a and b). An underlying facial bone dehiscence with crestal bone loss was diagnosed, and the treatment plan involved implant removal

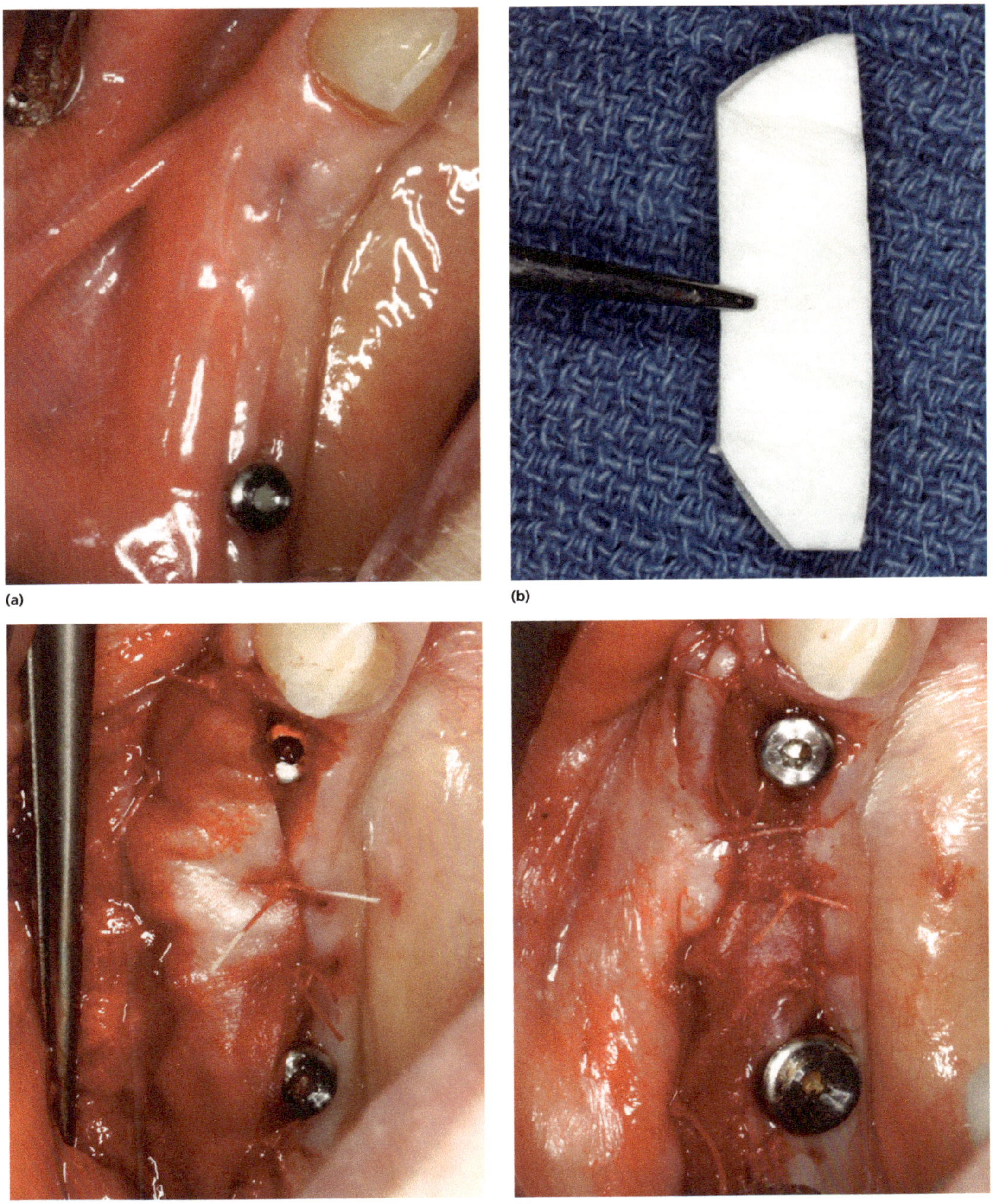

(a) (b) (c) (d)

Figure 8.9 (a) A view of a left mandibular first premolar site prior to second-stage implant uncovering, demonstrating a thick frenal attachment, minimal attached tissue, and minimal vestibular depth. (b) Porcine dermal matrix (Mucograft®, Geistlich Pharma, Wolhusen, Switzerland) was trimmed to fit the exposed split-thickness vestibular dissection. (c) Porcine dermal matrix saturated in rhPDGF ("off-label" use of GEM 21S®) was secured to the surrounding margins, including the wound base periosteum, with 5-0 polyglycolic sutures. (d) Frenoplasty and an anterior vertical releasing incision were completed and the mucosal portion of the split-thickness flap apically positioned and sutured to increase vestibular depth and attached tissue height. Portions of the porcine dermal matrix were left exposed for open wound healing, and the wound covered with periodontal dressing.

(Continued)

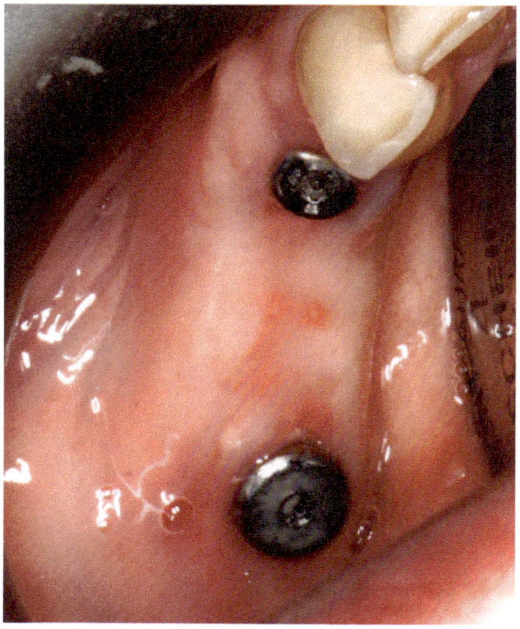

(e)

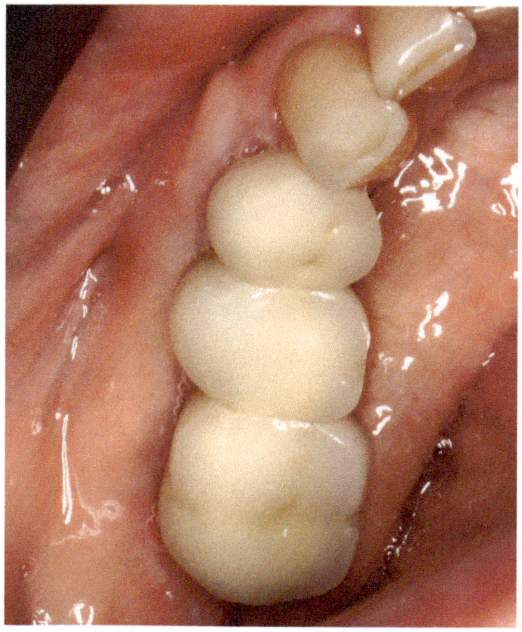

(f)

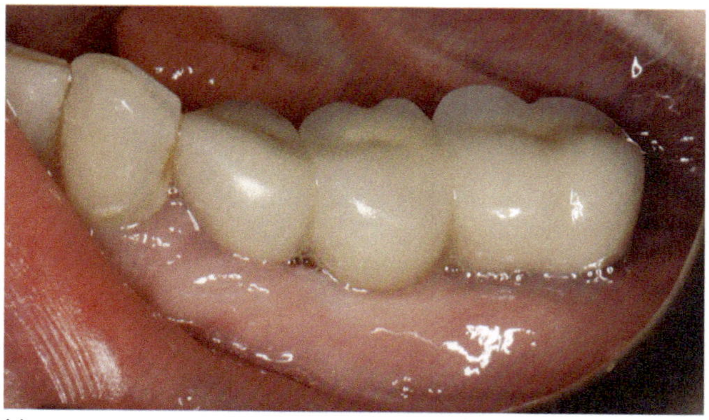

(g)

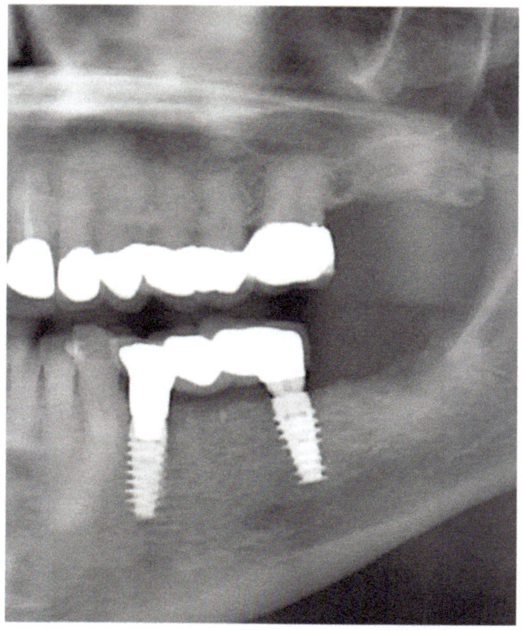

(h)

Figure 8.9 (Continued)
(e) The 12-week post-operative view demonstrating a wide attached tissue margin and healing. (f, g) The 6-month post-restoration occlusal and lateral views, showing maintenance of bone and soft tissue contours. (h) A panoramic radiograph taken 6 months after restoration demonstrating the implant position and bone levels. © Daniel R. Cullum.

and site development for improved soft tissue esthetics. The flap was dissected with a trapezoidal base and an anterior and posterior vertical release following the contour of the mucosal surface and freeing the epithelium and superficial connective tissue from the underlying layers of muscle and periosteum (Figure 8.10c). An inner flap then was elevated at the subperiosteal level revealing the facial bone dehiscence (Figure 8.10d). After implant removal (Figure 8.10e), over-grafting of the defect with "off-label" use of rhPDGF-enhanced (GEM 21S, Osteohealth, Shirley, NY), freeze-dried cortico-cancellous bone allograft (MinerOss®, BioHorizons, Birmingham, AL) was completed (Figure 8.10f). Tissue thickening was achieved with the addition of acellular dermal matrix (Alloderm®, LifeCell, Branchburg, NJ), and the flap repositioned with tension-free closure (Figure 8.10g and h). After site healing, a single implant was placed in the canine site and later used to support a cantilever replacing the lateral incisor. The final restoration and 24-month post-operative periapical radiographs are shown in Figure 8.10i and j.

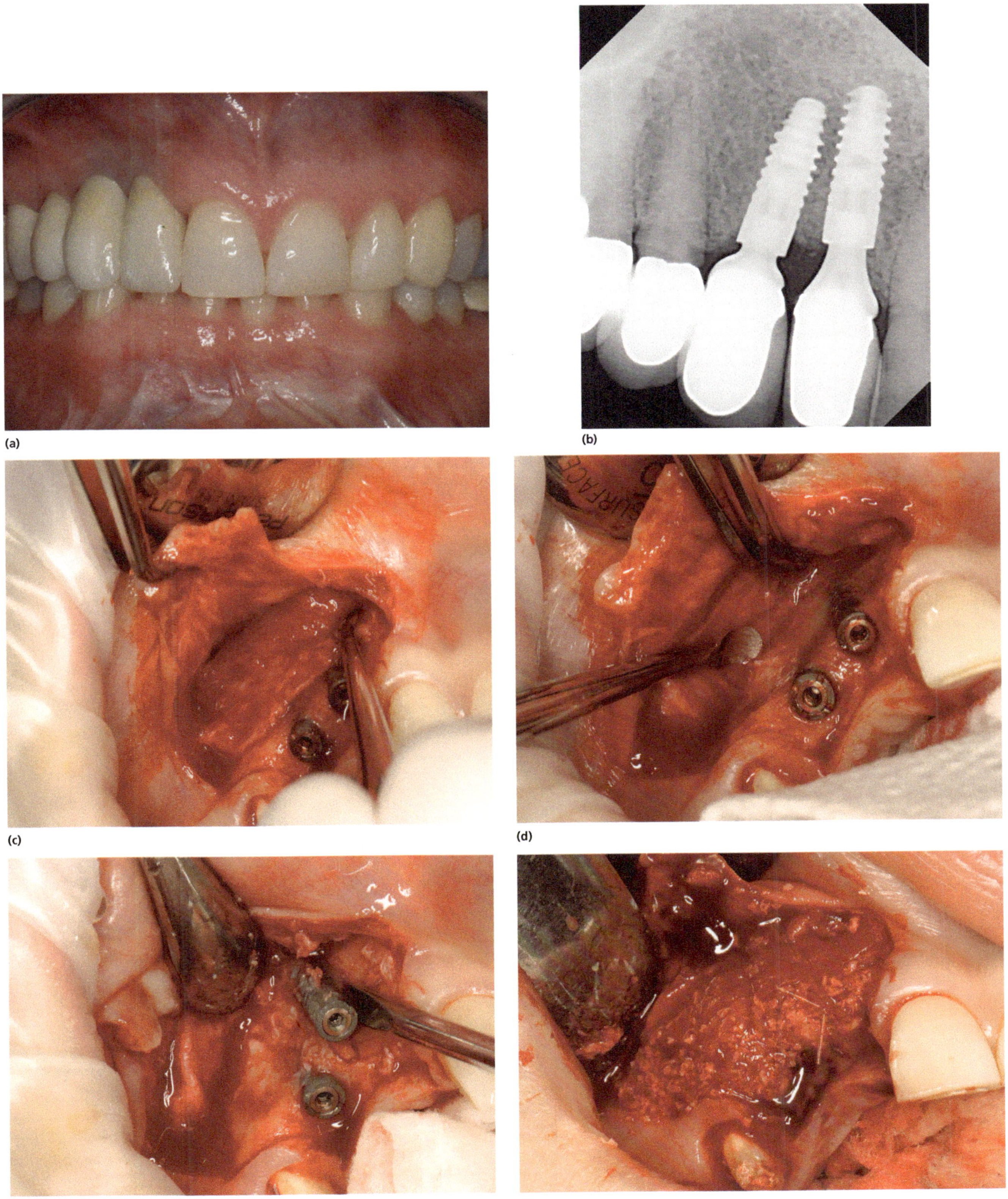

Figure 8.10 (a) The implant-retained crowns at the maxillary right canine and lateral incisor showed bone loss resulting in tooth form and soft tissue asymmetry and dark marginal tissue. (b) The pretreatment radiograph of these adjacent implants. (c) Flap dissection was completed following the contour of the mucosal surface and with a trapezoidal base and vertical releasing incisions. The epithelium and superficial connective tissues were dissected free from the underlying layers of muscle and periosteum. (d) A superficial split-thickness flap dissection illustrating the raised epithelial–connective tissue flap and the deeper muscle/periosteal component. (e) Luxation of the lateral incisor implant for removal. (f) Containment of combined (GEM 21S®) rhPDGF–xenograft within the muscle–periosteal component of the flap was aided by a resorbable collagen membrane. The slow-resorbing particulate graft was meant to provide volume at the maxillary buccal deficiency produced by removal of implant #7. A monocryl horizontal mattress suture from the base of the muscle–periosteal flap to the palatal flap provided stabilization of the inner flap.

(*Continued*)

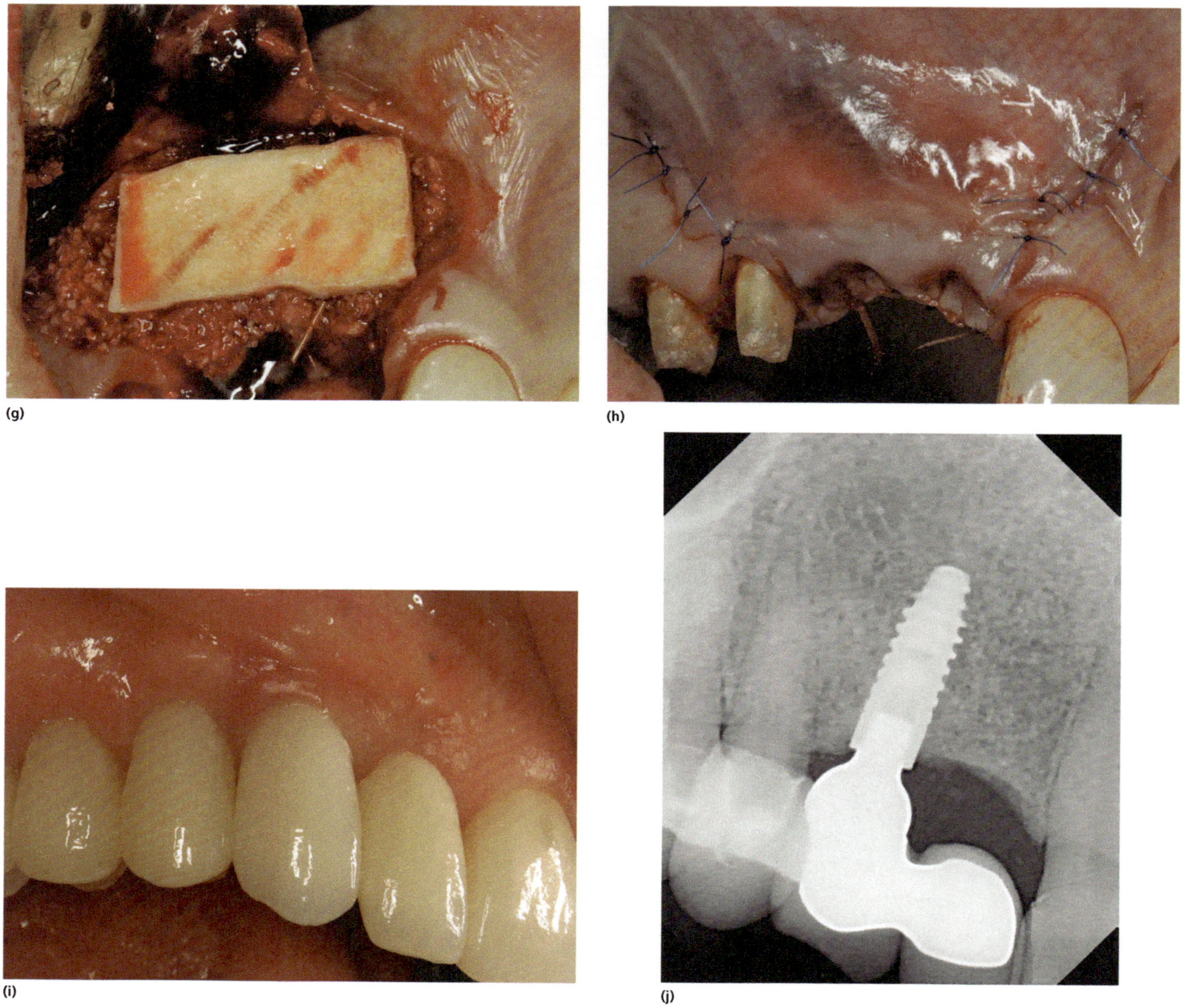

Figure 8.10 (Continued)
(g) An acellular dermal matrix graft was placed and later contoured and positioned to the buccal and crestal aspect to provide additional tissue thickness and barrier support to this large particulate graft. (h) The immediate post-operative image demonstrates tension-free wound closure. (i) The final restoration showed improved gingival esthetics. An implant-retained fixed partial denture at site #6 included an anterior cantilever at site #7. (j) The 2-year post-operative radiograph of the final restoration.

Tunnel flaps

Tunnel flaps are minimally invasive and offer optimal vascular support for soft tissue grafting providing bilaminar blood supply at both the outer and inner graft surfaces. In this scenario, autogenous connective tissue grafts do not require complete submergence under overlying flaps and can be used to increase the quality and thickness of the overlying tissue. Allograft material can be used in sites with ≥2 mm of existing keratinized tissue but, unlike autogenous connective tissue, it does need to be completely submerged.

In esthetic sites when tissue thickening is needed at a fragile gingival margin, a distant semilunar incision can be employed. Figure 8.11a illustrates an example of thin marginal tissue showing metallic translucency from the underlying healing abutment. Surgical correction prior to the restorative phase was critical to avoid any apical migration of the marginal tissue. A semilunar incision apical to the defect was used to create a supraperiosteal releasing incision with a 1/2 Allen Orban knife (Hu-Friedy, Chicago, IL) and a tunnel to receive the graft (Figure 8.11b and c).The papillae were included in this approach with supraperiosteal release over the ridge crest to allow the superficial marginal tissue to be mobilized coronally. A connective tissue graft was then harvested from the maxillary tuberosity with a "semilunar oblique" incision, de-epithelialized and adapted into the tunnel (Figure 8.11d and e). Horizontal mattress sutures were placed on both the mesial and distal of the recipient site to manipulate the graft within the tunnel. The initial purchase at each site penetrated both graft and overlying gingiva exiting at the palatal aspect of the adjacent tooth sulcus. The return suture was passed through the palatal mucosa in a horizontal mattress fashion exiting the buccal aspect of the previous sulcus to secure the graft in a coronal position (Figure 8.11f). Closure at the tuberosity donor site is demonstrated in Figure 8.11g. The

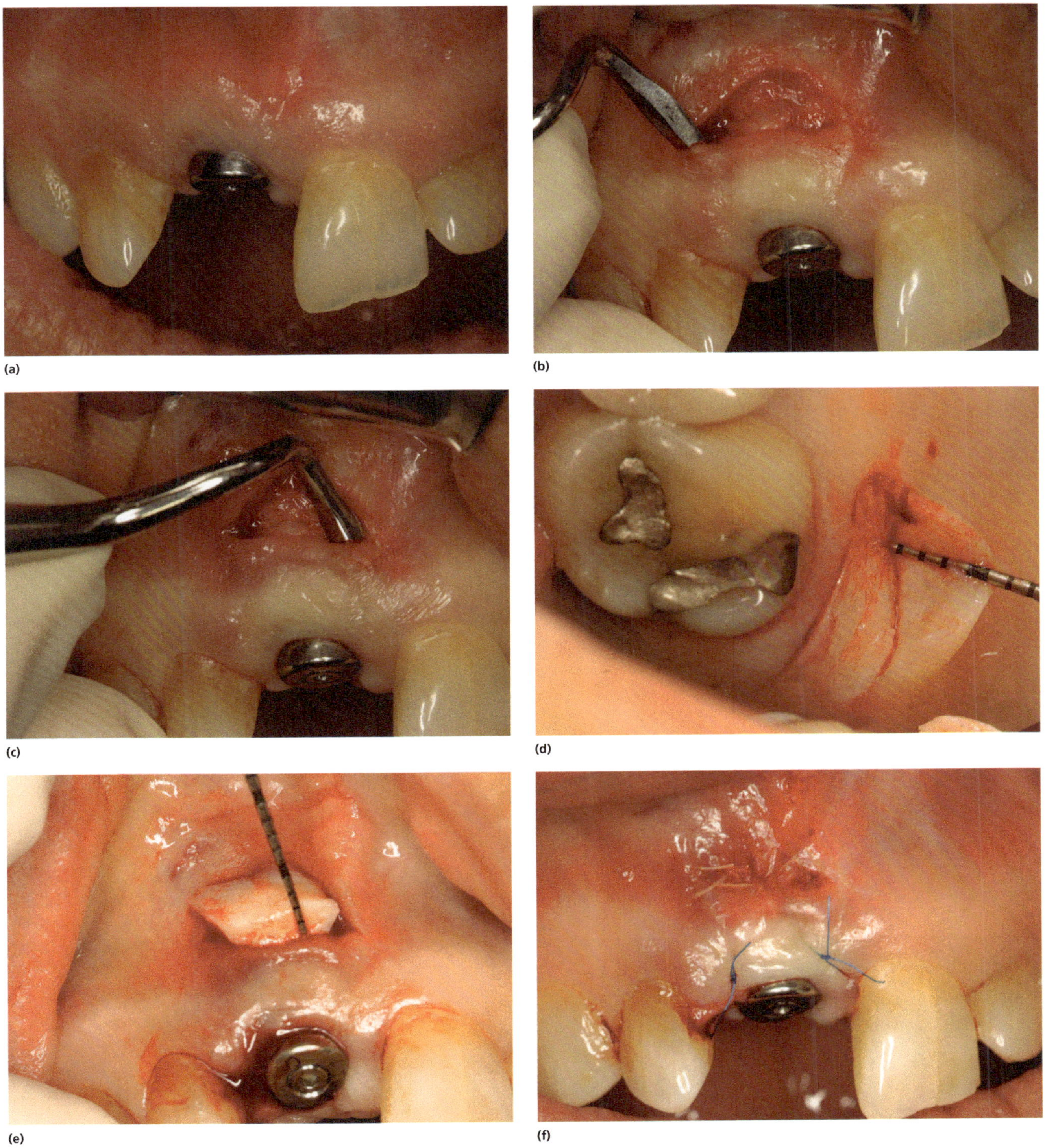

Figure 8.11 (a) The gingival margin at this right central incisor implant is thin facially and narrow vertically. The healing abutment showed through the soft tissue. An attempt to restore the implant at this stage would have resulted in an apical migration of the soft tissues. (b) A semilunar incision in the mucosa at the mucogingival junction was completed with a #15 blade and followed with a split-thickness dissection and elevation using an angled instrument (1/2 Allen Orban knife). (c) The split-thickness elevation continued to the adjacent tooth laterally and to the crest with release of the papillary tissue. (d) Donor site incision for a full-thickness tissue harvest from the left maxillary tuberosity. (e) The tuberosity tissue was trimmed to remove all epithelial remnants and placed into a subperiosteal tunnel at the facial aspect of the implant. (f) Coronal positioning of the semilunar flap and stabilization of the connective tissue graft were achieved with suspending 6-0 monofilament sutures.

(Continued)

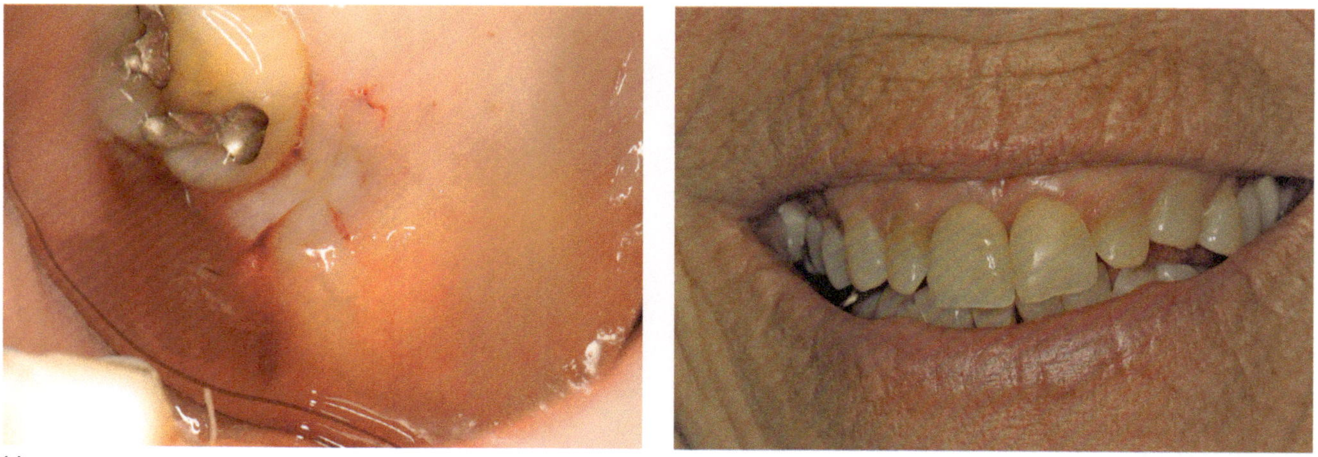

(g) (h)

Figure 8.11 (Continued)
(g) Closure of the maxillary tuberosity donor site. (h) The final implant restoration after 1 year.

graft-stabilizing sutures were maintained for 6 weeks. Consideration of the use of a non-flared (flat emergence profile) healing abutment also may help to reduce the risk of gingival recession during the immediate post-operative phase. The 1-year post-restoration view is seen in Figure 8.11h, demonstrating excellent tissue quality and gingival form.

Allograft material is uniform in thickness, unlimited in quantity, and requires no distant donor site. Histological assessment of sites treated with this material have verified enhanced connective tissue thickness being achieved.[54] Figure 8.12a illustrates a case with generalized recessions affecting several teeth in the right maxilla.

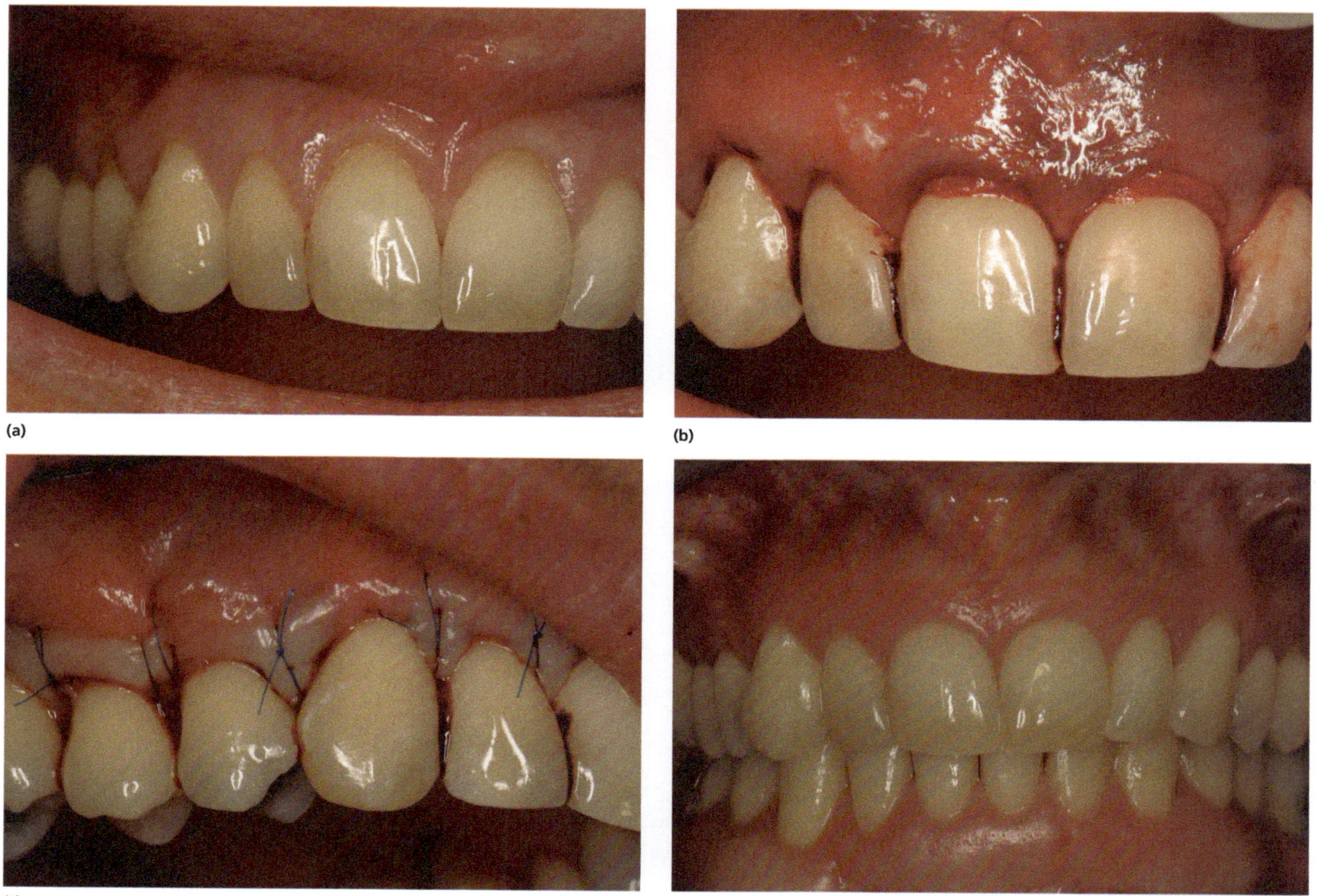

(a) (b) (c) (d)

Figure 8.12 (a) Generalized labial recession can be seen in this maxillary right quadrant. (b) An acellular dermal matrix graft was introduced into a supraperiosteal tunnel preparation. (c) Coronal positioning of the tunnel flap and stabilization of the graft were achieved with vertical mattress 6-0 monofilament suture. (d) The 5-year post-surgical follow-up.

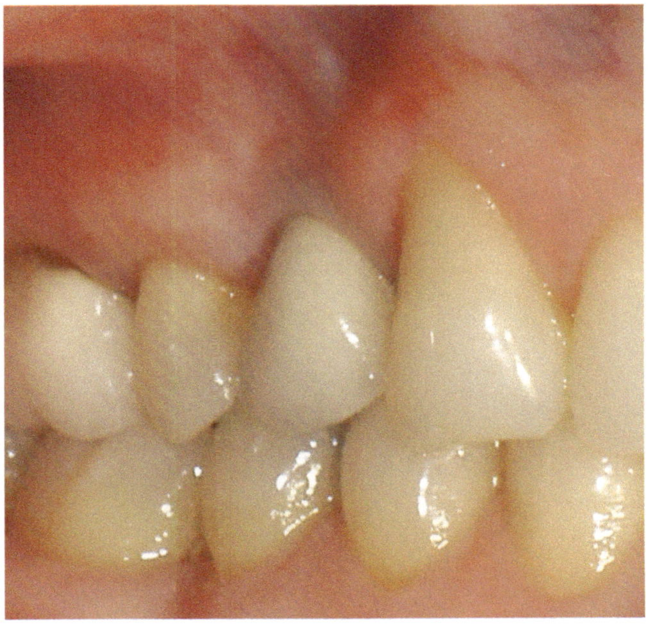

(a)

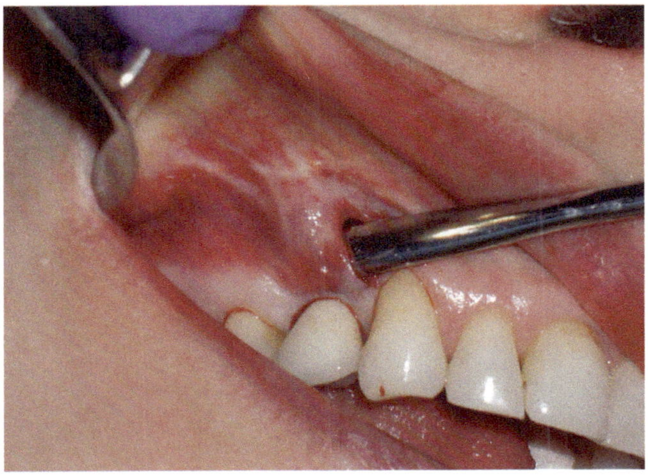

(b)

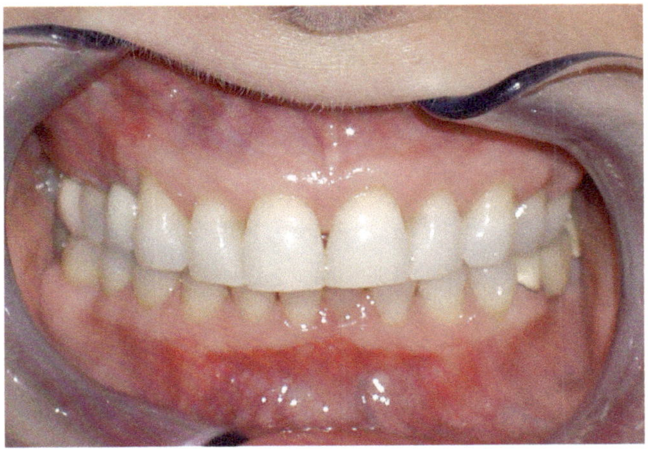

(c)

Figure 8.13 (a) A preoperative photograph showing a buccal soft tissue concavity at implant site #5 with marginal tissue translucency showing the darkness of the underlying metal abutment. (b) A subperiosteal tunnel was created over the deficient area with the use of a periosteal elevator. Alloderm was placed in the tunnel and sutured mesially and distally with a chromic gut horizontal mattress suture. The vertical incision was closed with interrupted sutures. (c) The 12-month situation after soft tissue allografting.

Following root preparation with periodontal curettes, soft tissue preparation was initiated through the sulcus with sharp dissection using a 1/2 Allen Orban knife. This was followed with blunt supraperiosteal dissection using an Allen periosteal elevator (Hu-Friedy, Chicago, IL) releasing the papillae from their underlying bone and extending apically approximately 10 mm. This was followed by sharp dissection with the 1/2 Allen Orban knife to provide flap mobility. No external vertical releasing incisions were used, and the acellular dermal matrix (Alloderm) was introduced through the sulcus of the mobilized labial flap (Figure 8.12b). Because exposure of dermal matrix allograft can lead to loss of graft material, the graft and flap should be sutured separately. The graft can be initially sutured with the subgingival double-back continuous sling suture first described by Allen.[55,56] After the graft is sutured, the tunnel margins can then be advanced to cover the graft completely, and secured with interrupted vertical mattress sling sutures with the knots on the facial aspect (Figure 8.12c). In the example, the sutures were left in situ for 6 weeks' healing. The 5-year stable outcome is shown in Figure 8.12d.

A tunnel approach with vertical releasing incisions was used for the placement of Alloderm to correct the localized bone and soft tissue deficiency over the implant seen in Figure 8.13. This tunnel can be accomplished in a supraperiosteal manner with sharp dissection of the mucosa and periosteum, but in this case a subperiosteal tunnel was created under the deficient area with limited periosteal dissection (Figure 8.13b) Alloderm was inserted into the tunnel and stabilized with sutures. The outcome after 12 months can be seen in Figure 8.13c.

Another application for soft tissue allograft is illustrated in a maxillary edentulous case planned for treatment with conventional fixed tooth-supported prosthodontics (Figure 8.14a). The material was folded to create a thicker graft, and the folded layers sutured tightly together to avoid dead space between them (Figure 8.14b). A midline vertical incision gave access for a subperiosteal tunnel created over the deficient area with limited dissection using a periosteal elevator (Figure 8.14c). The tunnel grafting attempted to reconstruct the impression of root eminences. Figure 8.14d illustrates the 1-year follow-up after restoration.

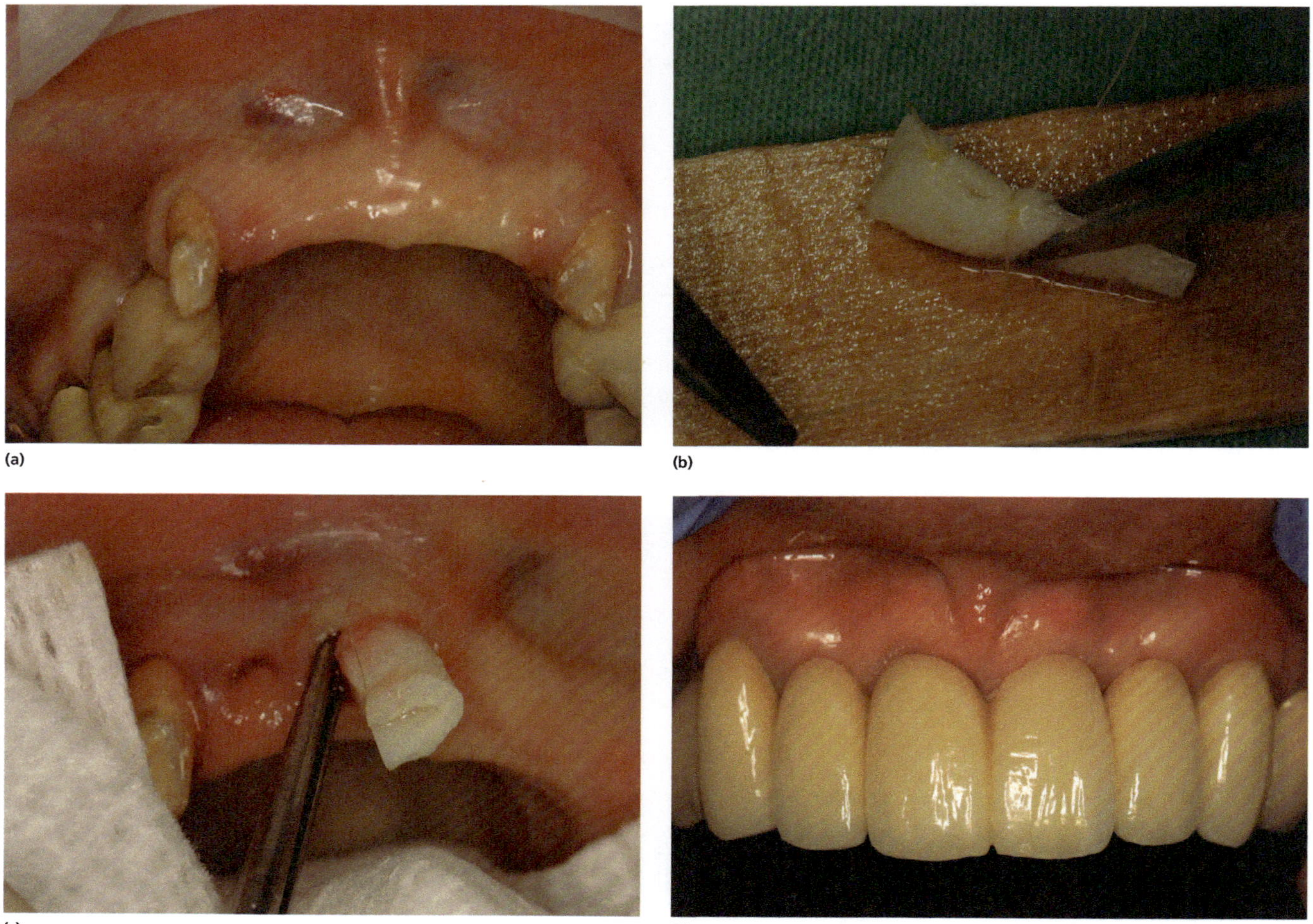

(a) (b) (c) (d)

Figure 8.14 (a) The preoperative view of a labial undercut and ridge dimension where pontic site development is needed. (b) A folded acellular dermal matrix graft stabilized with gut suture. (c) The acellular dermal matrix was introduced into a localized subperiosteal tunnel preparation. (d) The 1-year follow-up after pontic site development with acellular dermal matrix.

Vascular pedicle "plastic" techniques

The advantage with pedicle flaps is that they retain their own vascular supply. They can be positioned apically, coronally, laterally, or in a rotated fashion. Indications include repositioning adjacent keratinized tissue, attaining primary closure over an open extraction socket defect, or providing a bilaminar blood supply for a connective-tissue-enhancing procedure.

Apical-positioned flap

The apical-positioned flap is a straightforward procedure, which can be used during implant placement surgery or at second-stage implant uncovering when inadequate keratinized tissue exists at the site (Figure 8.15a). An apically positioned flap enhances the volume of keratinized and attached tissue, and also can help to increase vestibular depth. In the example shown, a split-thickness incision was made at the anticipated lingual position of the implant and carried through the interproximal region in a "papilla-sparing" fashion (Figure 8.15b). Implant site development was completed with an osteotome ridge expansion technique (see Chapter 16) with limited crestal exposure (Figure 8.15c). Implant placement was completed with temporary insertion of a healing cap. Beveled vertical releasing incisions were used and a split-thickness flap developed, maintaining the periosteal vascular supply (Figure 8.15d). Following implant placement, an immediate, screw-retained provisional restoration was fabricated (see Chapter 19) and inserted (Figure 8.15e and f). The soft tissue flap was apically positioned to the buccal to increase the height and facial volume of keratinized gingiva (Figure 8.15g). The immediate post-operative radiograph is seen in Figure 8.15h. Initial soft tissue healing is demonstrated after 2 weeks in Figure 8.15i. The final restoration and radiograph demonstrate an adequate quality and quantity of attached tissue and bone levels after 1 year (Figure 8.15j and k) and after more than 4 years (Figure 8.15l and m).

Coronal advanced flap

Coronal advanced flaps can be used to cover connective tissue grafts, to thicken the biotype, to provide an appearance of root eminence, and to mask tissue graying from underlying implant components. Coronal advanced tissue will retain its original color

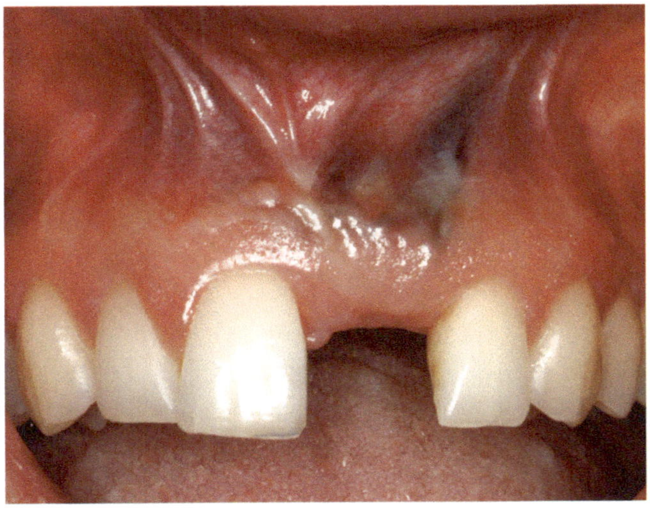
(a)

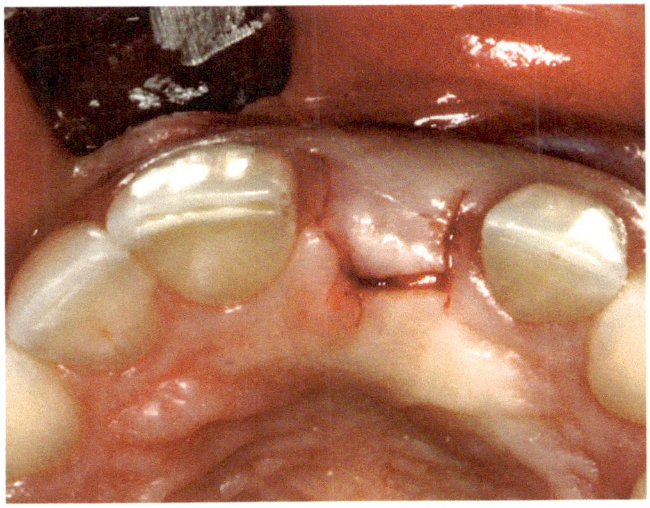
(b)

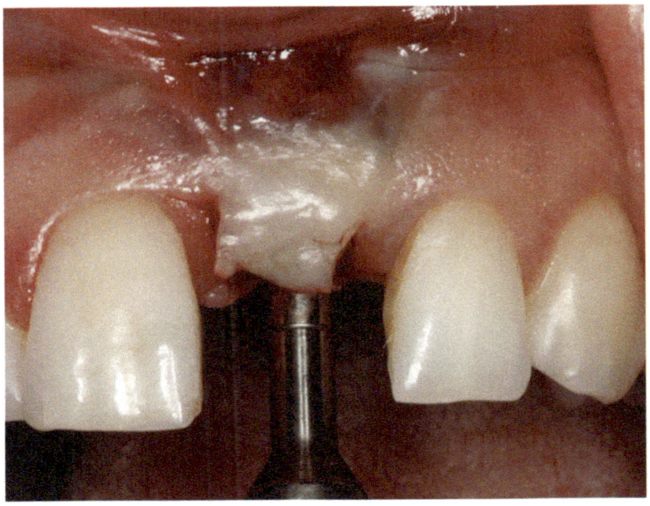
(c)

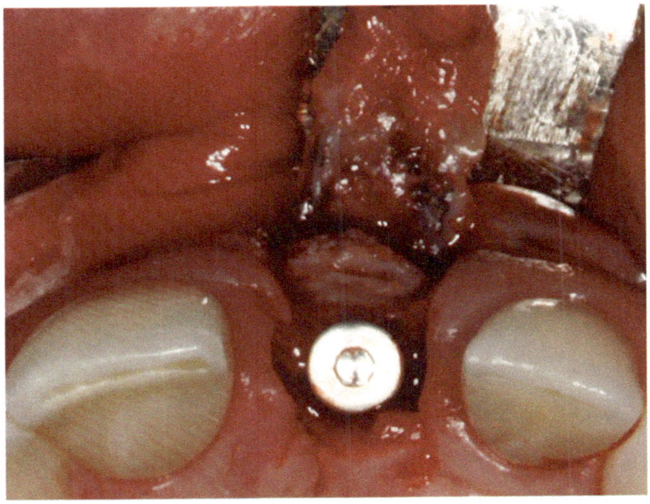
(d)

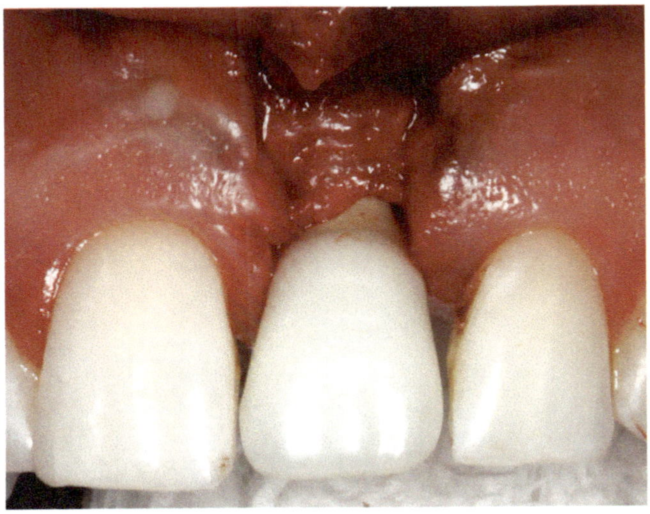
(e)

Figure 8.15 (a) This preoperative view demonstrates inadequate keratinized tissue and a metallic foreign body "tattoo" at the healed site. (Same patient after treatment in Figure 8.19.) (b) A papilla-sparing palatal incision was used for an apically positioned flap and implant placement. (c) Implant placement was completed with the osteotome ridge expansion technique (see Chapter 16). (d) Beveled soft tissue vertical incisions were completed with split-thickness dissection for apical flap positioning. (e, f) A screw-retained immediate provisional restoration was fabricated with a flat gingival emergence profile and the incisal edge was reduced to remove protrusive contacts (see Chapter 19).

(Continued)

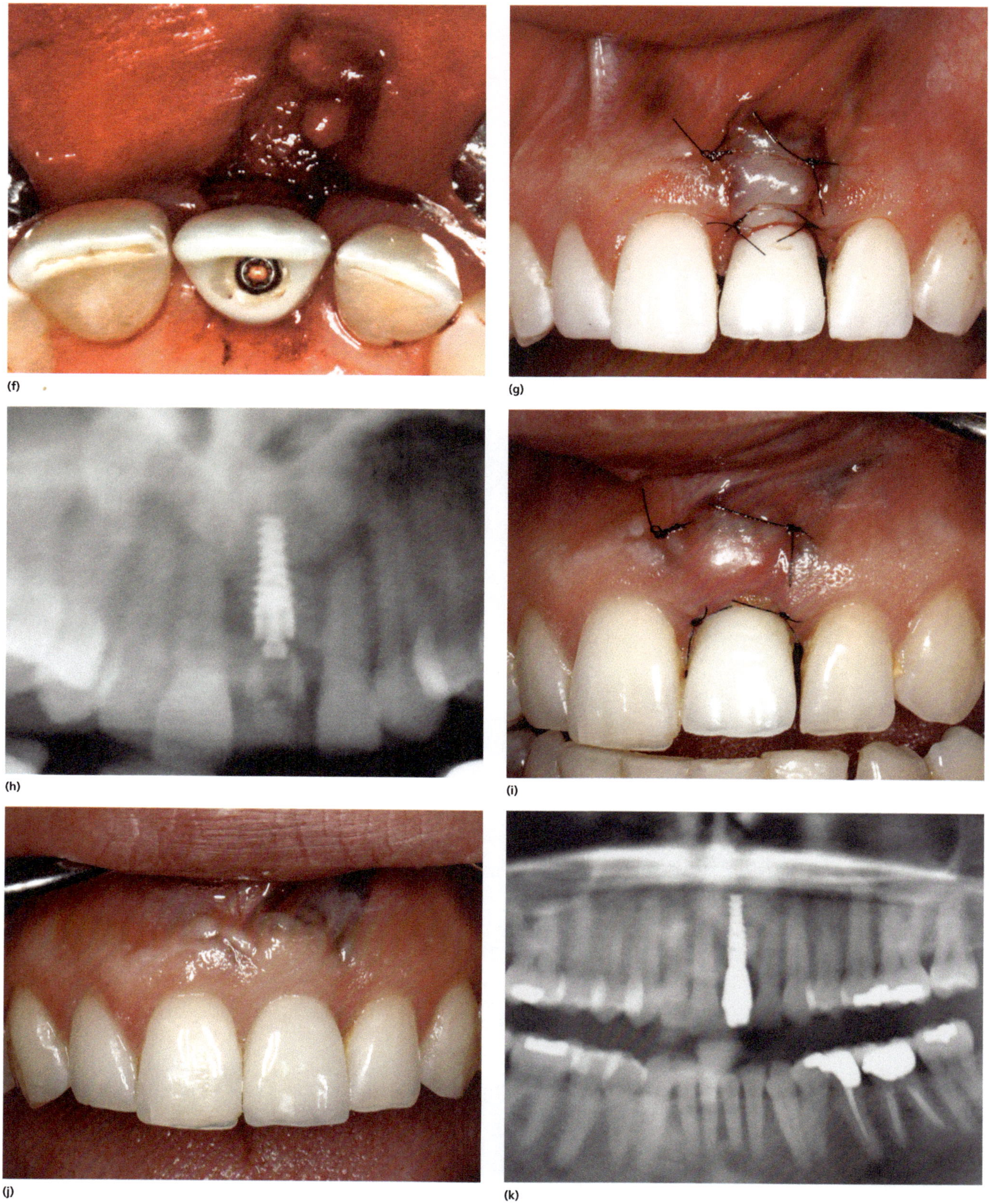

Figure 8.15 (Continued)
(g) The immediate provisional restoration was placed before the apically positioned flap was secured with 6-0 nylon sutures, ensuring the gingival margin placement to be 2 mm coronal to that of the contralateral tooth. (h) The immediate post-operative radiograph. (i) The 2-week post-operative view after immediate provisional restoration and apically positioned flap to increase the attached tissue margin. The 1-year clinical (j) and radiographic (k) images demonstrating the esthetic outcome and stable crestal bone levels.

(Continued)

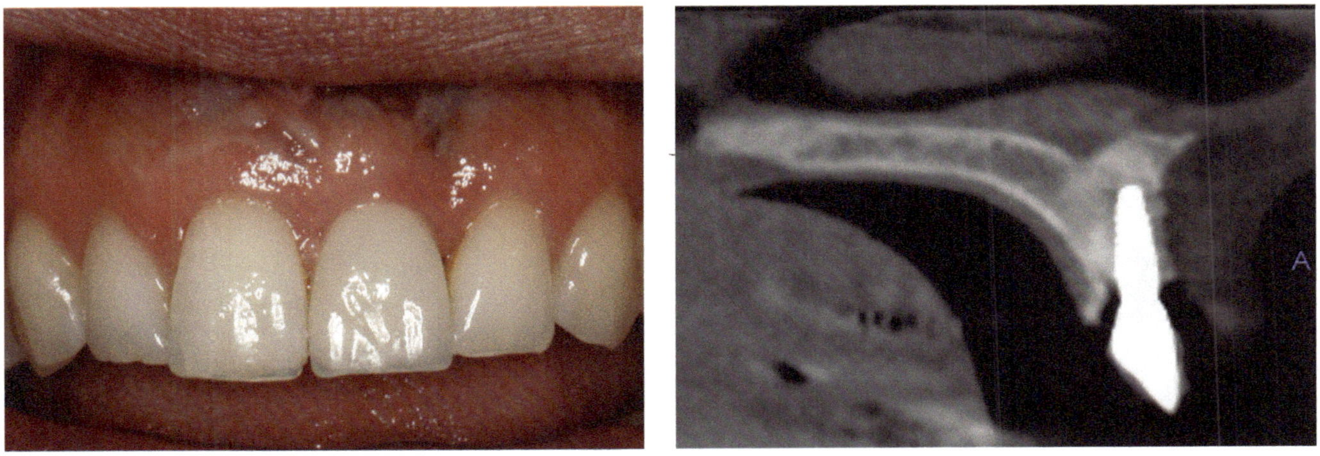

(l) (m)

Figure 8.15 (Continued)
The 4.5-year follow-up clinical (l) and CBCT cross-sectional radiographic (m) images. *Source*: Restoration by Tom Smart DDS. © Daniel R. Cullum.

and texture. The tooth recession classification of Miller[38] (Table 8.1) can help with flap design and assessment of surrounding hard and soft tissues with respect to the collateral blood supply. When repositioning keratinized tissue coronally, it is best to have healthy papilla tips 3–4 mm coronal to the desired new tissue margin in order to provide adequate lateral vascular support for the flap when positioned over an avascular tooth or implant surface. Root coverage can be successful if the restoration is ≤2 mm deep on the root surface and the desired gingival margin is 3 mm apical to the adjacent papilla tips. Figure 8.16 shows a case that initially presented with a class V restoration on the root surface of the maxillary right canine and recession defects also affecting the adjacent premolar tooth. The treatment plan included removal of the restoration with placement of provisional crowns at the ideal esthetic gingival position (Figure 8.16a). Root-plasty of the root surface is usually necessary to reduce the buccal prominence within the alveolar housing.

Table 8.1 Miller classification.[38] This classification, established for recession defects affecting natural teeth, can be used to predict soft tissue grafting outcomes with teeth and implants. Interproximal bone height is a crucial factor

Gingival recession	Level of receded tissue	Interproximal bone height	Prospect of root coverage
Class I	Coronal to the mucogingival junction	No loss	Excellent
Class II	Extends to or beyond the mucogingival junction	No loss	Excellent
Class III	Extends to or beyond the mucogingival junction	Loss or tooth malpositioned	Only partial coverage anticipated
Class IV	Extends to or beyond the mucogingival junction	Extreme loss or extreme malposition	Cannot be anticipated

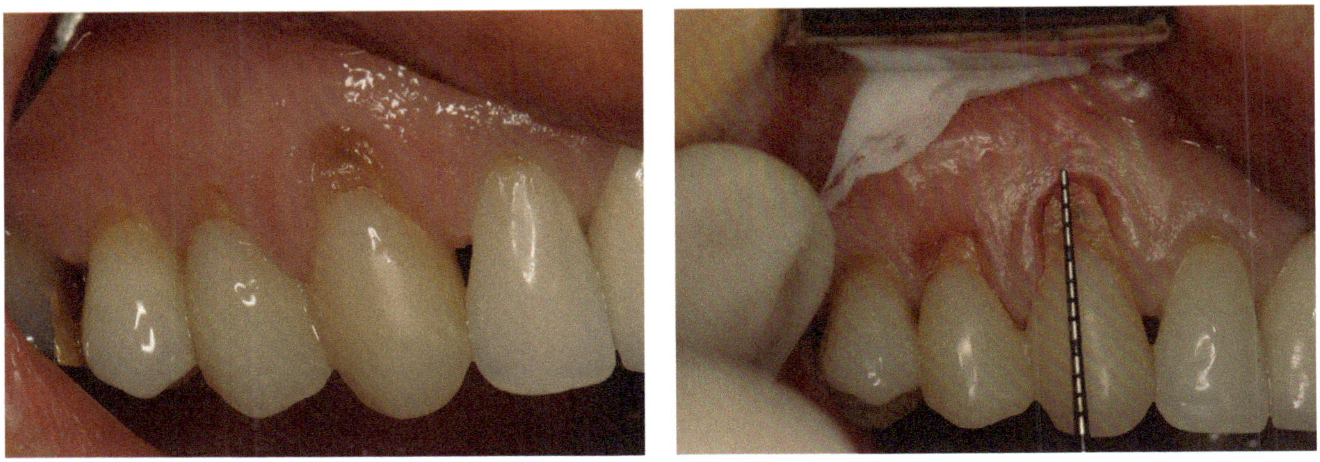

(a) (b)

Figure 8.16 (a) The patient's maxillary right first premolar and canine teeth after removal of the failing class V composite restorations and provisional crown restorations at the ideal gingival position in preparation for coronal advanced flap and connective tissue graft. (b) An intraoperative view after root preparation for a coronally advanced flap.

(Continued)

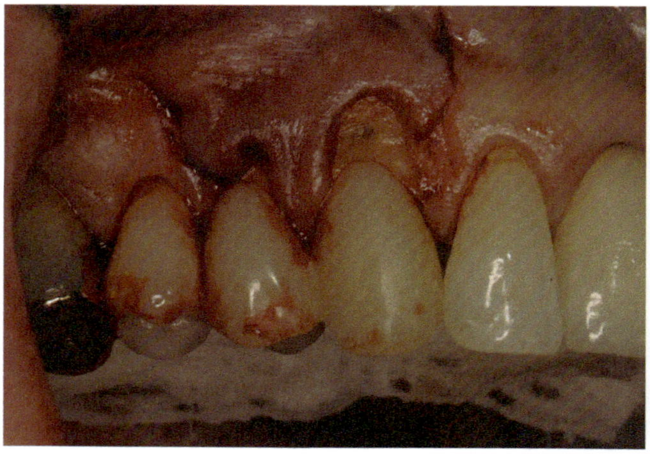

(c)

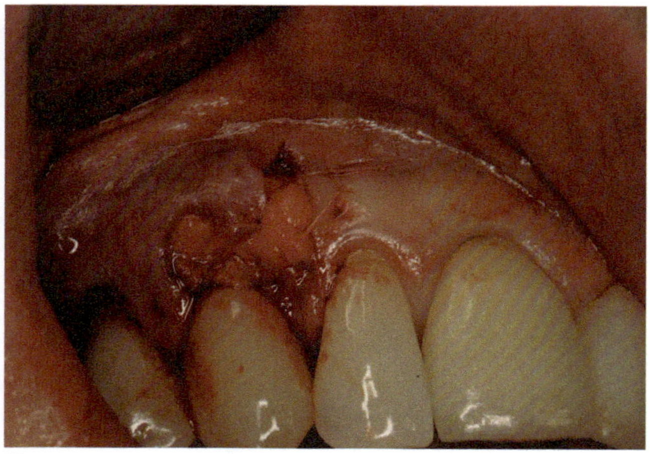

(d)

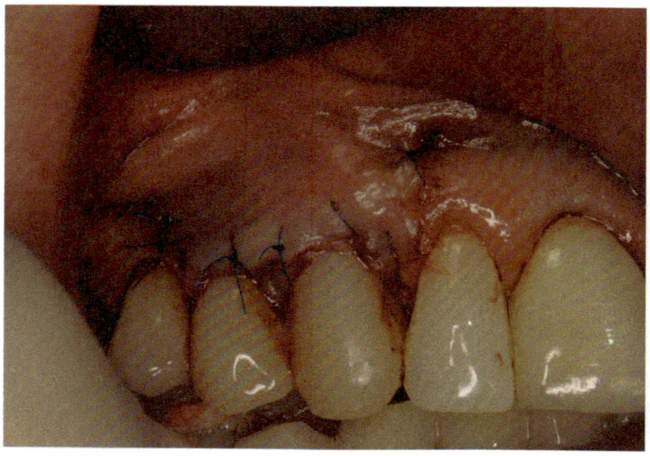

(e)

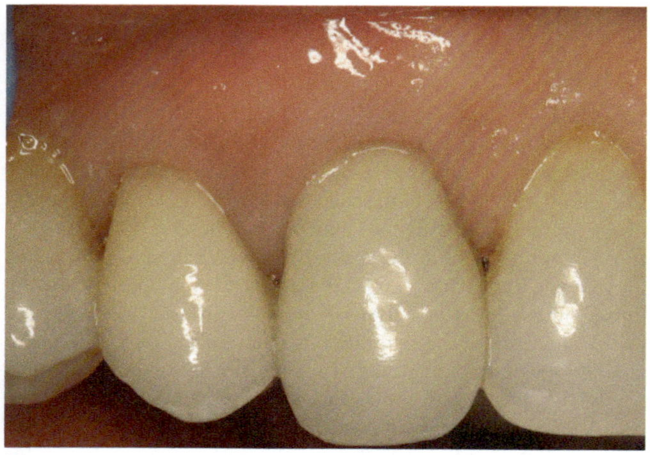

(f)

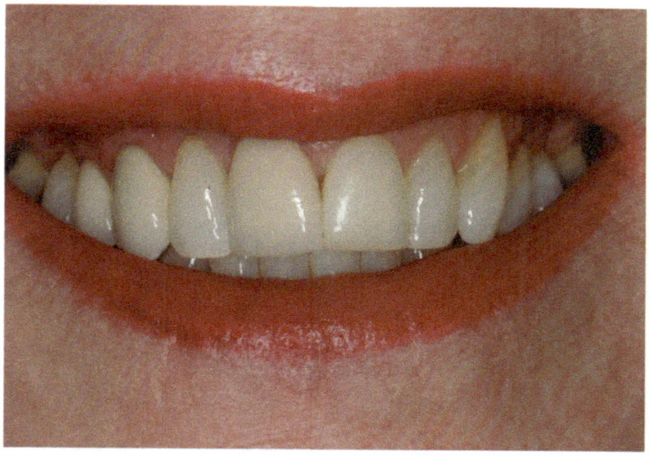

(g)

Figure 8.16 (Continued)
(c) The coronally advanced flap design included vertical releasing incisions at the terminal end of flap with the centeral/lateral papilla maintained to minimize vascular compromise to overlying flap. De-epithelialization was completed at the mesial of canine papilla in preparation for the new coronal position of mesial flap margin. (d) A connective tissue graft was placed into a tunnel preparation of the mobilized partial thickness mucoperiosteal flap, and stabilized with vertical mattress 6-0 plain gut sutures. (e) The coronally positioned flap was secured with 6-0 polypropylene sutures. (f) Final healing at 2 years following the definitive restorative treatment. (g) Full smile view of the final result after 2 years.

Direct adaptation of the connective tissue graft onto the root surface is necessary to eliminate possible voids, and ensure that the graft is secured without mobility, to avoid necrosis (Figure 8.16b). The coronally advanced flap design used in this case included vertical releasing incisions mesial and distal to the site with preservation of the interdental papillae to aid in flap vascularity and stability. A tunneling incision was used to release the papillae from underlying periosteum with blunt dissection at the supraperiosteal level to connect the mesial and distal flap margins to the tunneled papillary dissections. De-epithelialization was completed at the mesial papilla of the canine in preparation for the new coronal position of mesial flap margin. The flap was mobilized in a tension-free fashion over the de-epithelialized papilla adjacent to the defect (Figure 8.16c). To enhance thickness, a connective tissue graft was placed and secured with resorbable sutures (Figure 8.16d), and final closure was completed with 6-0 polypropylene sutures (Figure 8.16e). Two years after restorative treatment, the soft tissue levels demonstrate excellent health and contours (Figure 8.16f and g).

Lateral repositioned pedicle flap

When a soft tissue deficiency exists over an implant, and there is adequate gingiva at adjacent tooth sites, a lateral repositioned flap can be used to correct the deficiency. To overcome the implant esthetic defect shown in Figure 8.17a, a combined approach was used with a coronal advanced flap, a lateral rotated pedicle flap, and a connective tissue graft. An intrasulcular incision was completed for the coronal advanced flap and continued laterally with submarginal oblique incisions at the adjacent papillae.[57] The flap extended to the mesial and distal one tooth beyond the recession defect. The mesial vertical releasing incision was curvilinear to provide a broad trapezoidal base. In Figure 8.17b, arrows indicate the direction of movement of each flap component. The mesial component was released first by partial-thickness dissection, rotated over the recession defect on the implant and secured to the fixed distal component with 6-0 polypropylene monofilament suture (Figure 8.17c). The remaining distal component was released in a superficial-layer, split-thickness fashion, maintaining the angle of the dissection parallel to the overlying mucosa (Figure 8.17d). Figure 8.17e illustrates the overlying coronal advanced flap showing immobility even with the lip stretched. Connective tissue was harvested from the right posterior palate and placed under the combination flap. This addition of connective tissue was meant to establish thick gingiva to mask the underlying implant components. The graft was first stabilized with 5-0 chromic gut suture (Figure 8.17f) followed by the coronal advanced combination flap being secured with 6-0 monofilament suture (Figure 8.17g). The 4-year follow-up revealed tissue stability approximately 3 mm apical to the papilla tips (Figure 8.17h).

Palacci and Nowzari[49] introduced another technique to allow primary closure and create stable tissue anatomy around implant abutments by strategically rotating small pedicles from the larger palatal flap to fill the interproximal spaces of the wound. The flap is designed to allow the buccal aspect to be positioned apically to ensure adequate quality and quantity of keratinized tissue (Figure 8.18a and b). A "c"-shaped incision is made into the palatal flap to allow pedicles to move into the mesial and/or distal interproximal spaces created by the apically positioned buccal flap. The tissue flap is rotated into the desired position, maintaining vascular supply via the pedicle with suturing for tension-free primary soft tissue closure (Figure 8.18c). This surgical soft tissue manipulation can produce an enhanced peri-implant soft tissue contour that matches the natural gingival architecture. The clinical image is seen after 4 months' healing in Figure 8.18d.

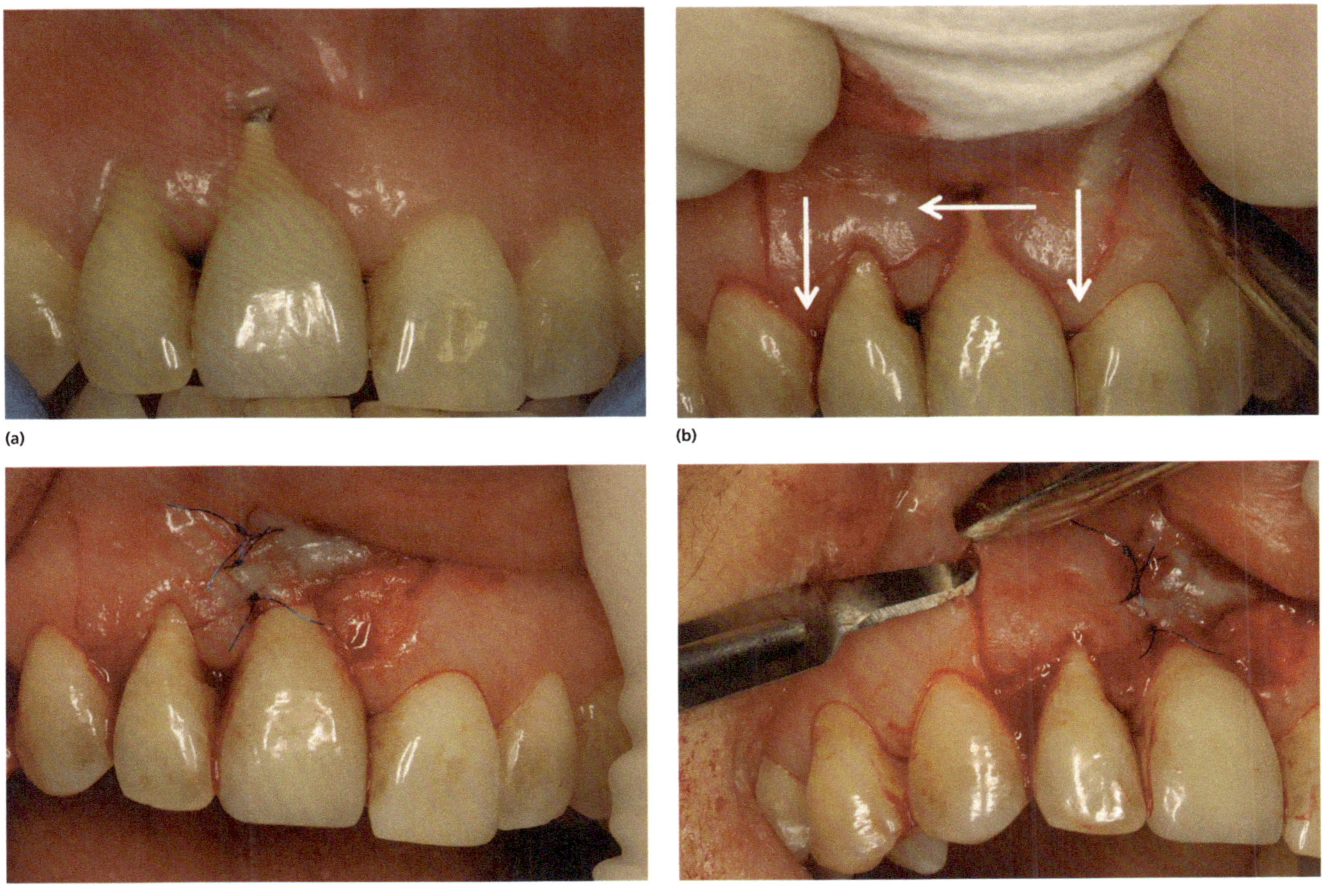
(a) (b) (c) (d)

Figure 8.17 (a) A recession defect resulting in implant esthetic deficiency at the right central incisor location. (b) The flap design allowed for coronal advancement and a lateral sliding pedicle flap. (c) A split-thickness lateral pedicle flap was rotated from the mesial aspect of maxillary central incisor and secured to the remaining fixed flap with independent 6-0 monofilament suture. (d) The distal aspect of the flap was released with the scalpel blade parallel to the outer mucosal plane in order to develop a superficial split-thickness flap.

(Continued)

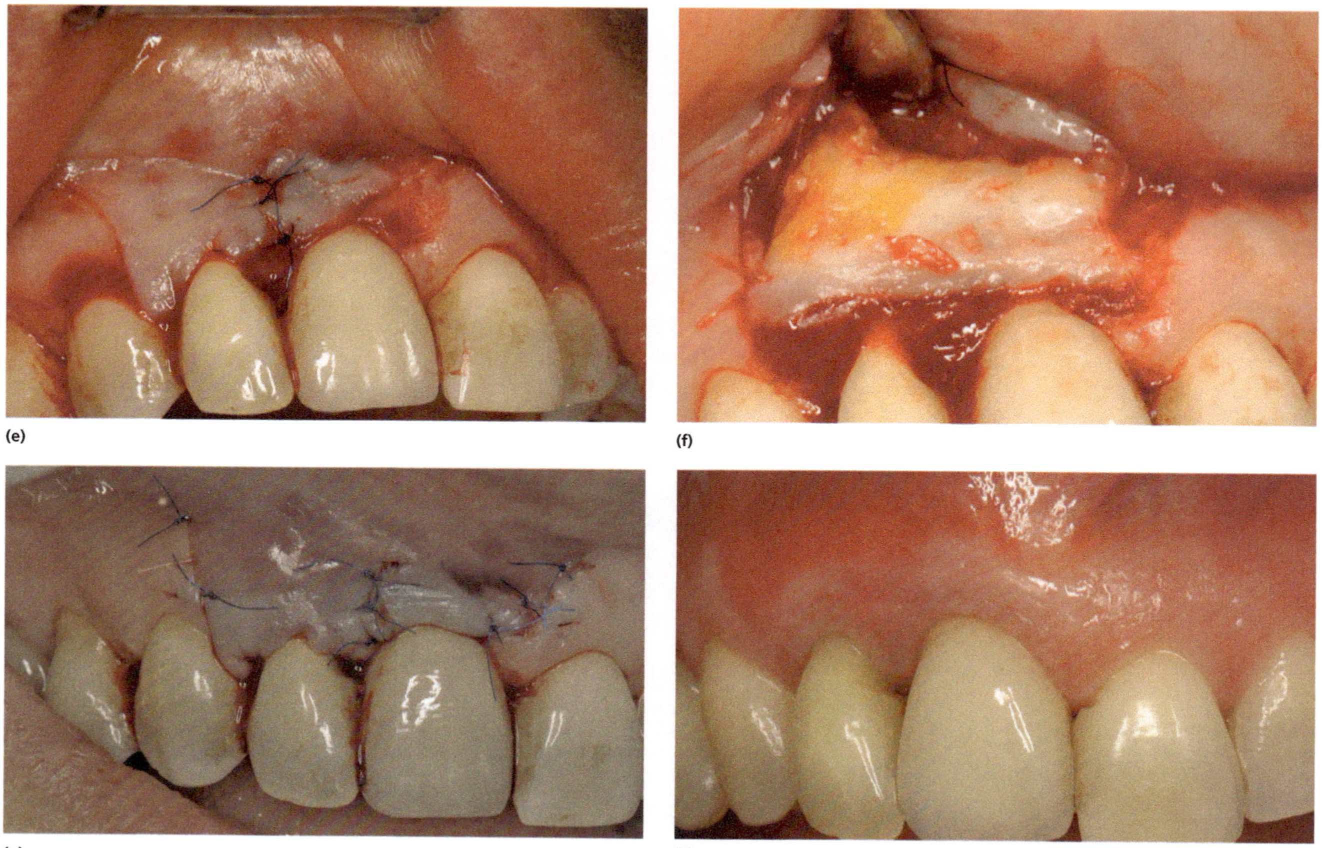

(e) (f) (g) (h)

Figure 8.17 (Continued)
(e) Passive positioning of the combined lateral positioned flap and coronally advanced flap. (f) The connective tissue graft was positioned and secured laterally with 5-0 resorbable suture. (g) The coronally advanced combined superficial split-thickness flap with full connective tissue graft coverage was secured with 6-0 monofilament suture. (h) A facial retracted view 4 years after the combined coronally and laterally positioned flaps and connective tissue grafting at the maxillary right central incisor site.

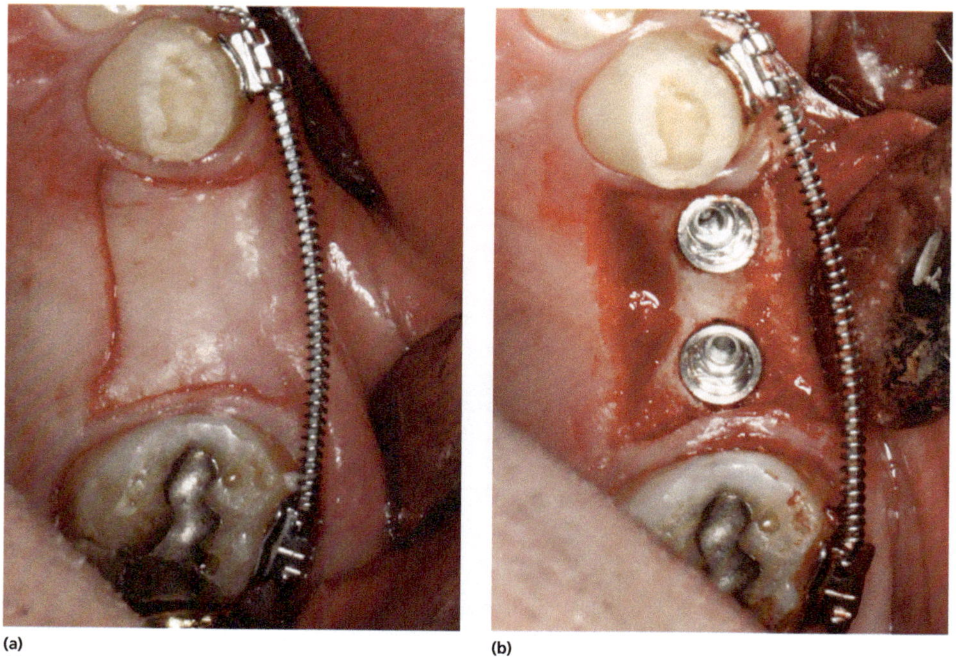

(a) (b)

Figure 8.18 (a) This flap was designed to allow the buccal aspect to be positioned apically to ensure adequate quality and quantity of keratinized tissue. (b) After implant placement, Palacci-type flaps were created with a "c"-shaped incision into the palatal flap to allow the pedicle to move into the mesial interproximal space.

(Continued)

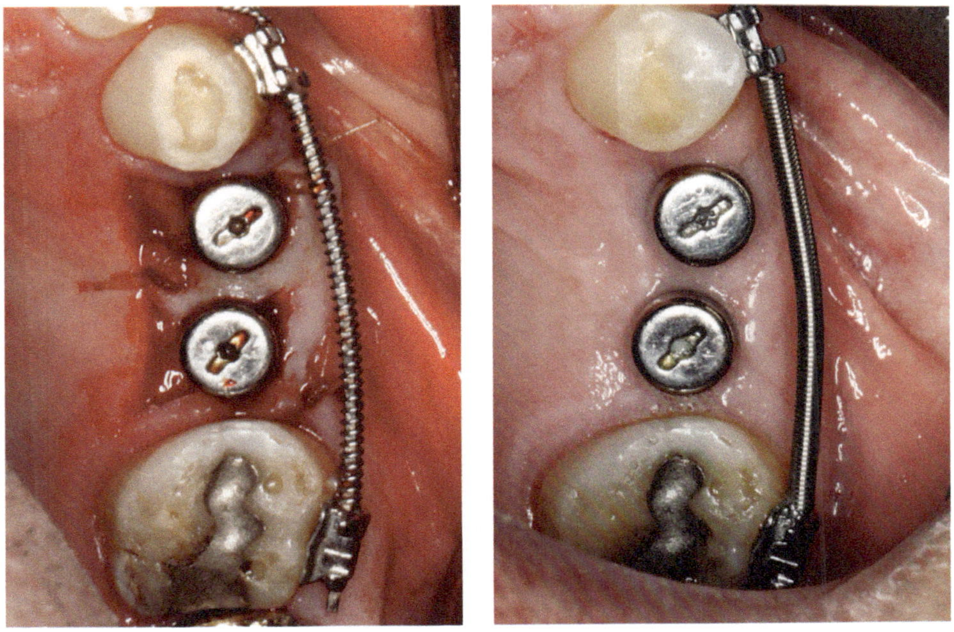

(c) (d)

Figure 8.18 (Continued)
(c) The soft tissue flap was rotated into the desired position, maintaining vascular supply, and sutured for tension-free soft tissue closure. (d) The clinical image is seen here after 4 months' healing and shows good peri-implant soft tissue contours. © Daniel R. Cullum.

Palatal pedicle flap

Khoury and Happe[58] described the palatal pedicle subepithelial connective tissue flap to cover maxillary defects. Palatal pedicle grafts can provide large amounts of connective tissue to cover larger grafted areas with incomplete mucosal coverage or in sites with high esthetic demand since their blood supply is maintained during and after the procedure.[59] Free connective tissue can be used for enhancing tissue thickness at a graft or implant site, but requires adequate periosteal and/or overlying flap coverage for revascularization. The specific anatomic depth and thickness of the palatal mucosa will dictate the amount of tissue available, and the design must optimize the pedicle thickness and vascular supply. A palatal pedicle flap design has the advantage of providing vascularized primary closure without significant elevation or advancement of a buccal flap for primary closure. In the esthetic zone, this flap design preserves soft tissue anatomy by maintaining the position of the mucogingival junction. Application of an anterior-based palatal pedicle flap design in a complex demand patient (high smile line, thin biotype, esthetic zone) with socket preservation grafting is demonstrated in Figure 8.19.

This patient presented with a failing endodontically treated maxillary left central incisor with significant inflammation and extrusion (Figure 8.19a). CBCT cross-sectional imaging demonstrated significant facial and palatal vertical bone loss (Figure 8.19b). Minimally invasive tooth removal and aggressive site debridement were followed by closed site evaluation, demonstrating a significant alveolar defect on the facial and interproximal aspects (Figure 8.19c–e). Interdental envelope flap release allowed for minimal flap exposure of the defect in preparation for a combined bone and soft tissue reconstruction (Figure 8.19f). A palatal mucosal incision was completed extending from the mesial of the left maxillary first molar to the distal papilla interface of the central incisor (Figure 8.19g). Palatal epithelial–connective tissue flap exposure can be seen after dissection along the superficial connective tissue plane to the height of the palatal vault. The anterior portion of the connective tissue and periosteum must be maintained as a pedicle with adequate thickness to ensure vascular supply. The incision design for the anterior-based pedicle is outlined with a dashed line in Figure 8.19h. Incision to bone was completed through the periosteum with subperiosteal elevation beginning at the distal free margin (indicated by the arrow in Figure 8.19h). The flap was mobilized to ensure enough tissue for complete defect coverage and an intact pedicle (Figure 8.19i). A collagen barrier (Cytoplast RTM™, Osteogenics, Lubbuc, TX) was trimmed and shaped for buccal and palatal coverage, saturated with venous blood, and placed into the facial subperiosteal pocket resting on the remaining marginal bone (Figure 8.19j). After particulate graft placement, the collagen barrier was closed over the crestal area in preparation for positioning of the pedicle flap (Figure 8.19k). The connective tissue pedicle was advanced to a position under the facial soft tissue and secured with a horizontal mattress suture. The interproximal and palatal areas were closed with 5-0 polyglycolic sutures (Figure 8.19l and m). The result after 4 months' healing can be seen in Figure 8.19n, while the implant-supported restoration with esthetic bone and gingival contours and the associated radiograph after 11 months are shown in Figure 8.15j and k. The final treatment results for this patient are seen in Figure 8.15a–k.

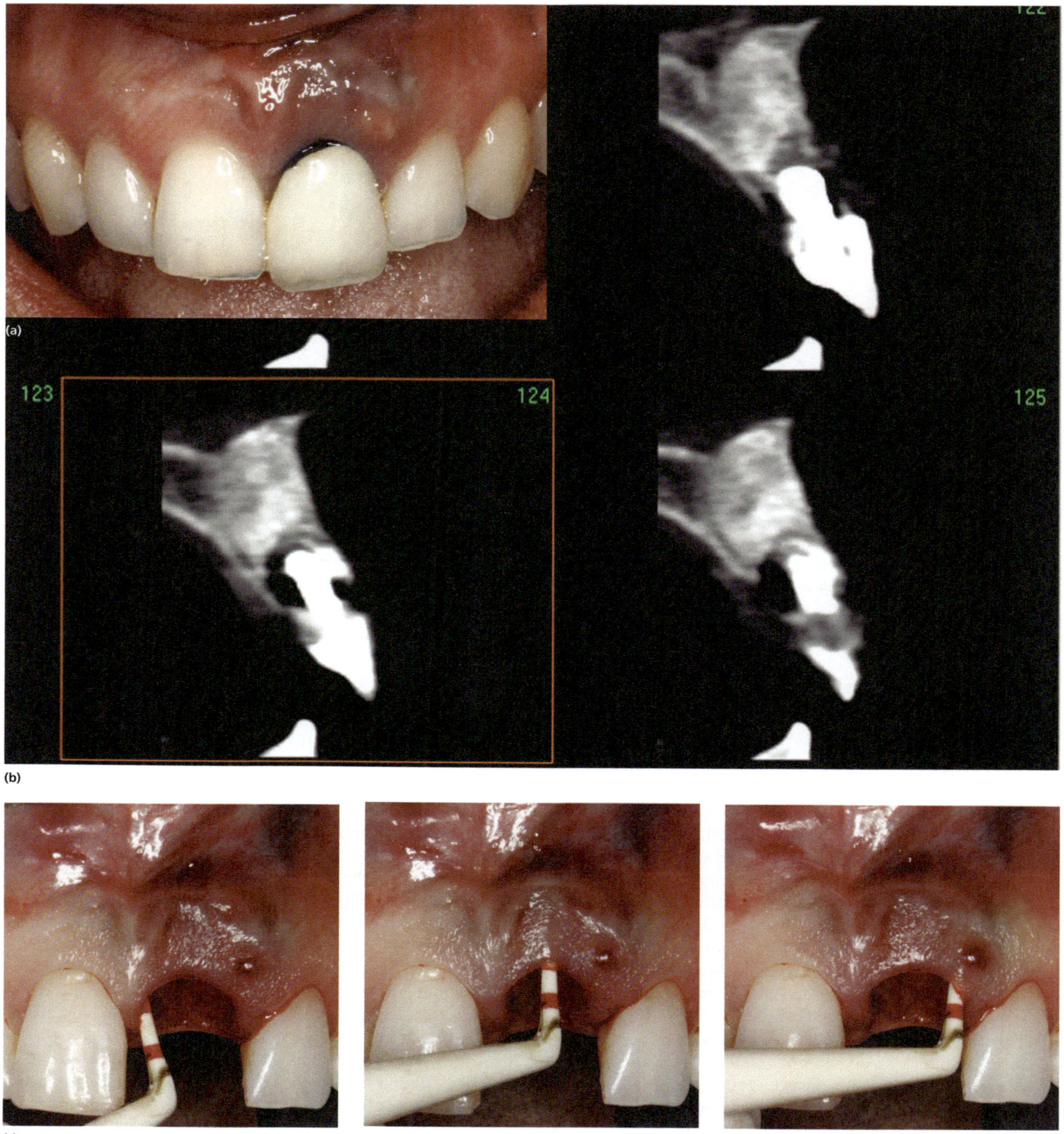

(a) (b) (c) (d) (e)

Figure 8.19 (a) A frontal view of a failing endodontically treated maxillary left central incisor with significant inflammation and extrusion. (b) The preoperative cross-sectional CBCT image demonstrated significant facial and palatal vertical bone loss. (c–e) Minimally invasive tooth removal and debridement was followed by closed site evaluation revealing a significant facial and distal defect extending into the interproximal region.

(Continued)

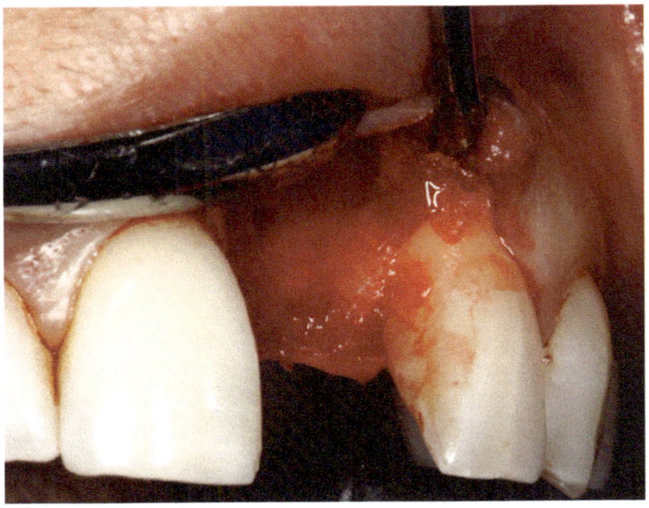

(f)

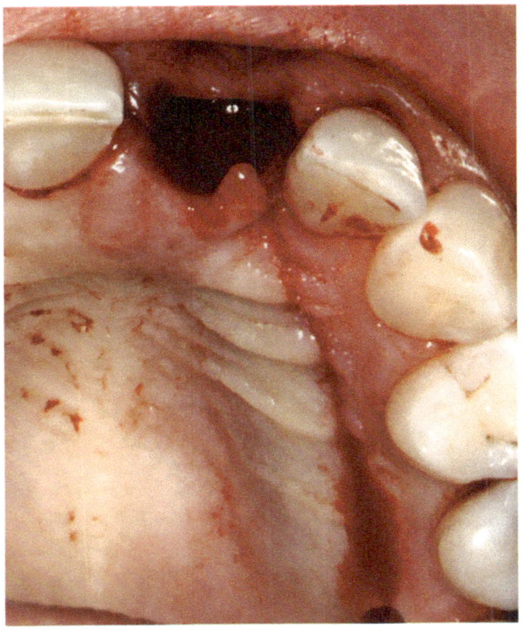

(g)

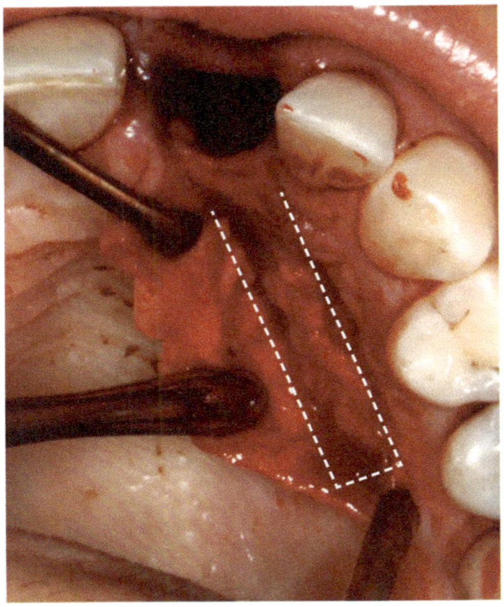

(h)

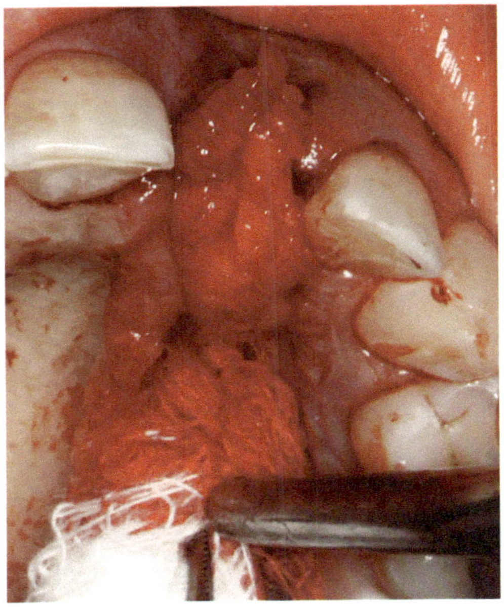

(i)

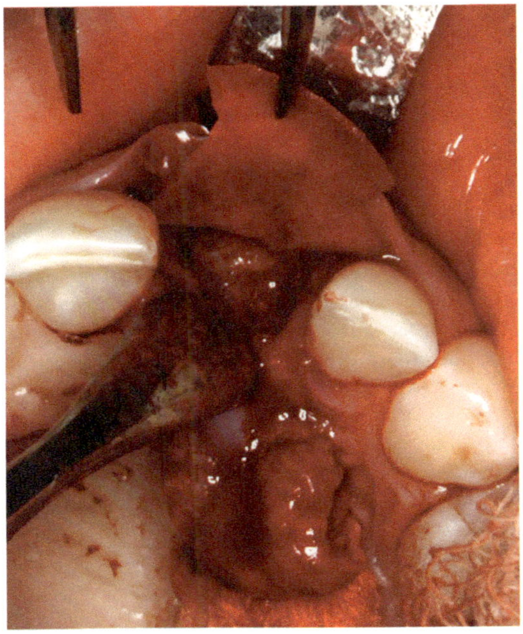

(j)

Figure 8.19 (Continued)

(f) An interdental incision allowed minimal flap exposure in preparation for combined bone and soft tissue reconstructions. (g) A palatal mucosal incision was completed extending from the mesial of the left maxillary first molar to the distal papilla interface of the central incisor. (h) Palatal flap exposure was completed with dissection along the superficial connective tissue plane to the height of the palatal vault. The anterior portion required maintenance of adequate thickness of the periosteal–connective tissue component to ensure vascular supply. The incision design for the anteriorly based pedicle is outlined by a dashed line. The incision was completed through the periosteum with subperiosteal elevation beginning at the distal free margin (indicated by the arrow). (i) The flap was mobilized to ensure subsequent complete defect coverage and an intact pedicle prior to grafting. (j) A collagen barrier was trimmed and shaped for buccal and palatal coverage, saturated with venous blood, and placed into the facial subperiosteal pocket resting on the adjacent bone margins.

(Continued)

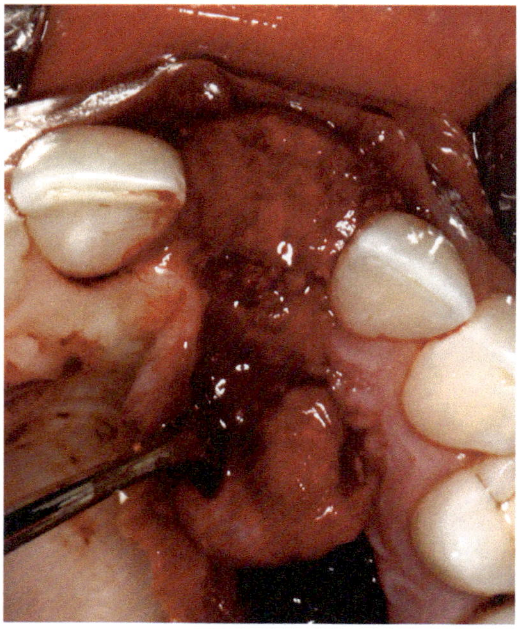

(k)

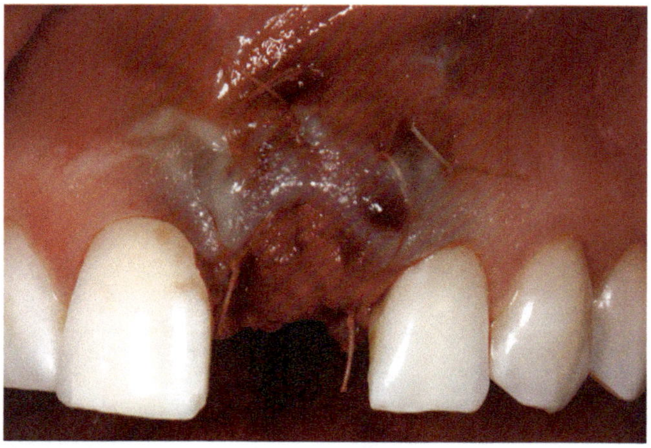

(l)

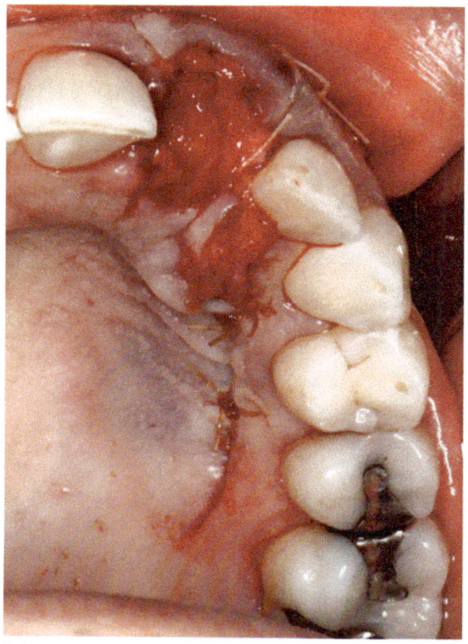

(m)

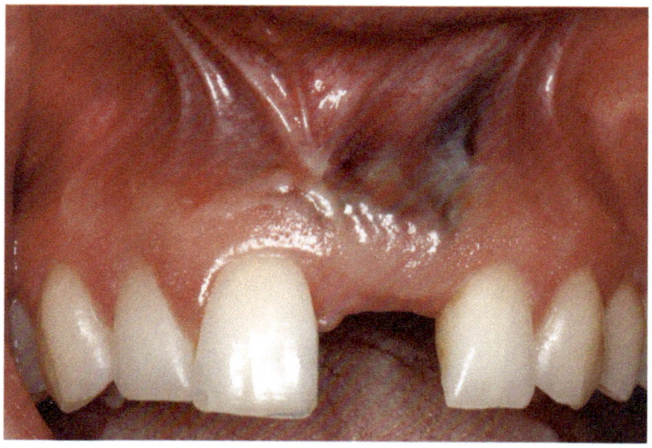

(n)

Figure 8.19 (Continued)
(k) After particulate graft placement, the collagen barrier was positioned over the crestal area in preparation for the pedicle flap. (l, m) The connective tissue pedicle was advanced and sutured to the facial soft tissue flap, and the interproximal and palatal areas closed with 5-0 polyglycolic sutures. (n) Frontal view showing healing after 4 months (same patient continued in Figure 8.15) © Daniel R. Cullum.

Conclusions

Peri-implant soft tissue plastic surgery represents a variety of mucogingival procedures developed originally for use with natural teeth and bone defects. These soft tissue plastic surgery techniques can have significant applications in implant reconstruction to enhance gingival biotype and the width and/or thickness of soft tissues with the goal of providing stable and esthetically pleasing implant-supported prostheses. In some instances it is optimal to complete soft tissue surgery before implant placement. An example would be the large edentulous site with inadequate attached gingiva requiring a full-thickness free gingival onlay graft. Alternatively, necessary soft tissue grafting can be done at the time of tooth extraction and socket preservation grafting, at implant placement, or with subsequent uncovering. The most commonly used peri-implant soft tissue plastic procedures include connective tissue grafts taken from the palate or tuberosity in combination with a variety of flap procedures to provide protection and vascular support. With efforts to refine surgical technique and minimize trauma, the approach can become minimally invasive with reduced pain and edema, number of procedures, duration of treatment, and/or cost. Given the high expectations of patients seeking implant treatment today, implant surgeons must be skilled in the use soft tissue procedures. Careful treatment planning, in concert with the restorative team members, and comprehensive surgical training/skill development will help ensure that the techniques are applied in a minimally invasive fashion.

References

1. Zucchelli G, Mele M, Mazzotti C, et al. Coronally advanced flap with and without vertical releasing incisions for the treatment of multiple recessions: a comparative controlled randomized clinical trial. J Periodontol 2009; 80: 1083–1094.
2. Salama H, Salama M, Garber D. The tunnel technique in the periodontal plastic treatment of multiple adjacent gingival recession defects: a review. Inside Dent 2008; 4(9).
3. Warren R, Grupe H. Repair of gingival defects by a sliding flap operation. J Periodontol 1956; 27: 290–295.
4. Pfeifer J, Heller R. Histologic evaluation of full and partial thickness lateral repositioned flaps. A pilot study. J Periodontol 1971; 42: 331–333.
5. Pini-Prato G, Baldi C, Pagliaro U, et al. Coronally advanced flap procedure for root coverage. Treatment of root surface: root planing versus polishing. J Periodontol 1999; 70: 1064–1076.
6. Maynard J, Wilson R. Physiologic dimensions of the periodontium significant to the restorative dentist. J Periodontol 1979; 50: 170–179.
7. Bouri A, Bissada N, Al-Zahrani M, et al. Width of keratinized gingiva and the health status of the supporting tissues around dental implants. Int J Maxillofac Implants 2008; 23: 323–326.
8. Zigdon H, Machtei E. The dimensions of keratinized mucosa around implants affect clinical and immunological parameters. Clin Oral Implants Res 2008; 19: 387–392.
9. Ten Cate A. Oral Histology. St. Louis, MO: Mosby, 1989, pp. 368–374.
10. Nevins M, Becker W, Kornman K. Proceedings of the World Workshop in Clinical Periodontics. Chicago, IL: American Academy of Periodontology, 1989, pp. vii, 1–21.
11. Claffey N, Shanley D. Relationship of gingival thickness and bleeding to loss of probing attachment in shallow sites following non-surgical periodontal therapy. J Clin Periodontol 1986; 13: 654–657.
12. Kan J, Rungcharassaeng K, Cosyn J. Immediate placement and provisionalization of maxillary anterior single implants: a 1-year prospective study. Int J Oral Maxillofac Implants 2003; 18: 31–39.
13. Zucchelli G. Mucogingival Surgery. Milan: Quintessenza, 2013, chapter 3, pp. 14–58.
14. Fu J, Yeh H, Tatarakis N, et al. Tissue biotype and its relation to the underlying bone morphology. J Periodontol 2010; 81: 569–574.
15. Hwang D, Wang H. Flap thickness as a predictor of root coverage: a systematic review. J Periodontol 2006; 77: 1625–1634.
16. Baumann G, Rapley J, Hallmon W, Mills M. The peri-implant sulcus. Int J Oral Maxillofac Implants 1993; 8: 273–280.
17. Nevins M, Nevins M, Camelo M, et al. Human histologic evidence of a connective tissue attachment to a dental implant. Int J Periodontics Restorative Dent 2008; 28: 111–121.
18. Nevins M, Camelo M, Nevins ML, et al. Connective tissue attachment to laser-micro-grooved abutments: a human histological case report. Int J Periodontics Restorative Dent 2012; 32: 385–392.
19. Nevins M, Nevins ML, Gobbato L, et al. Maintaining inter-implant crestal bone height via a combined platform-switched, Laser-Lok implant–abutment system: a proof-of-principle canine study. Int J Periodontics Rest Dent 2013; 33: 261–267.
20. Salvi G, Alietta M, Eick S, et al. Reversibility of experimental peri-implant mucositis compared with experimental gingivitis in humans. Clin Oral Implants Res 2012; 23: 182–190.
21. Lindhe J, Berglundh T, Ericsson I, et al. Experimental breakdown of peri-implant and periodontal tissues. A study in the beagle dog. Clin Oral Implants Res 1992; 3: 9–16.
22. Berglundh T, Gotfredsen K, Zitzmann N, et al. Spontaneous progression of ligature induced peri-implantitis at implants with different surface roughness: an experimental study in dogs. Clin Oral Implants Res 2007; 18: 655–661.
23. Tesmer M, Wallet S, Koutouzis T, Lundgren T. Bacterial colonization of the dental implant fixture–abutment interface: an *in vitro* study. J Periodontol 2009; 80: 1991–1997.
24. King G, Hermann J, Schoolfield D, et al. Influence of the size of the micro-gap on crestal bone levels in non-submerged dental implants: a radiographic study in the canine mandible. J Periodontol 2002; 73: 1111–1117.
25. Wilson T. The positive relationship between cement excess and peri-implant disease: a prospective clinical endoscopic study. J Periodontol 2009; 80: 1388–1392.
26. Degidi M, Nardi D, Piattelli A. One abutment at one time: non-removal of an immediate abutment and its effect on bone healing around subcrestal tapered implants. Clin Oral Implants Res 2001; 22: 1303–1307.
27. Prichard, JF. The etiology, diagnosis, and treatment of the intrabony defect. J Periodontol 1967; 38: 455–465.
28. Grunder U, Gracis S, Capelli M. Influence of the 3-D bone to implant relationship on esthetics. Int J Periodontics Rest Dent 2005; 25: 113–119.
29. Spray R, Black G, Morris H, et al. The influence of bone thickness on facial marginal bone response: stage I placement through stage 2 uncovering. Ann Periodontol 2000; 5: 119–128.
30. Linkevicius T, Apse P, Grybauskas S, et al. The influence of soft tissue thickness on crestal bone changes around implants: a 1-year prospective controlled clinical trial. Int J Oral Maxillofac Implants 2009; 24: 712–719.
31. Le B, Borzabadi-Farahani A. Labial bone thickness in area of anterior maxillary implants associated with crestal labial soft tissue thickness. Implant Dent 2012; 21: 406–410.
32. Tarnow D, Magner A, Fletcher P. The effect of distance from the contact point to the crest of bone on the presence or absence of the interproximal dental papilla. J Periodontol 1992; 63: 995–996.
33. Salama H, Salama M, Garber D, Adar P. The interproximal height of bone: a guidepost to esthetic strategies and soft tissue contours in anterior tooth replacement. J Pract Periodontics Aesthet Dent 1998; 10: 1131–1141.
34. Chung D, Oh T, Shotwell J, et al. Significance of keratinized mucosa in maintenance of dental implants with different surfaces. J Periodontol 2006; 77: 1410–1420.
35. Adibrad M, Shahabuei M, Sahabi M. Significance of the width of keratinized mucosa on the health status of the supporting tissues around implants supporting overdentures. J Oral Implantol 2009; 35: 232–237.
36. Evans C, Chen S. Esthetic outcomes of immediate implant placements. Clin Oral Implants Res 2008; 19: 73–80.
37. Levine R, Huynh-Ba G, Cochran D. Soft tissue augmentation procedures for mucogingival defects in esthetic sites. Int J Oral Maxillofac Implants 2014; 29(Suppl): 155–185.
38. Miller P. A classification of marginal tissue recession. Int J Periodontics Restorative Dent 1985; 5: 8–13.
39. Raetzke P. Covering localized areas of root exposure employing the "envelope" technique. J Periodontol 1985; 56: 397–402.
40. Abrahamsson I, Berglundh T, Glantz P, Lindhe J. The mucosal attachment at different abutments. An experimental study in dogs. J Clin Periodontol 1998; 25: 721–727.
41. Khoury F, Tunkel J. Bone augmentation and soft tissue management. In: Bone Augmentation in Oral Implantology, Khoury F, Antoun H, Missika P, eds. Chicago, IL: Quintessence, 2007, pp. 75–114.
42. Lazzara R, Porter S. Platform switching: a new concept in implant dentistry for controlling post-restorative crestal bone levels. Int J Periodontics Restorative Dent 2006; 26: 9–17.
43. Rodriquez-Ciurana X, Vela-Nebot X, Segala-Torres M, et al. The effect of inter-implant distance on the height of inter-implant bone crest when using platform-switched implants. Int J Periodontics Restorative Dent 2009; 29: 141–151.
44. Morris HF, Ochi S, Creum P, Orenstein IH, Winkler S. AICRG Part I: a 6-year multi-centered, multidisciplinary clinical study of a new and innovative implant design. J Oral Implantol 2004; 30: 125–133.
45. Wood D, Donnenfeld W, Hoag P, Rosenfeld L. Alveolar crest reduction following full and partial thickness flaps. J Periodontol 1972; 43: 141–144.
46. Greenwell H, Vance G, Munninger B, Johnston H. Superficial-layer split-thickness flap for maximal flap release and coronal positioning: a surgical technique. Int J Periodontics Restorative Dent 2004; 24: 521–527.
47. Santarelli G, Ciancaglini R, Companari F, et al. Connective tissue grafting employing the tunnel technique: a case report of complete root coverage in the anterior maxilla. Int J Periodontics Restorative Dent 2001; 21: 77–88.
48. Tozum T, Dini F. Treatment of adjacent gingival recessions with subepithelial connective tissue grafts and the modified tunnel technique. Quintessence Int 2003; 34: 7–13.
49. Palacci P, Nowzari H. Soft tissue enhancement around dental implants. Periodontol 2000 2008; 47: 113–132.
50. Nabers J. Extension of the vestibular fornix utilizing a gingival graft – a case report. Periodontics 1966; 4: 243–245.
51. Lorenzana E, Allen P. The single-incision palatal harvest technique. Strategy for esthetics and patient comfort. Int J Periodontics Rest Dent 2000; 20: 297–305.
52. Stimmelmaier M, Allen EP, Reichert T, Iglhaut G. Use of a combination epithelized-subepithelial connective tissue graft for closure and soft tissue augmentation of an extraction site following ridge preservation or implant placement: description of a technique. Int J Periodontics Restorative Dent 2010; 30: 375–381.

53. Kelly E. Changes caused by a mandibular removable partial denture opposing a maxillary complete denture. J Prosthet Dent 1972; 27: 140–150.
54. Cummings L, Kaldahl W, Allen E. Histologic evaluation of autogenous connective tissue and acellular dermal matrix grafts in humans. J Periodontol 2005; 76: 178–186.
55. Allen EP. Multiple tooth recession: papilla retention pouch procedure. In: Contemporary Oral Plastic Surgery Procedural Manual, Allen EP, ed. Dallas, TX: Center for Advanced Dental Education, 2004, pp. 9–16.
56. Allen EP. Subpapillary continuous sling suturing method for soft tissue grafting with the tunneling technique. Int J Periodontics Restorative Dent 2010; 30: 479–485.
57. Zucchelli G, De Santis M. Treatment of multiple recession-type defects in patients with esthetic demands. J Periodontol 2000; 71: 1506–1514.
58. Khoury F, Happe A. The palatal subepithelial connective tissue flap method for soft tissue management to cover maxillary defects: a clinical report. Int J Oral Maxillofac Implants 2000; 15: 415–418.
59. Mathews D. The pediculated connective tissue graft: a technique for improving unaesthetic implant restorations. Pract Proced Aesthet Dent 2002; 14: 719–724.
60. Sclar AT. Systematic evaluation of the esthetic implant patient. In: Soft Tissue and Esthetic Considerations in Implant Therapy. Chicago, IL: Quintessence, 2003, pp. 163–187.

CHAPTER 9

Minimally Invasive Implant Surgery Using Computer-Guided Technology

Gary Orentlicher,[1,2] Andrew Horowitz,[1,2] & Marcus Abboud[3]
[1]Private Practice, New York Oral, Maxillofacial and Implant Surgery, Scarsdale, NY, USA
[2]Division of Oral and Maxillofacial Surgery, White Plains Hospital, White Plains, NY, USA
[3]Department of Prosthodontics and Digital Technology, Stony Brook University, Stony Brook, NY, USA

Introduction

The concept of minimally invasive surgery is intended to reduce tissue trauma, resulting in decreased patient pain and swelling, thereby improving patient experiences post-operatively. Computer-guided implant planning and treatment workflows were developed to allow implant placement in a minimally invasive manner, with the intended additional benefit of improved accuracy. Dental implants have historically been placed with direct visualization of bone following elevation of soft tissue flaps. However, some clinicians have advocated implant placement using flapless surgery either with or without initial 3-D radiographic evaluation of the underlying anatomy. The clinical challenge of a "flapless" non-guided approach is significant, requiring careful 3-D position assessment, intuition, and experience. In the early 2000s computerized tomographic (CT) guided dental implant planning was introduced. Development and fabrication of corresponding surgical guides and implant-specific guided surgical instrumentation gave clinicians the ability to place dental implants using truly minimally invasive, flapless techniques without sacrificing accuracy, precision, or predictability.

History

Prior to the early 2000s, computerized axial tomography (CAT) imaging for dental purposes was performed in a hospital setting or in a private radiology facility using helical "medical" CT scanners. This technology was not widely adopted by the dental community because of cost, difficult access to machines in hospitals, and lack of familiarity and training in reading and interpreting images. Additionally, the cost/benefit ratio was a concern when the radiation dosage was considered. In 1998, Mozzo et al.[1] reported on the use of the first cone beam volumetric tomography (CBVT) or cone beam CT (CBCT) machine specifically designed for dentistry (New Tom 9000; Quantitative Radiology, Verona, Italy). This equipment allowed for less expensive, smaller, office-based machines with lower radiation doses, and resultant reduced image definition.[2–4] Since that time, multiple manufacturers have developed CBVT/CBCT machines for the dental market; either "medical" CT or CBVT/CBCT can be used for patient evaluation and treatment planning. Given the advantages and disadvantages of each, the decision as to which form of imaging to use in an individual patient case is up to the judgment of the clinician.

As early as the late 1980's, publications in the scientific literature began to appear discussing the use of DentaScan® (GE Healthcare, Waukesha, WI) in the preoperative evaluation of maxilla and mandible for dental implants.[5–8] In 1988, Columbia Scientific Inc. (CSI; Columbia, MD) introduced the "3-D/Dental" software. This software allowed radiologists to provide dental clinicians with reformatted, detailed cross-sectional anatomic images of a patient's alveolar ridges. In 1991, CSI combined multiple software products into the ImageMaster-101® software that allowed the placement of graphical implants virtually onto CT images. In July 1993, the first version of SimPlant® (Dentsply Implants Inc., York, PA) was released. With this software, the clinician could visualize the patient's axial, cross-sectional, and panoramic views on a single display screen and place virtual implants. In 1999, with the introduction of Simplant 6.0®, the ability to create 3-D reformatted images was added to the software.[9] In 2001, Materialise® (Leuven, Belgium) purchased CSI, and the SurgiGuide® technology for guided implant placement was introduced to the North American market in 2002. These guides required soft tissue incisions and bone exposure. Materialise Dental® was purchased by Dentsply® (York, PA, USA) in 2011. NobelBiocare® (Zurich, Switzerland) introduced the NobelGuide® technology workflow in 2005. The latter was the first comprehensive system with implant-specific instrumentation designed for flapless placement of dental implants. Software from other manufacturers, such as coDiagnostiX™ (Straumann®, Basel, Switzerland), VIP™ (BioHorizons®, Birmingham, AL), Invivo 5® (Anatomage®, San Jose, CA, USA), 360 imaging dps™ (360imaging®, Atlanta, GA, USA), and Implant Master™ (IDent®, Foster City, CA) are now available as well. Most major implant manufacturers have produced instrumentation for minimally invasive flapless placement of their implants through CT-generated surgical guides.

Computer-guided technology overview

When placing dental implants, surgeons commonly use surgical guides fabricated on articulated patient models. These guides can be simple (i.e. vacuforms with the buccal or palatal/lingual facings

Minimally Invasive Dental Implant Surgery, First Edition. Edited by Daniel R. Cullum and Douglas Deporter.

of the planned restorations) or more complex (i.e. 2 mm drill holes or metal tubes embedded in hard acrylic appliances that reproduce planned restorations). There is limited correlation between these appliances and the planned restoration or underlying bony anatomy. In contrast, computer-guided implant surgical guides correlate with these important treatment factors for evaluation and planning prior to surgery.

All implant surgical guides are developed based on a patient's intraoral anatomy and local references, such as the numbers and locations of teeth in the arch to be treated and/or in the opposing arch. As the length of the edentulous area increases, the surgeon has fewer anatomic references to use to predictably place implants with accuracy. In a fully edentulous patient, all local references other than soft tissue have been lost. Additionally, the predictable use of a traditional surgical guide becomes more difficult, as bone and soft tissues are lost from periodontal disease, bony atrophy, sinus pneumatization, and long-term denture wear.

Medical-grade CT scanners and in-office CBCT scanners allow the restorative dentist and surgeon to visualize a patient's bony anatomy in three dimensions. Visualization of the available bone for implant placement, soft tissue thicknesses, and locations of the maxillary sinuses and pertinent vital structures, such as the mandibular canals, are possible.[10–12] The images can be imported into one of the available proprietary software programs that allow the clinician to place implants "virtually" on a computer for treatment planning purposes. The type and dimensions of the planned implant, its position, its relationship to the planned restoration and adjacent teeth and/or other implants, and its proximity to vital anatomic structures can all be determined prior to surgery.[10–14] From the "virtual" treatment plan, computer-generated drilling guides can be fabricated. These surgical guides allow the clinician to place the implant(s) as planned in the "virtual" treatment plan. This process can allow more accurate and predictable implant placements,[15–19] and reduce potential patient morbidity.[20–23]

Most of the current software programs have similar workflows. In the most common workflow, the clinician creates a "scan prosthesis," which duplicates the planned final restoration. The patient wears this appliance while undergoing a CT or CBCT scan (Figure 9.1a and b). The Digital Imaging and Communications in Medicine (DICOM) images are then imported into the proprietary software program being used. The software can then be used to place implants "virtually" into their ideal positions related to the planned restoration and underlying bone (Figure 9.1c and d). The clinician then forwards the "virtual" treatment plan to a manufacturer for fabrication of a surgical guide (Figure 9.1e and f). Finally, the surgeon uses the prepared surgical guide with implant-specific drilling instrumentation to precisely place the implants according to the "virtual" treatment plan.

The most common computer-guided implant planning software platforms are Simplant, NobelClinician™, coDiagnostiX, VIP Software®, 360imaging dps, Invivo 5™, and IDent. Using the Simplant software platform, a number of dental implant manufacturers have developed surgical instrumentation for the placement of their implants through Simplant-based stereolithographically fabricated CT surgical guides (e.g. Astra Facilitate™; Ankylos Expertease™ (Dentsply, York, PA, USA); 3i Navigator® (Biomet3i®, Palm Beach Gardens, FL, USA); Camlog Guided System™ (Henry Schein®, Melville, NY, USA); Zimmer Guided Surgery™ (Zimmer Dental, Warsaw, IN, USA)). Other manufacturers have developed non-stereolithographic model technologies for the fabrication of surgical guides (e.g. Straumann coDiagnostiX – Straumann, Basel, Switzerland; IDent – Foster City, CA; EZ Guide® – Keystone Dental®, Burlington, MA). In these workflows, the patient is scanned with a barium radiographic appliance in position. Implant placement is planned "virtually" and the surgical guide is created by milling the radiographic appliance according to the digital CT-based treatment plan with the addition of guide sleeves for precise implant placement.

There is functionality common to most proprietary CT-based dental implant planning software programs, including importing and conversion of DICOM image data. However, Simplant requires processing and conversion of the DICOM data by an outside contractor with processing software (Simplant Master™) prior to importing the data into the clinician's Simplant Planner software for treatment planning. All of the software has the ability to: (i) make detailed linear and angular measurements; (ii) evaluate bony anatomy in cross-sectional, panoramic, and axial views; (iii) isolate, identify, and "draw in" the inferior alveolar nerve and other vital structures; (iv) visualize and isolate roots of teeth and implants; (v) "virtually" place, measure, and alter the position of dental implants in the bony images as related to the planned restorations and other anatomic structures; (vi) visualize accurate stock abutments; (vii) visualize, remove, rotate, and focus on detailed 3-D virtual reformations of the bony anatomy (termed "surface rendering"); and (viii) digitally upload the virtual treatment plan to a manufacturer for the fabrication of a surgical guide based on the virtual treatment plan.

Many software applications have incorporated newer digital technologies in their treatment planning workflow, such as the addition of "virtual" teeth, virtually created custom abutments, incorporation of optical scans of patient models and diagnostic wax-ups, stereolithographic production of master casts, and the preoperative milling of provisional restorations from virtual implant treatment plans (Figure 9.2).

Three types of computer-generated surgical guides are currently available: tooth-supported, mucosa-supported, and bone-supported. Tooth-supported guides are used in partially edentulous cases and are designed to rest on teeth for accuracy of guide fit. Mucosa-supported guides are designed to rest on the mucosa and are primarily used in fully edentulous cases. Bone-supported guides can be used in partially or fully edentulous cases, but are used primarily in the latter when significant ridge atrophy is present and good seating of a mucosa-supported guide is questionable. An extensive full-thickness flap is necessary when using bone-supported guides to expose the bone in the planned implant sites and in the adjacent areas for fully stable guide seating over the bony ridge.

When using a CT-guided surgery workflow, an accurate inter-arch bite registration is of utmost importance to ensure accurate scanning appliance positioning in the patient's mouth during the CT/CBCT scan (see Figures 9.11d and 9.12g). This minimizes potential error that can be carried through the treatment planning workflow. Additionally, an inter-arch bite registration should be used to ensure accurate surgical guide positioning during surgery (see Figures 9.11i and 9.12p).

Dental implant placement using CT-guided surgery with drill guides is known to enhance safety compared with "freehand" techniques,[24,25] while being compatible with conventional flap elevation surgery or flapless procedures.[26] All reports on the use of stereolithographic guides show some error in all dimensions between the virtual planning and actual implant positions obtained.[27] Data show that implants placed using mucosa-supported guides have lower mean deviations than those placed using bone-supported guides.[28] Tooth-supported guides have the

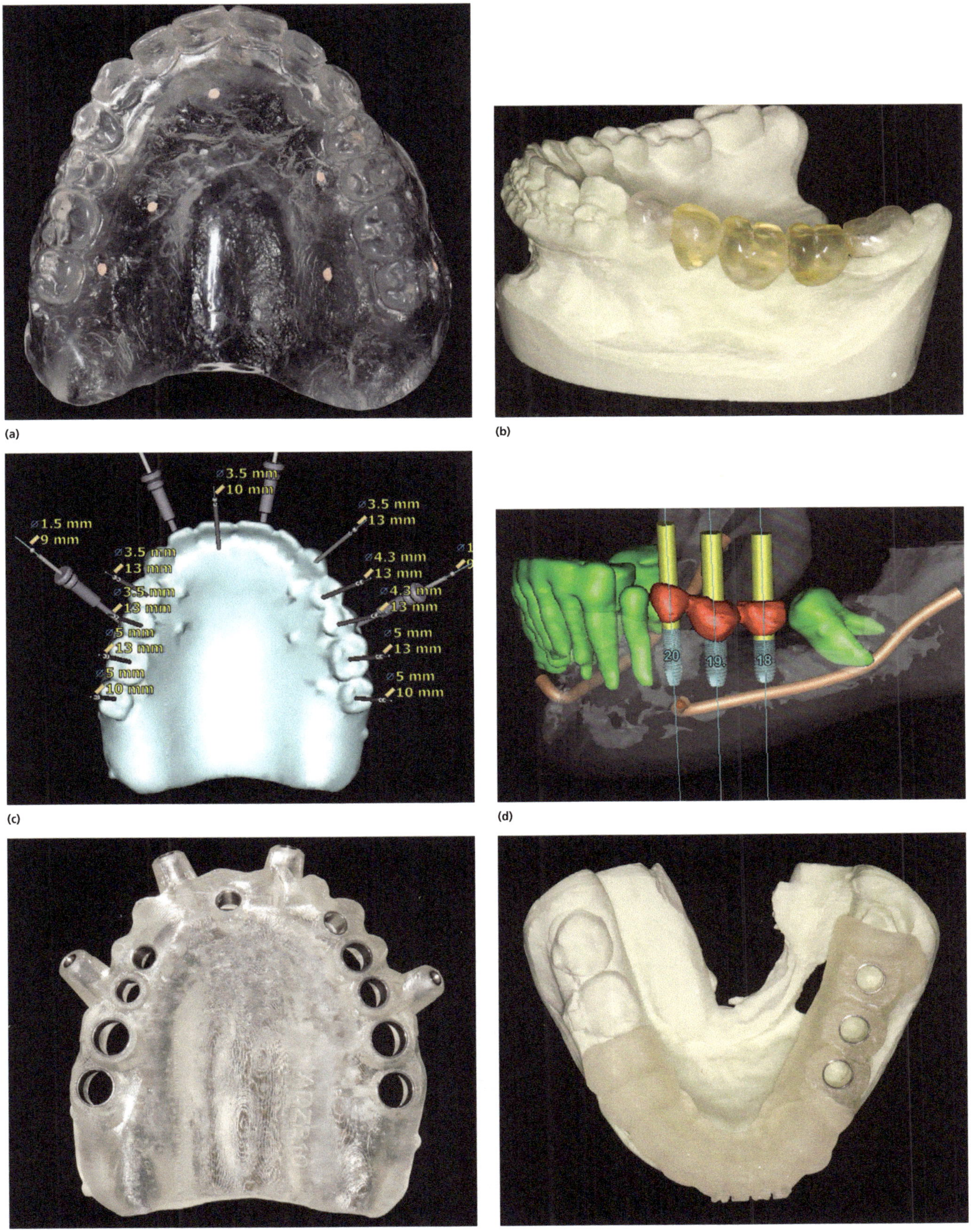

Figure 9.1 (a) Fully edentulous scanning appliance, NobelGuide. (b) Barium partially edentulous scanning appliance, Simplant. (c) Virtual treatment plan, NobelClinician. (d) Virtual treatment plan, Simplant Planner™. (e) Surgical guide produced from plan, NobelGuide. (f) Surgical guide produced from plan, Facilitate™.

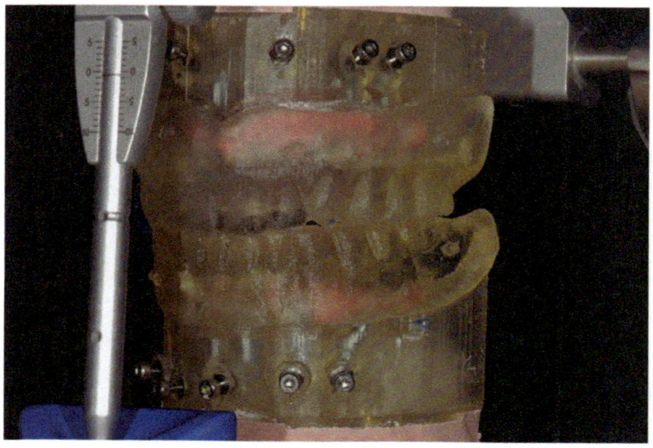

(a)

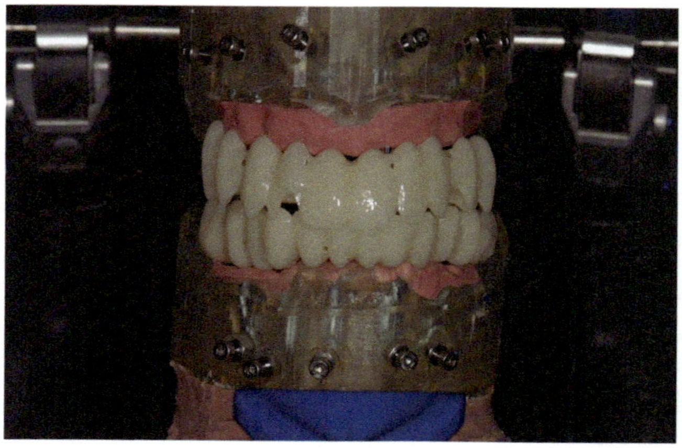

(b)

Figure 9.2 (a) Stereolithographically produced maxillary and mandibular master casts, mounted with stereolithographically produced dentures. Reproduced with permission of DENTSPLY Implants.
(b) Polymethylmethacrylate (PMMA) milled restorations on stereolithographically produced mounted master casts. Reproduced with permission of DENTSPLY Implants.

lowest measured deviation, likely because the teeth provide accurate "stops" for guide placement.[29] Considerations to further minimize error with surgical guides include using specific CT-guided drilling instrumentation, metal guide sleeves, and rigid screw or pin fixation for appliance stabilization to bone. Most systems use these fixation techniques to stabilize mucosa-supported guides; some use them to stabilize all guides.

Following CT-guided placement, an implant can be loaded immediately or not, based on the clinical situation and the clinician's choice. If immediate loading is planned, clinicians commonly place provisional acrylic restorations, not definitive restorations, for many reasons (see Chapter 4). Accurate prediction of the contours and anatomy of the healed gingiva is impossible, whether a case is done flapless or not. This is an issue for the entire implant team. Observation of tissue responses to the provisional restoration gives the restorative dentist invaluable information as to the gingival contours and esthetic requirements in preparation for the definitive restoration. Additionally, a small number of implant failures occur, regardless of whether an implant is placed with CT-guided or conventional surgery. Most surgery-related implant failures typically occur within the first 3–4 months after placement. Management of an implant failure, both surgically and restoratively, is best completed prior to insertion of the definitive restoration. According to Abrahamsson et al.,[30] changing from a healing abutment to a permanent abutment does not result in a change in the dimension and quality of the transmucosal attachment that develops and does not differ from the mucosal barrier that forms to a permanent abutment placed after surgery. Additionally, an acrylic occlusal surface or a composite restoration used for immediate loading has been found to have a better shock absorbing behavior and to reduce the forces of impact when compared with ceramic materials.[31]

Maximizing patient comfort by minimizing trauma is the rationale for using minimally invasive procedures. Flapless insertion of dental implants has been found to have success rates comparable to conventional implant placement procedures, while minimizing the potential complications with soft tissue elevation, such as bone loss, infection, dehiscence, and soft and/or hard tissue necrosis.[32–34] Surgical guidance for drill depth and angulation, in combination with a flapless technique, minimizes the potential injury to underlying anatomical structures during osteotomy preparation.

Flapless surgery is not advised in most Simplant cases without the use of fully guided, implant-specific manufacturer instrumentation. If instrumentation is not available, depth and angulation guidance of all osteotomies is possible, but accurate implant platform placement will require direct visualization of bone, necessitating elevation of a flap. Fully guided and flapless placement of implants is possible with NobelGuide™-, Straumann CARES™-, Navigator-, ExpertEase®-, Facilitate®-, and Materialise-fabricated NobelGuide-compatible surgical guides, and using other major implant manufacturers that have developed fully guided instrumentation for their implant systems.

When planning the use of fully CT-guided surgery, it is imperative that the clinician confirms the amount of attached gingiva in the planned implant site. If a thick zone of attached gingiva is present, most manufacturers have designed soft tissue "coring" drills or tissue punches for removing "islands" of soft tissue prior to fully guided implant placement. If the zone of attached gingiva in the planned implant surgical site is questionable, either small "mini-flaps" should be made to preserve the attached gingiva present, or soft tissue grafting should be planned preoperatively or post-operatively.

CT-based technologies available today have limitations requiring further investigation as to their effects on guided surgery outcomes. For example, the resolution and accuracy of specific CBCT machines compared with the "gold standard" of medical-grade CT scanners has been questioned.[35,36] A "calibration object" is marketed by NobelBiocare that allows calibration of an individual CBCT/CT machine to an acrylic object of known contour and density specific to the NobelGuide protocol. This calibration device improves precision of the stereolithographic fabrication of the NobelGuide.[37] (Figure 9.3) Production of a stereolithographic surgical guide/model reproduces the digitally planned dimensions of an object with a laser beam, selectively solidifying an ultraviolet-sensitive liquid resin. Stereolithographic materials have potential problems with light sensitivity, expansion, and/or shrinkage of the material. Exposure to light for extended periods or sterilization in a high-temperature autoclave causes distortion. Guided surgery techniques can generate increased heat at the osteotomy site, regardless of the irrigation system used, when compared with classic implant site preparation.[38]

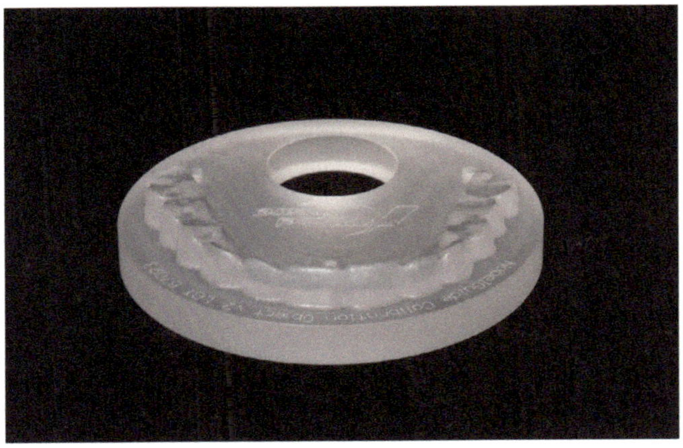

Figure 9.3 Calibration object (NobelBiocare).

Computerized-tomography-guided surgery indications

Because of the precision and accuracy necessary in minimally invasive implant placement, an argument could be made for the use of CT-guided implant surgery in most implant placement procedures. As with any technique, a cost/time/benefit determination must be made by the clinician based on the circumstances of the individual patient scenario. In certain cases, the increased treatment planning time, added expense, and additional patient radiation exposure may outweigh the clinical benefits. We have found that CT-guided technology is most beneficial to the patient and dental team in the following clinical circumstances:

- three or more implants in a row;
- fully edentulous patients;
- cases in which tilted implants are planned, including All-on-Four™;
- proximity to vital anatomic structures (nerves, sinuses, teeth, nasal floor, etc.);
- questionable bone volume;
- implant position that is critical to the planned restoration;
- flapless implant placement;
- multiple unit or full-arch cases, with or without extractions and immediate placement, in which immediate provisional restorations are planned;
- significant alteration of the soft tissue or bony anatomy by prior surgery or trauma;
- patients with physical, medical, and psychiatric co-morbidities.

Numbers and locations of implants

In cases in which multiple implants will be placed in a row, concepts of spacing and angulations, parallelism in all dimensions, proximity to anatomic structures, and relationships between implant positions and the planned restorations are significant considerations. CT/CBCT-guided surgery allows for the ideal placement of multiple implants according to the planned restoration(s), the relationships of implants to surrounding anatomy, and principles of ideal prosthodontic implant positioning and spacing (see Chapters 1 and 2) (Figure 9.4).

Differences in X-ray machines and radiographic techniques commonly lead to distortion of anatomic structures on conventional 2-D images, such as elongation, shortening, stretching, and contraction. Accurate 3-D evaluations and measurements of the relationships between a planned implant and the position of the mental nerve (Figure 9.5a), inferior alveolar nerve (Figure 9.5b), nasopalatine/incisive nerve (Figure 9.5c and d), maxillary sinuses (Figure 9.5e), and nasal floor (Figure 9.5f) are best visualized, evaluated, and measured by using CT-generated images. In cases in which there are questions of nerve or sinus proximity related to the patient's available bone, the additional accuracy of minimally invasive implant placement using CT-generated guides is a clear benefit to both the clinician and the patient. The goal of any treatment is to maximize patient outcomes while minimizing potential patient morbidities.

All proprietary implant planning software programs have functionality to isolate the tooth roots adjacent to edentulous areas for accurate placement of implants between and adjacent to tooth roots. Most programs have the ability to alter sensitivity to Hounsfield units or isovalues in order to virtually remove bone from around tooth roots, termed "segmentation" (Figure 9.6). These features are used in most cases in which implants are being placed adjacent to teeth. They are most beneficial when implants are placed in tight spaces due to root proximities or when tooth roots are extremely divergent or convergent (Figure 9.7). Many software programs can virtually isolate specific teeth and allow clinicians to virtually "extract" teeth and visualize the remaining bone in preparation for actual tooth extraction and immediate implant placement (Figure 9.8).

Anatomic restrictions that severely limit implant position or depth can be common. Clinical scenarios frequently require the placement of implants into areas with minimal bone leeway mesial-distally, buccal-lingually, or both. Tooth root proximities can require "threading the needle" with implant placement, a common problem with congenitally missing teeth (Figures 9.5a and d, 9.7, and 9.9). Scenarios of limited bone volume often create situations in which the patient's anatomy dictates implant placement.

Esthetic zone implant reconstruction, involving single or multiple implants, can be challenging dilemmas in implant dentistry. Thicknesses of crestal and buccal soft tissues and buccal and palatal cortical plates, buccal–lingual ridge dimensions, proximity to adjacent teeth, implant-to-root relationships, gingival and papilla support and contours, gingival exposure, smile lines, and implant angulations and emergence are just a few of the many considerations. Knowledge of the appropriate implant position based on the type of restoration planned (i.e. cement- or screw-retained) also is an important prosthetics-based consideration (see Chapters 1 and 2). Small variations in implant positions can lead to difficult restorative dilemmas in these cases. Proper implant position can be critical to the esthetic and functional success of the planned restoration. The use of minimally invasive CT/CBCT-guided technology in these difficult cases can lead to improved patient outcomes by positioning implants ideally based on individual patient needs[39] (Figure 9.10).

Immediate loading

The time required from implant placement to loading has been dramatically reduced by implant technologies and surface textures in use today. Immediate placement and immediate provisional restoration of implants are commonly performed. In some cases, teeth can be extracted, implants placed immediately, and provisional crowns delivered at the time of implant insertion or shortly thereafter (within 24 h). Concepts of cross-arch stabilization and loading of multiple implants have changed the way cases are treatment planned. Depending on the clinical circumstances and the experience and comfort level of the clinician, these concepts can be used to place single units, multiple units, or full arches of implants with a tissue incision or with a flapless approach.

Successful immediate or early implant loading has been described in many studies using the latest generation of implants.[40–42] Rigid cross-arch stabilization has been shown to allow immediate loading in edentulous ridges with 6–24 month implant survival rates of

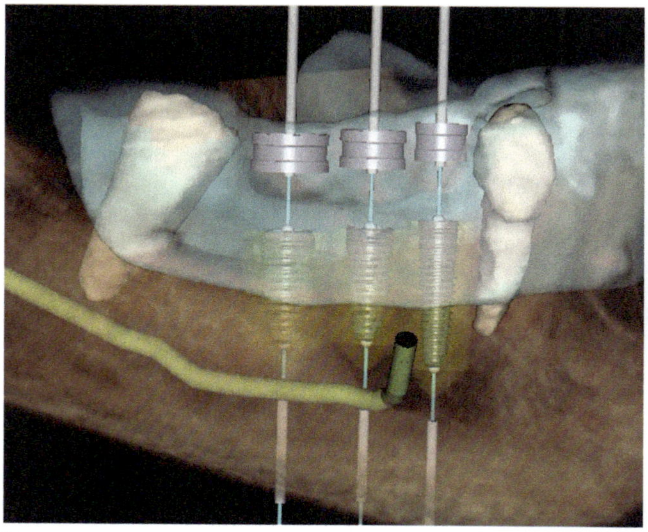

(a)

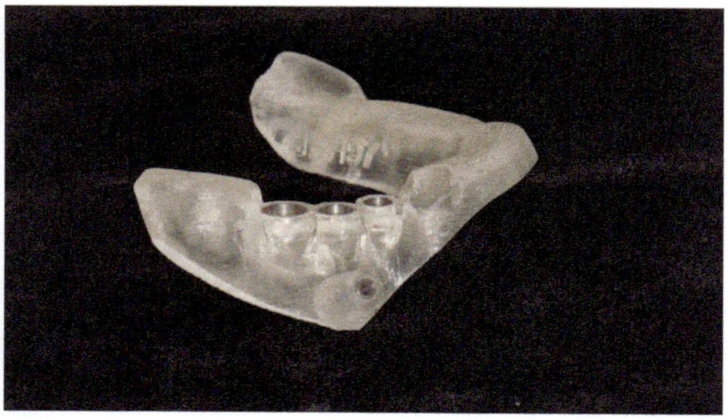

(b)

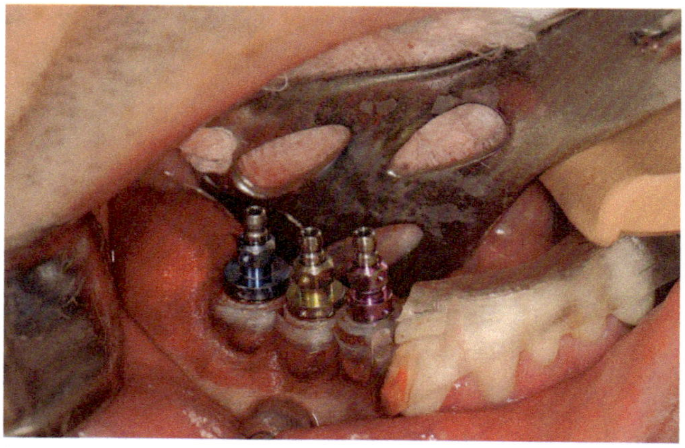

(c)

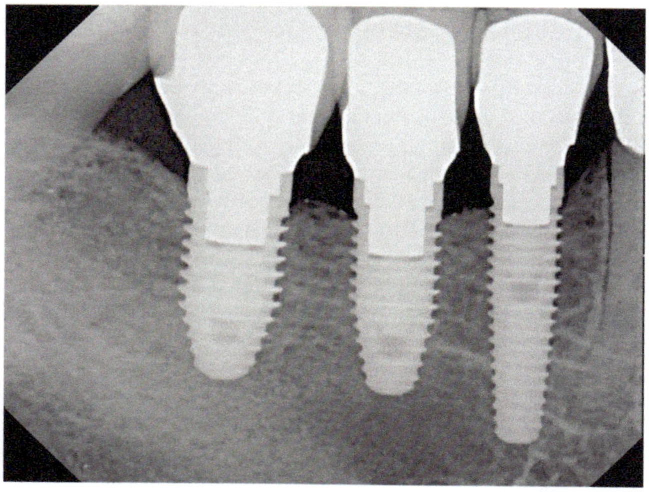

(d)

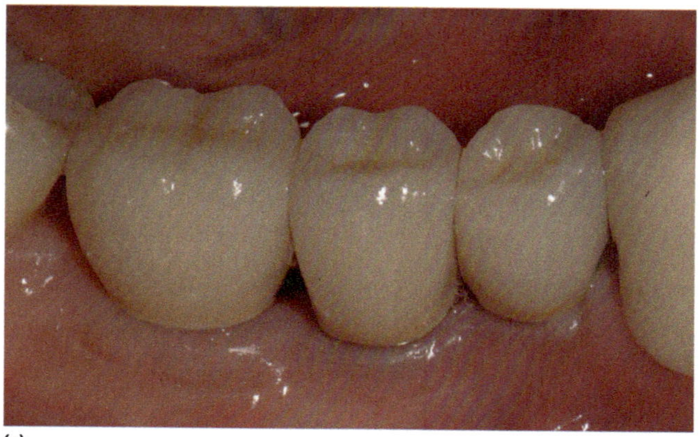

(e)

Figure 9.4 (a) Three implants in a row, virtual treatment plan (NobelClinician). (b) Surgical guide produced from plan in (a). (c) Three implants in place, placed fully guided, using Implant Mounts, minimally invasive flapless. (d) Definitive restorations, periapical radiograph. (e) Definitive individual restorations, plan in (a).

91–96.9%.[43–45] With the combination of new implant designs and surface technologies, immediate placement of an implant-supported restoration following surgery is now a predictable treatment option for single-tooth implants and implant-supported fixed prostheses.[46–49] Immediate loading of dental implants may have a positive effect on peri-implant tissue differentiation and bone formation.[50]

The fabrication of a provisional prosthesis immediately following implant placement surgery can be difficult, stressful, and costly to the restorative dentist because of the extended time needed immediately after surgery. This can be most difficult in immediate loading of fully edentulous patient cases. Numerous techniques for the fabrication of immediate provisional restorations have been developed. One common technique is the retro-fitting of an existing complete denture by providing relief in the areas of the implants and using acrylic to create a retentive framework, known as a "conversion prosthesis."[51] Another technique involves processing a laboratory-fabricated provisional prosthesis following implant placement by making a traditional implant-level impression at surgery. A new approach has recently been introduced involving the fabrication of a provisional restoration based on a virtual implant treatment plan prior to surgery. Immediately after

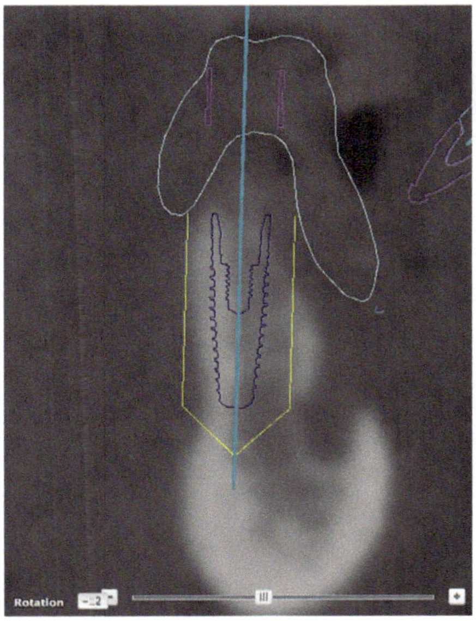

(a)

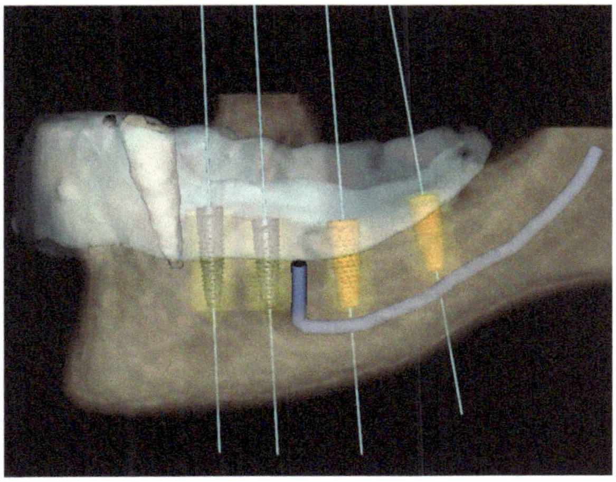
(b)

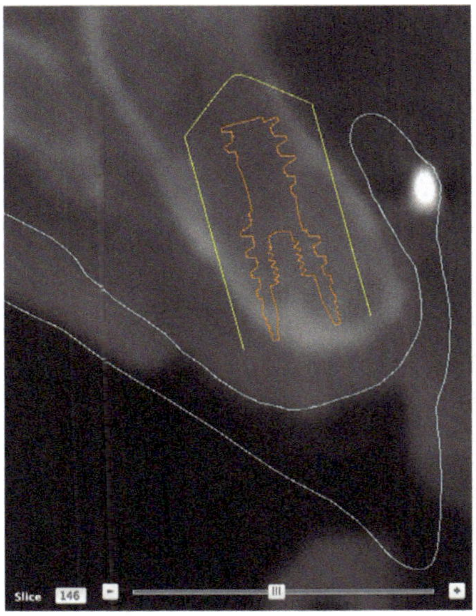

(c)

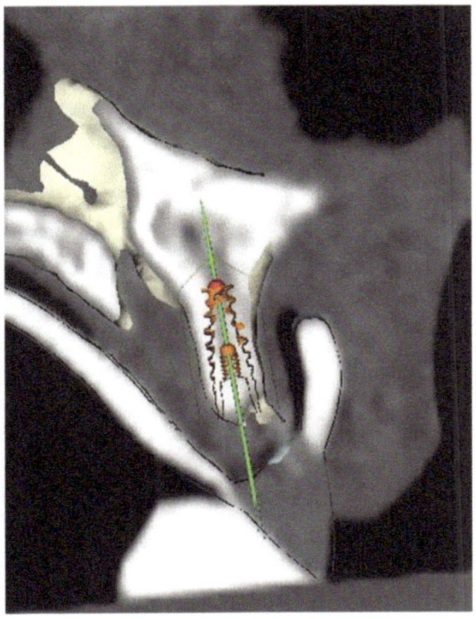
(d)

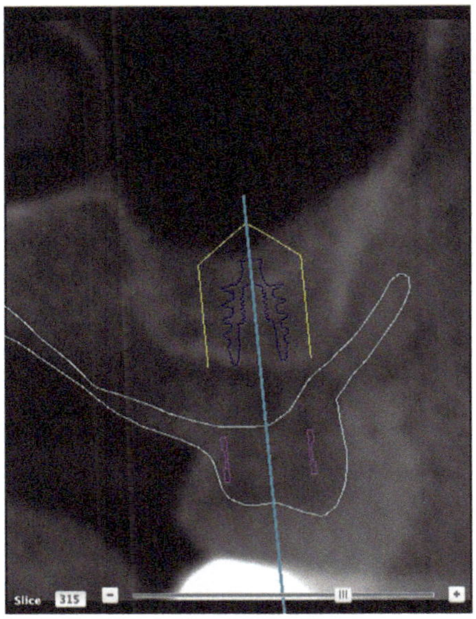

(e)

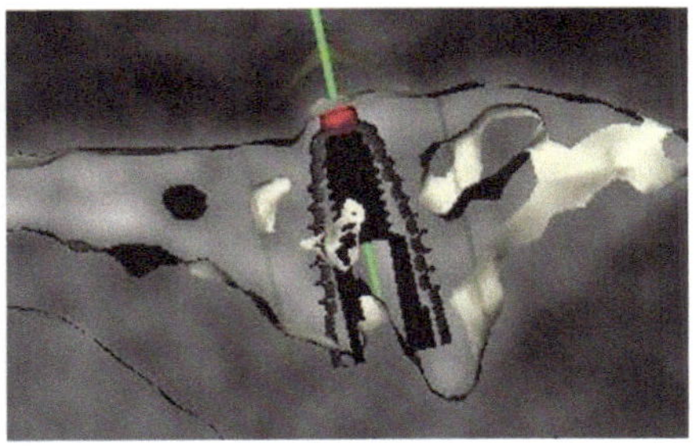
(f)

Figure 9.5 (a) Implant placed virtually in close proximity to the mental foramen, cross-sectional view. (b) Implants placed in proximity to the inferior alveolar nerve, lateral view, 3-D reformation. (c) Cross-sectional view of large incisive canal with virtual implant placement. (d) Cross-sectional view of large incisive canal with virtual implant placement in narrow ridge. (e) Virtual implant placement in proximity to the maxillary sinus. (f) Virtual implant placement in anterior nasal spine, severe atrophy.

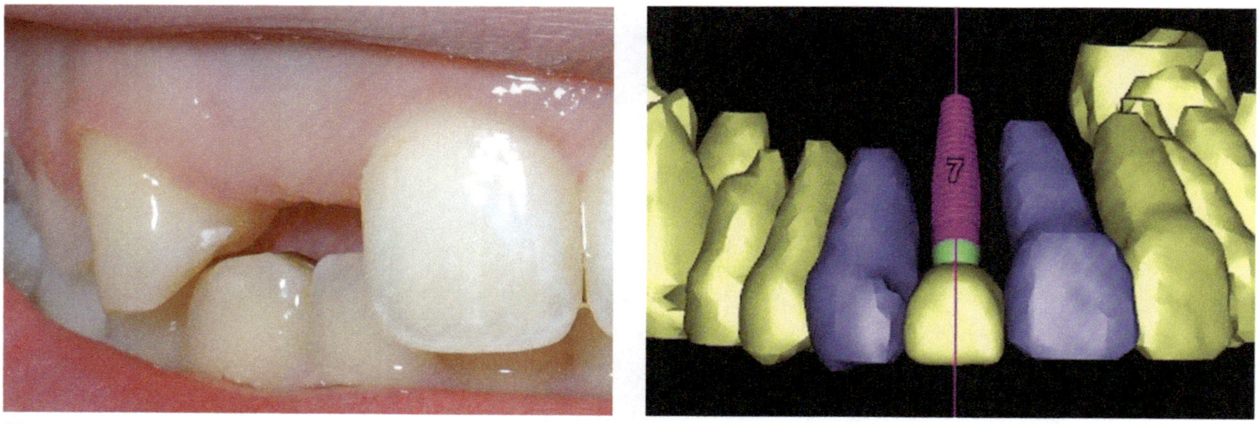

(a) (b)

Figure 9.6 (a) Congenitally missing right maxillary lateral incisor. (b) "Segmentation," altering software sensitivity to Hounsfield units or isovalues to virtually remove bone and visualize surrounding teeth.

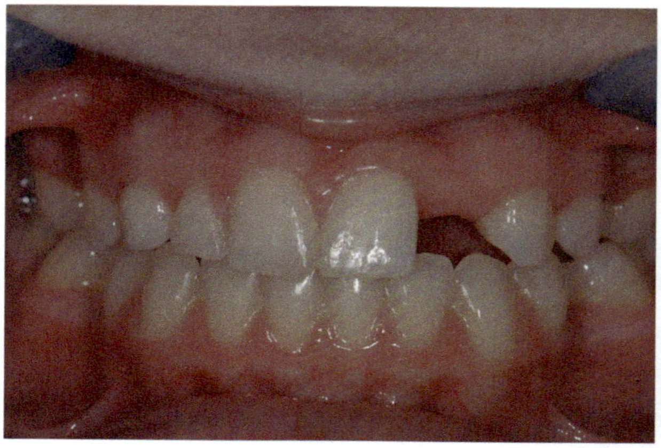

(a)

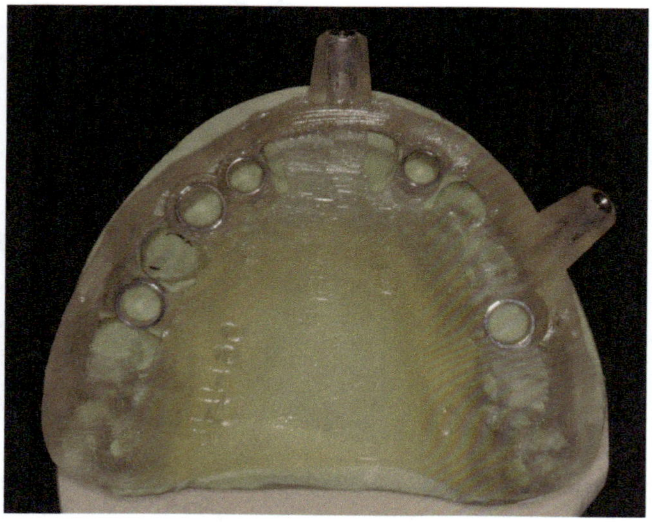

(b)

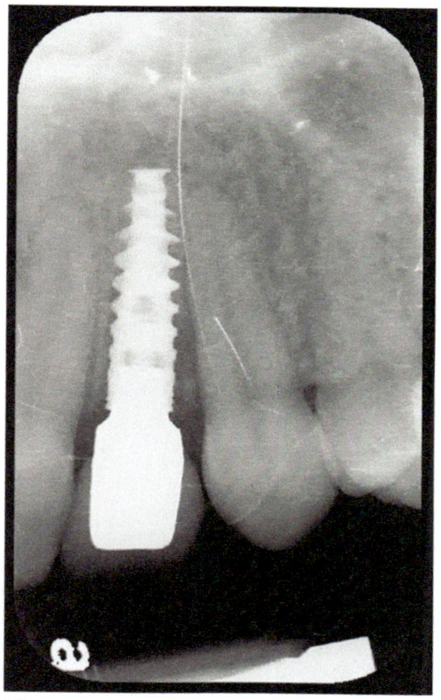

(c)

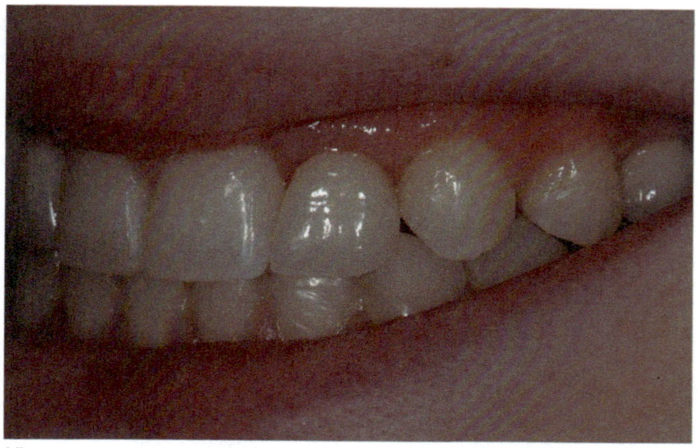

(d)

Figure 9.7 (a) Congenitally missing maxillary left lateral incisor. (b) Surgical guide used to place minimally invasive flapless implant. (c) Periapical radiograph of definitive implant restoration. Note the convergence of the roots of the adjacent teeth into the space. (d) Definitive restoration.

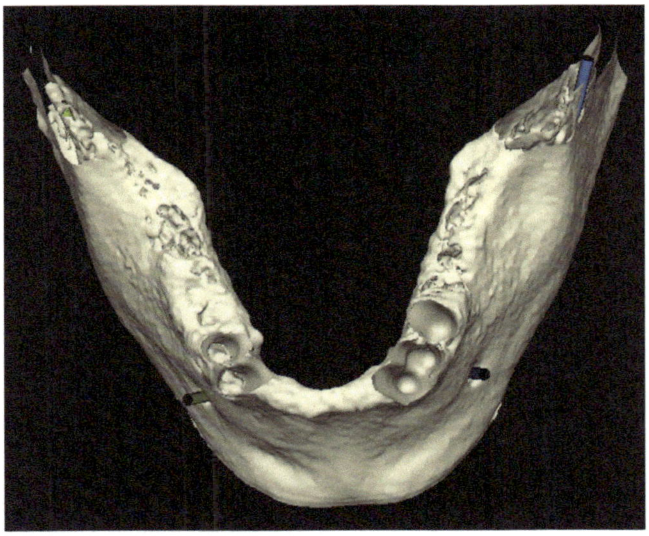

Figure 9.8 Virtual "extraction" of teeth for planning of extraction and immediate implant placement patient cases.

implant surgery, the insertion of a prefabricated provisional restoration allows a dramatic reduction in chair time together with improvement in function and esthetics. CT-guided surgery is necessary for this technique to transfer the preoperative implant plan to the intraoperative site with precision. A prefabricated provisional restoration can then be accurately placed with minimal modification.

In the edentulous mandible, immediate loading of implants was first advanced by Ledermann, Schnitman, and Tarnow, who were pioneers of this technique.[46,52–54] The immediate loading concepts of Schnitman and Tarnow involved loading a select few implants among a larger number of implants in edentulous mandibles. Wolfinger further advanced this concept, placing fewer implants all loaded at the same time.[55] Both concepts for immediate loading were reported to achieve long-term survival rates of 96.6–99.4% for screw-type implants in edentulous mandibles.[56–60] While Tarnow et al.[46] recommended that immediate loading must include at least five dental implants in edentulous mandibles, other clinicians have shown that three or four implants may be sufficient.[61,62]

A high degree of primary implant stability (high insertion torque value) is one of the prerequisites for successful immediate/early loading procedures.[63] Insertion torques, ranging from 25 to 50 N cm, and favorable Periotest™ or implant stability quotient measurements appear to be effective criteria for good primary stability and

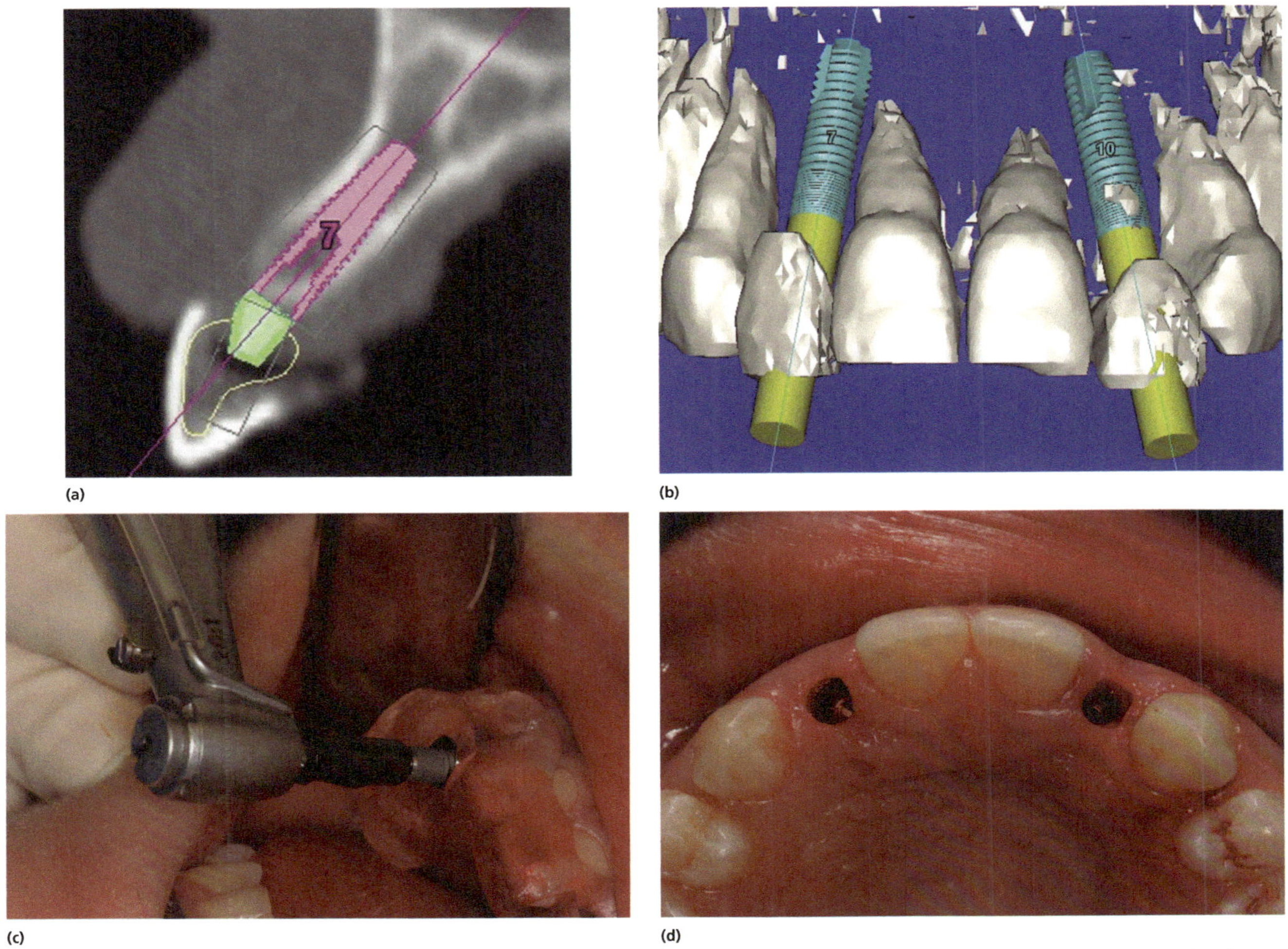

Figure 9.9 (a) Limited bone volume in a maxillary lateral incisor space. Note virtual angled abutment. (b) Virtual treatment plan (Facilitate). (c) Fully guided implant placement with Implant Mount. (d) Post-operative placement of implants, minimally invasive flapless.

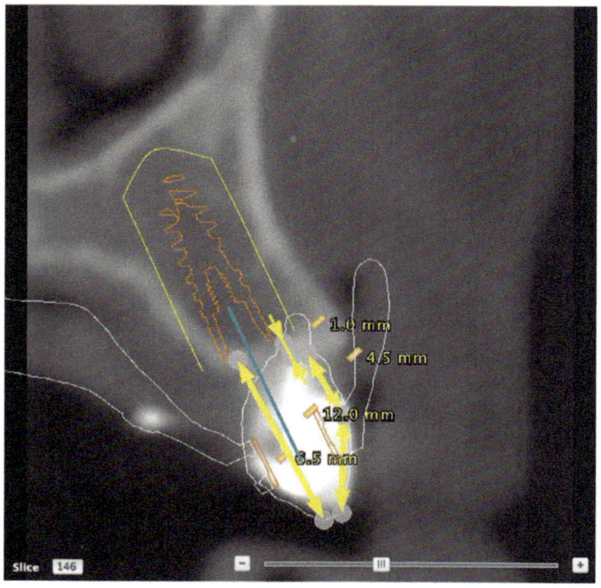

Figure 9.10 Virtual planning, congenitally missing upper right canine with overretained primary tooth. Note extensive measurements used to ideally plan the implant platform position.

possible immediate loading. Cumulative survival rates (CSRs) of 98.4% have been reported for immediately loaded implants placed with CT guidance.[64] This is comparable to reports of immediate loading of implants placed freehand, such as the 98.2% CSR after 6 months reported by Malo et al.,[62] the CSR of 96% (mean follow-up, 36 months) presented by Valente et al.,[65] or the results from a systematic review and meta-analysis of the Cochrane database. The latter found no statistically significant differences amongst immediately loaded (within 1 week), early loaded (between 1 week and 2 months), and conventionally loaded (after 2 months) implants.[63]

Although success rates with immediately loaded implants in the edentulous jaw are comparable to those with staged healing protocols, there are greater risks with the immediate load approach. A non-passive fit of the provisional restoration, screw loosening, prosthesis breakage, overloading, and/or parafunction can all lead to micromovement of the implants, resulting in potential failure.[66] Hence, proper case selection and patient awareness, education, and compliance are all critical factors for success.

A major advantage to using CT-guided surgery for immediately loaded implant cases is the ability to accurately fabricate a provisional restoration *prior* to implant insertion. After the virtual treatment plan is created (Figures 9.11a–d and 9.12a–h, j, and k), computer-generated surgical guides are fabricated by the manufacturer or dental laboratory from the virtual plan (Figures 9.11f and 9.12i and l). Using the fabricated surgical guide along with patient models, a dental laboratory then fabricates temporary restorations *prior* to implant placement (Figures 9.11g and h and 9.12m–o). The surgical guide is then used to place implants flaplessly, removing only a core of soft tissue in the planned implant site(s). Once the surgical guide is accurately secured in the patient's mouth it rarely is removed until all implants are inserted to proper depth and direction (Figures 9.11i and j and 9.12p–r). Abutments can be immediately placed on the implants, and provisional restorations can be inserted (Figures 9.11k–o and 9.12s–u). Definitive restorations are not fabricated until after osseointegration is complete (Figure 9.12v–x).

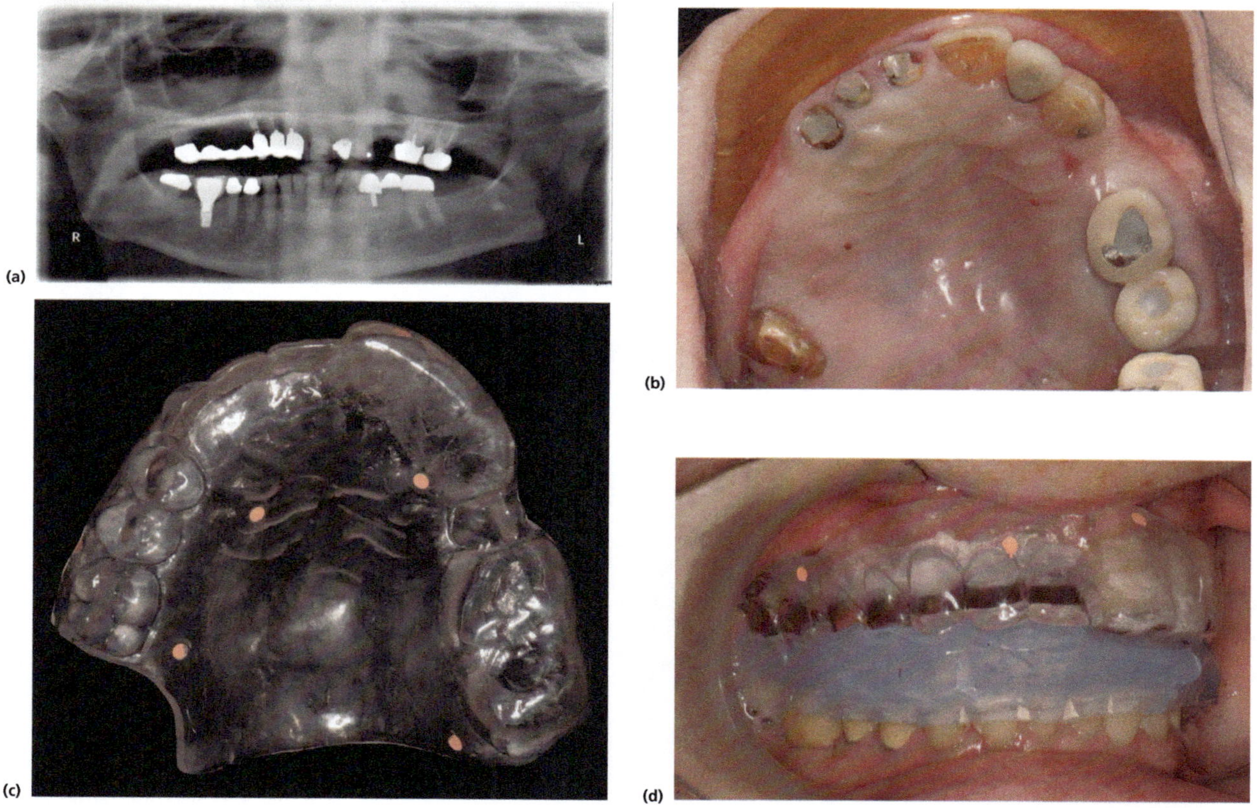

Figure 9.11 (a) Preoperative panoramic radiograph, 65-year-old female. Implants to be placed in the right maxilla with immediate provisional restoration. (b) Preoperative clinical situation, occlusal view. (c) Scanning appliance fabricated for patient to wear during a CBCT scan (NobelGuide). (d) Scanning appliance in place in patient's mouth, prior to CBCT scan. Note the bite registration in place for confirmation of appliance position.

(Continued)

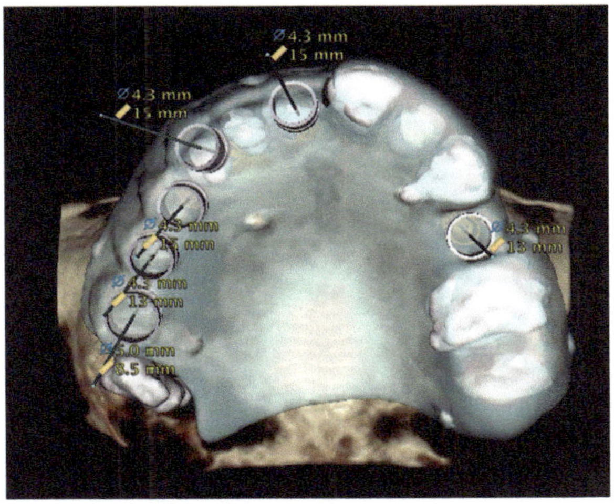

(e)

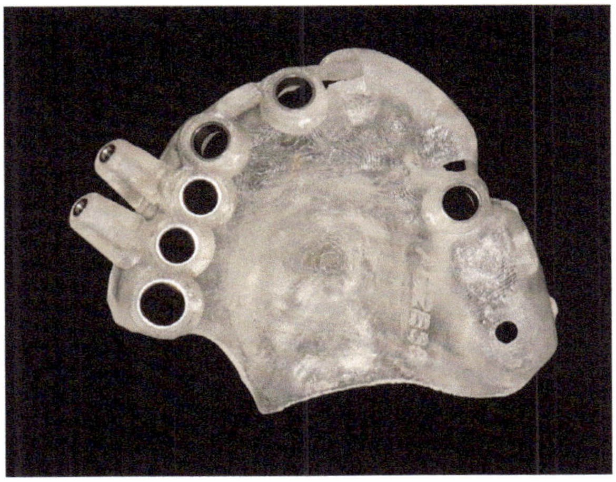

(f)

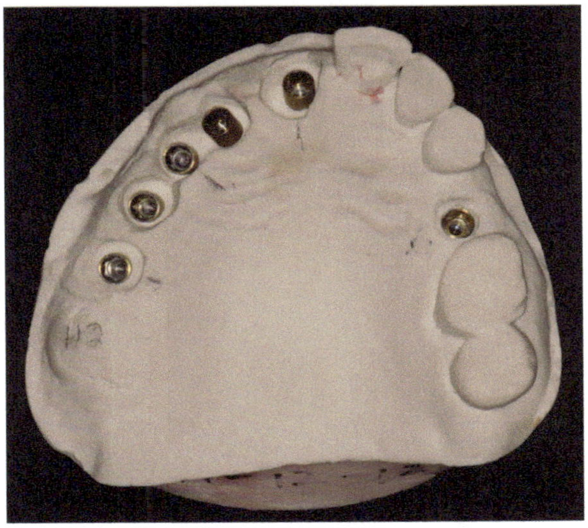

(g)

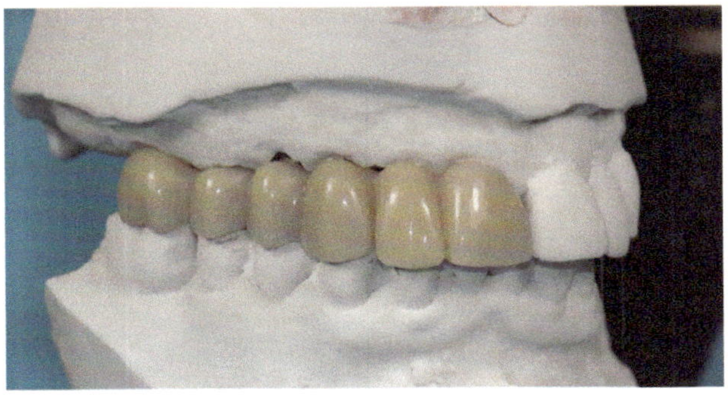

(h)

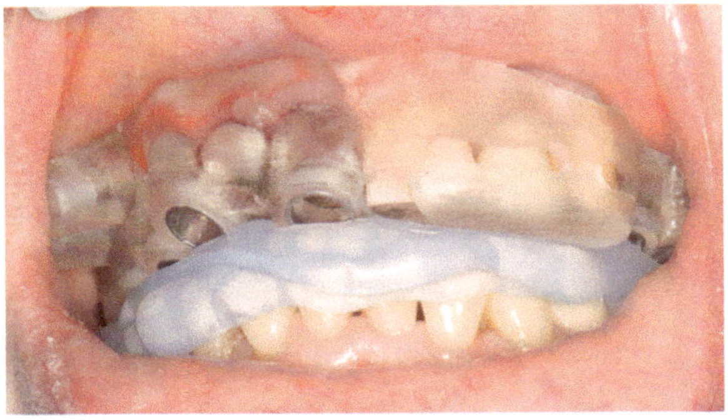

(i)

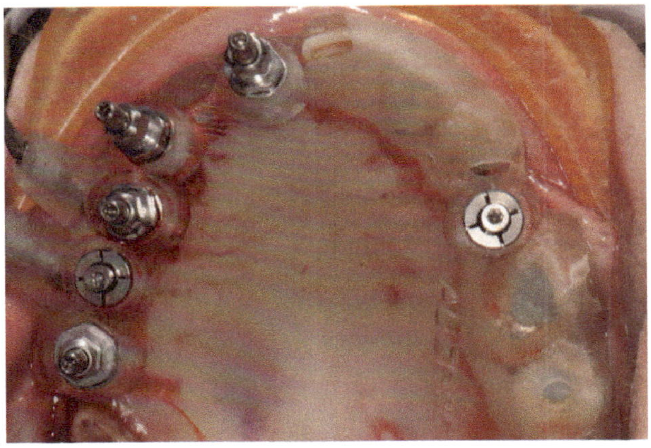

(j)

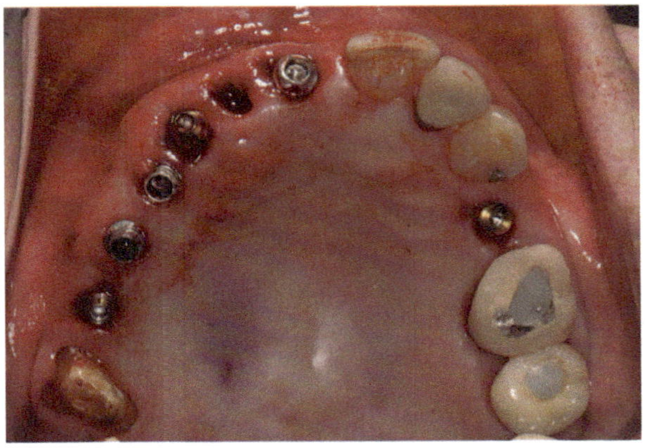

(k)

Figure 9.11 (Continued)
(e) Virtual treatment plan for patient (NobelClinician™). (f) Surgical guide produced based on virtual plan. (g) Master cast fabricated from surgical guide. (h) Provisional restoration fabricated prior to surgery, right lateral view. (i) Surgical guide in place at surgery. Note use of a bite registration to assure proper positioning of the surgical guide. (j) Fully guided implant placement, six implants, minimally invasive flapless. (k) Abutments in place immediately after implant placement, occlusal view.

(Continued)

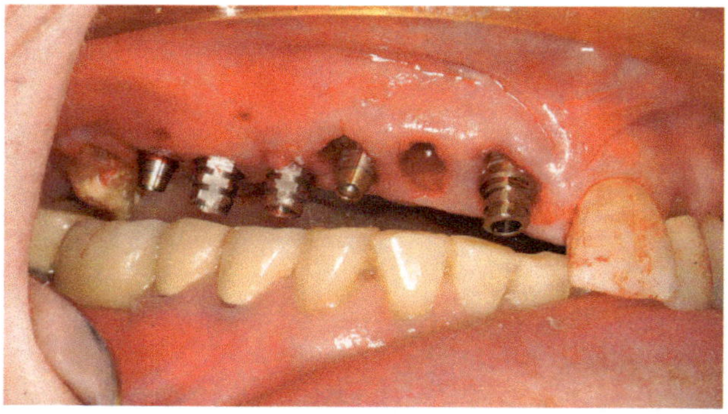

(l)

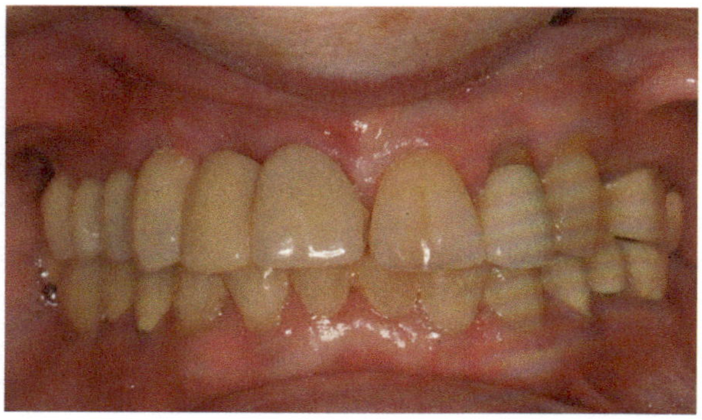

(m)

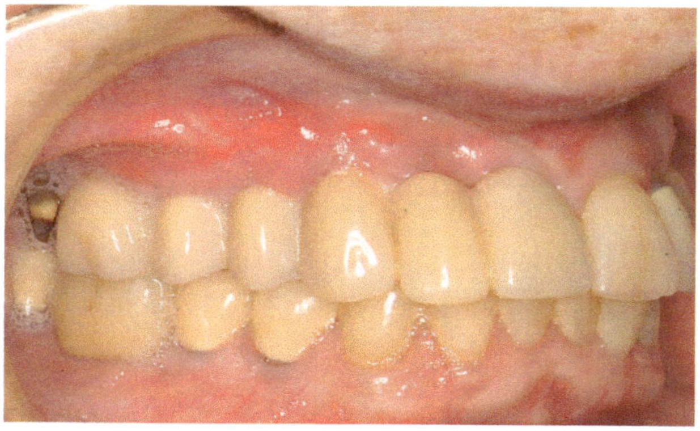

(n)

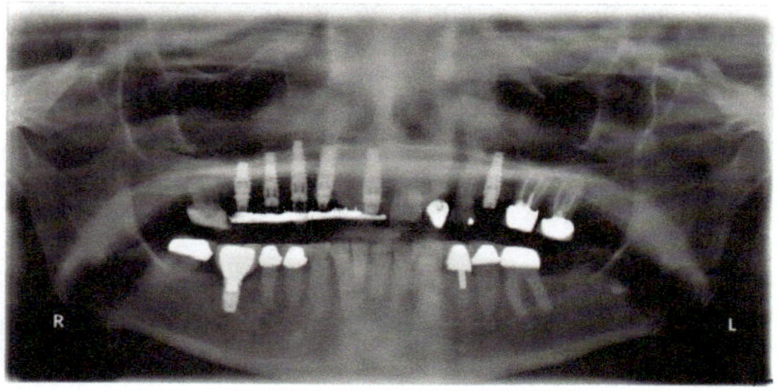

(o)

Figure 9.11 (Continued)
(l) Abutments in place immediately after implant placement, right lateral view. (m) Provisional restoration in place immediately after implant placement. Note: restoration was made prior to surgery. (n) Provisional restoration, immediately after surgery, lateral view. (o) Post-operative panorex, implants, and immediate provisional restoration in place.

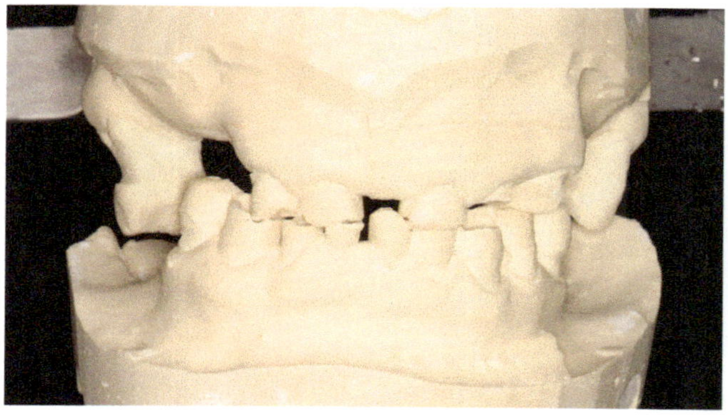

(a)

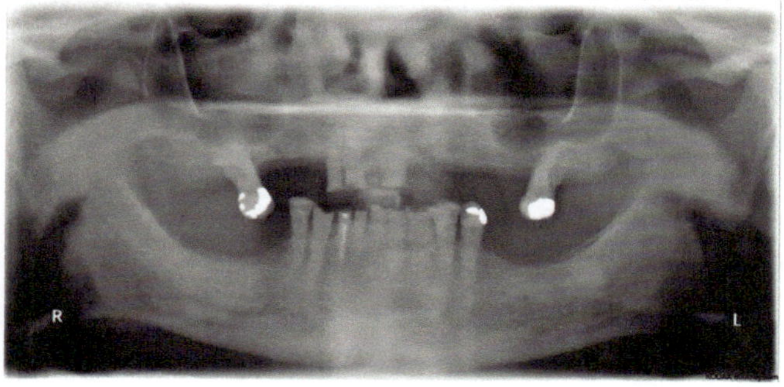

(b)

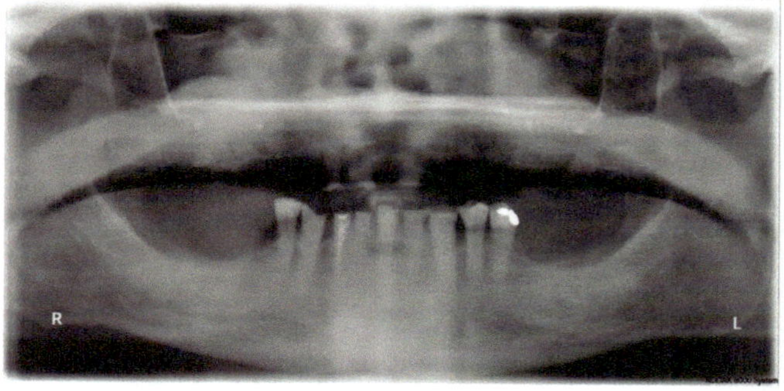

(c)

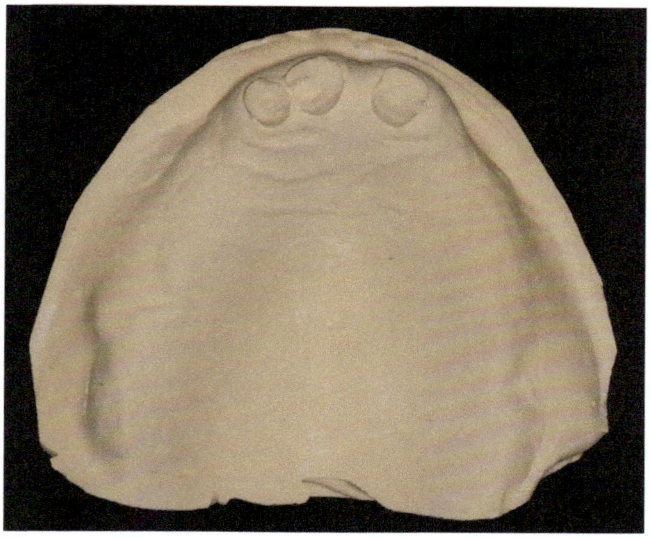

(d)

Figure 9.12 (a) A 68-year-old male, mutilated upper dentition, partially edentulous posterior mandible. (b) Preoperative panoramic radiograph. (c) Post-operative panorex after bilateral sinus lift grafts and extraction of posterior teeth. (d) Upper ridge, prior to implant planning.

(Continued)

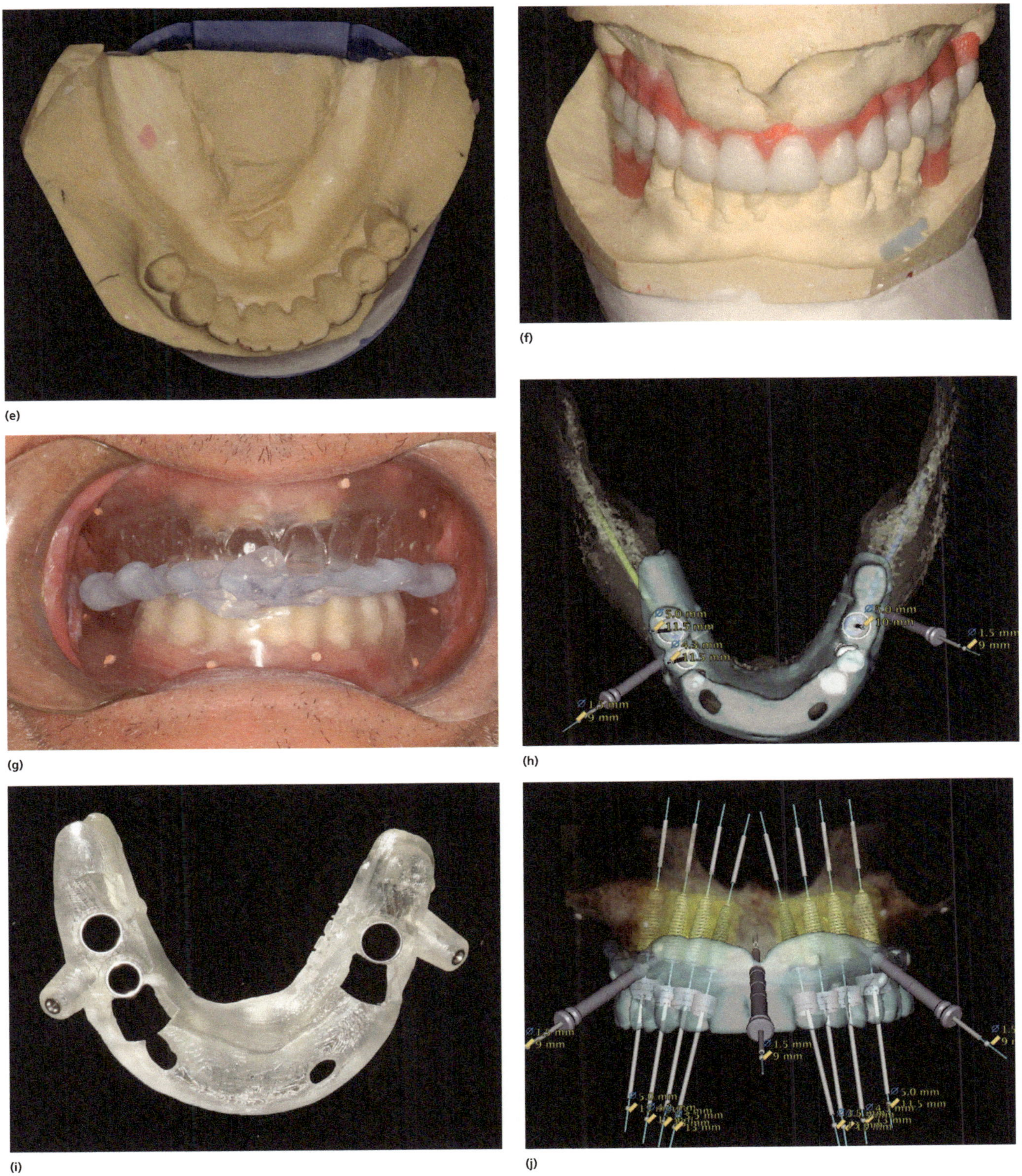

Figure 9.12 (Continued)
(e) Lower ridge, prior to implant planning. (f) Diagnostic wax-ups, maxilla and mandible. (g) Scanning appliances in place, maxilla and mandible, prior to CBCT scan. Note bite registration between the arches to confirm accurate positioning of scanning appliances. (h) Virtual treatment plan, mandibular arch. (i) Surgical guide fabricated from plan. (j) Virtual treatment plan, upper arch, frontal view.

(Continued)

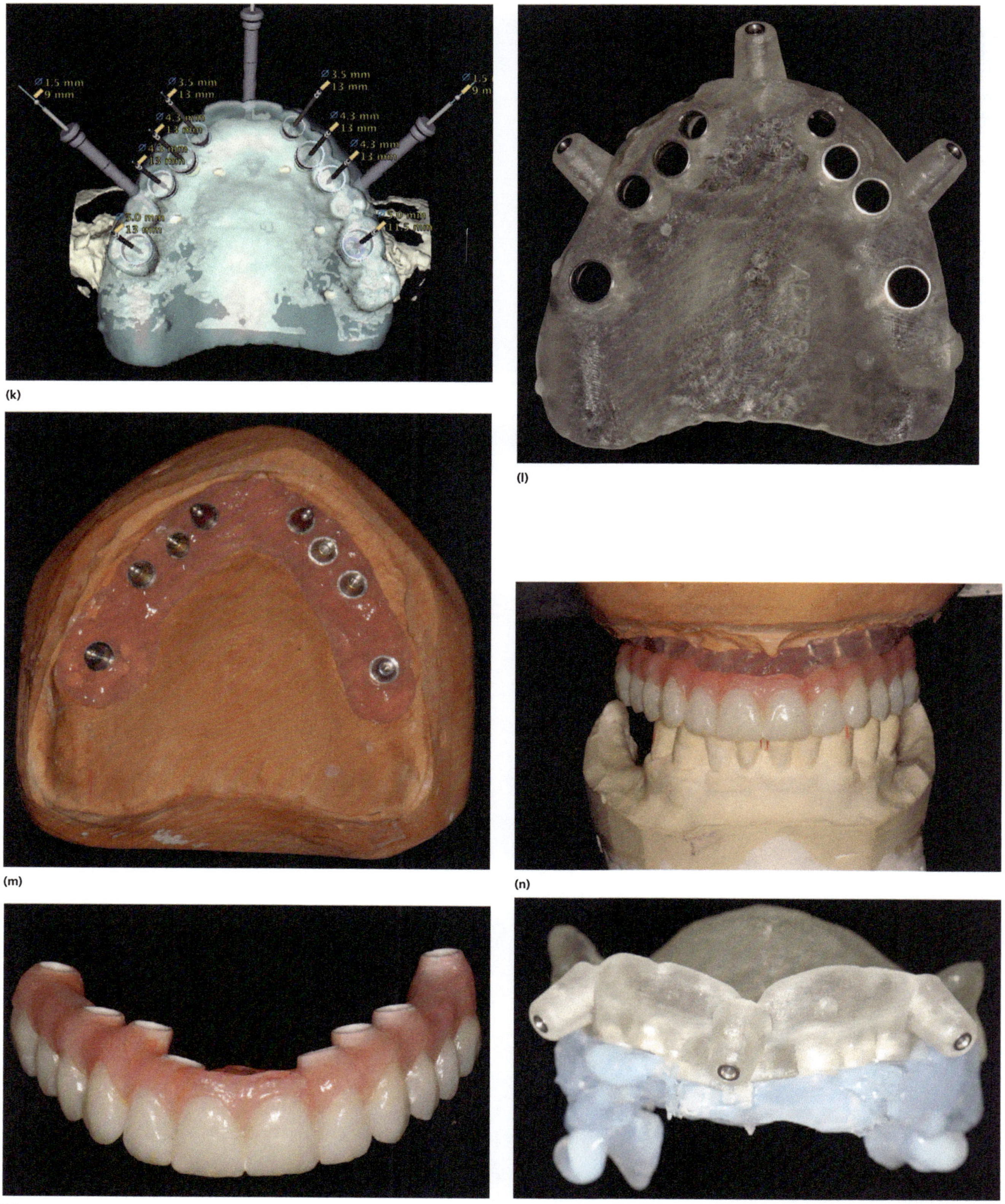

Figure 9.12 (Continued)
(k) Virtual treatment plan, upper arch, occlusal view. (l) Surgical guide fabricated from virtual treatment plan. (m) Master cast, upper arch fabricated preoperatively from surgical guide. (n) Provisional restoration on master cast, fabricated prior to surgery, for immediate load. (o) Provisional restoration, fabricated prior to surgery, for immediate load. (p) Surgical guide with bite registration. Note the bite registration was used to assure accurate positioning of the surgical guide.

(Continued)

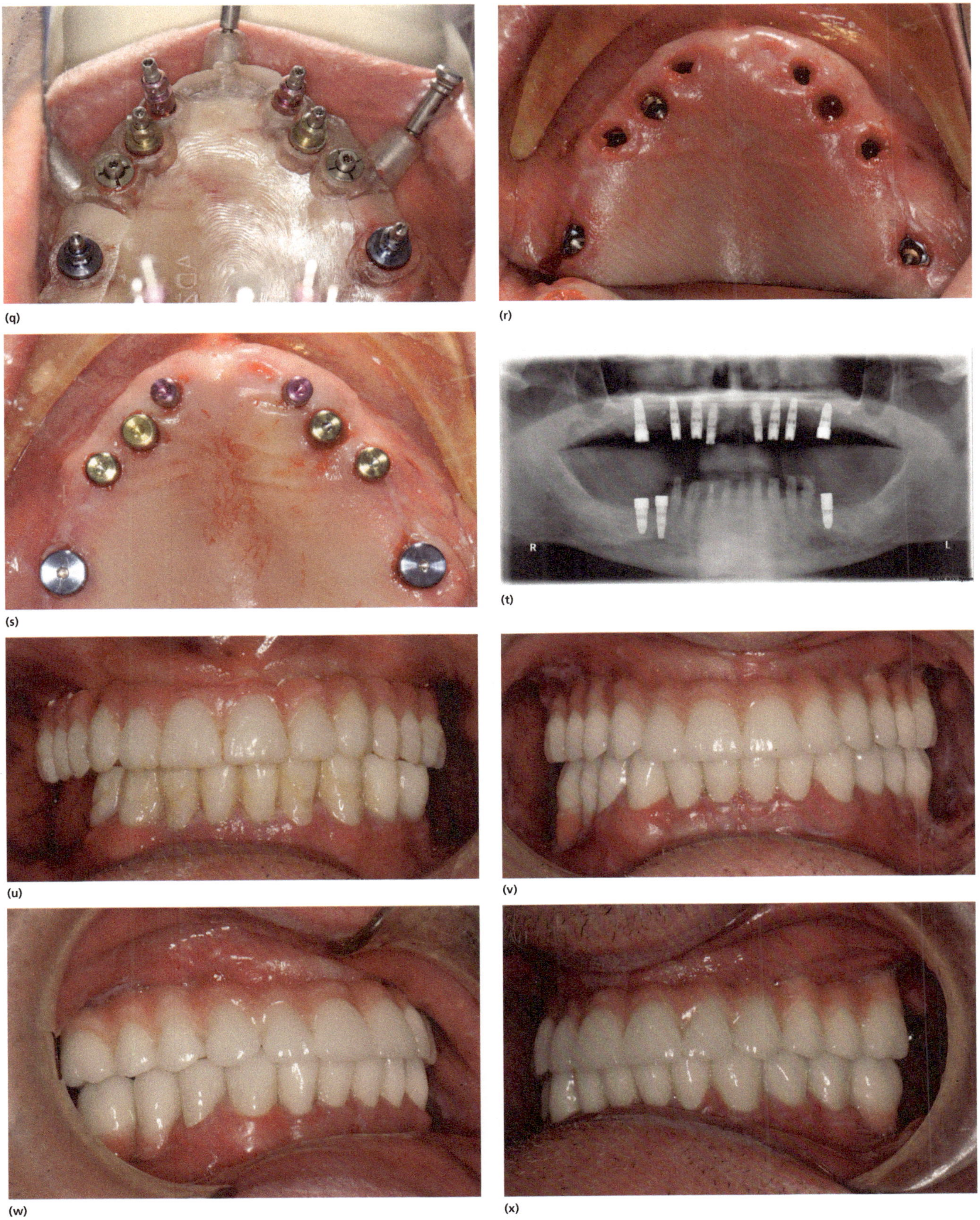

Figure 9.12 (Continued)

(q) Fully guided implant placement (eight total), minimally invasive flapless. (r) Surgical guide removed, eight implants in place. (s) Healing abutments in place immediately after implant placement to minimize tissue collapse. (t) Post-implant placement panoramic radiograph. (u) Provisional restoration inserted immediately after implant placement, maxilla, frontal view. (v) Definitive restoration, frontal view. (w) Definitive restoration, right lateral view. (x) Definitive restoration, left lateral view.

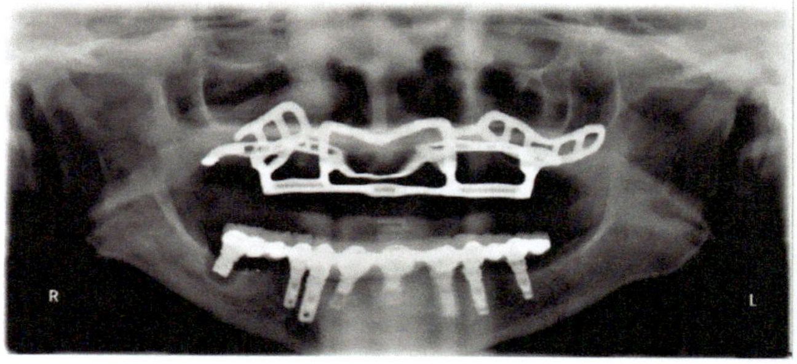

(a)

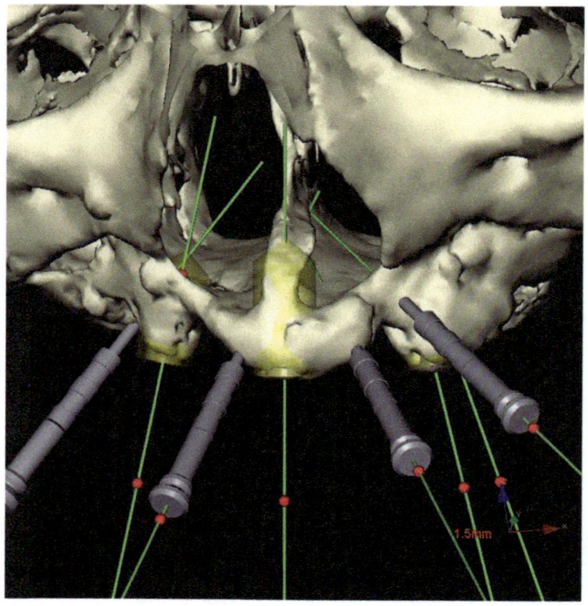

(b)

Figure 9.13 A 72-year-old female with failing maxillary subperiosteal implant. (b) Virtual treatment plan with four implants for overdenture fabrication patient.

Applications in complicated situations

In the daily practice of implant dentistry, questions will arise as to the quality and quantity of bone and soft tissue. Available space, implant distribution, implant positioning related to the planned restoration, and the proximity of implants to teeth and vital structures are a few of the issues that require pretreatment determination. Some patients require complex sequential treatment plans requiring multiple soft or hard tissue grafting and contouring procedures before and after implant placement. These patients are some of the most challenging cases for restorative dentists and surgeons. The diagnostic and treatment planning information provided to the clinician from a 3-D evaluation of the patient's anatomy using CT technologies can be instrumental in the successful management of such complicated cases.[67] Minimally invasive CT-guided flapless techniques can be used to place implants accurately into areas of distorted and compromised anatomy.

In most circumstances, "placing the implants where the bone is" has become a concept from the past. Soft tissue grafts, sinus lift grafts, block bone grafts, ridge splitting, lateral ridge augmentations, and alveolar distraction are a few of the procedures routinely performed today to prepare recipient sites prior to implant placement. Previous failed implants, including blade and subperiosteal implants, and the associated site damage can leave patients with challenging reconstructive defects (Figure 9.13). Traumatic injuries or benign or malignant pathology can result in the loss of bone, teeth, and soft tissue with resultant defects of varying sizes. Reconstructive procedures to treat these defects can leave areas of abnormal bony anatomy and scarred soft tissue (Figure 9.14) that complicate the achievement of a satisfactory implant restoration. Lateral block-onlay grafts can resorb a portion of their bone volume during healing and maturation and require accurate 3-D assessment and planning[68–70] (Figures 9.15 and 9.16).

Compromised patients

Pre- and post-operative radiation therapy potentially alters healing capacity in head and neck cancer patients. To increase bone vascularity prior to implant placement, the literature advocates courses of hyperbaric oxygen therapy in these patients.[71–74] Reducing trauma to bone is indicated in order to minimize the risk of osteoradionecrosis.[75] Bleeding, swelling, and alteration of blood supply to bone and soft tissue can be minimized by using CT-guided technologies, and success in placing implants in these patients has been reported.[76]

Patients with other medical problems, such as blood dyscrasias or significant cardiovascular disease, may rely on specific medication protocols that cannot be altered presurgically. Minimizing bleeding again is indicated in these patients. 3-D implant evaluation and planning with CT-guided implant placement will allow

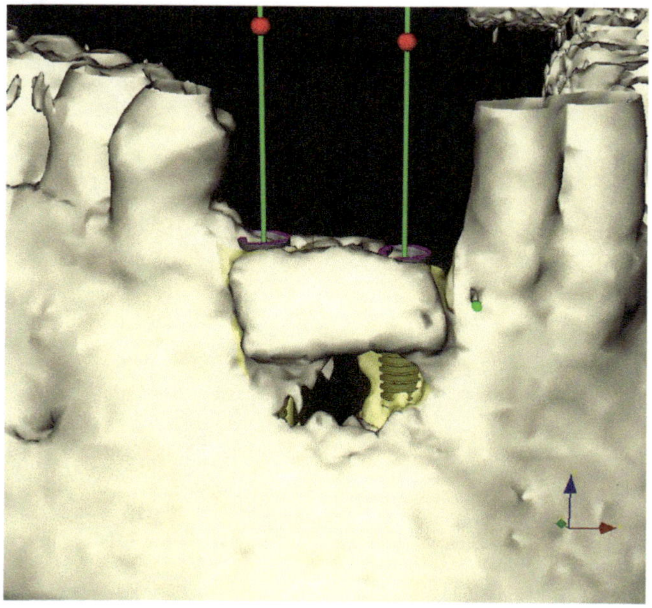

Figure 9.14 A 45-year-old male, trauma anterior mandible, alveolar distraction osteogenesis, two implants virtually placed.

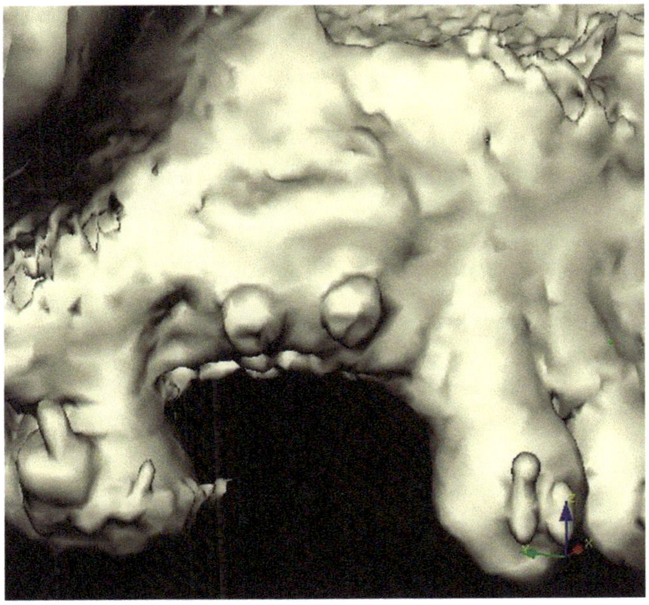

Figure 9.15 A 25-year-old female, block graft anterior maxilla.

for minimally invasive, flapless, minimally traumatic, and accurate implant placement.

Long periods in a dental chair can prevent some patients from seeking treatment because of orthopedic and spinal disorders or anxiety-related to stress and phobias. Additionally, wheelchair-bound patients can pose logistical treatment problems. These patients require extensive pretreatment planning and preparation. Without compromising quality, treatment must be performed quickly and efficiently, limiting surgical stress and treatment time.

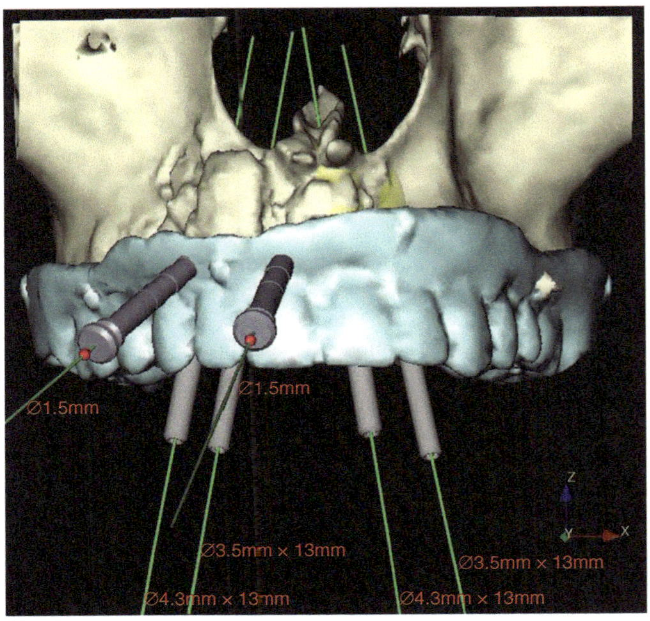

Figure 9.16 A 40-year-old male, block graft anterior maxilla, virtual treatment plan, four implants.

Implant-specific instrumentation

Initially, most guided surgery software programs and implant-specific guided surgery instrumentation kits were designed for the minimally invasive placement of cylindric (i.e. straight-walled) implants. Instrumentation for the placement of tapered implants is now available from some manufacturers. Some implant-specific instrument kits are designed only for the depth and direction of the initial pilot drills, typically 2.0 mm diameter burs, thus requiring the reflection of soft tissue flaps. Other more comprehensive systems (Figure 9.17) are designed for flapless implant placement using counter-bores and/or tissue punches, surgical guide stabilization abutments, pins and screws, drill guides (Figure 9.18a), an assortment of different diameter drills with drill stops designed for guided surgery (Figure 9.18b–e), and/or implant-specific carriers or mounts for implant placement through the surgical guide to the planned depth (Figure 9.18f–h). Additionally, some more sophisticated instrumentation systems have specific dental laboratory componentry designed for the fabrication of provisional restorations *prior* to implant placement.

Clinicians interested in using CT-guided surgery should be aware that guided surgical instrumentation has greater space requirements than conventional freehand implant surgical instrumentation. Guided surgical burs can be 7–13 mm longer than conventional non-guided burs, depending on the system used (Figure 9.18c and d). Patients' maximal inter-incisal openings can be problematic, especially when placing implants in posterior regions, between existing teeth, or with intact opposing dentitions. A thorough understanding of the system-specific instrumentation and componentry for guided surgery is essential.

Benefits to patients and clinicians

The clinician wants to place implants in a predictable fashion while considering the position of the planned dental restoration, as well as the patient's medical history, bone biology, and individual anatomy. The goal is for the implant(s) to be placed atraumatically and into the highest quantity and quality of bone, while minimizing the risk of involvement of surrounding vital structures and teeth. The patient wants implant-supported restorations that look and function like natural teeth for a lifetime. Patients want the treatment to be performed quickly, predictably, and successfully with minimal pain, swelling, stress, and complications, and with little interruption in their everyday lives.

The benefits to clinicians of using CT-based technologies are enormous. 3-D patient evaluation and implant planning allow examination of the patient's bony anatomy prior to making an incision. They allow detailed 1 : 1 measurements of the width and height of available bone in areas planned for implants. Exact identification of vital anatomic structures and dimensions of bone are possible. Distances between planned implants, angulations of adjacent implants, angulation differences from one side of an arch to the other, evaluation of prosthesis path of insertion issues, exact placement of screw chambers, and presurgical abutment selection can all be predetermined. Soft tissue thicknesses, evaluation for preoperative or intraoperative adjunctive augmentation procedures, and preoperative knowledge of the exact lengths and widths of the implants to be placed can help reduce intraoperative surprises.

If this technology increases the accuracy of implant placement, decreases potential surgical complications, and increases the predictability of implant case outcomes, then why is it not more widely used in dental implant placement? Considerable additional

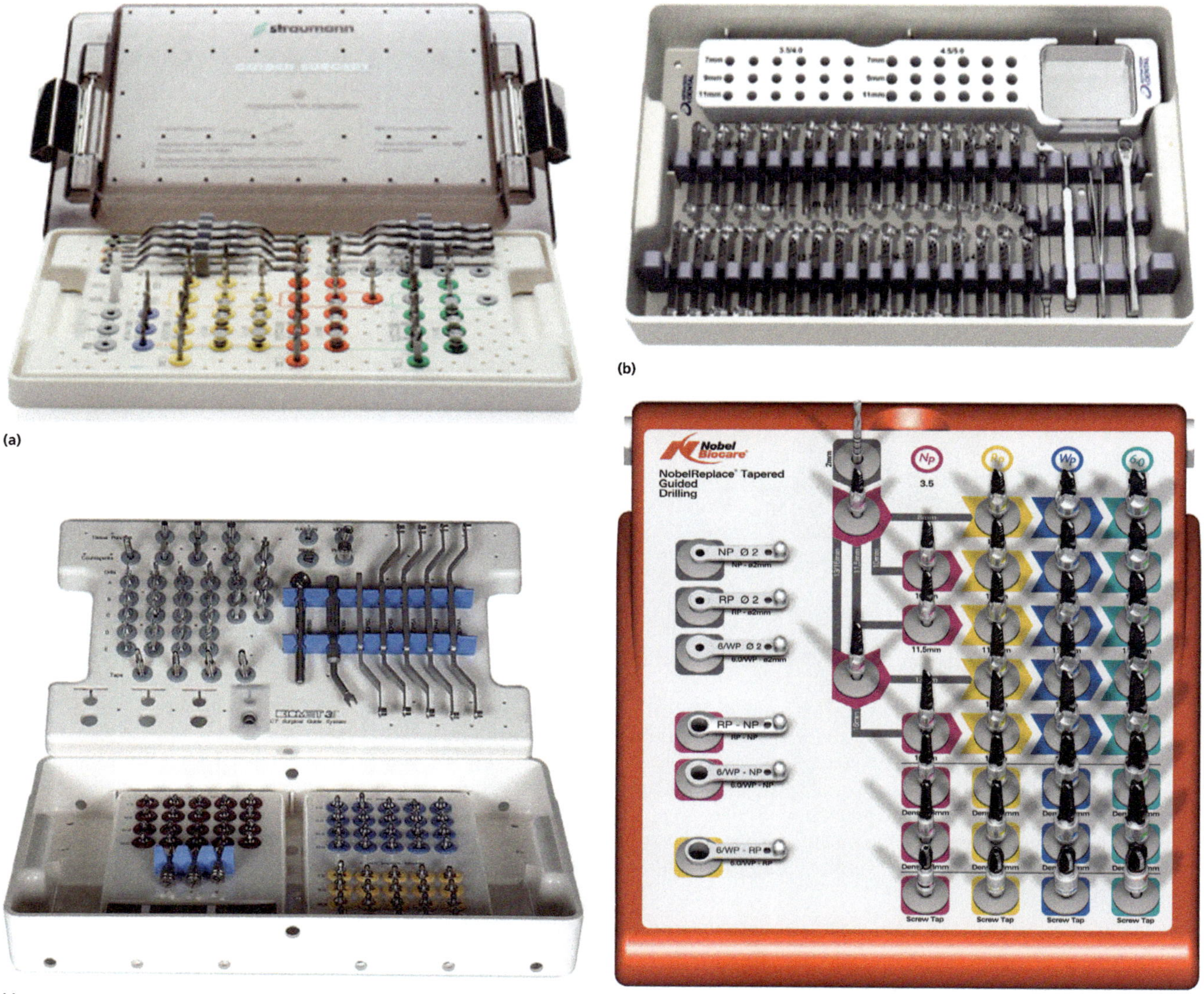

(a) (b) (c) (d)

Figure 9.17 (a) The Straumann guided surgery instrument tray. *Source:* Straumann USA, LLC its parents, affiliates or subsidiaries. Reproduced with permission of Straumann USA LLC. (b) The Astra® Facilitate™ instrument tray. *Source:* Reproduced with permission of DENTSPLY Implants. (c) The Biomet/3i® Navigator® instrument tray. *Source:* Biomet/3i® Navigator® instrument tray. Reproduced with permission of BIOMET/3i. (d) The NobelReplace™ tapered groovy instrument tray. *Source:* Nobel Biocare. Reproduced with permission of Nobel Biocare.

time is needed for the clinician to make impressions, work up the planned restoration with a diagnostic wax-up, fabricate a radiographic template for the patient to wear while having the CT/CBCT scan, ordering or taking the CT/CBCT scan, importing the CT/CBCT data into software, planning the case "virtually," ordering the surgical guide, and learning the techniques and equipment necessary to place implants through a surgical guide.

The treatment will require that the patient incurs additional costs for the laboratory work to fabricate the radiographic scan prosthesis, the CT/CBCT scan, and the surgical guide. The clinician will incur additional costs in the learning of new technologies, upgrading computer hardware, and purchasing new software programs and armamentaria. New technologies that must be learned, often with multiple-step workflows, can be difficult and expensive to incorporate into an existing practice. Many may fear that the case could be lost if additional costs are incurred by the patient. Furthermore, clinicians may be pleased with the level of success they have attained in treatment planning and placing implants without using computer-based technologies, and thus have no motivation to change.

We are reminded that implant patients seek treatment for *teeth*, not implants! Commonly, a patient's fears and questions relate to pain, swelling, and recuperation time. Many of the software products on the market have embedded tools that will help clinicians educate patients visually during a consultation about "virtual" technologies. Visual demonstration commonly allays patient fears and cost concerns. Furthermore, it facilitates discussion of the benefits of minimally invasive CT-guided flapless techniques and the possibility of placing immediate provisional restorations.

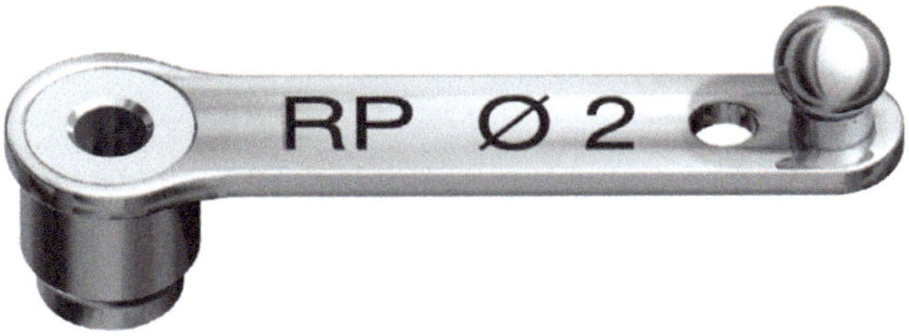

(a)

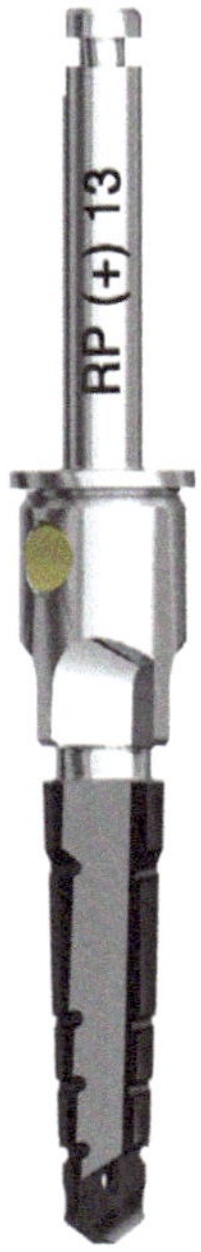

(b)

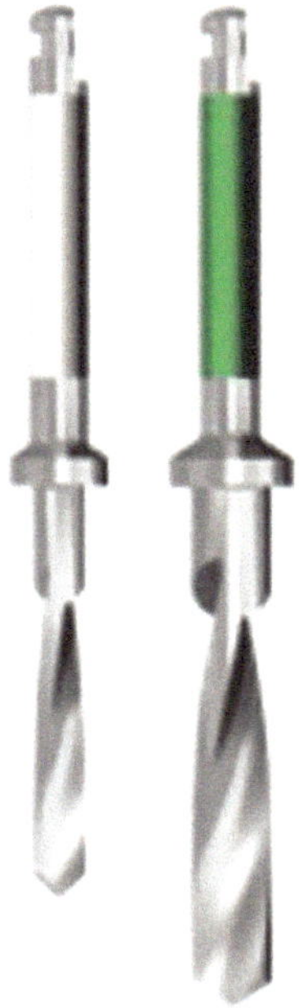

(c)

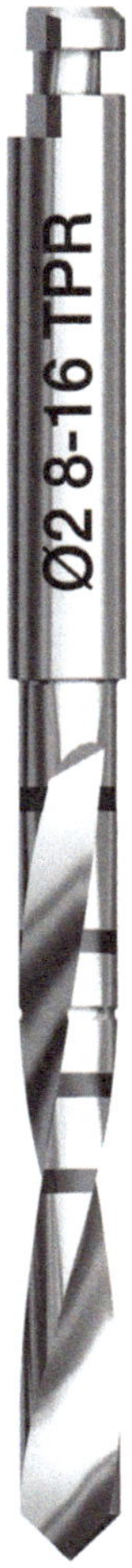

(d)

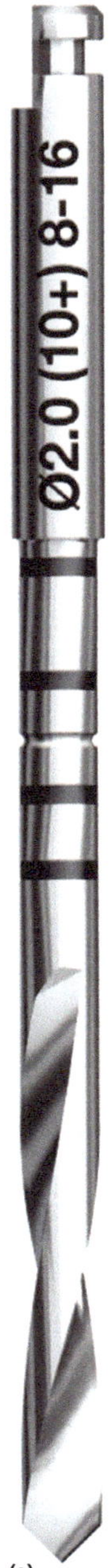

(e)

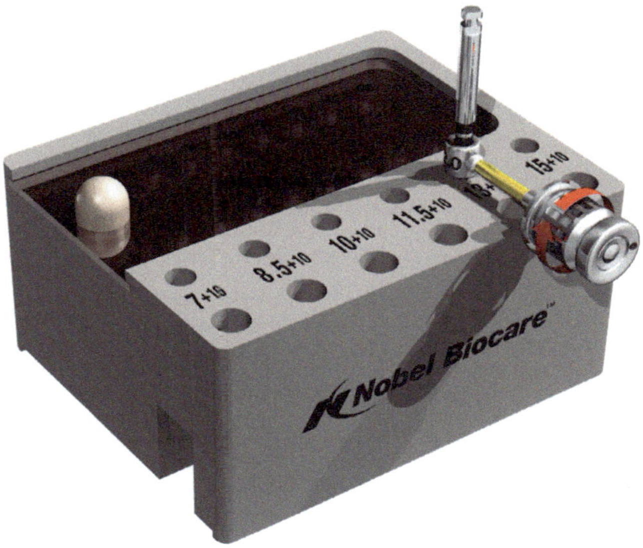

(f)

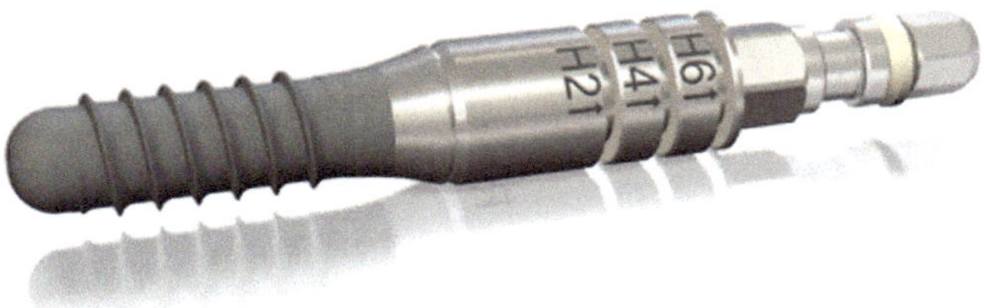

(g)

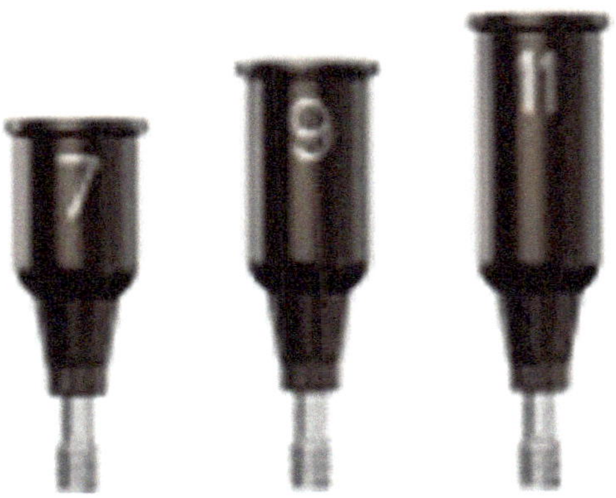

(h)

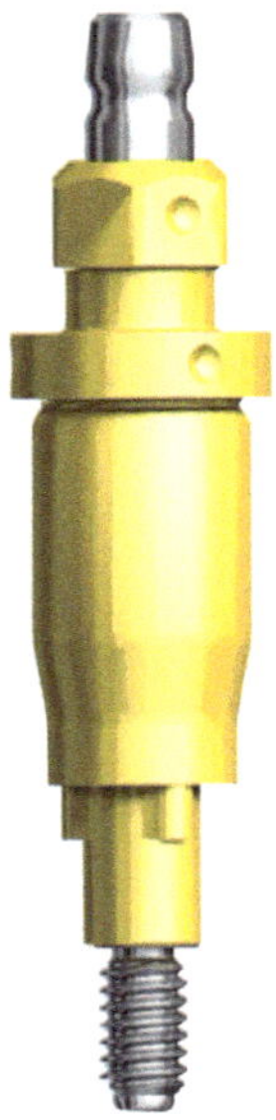

(i)

Figure 9.18 (a) Drill guide. *Source:* Nobel Biocare. Reproduced with permission of Nobel Biocare. (b) Guided tapered drill with integrated drill stop. *Source:* Nobel Biocare. Reproduced with permission of Nobel Biocare. (c) Guided straight drills with integrated drill stops, Facilitate. *Source:* Reproduced with permission of DENTSPLY Implants. (d) Conventional straight drill, 18 mm in length. *Source:* Nobel Biocare. Reproduced with permission of Nobel Biocare. (e) Guided straight drill, 28 mm in length. *Source:* Nobel Biocare. Reproduced with permission of Nobel Biocare. (f) Guided drill stop kit. *Source:* Nobel Biocare. Reproduced with permission of Nobel Biocare. (g) Implant with integrated Implant Mount, Straumann. *Source:* Straumann USA, LLC its parents, affiliates or subsidiaries. Reproduced with permission of Straumann USA LLC. (h) Implant mounts, Facilitate. *Source:* Reproduced with permission of DENTSPLY Implants. (i) Implant mount, NobelGuide. *Source:* Nobel Biocare. Reproduced with permission of Nobel Biocare.

Conclusions

New technologies based on 3-D patient evaluation for dental implants enhance accurate and predictable diagnosis, planning, and treatment, while facilitating communication between clinicians, the patient, and the dental laboratory. The implant surgeon must become proficient with CT interpretation, proprietary planning software, treatment workflow, and guided surgery instrumentation/techniques for successful patient outcomes. Established concepts of implant dentistry, prosthodontics, and surgery must be followed. CT-guided implant surgery facilitates the placement of dental implants into ideal positions according to a restorative-driven treatment plan based on the individual case requirements. Patients can be treated with a submerged or non-submerged technique or with immediate provisional restoration based on the intra- and post-operative findings. This choice involves individual case selection, planning, and the required level of experience and skill of the surgical and restorative teams. Planning software enhances patient awareness, education, and compliance and is an instrumental component of success. Clinicians should consider the additional investment in time and cost involved in using this proprietary software and computer-aided design/computer-aided manufacturing processing technologies. Successful integration of CT technology and CT-guided surgery into a dental implant practice can have a steep learning curve; however, the benefits to the patient and clinician are outstanding.

References

1. Mozzo P, Procacci C, Tacconi A, et al. A new volumetric CT machine for dental imaging based on the cone beam technique: preliminary results. Eur Radiol 1998; 8: 1558–1564.
2. Mah J, Hatcher D. Three-dimensional craniofacial imaging. Am J Orthod Dentofac Orthoped 2004; 126: 308–309.
3. Hashimoto K, Yoshinori A, Kazui I, et al. A comparison of a new, limited cone beam computed tomography machine for dental use with a multi-detector row helical CT machine. Oral Surg Oral Med Oral Path Oral Radiol Endo 2005; 95: 371–377.
4. Sukovic P. Cone beam computed tomography in craniofacial imaging. Orthod Craniofac Res 2003; 6(Suppl 1): 31–36.
5. Rothman SL, Chaftez N, Rhodes ML, Schwarz MS. CT in the preoperative assessment of the maxilla and mandible for endosseous implant surgery. Radiology 1988; 168: 171–175.
6. Casselman JW, Deryckere F, Hermans R, et al. Denta Scan: CT software program used in the anatomic evaluation of the mandible and maxilla in the perspective of endosseous implant surgery. Rofo 1991; 155(1): 4–10.
7. Villari N, Fanfani F. Diagnostic contribution of CT in implantology: use of a new Denta-Scan reconstruction program. Radiol Med 1992; 83: 608–614.
8. Tal H, Moses O. A comparison of panoramic radiography with computed tomography in the planning of implant surgery. Dentomaxillofac Radiol 1991; 20: 40–42.
9. SimPlant Sources. Web history – About CSI. Available at: http://sites.google.com/site/simplantisrael/simplantsources. Last accessed May 13, 2015.
10. Ramez J, Donazzan M, Chanavaz M, et al. The contribution of scanner imagery in implant surgery and sinus overflow using frontal oblique orthogonal reconstruction. Rev Stomatol Chir Maxillofac 1992; 93: 212–214.
11. Pattijn V, van Cleynenbreugel T, vander Sloten J, et al. Structural and radiological parameters for the nondestructive characterization of trabecular bone. Ann Biomed Eng 2001; 29: 1064–1073.
12. Sonick M, Abrahams J, Faiella R. A comparison of the accuracy of periapical, panoramic, and computerized tomographic radiographs in locating the mandibular canal. Int J Oral Maxillofac Implants 1994; 9: 455–460.
13. Todd A, Gher M, Quintero G, Richardson AC. Interpretation of linear and computed tomograms in the assessment of implant recipient sites. J Periodontol 1993; 64: 1243–1249.
14. Gehr ME, Richardson AC. The accuracy of dental radiographic techniques used for evaluation of implant fixture placement. Int J Periodontics Restorative Dent 1995; 15: 268–283.
15. Van Steenberghe D, Glauser R, Blombäck U, et al. A computed tomographic scan derived customized surgical template and fixed prosthesis for flapless surgery and immediate loading of implants in fully edentulous maxillae. A prospective multicenter study. Clin Implant Dent Relat Res 2005; 7(Suppl 1): s111–s120.
16. Ganz, SD. Pre-surgical planning with CT-derived fabrication of surgical guides. J Oral Maxillofac Surg 2005; 63(Suppl 2): 59–71.
17. Rosenfeld AL, Mandelaris GA, Tardieu PB. Prosthetically directed implant placement using computer software to ensure precise placement and predictable prosthetic outcomes. Part 3: stereolithographic drilling guides that do not require bone exposure and the immediate delivery of teeth. Int J Periodontics Restorative Dent 2006; 26: 493–499.
18. Vrielinck L, Politis C, Schepers S, et al. Image-based planning and clinical validation of zygoma and pterygoid implant placement in patients with severe bone atrophy using customized drill guides. Preliminary results from a prospective clinical follow-up study. Int J Oral Maxillofac Surg 2003; 32: 7–14.
19. Sarment DP, Sukovic P, Clinthorne N. Accuracy of implant placement with a stereolithiographic surgical guide. Int J Oral Maxillofac Implants 2003; 18: 571–577.
20. Hahn, J. Single stage, immediate loading, and flapless surgery. J Oral Implantol 2000; 26: 193–198.
21. Campelo L, Dominguez Camara J. Flapless implant surgery: a 10-year clinical retrospective analysis. Int J Oral Maxillofac Implants 2002; 17: 271–276.
22. Becker W, Goldstein M, Becker BE, Sennerby L. Minimally invasive flapless implant surgery: a prospective multicenter study. Clin Implant Dent Relat Res 2005; 7(Suppl 1): s21–s27.
23. Becker W, Wikesjo U, Sennerby L, et al. Histologic evaluation of implants following flapless and flapped surgery: a study in canines. J Periodontol 2006; 77: 1717–1722.
24. Komiyama A, Pettersson A, Hultin M, et al. Virtually planned and template-guided implant surgery: an experimental model matching approach. Clin Oral Implants Res 2010; 22: 308–313.
25. Wagner A, Wanschitz F, Birkfellner W, et al. Computer-aided placement of endosseous oral implants in patients after ablative tumour surgery: assessment of accuracy. Clin Oral Implants Res 2003; 14: 340–348.
26. Casap N, Tarazi E, Wexler A, et al. Intraoperative computerized navigation for flapless implant surgery and immediate loading in the edentulous mandible. Int J Oral Maxillofac Implants 2005; 20: 92–98.
27. D'Haese J, Van De Velde T, Komiyama A, et al. Accuracy and complications using computer-designed stereolithographic surgical guides for oral rehabilitation by means of dental implants: a review of the literature. Clin Implant Dent Relat Res 2012; 14: 321–335.
28. Arisan V, Karabuda ZC, Ozdemir T. Accuracy of two stereolithographic guide systems for computer-aided implant placement: a computed tomography-based clinical comparative study. J Periodontol 2010; 81: 43–51.
29. Ozan O, Turkyilmaz I, Ersoy AE, et al. Clinical accuracy of 3 different types of computed tomography-derived stereolithographic surgical guides in implant placement. J Oral Maxillofac Surg 2009; 67: 394–401.
30. Abrahamsson I, Berglundh T, Sekino S, Lindhe J. Tissue reactions to abutment shift: an experimental study in dogs. Clin Implant Dent Relat Res 2003; 5: 82–88.
31. Gracis S, Nicholls J, Chalupnik J, Yuodelis R. Shock-absorbing behavior of five restorative materials used on implants. Int J Prosthodont 1991; 4: 282–291.
32. Arisan V, Karabuda CZ, Ozdemir T. Implant surgery using bone- and mucosa-supported stereolithographic guides in totally edentulous jaws: surgical and post-operative outcomes of computer-aided vs. standard techniques. Clin Oral Implants Res 2010; 21: 980–988.
33. Becker W, Goldstein M, Becker BE, Sennerby L. Minimally invasive flapless implant surgery: a prospective multicenter study. Clin Implant Dent Relat Res 2005; 7(Suppl 1): s21–s27.
34. Cannizzaro G, Torchio C, Leone M, Esposito M. Immediate versus early loading of flapless-placed implants supporting maxillary full-arch prostheses: a randomised controlled clinical trial. Eur J Oral Implantol 2008; 1: 127–139
35. Van Assche N, van Steenberghe D, Guerrero ME, et al. Accuracy of implant placement based on pre-surgical planning of three-dimensional cone-beam images: a pilot study. J Clin Periodontol 2007; 34: 816–821.
36. Abboud M, Calvo Guirado J, Orentlicher G, Wahl G. Comparison of the accuracy of cone beam computed tomography and medical computed tomography: implications for clinical diagnostics with guided surgery. Int J Oral Maxillofac Implants 2013; 28: 536–542.
37. Wouters V, Mollemans W, Schutyser, F. Calibrated segmentation of CBCT for digitization of dental prostheses. Int J Comput Assist Radiol Surg 2011; 6: 609–616.
38. Misir A, Sumer M, Yenisey M, Ergioglu E. Effect of surgical drill guide on heat generated from implant drilling. J Oral Maxillofac Surg 2009; 67: 2663–2668.
39. Orentlicher G, Goldsmith D, Abboud M. Computer guided planning and placement of dental implants. In: Digital Technologies in Oral and Maxillofacial Surgery, Atlas of Oral and Maxillofacial Surgery Clinics, Orentlicher G, ed. Philadelphia, PA: Elsevier, 2012, pp. 53–79.
40. Gapski R, Wang H, Mascarenhas P, Lang N. Critical review of immediate implant loading. Clin Oral Implants Res 2003; 14: 515–527.

41. Ogawa T, Nishimura I. Different bone integration profiles of turned and acid-etched implants associated with modulated expression of extracellular matrix genes. Int J Oral Maxillofac Implants 2003; 18: 200–210.
42. Zechner W, Tangl S, Furst G, et al. Osseous healing characteristics of three different implant types. Clin Oral Implants Res 2003; 14: 150–157.
43. Lorenzoni M, Pertl C, Zhang K, Wegscheider WA. In-patient comparison of immediately loaded and non-loaded implants within 6 months. Clin Oral Implants Res 2003; 14: 273–279.
44. Jaffin R, Kumar A, Berman C. Immediate loading of dental implants in the completely edentulous maxilla: a clinical report. Int J Oral Maxillofac Implants 2004; 19: 721–730.
45. Gatti C, Haefliger W, Chiapasco M. Implant-retained mandibular overdentures with immediate loading: a prospective study of ITI implants. Int J Oral Maxillofac Implants 2000; 15: 383–388.
46. Tarnow D, Emtiaz S, Classi A. Immediate loading of threaded implants at stage 1 surgery in edentulous arches: ten consecutive case reports with 1- to 5-year data. Int J Oral Maxillofac Implants 1997; 12: 319–324.
47. Chatzistavrou M, Felton D, Cooper L. Immediate loading of dental implants in partially edentulous patients: a clinical report. J Prosthodont 2003; 12: 26–29.
48. Glauser R, Lundgren AK, Gottlow J, et al. Immediate occlusal loading of Brånemark TiUnite implants placed predominantly in soft bone: 1-year results of a prospective clinical study. Clin Implant Dent Relat Res 2003; 5(Suppl 1): 47–56.
49. Abboud M, Koeck B, Stark H, et al. Immediate loading of single-tooth implants in the posterior region. Int J Oral Maxillofac Implants 2005; 20: 61–68.
50. Vandamme K, Naert I, Geris L, et al. Histodynamics of bone tissue formation around immediately loaded cylindrical implants in the rabbit. Clin Oral Implants Res 2007; 18: 471–480.
51. Zitzmann N, Marinello C. Treatment plan for restoring the edentulous maxilla with implant-supported restorations: removable overdenture versus fixed partial denture design. J Prosthetic Dent 1999; 82: 188–196.
52. Ledermann P. Bar-prosthetic management of the edentulous mandible by means of plasma-coated implantation with titanium screws. Dtsch Zahnarztl Z 1979; 34: 907–911.
53. Ledermann D. 6-year clinical trial with titanium plasma-coated ITI (Internationales Team für Implantologie) screw implants in the mandibular interforaminal region. SSO Schweiz Monatsschr Zahnheilkd 1983; 93: 1070–1089 (in German).
54. Schnitman P, Wohrle P, Rubenstein J, et al. Ten-year results for Brånemark implants immediately loaded with fixed prostheses at implant placement. Int J Oral Maxillofac Implants 1997; 12: 495–503.
55. Wolfinger G, Balshi T, Rangert B. Immediate functional loading of Brånemark system implants in edentulous mandibles: clinical report of the results of developmental and simplified protocols. Int J Oral Maxillofac Implants 2003; 18: 250–257.
56. Horiuchi K, Uchida H, Yamamoto K, Sugimura M. Immediate loading of Brånemark system implants following placement in edentulous patients: a clinical report. Int J Oral Maxillofac Implants 2000; 15: 824–830.
57. Ganeles J, Rosenberg M, Holt R, Reichman L. Immediate loading of implants with fixed restorations in the completely edentulous mandible: report of 27 patients from a private practice. Int J Oral Maxillofac Implants 2001; 16: 418–426.
58. Aalam A, Nowzari H, Krivitsky A. Functional restoration of implants on the day of surgical placement in the fully edentulous mandible: a case series. Clin Implant Dent Relat Res 2005; 7: 10–16.
59. Degidi M, Piattelli A, Felice P, Carinci F. Immediate functional loading of edentulous maxilla: a 5-year retrospective study of 388 titanium implants. J Periodontol 2005; 76: 1016–1024.
60. Brånemark P, Engstrand P, Ohrnell L, et al. Brånemark Novum: a new treatment concept for rehabilitation of the edentulous mandible. Preliminary results from a prospective clinical follow-up study. Clin Implant Dent Relat Res 1999; 1: 2–16.
61. De Bruyn H, Kisch J, Collaert B, et al. Fixed mandibular restorations on three early-loaded regular platform Brånemark implants. Clin Implant Dent Relat Res 2001; 3: 176–184.
62. Malo P, Rangert B, Nobre M. "All-on-Four" immediate-function concept with Brånemark system implants for completely edentulous mandibles: a retrospective clinical study. Clin Implant Dent Relat Res 2003; 5(Suppl 1): 2–9.
63. Esposito M, Grusovin M, Achille H, et al. Interventions for replacing missing teeth: different times for loading dental implants. Cochrane Database Syst Rev 2009: CD003878.
64. Abboud M, Wahl G, Guirado JLC, Orentlicher G. CT guided implant surgery with immediate loading: comparison and outcomes of two technologies. Int J Oral Maxillofac Implants 2012; 27: 634–643.
65. Valente F, Schiroli G, Sbrenna A. Accuracy of computer-aided oral implant surgery: a clinical and radiographic study. Int J Oral Maxillofac Implants 2009; 24: 234–242.
66. Misch CM. Immediate loading of definitive implants in the edentulous mandible using a fixed provisional prosthesis: the denture conversion technique. J Oral Maxillofac Surg 2004; 62: 106–115.
67. Orentlicher G, Goldsmith D, Horowitz A. Applications of 3-dimensional virtual computerized tomography technology in oral and maxillofacial surgery: current therapy J Oral Maxillofac Surg 2010; 68: 1933–1959.
68. Johansson B, Grepe A, Wannfors K, Hirsch JM. A clinical study of changes in the volume of bone grafts in the atrophic maxilla. Dentomaxillofac Radiol 2001; 30: 157–161.
69. Verhoeven J, Ruijter J, Cune M, et al. Onlay grafts in combination with endosseous implants in severe mandibular atrophy; one year results of a prospective, quantitative radiological study. Clin Oral Implants Res 2000; 11: 583–594.
70. Smolka W, Eggensperger N, Carollo V, et al. Changes in the volume and density of calvarial split bone grafts after alveolar ridge augmentation. Clin Oral Implants Res 2006; 17: 149–155.
71. Marx R. Osteoradionecrosis: a new concept of its pathophysiology. J Oral Maxillofac Surg 1983; 41: 283–288.
72. Marx R, Ames J. The use of hyperbaric oxygen therapy in bony reconstruction of the irradiated and tissue-deficient patient. J Oral Maxillofac Surg 1982; 40: 412–420.
73. Granström G. Placement of dental implants in irradiated bone: the case for using hyperbaric oxygen. J Oral Maxillofac Surg 2006; 64: 812–818.
74. Granström G: Radiotherapy, osseointegration, and hyperbaric oxygen therapy. Periodontol 2000 2003; 33: 145–162.
75. Koga D, Salvajoli J, Alves F. Dental extractions and radiotherapy in head and neck oncology: review of the literature. Oral Dis 2008; 14: 40–44.
76. Horowitz A, Orentlicher G, Goldsmith D. Case report – computerized implantology for the irradiated patient. J Oral Maxillofac Surg 2009; 67: 619–623.

SECTION III

Optimizing Anatomical Limits with Short, Narrow and Angled Implants

CHAPTER 10

Short Implants

Douglas Deporter
Discipline of Periodontics, Faculty of Dentistry, University of Toronto, Toronto, ON, Canada

Introduction

There is currently much attention being given to the use of short dental implants in edentulous sites having minimal bone height, and/or to make implant surgery less invasive. Historically, long implants (i.e. >10 mm in mandible and >13 mm in maxilla) were preferred based on early data using threaded implants with machine-turned surfaces.[1–4] The use of long implants, however, had limitations, in that many sites had insufficient bone, making it necessary to invoke supportive surgical procedures meant to increase alveolar ridge height. These procedures were invasive, often beyond the abilities of many clinicians and costly, and their outcomes unpredictable, with the exception of open sinus grafting.[5] Long implants also increased risk of damage to vital structures, such as the mandibular neurovascular bundle, or penetration of mandibular lingual cortical plate with life-threatening bleeding implications. Innovations in dental implant designs, including surface treatments that promote greater bone-to-implant contact,[6] macrogeometry and prosthetic connection, and alterations in surgical technique meant to improve initial implant stability, have increased the usefulness of short implants. Reliable short implant designs will offer the most efficient way to overcome anatomical barriers with minimal invasiveness, greater safety, applicability by a wider range of practitioners, and an economic benefit for patients. The purpose of this chapter is to review recent data on the use of short implants and to highlight ways to maximize successful treatment outcomes.

Literature review

For many years, the definition of "short dental implant" was one with a length of ≤10 mm, but this definition was refined in a widely quoted paper by Renouard and Nisand.[7] These clinicians suggested that a short implant has a "designed intrabony length" (DIL) of ≤8 mm. The DIL is the length of implant intended to engage bone and remain in contact with bone once the implant becomes functional (i.e. the surface of implant root meant to achieve and maintain "osseointegration"), and does not include the length of implant collar segment meant to accommodate peri-implant soft tissues. This new definition was accepted by the State of Science on Implant Dentistry workshop (SSID Conference) sponsored by the Academy of Osseointegration, in Chicago, Illinois, in August of 2006. Since that time, considerable efforts have been directed toward understanding if and how dental implants of lengths ≤8 mm can be used successfully. It would appear that multiple factors besides implant length are at play, including:

1 implant surface topography;
2 implant diameter;
3 surgical preparation of the osteotomy;
4 operator experience;
5 initial implant stability;
6 progressive early implant loading;
7 crestal bone loss after onset of function; and
8 mechanical overload.

Implant surface topography

Albrektsson and Wennerberg[6] reviewed dental implant surface topographies and classified them as minimally rough, moderately rough, or rough. The early poor outcomes with truly short implants were thought to be due primarily to the fact that implants being used had machine-turned (i.e. minimally rough) surfaces that did not provide adequate functional surface area in their crestal regions,[8] resulting in a weak bone-to-implant interface.[9,10] As a result, they had minimal resistance to tensile forces arising from off-axis loading of crestal bone,[11,12] which may have led to crestal bone microfractures due to bone compression, subsequent bone loss, and finally implant loosening[13] (Figure 10.1).

Pierrisnard et al.[14] presented data from 3-D finite element analysis (FEA) modeling of machine-turned implants that suggested that forces experienced by dental implants are likely to be concentrated to the most coronal three to five threads (the "functional surface area"[8]) and that this situation should not vary by increasing implant length. In support of this speculation, in a dog study designed to measure removal torque of osseointegrated, machine-turned implants, Bernard et al.[15] reported that increasing implant length from 7–10 mm had no significant impact on the strength of the bone-to-implant interface. Interestingly, Renouard and Nisand[7] were able to use the original machine-turned, Brånemark-type threaded implant in lengths of 7 mm with success, and they attributed their outcomes not to implant design, but rather to modifications in osteotomy site preparation meant to increase initial implant stability. This suggested that a surgical technique (various modifications have been recommended) specific for use with short implants could be an important factor in success. More will be said of this later.

Truly rough implant surfaces ($S_a \geq 20\mu m$), like those plasma-sprayed with titanium or hydroxyapatite, were sometimes used with short lengths[16] but are currently not widely used because of risk of exposure of these surfaces to bacterial plaque, progressive bone loss, and late implant failure.[17,18] Consequently, moderately rough ($S_a \leq 2\mu m$) dental implants have become the ones most commonly used. Examples include implants with surface treatments created by acid-etching, particle-blasting with or without additional acid-etching, and those with thickened oxide surface layers (e.g. TiUnite®). All of these moderately rough surfaces appear to work equally well if employed properly (e.g. Figure 10.2). Like rough surfaces, moderately rough surfaces promote faster integration and result in more extensive and stronger bone-to-implant interfaces than machine-turned surfaces.[9,10,19] However, they

Minimally Invasive Dental Implant Surgery, First Edition. Edited by Daniel R. Cullum and Douglas Deporter.

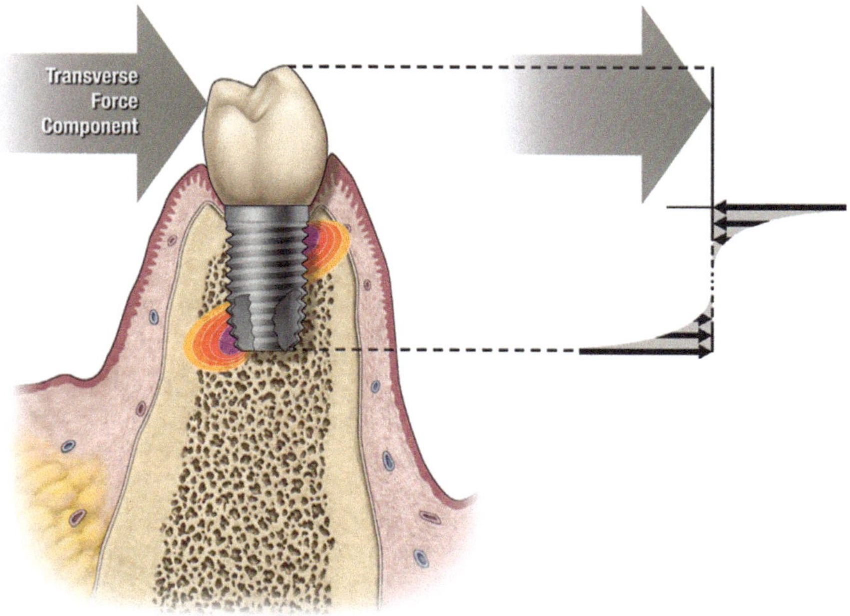

Figure 10.1 Transverse loading of threaded implants can cause high stress concentration in crestal bone (and the diagonally opposite apical region) on downstream (i.e. compressive) surfaces which can lead to crestal bone microfractures and resorption. *Source:* Hagi et al. 2004.[13] Reproduced with permission of the American Academy of Periodontology.

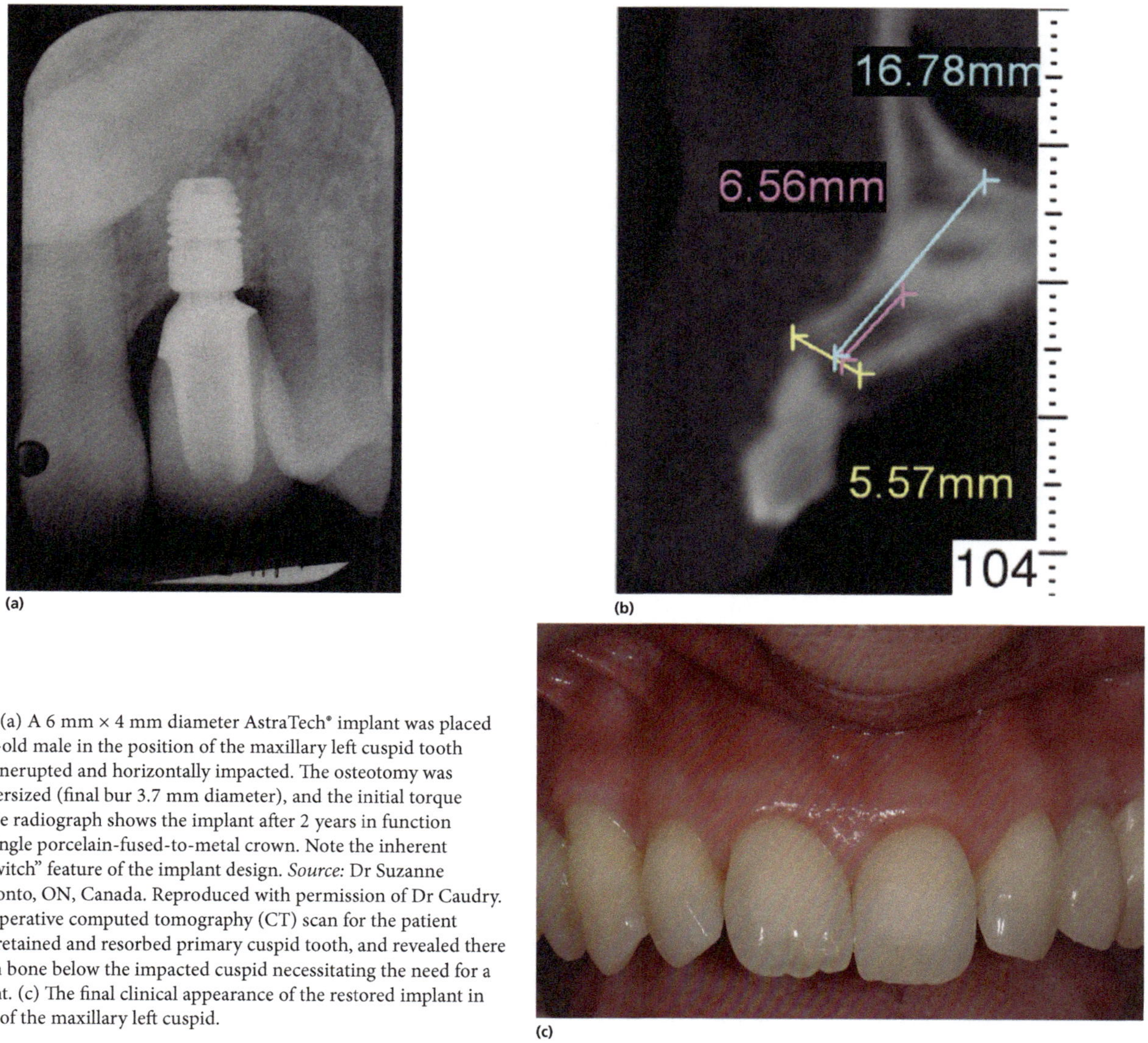

Figure 10.2 (a) A 6 mm × 4 mm diameter AstraTech® implant was placed in a 40-year-old male in the position of the maxillary left cuspid tooth which was unerupted and horizontally impacted. The osteotomy was slightly undersized (final bur 3.7 mm diameter), and the initial torque 25 N cm. The radiograph shows the implant after 2 years in function carrying a single porcelain-fused-to-metal crown. Note the inherent "platform-switch" feature of the implant design. *Source:* Dr Suzanne Caudry, Toronto, ON, Canada. Reproduced with permission of Dr Caudry. (b) The preoperative computed tomography (CT) scan for the patient showed the retained and resorbed primary cuspid tooth, and revealed there to be <7 mm bone below the impacted cuspid necessitating the need for a short implant. (c) The final clinical appearance of the restored implant in the position of the maxillary left cuspid.

are thought to be less at risk if they suffer some crestal bone loss with exposure of roughened surface to dental plaque.

Many clinicians,[20–24] but not all,[25] have reported good clinical results with moderately rough implants in both standard and short lengths. In their recent meta-analysis of published reports on over 19,000 implants, Pommer et al.[26] concluded that short rough and moderately rough implants performed better than short machine-turned implants, although it is important to note that the length range considered short was 7–10 mm, making many of the implants ineligible for consideration using the definition of Renouard and Nisand.[7] Telleman et al.[27] also published a meta-analysis of studies reporting on the performance of short implants primarily in posterior regions of partially edentulous patients. The implant lengths included were 5, 7, 8, 8.5, 9, and 9.5 mm. It was concluded that there was a small tendency for failure to increase as implant length decreased. There were too few 5 mm implants included, but the survival rates for 6 mm, 7 mm, 8 mm, and 8.5 mm implants were 97.4%, 97.6%, 98.4%, and 98.8% respectively. Significantly better outcomes were found for all categories of short implant in posterior mandible versus posterior maxilla, and in non-smokers versus smokers (≥15 cigarettes/day). A higher failure rate for short implants in posterior maxilla was also reported by Pommer et al.[26] This is likely explained by the fact that bone in posterior maxilla is primarily cancellous,[28] making good initial implant stability more of an issue. Implant macrodesign may play a role with short implants in cancellous bone. Misch et al.[29] reported that altering implant thread pitch (i.e. number of threads per unit implant length) and thread depth could improve initial stability and success with shorter implants in cancellous bone. They suggested that short implants with a greater number of threads, and therefore greater surface area, could favorably affect outcomes in posterior jaw sites.

Fugazzotto et al.[21] presented data at times zero to 84 months for a group of patients treated using the manufacturer's (Straumann ITI, Basel, Switzerland) surgical protocol with rough (titanium plasma spray-coated) or moderately rough (particle-blasted/acid-washed) implants in lengths of 9 mm or less. Implants were placed only in posterior maxilla, and used to support single crowns. A total of 979 implants were placed, 839 (85.7%) of which were short (7–8 mm) with 69.2% of wide diameter (4.8 mm). Only 10 (1.2%) short implants were lost, all 8 mm in length. Eight failed within the first 2 years, and two failed after 5 years, perhaps explained by the FEA studies of others.[30] The latter investigators suggested that occlusal overload may be the most important stress concentration factor for single posterior implant crowns supported by short (7 mm long × 5 mm diameter) threaded implants. Whether the late failures in Fugazzotto et al.'s report were rough or moderately rough implants was not stated. While longer term follow-up, including evaluation of crestal bone changes, is needed, the results do appear to support the use of short, wide, rough to moderately rough threaded implants in posterior maxilla even when restored with single crowns.

Lai et al.[31] recently reported 5- to 10-year retrospective outcomes with short, moderately rough threaded implants placed in posterior jaw locations, and later used to support single crowns. A total of 168 patients received 231 implants (i.e. 1.4 implants per patient) using a hand ratchet without pre-tapping to ensure good initial stability. Implant lengths were either 6 or 8 mm (85.7% of implants used) with diameters of either 4.1 (78.8% of implants used) or 4.8 mm, and posterior maxilla and posterior mandible were more or less equally represented. Mean functional time was 7.2 years, and the 5- to 10-year survival rates were both calculated to be about 98%. Furthermore, mean crestal bone loss was insignificant after year 1.

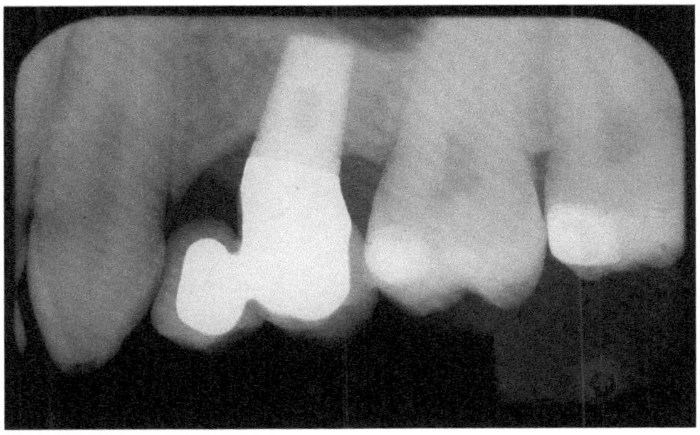

Figure 10.3 This radiograph shows the 5-year follow-up for a 7 mm long SPS implant that has been supporting a mesial cantilever in a patient with oligodontia. No sinus grafting was completed.

However, biological complications, such as peri-implant mucositis and peri-implantitis, affected 7.8% of implants, which would lower the success rate accordingly.

In a discussion about short implants, mention is due to sintered porous-surfaced (SPS) press-fit implants. These have been shown to perform well in lengths of 7 mm or less[32–35] with or without splinting to other implants[36] (Figure 10.3). Indeed, when comparing lengths of 7, 9, and 12 mm all with 4.1 mm diameters, there was no benefit to using an SPS implant longer than 7 mm based on implant stability determined with the Periotest® device.[37]

Deporter et al.[33] reported 10-year results from a prospective human clinical trial in which non-splinted SPS implants were used to retain mandibular overdentures (Figure 10.4). Implant lengths used were 7, 8, 9, and 10 mm; all had 2 mm transgingival machined collars, making their DILs 5, 6, 7, or 8 mm. The best performance after 10 years was with the shortest implant (i.e. 7 mm with 5 mm DIL), and this remained the case after 20 years in function.[38]

After 10 years of function in posterior mandible of partially edentulous patients, Deporter et al.[39] reported mean cumulative crestal bone loss of 1.2 mm for SPS implants (Figure 10.5). Because of their preference for highly vascular bone (types III and IV), SPS implants also perform well in posterior maxilla where short implants are often needed to avoid open sinus grafting[34,40] (Figure 10.6; see also Chapter 15). Current designs of SPS implants have a platform-switch feature to help to further reduce crestal bone loss (OT-3 implants, OT Medical, Bremen, Germany). However, as with rough-surfaced threaded implants, SPS implants must not come into contact with bacterial plaque.[41] The sintered surface segment must be fully submerged in bone, and buccal bone thickness after osteotomy preparation should not be <2 mm,[42] or augmentation is required at the time of implant placement. This is crucial to minimize risk of buccal bone loss and exposure of sintered surface to bacterial plaque.

Wide-diameter implants

The second factor that may affect performance of short implants is their diameter. FEA modeling studies have suggested that wider (i.e. ≥4.5 mm[7]) diameter threaded dental implants can reduce stress on crestal bone compared with those of standard diameter,[43,44] and this result was supported by morphometric data from animal experiments.[45] Further, in a 3-D FEA study of five different and primarily moderately rough threaded implant systems with diameters

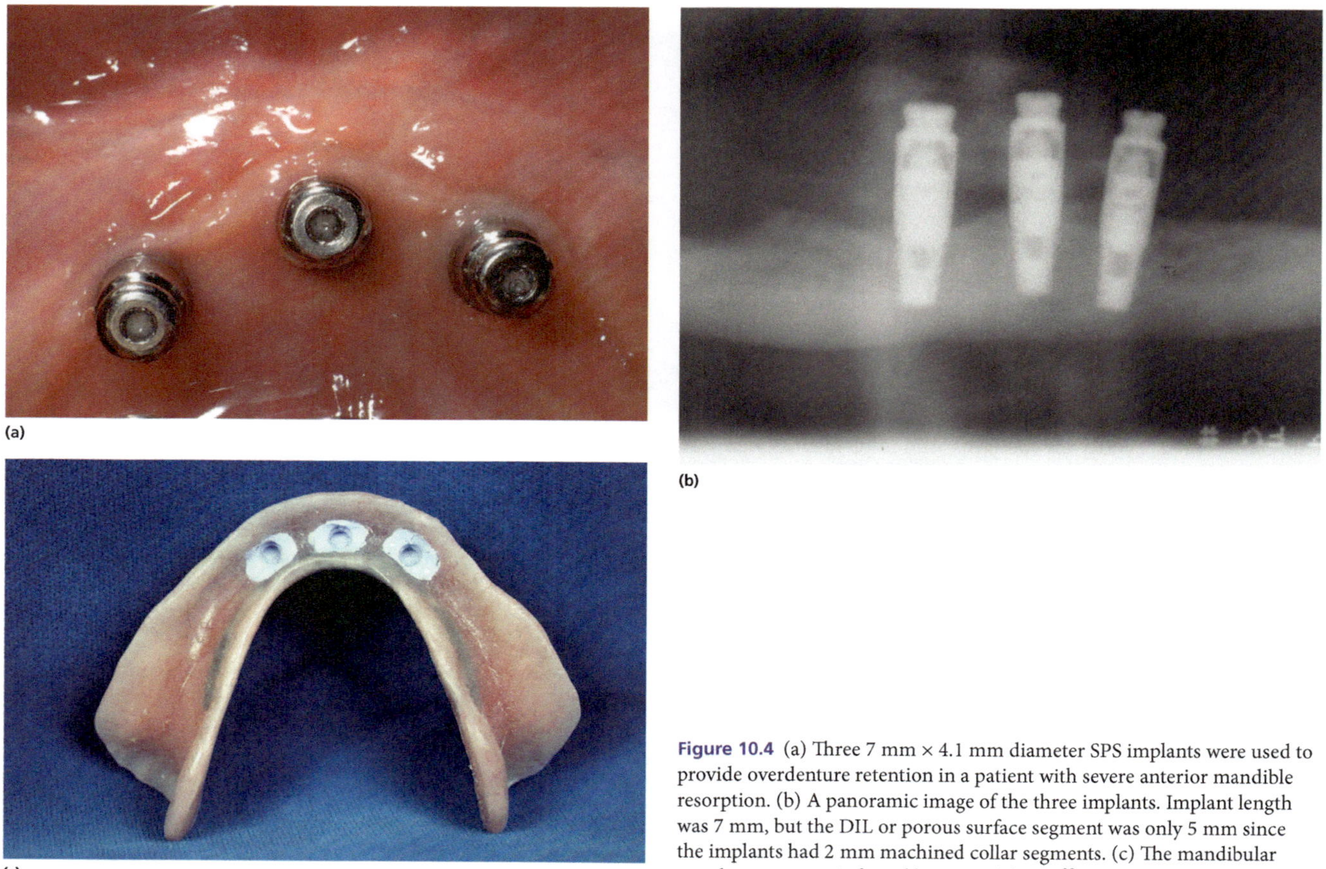
(a)
(b)
(c)

Figure 10.4 (a) Three 7 mm × 4.1 mm diameter SPS implants were used to provide overdenture retention in a patient with severe anterior mandible resorption. (b) A panoramic image of the three implants. Implant length was 7 mm, but the DIL or porous surface segment was only 5 mm since the implants had 2 mm machined collar segments. (c) The mandibular overdenture was reinforced by a metal frame.[33]

3.3–4.5 mm and lengths of 7.5–12 mm, Baggi et al.[46] found that increasing implant diameter decreased stresses in crestal cortical bone, but not in cancellous bone. More favorable stress distribution in cancellous bone was achieved by increasing implant length rather than increasing implant diameter, suggesting that short implants with wider diameters may be more appropriate for mandibular than for maxillary sites. This suggestion has not been confirmed clinically to date. However, human clinical studies have shown a benefit of increased diameter in reducing crestal bone loss.[46] Reducing stresses received by crestal bone will lessen the likelihood of bone microfractures and resultant crestal resorption. Newer implant designs have other design features, such as coronal microthreads or laser microgrooves,

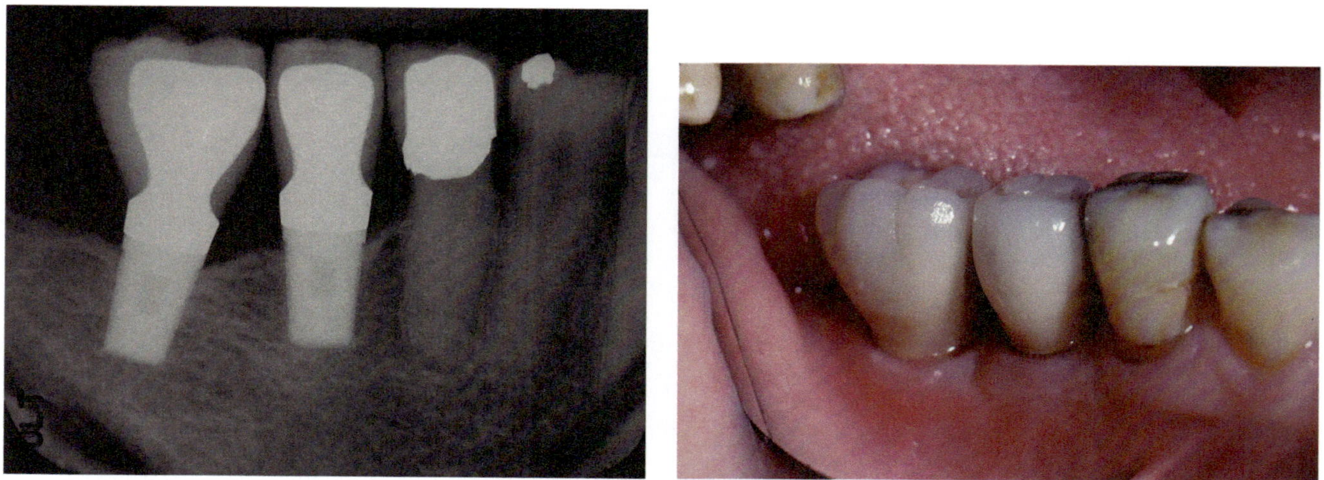
(a)
(b)

Figure 10.5 (a) The radiograph shows two 7 mm × 4.1 mm SPS implants that have been in function carrying single crowns for >10 years. Overall implant length was 7 mm, but the DIL was 6 mm as they had 1 mm machined collars. Crestal bone remodeling is limited to the machined collar regions. (b) The opposing dentition was of natural teeth. *Source*: Restorations provided by Dr Reynaldo Todescan, Toronto, ON, Canada. Reproduced with permission of Dr Todescan.

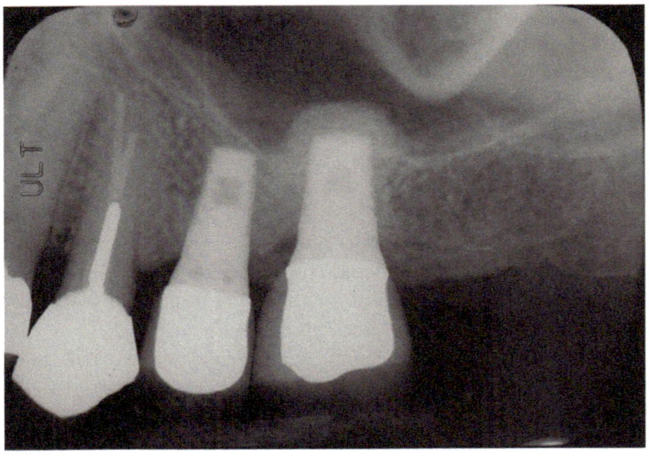

Figure 10.6 The radiograph shows two SPS implants used to replace posterior maxillary teeth after 13 years in function. The mesial implant was 7 mm (5 mm DIL) × 4.1 mm, while the distal implant was 7 mm (5 mm DIL) × 5 mm, and required a localized, osteotome-mediated, sinus floor elevation of approximately 3 mm at the time of implant placement. *Source*: Restorations provided by Dr Richard Cameron. Reproduced with permission of Dr Cameron.

also thought to provide lower (i.e. more physiological) stress levels to crestal bone (see " Minimizing crestal bone loss" section).

Clinical investigations have shown no negative impact with the use of wider diameter implants.[24,47–49] Tawil and Younan[47] actually reported improved performance with increased implant diameter. These clinicians reported data on 27 machine-turned implants of length 7 mm (diameters 3.75, 4.0, or 5.0 mm) after 12–92 months' function. Five implants (18.5%), all with diameters 3.75 or 4.0 mm failed, while all 5 mm diameter implants survived. Pommer et al.,[26] in their systematic review of literature, could find no relationship between diameter and implant failure after at least 1 year in function. However, success with machine-turned implants again often required modified surgical protocols, as will be discussed shortly. Short, ultrawide implants also can be used as immediate molar implants in situations where infection is not an issue and buccal cortex remains intact following tooth extraction and site preparation.[50] (See also Chapter 18.) However, these implants do come with the risk of buccal bone loss if the buccal bone is compromised during osteotomy preparation and ends up <2 mm in thickness.

Deporter et al.[35] reported on the use of 5 mm long by 5 mm diameter SPS implants which they termed "ultrashort." The implant had a 1 mm machined collar, making its DIL 4 mm (Figures 10.7 and 10.8). When used in posterior mandible, this implant was 100% successful,

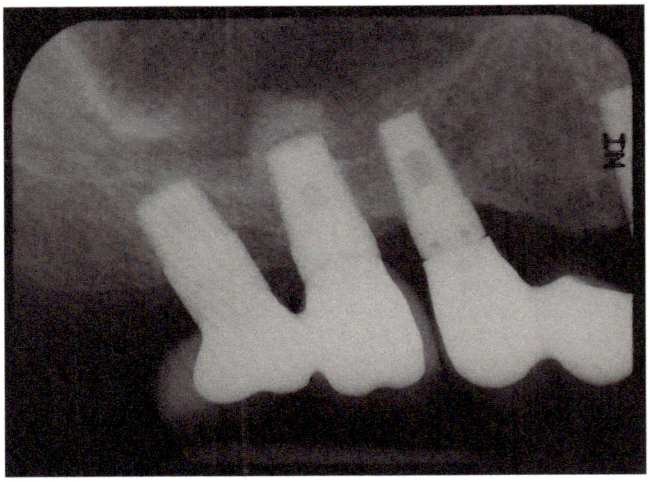

(a)

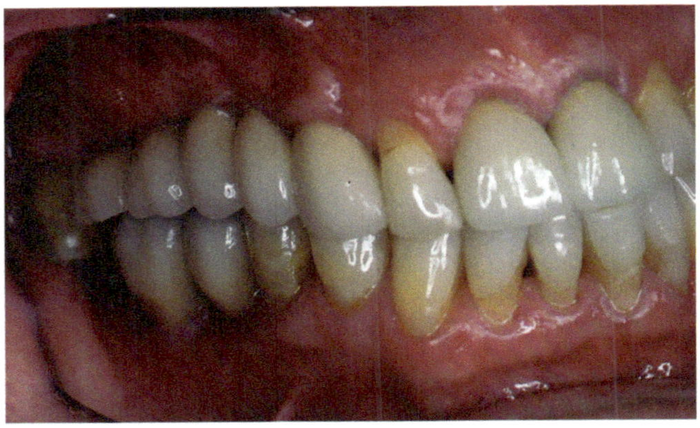

(b)

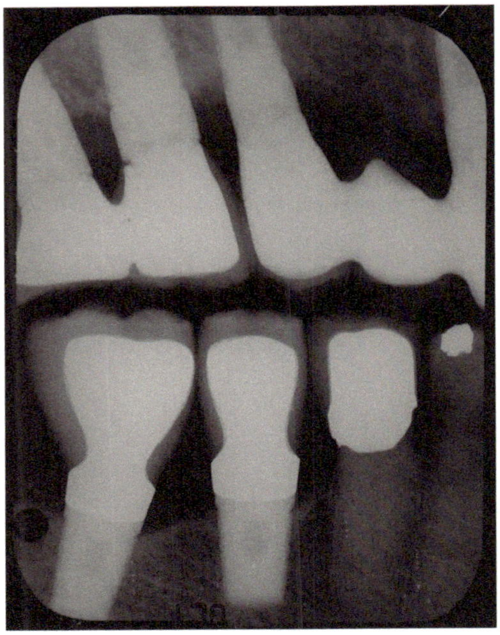

(c)

Figure 10.7 (a) This patient received three short SPS implants to restore his maxillary right posterior segment. The most distal implant was an ultrashort (5 mm × 5 mm), and it was splinted to a 7 mm long × 5 mm diameter. The most mesial implant was a 7 mm × 4.1 mm diameter implant, and was part of a three-unit prosthesis supported by two implants. The radiograph were taken after >10 years in function with the implant prostheses, and the opposing arch consisted of implants and natural teeth. (b) The clinical picture of the final restorations. (c) This vertical bitewing radiograph shows the opposing arch for the maxillary implants seen in (a) at the same recall appointment. *Source*: Restorations provided by Dr Reynaldo Todescan, Toronto, ON, Canada. Reproduced with permission of Dr Todescan.

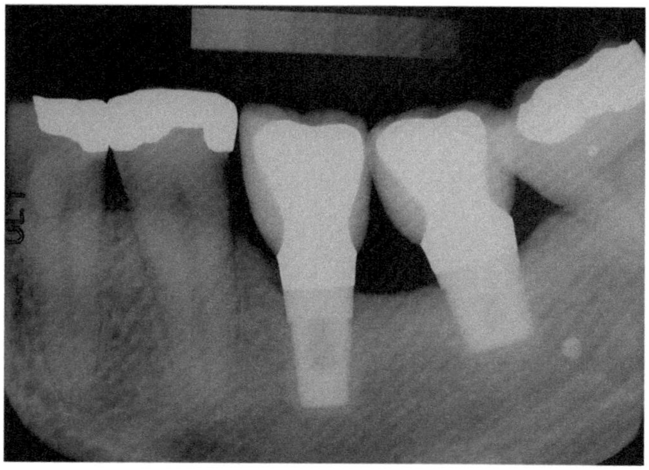

Figure 10.8 This radiograph shows the >13-year follow-up for two SPS implants in the posterior mandible. The mesial implant was 7 mm × 4.1 mm with a 2 mm machined collar (i.e. 5 mm DIL), while the distal implant was an ultrashort implant (5 mm × 5 mm with 1 mm machined collar; i.e. 4 mm DIL). Note also the lamina dura-like density outlining the 7 mm implant. These non-splinted implants have functioned against a natural dentition. *Source*: Restorations provided by Dr Reynaldo Todescan, Toronto, ON, Canada. Reproduced with permission of Dr Todescan.

an outcome also reported by Lombardo et al.[51] However, as with other very short implant designs, lower survival rates were achieved for posterior maxilla,[35,52] failures being primarily in cigarette smokers.

Esposito et al.[53] recently published early results of a randomized prospective study in which 5 mm long, wide-diameter (6 mm), moderately rough threaded implants were placed in resorbed posterior maxilla or mandible. The investigators compared these short, wide implants with similar but longer (10–13 mm) standard diameter (4 mm) implants placed in resorbed sites that had been previously grafted to increase alveolar ridge height. After 1 year in function, the two implant treatments showed similar results. Two long implants (an 8.5 mm in mandible and a 13 mm in maxilla) and one short (in maxilla) failed. However, the short, wide implants had significantly less mean crestal bone loss (1.30 versus 1.48 mm). This outcome appears to support the FEA results of Baggi et al.[46] mentioned previously. Nevertheless, 1.3 mm of bone loss with an implant of 5 mm DIL represents 26% of overall implant length, and as crestal bone loss occurs, increased stresses are experienced by the remaining bony housing.[54] Therefore, further long-term data will be needed to verify that this bone loss does not become progressive or that the implants suffer from mechanical overload. Urdaneta et al.[55] provided retrospective data from 291 patients who had received 211 ultrashort (5 or 6 mm) 5 mm diameter, locking-taper, hydroxyapatite-coated, threaded implants (Integra-CP®, Bicon Corp., Boston, MA), 94.6% of which were restored with single crowns. Most were placed in posterior mandible, and only five implants were lost. However, all implants had not passed 1 year in function at the time of the report, and no marginal bone loss data were provided. Examples of this type of implant are shown in Figure 10.9.

Using wider diameter (>4.5 mm) dental implants may have benefit when combined with short implant length, especially in posterior mandible where proximity to the neurovascular bundle is a concern. However, it is important to note that most edentulous sites with advanced vertical bone loss also show reduced alveolar ridge width. Implants with diameter of ≥5 mm require bucco-lingual/palatal alveolar ridge width of at least 8 mm, which is a rare occurrence in sites with co-existing vertical ridge deficiencies. This again would necessitate pre-implant grafting that could be considered invasive. Rossi et al.[56] reported 2-year data from a prospective study of 35 patients with 40 single-stage, 6 mm long moderately rough (SLActive®, Straumann, Waldenburg, Switzerland) threaded implants of diameters 4.1 and 4.8 mm. Most (63%) implants were placed in posterior mandible and in dense bone. Two 4.1 mm diameter implants (5%) failed to integrate, one in each of two patients, both of whom were smokers (≥10 cigarettes/day). The remaining implants were allowed only 6 weeks initial healing before their permanent restorations were begun, with an attempt to insert the restorations, all single crowns, by the seventh week. All of the restored implants were still present at 2 years in function, and the mean crestal bone loss between insertion and 2 years was 0.75 ± 0.71 mm, and as such was limited to the machined collar segment of the implants.

Arlin[24] had earlier reported a 2-year survival rate of 94% for 6 mm long SLA Straumann implants used primarily in posterior mandible, but had not provided crestal bone loss measurements. However, with longer periods of function (>5 years), he has found that there is an

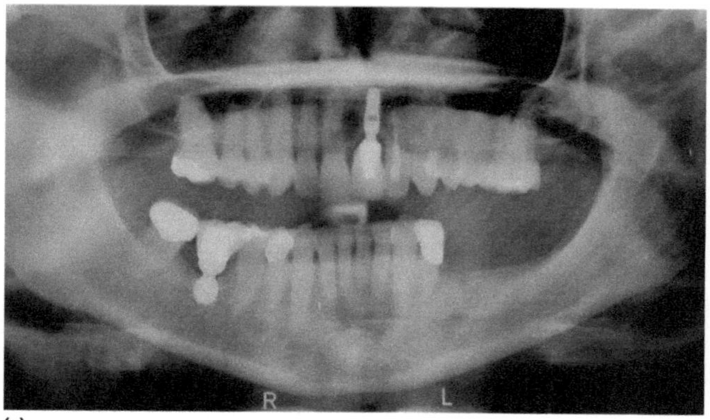

(a)

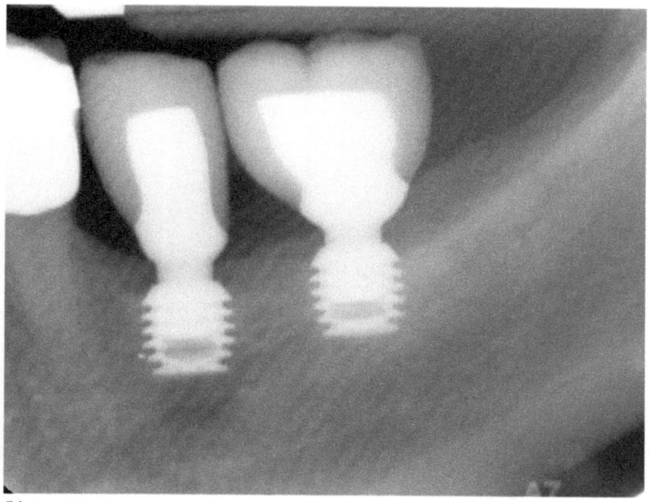

(b)

Figure 10.9 (a) The patient presented requiring restoration of the left posterior mandible with short dental implants. The right mandibular first molar was already replaced with a short implant (Bicon Corp., Boston, MA), and the same device was planned for the left mandible. (b) Radiographic view after restoration of ultrashort implants at the left posterior mandible (Bicon Corp., Boston, MA). *Source:* Dr Clarence C. Lindquist, DDS, Chevy Chase, MD. Reproduced with permission of Dr Lindquist.

increasing risk of implant loosening and failure likely due to mechanical overload (Arlin, 2013, personal communication). A sample case of late failure with this implant model possibly related to mechanical overload is shown in Figure 10.10. The patient was a 52-year-old female with controlled type II diabetes. At the time of implant placement the insertion torque was >40 N cm. The implant was 6 mm long × 4.8 mm wide and had the SLA surface. It functioned well for >7 years, but then became symptomatic, and a radiograph suggested a narrow peri-implant radiolucency (Figure 10.10b). No clinical or radiographic evidence of infection or extensive bone loss were observed, but the implant was clinically mobile and removed.

Recently, Slotte et al.[57] used 4 mm long by 4.1 mm diameter moderately rough (SLActive® tissue level) prototype implants in posterior mandible of partially edentulous patients. Using single-stage surgery, they placed one implant for each missing tooth in 32 patients, mean age 64 years. No known patients with parafunction were included. Ridge contouring was used to establish a flat bone surface of sufficient width (≥6.1 mm). In total, 100 implants were placed, of which three did not attain primary stability at surgery and four were lost before loading. The remaining 93 implants in 26 patients received screw-retained and splinted, fixed partial dentures 10–12 weeks after implant placement. Great care was taken in prosthesis design and insertion to ensure freedom in centric occlusion, avoiding steep cusp slopes and extreme occlusal working contacts. No cantilevers were employed, but the average crown-to-root ratio was 2.5. Periapical radiographs were taken at 6 months and 1 and 2 years, and the prostheses were removed at 1 and 2 years to allow optimal clinical assessment. Between 1 and 2 years, one patient insisted that all of her successful implants be removed and another patient died. Notwithstanding these two patients, implant survival was 95.7% after 1 year and 92.3% after 2 years. Mean crestal bone loss was 0.43 mm (range 0.31–0.59 mm) during year 1 and 0.11 mm (range 0.01–0.43mm) during year 2; that is, within accepted success criteria.[58] Longer term follow-up of these patients will be important given Arlin's suggestion that late failure of short, moderately rough, threaded implants may result from mechanical overload.

Gulje et al.[59] used 6 mm long by 4 mm diameter particle-blasted implants (Astra Tech OsseoSpeed™) with coronal microthreads in severely resorbed anterior mandible to retain overdentures. Twelve patients each received four implants placed using a submerged technique in the inter-foraminal region of mandible. For their restoration, the implants were splinted together with a bar to prevent overloading. After 1 year in function, the implant survival rate was 96% and mean crestal bone loss was negligible (0.1 mm); this positive outcome is possibly related to the presence of the coronal microthreads. One example of this implant type was shown in Figure 10.2, but a second example can be seen in Figure 10.11.

In the studies by Slotte et al.[57] and by Gulji et al.,[59] the investigators used only splinted prostheses to promote more uniform force distribution[60] and minimize crestal bone loss. Lack of splinting may contribute to late failure of very short threaded implants, but this needs further investigation. Short SPS implants of 4.1 mm diameter in ultrashort lengths (5.5 mm) have been used for single crowns as well as for splinted prostheses (Figures 10.12 and 10.13), but no prospective clinical trial data on a reasonable sample of patients/implants have been provided to date.

Modifications in osteotomy preparation for short implant placement

As already mentioned, some investigators have reported good success with short threaded implants of standard diameter with minimal surface roughness with the use of slightly undersized osteotomies to improve initial implant stability.[23,61–63] There are likely limits as to how undersized an osteotomy can be without having untoward local effects on bone healing.[64,65] Using disposable surgical burs also may be of benefit as this ensures the most precise drilling and avoids the risk of overheating bone with dull burs. Degidi et al.[66] reported a significant correlation between final bur diameter and initial implant stability measured by resonance frequency. Avoiding countersinking also may be important, especially in less dense bone.[67,68] With this approach, Renouard and Nisand[23] achieved statistically similar outcomes in posterior maxilla with short, machine-turned (7.4% failure) and short, moderately rough threaded implants (2.4% failure; TiUnite, Nobel Biocare AB, Gothenburg, Sweden) in both standard and wider diameters (Figure 10.14). However, 77% of the implants used were 8.5 mm long; that is, not truly short by their own definition. Mean bone loss after 2 years function was 0.44 mm when all implants (54 machined,

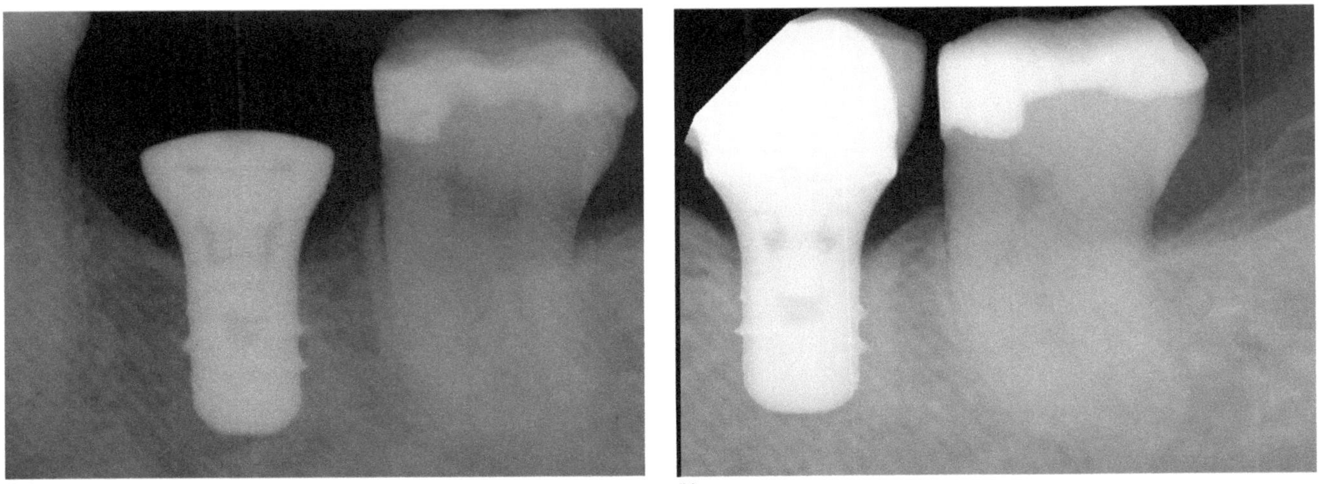

(a) (b)

Figure 10.10 (a) A 6 mm moderately rough implant was used to replace a mandibular first molar tooth. *Source:* Dr Murray Arlin, Toronto, ON, Canada. Reproduced with permission of Dr Arlin. (b) After >7 yrs in function, the implant became symptomatic. A thin radiolucent line can be seen along the mesial aspect of the implant.

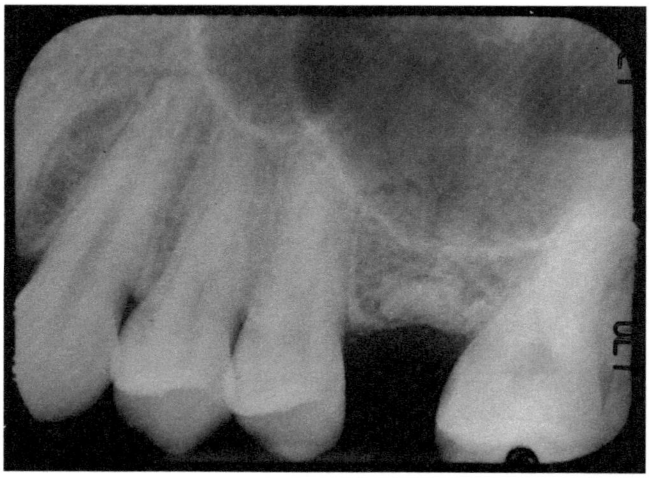

(a)

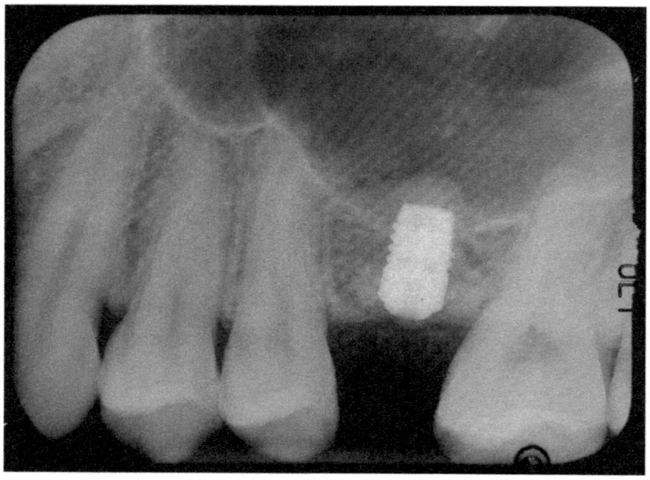

(b)

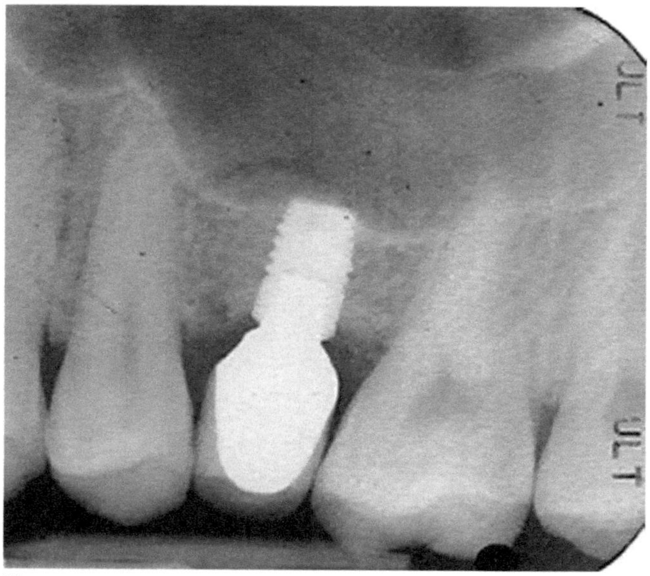

(c)

Figure 10.11 (a) The maxillary first molar was extracted and its socket preserved with grafting. (b) Delayed implant (6 mm × 4 mm AstraTech) placement included a small indirect sinus floor elevation. (c) The radiographic appearance after 2 years in function. *Source*: Dr Suzanne Caudry, Toronto, ON, Canada. Reproduced with permission of Dr Caudry.

42 TiUnite) were considered together. Four implants (details on length and surface finish not provided) showed >2.5 mm bone loss (i.e. ~30% of implant length), but were not considered failures.

Anitua et al.[69] also suggested that slow drilling speeds (50 rpm), apically self-tapping implants, and coating short, moderately rough implants with growth factors may help outcomes. In posterior maxilla, using hand osteotomes to develop implant sites does not appear to be of benefit in increasing bone–implant contact.[70,71] Osteotomes may be of benefit in increasing initial implant stability,[72] although this benefit disappears with time compared with implant sites prepared with burs.[73] One report addressed a possible negative impact of computer-generated surgical guides for short implant placement.[74] Of thirty-eight 6 mm particle-blasted implants thus placed, seven (18.4%) failed to integrate, and the authors suggested that these early failures may have been due to inadequate cooling provided by the external saline irrigation used.

Initial implant stability

Achieving good initial implant stability is dependent on a number of factors, including bone density and implant length/diameter. Ostman et al.[75] reported inadequate initial stability to be a risk in lower density bone in humans, and this conclusion was supported by Marquezan et al.[76] in their review of the topic. These investigators also noted that increasing implant diameter increased initial stability, while increasing implant length decreased it, perhaps due to over-instrumentation for placement of longer implants.

Placing short cylindrical implants in undersized osteotomies by using surgical burs of smaller diameter than the implant is one strategy to overcome their geometric disadvantage.[23,66] Tapered implant designs and self-tapping implants also may have benefit in lower density bone as they result in greater initial stability than cylindrical designs.[77] Using hand osteotomes, either alone or in combination with drilling in the maxilla, also may improve initial implant stability. Primary implant stability in bone of low density, as measured using resonance frequency analysis, was higher following osteotome preparation compared with conventional drilling, and mean insertion torque values also were higher at osteotome-prepared sites.[72] Finally, placing short implants with hand ratchets without pre-tapping also may be effective in achieving adequate initial stability.[31]

Submerged implant healing can be recommended in sites where good initial implant stability is questionable. Jung et al.[78] used a dog model to compare submerged healing with moderately rough threaded implants that had been placed either with standard technique or in such a way that implants showed lack of initial stability. Digital manipulation was used to ensure that the latter group of implants displayed rotational and vertical movements. Both control and unstable implants became osseointegrated based on histometric analyses of retrieved specimens. Some investigators used submerged healing in their clinical studies with short threaded implants,[47,59] while others did not.[23,53,56] Altering bone healing with growth factors, such as platelet-derived growth factor or recombinant human bone morphogenetic protein-2 added to implant surfaces[69,79] or into the final osteotomy site before implant seating, might be another route in optimizing ultimate stability with short implants, but this idea has yet to be fully investigated.

Progressive early implant loading

Some clinicians who report good outcomes with short implants employ provisional prostheses or simply healing abutments to introduce gradual loading meant to produce a reactive increase

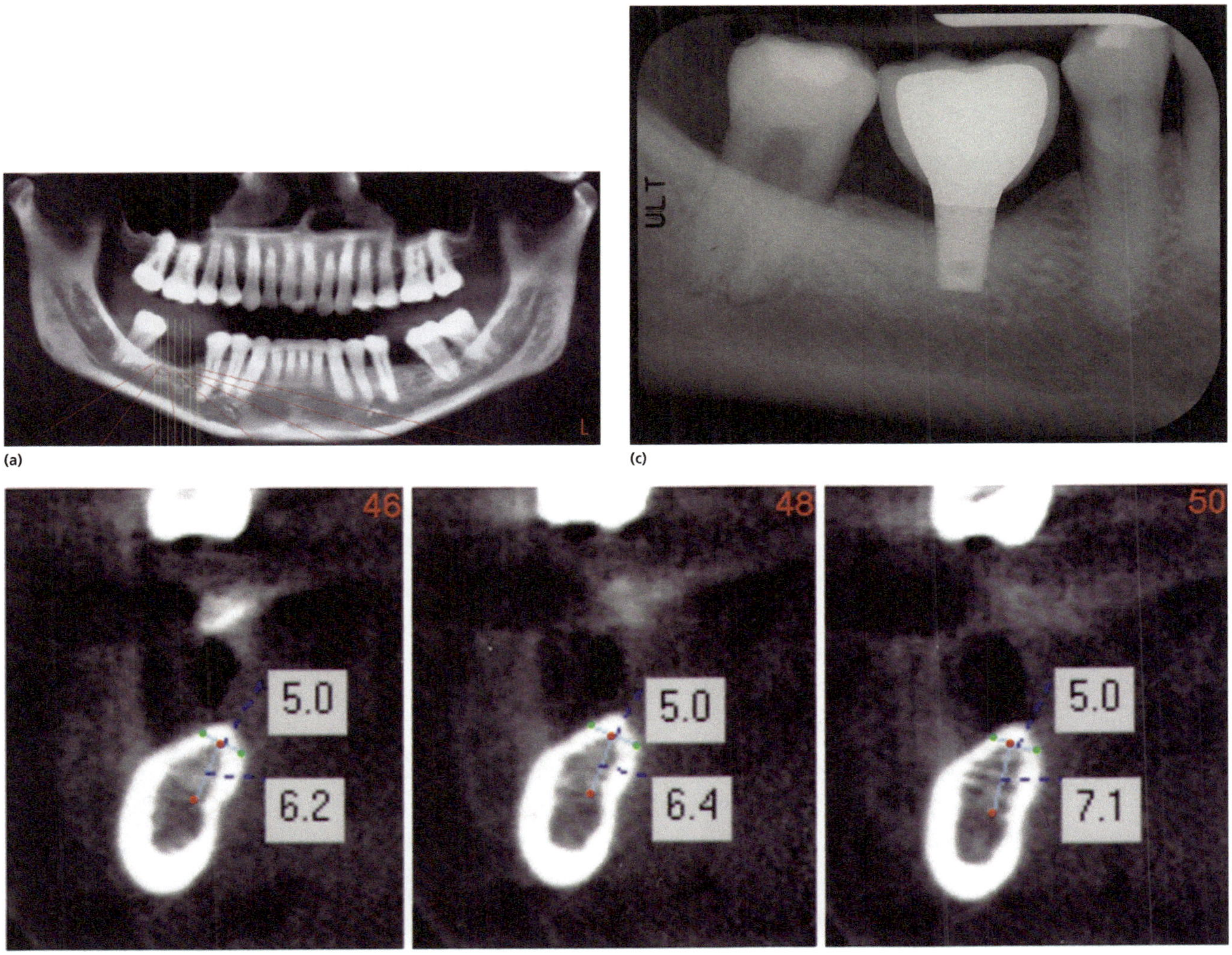

(a) (c) (b)

Figure 10.12 (a) The preoperative panoramic radiograph showing the sites from which the CT scan slices were taken. (b) The intended implant site had 6–7 mm of bone above the mandibular canal. (c) A 5.5 mm SPS implant (4 mm DIL) and diameter 4.1 mm was placed using single-stage protocol and restored after 8 weeks' initial site healing. The radiograph shown was taken after 4 years in function with a single, anatomically correct molar crown. *Source:* Restoration provided by Dr Reynaldo Todescan, Toronto, ON, Canada. Reproduced with permission of Dr Todescan.

in bone density at the implant–bone interface.[80] This was the approach taken by Esposito et al.[53] in their study of 5 mm long × 6 mm diameter threaded implants. Implants were used in groups of two or more, allowed submerged healing, and then connected with provisional splinted prostheses for 4 months before delivery of final splinted prostheses. The same investigators used a progressive loading protocol for 7 mm long, moderately rough threaded implants (NanoTite®, Biomet 3i, Palm Beach, Fl.) placed in posterior mandible.[81] In contrast, Renouard and Nisand[23] did not use provisional prostheses in their study of short, machine-turned or moderately rough (TiUnite) threaded implants. However, they did use a single-stage surgical protocol by adding healing or definitive abutments at implant placement. The healing interval before undertaking prosthesis fabrication was either 3 (TiUnite) or 6 months (machine-turned), and probable inadvertent progressive loading would have occurred during this healing phase, perhaps providing the necessary reactive bone response to optimize bone-to-implant interface density. While progressive loading has been proposed for all threaded designs,[82] it may be particularly relevant for short implants,[30] but no definitive prospective, controlled clinical studies have investigated this possibility.

Minimizing crestal bone loss

Crestal bone loss around endosseous dental implants is the cumulative outcome of many contributing factors, including surgical trauma at implant placement and re-entry, final buccal bone thickness following osteotomy preparation, implant design, length, and diameter, patient habits and general health, prosthetic design, method of prosthesis retention, and more.[83] Most dental implant designs display some initial bone loss or remodeling to allow for the establishment of a "biologic width"; that is, a minimal thickness of fibrous connective tissue meant to form a mucosal barrier separating bone from oral epithelium and bacterial plaque.[84–86] Ideally, this biologic width remodeling will affect only the transgingival collar segment of implants and not the DIL (i.e. osseointegrated implant

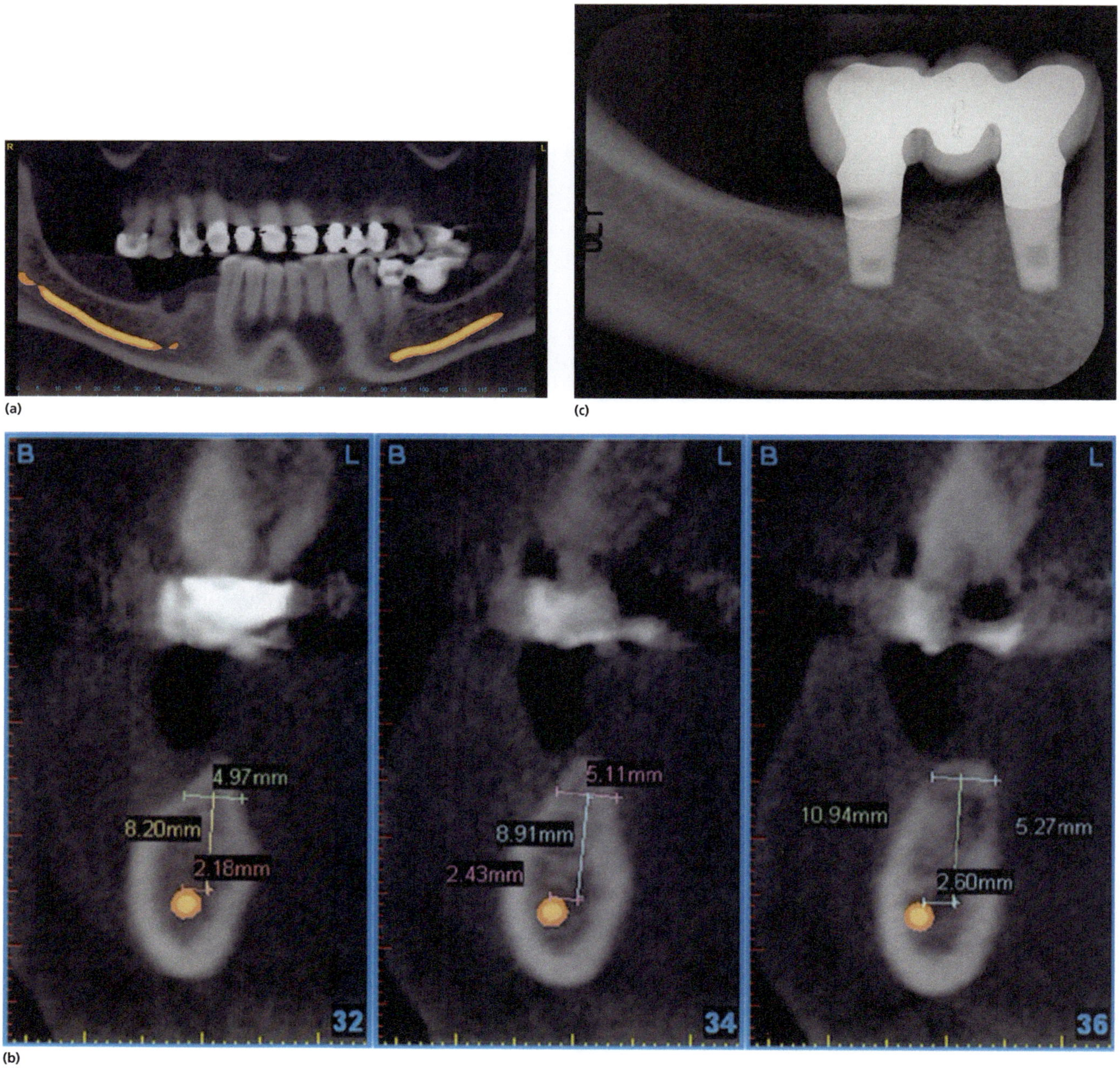

Figure 10.13 (a) The preoperative panorex of a patient requesting an implant-supported restoration in the right posterior mandible. The position of the mandibular canal is colored orange. (b) The CT slices for the intended implant site. An ultrashort (4 mm DIL) SPS implant was used in the distal site while a 7 mm long (5 mm DIL) × 4.1 mm SPS implant was used anteriorly to support this fixed implant-supported three-unit prosthesis. (c) This radiograph was taken after 2 years of implant function. *Source*: Restoration done by Dr Reynaldo Todescan, Toronto, ON, Canada. Reproduced with permission of Dr Todescan.

surface) with its moderately rough to rough surface topography. Three innovative implant design modifications have been directed towards minimizing this DIL-associated crestal bone loss. These include machined coronal microthreads, laser-ablated coronal microgrooves added to the implant neck region, and/or "platform switching." Laser microgrooves and their possible benefits have been described in detail in Chapter 6.

Machined coronal microthreads were first employed in the AstraTech threaded implant device (Figures 10.2 and 10.11). Microthreads appear to offer advantages in minimizing crestal bone loss with additional increased linear length of coronal implant surface available for biologic width accommodation and to allow the reduction of stress transfer in the coronal region.[87] This lower level of stress transfer to crestal bone is less likely to cause bone microfractures and also will reduce the probability for stress-shielding and disuse atrophy of crestal bone as may occur with traditional polished implant collars.[88] Both clinical[89,90] and animal[91] studies have documented good retention of crestal

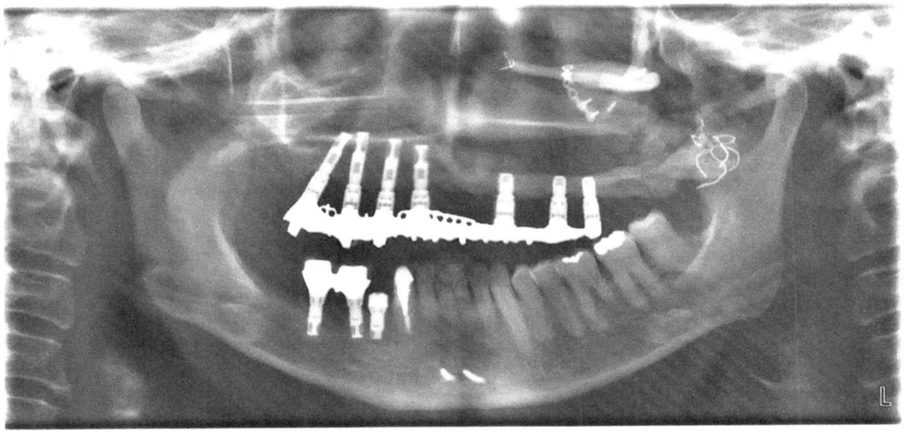

Figure 10.14 This patient had a major jaw resection to eradicate a tumor, leaving minimal bone in the left maxilla. Three 7 mm × 3.75 mm diameter machined implants were placed in grafted bone using a submerged technique as part of a full-arch prosthesis. The panoramic film was taken after 19 years of continuous function. *Source:* Dr Franck Renouard. Reproduced with permission of Dr Renouard.

bone for implants with incorporated microthreads. In a 5-year prospective study of 40 implants with microthreads in 40 patients, Wennström et al.[90] reported that mean cumulative bone loss over 5 years was only 0.11 mm and that about 50% of implants demonstrated zero loss (note that these implants also incorporated platform switching in their design). In a group of 68 patients, Shin et al.[92] compared crestal bone changes in relation to three threaded implant devices, all with different neck designs. One design had coronal microthreads finished with a moderately rough surface. A second design had a particle-blasted flared collar without microthreads, while the third design had a parallel-sided polished collar, again without microthreads. Over the 1 year in function study period, the least crestal bone loss (mean 0.18 mm) was seen with the implant incorporating microthreads, while the greatest bone loss (mean 1.32 mm) was seen with the polished collar design. Lee et al.[93] compared two threaded implant designs from one manufacturer, both with particle-blasted surfaces and platform switching but differing in that one design also had coronal microthreads. The two implant types were placed adjacent to each other in 17 partially edentulous patients, and marginal bone loss was evaluated radiographically over a 3-year period. Bone loss with the microthreaded design was significantly less ($p < 0.01$).

The concept of platform switching as a means of reducing peri-implant crestal bone loss was first noted by Lazzara and Porter.[94] It was defined as the inward horizontal repositioning of the implant–abutment interface ("microgap") by employing a prosthetic abutment approximately 0.5 mm smaller in diameter than the implant itself. This not only shifted the bacteria-inhabited microgap 0.5 mm away from bone around the entire implant periphery, but also created a horizontal component for total linear length of implant collar surface needed for biologic width accommodation.[95] Less bacterial-induced soft tissue inflammation and a reduced requirement for vertical length (by adding horizontal length) of implant surface needed for biologic width will both help to limit crestal bone loss. Platform switching also may have a mechanical advantage by reducing crestal bone stresses.[46,96] Others have confirmed the clinical benefits of platform switching in reducing crestal bone loss,[97–99] but also in improving esthetics by providing better soft tissue support,[100] in minimizing the effect on bone of repeated dis/reconnection of abutments and implants,[101] and in limiting bone loss due to less than ideal proximity of implant-to-implant[102] and implant to natural tooth root.[103] Platform switching, when specifically used with short dental implants, has not been reported with the exception of ultrawide implants,[104] but should only be of benefit since as little as 1 mm of bone loss on a 5 mm long implant will reduce the effective osseointegration by 20%.[53]

Mechanical overload

There can be various reasons why a short implant could suffer mechanical overload and loss of integration. Short implants generally result in long crown-to-implant root ratios (*C*/*R*). As stressed by Fugazzotto,[49] one of the original arguments for using long dental implants was the assumption that they would provide a more favorable *C*/*R*. This assumption was extrapolated from the known impact of *C*/*R* on natural teeth.[105] However, a number of investigators have since shown that *C*/*R* does not appear to be a major contributor to peri-implant crestal bone loss and/or implant failure[36,106–108] with successfully integrated implants. Indeed, one group of investigators reported an inverse relationship; that is, increasing *C*/*R* resulted in less crestal bone loss.[109] However, the majority of implants used in these studies were of standard length, rather than truly short lengths, were primarily placed in posterior mandible where bone tends to be denser, were splinted, and/or were left for protracted initial healing intervals (e.g. 12 months by Schneider et al.[109]) before loading. Splinted implant restorations are known to provide more uniform stress distribution.[110,111]

Rokni et al.'s database[36] comprised a group of patients treated with SPS implants, many of which were 7 mm in length and non-splinted. It was reported that *C*/*R* had no impact on crestal bone levels. Likewise, Tawil et al.[112] found that crestal bone loss was not affected with short, machine-turned threaded implants that had been placed with altered surgical technique so as to improve initial implant stability. However, short implants were considered to be those ≤10 mm in length, were mostly (88.5%) placed in posterior mandible, and again mostly (87%) splinted. Clearly, more data on the impact of *C*/*R* from prospective, long-term studies with truly short (≤8 mm DIL) implants need to be collected.[112] Cases have been reported of short implants simply losing integration after many years in function without signs of crestal bone loss, suggesting mechanical overload as the etiology (Figures 10.10 and 10.15). Gabet et al.[113] offered an explanation for this outcome at the bone–implant interface. A successfully integrated dental implant is connected to a network of peri-implant cancellous bone trabeculae, which are connected to the outer bone cortices.[19] Once an implant is osseointegrated, peri-implant trabeculae are the principal means of stress distribution. Using an animal model including induced

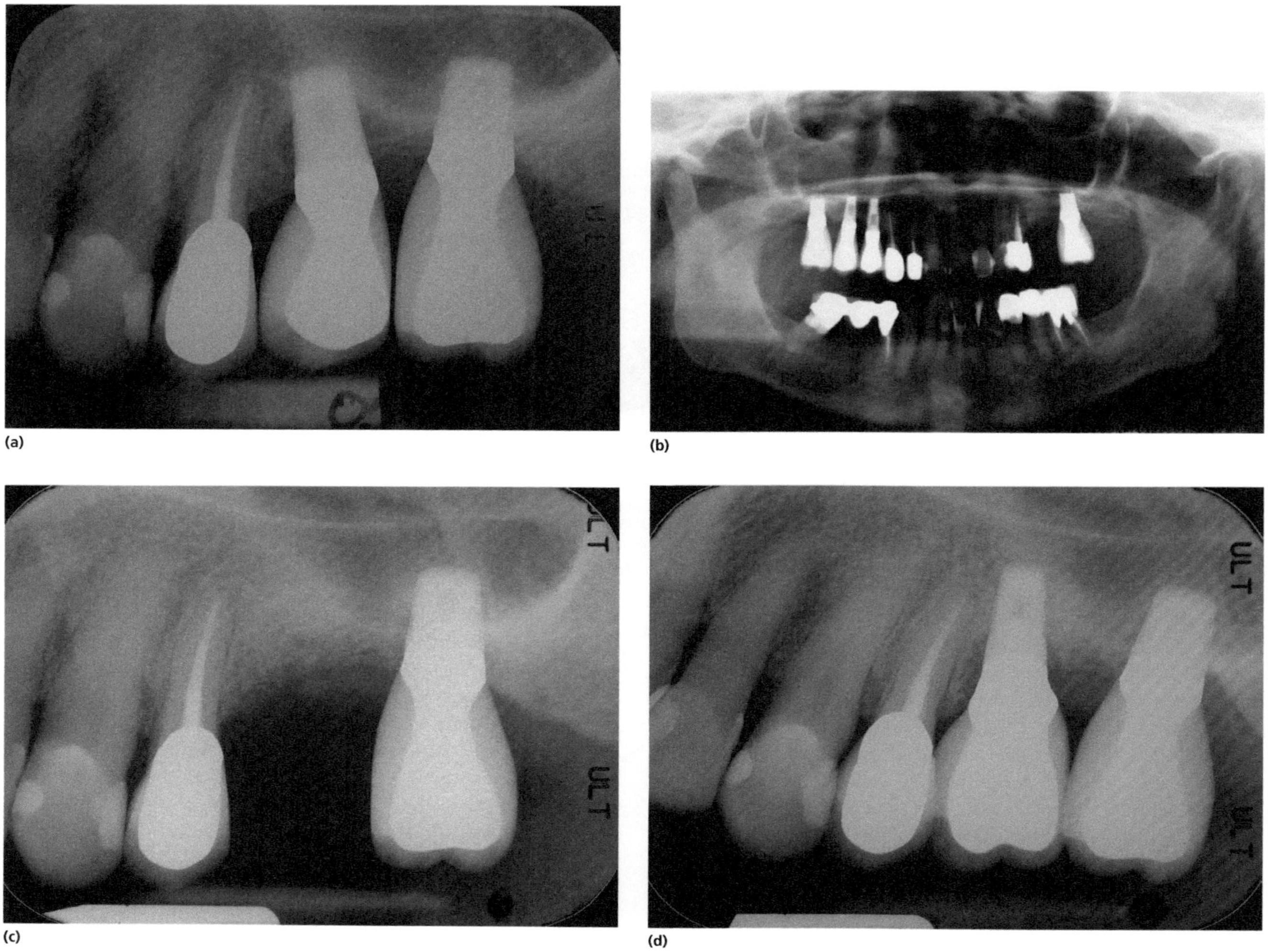

Figure 10.15 (a) The left posterior maxilla received two SPS implants, the more distal of which was "ultrashort" (5 mm × 5 mm with 4 mm DIL). The more mesial implant was 7 mm × 5 mm diameter. Both implants were restored using single crowns by Dr Reynaldo Todescan, Toronto, ON. This radiograph was taken after 7 years in function. The mesial implant has suffered peri-implant bone loss and was determined to be hopeless. (b) The failing implant seen in (a) was extracted and its socket grafted to preserve and develop bone for a replacement implant. (c) During the time needed for site healing, the "ultrashort" distal implant was left free-standing. In this radiograph taken shortly before the replacement implant surgery, a thin radiolucency can be seen surrounding the ultrashort implant length in the regenerated bone. The original native subantral bone height was approximately 2 mm. (d) After site healing, a replacement implant (7 mm × 4.1 mm diameter) was placed and restored with a single crown. At this time, the distal implant had become symptomatic and was removed.

osteoporosis compared with similar animals subsequently administered parathyroid hormone to increase bone density (i.e. to increase trabecular thickness), Gabet et al.[113] concluded that osseointegrated implants may fail under excessive load because of bending forces affecting weak trabeculae in the immediate (0.5–1.0 mm) peri-implant vicinity. Sotto-Maior et al.[30] suggested that occlusal overload may be the most important stress concentration factor for single posterior implant crowns supported by short (7 mm long × 5 mm diameter) threaded implants. Tawil et al.[112] showed a case of a two-unit fixed, implant-supported prosthesis in posterior mandible in which the more distal, short (7 mm × 3.75 mm diameter), machined implant lost integration after 7 years. No radiographic evidence of bone loss or infection was found.

A case study of implant failure probably due to mechanical overload is demonstrated in Figure 10.15. This patient received SPS implants bilaterally in her posterior maxilla in 1998. The most distal implants on each side were ultrashort (5 mm × 5 mm with 4 mm DIL). There was approximately 2 mm of remaining subantral bone at these two sites; therefore, the ultrashort implants were largely seated into bovine xenograft material following indirect sinus elevation. The implants were allowed 6 (left side) to 8 months (right side) of submerged healing, and ultimately received nonsplinted crowns. The *C*/*R* for the two ultrashort implants was 3 : 1. The ultrashort implant in right maxilla has continued to function without issue (Figure 10.15b). However, in 2008 after 9 years in function, the more mesial implant (7 mm × 5 mm diameter) on the right side became symptomatic. Review of the records indicated that an isolated 6 mm palatal pocket with bleeding on probing had been detected on this implant 6 months following crown insertion. The pocket could not be detected on later visits. At the 2008 recall, extensive peri-implant bone loss could be seen on the radiograph (Figure 10.15a), and the implant was scheduled for removal and replacement. After removal of the failed implant, the posterior "ultrashort" implant restoration remained during the healing interval (Figure 10.15b and c), possibly resulting in mechanical overload during the extended (>1 year) healing period. Shortly after the anterior replacement implant went into function, the "ultrashort" implant lost its integration and had to be removed (Figure 10.15d). There had been no radiographic changes; on implant removal, its socket lining was observed to be whitish and granular with almost no bleeding, suggesting a predominance of incorporated xenograft particles. In retrospect, it may have been wiser to have removed the screw-retained crown from this implant and replaced it with a healing abutment for the treatment interval.

Conclusions

Accumulating data support the conclusion that short (DIL ≤8mm) dental implants can be of value provided that certain key factors in implant design and surgical and prosthetic management are respected. Most data available suggest that short threaded implants likely perform better in posterior mandible than posterior maxilla because of differences in bone density at these two sites. Good initial implant stability is crucial, and may be improved with slightly undersized osteotomies, avoiding countersinking, and/or placing the implants using hand ratchets without pre-tapping in less dense bone. Every attempt should be made to minimize crestal bone loss through the use of wider diameter implants, platform switching, implant neck design features such as microthreads or laser microgrooves, splinted prostheses (or tooth-protected sites with single implant crowns), and/or progressive implant loading protocols. Nevertheless, the number of long-term clinical studies with truly short implants including close monitoring of the possibility of progressive late bone loss is limited. For the present, clinicians wishing to employ short threaded implants might be wise to employ the considerations reviewed in this chapter.

References

1. Van Steenberghe D, Lekholm U, Bolender C, et al. The applicability of osseointegrated oral implants in the rehabilitation of partial edentulism: a prospective multicenter study of 558 fixtures. Int J Oral Maxillofac Implants 1990; 5: 272–281.
2. Wyatt C, Zarb G. Treatment outcomes of patients with implant-supported fixed partial prostheses. Int J Oral Maxillofac Implants 1998; 13: 204–211.
3. Winkler S, Morris H, Ochi S. Implant survival to 36 months as related to length and diameter. Ann Periodontol 2000; 5: 22–31.
4. Weng D, Jacobson Z, Tarnow D, et al. A prospective multicenter clinical of 3i machined-surface implants. Results after 6 years of follow-up. Int J Oral Maxillofac Implants 2003; 18: 417–423.
5. Geurs N, Wang I-C, Shulman L, Jeffcoat M. Retrospective radiographic analysis of sinus graft and implant placement procedures from the Academy of Osseointegration Consensus Conference on Sinus Grafts. Int J Periodontics Restorative Dent 2001; 21: 517–523.
6. Albrektsson T, Wennerberg A. Oral implant surfaces: part I: review focusing on topographic and chemical properties of different surfaces and *in vivo* responses to them. Int J Prosthodont 2004; 17: 536–543.
7. Renouard R, Nisand D. Impact of implant length and diameter on survival rates. Clin Oral Implants Res 2006; 17(Suppl 2): 35–51.
8. Misch CE. Short versus long implant concepts – functional surface area. Dent Today 1999; 18(8): 60–65.
9. Wennerberg A, Ektessabi A, Albrektsson T, et al. A 1-year follow-up of implants of differing surface roughness placed in rabbit bone. Int J Oral Maxillofac Implants 1997; 12: 486–494.
10. Klokkevold P, Johnson P, Dadgostari S, et al. Early endosseous integration enhanced by dual acid etching of titanium: a torque removal study in the rabbit. Clin Oral Implants Res 2001; 12: 350–357.
11. Rangert B, Krogh P, Langer B, van Roekel N. Bending overload and implant fracture. A retrospective clinical analysis. Int J Oral Maxillofac Implants 1995; 10: 326–334.
12. Pilliar R, Shagal G, Meguid S, et al. Threaded vs porous-surfaced implants as anchorage units for orthodontic treatment: 3-D finite element analysis of peri-implant bone tissue stresses. Int J Oral Maxillofac Implants 2006; 21: 879–889.
13. Hagi D, Deporter DA, Pilliar RM, et al. A targeted review of study outcomes with short (≤7 mm) endosseous dental implants placed in partially edentulous patients. J Periodontol 2004; 75: 798–804.
14. Pierrisnard L, Renouard F, Renault P, Barquins M. Influence of implant length and bicortical anchorage on implant stress distribution. Clin Implant Dent Relat Res 2003; 5: 254–262.
15. Bernard J-P, Szmukler-Moncler S, Pessotto S, et al. The anchorage of Brånemark and ITI implants of different lengths. I. An experimental study in the canine mandible. Clin Oral Implants Res 2003; 14: 593–600.
16. Ten Bruggenkate C, Asikainen P, Foitzik C, et al. Short (6 mm) non-submerged dental implants: results of a multicenter clinical trial of 1 to 7 years. Int J Oral Maxillofac Implants 1998; 13: 791–798.
17. Astrand P, Engquist B, Anzen B, et al. A three-year follow-up report of a comparative study of ITI® Dental implants and Brånemark system implants in the treatment of the partially edentulous maxilla. Clin Implant Dent Relat Res 2004; 6: 130–141.
18. Elkhoury J, McGlumphy E, Tatakis D, Beck M. Clinical parameters associated with success and failure of single-tooth titanium plasma-sprayed cylindric implants under stricter criteria: a 5-year retrospective study. Int J Oral Maxillofac Implants 2005; 20: 687–694.
19. Davies J. Understanding peri-implant endosseous healing. J Dent Educ 2003; 67: 932–949.
20. Khang W, Feldman S, Hawley CE, Gunsolley J. A multi-center study comparing dual acid-etched and machined-surfaced implants in various bone qualities. J Periodontol 2001; 72: 1384–1390.
21. Fugazzotto P, Beagle J, Ganeles J, et al. Success and failure rates of 9 mm or shorter implants in the replacement of missing maxillary molars when restored with individual crowns: preliminary results 0 to 84 months in function. A retrospective study. J Periodontol 2004; 75: 327–332.
22. Nedir R, Bischof M, Briaux J-M, et al. A 7-year life table analysis from a prospective study of ITI implants with special emphasis on the use of short implants. Results from a private practice. Clin Oral Implant Res 2004; 15: 150–157.
23. Renouard F, Nisand D. Short implants in the severely resorbed maxilla: a 2-year retrospective clinical study. Clin Implant Dent Relat Res 2005; 7: s104–s110.
24. Arlin M. Short dental implants as a treatment option: results from an observational study in a single private practice. Int J Oral Maxillofac Implants 2006; 21: 769–776.
25. Olate S, Lyrio M, de Moraes M, et al. Influence of diameter and length of implant on early dental implant failure. J Oral Maxillofac Surg 2010; 68: 414–419.
26. Pommer B, Frantal S, Willer J, et al. Impact of dental implant length on early failure rates: a meta-analysis of observational studies. J Clin Periodontol 2011; 38(9): 856–863.
27. Telleman G, Raghoebar G, Vissink A, et al. A systematic review of the prognosis of short (<10 mm) dental implants placed in the partially edentulous patient. J Clin Periodontol 2011; 38: 667–676.
28. Sogo M, Ikebe K, Yang T-C, et al. Assessment of bone density in the posterior maxilla based on Hounsfield units to enhance the initial stability of implants. Clin Implant Dent Relat Res 2012; 14(Suppl 1): e183–e187.
29. Misch CE, Steigenga J, Barboza E, et al. Short dental implants in posterior edentulism: a multicenter retrospective 6-year case series study. J Periodontol 2006; 77: 1340–1347.
30. Sotto-Maior B, Senna P, da Silva W, et al. Influence of crown-to-implant ratio, retention system, restorative material, and occlusal loading on stress concentrations in single short implants. Int J Oral Maxillofac Implants 2012; 27: e13–e18.
31. Lai H-C, Si M-S, Zhuang L-F, et al. Long-term outcomes of short dental implants supporting single crowns in posterior region: a clinical retrospective study of 5–10 years. Clin Oral Implants Res 2013; 24: 230–237.
32. Deporter D, Todescan R, Caudry S. Simplifying management of the posterior maxilla using short porous-surfaced dental implants and simultaneous indirect sinus elevation. Int J Periodontics Restorative Dent 2000; 20: 477–485.
33. Deporter D, Watson P, Pharoah M, et al. Ten-year results of a prospective study using porous-surfaced dental implants and a mandibular overdenture. Clin Implant Dent Relat Res 2002; 4: 183–189.
34. Deporter D, Caudry S, Kermalli J, Adegbembo A. Further data on the predictability of the indirect sinus elevation procedure used with short sintered porous-surfaced dental implants. Int J Periodontics Restorative Dent 2005; 25: 585–593.
35. Deporter D, Ogiso B, Sohn D-S, et al. "Ultrashort" sintered porous-surfaced dental implants used to replace posterior teeth: a case series report. J Periodontol 2008; 79: 1280–1286.
36. Rokni S, Todescan R, Watson P, et al. An assessment of crown-to-root ratios with short sintered porous-surfaced implants supporting prostheses in partially edentulous patients. Int J Oral Maxillofac Implants 2005; 20: 69–76.

37. Deporter D, Todescan R, Riley N. Porous-surfaced dental implants in the partially edentulous maxilla. Assessment of subclinical mobility. Int J Periodontics Restorative Dent 2002; 22: 185–192.
38. Deporter D, Pharoah M, Yeh S, et al. Performance of titanium alloy sintered porous-surfaced (SPS) implants supporting mandibular overdentures during a 20-year prospective study. Clin Oral Implants Res 2014; 25: e189–e195.
39. Deporter D, Kermalli J, Todescan R, Atenafu E. Performance of sintered porous-surfaced press-fit implants after 10 or more years of function in the partially edentulous posterior mandible. Int J Periodontics Restorative Dent 2012, 32: 563–570.
40. Deporter, D. Dental implant design and optimal treatment outcomes. Int J Periodontics Restorative Dent 2009; 29: 625–633.
41. Deporter, D. Harnessing advantages and avoiding risks with sintered porous-surfaced dental implants. J Clin Pract Oral Implantol 2010; 1(2): 17–24.
42. Qahash M, Susin C, Polimeni G, et al. Bone healing dynamics at buccal peri-implant sites. Clin Oral Implants Res 2008; 19: 166–172.
43. Himmlova L, Dostalova T, Kacovsky A, Konvickova S. Influence of implant length and diameter on stress distribution: a finite element analysis. J Prosthetic Dent 2004; 91: 20–25.
44. Anitua E, Tapia R, Luzuriaga F, Orive G. Influence of implant length, diameter and geometry on stress distribution: a finite element analysis. Int J Periodontics Restorative Dent 2010; 30: 89–95.
45. Brink J, Meraw S, Sarment D. Influence of implant diameter on surrounding bone. Clin Oral Implant Res 2007; 18: 563–568.
46. Baggi L, Cappelloni I, Di Girolamo M, et al. The influence of implant diameter and length on stress distribution of osseointegrated implants related to crestal bone geometry: a three-dimensional finite element analysis. J Prosthetic Dent 2008; 100: 422–431.
47. Tawil G, Younan R. Clinical evaluation of short, machine-surface implants followed for 12 to 92 months. Int J Oral Maxillofac Implants 2003; 18: 894–901.
48. Gentile M, Chuang S-K, Dodson T. Survival estimates and risk factors for failure with 6 × 5.7 mm implants. Int J Oral Maxillofac Implants 2005; 20: 930–937.
49. Fugazzotto P. Shorter implants in clinical practice: rationale and treatment results. Int J Oral Maxillofac Implants 2008; 23: 487–496.
50. Vandenweghe S, Ackermann A, Bronner J, et al. A retrospective, multicenter study on a novo wide-body implant for posterior regions. Clin Implant Dent Relat Res 2012; 14: 281–292.
51. Lombardo G, Corrocher G, Trevisiol L, et al. Impianti ultracorti a sinterizzata: analisi della stabilità dell'osso crestale a distanza di 2 anni dal carico. Implantologia 2010; 2: 13–30.
52. Perelli M, Abundo R, Corrente G, Saccone C. Short (5 and 7 mm long) porous implants in the posterior atrophic maxilla: a 5-year report of a prospective single-cohort study. Eur J Oral Implantol 2012; 5: 265–272.
53. Esposito M, Pellegrino G, Pistilli R, Felice P. Rehabilitation of posterior atrophic edentulous jaws: prostheses supported by 5 mm short implants or by longer implants in augmented bone? One-year results from a pilot randomized clinical trial. Eur J Oral Implantol 2011; 4: 21–30.
54. Yoon K-H, Kim S-G, Lee J-H, Suh S-W. 3-D finite element analysis of changes in stress levels and distributions for an osseointegrated implant after vertical bone loss. Implant Dent 2011; 20: 354–359.
55. Urdaneta R, Daher S, Leary J, et al. The survival of ultrashort locking-taper implants. Int J Oral Maxillofac Implants 2012; 27: 644–654.
56. Rossi F, Ricci E, Marchetti C, et al. Early loading of single crowns supported by 6-mm-long implants with a moderately rough surface: a prospective 2-year follow-up cohort study. Clin Oral Implants Res 2010; 21: 937–943.
57. Slotte C, Gronningsaeter A, Halmoy A-M, et al. Four-millimeter implants supporting fixed partial dental prostheses in the severely resorbed posterior mandible: two-year results. Clin Implant Dent Relat Res 2012; 14(Suppl 1): e46–e58.
58. Albrektsson T, Zarb G, Worthington P, Eriksson A. The long-term efficiency of currently used dental implants. A review and proposed criteria of success. Int J Periodontics Restorative Dent 1986; 1: 11–25.
59. Gulje F, Raghoebar G, Ter Meulen J-W, et al. Mandibular overdentures supported by 6-mm dental implants: a 1-year prospective cohort study. Clin Implant Dent Relat Res 2012; 14: e359–e366.
60. Clelland N, Seidt J, Daroz L, McGlumphy E. Comparison of strains for splinted and nonsplinted implant prostheses using three-dimensional image correlation. Int J Oral Maxillofac Implants 2010; 25: 953–959.
61. Calandriello R, Tomatis M, Rangert B. Immediate functional loading of Brånemark System® implants with enhanced initial stability: a prospective 1- to 2-year clinical and radiographic study. Clin Implant Dent Relat Res 2003; 5(Suppl 1): 10–20.
62. Ostman P-O, Hellman M, Sennerby L. Immediate occlusal loading of implants in the partially edentulous mandible: a prospective 1-year radiographic and 4-year clinical study. Int J Oral Maxillofac Implants 2008; 23: 315–322.
63. Blanco J, Alvarez E, Munoz F, et al. Influence on early osseointegration of dental implants installed with two different drilling protocols: a histomorphometric study in rabbit. Clin Oral Implant Res 2010; 22: 92–99.
64. Tabassum A, Meijer G, Walboomers X, Jansen J. Biological limits of the undersized surgical technique: a study in goats. Clin Oral Implant Res 2011; 22: 129–134.
65. Nevins M, Nevins ML, Schupbach P, et al. The impact of bone compression on bone-to-implant contact of an osseointegrated implant: a canine study. Int J Periodontics Restorative Dent 2012; 32: 637–645.
66. Degidi M, Daprile G, Piattelli A, Carinci F. Evaluation of factors influencing resonance frequency analysis values, at insertion surgery, of implants placed in sinus-augmented and non-grafted sites. Clin Implant Dent Relat Res 2007; 9: 144–149.
67. Vidyasagar L, Salms G, Apse P, Teibe U. The influence of site preparation (countersinking) on initial dental implant stability. An *in vitro* study using resonance frequency analysis. Stomatologija Baltic Dent Maxillofac J 2004; 6: 14–16.
68. Das Neves F, Fomes D, Bernardes S, et al. Short implants: an analysis of longitudinal studies. Int J Oral Maxillofac Implants 2006; 21: 86–94.
69. Anitua E, Orive G, Aguirre J, Andia I. Five-year clinical evaluation of short dental implants placed in posterior areas: a retrospective study. J Periodontol 2008; 79: 42–48.
70. Buchter A, Kleinheinz J, Wiesmann H, et al. Interface reaction at dental implants inserted in condensed bone. Clin Oral Implants Res 2005; 16: 509–517.
71. Shalabi M, Wolke J, Ruijter A, Jansen J. Histological evaluation of oral implants inserted with different surgical techniques into the trabecular bone of goats. Clin Oral Implants Res 2007; 18: 489–495.
72. Nobrega A, Norton A, Silva JA, et al. The osteotome versus conventional drilling technique for implant site preparation: a comparative study in the rabbit. Int J Periodontics Restorative Dent 2012; 32: e109–e115.
73. Shayesteh Y, Khojasteh A, Siadat H, et al. A comparative study of crestal bone loss and implant stability between osteotome and conventional implant insertion techniques: a randomized controlled clinical trial study. Clin Implant Dent Relat Res 2013; 15(3): 350–357.
74. Kennedy K, Jones E, Kim D-G, et al. A prospective clinical study to evaluate early success of short implants. Int J Oral Maxillofac Implants 2013; 28: 170–177.
75. Ostman P-O, Hellman M, Wendelhag I, Sennerby L. Resonance frequency analysis measurements of implants at placement surgery. Int J Prosthodont 2006; 19: 77–83.
76. Marquezan M, Osorio A, Sant'Anna E, Souza M, Maia L. Does bone mineral density influence the primary stability of dental implants? A systematic review. Clin Oral Implants Res 2012; 23: 767–774.
77. O'Sullivan D, Sennerby L, Meredith N. Influence of implant taper on the primary and secondary stability of osseointegrated titanium implants. Clin Oral Implant Res 2004; 15: 474–480.
78. Jung U-W, Kim S, Kim Y-H, et al. Osseointegration of dental implants installed without mechanical engagement: a histometric analysis in dogs. Clin Oral Implants Res 2011; 00: 1–5.
79. Simon Z, Deporter D, Pilliar R, Clokie C. Heterotopic bone formation around sintered porous-surfaced Ti-6A1-4V implants coated with native bone morphogenetic proteins. Implant Dent 2006; 15: 265–274.
80. Stanford C, Brand R. Toward an understanding of implant occlusion and strain adaptive bone modeling and remodeling. J Prosthetic Dent 1999; 81: 553–561.
81. Felice P, Checchi B, Pistilli R, et al. Bone augmentation versus 5-mm dental implants in posterior atrophic jaws. Four-month post-loading results from a randomized controlled clinical study. Eur J Oral Implantol 2009; 2: 267–281.
82. Misch C. Progressive bone loading. In: Contemporary Implant Dentistry, 2nd ed., MischC, ed. St. Louis, MO: Mosby, 1999, pp. 595–608.
83. Ketabi M, Pilliar R, Deporter D. Factors driving peri-implant crestal bon loss: a concise literature review and discussion: part I. J Implant Adv Clin Dent 2009; 1(2): 19–27.
84. Abrahamsson I, Berglundh T, Wennstrom J, Lindhe J. The peri-implant hard and soft tissues at different implant systems. A comparative study in the dog. Clin Oral Implants Res 1996; 7: 212–219.
85. Berglundh T, Lindhe J. Dimension of the peri-implant mucosa. Biological width revisited. J Clin Periodontol 1996; 23: 971–973.
86. Deporter D, Al-Sayyed A, Pilliar RM, Valiquette N. "Biologic width" and crestal bone remodeling with sintered porous-surfaced dental implants. A study in dogs. Int J Oral Maxillofac Implants 2008; 23: 544–550.
87. Hansson S. The implant neck: smooth or provided with retention elements. A biomechanical approach. Clin Oral Implant Res 1999; 10: 394–405.
88. Wiskott H, Belser U. Lack of integration of smooth titanium surfaces: a working hypothesis based on strains generated in the surrounding bone. Clin Oral Implant Res 1999; 10: 429–444.
89. Palmer R, Palmer P, Smith B. A 5-year prospective study of Astra single tooth implants. Clin Oral Implant Res 2000; 11: 179–182.
90. Wennström J, Ekestubbe A. Gröndahl K, et al. Implant-supported single-tooth restorations. A 5 year prospective study. J Clin Periodont 2005; 32: 567–574.
91. Abrahamsson I, Berglundh T. Tissue characteristics at micro-threaded implants: an experimental study in dogs. Clin Implant Dent Relat Res 2006; 8: 107–113.

92. Shin Y, Han C, Heo S, et al. Radiographic evaluation of marginal bone level around implants with different neck designs after 1 year. Int J Oral Maxillofac Implants 2006; 21: 789–794.
93. Lee D, Choi Y, Park K, et al. Effect of micro-thread on the maintenance of marginal bone level: a 3-year prospective study. Clin Oral Implant Res 2007; 18: 465–470.
94. Lazzara R, Porter S. Platform switching: a new concept in implant dentistry for controlling post-restorative crestal bone levels. Int J Periodontics Restorative Dent 2006; 26: 9–17.
95. Vela-Nebot X, Rodríguez-Ciurana X, Rodado-Alonso C, Segalà-Torres M. Benefits of an implant platform modification technique to reduce crestal bone resorption. Implant Dent 2006; 15: 313–320.
96. Maeda Y, Miura J, Taki I, Sogo M. Biomechanical analysis on platform-switching: is there any biomechanical rationale? Clin Oral Implant Res 2007; 18: 581–584.
97. Cappiello M, Luongo R, Di Lorio D, et al. Evaluation of peri-implant bone loss around platform-switched implants. Int J Periodontics Restorative Dent 2008; 28: 347–355.
98. Cannullo L, Fedele G, Iannello G, Jepsen S. Platform switching and marginal bone-level alterations: the results of a randomized-controlled trial. Clin Oral Implants Res 2010; 21: 115–121.
99. Calvo-Guirado J, Gomez-Moreno G, Lopez L, et al. Crestal bone loss evaluation in Osseotite expanded platform implants: a 5-year study. Clin Oral Implants Res 2011; 22: 1409–1414.
100. Gardner D. Platform switching as a means to achieving implant esthetics. N Y State Dent J 2005; 71: 34–37.
101. Rodriguez-Ciurana X, Vela-Nebot X, Mendez V, et al. The effect of abutment dis/reconnection on peri-implant bone resorption: a radiologic study of platform-switched and non-platform-switched implants in animals. Clin Oral Implants Res 2013; 24(3): 305–311.
102. Rodriguez-Ciurana X, Vela-Nebot X, Mendez V, et al. The effect of inter-implant distance on the height of the inter-implant bone crest when using platform-switched implants. Int J Periodontics Restorative Dent 2009; 29: 141–151.
103. Vela X, Mendez V, Rodriguez X, et al. Crestal bone changes on platform-switched implants and adjacent teeth when the tooth-implant distance is less than 1.5 mm. Int J Periodontics Restorative Dent 2012; 32: 149–155.
104. Vandeweghe S, De Bruyn H. A within-implant comparison to evaluate the concept of platform switching. A randomized, controlled study. Eur J Oral Implantol 2012; 5: 253–262.
105. Grossman Y, Sadan A. The prosthodontic concept of crown-to-root ratio: a review of the literature. J Prosthetic Dent 2005; 93: 559–562.
106. Blanes R. To what extent does the crown-to-root ratio affect the survival and complications of implant-supported reconstructions? A systematic review. Clin Oral Implants Res 2009; 20(Suppl 4): 67–72.
107. Salvi G, Bragger U. Mechanical and technical risks in implant therapy. Int J Oral Maxillofac Implants 2009; 24(Suppl): 69–85.
108. Blanes R, Bernard J, Blanes Z, Belser U. A 10-year prospective study of ITI dental implants placed in the posterior region. II. Influence of the crown-to-implant ratio and different prosthetic treatment modalities on crestal bone loss. Clin Oral Implants Res 2007; 18: 707–714.
109. Schneider D, Witt L, Hammerle C. Influence of the crown-to-root length ratio on the clinical performance of implants supporting single crown restorations: a cross-sectional retrospective 5-year investigation. Clin Oral Implants Res 2012; 23: 169–174.
110. Guichet D, Yoshinobu D, Caputo A. Effect of splinting and interproximal contact tightness on load transfer by implant restorations. J Prosthetic Dent 2002; 87: 528–535.
111. Kim Y, Oh T-J, Misch C, Wang H-L. Occlusal considerations in implant therapy; clinical guidelines with biomechanical rationale. Clin Oral Implants Res 2005; 16: 26–35.
112. Tawil G, Aboujaoude N, Younan R. Influence of prosthetic parameters on the survival and complication rates of short implants. Int J Oral Maxillofac Implants 2006; 21: 275–282.
113. Gabet Y, Kohavi D, Voide R, et al. Endosseous implant anchorage is critically dependent on mechanostructural determinants of peri-implant bone trabeculae. J Bone Miner Res 2010; 25: 575–583.

CHAPTER 11

Narrow Implants

Joerg Neugebauer,[1] Douglas Deporter,[2] and Daniel R. Cullum[3]
[1]Department of Craniomaxillofacial and Plastic Surgery, University of Cologne, Cologne, Germany
[2]Discipline of Periodontics, Faculty of Dentistry, University of Toronto, Toronto, ON, Canada
[3]Private Practice Coeur d'Alene, ID; Loma Linda University Department of OMS, Loma Linda, CA; UCLA Department of OMS, Los Angeles, CA, USA

Introduction

Narrow-diameter dental implants (NDIs) have been defined as those with diameters ≤3.5 mm.[1] Those with diameters ≤2.7 mm have also been termed "mini" dental implants (MDIs).[2] Both have been proposed for sites where considerable loss of bucco-lingual ridge width prevents the placement of standard-diameter implants (SDIs); that is, those having diameters of at least 3.75 mm. NDIs also can prove useful in narrow inter-radicular sites between two teeth, such as with single mandibular incisors or maxillary lateral incisors,[3,4] or in sites with congenitally missing lateral incisors and underdeveloped bucco-palatal ridge width.[5] Traditionally, sites with reduced bucco-lingual palatal ridge width were approached with pre-implant surgical augmentation using autogenous block grafts or guided bone regeneration procedures followed by delayed SDI placement. Alternatively, SDIs have been placed using ridge-splitting procedures at the time of implant placement. While these procedures to increase alveolar ridge width are all widely used, they do increase the complexity, trauma, invasiveness, and sometimes the cost of treatment. Therefore, NDIs can offer clear advantages for the clinician and patient favoring minimally invasive treatment.

Literature review

MDIs and NDIs were initially used as transitional implants rather than for the support of final prosthetic restorations. For example, Froum et al.[6] used immediately loaded, 1.8 mm diameter threaded implants to support fixed temporary prostheses during the time required for permanent SDIs to become osseointegrated with submerged, undisturbed healing. Others recommended the use of NDIs to give some support to transitional mandibular overdentures.[7] This, of course, was generally before the concept of immediate loading of SDIs came into existence. However, it was subsequently observed that NDIs might be considered in certain situations to support definitive prostheses as well.

In a retrospective report, Olate et al.[8] documented an inverse relationship between implant diameter and early implant failure (i.e. before implant loading) following submerged site healing. Implants of 3.5 mm diameter failed at a rate of 5.1% compared with 2.7% for larger diameter implants, although a significant cofactor may have been bone density. Baqain et al.[9] reported a similar inverse relationship in a prospective study of early implant failure. Not surprisingly then, Quesada-Garcia et al.[10] reported that implant diameter had a significant impact on implant stability as measured by resonance frequency (measured in implant stability quotient (ISQ) units) after 12 weeks of site healing. NDIs had the smallest ISQ values, while implants placed in maxilla had significantly lower ISQ values than those placed in mandible. Others have shown when using 3.5 mm diameter implants that there is a strong correlation between crestal cortical bone thickness (determined by computed tomography (CT) imaging) and initial implant stability (measured by resonance frequency analysis as ISQ values).[11] These results showed significantly higher implant stability (ISQ values) with NDIs in mandible compared with maxilla, as confirmed by others.[10] Thickness of cortical bone was actually found to be more important than implant length in achieving initial implant stability with NDIs.[11] Review papers investigating outcomes with functional NDIs generally show high survival rates (>90%), likely reflecting careful case selection, operator experience, and appropriate bone density.[1,12]

The main concern with NDIs is that reduced implant diameter will increase the strain on crestal bone with the possibility of mechanical overload and loss of crestal bone and osseointegration. Anitua et al.[13] studied the impact on stress to peri-implant bone with implant diameters of 2.5–5.0 mm using 3-D finite element analysis (FEA) studies. Increasing implant diameter from 2.5 to 3.3 mm reduced bone stresses by 30.7%. Likewise, the maximum stress on bone with implant diameter 3.3 mm was 28.2% higher than with 4.0 mm diameter. However, implant diameter may have different effects in the maxilla than in the mandible. Some FEA studies suggest that increasing implant diameter reduces crestal bone stresses in mandible, while in maxilla the bone stress is reduced with longer implant lengths.[14,15] Regardless of implant diameter, bone stress was always greatest in the cortical bone around the implant neck and decreased more apically. Decrease in cortical bone thickness may lead to increased bone stresses.[15] The greatest stress was always seen in the most coronal five to six threads regardless of implant diameter.[13,16] Insertion depth may also play a role, with strain on crestal bone decreasing as implant insertion depth increases (from supracrestal to crestal to subcrestal implant positioning).[14,17] One FEA study suggested that, to minimize unfavorable bone and implant stresses, NDIs should be inserted so that the most coronal threads are positioned well below the cortical bone crest.[18] Clinically, however, the role of biologic width and remodeling secondary to implant–abutment connection, macrodesign, crestal microthreads, and laser surface treatment would have to be considered for the long-term stability of the peri-implant bone and soft tissue.

Minimally Invasive Dental Implant Surgery, First Edition. Edited by Daniel R. Cullum and Douglas Deporter.

An appropriate situation for consideration of NDIs appears to be in the retention of mandibular overdentures in completely edentulous patients with adequate alveolar ridge height but unfavorable bucco-lingual ridge width. Zinsli et al.[19] reported outcomes of a prospective study that included 298 rough- (titanium plasma spray (TPS)-coated) surfaced NDIs (3.3 mm), the majority (77%) being used to support either maxillary or mandibular overdentures. While implants were placed using non-submerged healing, they were not directly loaded by provisional prostheses. For maxillary overdentures, NDIs were used in combination with SDIs, while 53 of 74 (71.6%) mandibular overdentures were retained only by NDIs. This makes sense, since higher crestal stresses are known to affect implants of any diameter placed in maxilla compared with mandible.[14] In the study by Zinsli et al.[19], the cumulative survival rate for NDIs after 6 years in function was 96.6%. Most failures were due to peri-implantitis, suggesting that the TPS surface could have been more of an issue in failure than implant diameter was. However, crestal bone loss could be the result of occlusal load distribution leading to exposure of the TPS surface to bacterial plaque and further development of peri-implant disease. Morneburg and Proschel[20] undertook a prospective study in which 67 fully edentulous patients each received two 2.5 mm diameter moderately rough (sand-blasted and calcium phosphate-coated) threaded implants of lengths 9, 12, or 15 mm. The traditional two-stage implant placement protocol was used and implants placed in the intraforaminal region of anterior mandible. Following 3–4 months' submerged healing, implants were uncovered and used to support complete mandibular overdentures retained by either magnets or O-rings. After an average functional time of 6 years, the implant survival rate was again favorable at 95.5%.

Sohrabi et al.[12] recently reviewed published work on the use of NDIs and MDIs, and found that shorter implants (≤13 mm) were more likely to fail under loading than longer (>13 mm) ones. They concluded, therefore, that long NDIs or even MDIs can be considered for retention of complete mandibular overdentures, even with the use of flapless surgery, the latter approach being intended to reduce surgical trauma and patient apprehension, especially in older individuals with medical issues. Short implant length may explain the recent poor outcomes with NDIs reported by Wang et al.[21] These clinicians used 2.2 or 2.4 mm diameter implants to support provisional fixed temporaries. Thirty-one implants of lengths 7, 10, or 14 mm were used in 10 patients, and 51.5% were placed in type III bone.[22] While implant survival was 93.5% at 1 year, implant success based on crestal bone loss was only 38.7%. Mean bone loss at 1 year was 1.19 mm (range 0–3.5 mm). Recently, Elsyad et al.[23] included immediate loading in the treatment protocol for mandibular overdentures despite the fact that this approach could lead to inhibition of osseointegration secondary to implant micromovements. For example, Grassi et al.[24] published a case report showing formation of a fibrous connective tissue interface with implant surface in deep, narrow, infrabony coronal bone defects affecting immediately loaded NDIs.

Elsyad et al.[23] placed four 1.8 mm diameter, moderately rough (sand-blasted/acid-etched) implants in the intraforaminal regions of 28 fully edentulous patients. Implant lengths of 12–18 mm (majority ≥14 mm) were used along with a flapless one-stage protocol. To ensure maximum initial implant stability, bone drilling was limited to the coronal half of the osteotomy only, and followed by self-tapping implants inserted manually and finalized with a torque wrench. Previously, newly fabricated full dentures were then modified to receive O-ring attachments and delivered the same day. Follow-up examinations were conducted at 6, 12, 24, and 36 months, and included radiographs taken with customized acrylic bite blocks to ensure standardization amongst serial radiographs of the same implant. Thus, both implant survival and success (based on crestal bone loss of <1.5 mm) could be calculated. Survival after 3 years in function was 96.4%, and the four failed implants were either 12 or 14 mm in length (i.e. the shorter two lengths used). Based on crestal bone loss, the 3-year implant success rate was 92.9%.

With regard to more widespread use of NDIs, a number of investigators have reported outcomes of clinical trials. Most employed long NDIs, since short implant length is known to predispose NDIs to failure.[12,25] Vigolo et al.[26] reported 7-year results from a study of 3227 implants that had been placed in 683 patients. Of these implants, 192 were NDIs with a moderately rough surface, diameters of either 2.9 or 3.25 mm, and were allowed submerged implant site healing. Ninety-four of the NDIs were used to replace single teeth, while the other 98 were used to support fixed partial prostheses along with SDIs. No partial restorations employed only NDIs for support. After 7 years in function, the survival rate of NDIs was 95.3%. Nine NDIs were lost either at re-entry or during the first 6 months of function. Survival was basically the same as the 3035 SDIs used in the same study (94.3%). It is important to note, however, that one prosthodontist had restored all of the patients, and he had been careful to avoid premature contacts in all eccentric movements; that is, to avoid off-axis loading of implants. Romeo et al.[27] reported data from a study in which they compared outcomes with NDIs (3.3 mm diameter) versus SDIs (4.1 mm). Cases which had prostheses that were supported by a combination of NDIs and SDIs were excluded. Over a 7-year period, 188 partially edentulous patients were treated with 330 rough (TPS-coated), threaded implants of which 122 placed in 68 patients were NDIs. These NDIs were used to support 45 fixed partial prostheses and 23 single crowns. Implant failures and biological failures (infection requiring intervention) with the NDIs were similar to those with SDIs. The cumulative success rates (based on implant loss and excessive crestal bone loss) for NDIs were 96.1% in maxilla and 92% in mandible. As in the study by Zinsli et al.[19] using the same implant type, most failures were linked to peri-implantitis. There did not appear to be an effect of diameter on crestal bone loss when NDI data were compared with SDI data.

Degidi et al.[28] reported retrospective data on outcomes with 510 NDIs. Implant diameters ranged from 3.0 to 3.5 mm, and the majority of implants had either rough or moderately rough surfaces.[29] A major question addressed by the investigators was whether immediate restoration without loading (IRWL) would impact negatively on survival. Therefore, 255 of the 510 implants received IRWL, while the others did not. The data were reported after only a mean of 20 months' function, and by that time three implants had been lost. Slightly more bone loss occurred in the IRWL implant group, and greater bone loss was observed for both groups of implants (IRWL and delayed loading) with diameters <3.4 mm and lengths of ≤13 mm, so that longer term follow-up will be needed from these investigators. The 1-year results from other investigators using moderately rough 3 mm diameter NDIs in prospective study designs incorporating IRWL also showed favorable outcomes.[30,31] However, these investigators did limit treatment to single maxillary or mandibular incisor sites. Other studies that limited usage of moderately rough NDIs to replacement of single incisor teeth include those by Reddy et al.,[32] Zarone et al.,[5] and Andersen et al.[33] Success rates after 1–3 years ranged from 93.8% to 96.7%.

Other published studies have included longer term follow-up with NDIs, including those used in partially edentulous patients.

Arisan et al.[34] evaluated the performance of a group of 316 moderately rough NDIs (3.3 or 3.4 mm diameters) placed in 139 patients after 5–10 years using retrospective data. Prosthetic treatments provided included 31 single crowns, 65 fixed partial dentures (FPDs), and 24 overdentures. In total, 65% of the FPDs were supported only by NDIs, while 35% were supported by a combination of NDIs and SDIs. All overdentures were used exclusively with NDIs. The cumulative implant success rate based on implant loss and excessive bone loss was 91.4% at 10 years. Crestal bone loss was measured from panoramic radiographs; therefore, the data must be viewed with caution, but they did indicate greater bone loss in posterior versus anterior sites and in smokers (≤10 cigarettes/day) versus non-smokers. NDI failures in smokers mostly occurred between 3 and 5 years, and at the end of the study their survival rate was only 73.6%. In another paper, Malo and Nobre[35] reported retrospective results up to 11 years with 3.3 mm diameter NDIs that had been used exclusively in posterior sites in either jaw. The majority of implants replaced bicuspid teeth; and in the examples shown, all were in protected sites with natural teeth mesially and distally to the implant prostheses. Two hundred and forty-seven implants were used in 147 patients, most to replace single teeth (mostly bicuspids) or support short-span FPDs. The cumulative survival after a median (range 1–11 years) functional time of 6 years was 95%. Interestingly, however, failures were significantly higher when NDIs supported posterior FPDs than when they replaced single posterior teeth, perhaps related to the more favorable loading likely to occur when a single bicuspid tooth has the benefit of adjacent natural teeth. Particularly in situations where NDIs are meant to act as the distal-most abutment, occlusal overload leading to either implant failure or fracture may be an increased risk.[36]

The risk of implant fracture increases with decreasing implant diameter[37] and is particularly high if NDIs have diameters <3 mm,[38] but fractures of NDIs ≥3 mm in diameter do occur. Fractures of 3.3 mm diameter, rough-surfaced implants were reported to have occurred with a frequency of 3–9%.[19,27] Some authors have stated that NDIs (including MDIs) used with fixed restorations should always be splinted with other implants except when used to replace maxillary and mandibular lateral incisors.[39] For posterior implant-supported FPDs, one implant per tooth, narrow occlusal tables, and minimal cusp heights may help to reduce crestal bone overload of NDIs/MDIs.[40]

Shatkin and Petrotto[41] reported retrospective outcomes with 5640 NDIs ranging in diameters from 1.8 to 3 mm. The implants had been placed in 1260 patients over a 12-year period. At the time of the report, mean follow-up was 3.5 years and the survival rate 92.1%. Those implants retaining full maxillary overdentures fared the worst (survival 85.2%), and generally those supporting fixed prostheses fared better than those used with removable prostheses (94.7% versus 88.4%). For implant placement, these clinicians recommended using a 1.2 mm pilot bur (i.e. approximately half the implant diameter) and different bur penetration depths depending on bone quality. For very dense bone, a pilot hole depth of 80% of the intended implant length was used, while pilot hole depths of 60% and 50% of the intended implant lengths were used for moderately dense and low-density bone. Interestingly, gender played a role, with lower survival in men (90.8%) versus women (93.0%), which is likely related to different levels of stress generated during function.

Clinical results

The lead author (JN) was involved in NDI evaluation at the University of Cologne. A total of 422 patients and 1529 implants were placed between April 2002 and December 2009 and demonstrated a high survival rate, especially in combination with various grafting techniques. A large number of NDIs were placed to reduce the volume and morbidity of grafting needed, or to avoid grafting techniques altogether. The NDIs showed a cumulative success rate of 97.2% (n = 69) for the 3.0 mm diameter and 99.8% (n = 504) for the 3.4 mm diameter. In comparison, the success rate for the SDIs was 99.2% (n = 8369) and 100% (n = 110) for wide-body implants after an observation period of up to 4 years.[42]

Clinical applications of narrow-diameter dental implants

NDIs are appropriate for use where horizontal augmentation procedures would otherwise be needed to augment bucco-lingual ridge width and the patient is unwilling to accept this more invasive and costly approach. Surgical planning requires a minimum facial bone thickness of about 1.5–2 mm or more after osteotomy preparation to promote a stable long-term result. Application of NDIs for the retention of mandibular overdentures is demonstrated in Case11.1 (Figure 11.1). Completely edentulous patients with adequate mandibular

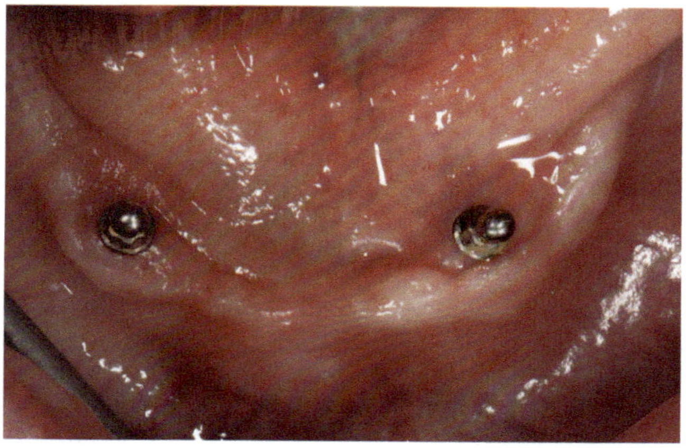

(a)

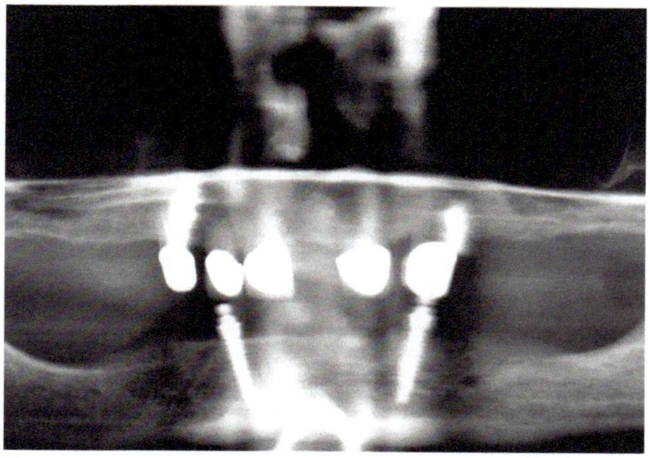

(b)

Figure 11.1 NDI-supported mandibular overdenture. (a) Clinical outcome with two NDI one-piece implants (mini1Sky-implant D2.8, L 14 mm) with integrated ball attachment after 30 months in function. (b) Radiograph of NDI in the anterior mandible to support the removable prosthesis alveolar ridge height but unfavorable bucco-lingual ridge width can be considered candidates for an overdenture retained by two NDIs placed in the mandibular canine regions. The patient shown demonstrates the clinical outcome of this treatment using one-piece NDIs with integrated ball attachments after 30 months in function.

After a detailed diagnosis, preferably including cone beam CT (CBCT), the amount of available bone will help determine the most appropriate implant diameters and positions. Case 11.2 demonstrates application of NDIs for replacement of two missing mandibular molars in sites with significant facial bone loss (Figure 11.2). In such situations, if possible, implant threads should be covered with native bone and augmented with autologous particulate bone (Figure 11.2d) or particulate xenograft.

NDIs also may be indicated in situations where bone grafting procedures have previously failed or are at risk of failing because of local site conditions. For example, grafting in anterior mandible is always risky owing to the high mobility of lip muscles leading to an increased risk of wound dehiscence and graft infection. Also, very dense and avascular bone can sometimes be encountered in anterior mandible and may compromise graft revascularization.

Replacement of maxillary lateral incisors, mandible single incisors, or bicuspid teeth also are indications for use of NDIs, assuming that these single-tooth implants will be protected by mesial and distal contiguous natural teeth. However, small edentulous sites require special attention with treatment planning. Case 11.3 documents the replacement of a maxillary lateral incisor implant (Figure 11.3). The mesio-distal dimensions are important for maintenance of interproximal bone and physiological soft tissue contours. Treatment planning must also anticipate the proximity of the implant apex to adjacent tooth roots (Figure 11.3d).

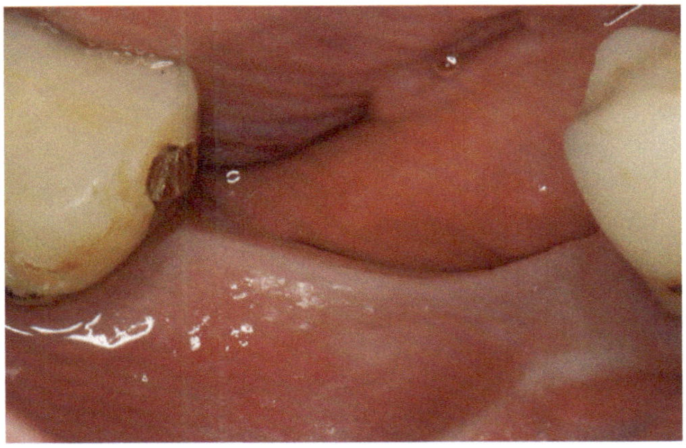

(a)

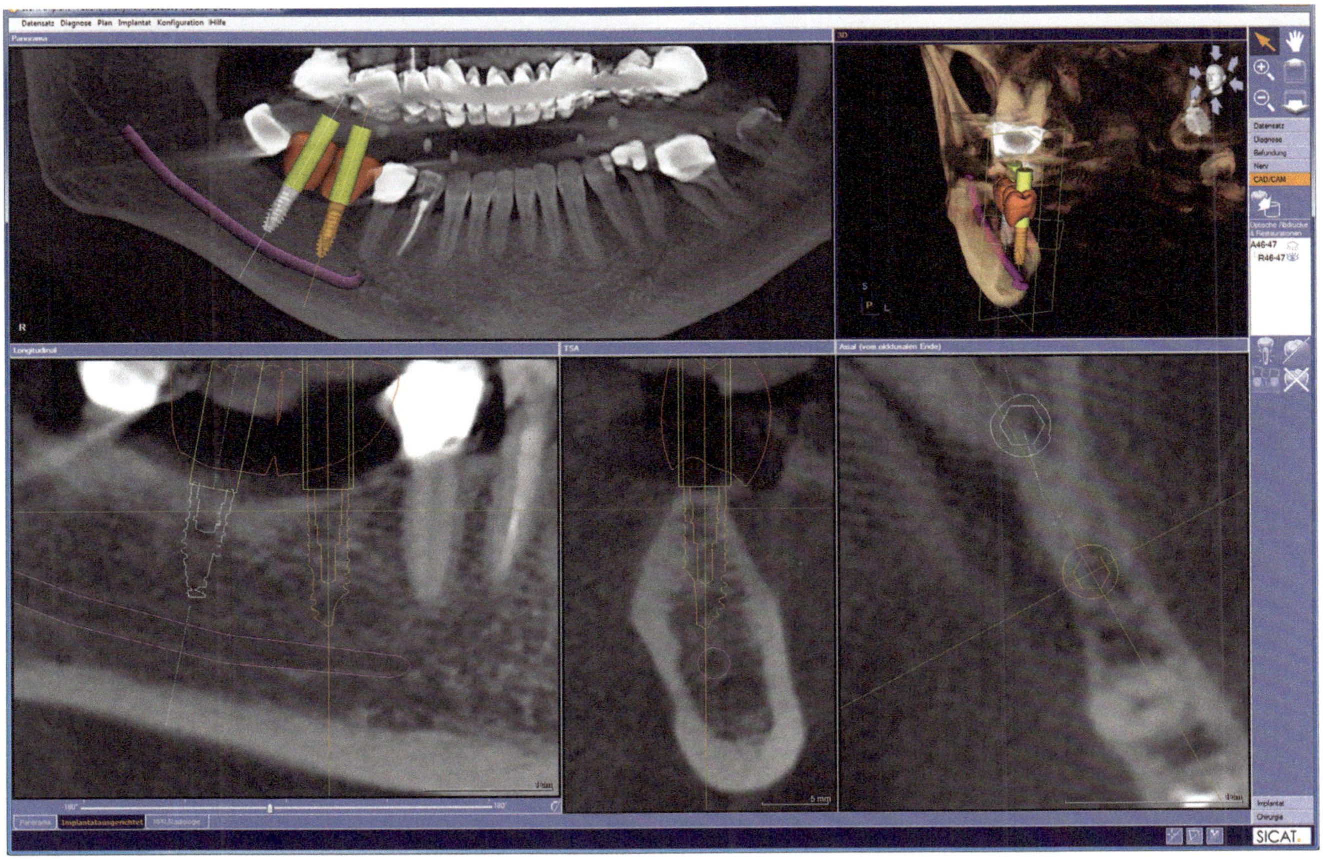

(b)

Figure 11.2 NDI reconstruction of horizontal bone defect at adjacent molar teeth. (a) Loss of the first and second mandibular molars has resulted in significant atrophy of the edentulous alveolar ridge. (b) A CBCT scan allowed for virtual implant planning.

(Continued)

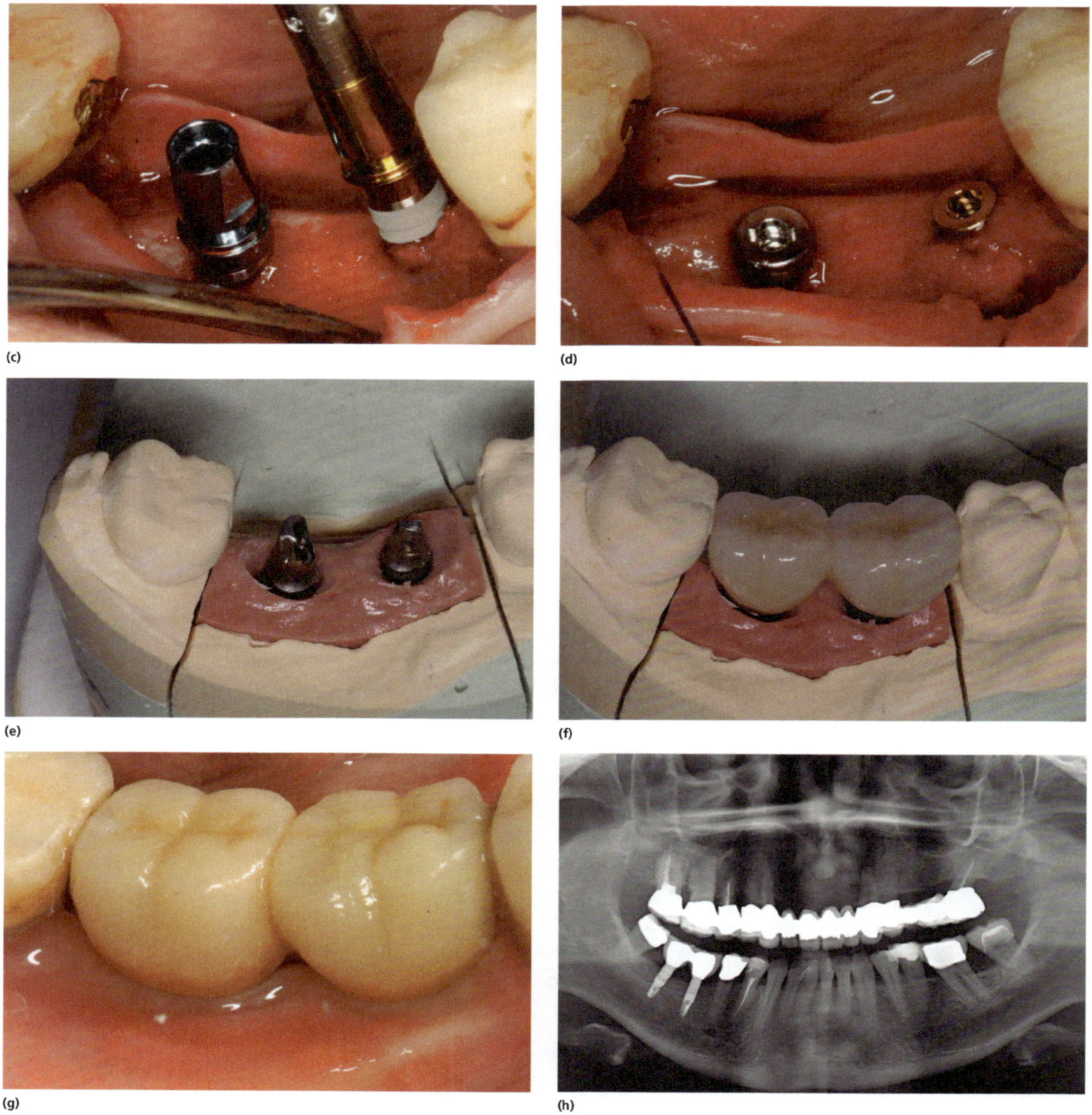

Figure 11.2 (Continued)
(c) NDI placement was undertaken using a 3.0 mm diameter, 11 mm length implant for first molar and a 3.4 mm diameter, 11 mm length implant for the second molar. Buccal bone is thin but intact. (d) The thin buccal bone has been augmented with autologous particulate bone. (e) Individualized abutments were prepared for splinted porcelain-fused-to-metal crowns. (f) Splinted porcelain-fused-to-metal crowns were prepared with tooth analog designs. (g) Clinical appearance after placement of splinted crowns 6 months after placement. (h) A panoramic radiograph of the NDI-supported restoration after 2.5 years.

Case 11.4 demonstrates the use of NDIs for reconstruction with two adjacent implants for missing maxillary central and lateral incisors in a site with reduced horizontal bone volume (Figure 11.4). The prosthetic management will be discussed in the next section.

NDIs must be used with caution for FPD restorations, especially in posterior jaw sites, where natural teeth do not exist distal to the planned prosthesis. They should also be avoided in resorbed posterior maxillary sites where long implant lengths cannot be used. Consideration should also be given to possible future tooth loss that could have adverse effects on an NDI-supported prosthesis because of an increased load altering a previously stable restoration.

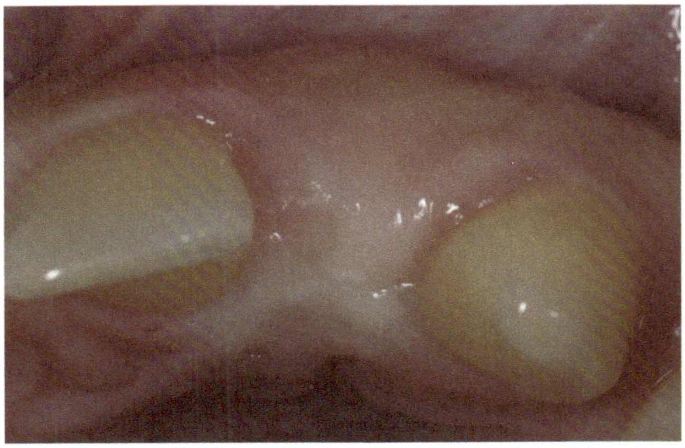

(a)

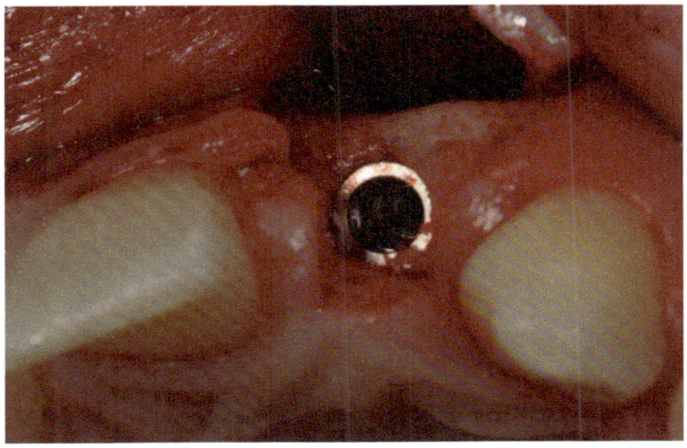

(b)

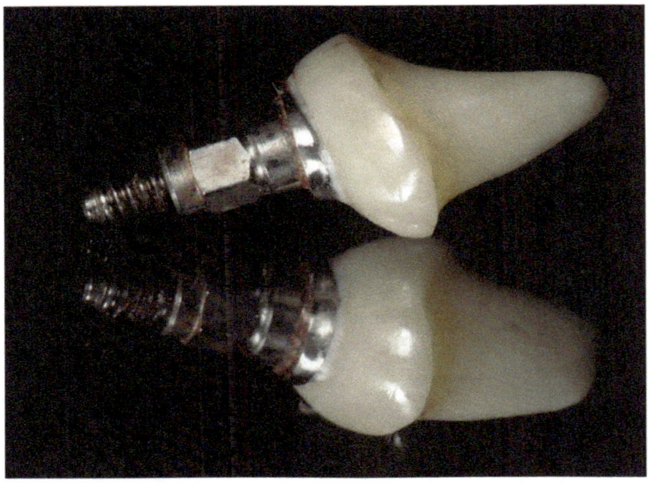

(c)

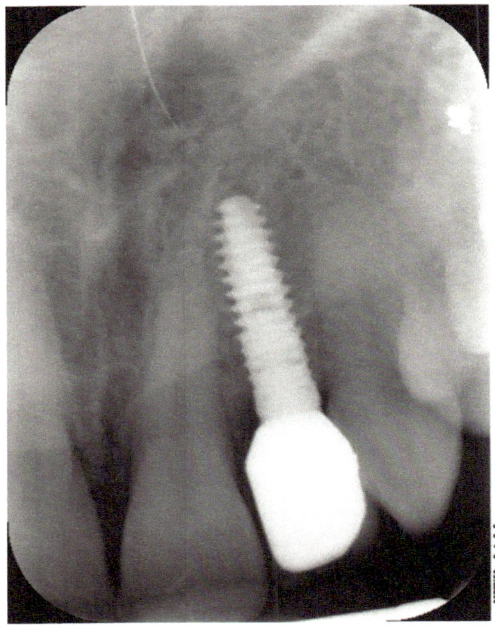

(d)

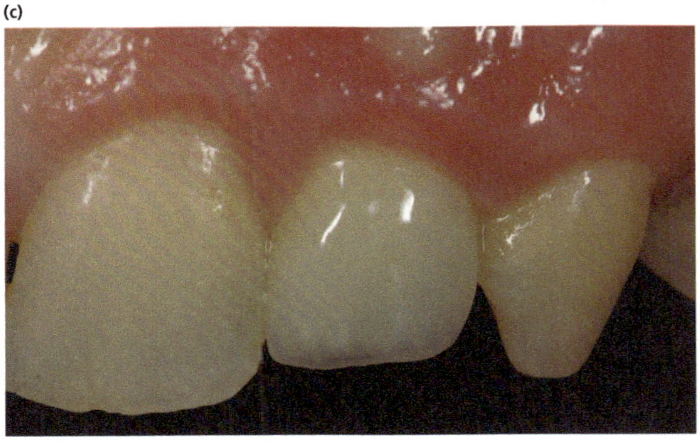

(e)

Figure 11.3 Esthetic zone NDI reconstruction of maxillary lateral incisor. (a) Congenital aplasia of left lateral incisor with adequate bucco-palatal bone volume but narrow mesio-distal dimension. (b) Placement of 3.0 mm diameter NDI (13 mm length) with internal implant abutment connection. (c) Custom titanium abutment with ceramic veneering to form a significant transgingival emergence profile. (d) A post-restoration image of the final restoration. (e) Restoration with a full ceramic crown showing stable peri-implant soft tissues after 1.5 years.

NDIs in combination with minimally invasive techniques like ridge expansion demand a high level of experience by the surgeon (see Chapter 16). The combination of NDIs and reduced bone volume could increase the risk of failures. Case 11.5 presents a multidisciplinary approach with orthodontic site development in a patient with congenitally missing lower central incisors (Figure 11.5). The lateral incisors were moved into the central incisor positions to avoid having two adjacent implants and to utilize the residual bone volume after tooth movement (Figure 11.5a and b). The residual bucco-lingual bone width of 4 mm was then expanded with piezosurgery-assisted bone sectioning and mechanical screw ridge expanders (Meisinger, USA) (Figure 11.5c and d). The buccal bone thickness of the expanded ridge in passive position after removal of the screw expanders is visualized in Figure 11.5f. Insertion of two-piece 3.0 mm NDIs was completed with a transgingival healing protocol (Figure 11.5g). Post-expansion bone volume is demonstrated in Figure 11.5h and i. The clinical and radiographic outcomes 12 months after implant placement are shown in Figure 11.5j and k.

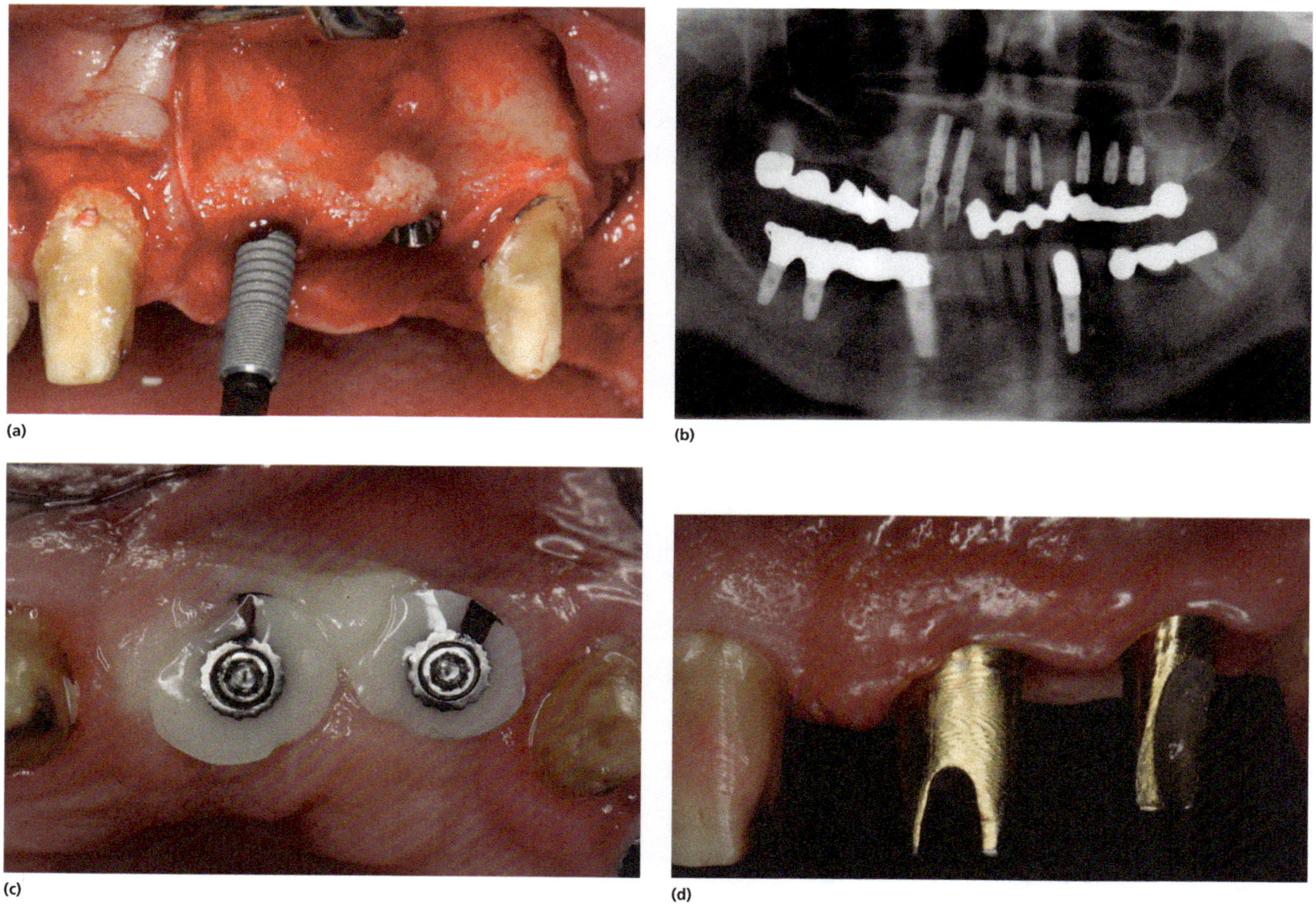

(a) (b) (c) (d)

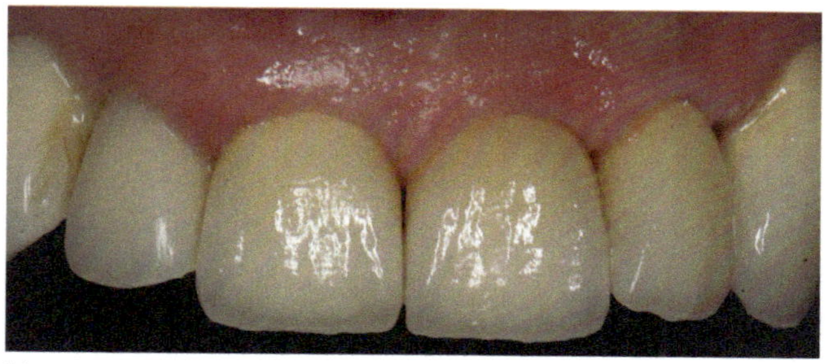

(e)

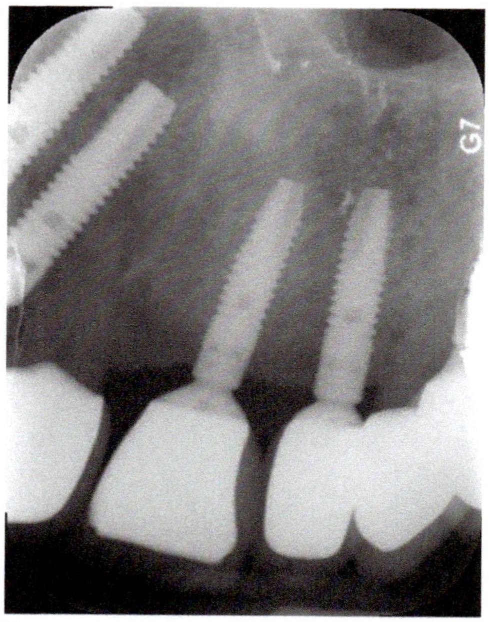

(f)

Figure 11.4 Adjacent NDIs with reduced horizontal bone volume. (a) Two NDI implants (diameter 3.0 mm) were placed in the anterior maxilla for left central and lateral incisors. (b) A post-operative radiograph following implant placement. (c) Custom temporary abutments (prepared by index registration at implant placement) were used as gingiva formers to develop the emergence profile and soft tissue contours. (d) Custom final abutments were prepared to maintain the soft tissue contours. (e) The final crowns have provided an esthetically pleasing result despite the wide emergence profiles on the custom abutments. (f) Periapical radiographs of implant bone level 2.5 years after prosthetic loading.

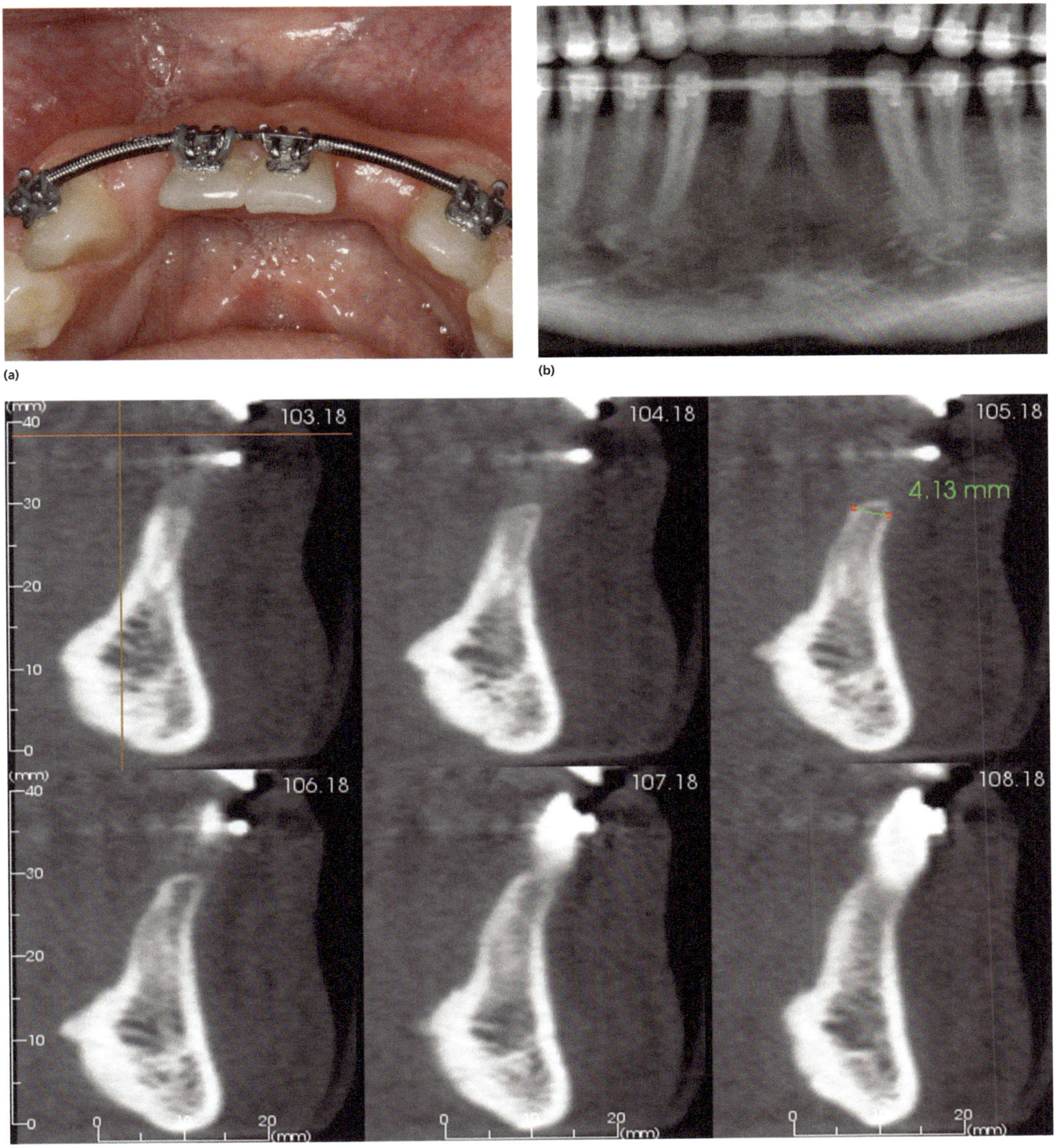

(c)

Figure 11.5 Application of NDIs for lower lateral incisors in combination with orthodontic site development and ridge expansion. (a) Preoperative view of edentulous lower lateral incisor sites after orthodontic repositioning of the lateral incisors into the central incisor positions to avoid having two adjacent implants. (b) Preoperative radiograph. (c) Preoperative axial CBCT of mandibular right lateral incisor demonstrating pre-implant bone dimensions.

(Continued)

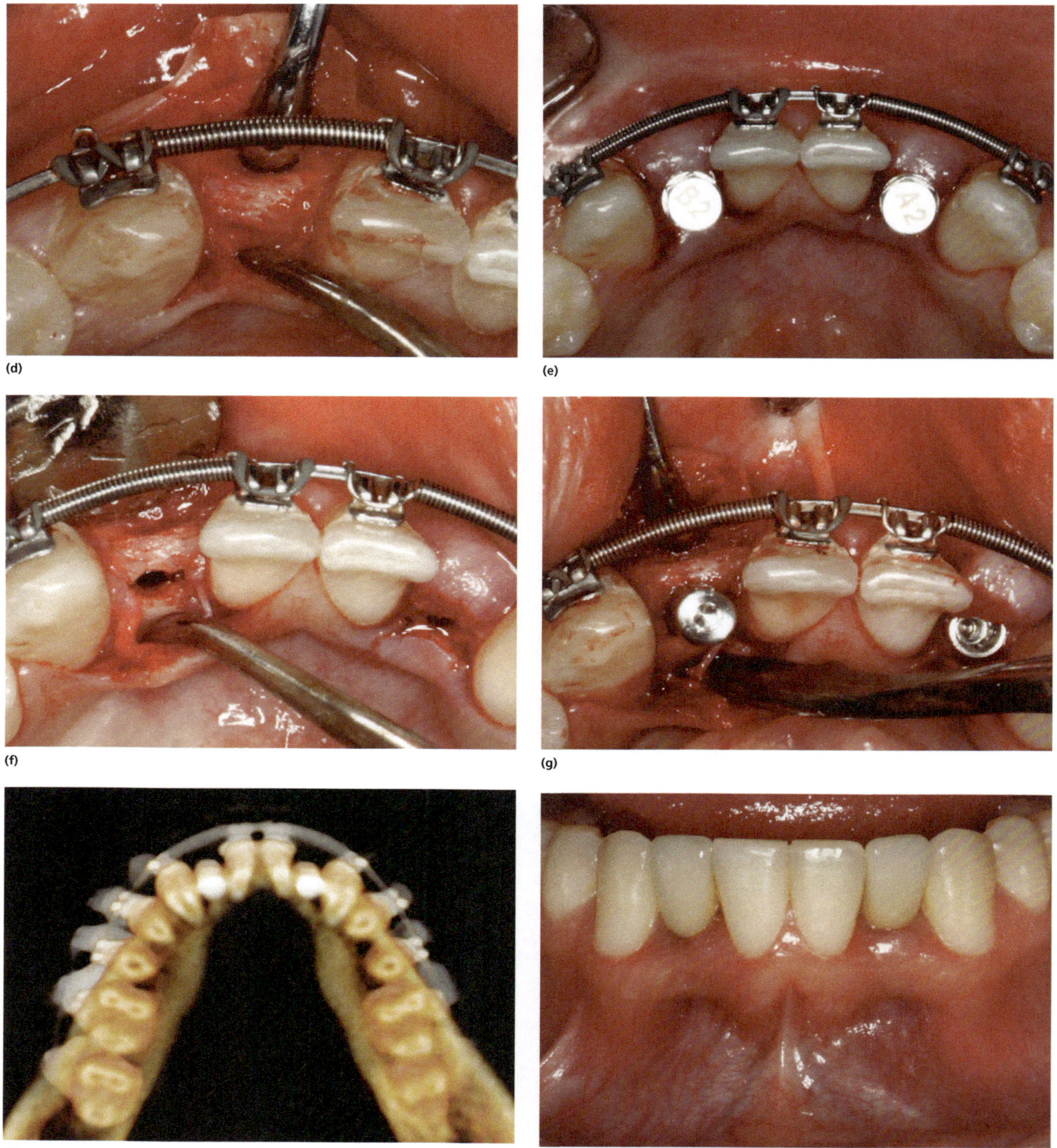

(d) (e) (f) (g) (h) (i)

Figure 11.5 (Continued)
(d) Ridge dimensions on surgical exposure for implant placement. (e) Screw expanders in position after piezosurgery ridge sectioning. (f) Expanded ridge in passive position. (g) 3.0 mm diameter implants in position demonstrating expanded ridge contour and intact buccal plate. (h) Post-operative CBCT image demonstrating implant placement and intact buccal bone. (i) Post-restoration facial view (12 months after implant placement).

(Continued)

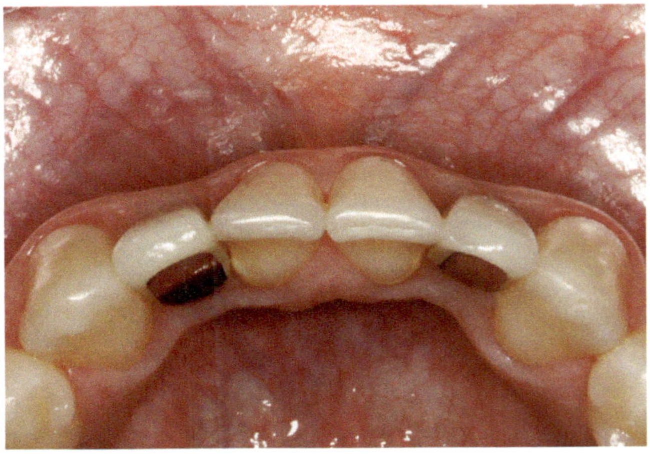

(j)

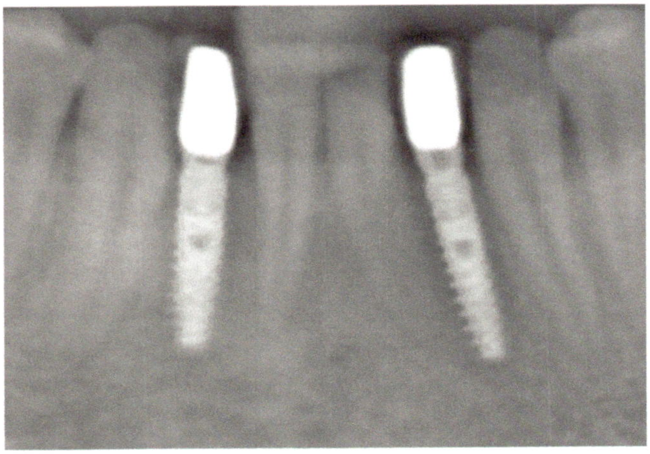

(k)

Figure 11.5 (Continued)
(j) Post-restoration occlusal view. (k) Post-restoration radiograph. © Daniel R. Cullum.

Prosthetic considerations

Prosthetic challenges with NDIs arise in the development of appropriate emergence profiles to reproduce the root and crown anatomy of the tooth being replaced. The larger the final crown of the restoration, the greater the horizontal emergence that must be developed. The challenge is to develop the emergence in the typical 3 mm of vertical height of the biologic width ending with a predictable facial gingival margin (see Chapters 1 and 4). With increasing amounts of horizontal bone loss, the buccal cantilever of the restoration will be increased to return the anatomy to normal contour (Figure 11.3c). The interproximal dimensions will be dependent on the adjacent teeth for bone and soft tissue support. The interproximal dimensions must extend laterally to give the appearance of an appropriate root dimension (Figure 11.3c–e). The crown and abutment contours are best developed in the provisional phase (Figure 11.4c) and need to be convex to support the tissue and allow for adequate cleansability. These contours must be duplicated in the final restoration (Figure 11.3c), both for esthetics and hygiene maintenance by the patient (see Chapter 4).

For patients treated with NDIs it is important that home care and oral hygiene are closely monitored. Fixed prosthetic restorations with a wide emergence profile can have long soft tissue contacts with deeper probing depths. This could lead to the accumulation of anaerobic bacteria and an increased risk of developing peri-implant disease.

Edentulous sites with significant alveolar atrophy often display a reduced zone of attached keratinized gingiva or a mobile remnant on the ridge crest. Following implant placement, the mobile gingiva can become inflamed. This often occurs at the transition zone of the superstructure as a result of a "pumping" effect, which can lead to bone and soft tissue loss or peri-implant disease. Soft tissue enhancement with connective tissue grafting, lateral pedicle flap, and/or a vestibuloplasty could be necessary.

Conclusions

NDIs can be an option to provide minimally invasive implant treatment. As with any implant application, success requires adequate interproximal and bucco-lingual bone volume, just a smaller volume for a narrower implant. NDIs come with limitations, including higher stress concentration in peri-implant crestal bone, a deeper sulcus from an NDI emergence to a standard crown size, and consideration of splinted restoration designs that avoid eccentric loading. Optimal implant placement, including alignment and insertion depth, is important owing to the minimal dimensions of the recipient site and adjacent anatomy. Overengineering restorative designs with greater numbers of implants should be considered. Success with NDIs to support a complete removable mandibular prosthesis is more predictable with an opposing edentulous maxilla and implant lengths >14 mm. NDI applications for replacement of maxillary lateral incisors and mandibular incisors are predictable provided that adequate interproximal (1.5 mm) and facial (2 mm) bone dimensions can be maintained.

References

1. Renouard F, Nisand D. Impact of implant length and diameter on survival rates. Clin Oral Implants Res 2006; 17(Suppl 2): 35–51.
2. Gleiznys A, Skirbutis G, Harb A, et al. New approach towards mini dental implants and small-diameter implants: an option for long-term prostheses. Stomatologija Baltic Dent Maxillofac J 2012; 14: 39–45.
3. Davarpanah M, Martinez H, Tecucianu J, et al. Small-diameter implants: indications and contraindications. J Esthetic Dent 2000; 12: 186–194.
4. Froum S, Cho S, Cho Y, et al. Narrow-diameter implants: a restorative option for limited interdental space. Int J Periodontics Restorative Dent 2007; 27: 449–455.
5. Zarone F, Sorrentino R, Vaccaro F, Russo S. Prosthetic treatment of maxillary lateral incisor agenesis with osseointegrated implants: a 24–39-month prospective clinical study. Clin Oral Implants Res 2006; 17: 94–101.
6. Froum S, Emtiaz S, Bloom M, et al. The use of transitional implants for immediate fixed temporary prostheses in cases of implant restorations. Pract Periodontics Aesthet Dent 1998; 10: 737–746.
7. Ahn M-R, An K-M, Choi J-H, Sohn D-S. Immediate loading with mini dental implants in the fully edentulous mandible. Implant Dent 2004; 13: 367–372.
8. Olate S, Negreiros M, de Moraes M, et al. Influence of diameter and length of implant on early dental implant failure. J Oral Maxillofac Surg 2012; 68: 414–419.
9. Baqain Z, Moqbel W, Sawair F. Early dental implant failure: risk factors. Br J Oral Maxillofac Surg 2012; 50: 239–243.
10. Quesada-Garcia P, Prados-Sanchez E, Olmedo-Gaya V, et al. Dental implant stability is influenced by implant diameter and localization and by the use of plasma rich in growth factors. J Oral Maxillofac Surg 2012; 70: 2761–2767.
11. Miyamoto I, Tsuboi Y, Wada E, et al. Influence of cortical bone thickness and implant length on implant stability at the time of surgery – clinical, prospective, biomechanical and imaging study. Bone 2005; 37: 776–780.

12. Sohrabi K, Mushantat A, Esfandiari S, Feine J. How successful are small-diameter implants? A literature review. Clin Oral Implants Res 2012; 23: 515–525.
13. Anitua E, Tapia R, Luzuriaga F, Orive G. Influence of implant length, diameter, and geometry on stress distribution: a finite element analysis. Int J Periodontics Restorative Dent 2010; 30: 89–95.
14. Baggi L, Cappelloni I, Di Girolamo M, et al. The influence of implant diameter and length on stress distribution of osseointegrated implants related to crestal bone geometry: a three-dimensional finite element analysis. J Prosthetic Dent 2008; 100: 422–431.
15. Guan H, van Staden R, Loo Y-C, et al. Influence of bone and dental implant parameters on stress distribution in the mandible: a finite element study. Int J Oral Maxillofac Implants 2009; 24: 866–876.
16. Pierrisnard L, Renouard F, Renault P, Barquins M. Influence of implant length and bicortical anchorage on implant stress distribution. Clin Implant Dent Relat Res 2003; 5: 254–262.
17. Chou H-Y, Muftu S, Bozkaya D. Combined effects of implant insertion depth and alveolar bone quality on peri-implant bone strain induced by wide-diameter, short implant and a narrow-diameter, long implant. J Prosthetic Dent 2010; 104: 293–300.
18. Qian L, Todo M, Matsushita Y, Koyano K. Effects of implant diameter, insertion depth, and loading angle on stress/strain fields in implant/jawbone systems: finite element analysis. Int J Oral Maxillofac Implants 2009; 24(5): 877–886.
19. Zinsli B, Sagesser T, Mericske E, Mericske-Sterne R. Clinical evaluation of small-diameter ITI implants: a prospective study. Int J Oral Maxillofac Implants 2004; 19: 92–99.
20. Morneburg T, Proschel P. Success rates of microimplants in edentulous patients with residual ridge resorption. Int J Oral Maxillofac Implants 2008; 23: 270–276.
21. Wang H-L, Okayasu K, Ju J-H, et al. The success rate of narrow body implants used for supporting immediate provisional restorations: a pilot feasibility study. Implant Dent 2012; 21: 467–473.
22. Lekholm U, Zarb G. Patient selection. In: Tissue-Integrated Prostheses: Osseointegration in Clinical Dentistry, BrånemarkP-I, AlbrektssonT, ZarbG, eds. Chicago, IL: Quintessence, 1985, pp. 199–210.
23. Elsyad M, Gebreel A, Fouad M, Elshoukouki A. The clinical and radiographic outcome of immediately loaded mini implants supporting a mandibular overdenture. A 3-year prospective study. J Oral Rehabil 2011; 38: 827–834.
24. Grassi R, Rebaudi A, Trisi P, et al. Bone loss around immediately loaded transitional implants: histologic and microcomputed tomographic analysis – a case report. Int J Periodontics Restorative Dent 2012; 32: e195–e203.
25. Saadoun A, Le Gall M. An 8-year compilation of clinical results obtained with Steri-Oss endosseous implants. Compend Contin Educ Dent 1996; 17: 669–674.
26. Vigolo P, Givani A, Majzoub Z, Cordioli G. Clinical evaluation of small-diameter implants in single-tooth and multiple-implant restorations: a 7-year retrospective study. Int J Oral Maxillofac Implants 2004; 19: 703–709.
27. Romeo E, Lops D, Amorfini L, et al. Clinical and radiographic evaluation of small-diameter (3.3 mm) implants followed for 1–7 years: a longitudinal study. Clin Oral Implants Res 2006; 17: 139–148.
28. Degidi M, Piattelli A, Carinci F. Clinical outcome of narrow diameter implants: a retrospective study of 510 implants. J Periodontol 2008; 79: 49–54.
29. Albrektsson T, Wennerberg A. Oral implant surfaces: part I: review focusing on topographic and chemical properties of different surfaces and *in vivo* responses to them. Int J Prosthodont 2004; 17: 536–543.
30. Galindo-Moreno P, Nilsson P, King P, et al. Clinical and radiographic evaluation of early loaded narrow diameter implants – 1-year follow-up. Clin Oral Implants Res 2012; 23: 609–616.
31. Oyama K, Kan J, Rungcharassaeng K, Lozada J. Immediate provisionalization of 3.0 mm diameter implants replacing single missing maxillary and mandibular incisors: 1-year prospective study. Int J Oral Maxillofac Implants 2012; 27: 173–180.
32. Reddy M, O'Neal J, Haigh S, et al. Initial clinical efficiency of 3 mm implants immediately placed into function in conditions of limited space. Int J Oral Maxillofac Implants 2008; 23: 281–288.
33. Andersen E, Saxegaard E, Knutsen M, Haanaes H. A prospective clinical study evaluating the safety and effectiveness of narrow-diameter threaded implants in the anterior region of the maxilla. Int J Oral Maxillofac Implants 2001; 16: 217–224.
34. Arisan V, Bolukbasi N, Ersanli S, Ozdemir T. Evaluation of 316 narrow diameter implants followed for 5–10 years: a clinical and radiographic retrospective study. Clin Oral Implants Res 2010; 21: 296–307.
35. Malo P, Nobre M. Implants (3.3 mm diameter) for the rehabilitation of edentulous posterior regions: a retrospective clinical study with up to 11 years of follow-up. Clin Implant Dent Relat Res 2011; 13: 95–103.
36. Cehreli M, Akca K. Narrow-diameter implants as terminal support for occlusal three-unit FPDs: a biomechanical analysis. Int J Periodontics Restorative Dent 2004; 24: 513–519.
37. Quek C, Tan K, Nicholls J. Load fatigue performance of a single-tooth implant abutment system: effect of diameter. Int J Oral Maxillofac Implants 2006; 21: 929–936.
38. Allum S, Tomlinson R, Joshi R. The impact of loads on standard diameter, small diameter and mini implants: a comparative laboratory study. Clin Oral Implants Res 2008; 19: 553–559.
39. Anitua E, Errazquin J, de Pedro J, et al. Clinical evaluation of Tiny® 2.5- and 3.0-mm narrow-diameter implants as definitive implants in different clinical situations: a retrospective cohort study. Eur J Oral Implantol 2010; 3: 315–322.
40. Flanagan D. Fixed partial dentures and crowns supported by very small diameter dental implants in compromised sites. Implant Dent 2008; 17: 182–191.
41. Shatkin T, Petrotto C. Mini dental implants: a retrospective analysis of 5640 implants placed over a 12-year period. Compend Contin Educ Dent 2012; 33(Spec 3): 2–9.
42. Karapetian V, Roels M, Neugebauer J, Zoller J. Survival rate of 469 implants of two different diameter-reduced implant systems over a 7.75 year period. Poster presentation P212, Annual Meeting of the Academy of Osseointegration, 2010, Orlando, FL, March 4–6.

CHAPTER 12

Minimally Invasive Complete Arch Treatment: The Versatility of Angled Implants

Ole T. Jensen[1] & Daniel R. Cullum[2]
[1]University of Utah, School of Dentistry, Salt Lake City, UT, USA
[2]Private Practice, Coeur d'Alene, ID; Loma Linda University Department of OMS, Loma Linda, CA; UCLA Department of OMS, Los Angeles, CA, USA

Introduction

The use of angulation in dental implant placement remains controversial, yet the very first screw-form implants placed by Brånemark in 1965 were all off-axis, with most placed at about a 30° angulation relative to the plane of occlusion. These implants lasted until the death of the patient in 2009, and remain a historical measuring reference when discussing advantages and disadvantages of off-axis implant placement.[1]

There are several intuitive theories for the causes of implant-to-bone interface failure that have not borne out to be true over time. An example of this is the cantilever bridge with excess forces being thought to lead to crestal bone loss or failure of osseointegration. However, with cross-arch stabilization, the prosthesis and its framework or fastening screws appear to fail long before the bone-to-implant interface of the supporting implant.[2] Bone quality, length of cantilever extension, parafunctional loading, and brachiocephalic facial type are parameters thought to influence risk with prosthesis loading and cross-arch stabilization. Another intuitive theory proposed that four to six implants placed into the mandibular parasymphysis would cause fatigue bone loss or bone fractures posteriorly where jaw height and strength were compromised by bone atrophy. However, instead of developing mandibular fractures, bone strain on the anterior implants was transmitted posteriorly, leading to bone apposition over time.[3] A third theory proposed that angulation of implants would result in findings consistent with angled natural teeth, leading to angular bone defects and susceptibility to peri-implantitis. Unlike clinical findings in tooth-borne restorative dentistry, this has not been shown to be true for osseointegrated dental implants.[4–6]

In summary, there is little evidence that angulation of bone screws placed into jaws or weight-bearing long bones such as the femur will lead to implant-to-bone interface failure. Dental implants placed off-angle survive long term even with single tooth restorations. With splinted reconstructions on multiple implants, implant-to-bone interface failure is rare after osseointegration, although there are reports of implant fracture or componentry failure.[7] Nevertheless, the argument against non-axial implant placement remained until the late 1990s when it was rediscovered that there are distinct advantages to angled implant placement, particularly in the complete arch immediate function setting.[8–10] In the interval, thousands of restorative procedures had been planned and completed using angled implant placement.[11,12] From this evidence and experience, various advantages for angled implants have been proposed, including:

1. achieving biomechanical fixation into cortical bone;
2. facilitating splinted complete arch immediate function;
3. improving biomechanical distribution for complete arch restoration;
4. economy of implant placement for the complete arch;
5. increasing implant resistance form;
6. avoiding vital structures;
7. avoiding bone grafting;
8. increasing use of immediate function;
9. increasing patient acceptance of treatment; and
10. psycho-social benefits.

Achieving biomechanical fixation into cortical bone

For both maxilla and mandible, cortical bone is often necessary to achieve maximal primary stability and insertion torque with dental implants. Implant insertion torque correlates to bone mineral density and bone-to-implant contact in type I cortical bone. Bone of this nature is commonly found in both arches, and often can be used by angling an implant to engage cortical bone apically. Complete arch restoration cannot always proceed with immediate function using an axial implant placement strategy, particularly in the atrophic maxilla;[13] however, angled implant placement can help to facilitate this desired outcome.

Facilitating splinted complete arch immediate function

Implants placed with sufficient insertion torque (e.g. 120 N cm composite insertion torque for four implants) often can best be achieved with angled implant placement. Atrophy in both jaws can make complete arch immediate function difficult owing to limited residual bone. In the maxilla, absence of subnasal bone and anterior sinus location can compromise vertical implant

Minimally Invasive Dental Implant Surgery, First Edition. Edited by Daniel R. Cullum and Douglas Deporter.

placement. However, by angling anterior implants to the posterior and/or posterior implants to the anterior to engage the lateral pyriform rim, immediate function is frequently possible as insertion torque will be gained apically in cortical bone.[14]

Improving biomechanical distribution

The concept of increased anterior–posterior (A–P) spread (i.e. the linear distance between front and back implants) is important for reducing biomechanical stress on both the implants and the prosthesis in full-arch reconstructions. With adequate bone height, mandibular implant placement in the molar region above the inferior alveolar nerve allows maximum A–P spread (Figure 12.1a). With further bone atrophy in the jaws, A–P spread can be improved by implant angulation (Figures 12.1b–d and 12.2a and b), more so with a V- than U-shaped arch form. Increasing the A–P spread results in greater prosthetic stability with a reduced length

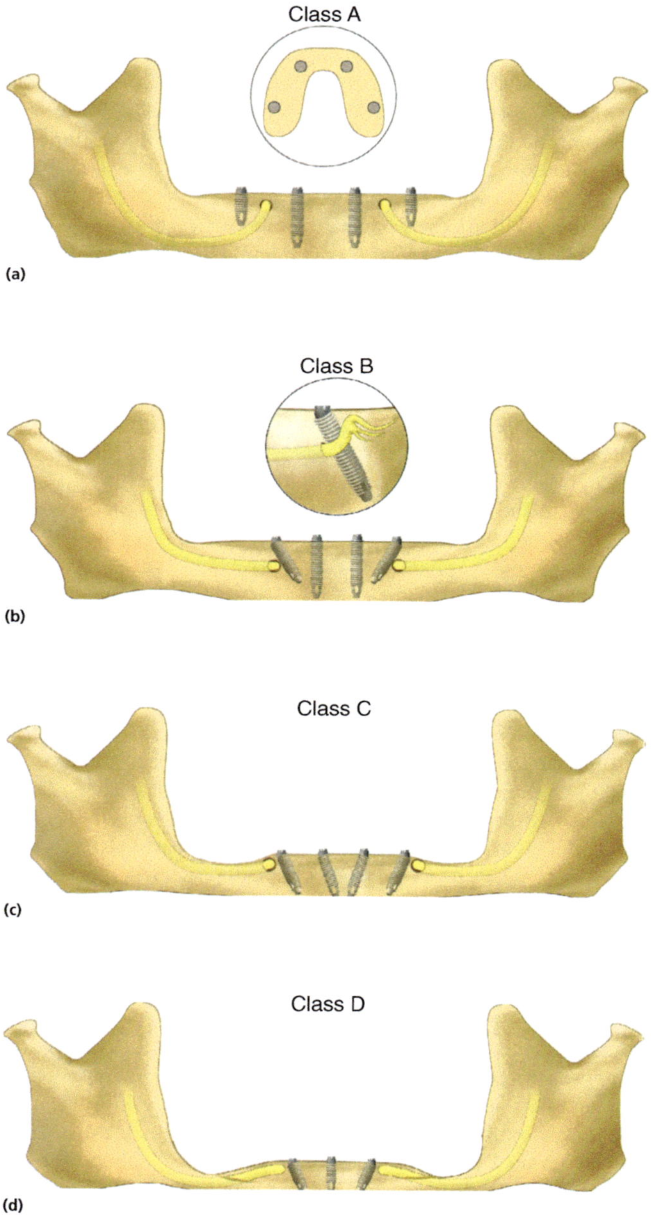

Figure 12.1 (a–d) Immediate-function site classification based on cortical bone fixation for the mandible according to availability of bone and required implant placement strategies. All cases are immediately loaded in this classification.

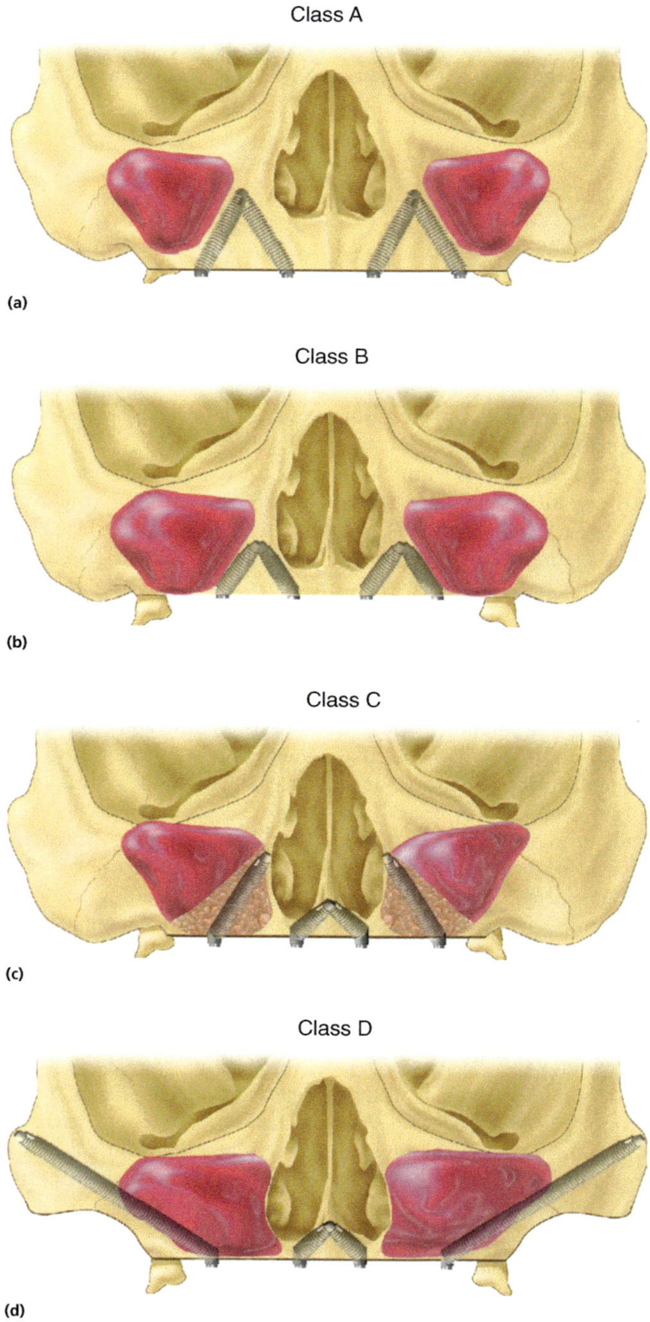

Figure 12.2 (a–d) Immediate-function site classification based on cortical bone fixation for the maxilla classified according to availability of bone and required implant placement strategies. All cases are immediately loaded in this classification with the trans-sinus graft material for the class C maxilla suggested as bone morphogenetic protein-2/absorbable collagen sponge–allograft in a 50% mixture by volume.

of cantilever extension in the prosthesis.[15] Angulation of implants makes favorable A–P spreads increasingly possible, especially when there is gross osseous deficiency.

Economy of implant placement

The number of implants used in a complete arch restoration is necessarily reduced when angled implants are employed. Typically, four implants placed at a 30° angle to the occlusal plane will make the placement of additional implants impossible. Two angled implants placed in the front of the arch will traverse the alveolus from the lateral incisor to cuspid region, while two angled implants placed posteriorly will traverse the molar–second premolar region. The four implants placed in this fashion form an M-shaped configuration (M-4) (Figure 12.2a). Additional implants do not add significant biomechanical advantage for this modality of complete arch treatment. However, for patients with risk of excess loading (bruxism or clenching habit) and a brachiocephalic facial type, additional posterior implants and reduced cantilever lengths are recommended in the molar regions by means of a six-implant-supported prosthesis.[16]

Increasing resistance form by angulation

Particularly when immediate function is employed, increasing resistance form with angled implants results in greater surface area due to increased implant surface contact with bone. Implants angled at 30° have 50% greater length in contact with bone than implants placed axially. The composite torque value for four implants is also likely to be higher with longer implant to bone contact. Long implants that are angled in a complex osseous conformation once splinted provide secondary stabilization due to an increased resistance form analogous to the secondary stabilization of prosthesis splinting.[17]

Avoiding vital structures

The use of implant angulation came about in an effort to avoid the maxillary sinus and the mandibular inferior alveolar nerve. When the maxillary sinus extends far to the anterior, vertical placement is often not possible without sinus bone grafting. Typically, however, there is a triangular-shaped segment of bone beneath the sinus that can be engaged if the implant is angled forward beneath the sinus cavity. This usually allows for the posterior implant to be placed 5–8 mm further to the posterior (Figure 12.2a and b). In mandible, if there is 4–5 mm of bone above the nerve canal behind the mental foramen, there may not be enough bone for axial implant placement even with short implants. However, if the posterior implant is angled at 30° from behind the mental foramen to the anterior, it will just miss the nerve and allow for the implant platform position to be 5–8 mm further to the posterior (Figure 12.1b). These strategies increase A–P spread even as they avoid vital structures.[18,19]

Avoiding bone grafting

The need for sinus bone grafting can be significantly reduced with the use of angled implants (Figures 12.2a and b and 12.3). Similarly, guided bone regeneration for site augmentation is less frequently needed as locations can usually be selected for angled implants,

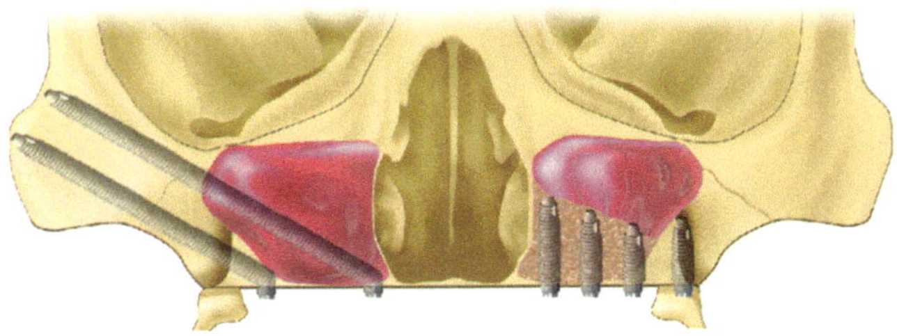

Figure 12.3 A class D maxilla depicting a traditional delayed sinus grafting and guided bone regeneration approach with an alternative treatment option using "quad zygomatic" fixtures.

thus avoiding bone grafting. Transalveolar angled placement from palatal to buccal in the maxilla can be done in a narrow alveolus without grafting as the majority of the implant length will be in bone.[20] Additionally, any exposed implant threads will be located on the palatal rather than the buccal. With increasing atrophy and sinus pneumatization, trans-sinus angled implant placement can be used with limited sinus membrane dissection to engage cortical bone. With limited implant exposure and sufficient anchorage, trans-sinus implants need not always be grafted. However with significant implant exposure, grafting with recombinant human bone morphogenetic protein-2/absorbable collagen sponge–bone allograft in a 50% mixture by volume is recommended (Figure 12.2c). In the mandible, an hourglass anatomy can usually be circumvented by angling to avoid the alveolar constriction either posteriorly (Figure 12.1c) or anteriorly.[21,22]

Increasing use of immediate function

There is greater likelihood for employing immediate function when implants are placed at an angle as the chance for adequate insertion torque is increased, particularly when implants can be fixed apically into cortical bone. In maxilla, cortical bone is found in the paranasal region, particularly at the lateral pyriform rim above the nasal fossa and at the nasal crest. The mandible almost always has availability of cortical bone, so that angled implants here are not as important for immediate function, but they may still play an important role in establishing adequate prosthetic support by increasing the A–P spread.[23]

Increasing patient acceptance to treatment

Patient acceptance of implant treatment can be improved by reducing the need for extensive multi-staged surgical and prosthetic treatments. Implant angulation offers the potential for immediate loading even with simultaneous multiple extractions. Angled implant placement can often avoid situations where previously extensive bone grafting was necessary to fulfill osseointegration criteria. Thus, patients are more willing to proceed with treatment having less potential morbidity and a reduced cost.[24]

Favorable psycho-social factors

Psychosocial factors can play an important role for patients seeking a seamless transition from a dentate state to an immediate function

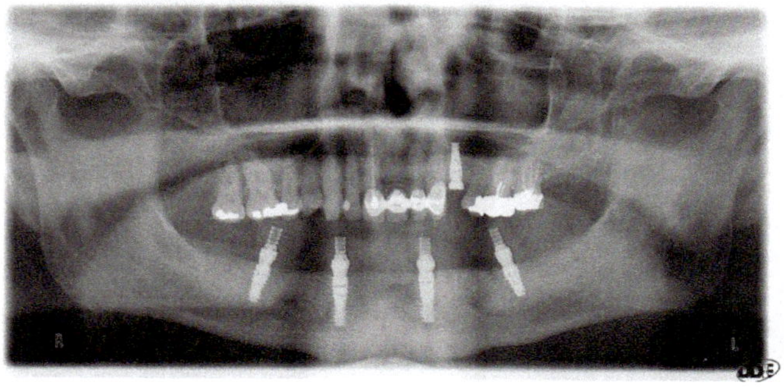

Figure 12.4 Panoramic image of a class A patient who had excellent bone available in the mandible for vertical implant placement above the nerve.

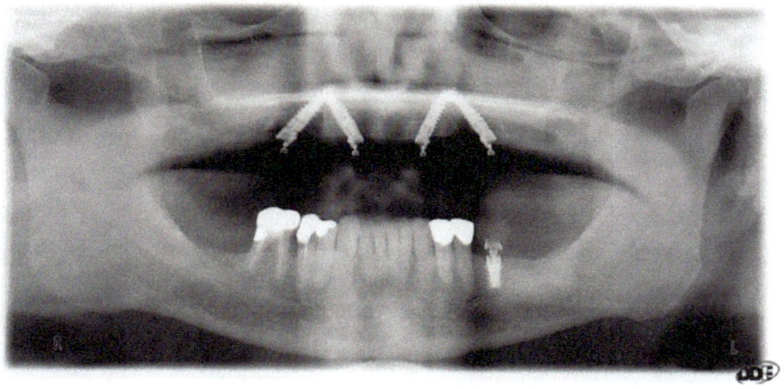

Figure 12.6 Treatment of a class B maxilla with an angled M-4 placement is demonstrated in this panoramic radiograph.

implant-supported prosthesis. Patients desire treatment that will improve function and esthetics. Temporary removable dentures can be avoided, minimizing upset to daily life, an important consideration for both clinician and patient. Angled implants provide a distinct advantage toward achieving an implant-supported immediate-function prosthesis.[25]

Discussion

Angled implant placement with immediate function must be based upon anatomic morphology within the setting of a fixed cross-arch stabilized prosthesis. A site classification for immediate function based on cortical fixation of implants has been published[26] (Figures 12.1 and 12.2). The basis of this classification is that typical variants of bone availability found in both jaws will be manageable with approximately four different angulation approaches to achieve successful osseointegration. An example of the classification is presented in a panoramic image of a class A patient who had excellent bone available in the mandible (Figure 12.4). In this patient, posterior implants emerged at the first molar positions and the A–P spread exceeded 20 mm. Figure 12.5 demonstrates a class A patient 1 year after restoration, with the final prosthesis treatment including extraction and immediately loaded, angled implants in the mandible.

With early atrophy and sinus pneumatization, the available bone housing in maxilla is reduced. Treatment of a class B maxilla with an angled M-4 placement is demonstrated on the panoramic radiograph in Figure 12.6. In the mandible with horizontal and vertical changes, the residual posterior bone height can prevent placement of short implants. Figure 12.7 shows the use of immediate angled implants in a class C mandible with vertical anterior osteoplasty for adequate prosthetic space, to avoid grafting and allow an immediate loading protocol.

As further atrophy occurs, the classification describes variations of angled implant placement with decreasing A–P spread. One thing notable in the maxillary classification is the considered use of nasal crest cortex for placement of "vomer" implants.[23] These 30° angled anterior implants engage cortical bone above the nasal floor in the midline sometimes up to the junction of the vomer. Vomer implants are used anteriorly in highly atrophic cases with

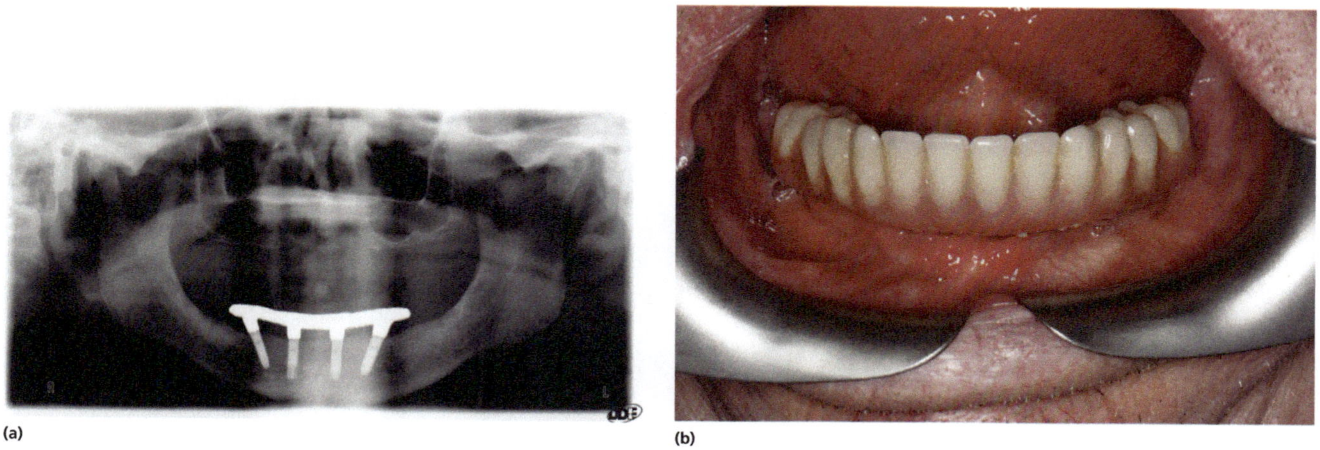

(a) (b)

Figure 12.5 Panoramic radiograph and clinical images demonstrate a class A patient 1 year after final restoration with angled immediate-loading implant placement in the mandible. *Source*: Restoration: Earl Ness, DDS, MS. © Daniel R. Cullum.

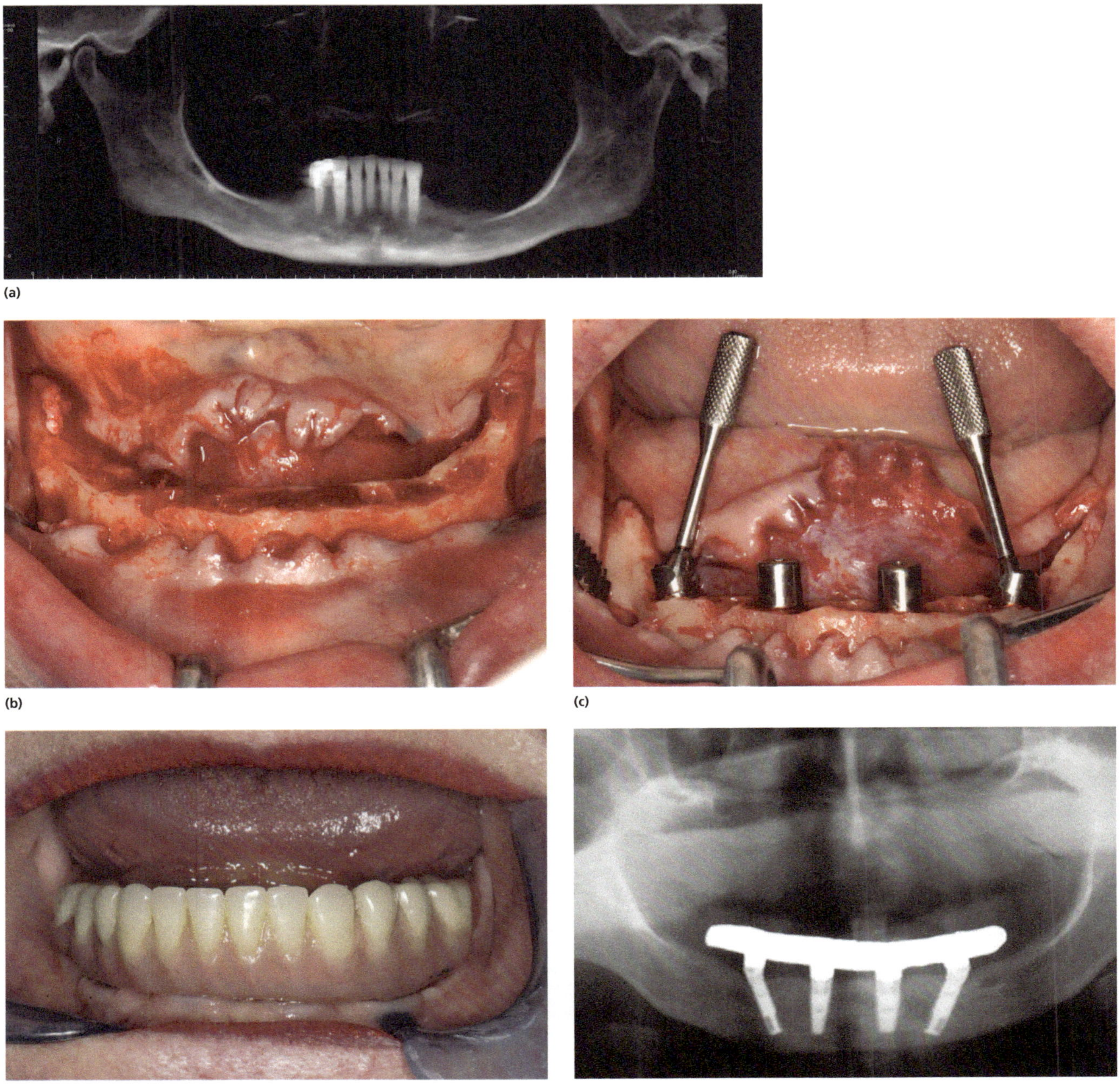

(a) (b) (c) (d) (e)

Figure 12.7 (a–e) A patient with a class B/C mandible can be seen with severe posterior bone loss and a failing anterior dentition. Angled immediate implant placement in the mandible was completed to avoid grafting and allow an immediate loading protocol. After extraction, vertical bone was reduced in the anterior region to allow adequate prosthetic space for the restoration. Angled distal implants and angled multi-unit abutments were placed to increase the A–P spread followed by placement of a "direct pick-up," immediate provisional prosthesis. Clinical and radiographic images after 5 years demonstrate the stability of this treatment. *Source*: Restoration: Earl Ness, DDS, MS. © Daniel R. Cullum.

either trans-sinus or zygomatic implants placed posteriorly in a four-implant scheme (Figure 12.8).

Other implant considerations for the maxilla include implant placement into the pterygoid process and/or the zygoma. Pterygoid implants are usually angled forward about 20°s, whereas zygomatic implants are angled laterally about 45°s. These implant locations are not ideal either prosthetically or surgically, but are required in settings of severe bone deficiency, especially when mid maxillary bone is absent. Implants placed in these locations, sometimes in conjunction with vomer implants, provide a six-implant scheme comprised of essentially extramaxillary implants[27,28] (Figure 12.9).

A further location in the maxilla that can be used with angled implant placement is the tuberosity, where enlargement of the sinus can leave a small, oblique bone reserve. Figure 12.10 demonstrates the use the maxillary tuberosity after loss of a short implant supporting a fixed restoration.

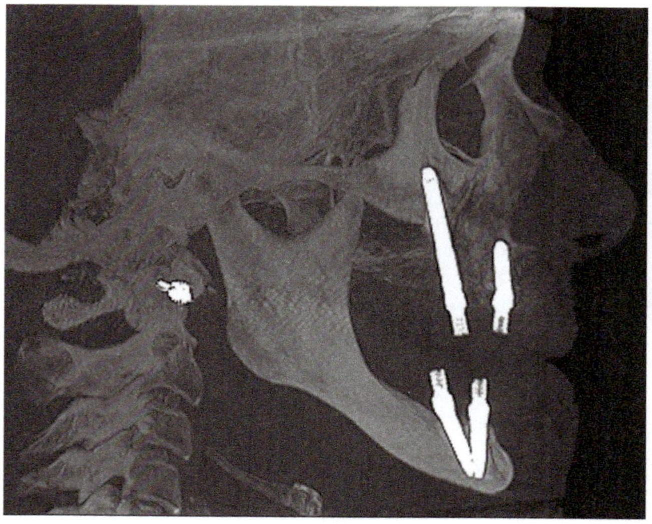

Figure 12.8 A cephalometric radiograph of a patient with a class D maxilla treated with vomer implants placed anteriorly into the nasal crest, and zygomatic implants placed in the posterior.

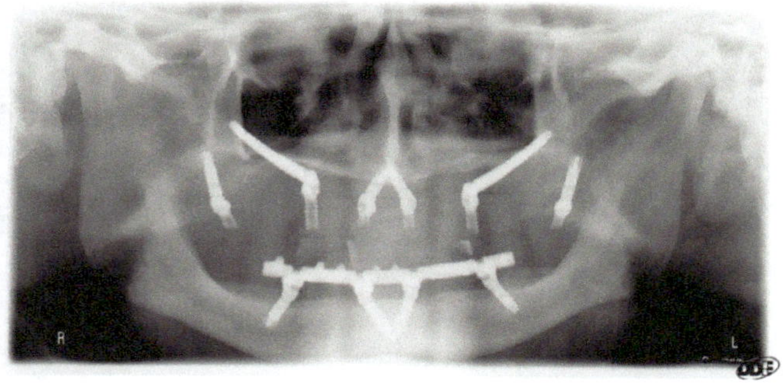

Figure 12.9 "Extramaxillary" implant placement of two anterior vomer implants placed into the nasal crest, two zygomatic implants placed into the zygomas, and two pterygoid implants placed into the pterygomaxillary sutures. The mandibular treatment demonstrates posterior angulation of the anterior fixtures and anterior angulation of the posterior fixtures to emerge through a wider alveolar crest avoiding the narrow undercut regions.

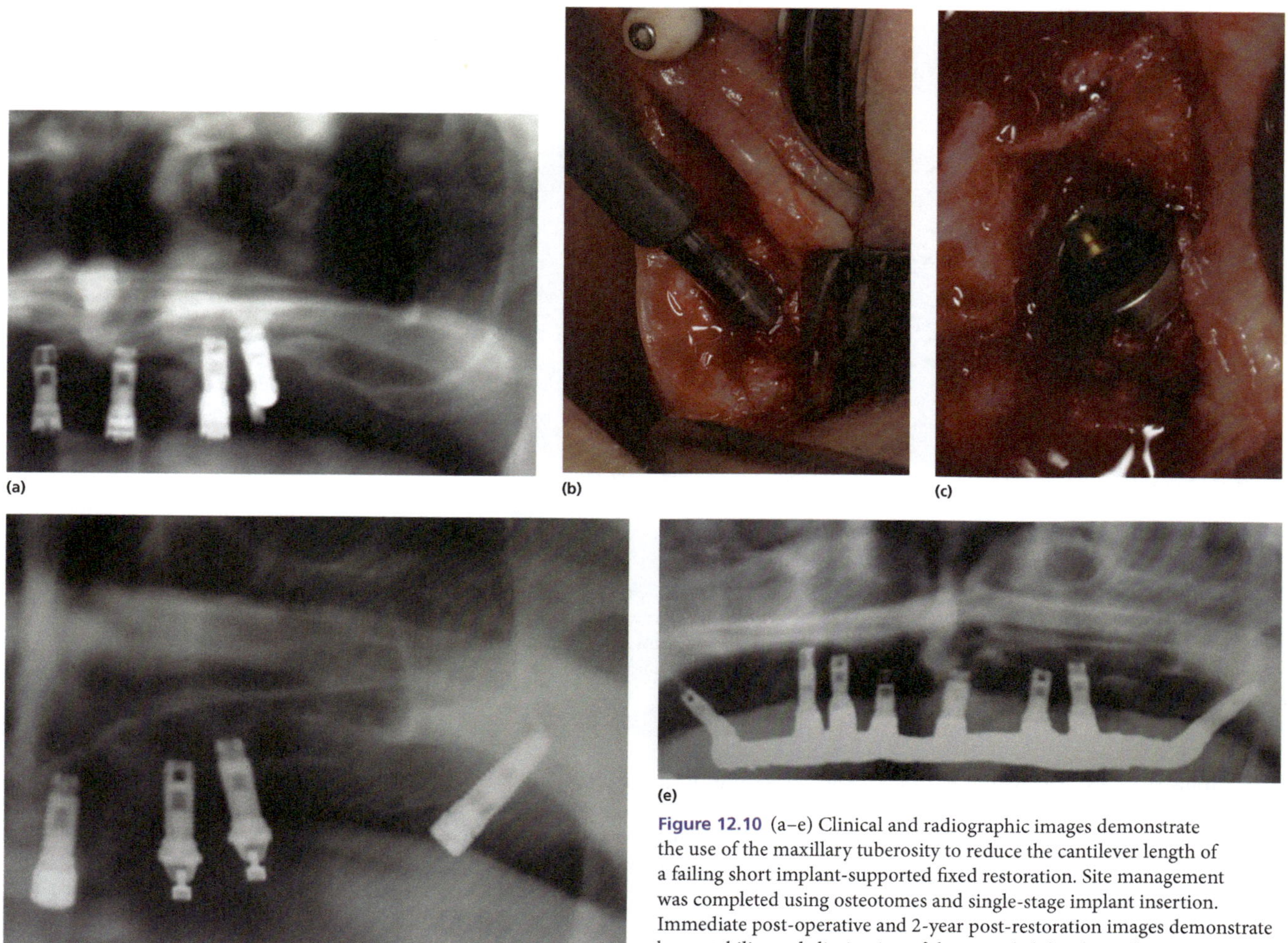

(a) (b) (c) (d) (e)

Figure 12.10 (a–e) Clinical and radiographic images demonstrate the use of the maxillary tuberosity to reduce the cantilever length of a failing short implant-supported fixed restoration. Site management was completed using osteotomes and single-stage implant insertion. Immediate post-operative and 2-year post-restoration images demonstrate bone stability and elimination of the extended distal cantilever. *Source*: Restoration: Earl Ness, DDS, MS. © Daniel R. Cullum.

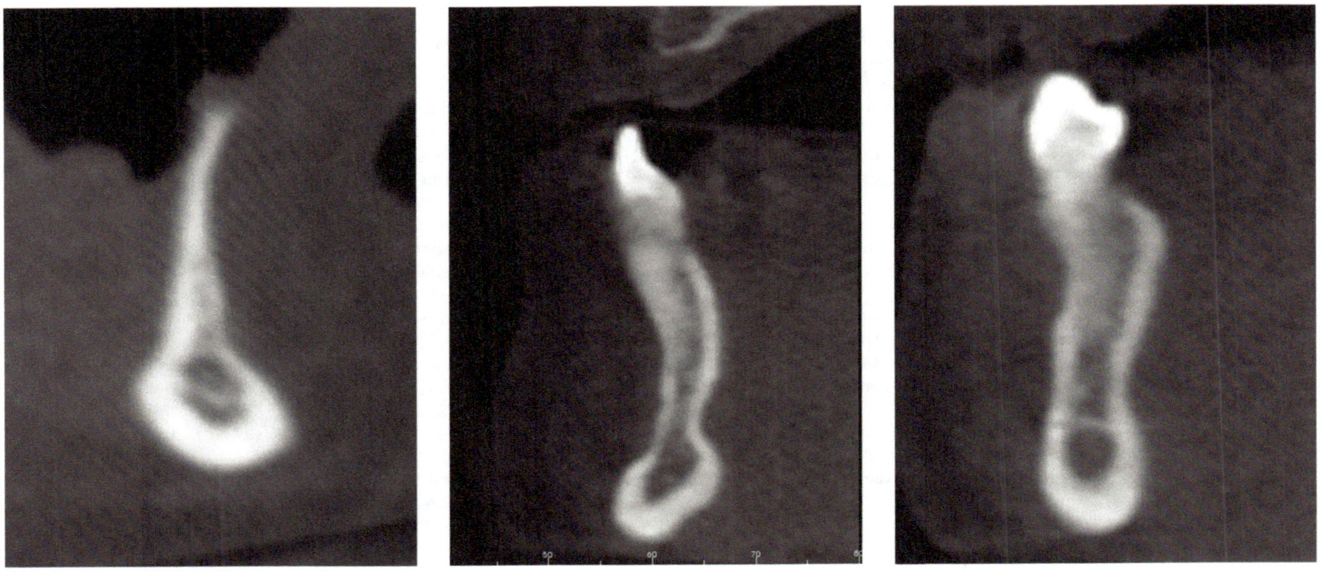

(a) (b) (c)

Figure 12.11 (a–c) Anatomic variants of limited bone volume include thin bucco-lingual dimension and areas of alveolar constriction in the mandible, as shown in the incisor zone. Tilted implants can be used to avoid a thin area and engage bone in a wider area. © Daniel R. Cullum.

Anatomic variants in the mandible include a severe thin horizontal bone volume (Figure 12.11a) or an hourglass morphology usually presenting as severe mid alveolar constriction (Figure 12.11b). The constriction can exist around the complete arch, but usually is limited to the anterior region with a wider osseous housing in the bicuspid zone (Figure 12.11c). In this setting, anterior implants can be placed angled posteriorly into the wider alveolar bone. When there is midline bone available for the hourglass mandible, anterior fixtures can be tilted forward to engage the wider bone in the midline (Figure 12.9). Implants in these cases can then be placed without bone grafting and without using a delayed placement strategy by angling implants into zones of available bone.[21]

There are multiple justifications for using an angled implant strategy for immediate function or to avoid vital structures. There has been no substantial evidence presented that angulation in splinted constructions has either deleterious biomechanical or biological consequences to bone. Bone loss appears about equal over time in patients treated with either straight or angled implants.[4–6] Placement of angled implants is a technically demanding procedure. However, when mastered, the approach offers significant advantages, and is becoming the preferred technique for many surgeons.

Conclusions

The 10 factors supporting the use of angled implant placement presented in this chapter are based on the comparative simplicity and versatility of angled implant placement versus the multiple surgery/multiple implant/multiple bridge approach when a ceramo-metal prosthesis is prescribed. Traditional reconstructions with treatment plans using vertical placement of dental implants often require extensive guided bone regeneration, short implants, and/or sinus grafting, and may also require secondary soft tissue procedures. The simplicity of angled implant placement and immediate loading concepts can obviate the need for staged, complex, and often expensive treatment, making access to care more likely for patients. Angled implants can also serve patients with failing implant reconstructions, allowing strategic placement and positioning to avoid lengthy retreatment scenarios. The use of angled implants adds great versatility to the clinician's armamentarium, effecting a more simplified and accessible treatment, particularly for complete arch immediate function.

References

1. Adell R, Lekholm U, Rockler B, Brånemark PI. A 15-year study of osseointegrated implants in the treatment of the edentulous jaw. *Int J Oral Surg* 1981; 10: 387–416.
2. Lindquist LW, Rockler B, Carlsson GE. Bone resorption around fixtures in edentulous patients treated with mandibular fixed tissue-integrated prostheses. *J Prosthet Dent* 1988; 59: 59–63.
3. Chen JC, Beaupre GS, Carter DR. An approach to quantifying bone overloading and hypertrophy with applications to multiple experimental studies. *Bone* 2010; 46: 322–299.
4. Ata-Ali J, Peñarrocha-Oltra, Candel-Marti E. Peñarrohca-Diago M. Oral rehabilitation with tilted dental implants: a metanalysis. Med Oral Patol Oral Bucal 2012; 17: e582–e587.
5. Menini M, Signori A, Tealdo T, et al. Tilted implants in the immediate loading rehabilitation of the maxilla: a systematic review. J Dent Res 2012; 91: 821–827.
6. Testori T, Del Fabbro M, Capelli M, et al. Immediate occlusal loading and tilted implants for the rehabilitation of the atrophic edentulous maxilla: 1-year interim results of a multicenter prospective study. Clin Oral Implants Res 2008; 19: 227–232.
7. Jemt T. Failures and complications in 391 consecutively inserted fixed prostheses supported by Brånemark implants in edentulous jaws: a study of treatment from time of prosthesis placement to first annual checkup. Int J Oral Maxillofac Implants 1991; 6: 270–276.
8. Mattsson T, Kondell PA, Gynther GW, et al. Implant treatment without bone grafting in severely resorbed edentulous maxillae. J Oral Maxillofac Surg 1999; 57: 281–287.
9. Krekmanov L, Kahn M, Rangert B, Lindstrom H. Tilting of posterior mandibular and maxillary implants for improved prosthesis support. Int J Oral Maxillofac Implants 2000; 15: 405–414.
10. Aparacio C. Perales P, Rangert B. Tilted implants as an alternative to maxillary sinus grafting: a clinical radiologic and periotest study. Clin Implant Dent Relat Res 2001; 3: 39–49.

11. Agliardi E, Panigatti S, Clerico M, et al. Immediate rehabilitation of the edentulous jaws with full fixed prostheses supported by four implants: interim results of a single cohort prospective study. Clin Oral Implants Res 2010; 21: 459–465.
12. Graves S, Mahler BA, Javid B, et al. Maxillary all-on-four therapy using angled implants: a 16-month clinical study of 1110 implants in 276 jaws. Oral Maxillofac Surg Clin North Am 2011; 23: 277–287.
13. Jensen OT, Adams MW. The maxillary M-4: a technical and biomechanical note for all-on-four management of severe maxillary atrophy – report of three cases. J Oral Maxillfac Surg 2009; 67: 1739–1744.
14. Jensen OT, Adams MW, Smith E. Paranasal bone: the prime factor affecting the decision to use trans-sinus vs zygomatic implants for biomechanical support for immediate function in maxillary dental implant reconstruction. Oral Craniofac Tissue Eng 2012; 2: 198–206.
15. Brunski JB. Biomechanics. In: Osseointegration in Dentistry: An Overview, 2nd ed., WorthingtonP, LangBR, RubinsteinJE, eds. Chicago, IL: Quintessence, 2003, pp. 64–65.
16. Parel SM, Phillips WR. A risk assessment treatment planning protocol for the four implant immediately loaded maxilla: preliminary findings. J Prosthet Dent 2011; 10: 359–366.
17. Jensen OT, Adams MW. Secondary stabilization of maxillary M-4 treatment with unstable implants for immediate function: biomechanical considerations and report of 10 cases after 1 year in function. Oral Craniofac Tissue Eng 2012; 2: 294–302.
18. Jensen OT, Adams MW, Cottam JR, et al. The all-on-four shelf: maxilla. J Oral Maxillofac Surg 2010; 68: 2520–2527.
19. Jensen OT, Adams MW. All-on-four treatment of highly atrophic mandible with mandibular V-4: report of 2 cases. J Oral Maxillofac Surg 2009; 67: 1503–1509.
20. Testori T, Mandelli F, Mantovani M, et al. Tilted trans-sinus implants for the treatment of maxillary atrophy: case series of 35 consecutive patients. J Oral Maxillofac Surg 2013; 71: 1187–1194.
21. Butura CC, Galindo DF, Adams MW, Jensen OT. Hourglass mandibular anatomic variant incidence and treatment considerations for all-on-four implant therapy: report of 10 cases. J Oral Maxillofac Surg 2011; 69: 2135–2143.
22. Brånemark PI, Adell R, Albrektsson T, et al. An experimental and clinical study of osseointegratied implant penetrating the nasal cavity and maxillary sinus. J Oral Maxillofac Surg 1984; 42: 497–505.
23. Jensen OT, Cottam JR, Ringeman JL, Adams MW. Angled dental implant placement into the vomer/nasal crest of atrophic maxillae for all-on-four immediate function: a 2-year clinical study. Oral Craniofac Tissue Eng 2012; 2: 66–71.
24. Romaos GE, Nentwig GH. Immediate functional loading in the maxilla using implant with platform-switching: five year results. Int J Oral Maxillofac Implants 2009; 24: 1106–1112.
25. Babbush CA. Post-treatment quantification of patient experiences with full-arch implant treatment using a modification of the OHIP-14 questionnaire. J Oral Implantol 2012; 38: 251–260.
26. Jensen OT. Complete arch site classification for all-on-four immediate function. J Prosthet Dent; 2014; 112(4): 741–751.e2.
27. Bedrossian E, Rangert B, Strumpel L, Indresano T. Immediate function with zygomatic implants: a graft-less solution for the patient with mild to advanced atrophy of the maxilla. Int J Oral Maxillofac Implants 2006; 21: 937–942.
28. Graves SL. The pterygoid plate implant: a solution for restoring the posterior maxilla. Int J Periodontics Restorative Dent 1994; 14: 512–523.

CHAPTER 13

Wedge Implants and Piezoelectric Surgery: A Minimally Invasive Implant Concept for the Treatment of Narrow Alveolar Ridges

Tomaso Vercellotti[1,2] & Claudio Stacchi[3]
[1]Private Practice, Genoa, Italy
[2]University College of London, Eastman Dental Institute, London, UK
[3]Department of Medical, Surgical and Health Sciences, University of Trieste, Trieste, Italy

Introduction

Tooth loss rapidly results in significant alveolar ridge remodeling. This bone resorptive process begins immediately after tooth extraction and ultimately results in an average 40–60% decrease in the horizontal and vertical dimensions of the alveolar ridge during the first 2 years, and mostly within the first 3 months.[1–3] It is now known that crestal remodeling is largely limited to bundle bone resorption,[4] making it most evident on the buccal aspect, especially in patients with thin periodontal biotypes where significant buccal hard and soft tissue recessions can occur during socket healing. Furthermore, ridge resorption continues with time as a result of a combination of anatomic, metabolic, and mechanical determinants,[5] including the use of complete or partial removable dentures.[6] Thus, it is common to encounter severely atrophic ridges when planning an implant-supported rehabilitation.

It is generally accepted that a dental implant should have a thickness of at least 2 mm of bone covering the buccal aspect to ensure stability and minimal risk of dehiscence of hard and soft tissues over time. If adequate ridge width preoperatively will not result in a sufficiently thick buccal bone plate after implant placement, ridge expansion and/or augmentation grafting will become necessary, and a variety of such approaches have been suggested and used with success (see also Chapters 16 and 17). In a recent review paper, Milinkovic and Cordaro[7] reported that staged guided bone regeneration (GBR) showed a subsequent implant survival rate (ISR) of 100% and a complication rate (CR) of 11.9%. In contrast, bone block grafts resulted in a 98.4% ISR and 6.3% CR, and ridge expansion/splitting showed a 97.4% ISR and 6.8% CR. However, as the authors stated, they found only a few suitable papers that could be included in their review (five for staged GBR, eight for bone blocks, and six for ridge expansion), and most included results for small groups of patients. Likewise, Esposito et al.[8] concluded that, even if the surgical techniques used for horizontal bone augmentation appear to give good clinical results, the evaluation on their predictability is still based on few trials including few patients, sometimes having a short follow-up, and often being judged as having high risk of bias. Various techniques can reconstruct bone horizontally, but it is unclear which is the most efficient. Furthermore, procedures such as GBR, bone block grafting, and ridge expansion are advanced techniques needing an extensive surgical background and an adequate learning curve to achieve optimal results. Therefore, it may be unrealistic to expect the same success for every clinician employing these surgical options.

Ultrasonic bone surgery has gained broad application since first introduced in implant-related osteotomies.[9] The beneficial effects of safety, precision, and reduced risk of damage at adjacent structures have made this technology an integral part of the armamentarium for dental implant reconstruction. Applications with bone harvesting, implant site preparation, and precise osteotomies can facilitate procedures reducing lateral thermal damage and enhancing wound healing.[10] These are significant convenience and safety advantages with ultrasonic implant site preparation compared with rotary instruments or micro-saws.[11]

In the early days of implant dentistry, attempts to treat narrow ridges with blade-vent implants were often problematic. However, we have revisited this concept and in this chapter describe a new implant designed to achieve osseointegration for specific use in narrow ridges. This implant has a bucco-lingual dimension of only 1.8 or 2.9 mm, and its wedge shape makes its positioning possible with minimal site preparation. A piezoelectric bone-cutting system with dedicated tips is used to perform a precise and conservative osteotomy followed by press-fit implant insertion using a specific magnetic mallet. The use of this implant may allow for an effective and minimally invasive treatment of narrow edentulous ridges, with significant advantages for the patient that include reduced morbidity, simplified treatment, cost reduction, and shorter duration of therapy.

Ultrasonic bone surgery: an overview

In 1938, Pohlman introduced ultrasound to medical practice with the successful application of ultrasonic physiotherapy at the Charité Hospital in Berlin. In the 1940s, extensive experimentation was conducted using ultrasound for diagnostic purposes

Minimally Invasive Dental Implant Surgery, First Edition. Edited by Daniel R. Cullum and Douglas Deporter.

and for treatment of different pathologies. Catuna reported the first use of ultrasonics as a cutting method for dental application in 1953.[12] In the following decades, a few attempts were made to perform osteotomies using ultrasonic energy;[13–16] however, limitations with sufficient cutting power and potential overheating with bone damage were evident. A review on bone-cutting instruments by Giraud et al.[17] in 1991 classified ultrasound as an "unconventional" bone-cutting device that needed further technological improvements and scientific studies to enter into routine clinical use.

In 2000, Vercellotti published the first case report on a ridge expansion in the upper jaw where the osseous surgery was completed with a specifically designed ultrasonic device.[9] This innovative "Piezosurgery®" device used ultrasonic microvibrations to cut bone in a safe and predictable way, overcoming the limits of the instruments previously used in osseous surgery (Figure 13.1). The advantages of piezoelectric osseous surgery include the micrometric cutting motion (leading to a precise and controllable surgical action), selective action on mineralized tissues, the cavitation effect, and enhanced bone healing of the ultrasonic cut. The amplitude of the microvibrations of the tip range from 20 to 200 μm (which can vary depending on the device) and the frequency is 25,000–30,000 hits per second on the bone surface. These parameters give improved surgical control compared with conventional instruments such as rotary burs and saw blades. Every single impact of the working tip on bone is so minimal that it has an insignificant influence on the operator's control of the handpiece. Furthermore, the ideal force needed for the handpiece to obtain maximum cutting efficiency is around 1–3 N,[18,19] significantly lower than the load needed for conventional drills (15–20 N). These factors allow for increased surgical control and sensitivity.

The precision of the ultrasonic cut preserves osseous architecture, especially the trabecular integrity of cancellous bone, which loses its typical structure after conventional osteotomies performed with burs or saws.[20] With conventional instruments, cancellous bone spaces can be occluded with osseous debris, creating a mechanical obstacle for restoring the peripheral blood supply.[21] Blood perfusion and cell migration from the marrow spaces may be facilitated by preserving the integrity of the cancellous bone structure and enhancing the quality and the rate of the bone healing process.[22,23] Selective cutting is an important characteristic of piezoelectric bone surgery. The frequency of oscillation of the ultrasonic tips used for osteotomy ranges between 22 and 30 kHz, making it possible to prevent accidental damage to soft tissues and nerves; however, when frequencies over 50 kHz are used there is an increased risk of soft tissue injury. *In vitro* and *in vivo* studies[24,25] showed that accidental contact with a nerve structure during osseous surgery with an ultrasonic device will cause only a roughening of the epineurium without affecting the deeper structures.

The cavitation effect with ultrasonic bone surgery is a biophysical effect generated in saline by the microvibrations of the tip resulting in the formation and immediate implosion of gas bubbles in the proximity of the bone cut.[26] It typically occurs when a fluid is subjected to a rapid change in pressure, leading to the formation of lower pressure cavities within the liquid. In piezoelectric surgery, this constant growth and collapse of bubbles into many minute fractions (microscopic gas bubbles) has important effects. The cavitation phenomenon creates a virtually bloodless surgical site, improving visibility in the working area compared with conventional bone cutting instruments. Cavitation also has an antibacterial action by fragmenting the cellular membranes of bacteria[27] and cleansing the osteotomy surfaces. Cavitation results in effective removal of bone debris and tissue remnants from the site, exposing marrow spaces and favoring a rapid migration of osteoprogenitor cells into the fresh wound.

Several studies have shown a positive effect of ultrasonic osseous surgery on the rate of bone healing compared with traditional bone-cutting techniques. For example, a preclinical

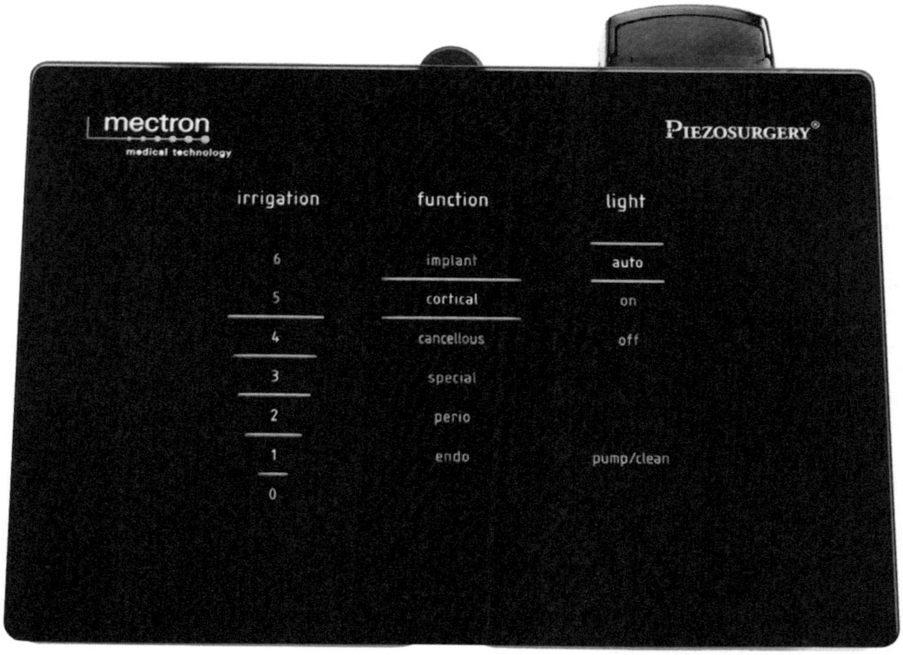

Figure 13.1 Mectron Piezosurgery device.

animal study[28] comparing diamond burs, carbide burs, and piezoelectric inserts in periodontal osseous surgery demonstrated that the ultrasonic bone cut provided a more favorable osseous repair and remodeling. Preti et al.[29] also compared ultrasonic implant site preparation with traditional rotary protocols in an animal model and demonstrated a higher concentration of inflammatory cells in samples taken from the drilled sites. Also, bone around implant sites inserted using an ultrasonic technique showed an earlier increase in BMP-4 and TGF-β2 proteins as well as a reduction in pro-inflammatory cytokines. In a human randomized controlled clinical trial, Stacchi et al.[30] reported that ultrasonic implant site preparation resulted in a smaller decrease in implant stability quotient (ISQ) in the early phases of healing and in a faster return to an increased stability pattern when comparing outcomes with traditional drilling technique. Ultrasonic implant site preparation also was tested in a recent multicenter clinical study including a large number of patients and was shown to be a reliable alternative to a conventional drilling technique.[31]

These findings have helped to expand the use of ultrasonic bone surgery from oral and maxillofacial surgery to orthopedics, ENT, neurosurgery, plastic surgery, cardio-thoracic surgery, and veterinary medicine with positive clinical outcomes. Continued basic research is needed on the mechanisms of piezoelectric bone surgery, including cavitation and the direct mechanical and thermal effects that occur. Further evaluation of ultrasonic tissue effects *ex vivo* and *in vivo* should target the definition of damage and removal mechanisms, and give indications for future technological improvements to optimize performance and safety during daily clinical applications.

Proper site preparation is a fundamental part in successful implant site preparation, even more so with the required dimensions for insertion of wedge implants. The osteotomy needs to be precise and narrow bucco-lingually in order to optimize implant stability and preserve the maximum amount of bone. This makes ultrasonic implant site preparation rather than rotary instruments or micro-saws the safest and most convenient option for these requirements.

Minimally invasive treatment of narrow ridges

When an atrophic ridge has an insufficient bucco-lingual width for a standard implant placement, one possibility to avoid a regenerative procedure is to choose an implant with reduced dimensions. Companies making the most commonly used implant systems offer a wide range of diameters for cylindrical and tapered implants, but the minimum diameter is usually about 3.0 mm (see also Chapter 11). These implants require a minimum crestal width of 5–6 mm for placement to allow sufficient bone covering on the buccal and lingual aspects. Furthermore, manufacturers often recommend limiting the use of these reduced-diameter implants to small anterior sites, owing to their reduced biomechanical characteristics. For these reasons, clinical applications of narrow-diameter implants are limited.

In the late 1960s, Linkow introduced the blade implant for treatment of the narrow ridge.[32] The blade design had a broad bone interface and an extremely narrow profile. A variety of shapes were provided so as to have an implant suitable for different clinical situations. The implants were inserted in a groove cut with a bur or saw blade and then tapped into their final position. According to Linkow and Cherchéve, the blade implant had several advantages:[33]

> Its broad face prevents it from being rotated on its axis by undue lateral stresses. The implant may be very long, and its wide shoulders bear two, rather than the standard one, abutment posts. A single blade implant may support a long-span prosthesis. If an implant is needed in an area of the jaw that curves, the implant may be bent to follow the curve without weakening it. The blade may be tall or short to fit the alveolar bone height or specially cut to fit an atypical site.

These interesting features led to an enthusiastic beginning; however, problems emerged, as the procedure was highly technique-sensitive. Implant failures were common due to biomechanical problems, biological incompatibility and infection. Accordingly, use of the technique remained limited to a small group of clinicians and limited clinical data was accumulated. We conducted a literature search of papers published on blade implants from 1968 to 2014, and this showed that most studies were confined to the lower categories of scientific evidence (Tables 13.1 and 13.2).

For many years, blade-form dental implants were classified by the US Food and Drug Administration (FDA) as class III medical devices, a designation intended for high-risk devices needing close regulation. This was the consequence of the limited knowledge and few studies regarding their clinical behavior. However, in July 2013, an FDA regulatory review panel re-examined the available evidence on safety and effectiveness and reclassified blade-form dental implants as class II medical devices. As a result, the FDA no longer requires pre-market approval before new models are introduced.

Table 13.1 Literature for blade implant studies

	Abstracts 1968–2014
Human studies	122
Animal, *in vitro*, ex vivo	40
Total	162

Table 13.2 Blade implants – level of scientific evidence

Expert opinions	77
Case reports	24
Case series	13
Case–control	5
Cohort	2
Randomized clinical trials	1
Systematic reviews	0
Total	162

Wedge implant design

Some years ago, Vercellotti explored the possibility of combining a blade-form implant with the "new" ultrasonic bone-cutting device to simplify treatment of the narrow ridge. Working with Alberto Rebaudi, and later Francesco Oreglia and Claudio Stacchi, a number of implant prototypes were tested, resulting ultimately in the Rex® wedge implant design made from Ti–6Al–4V (Eli grade 5). Available implant lengths are 9, 11, 13, and 15 mm, while mesio-distal widths are either 4 or 5 mm. It is recommended that the longest length and 5 mm diameter be used wherever possible to increase bone-to-implant contact. The main advantage is that the bucco-lingual thickness is only either 1.8 or 2.9 mm. The implant surface treatments under testing include machine-turned, particle blasted/acid-washed, and titanium plasma-sprayed.

The wedge shape offers advantages in treatment of narrow bucco-lingual ridges that include reliable stabilization of the implant on press-fit insertion and a coincident expansion effect on the buccal and lingual bone walls of the edentulous ridge. During this expansion, the wedge shape distributes pressure to the cortical bone over the entire mesio-distal length of the implant. In contrast, a cylindrical implant concentrates this pressure over a much smaller area, increasing the risk of cortical bone fracture. After a variety of laboratory tests and finite element analyses, it was determined that a minimum bucco-lingual implant width of 1.8 mm was necessary to ensure an adequate mechanical resistance to fracture load. This meant that the wedge implant width could be approximately 40% thinner than the smallest of the available narrow-diameter implants available for clinical use. In contrast, the mesio-distal size of a wedge implant can be 4 or 5 mm; that is, identical to conventional implants and, therefore, suitable even for single-tooth replacements.

A macrogeometry was developed to maximize the benefits of the wedge shape, including two longitudinal wings to ensure good implant stabilization in the mesio-distal plane and a series of splines and protrusions on the implant body to enhance bone-to-implant surface contact and stress distribution to bone (Figure 13.2). Occlusal load is transferred to bone as compressive, tensile, and shear forces.[34] The implant-to-bone interface is strongest in response to compressive loads, 30% weaker to tensile forces, and 65% weaker to shear forces.[35] Traditional blade implants transfer occlusal loads to bone mainly as tensile and shear forces, while the design of the wedge implant macrogeometry is intended to transfer occlusal loads to bone as compressive forces in a pattern similar to screw implants (unpublished data).

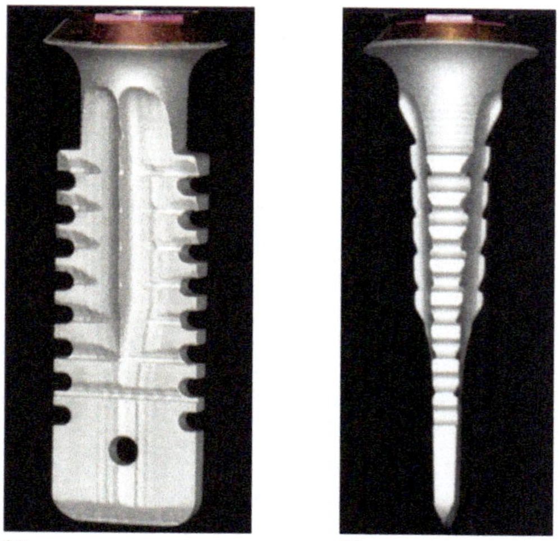

(a) (b)

Figure 13.2 First prototype of Rex® implant: (a) bucco-lingual surface view; (b) mesio-distal surface view.

Wedge implant site preparation

Osteotomy preparation for the Rex wedge implant is via piezoelectric bone surgery as this allows greater surgical control for the operator and creates a thinner, precise, and selective bone cut. Furthermore, reduced bleeding at the surgical site and an enhanced bone healing response allow for a safe and predictable surgical treatment and a high success rate. The shape of the desired preparation is a longitudinal osteotomy shaped to the length and thickness of the chosen wedge implant (Rex Implants, LLC). Specially designed instruments include depth gauges (Figure 13.3) and four ultrasonic tips (W1, W2, W3, and W4) meant for use with the Mectron Piezosurgery device set to "Implant" mode (Figures 13.3).

The surgical protocol presented here applies to the 1.8 mm wedge implant design currently available. After site evaluation to confirm adequate horizontal dimension, mesio-distal positioning is determined based on the desired prosthetic position of the final restoration (Figure 13.4a). The bucco-lingual/palatal dimension is limited by the remaining bone volume. The first Piezosurgery insert (W1) is used to prepare an initial central osteotomy corresponding to the desired implant axis and two shallower osteotomies to determine the mesio-distal limits of the implant site (Figure 13.4b). An indicator pin is used to check the 3-D position of the implant axis using a surgical guide (Figure 13.4c). The second Piezosurgery insert, a sharp micro-saw (W2), is used to join the three vertical osteotomy cuts (Figure 13.4d). The third insert, or smoothing chisel (W3), is used to refine the implant site and remove any surface irrregularities (Figure 13.4e). A depth gauge is used to check the site for length and width (Figure 13.4f). A fourth and final piezo insert, a sharp file (W4), is used to complete preparation of the osteotomy to maintain the maximum cortical bone thickness with slight underpreparation necessary to achieve primary implant stability (Figure 13.4g). Also, the cavitation effect of the saline solution produces implant site debridment and cell stimulation. The final implant position depends on the design characteristics of the implant selected, which can be either tissue level or bone level, and the implant is inserted with a special carrier (Figure 13.4h). The Rex mallet with selective electronic control facilitates implant insertion using the carrier as shown in Figure 13.4i.

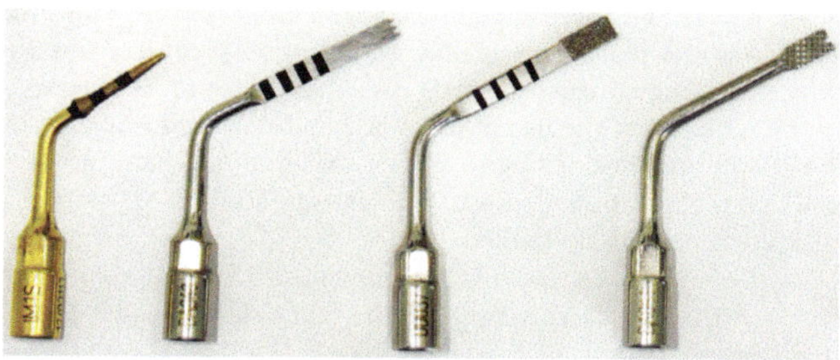

Figure 13.3 Piezosurgery inserts W1, W2, W3, and W4 (left to right) have been designed to allow the preparation of a precise osteotomy for the Rex® implant with the Mectron Piezosurgery device set to "Implant" mode.

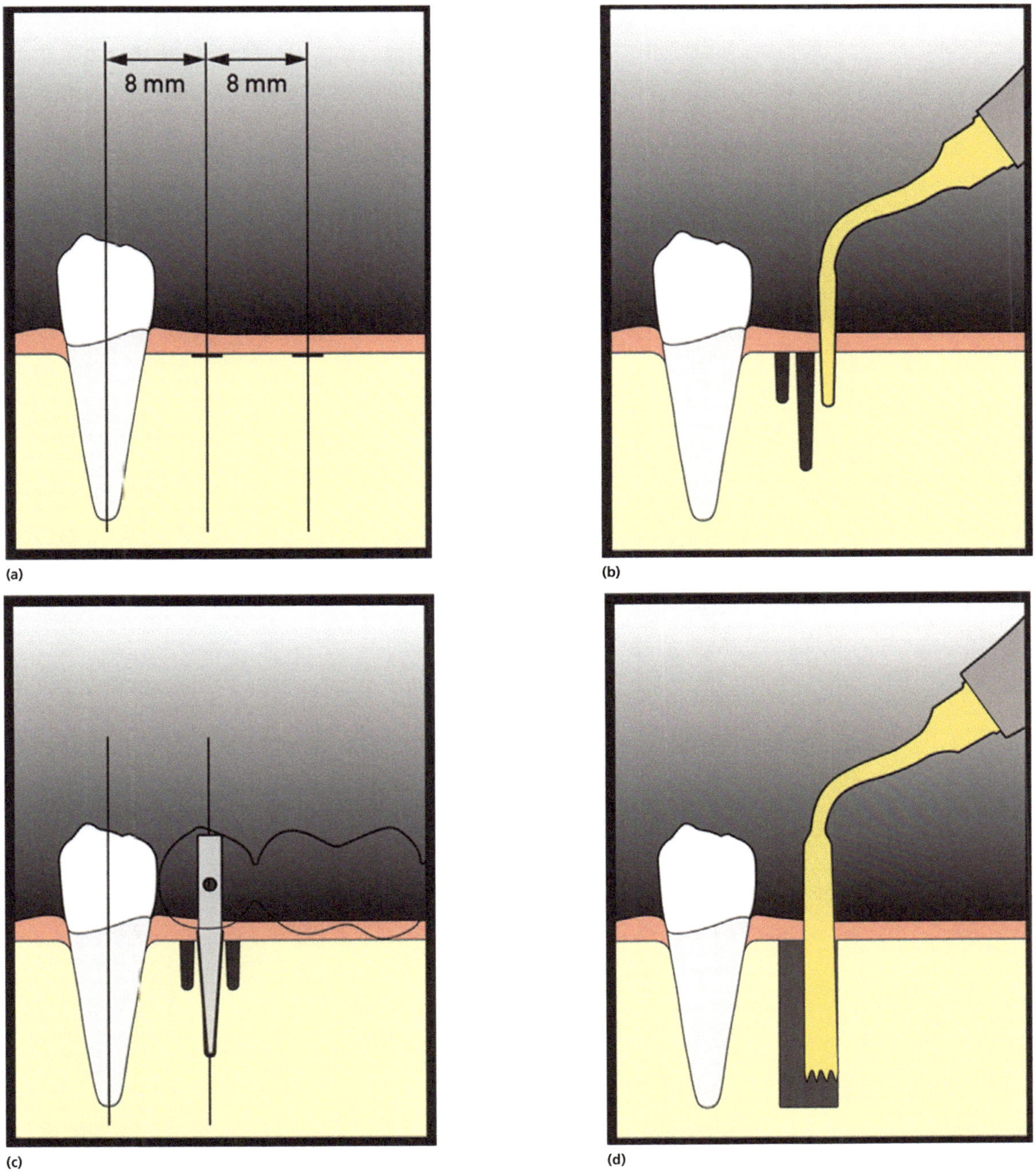

Figure 13.4 (a) Implant site positioning is planned following the desired prosthetic mesial–distal positioning of the final restoration. (b) The first Piezosurgery insert (W1) is used to prepare an initial central osteotomy corresponding to the desired implant axis. Two additional shallower osteotomies are completed to determine the mesio-distal limits of the implant site. (c) 3-D implant position is confirmed with an indicator pin and a surgical guide. (d) The second Piezosurgery insert, a sharp micro-saw (W2), is used to join the three vertical osteotomy cuts. *(Continued)*

Clinical case studies

Case study 13.1

An elderly female patient presented with a fractured left mandibular first premolar with adjacent edentulous second premolar and first molar sites (Figure 13.5a). The alveolar dimensions can be seen on periapical and cross-sectional computed tomographic (CT) images with narrow crestal volume and low-density cancellous bone (Figure 13.5b and c). Owing to the patient's advanced age, she did not want to proceed with a lateral augmentation procedure. The first molar was replaced with a narrow design Rex wedge implant, and an immediate cylindrical endosseous implant was placed at the first premolar site, planning for an implant-supported bridge to replace the three missing teeth. Surgical exposure with a partial-thickness flap at the site can be seen in Figure 13.5d with a significant horizontal bone defect. Piezoelectric site development was completed as described previously (Figure 13.5e). The final wedge implant site preparation was confirmed with a depth gauge (Figure 13.5f). A

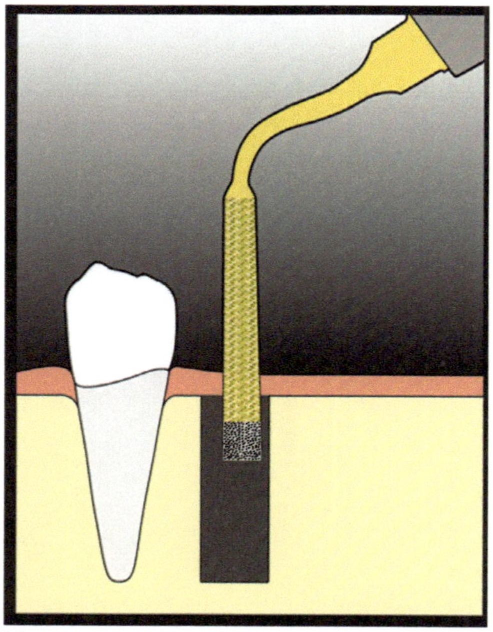

(e)

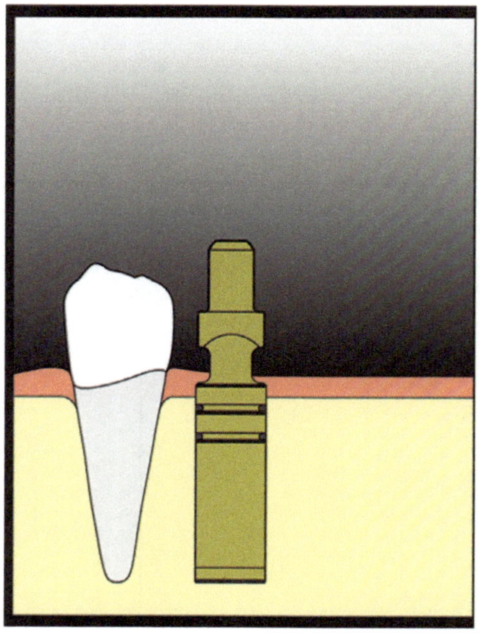

(f)

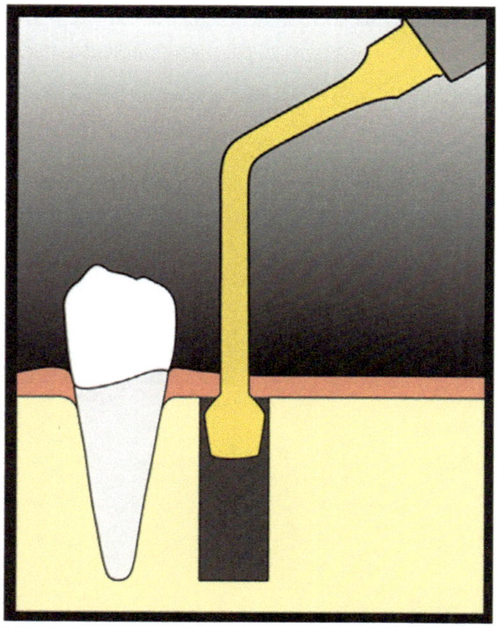

(g)

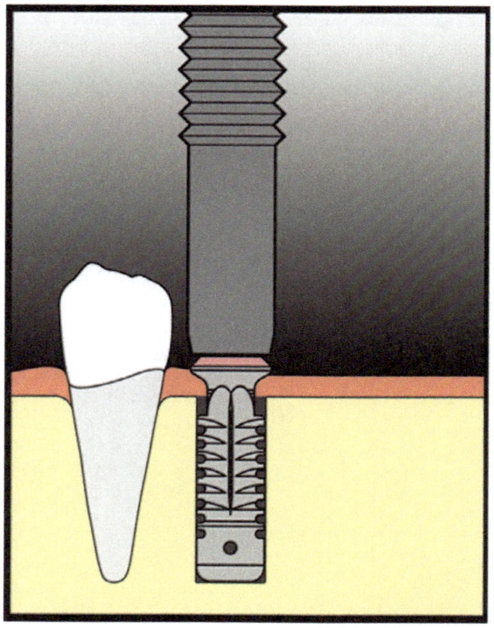

(h)

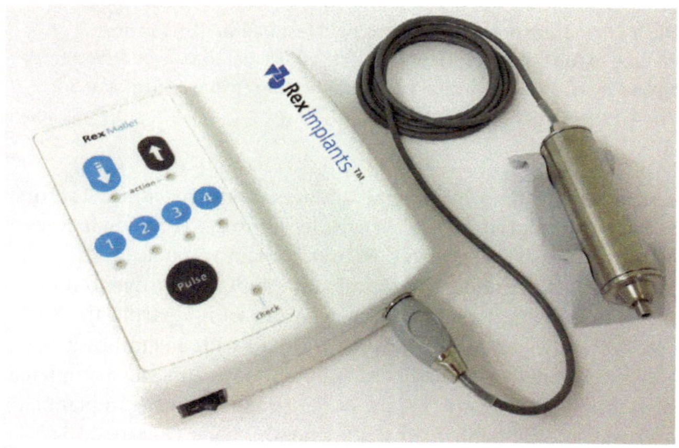

(i)

Figure 13.4 (Continued)
(e) The third insert, a smoothing chisel (W3), is used to refine the implant site surfaces and remove any irregularities. (f) A depth gauge is used to check the implant site preparation in length and width. (g) The fourth insert (W4) is a sharp file used a to complete preparation of the osteotomy to maintain the maximum cortical bone thickness with slight underpreparation necessary to achieve primary implant stability. (h) A special carrier is connected to the wedge implant to facilitate the surgical insertion. (i) The Rex mallet™ uses selective electronic control to optimize the surgical strikes and facilitate a "press-fit" implant insertion.

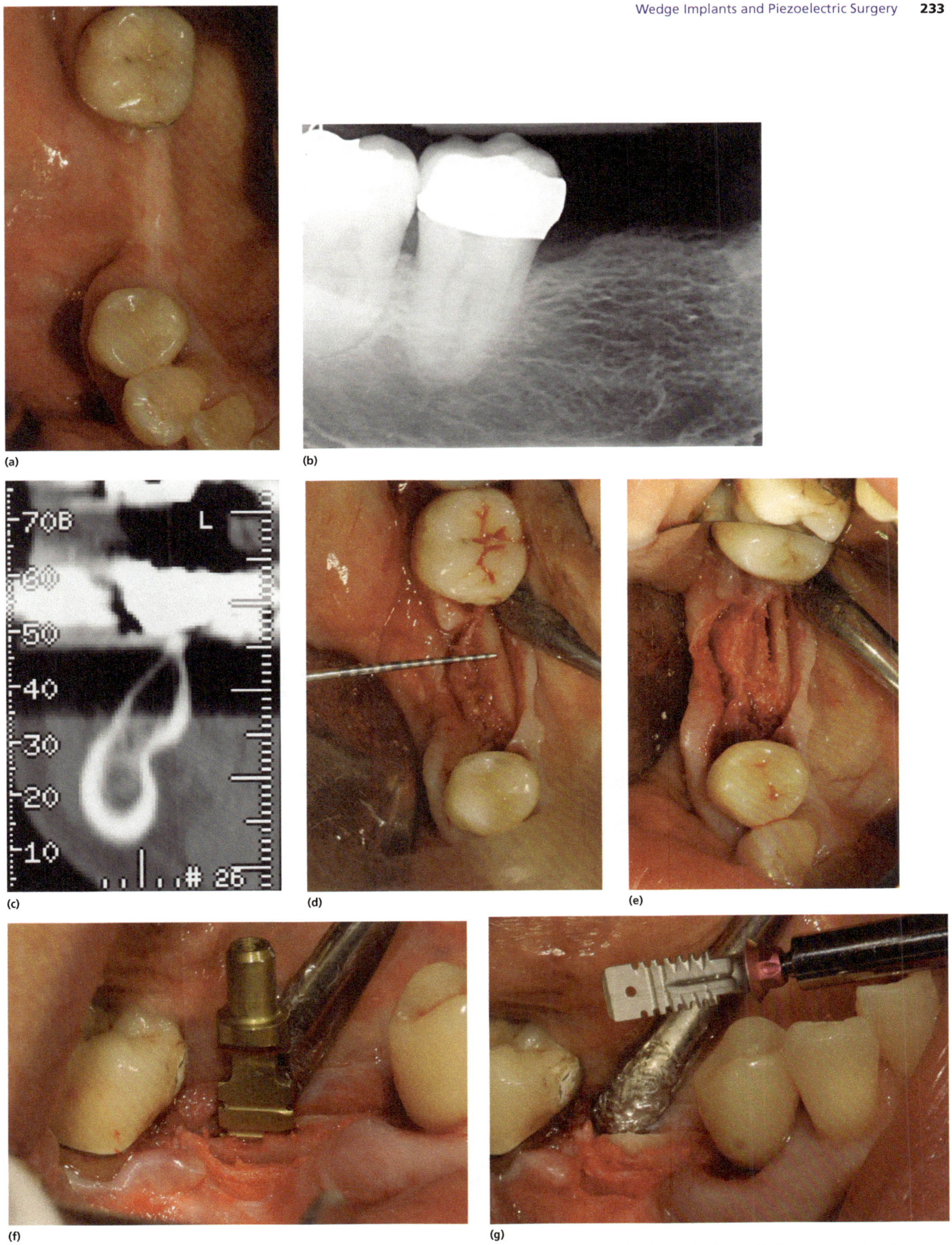

Figure 13.5 (a) Clinical findings at a long-standing edentulous second premolar and first molar sites and a fractured left mandibular first premolar. The patient required a simple narrow ridge treatment because of advanced age. (b, c) Periapical and CT cross-sectional images show the narrow crestal volume and low-density cancellous bone in the molar region. (d) Partial-thickness flap exposure of the atrophic ridge shows the minimal crestal bone width (2 mm). (e) Piezoelectric surgery is completed for implant site preparation. (f) Depth gauge insertion is used to verify implant site preparation. (g, h) The Rex® implant (small prototype 9 mm length × 4 mm width × 1.3 mm thickness).

(*Continued*)

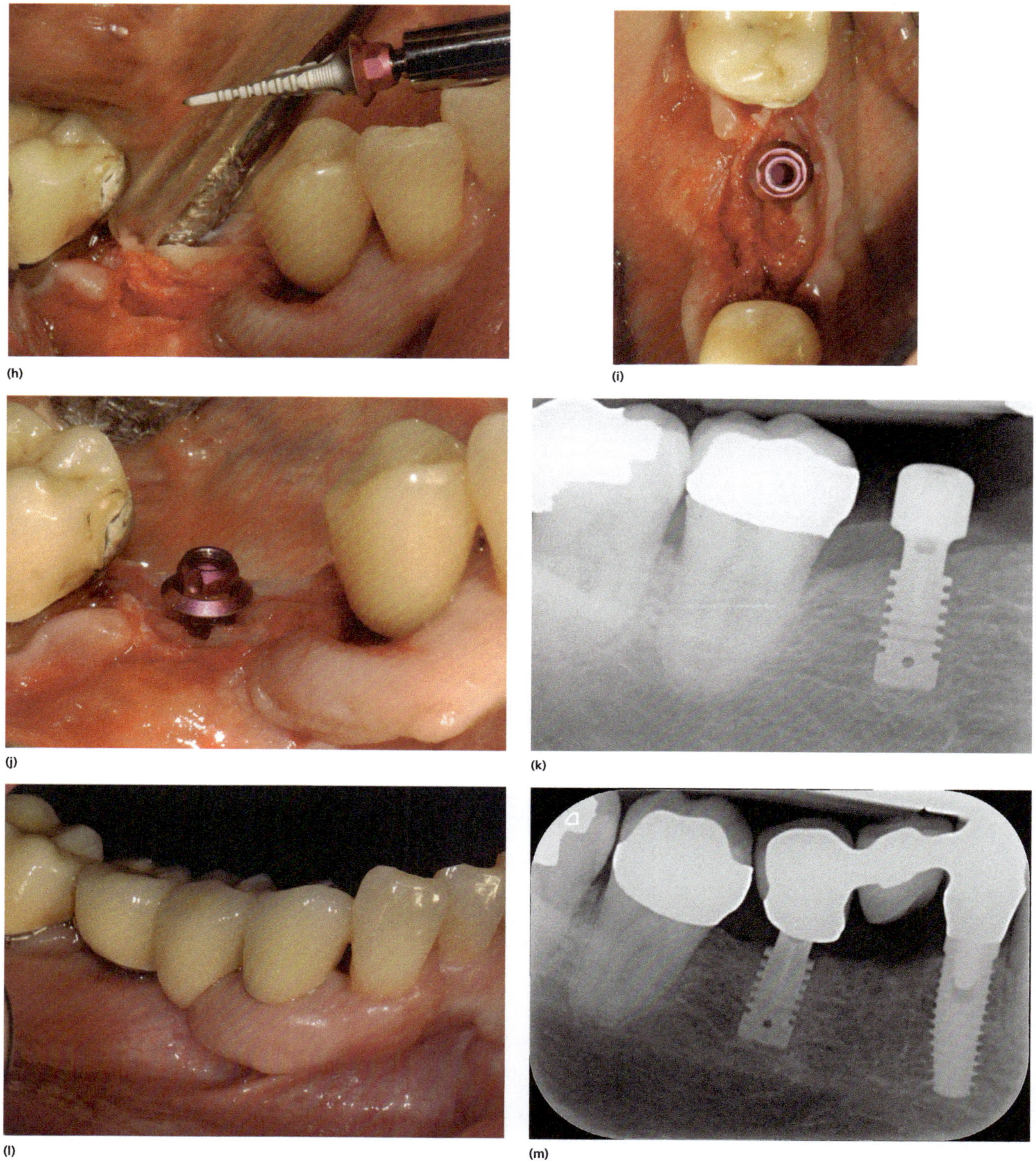

Figure 13.5 (Continued)
(i, j) Occlusal and lateral views after insertion of the Rex® implant. (k) A periapical radiograph demonstrates the Rex® implant after the osseointegration period of 3 months. (l) The definitive restoration of the wedge implant is with a three-unit bridge. Limited keratinized gingiva was present around the Rex® implant as the patient declined recommended mucogingival surgery. (m) Periapical radiograph after 4 years demonstrates successful clinical result.

small prototype of the Rex implant (9 mm length × 4 mm width × 1.3 mm thickness) can be seen in Figure 13.5g and h. The implant was inserted (Figure 13.5i and j) and the 3-month post-operative periapical radiograph demonstrates implant position and healing after osseointegration (Figure 13.5k). The definitive restoration can be seen in Figure 13.5l. Limited keratinized gingiva was present around the Rex implant as the patient declined recommended mucogingival surgery. The implant-supported restoration can be seen on periapical radiograph after 4 years with acceptable peri-implant bone levels and a successful restoration (Figure 13.5m).

Case study 13.2

An 81-year-old patient presented requiring implants to replace a failed prosthesis in the maxillary left posterior region (Figure 13.6a and b). The prosthesis was sectioned and the carious second bicuspid root removed. Preoperative cross-sectional CT images showed advanced horizontal bone loss in the left maxilla, confirming that the ridge was too thin for traditional dental implant placement (Figure 13.6c–e). Three Rex implants were inserted (following the described protocol) with non-submerged healing to replace the missing left cuspid and both bicuspids. The post-operative clinical findings can be seen after 2 weeks in Figure 13.6f, and again at 3 months in Figure 13.6g. Bucco-lingual and mesio-distal implant stability measurements were taken at 3 months with the Ostell® device, and shown to be acceptable (ISQ 53 for bucco-lingual and for ISQ 72 mesio-distal). Radiographs taken at the time of the final impressions (Figure 13.6h) and 1 year after restoration (Figure 13.6i) confirmed a successful treatment outcome. A clinical view of the final provisional prosthesis after 3 months can be seen in Figure 13.6j.

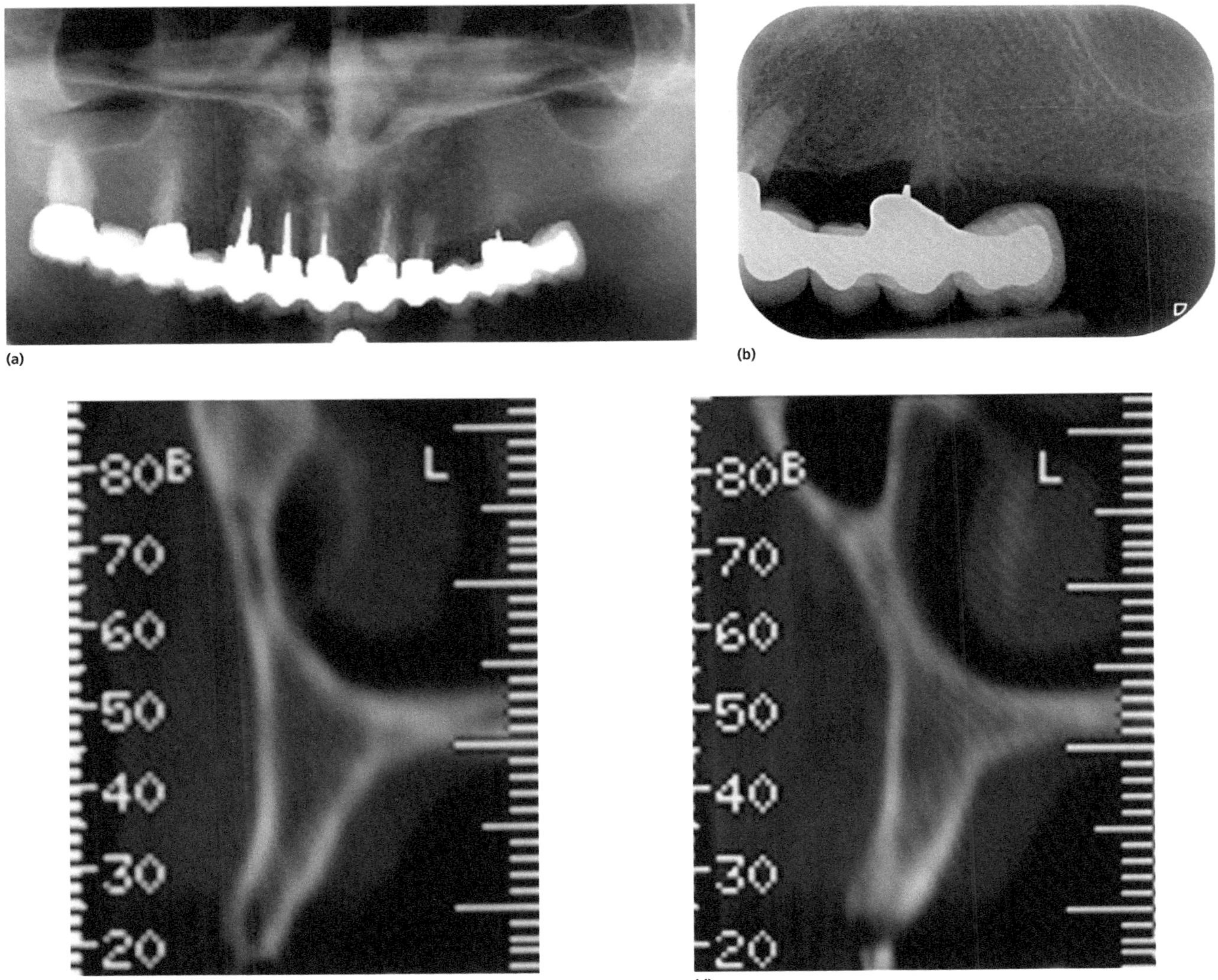

Figure 13.6 (a) A panoramic radiograph demonstrates a failing tooth-supported fixed prosthesis in this 81-year-old patient necessitating implant rehabilitation of the left upper arch. (b) The periapical radiograph shows the small root tip in the canine–premolar region. The prosthesis was sectioned and the root removed. (c–e) Presurgical CT scan of the three implant sites showed a very thin edentulous ridge (circa 3–4 mm) characterized by low-density cancellous bone. *(Continued)*

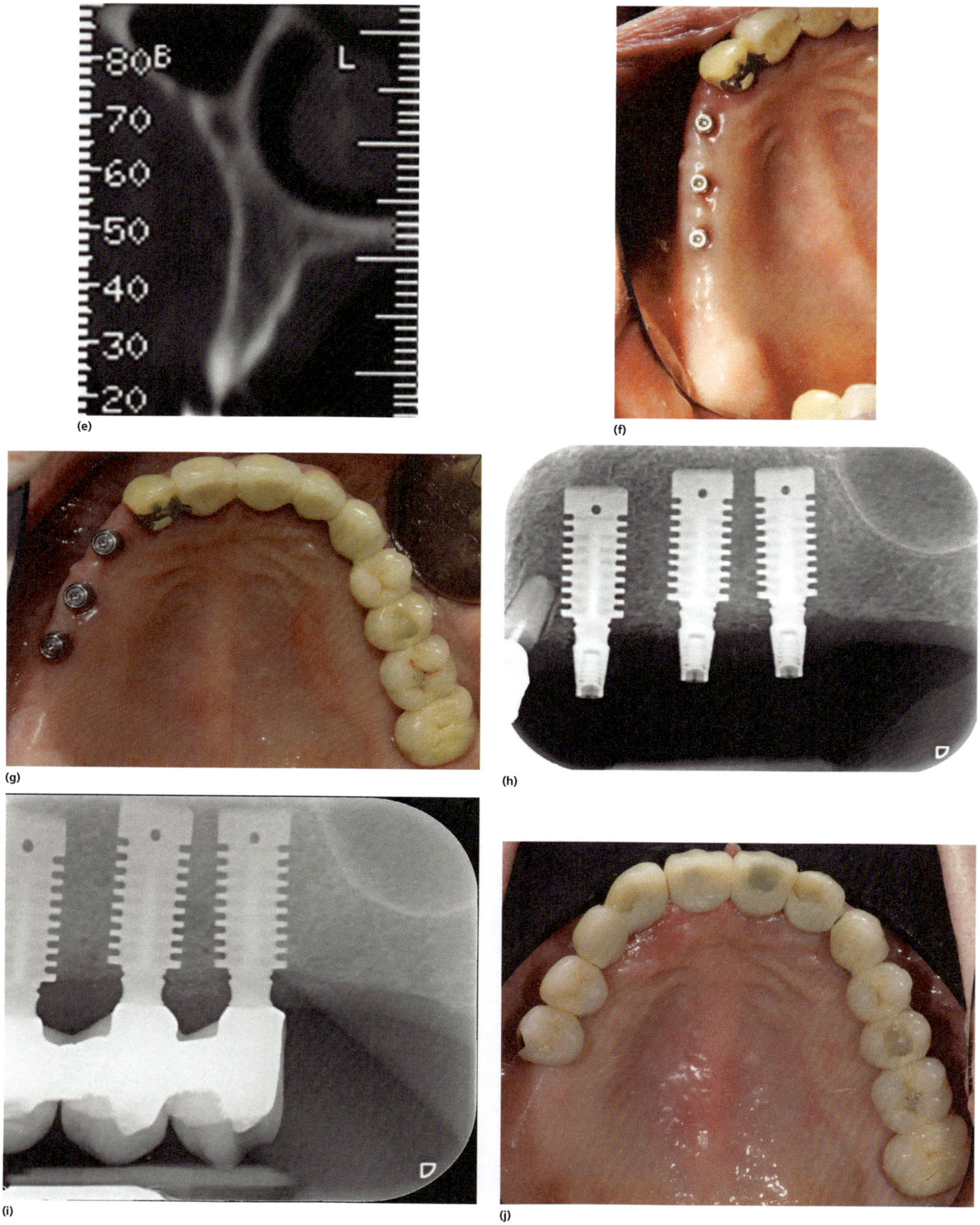

Figure 13.6 (Continued)
(f) Wedge implants were inserted and soft tissue healing can be seen 2 weeks post-op. (g) The clinical findings 3 months post-op with ISQ confirming implant stability. (h) Periapical radiograph of the transfer abutment check for prosthetic impression. (i) At 1 year after loading, the definitive restoration and the implant bone levels are intact on the periapical radiograph. (j) A clinical view of the final restoration can be seen after 3 months.

Conclusions

This chapter has presented an overview of the minimally invasive principles of ultrasonic bone surgery and the concept of a thin, press-fit wedge-shaped endosseous implant. The design principles and macrogeometry of the wedge implant may have future benefit as a minimally invasive alternative for management of edentulous sites with minimal bucco-lingual width. Implant site preparation is completed exclusively with use of specially designed Piezosurgery inserts, and is significantly different from that used for traditional endosseous cylindrical and tapered implant designs. This treatment concept may have significant clinical advantages with appropriate case selection. While the clinical applications of piezoelectric bone surgery are established, work with the wedge implant is preliminary, and will require carefully planned prospective clinical testing before it can be proposed for widespread clinical use. As with all implant procedures, the use of wedge implants requires careful patient evaluation and treatment planning to optimize clinical results and minimize the risk of complications.

References

1. Amler MH. The time sequence of tissue regeneration in human extraction wounds. Oral Surg Oral Med Oral Pathol 1969; 27: 309–318.
2. Johnson K. A study of the dimensional changes occurring in the maxilla following tooth extraction. Aust Dent J 1969; 14: 241–254.
3. Schropp L, Wenzel A, Kostopoulos L, Karring T. Bone healing and soft tissue contour changes following single-tooth extraction: a clinical and radiographic 12-month prospective study. Int J Periodontics Restorative Dent 2003; 23: 313–323.
4. Araújo MG, Lindhe J. Dimensional ridge alterations following tooth extraction. An experimental study in the dog. J Clin Periodontol 2005; 32: 212–218.
5. Gupta A, Tiwari B, Goel H, Shekhawat H. Residual ridge resorption: a review. Indian J Dent Sci 2010; 2: 7–11.
6. Tallgren A. The continuing reduction of the residual alveolar ridges in complete denture wearers: a mixed-longitudinal study covering 25 years. J Prosthetic Dent 2003; 89: 427–435.
7. Milinkovic I, Cordaro L. Are there specific indications for the different alveolar bone augmentation procedures for implant placement? A systematic review. Int J Oral Maxillofac Surg 2014; 43: 606–625.
8. Esposito M, Grusovin MG, Felice P, et al. The efficacy of horizontal and vertical bone augmentation procedures for dental implants – a Cochrane systematic review. Eur J Oral Implantol 2009; 2: 167–184.
9. Vercellotti T. Piezoelectric surgery in implantology: a case report – a new piezoelectric ridge expansion technique. Int J Periodontics Restorative Dent 2000; 20: 358–365.
10. Vercellotti T, Nevins ML, Kim DM, et al. Osseous response following resective therapy with piezosurgery. Int J Periodontics Restorative Dent 2005; 25: 543–549.
11. Parmar D, Mann M, Walmsley AD, Lea SC. Cutting characteristics of ultrasonic surgical instruments. Clin Oral Implants Res 2011; 22: 1385–1390.
12. Catuna MC. Sonic energy: a possible dental application, preliminary report on ultrasonic cutting method. Ann Dent 1953; 12: 100–101.
13. Mazorow HB. Bone repair after experimentally produced defects. J Oral Surg 1960; 18: 107–115.
14. McFall TA, Yamane GM, Burnett GW. Comparison of the cutting effect on bone of an ultrasonic cutting device and rotatory burs. J Oral Surg Anesth Hosp Dent Serv 1961; 19: 200–209.
15. Horton JE, Tarpley TM Jr, Wood LD. The healing of surgical defects in alveolar bone produced with ultrasonic instrumentation, chisel, and rotary bur. Oral Surg Oral Med Oral Pathol 1975; 39(4): 536–546.
16. Aro H, Kallioniemi H, Aho AJ, Kellokumpu-Lehtinen P. Ultrasonic device in bone cutting. A histological and scanning electron microscopical study. Acta Orthop Scand 1981; 52(1): 5–10.
17. Giraud JY, Villemin S, Darmana R, et al. Bone cutting. Clin Phys Physiol Meas 1991; 12: 1–19.
18. Walmsley A, Lea S. Cutting characteristics of ultrasonic surgical instruments. Clin Oral Implants Res 2011; 22: 1385–1390.
19. Claire S, Lea SC, Walmsley AD. Characterization of bone following ultrasonic cutting. Clin Oral Investig 2013; 17: 905–912.
20. Maurer P, Kriwalsky MS, Veras RB, et al. Micro-morphometrical analysis of conventional osteotomy techniques and ultrasonic osteotomy at the rabbit skull. Clin Oral Implants Res 2008; 19: 570–575.
21. Schweiberer L, Dambe LT, Eitel F, Klapp E. Revascularization of the tibia after conservative and surgical fracture fixation. Hefte Unfallheilkd 1974; 119: 18–26 (in German).
22. Soldner E, Herr G. Knochen, knochentransplantate und knochenersatzmaterialien. Grundlagen, aktueller stand und neue entwicklungen. Trauma Berufskrankh 2001; 3: 256–269.
23. Rundle CH, Wang H, Yu H, et al. Micro-array analysis of gene expression during the inflammation and endochondral bone formation stages of rat femur fracture repair. Bone 2006; 38: 521–529.
24. Metzger MC, Bormann KH, Schoen R, et al. Inferior alveolar nerve transposition: an *in vitro* comparison between piezosurgery and conventional bur use. J Oral Implantol 2006; 32: 19–25.
25. Schaeren S, Jaquiéry C, Heberer M, et al. Assessment of nerve damage using a novel ultrasonic device for bone cutting. J Oral Maxillofac Surg 2008; 66: 593–596.
26. Riesz P, Berdahl D, Christman CL. Free radical generation by ultrasound in aqueous and nonaqueous solutions. Environ Health Perspect 1985; 64: 233–252.
27. Walmsley AD, Walsh TF, Laird WR, Williams AR. Effects of cavitational activity on the root surface of teeth during ultrasonic scaling. J Clin Periodontol 1990; 17: 306–312.
28. Vercellotti T, Nevins M, Kim D, et al. Osseous response following respective therapy with piezosurgery. Int J Periodontics Restorative Dent 2005; 25: 543–549.
29. Preti G, Martinasso G, Peirone B, et al. Cytokines and growth factors involved in the osseointegration of oral titanium implants positioned using piezoelectric bone surgery versus a drill technique: a pilot study in minipigs. J Periodontol 2007; 78: 716–722.
30. Stacchi C, Vercellotti T, Torelli L, et al. Changes in implant stability using different site preparation techniques: twist drills versus Piezosurgery. A single-blinded, randomized, controlled clinical trial. Clin Implant Dent Relat Res 2013; 15: 188–197.
31. Vercellotti T, Stacchi C, Russo C, et al. Ultrasonic implant site preparation using Piezosurgery: a multicenter case series study analyzing 3,579 implants with a 1- to 3-year follow-up. Int J Periodontics Restorative Dent 2014; 34: 11–18.
32. Linkow LI. The blade-vent: a new dimension in endosseous implantology. Dent Concepts 1968; 11: 3–12.
33. Linkow LI, Cherchéve R. Theories and Techniques of Oral Implantology, vol. 1, St. Louis, MO: Mosby, 1970.
34. Reilly DT, Burstein AH. The elastic and ultimate properties of compact bone tissue. J Biomech 1975; 8: 393–405.
35. Guo EX. Mechanical properties of cortical bone and cancellous bone tissue. In: Bone Mechanics Handbook, CowinSC, ed. Boca Raton, FL: CRC Press, 2001, pp. 10/1–10/23.

SECTION IV

Implant Site Development

CHAPTER 14

Single-Stage Implant Placement and Simultaneous Grafting: The "Esthetic Contour Graft"

Bach T. Le[1] **& Sze Wing Cynthia Au Yeung**[1,2]
[1]Division of Oral & Maxillofacial Surgery, The Herman Ostrow School of Dentistry of USC, Los Angeles County/USC Medical Center, Los Angeles, CA, USA
[2]Private Practice, Los Angeles, CA, USA

Introduction

The extraction of teeth can result in up to 50% alveolar ridge width loss within the first year.[1–6] Achieving an ideal esthetic outcome is challenging when even moderate bone and soft tissue defects exist.[7–9] Various techniques and site development protocols have been described for the management of these common post-extraction defects. Traditional protocols involve an initial site development procedure to augment bone volume followed by a second procedure to place a dental implant. If needed, soft tissue augmentation also can be performed to improve gingival contours. However, the required prolonged treatment time involving multiple surgeries with associated costs and morbidity can pose clear obstacles for many patients. In this chapter, we will discuss single-stage implant placement with simultaneous bone grafting for properly selected cases as an alternative to traditional methods. Minimally invasive dental implant surgery refers to surgery that can be done through smaller incisions with the fewest surgical interventions possible. One of the main goals of minimally invasive surgery is to reduce physical trauma at the surgical site and psychological trauma to the patient. Multiple surgical interventions with repeated flap elevations can result in bone and tissue loss and significant scarring. Single-stage implant placement with simultaneous grafting allows the clinician to treat sites with mild to moderate defects with a single surgical procedure, and can be performed immediately at the time of tooth extraction or in a healed extraction socket with a tissue defect.

Single-stage implants with simultaneous guided bone regeneration: "esthetic contour graft"

Localized osseous defects are common following bone remodeling after tooth loss.[1–6] Guided bone regeneration (GBR) has been proven experimentally and clinically to promote osseous regeneration and to preserve a large percentage of grafted material.[10–13] Traditional GBR procedures are performed as a staged approach with a second surgical intervention to place the implant. If simultaneous bone grafting is performed, it is usually followed by submerged implant site healing beneath the repositioned soft tissue flap. Le and Burstein[14] described a bone-grafting procedure done simultaneously with implant placement and non-submerged healing by adding a healing abutment. This approach offers several advantages. The single-stage protocol minimizes compression and migration of particulate graft material, and allows the bony and soft tissue architecture to develop around the healing abutment during site healing. A large-diameter healing abutment will provide some tenting of the peri-implant soft tissues and result in less apical migration of the graft material. This improves the prognosis for retaining the greatest width and height of the remaining crestal bone. Grafting at the time of implant placement also takes advantage of the regional acceleratory phenomenon[15] that is induced by the trauma of implant placement, helping to accelerate healing.

Le and Borzabadi-Farahani[16] assessed the outcome of single-stage, non-submerged implant placement with simultaneous augmentation of vertical buccal bone dehiscence defects using a mineralized particulate allograft (Puros® Cancellous, Zimmer Dental) covered with a collagen membrane (Ossix Plus®, OraPharma Inc.). The vertical buccal defects were classified as small (<3 mm in height), medium (3–5 mm in height), or large (>5 mm in height). The initial defects were recorded by measuring the amount of implant rough surface exposure after implant placement. To assess site healing, sectional cone beam computed tomography scans were obtained at 36 months post-grafting. Evaluation of the sites of the original defects showed bone regeneration of 100% and 79.3% of small and medium-size vertical dehiscences respectively. Large-sized defects showed only partial improvement.

Jensen et al.[17] analyzed the long-term stability of bone contour augmentation in the esthetic zone used with early implant placement (i.e. 6–8 weeks of healing after tooth extraction) assessed using biopsies harvested after various time intervals. Implant placement was performed with simultaneous contour augmentation using a combination of autogenous bone (placed in direct contact with the exposed implant surface) and deproteinized bovine bone mineral (DBBM) covered with a double layer of collagen barrier membrane. Biopsies collected after 14–80 months of healing were subjected to histologic and histomorphometric analysis. These biopsies consisted of 32.0 ± 9.6% retained DBBM particles and 40.6 ± 14.6% bone; 70.3 ± 14.5% of the DBBM particle surfaces were covered with bone. The investigators concluded that their study confirmed previous findings that osseointegrated DBBM particles do not undergo significant resorption and substitution over time, and that this low substitution rate is likely the reason for the long-term clinical and radiographic stability of contour augmentations done using this procedure.

Minimally Invasive Dental Implant Surgery, First Edition. Edited by Daniel R. Cullum and Douglas Deporter.

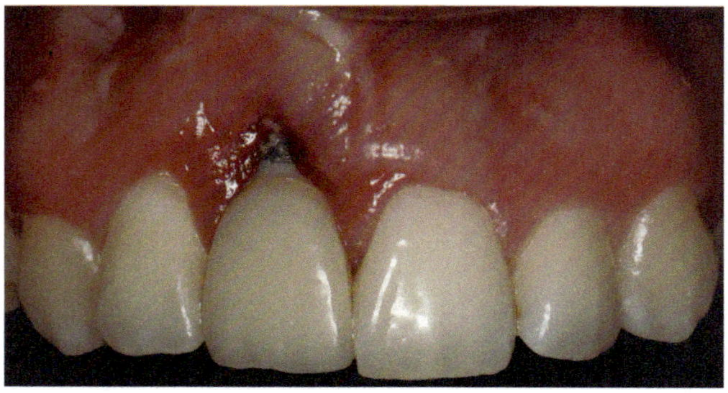

Figure 14.1 Failed guided tissue regeneration done with simultaneous implant placement may lead to exposed implant threads or crown margins. © Bach T. Le.

One of the primary goals of the "esthetic contour graft" is the successful placement and long-term maintenance of bone graft material in labial crestal contouring of the peri-implant region. This region is largely responsible for the labial soft tissue contour and long-term stability of the gingival margin level. With GBR, graft migration and resorption from this area can result in unesthetic tissue recession (Figure 14.1). The success of the "esthetic contour graft" concept is dependent on multiple variables, including defect configuration, flap design, space maintenance, graft material, membrane selection, and implant position. Each of these principles plays a critical role and will be discussed separately.

Defect configuration

With traditional GBR, migration of graft particles during site healing often results in unfavorable healing and soft tissue collapse/recession. The challenge in maintaining the graft particles in position depends on a number of critical factors related to defect configuration.

Width of edentulous span

Single tooth defects have a much better esthetic prognosis than multiple teeth defects[7] since particulate grafts placed in wider edentulous spans are more prone to migration due to the wider flap elevation required. Wider defects often require the use of a containment barrier or space maintenance device, such as a mesh or a membrane with tacks, to contain bone graft material.

Number of walls

New bone formation mainly depends on the surface area of exposed bone and bone marrow since the osteogenic and angiogenic cells that form new bone reside in the bone marrow.[18] The number of bony walls available in a defect has significant influence on the success of a GBR procedure. With more bone walls available, the healing potential of a given defect increases.[19] Three-wall bone defects (e.g. extraction sockets) have better healing potential than two-wall defects, which are frequently found in post-extraction sites, and also have good potential for bone regeneration. One-wall defects, however, are more challenging as there is a greater distance for osteogenic cells to bridge. Three- to four-wall defects also have a better prognosis for graft containment and space maintenance. Defects with fewer walls often require subsequent grafting procedures to attain an optimal result.

Type of defect

Horizontal defects with bony concavities will contain graft material better, improving the prognosis compared with defects having no concavities. Defects with vertical components are the most difficult, requiring the use of space maintenance devices such as titanium mesh[20,21] or tenting screws.[22] Distraction osteogenesis and segmental osteotomies also have been prescribed for the management of these defects.[23,24]

Flap design

Minimizing flap exposure to maximize vascular supply to the surgical site while creating adequate access for graft placement can be challenging. For small ridge defects (<2 mm), a flapless approach or sulcular incision may be adequate, but for larger defects an open-book flap design[14] can be used to enhance visualization and access (Figure 14.2). It is crucial to achieve tension-free adaptation of wound margins during wound closure, and this may require incising the periosteum of the flap before repositioning it. In addition to

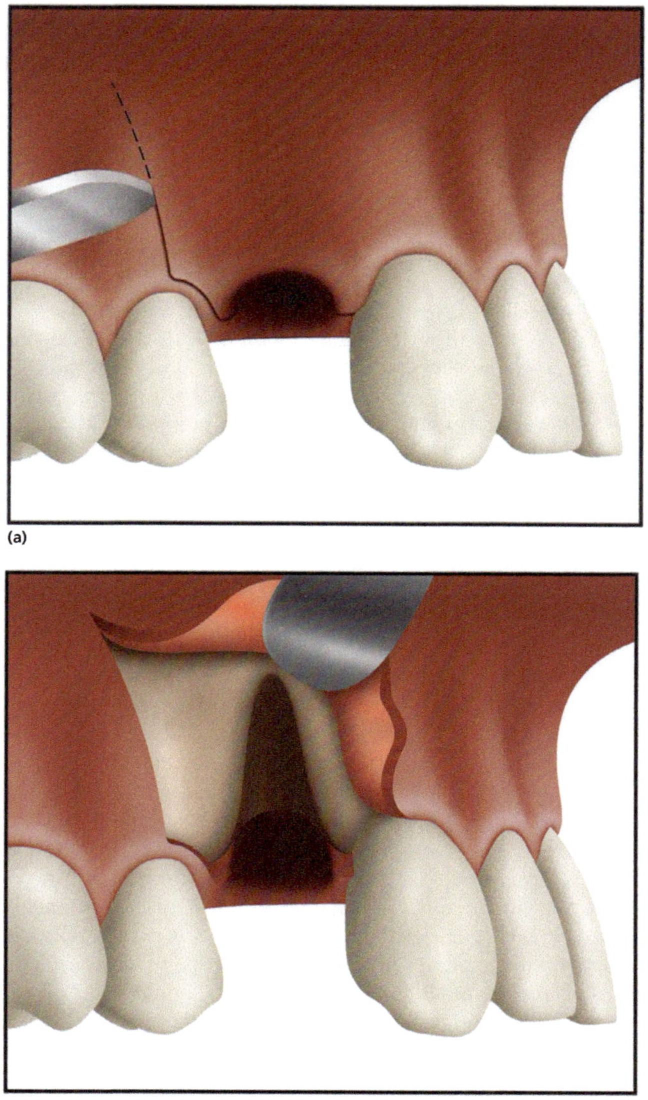

(a)

(b)

Figure 14.2 (a, b) "Open-book" flap design. © Bach T. Le.

allowing primary tension-free wound closure, scoring of the periosteum promotes angiogenesis by creating bleeding into the graft.[25]

Surgical technique

Grafting of labial wall defects using GBR with or without flap elevation has been described to correct post-extraction defects.[26] Although flapless surgery can be easier to perform, bone regeneration will be limited, and graft materials may be more readily resorbed beyond the confines of the labial defect wall during remodeling.[27] As a result, acceptable anatomic contours may not be achieved, and future bone grafting may still be needed. When labial wall defects are present, grafting with an open flap approach is recommended as it will yield more predictable outcomes.[14,28–30]

The open-book flap is developed with a crestal incision made slightly lingual to the ridge midline to preserve an adequate amount of labial keratinized tissue in the flap (Figure 14.3a and b). This is followed by a distal, curvilinear, vertical incision that follows the gingival margin of the distal proximal tooth. A wide subperiosteal reflection is made to expose two to three times the treatment area, and the papilla is reflected on the mesial side of the edentulous site (Figure 14.3b). During implant placement, the implant's restorative platform is positioned at the desired level for future prosthetic restoration (Figure 14.3c). The peri-implant soft tissue is released and advanced by scoring the periosteum so that tension-free closure can be achieved around the neck of the implant. This is done because moderate graft resorption will occur if there is an inadequate tissue seal around the implant neck or if tension-free closure is not achieved. To reduce intraoperative bleeding at the graft site, the periosteal release should be the last step before graft placement. Mineralized bone allograft material is packed into the defect and overcontoured by approximately 20–30% to compensate for the anticipated apical migration and partial resorption of the material. Prior to use, the allograft material should be hydrated according to the manufacturer's directions and mixed with the patient's blood, which serves as a coagulant. After graft placement (Figure 14.3d), the material is covered with a resorbable membrane, and a wide healing abutment is connected to the implant. A variation of Palacci's papilla regeneration technique[31] helps to release the tissue tension around the healing abutment, and to augment the interdental height of the soft tissue papilla (Figure 14.3e and f). This creates a tenting effect over the allograft and, together with the healing abutment, helps to hold the particulate material in place. Tissue contours 2 years after final restoration can be seen in Figure 14.3g.

Perforating the recipient bone bed is recommended by some surgeons to enhance healing. By perforating the cortical bone with a small round bur, the marrow cavity is opened and bleeds into the defect. Animal studies have shown that such perforations improve healing in a membrane-protected defect.[32,33] Larger perforations were associated with prompter bone formation.[32] However, the senior author of this chapter does not routinely perforate the recipient bone bed and has not seen a difference in outcomes.

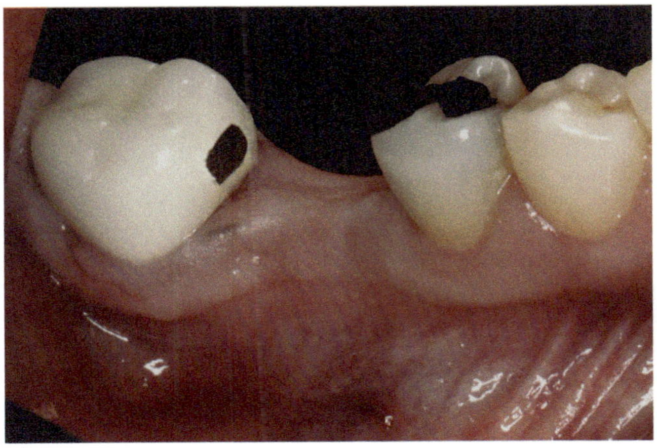

(a)

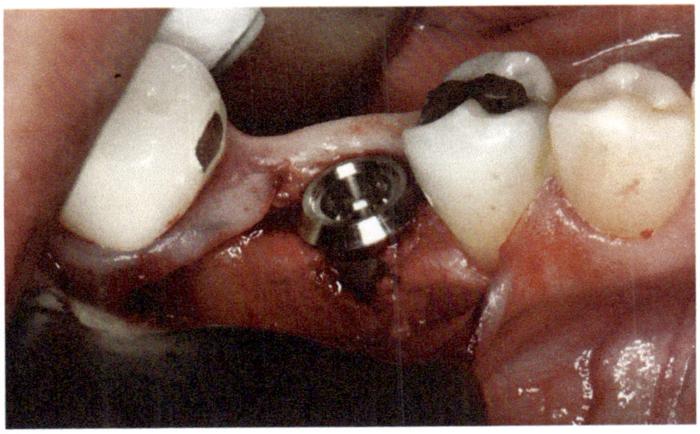

(c)

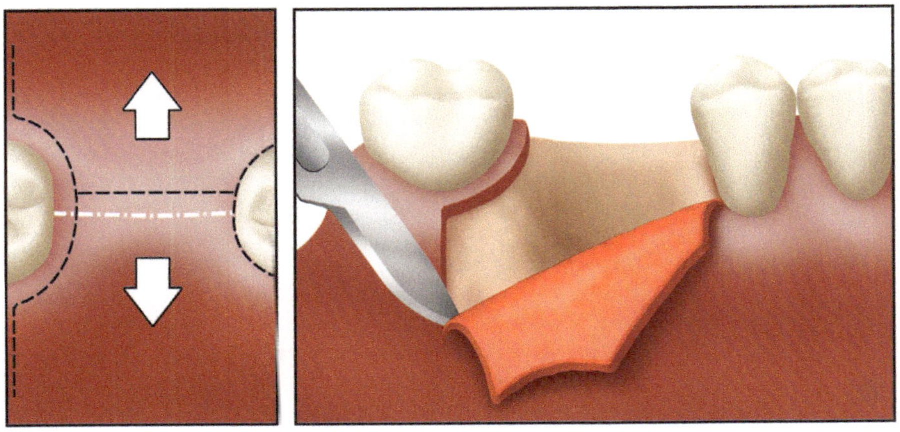

(b)

Figure 14.3 (a) A preoperative defect to be managed with the "esthetic contour grafting technique." (b, c) A crestal incision was made slightly towards the lingual to capture the available keratinized tissue in the labial flap.

(Continued)

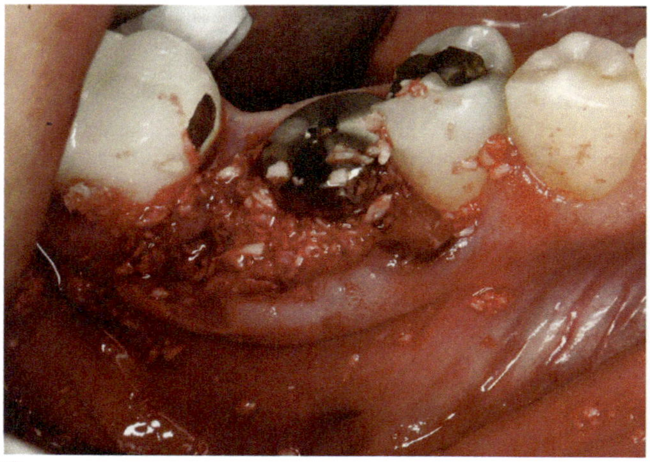
(d)

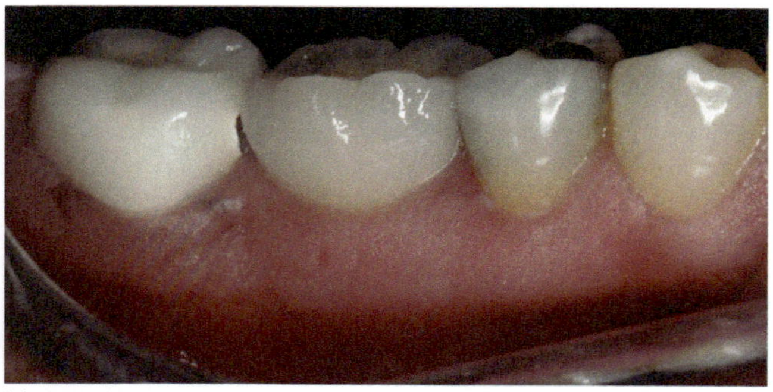
(g)

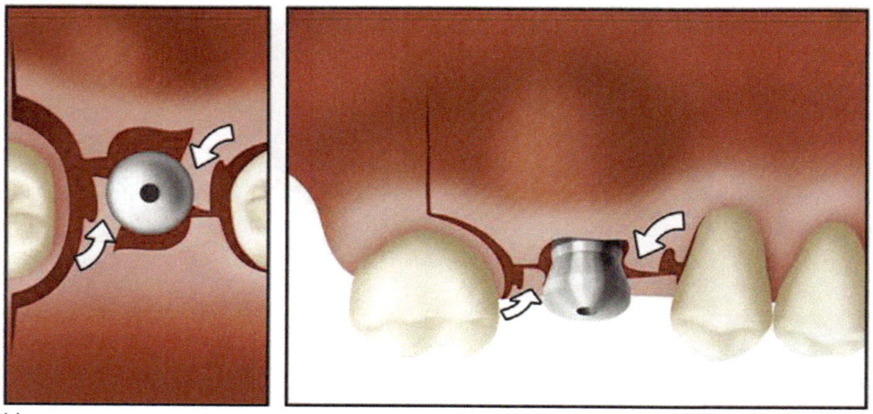
(e)

Figure 14.3 (Continued)
(d) Human mineralized bone allograft was packed into the defect and overcontoured by approximately 20–30%. (e) A variation of Palacci's papilla regeneration technique helped to release tissue tension around the healing abutment. (f) The soft tissues were positioned around the healing abutment using a sling suture. (g) The alveolar ridge form and peri-implant soft tissues at the 2-year follow-up. © Bach T. Le.

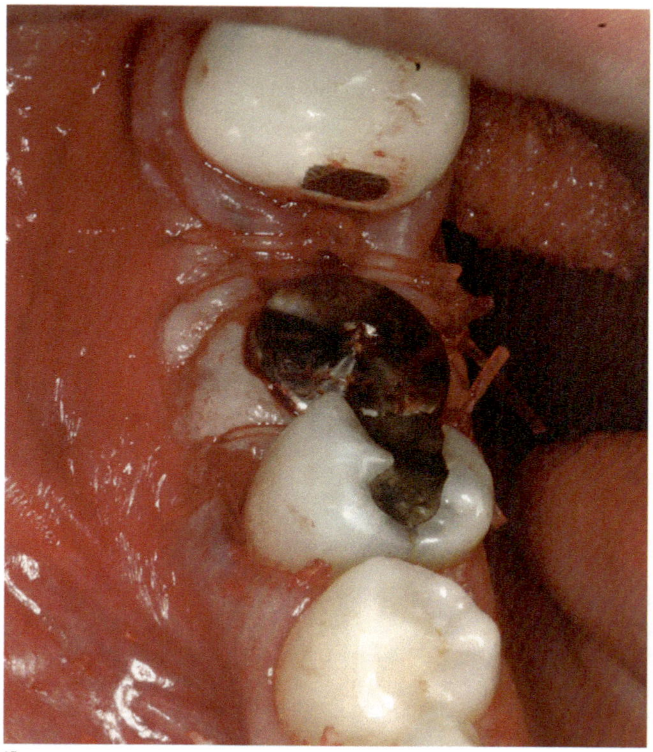
(f)

Bone graft materials

Various bone graft materials can be used successfully for GBR procedures. An ideal bone graft material would be osteogenic, osteoinductive, osteoconductive, biocompatible, have good handling properties, provide adequate mechanical support to prevent collapse of covering membranes and overlying soft tissues, avoid the need for donor sites and associated morbidity, be of low cost, and resist resorption. Unfortunately, no such graft material exists at present. Therefore, clinicians often combine two or more materials to obtain a predictable outcome. Autogenous bone has been considered the gold standard for bone grafting owing to its biocompatibility and osteogenic properties. Other bone grafting materials present in the market include allografts (fresh frozen bone, freeze-dried bone allograft (FDBA), demineralized, freeze-dried bone allograft (DFDBA)), xenografts (bovine or equine bone minerals; DBBM), coral minerals, algae minerals, alloplastic materials (e.g. calcium phosphates, polymers, bioactive glass), and genetically engineered, bone morphogenic proteins (BMPs) and other biologics (see also Chapter 7). At present, the most widely used materials are autogenous bone, FDBA, and DBBM.

Autogenous bone

Autogenous bone has osteogenic, osteoinductive, and osteoconductive properties. It can be harvested from intraoral or extraoral donor sites, and depending on the donor site location can be primarily cortical, cortico-cancellous, or cancellous. Intraoral donor sites include chin, mandibular ramus/body, maxillary tuberosity, anterior nasal spine, and zygomatic body. Extraoral donor sites include anterior iliac crest, posterior iliac crest, tibia, calvaria, and fibula. Choice of the donor site depends on the size and dimension of the defect being treated, as well as the clinician's preference and consideration of patient morbidity. Particle size of autogenous bone graft material is a factor since smaller particles have increased surface area, allowing more growth factors to be exposed to osteoprogenitor cells.[34]

Allografts

FDBAs have been utilized with success in GBR procedures.[35,36] Studies using histologic analyses of grafted sites have shown adequate bone formation for implant osseointegration.[22,37–39] Allografts are available as cortical, cortico-cancellous, or cancellous bone and can be demineralized or not. The demineralization of allograft materials, if carefully performed, exposes bone inductive proteins located in the bone matrix[40] so that crude protein extracts from DFDBA contain immunoreactive BMPs.[41] However, in a study in mandibles of minipigs, Buser et al.[42] concluded that DFDBA had only osteoconductive properties. Moreover, DFDBA has decreased mechanical stability compared with FDBA. When compared with DFDBA or bovine xenografts, mineralized allografts (FDBA) have been shown to have higher mean bone density as well as fewer residual particles after site healing.[43] Also, our clinical experiences suggest that FDBA may tolerate wound exposure better than other bone grafts;[22] therefore, when using allograft, we prefer FDBA over DFDBA.

Xenografts

The most commonly used xenograft in GBR is bovine bone matrix. In its preparation, every effort is made to remove the organic components by chemical treatment with strong alkaline solution, heat treatment to 300–1000 °C, or a combination of these methods. The resulting mineralized bone matrix is considered to be a safe xenograft with minimal risk of disease transmission.[44] In a study by Schwartz et al.,[45] small amounts of protein were found in bovine xenograft material, but these may represent transforming growth factor-beta (TGF-β) and BMP-2 as they were found to be osteoinductive in the nude mouse model when combined with inactive DFDBA.

In an animal model, Araújo and coworkers demonstrated that bovine bone matrix delayed bone healing in fresh extraction sockets.[46,47] Only minute amounts of newly formed bone appeared in the grafted sockets after 2 weeks of healing, while large amounts of woven bone had formed in the non-grafted sites. After a 3-month healing period, the newly formed hard tissue in extraction sockets grafted with the bovine material contained a large number of the graft particles that were surrounded by immature woven bone. Indeed, the general consensus is that mineralized bovine bone xenograft is slowly, if ever, resorbed, and histologic assessment of biopsies from augmented sinuses in humans showed remaining bovine bone particles up to 10 years post-operatively.[48] Although, as noted, some have found inhibitory effects with bovine bone matrix used in socket preservation, others have found it to be effective in preserving post-extraction alveolar ridge anatomy with adequate bone formation to allow subsequent successful implant placement.[49,50] Bovine bone matrix can be utilized for grafting sockets if its properties are understood. Given that the material is only osteoconductive, longer time intervals are likely needed between grafting and implant placement to allow for successful osseointegration.

Barrier membranes

An ideal barrier membrane for GBR should be biocompatible, easy to handle, resorbable to avoid the necessity of an extra procedure for removal, maintain space, have tissue integration, provide cell occlusion, and have minimal susceptibility to complications.[51] The two main categories of barrier membranes are non-resorbable and resorbable membranes. Non-resorbable membranes are generally made from polytetrafluoroethylene (PTFE), while resorbable membranes include polymer membranes and collagen membranes made from a variety of sources. Ridge preservation can be performed with or without barrier membranes.[52–57] A systematic review of available research to determine if a barrier membrane helped prevent resorption of autogenous onlay grafts concluded that more evidence is needed.[57] Guided tissue regeneration and GBR can be successfully performed using either resorbable or non-resorbable membranes.[58–61]

Non-resorbable membranes, particularly those made from expanded PTFE, have significant risk of premature membrane exposure.[62] They also have higher irritation and infection rates compared with resorbable membranes.[63] The advantages and use of non-expanded PTFE as an open barrier technique are discussed in detail in Chapter 5. Collagen membranes are the most widely used resorbable membranes, and are derived from modified bovine products (tendon, dermis, or pericardium), calf skin, or porcine dermis using type I collagen or a combination of type I and type III collagen.[64] Collagen materials also possess additional advantages, including hemostasis, easy manipulation, are better tolerated if exposed, and a second surgery is not necessary for membrane removal.

The role of bone and soft tissue augmentation

One of the keys to giving an implant restoration the esthetic illusion of a natural tooth is to create the ideal emergence profile.[65] A critical part of the emergence profile is based on the type of tissue surrounding the implant and whether any defects in the underlying bone are present. Even when there is adequate bone to place implants, irregular ridge anatomy that is not corrected can result in an unnatural appearance of the final restoration (Figure 14.4).

Goaslind et al.[66] described two gingival biotypes commonly found in the natural dentition: thick and thin (Figure 14.5). It has been suggested that a thicker soft tissue biotype is associated with less tissue recession, higher crestal bone levels, and better aesthetics.[67,68] Thus, thick soft tissue may be protective against crestal bone loss.[67] Gingival recession is always associated with alveolar bone dehiscence, but cannot occur in the presence of an intact labial wall.[69–74] Jung et al.[68] suggested that soft tissue thickness of at least 2 mm is ideal to achieve natural esthetics when using different

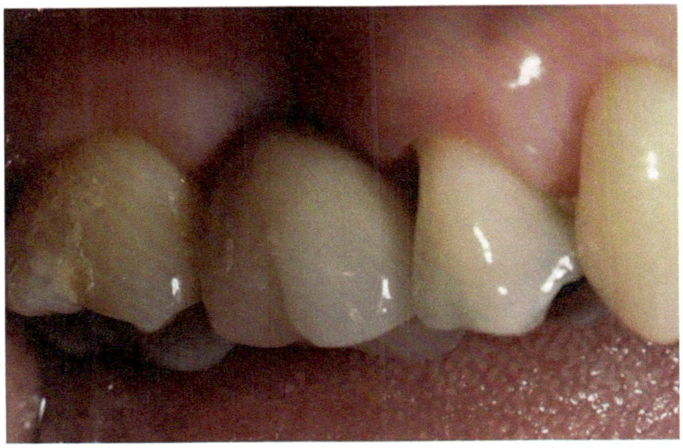

Figure 14.4 An implant-supported restoration showed unnatural ridge contour due to collapse of the buccal alveolar ridge. © Bach T. Le.

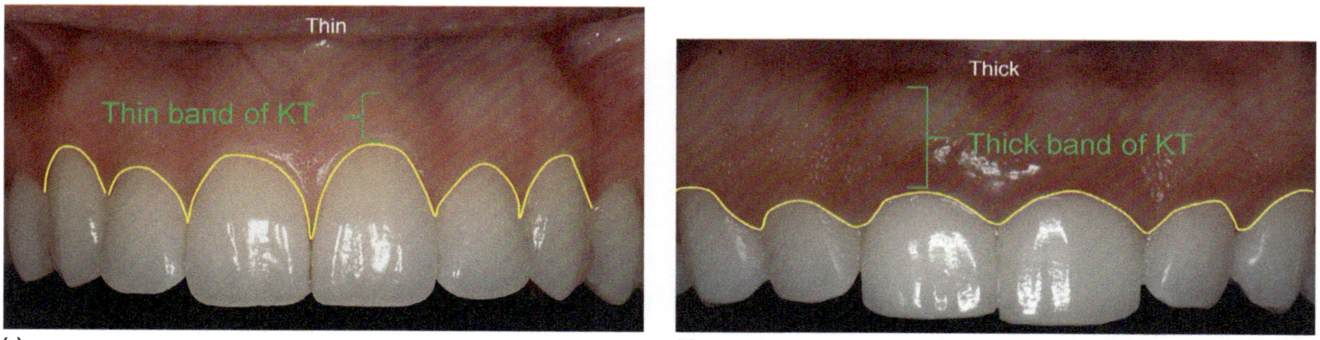

(a) (b)

Figure 14.5 Most patients will fall into two categories: (a) slender teeth with thin gingiva and high scalloped periodontium or (b) square teeth with thick gingiva and blunted periodontium. KT: keratinized tissue. © Bach T. Le.

abutment materials. As a result of these findings, many authors have recommended the routine use of connective tissue grafting in the esthetic zone to thicken the crestal labial soft tissue to 2 mm.[75,76]

Use of an "esthetic contour graft" at the time of implant placement may avoid the need for secondary soft tissue augmentation because it augments the underlying bone, helping to restore the natural soft tissue architecture. Clinical observation of labial soft tissue thickening is often noted after successful grafting with particulate allograft and collagen membrane at the time of implant placement. This new concept of "bone-driven tissue transformation" may replace the need for soft tissue augmentation in many instances and is demonstrated in Figure 14.6a–f and after 5 years in Figure 14.6g–i.

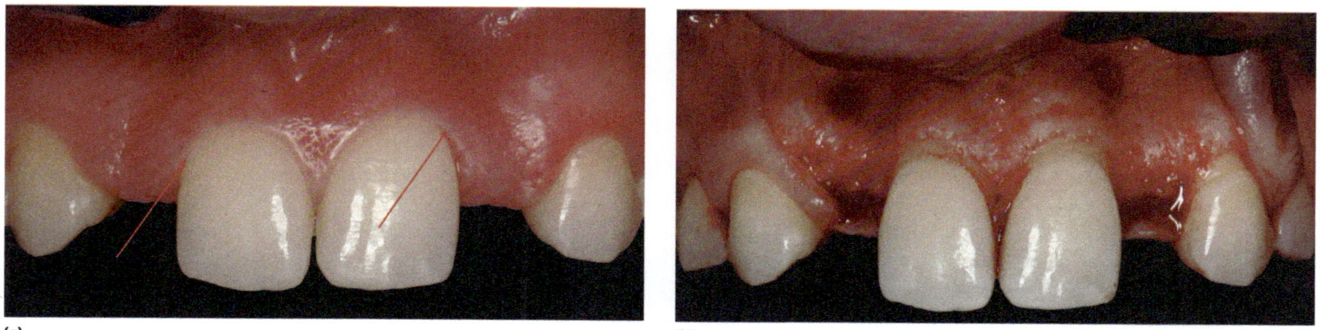

(a) (b)

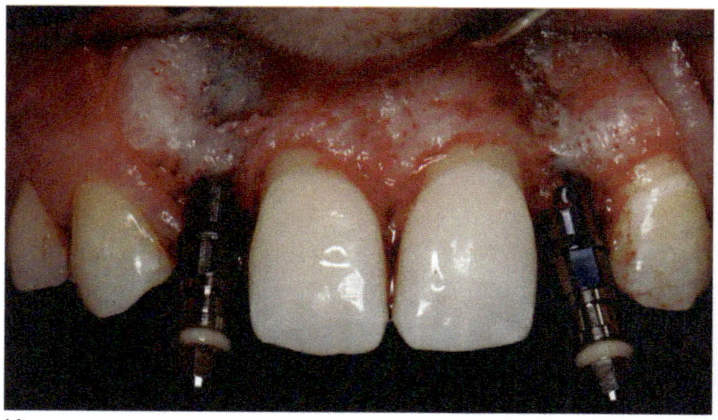

(c)

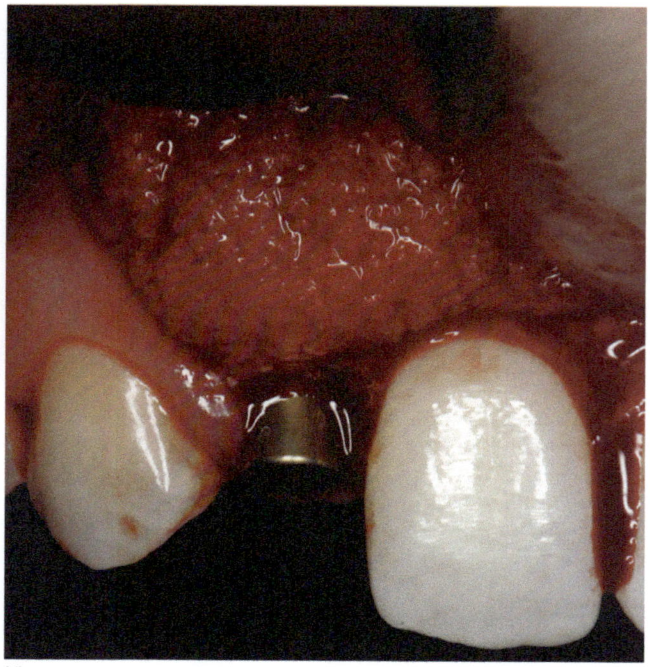

(d)

Figure 14.6 (a) The preoperative situation in a patient with congenitally missing maxillary lateral incisors. The arrows denote thin soft tissues and compromised underlying bone support. (b) An open-book flap design was used. (c) The implant placement resulted in thin residual buccal bone and visible metallic translucency. (d) An esthetic contour graft was used to augment the deficient buccal bone.

(Continued)

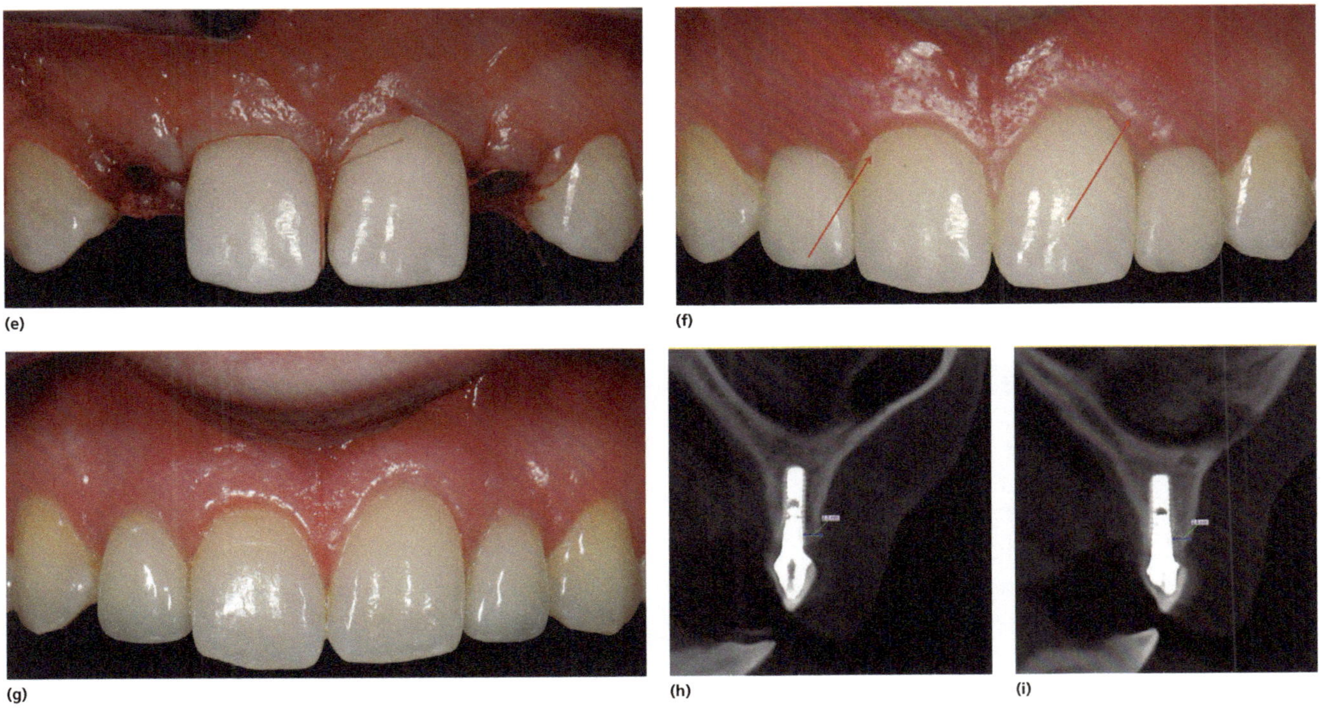

Figure 14.6 (Continued)
(e) The flap was repositioned for non-submerged implant healing. (f) Provisional restorations were used to "groom" the soft tissues; the arrows show the increased tissue thickness compared with the preoperative presentation. (g–i) The final restoration and cross-sectional CT images at 5 years. © Bach T. Le.

Studies have confirmed that the thickness of bone around implants can affect the overlying soft tissue profile. Le and Borzabadi-Farahani[77] showed a high correlation between labial crestal soft tissue thickness and underlying bone thickness with maxillary anterior implants, demonstrating that soft tissue thickness can be heavily influenced by the labial bone thickness (Figure 14.7). In other words, the thicker the bone, the thicker the crestal labial soft tissue around implants and vice versa. **Based on these findings, soft** tissue augmentation may not be necessary if adequate labial crestal bone thickness (>2 mm) exists or can be created.

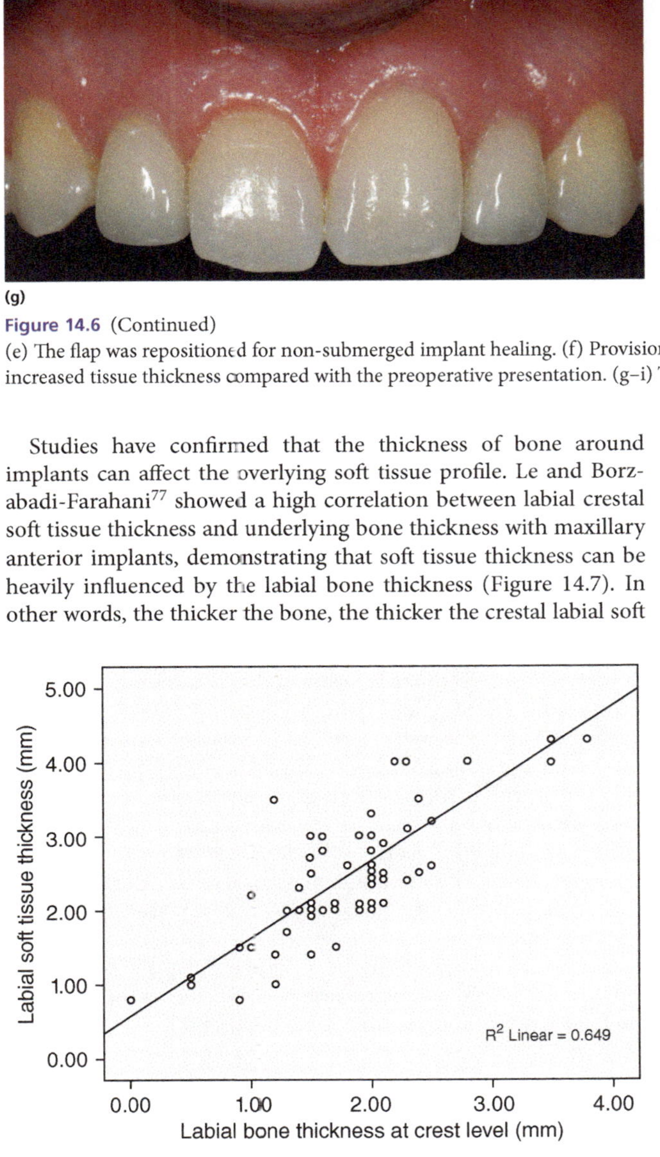

Figure 14.7 The labial soft tissue thickness and bone thickness around anterior maxillary implants; a linear correlation can be seen between the labial crestal soft tissue thickness and underlying bone thickness. *Source:* Le B, Borzabadi-Farahani A. Labial bone thickness in area of anterior maxillary implants associated with crestal labial soft tissue thickness. Implant Dent 2012; 21: 406–410. Reproduced with permission of Wolters Kluwer Health.[77]

Different opinions exist as to whether a lack of keratinized tissue may jeopardize the maintenance of soft tissue health around dental implants.[78–80] Some authors have reported that implants with a width of <2 mm of peri-implant keratinized mucosa are associated with increased buccal soft tissue recession, increased alveolar bone loss, more plaque accumulation, increased bleeding, and poorer soft tissue health,[81–83] while others have not found similar correlations.[84,85] Despite these observations, soft tissue augmentation at implant sites may need to be considered in some clinical situations where adequate crestal bone thickness cannot be achieved to facilitate successful restorative procedures, and to help maintain oral hygiene (see Chapter 8).

Implant position and labial soft tissue thickness

Dental implant therapy should be prosthetically driven and not primarily bone driven. To this end, the implant must be accurately placed in a 3-D (mesio-distal, labio-lingual/palatal, and apico-coronal) position with the goal of achieving a proper emergence profile for the final restoration. When the implant position is not accurate, the esthetic result is often compromised. Implants placed too deep apico-coronally or too labially often result is an unnaturally long restoration (Figure 14.8). In addition, implant position has been shown to have a direct influence on peri-implant bone and soft tissue thickness.[86]

Le et al.[87] studied the relationship between crestal labial soft tissue thickness and implant bucco-lingual angulation. The bucco-lingual angulation was recorded as cingulum-, incisally-, or labially-angled

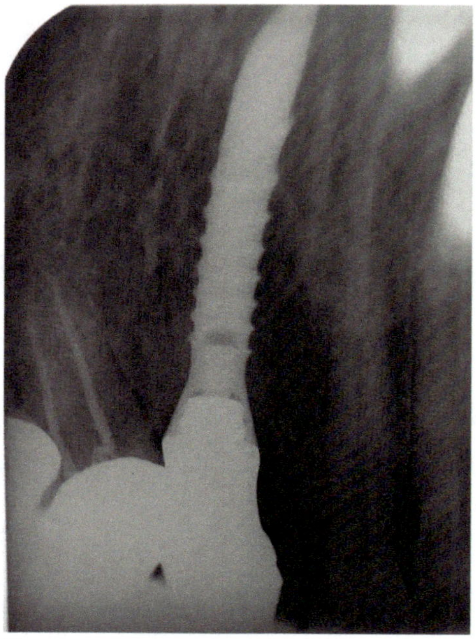

(a)

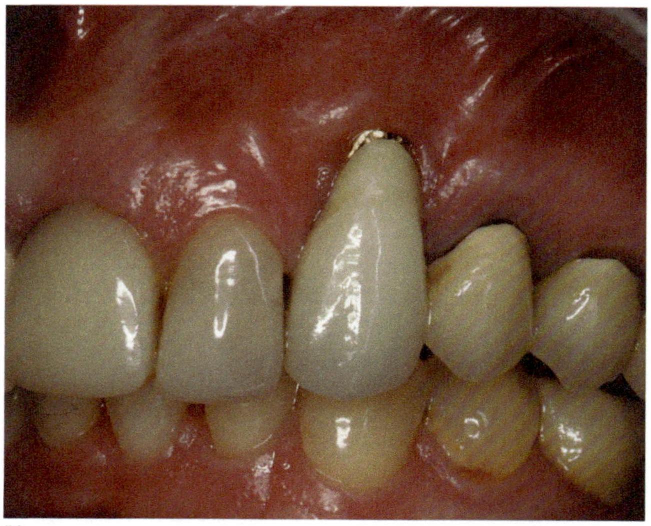

(b)

Figure 14.8 Implants if placed too deeply in (a) an apicocoronal position or (b) too labially often result in an unnaturally long restoration. © Bach T. Le.

based on the position of the screw access hole of the provisional restoration (Figure 14.9). The implant labial bone thickness was measured at the crestal and mid-implant levels using sectional cone beam computed tomography scans. Of implants with cingulum, incisal, and labial angulations, 3.4%, 20%, and 53.3% respectively had crestal labial soft tissue thickness of <2 mm. A significant association between crestal labial soft tissue thickness and implant bucco-lingual angulation was noted when implant labial bone thickness at crestal level was <2 mm ($p < 0.01$). The investigators concluded that implants with labial angulations carry a higher risk of soft tissue complications when the crestal implant labial bone thickness is <2 mm.

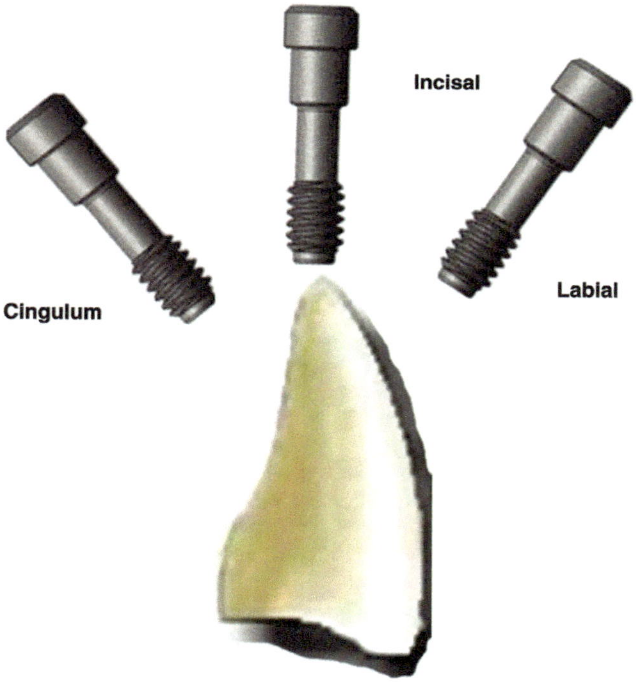

Figure 14.9 Implant angulation versus crestal labial soft tissue thickness. Significant differences were detected between crestal labial soft tissue thicknesses for implants with cingulum versus incisal angulation, as well as for implants with cingulum versuss labial angulations ($p < 0.01$). *Source:* Le B and Borzabadi-Farahani A 2014.[87] Reproduced with permission of Elsevier.

Conclusions

The goals of minimally invasive dental implant therapy include minimizing surgical interventions and achieving shorter healing times, while producing predictable and long-term functional and esthetic results. The decision on which technique to employ should be based on the comfort level of the surgeon, as this will dramatically affect the outcome. Failed guided tissue regeneration done with simultaneous implant placement may lead to exposed implant threads or crown margins. Single-stage implant placement and simultaneous grafting with particulate bone graft and membrane coverage is more predictable on alveolar ridges with small to medium-sized horizontal and vertical labial wall defects. The technique becomes more unreliable and more technique-sensitive as the length of the edentulous span increases and if multiple implants are being placed. In wide spans, tenting screws are needed to prevent collapse of the tissue and graft resorption. The use of a limited flap design to maintain vascular supply, optimize attached tissue and vestibular depth, and to ensure tension-free closure are important for the success of this technique.

References

1. Cardaropoli G, Araújo M, Lindhe J. Dynamics of bone tissue formation in tooth extraction sites. An experimental study in dogs. J Clin Periodontol 2003; 30: 809–818.
2. Pietrokovski J, Massler M. Alveolar ridge resorption following tooth extraction. J Prosthetic Dent 1967; 17: 21–27.
3. Araújo M, Wennström J, Lindhe J. Modeling of the buccal and lingual bone walls of fresh extraction sites following implant installation. Clin Oral Implants Res 2006; 17: 606–614.

4. Schropp L, Wenzel A, Kostopoulos L, Karring T. Bone healing and soft tissue contour changes following single-tooth extraction: a clinical and radiographic 12-month prospective study. Int J Periodontics Restorative Dent 2003; 23: 313–323.
5. Covani U, Ricci M, Bozzolo G, et al. Analysis of the pattern of the alveolar ridge remodeling following single tooth extraction. Clin Oral Implants Res 2011; 22: 820–825.
6. Van der Weijden F, Dell'Acqua F, Slot DE. Alveolar bone dimensional changes of post-extraction sockets in humans: a systematic review. J Clin Periodontol 2009; 36: 1048–1058.
7. Belser U, Schmid B, Higginbottom F, et al. Outcome analysis of implant restorations located in the anterior maxilla: a review of the recent literature. Int J Oral Maxillofac Implants 2004; 19(Suppl): 30–42.
8. Kan J, Rungcharassaeng K. Inter-implant papilla preservation in the esthetic zone: a report of six consecutive cases. Int J Periodontics Restorative Dent 2003; 23: 249–259.
9. Priest G. The esthetic challenge of adjacent implants. J Oral Maxillofac Surg 2007; 65: 2–12.
10. Becker W, Dahlin C, Becker B, et al. The use of e-PTFE barrier membranes for bone promotion around titanium implants placed into extraction sockets: a prospective multicenter study. Int J Oral Maxillofacial Implants 1994; 9: 31–40.
11. Buser D, Ruskin J, Higginbotton F, et al. Osseointegration of titanium implants in bone regenerated in membrane-protected defects: a histologic study in the canine mandible. Int J Oral Maxillofac Implants 1995; 10: 666–681.
12. Dahlin C, Gottlow J, Linde A, Nyman S. Healing of maxillary and mandibular defects using a membrane technique. An experimental study in monkeys. Scand J Plast Reconstr Surg Hand Surg 1990; 24: 13–19.
13. Mellonig J, Nevins M, Sanchez R. Evaluation of a bioabsorbable physical barrier for guided bone regeneration. Part II. Material and a bone replacement graft. Int J Periodontics Restorative Dent 1998; 18: 139–149.
14. Le B, Burstein J. Esthetic grafting for small volume hard and soft tissue contour defects for implant site development. Implant Dent 2008; 17: 136–141.
15. Frost HM. The regional acceleratory phenomenon: a review. Henry Ford Hosp Med J 1983; 31: 3–9.
16. Le BT, Borzabadi-Farahani A. Simultaneous implant placement and bone grafting with particulate mineralized allograft in sites with buccal wall defects: a three-year follow-up and review of literature. J Craniomaxillofac Surg 2014; 42: 552–559.
17. Jensen S, Bosshardt D, Gruber R, Buser D. Long-term stability of contour augmentation in the esthetic zone. Histologic and histomorphometric evaluation of 12 human biopsies 14 to 80 months after augmentation. J Periodontol 2014; 10: 1–15.
18. Schenk R, Buser D, Hardwick W, Dahlin C. Healing pattern of bone regeneration in membrane-protected defects: a histologic study in the canine mandible. Int J Oral Maxillofac Implants 1994; 9: 13–29.
19. Sculean A, Nikolidakis D, Schwarz F. Regeneration of periodontal tissues: combinations of barrier membranes and grafting materials – biological foundation and preclinical evidence: a systematic review. J Clin Periodontol 2008; 35: 106–116.
20. Louis PJ, Gutta R, Said-Al-Naief N, et al. Reconstruction of the maxilla and mandible with particulate bone graft and titanium mesh for implant placement. J Oral Maxillofac Surg 2008; 66: 235–245.
21. Louis P. Vertical ridge augmentation using titanium mesh. Oral Maxillofac Surg Clin North Am 2010; 22: 353–368.
22. Le B, Rohrer M, Prassad H. Screw "tent-pole" grafting technique for reconstruction of large vertical alveolar ridge defects using human mineralized allograft for implant site preparation. J Oral Maxillofac Surg 2010; 68: 428–435.
23. Jensen O, Cockrell R, Kuhike L, et al. Anterior maxillary alveolar distraction osteogenesis: a prospective 5-year clinical study. Int J Oral Maxillofac Implants 2002; 17: 52–68.
24. Jensen O. Segmental alveolar split combined with dental extractions and osteotome sinus floor intrusion in posterior maxilla using BMP-2/ACS allograft for alveolar reconstruction: technical note and report of three cases. J Oral Maxillofac Surg 2014; 71: 2040–2047.
25. Wang H, Boyapati L. "PASS" principles for predictable bone regeneration. Implant Dent 2006; 15: 8–17.
26. Elian N, Cho SC, Froum S, et al. A simplified socket classification and repair technique. Pract Proced Aesth Dent 2007; 19: 99–104.
27. Kan J, Rungcharassaeng K, Sclar A, Lozada J. Effects of the facial osseous defect morphology on gingival dynamics after immediate tooth replacement and guided bone regeneration: 1-year results. J Oral Maxillofac Surg 2007; 65: 13–19.
28. Spray J, Black C, Morris H, et al. The influence of bone thickness on facial marginal bone response: stage 1 placement through stage 2 uncovering. Ann Periodontol 2000; 5: 119–128.
29. Covani U, Cornelini R and Barone A. Buccal bone augmentation around immediate implants with and without flap elevation: a modified approach. Int J Oral Maxillofac Implants 2008; 23: 841–846.
30. Le BT, Kim E. Effectiveness of single-staged implant placement with simultaneous grafting using mineralized allograft. J Oral Maxillofac Surg 2009; 67(9): 57.
31. Palacci P, Nowzari H. Soft tissue enhancement around dental implants. Periodontol 2000 2008; 47: 113–132.
32. Nishimura I, Shimizu Y, Ooya K. Effects of cortical bone perforation on experimental guided bone regeneration. Clin Oral Implants Res 2004; 15: 293–300.
33. Slotte C, Lundgren D, Sennerby L, Lundgren A. Surgical intervention in endochondral and membranous bone: intra-individual comparisons in the rabbit. Clin Implant Dent Relat Res 2003; 5: 263–268.
34. Pallesen L, Schou S, Aaboe M, et al. Influence of particle size of autogenous bone grafts on the early stages of bone regeneration: a histologic and stereologic study in rabbit calvarium. Int J Oral Maxillofac Implants 2002; 17: 498–506.
35. Lyford R, Mills M, Knapp C, et al. Clinical evaluation of freeze-dried block allografts for alveolar ridge augmentation: a case series. Int J Periodontics Restorative Dent 2003; 23: 417–425.
36. Block M, Degen M. Horizontal ridge augmentation using human mineralized particulate bone: preliminary results. J Oral Maxillofac Surg 2004; 62: 67–72.
37. Minichetti J, D'Amore J, Hong A. Three-year analysis of tapered screw-vent implants placed into extraction sockets grafted with mineralized bone allograft. J Oral Implant 2005; 31: 283–293.
38. Wang H, Tsao Y. Mineralized bone allograft-plug socket augmentation: rationale and technique. Implant Dent 2007; 16: 33–41.
39. Block M, Finger I, Lytle R. Human mineralized bone in extraction sites before implant placement: preliminary results. J Am Dent Assoc 2002; 133: 1631–1638.
40. Schwartz Z, Mellonig J, Carnes D Jr, et al. Ability of commercial demineralized freeze-dried bone allograft to induce new bone formation. J Periodontol 1996; 67: 918–926.
41. Shigeyama Y, D'Errico JA, Stone R, Somerman MJ. Commercially-prepared allograft material has biological activity *in vitro*. J Periodontol 1995; 66: 478–487.
42. Buser D, Hoffmann B, Bernard JP, et al. Evaluation of filling materials in membrane-protected bone defects. A comparative histomorphometric study in the mandible of miniature pigs. Clin Oral Implants Res 1998; 9: 137–150.
43. Froum S, Wallace S, Elian N, et al. Comparison of mineralized cancellous bone allograft (Puros) and anorganic bovine bone matrix (Bio-Oss) for sinus augmentation histomorphometry at 26 to 32 weeks after grafting. Int J Periodontics Restorative Dent 2006; 26: 543–551.
44. Wenz B, Oesch B, Horst M. Analysis of the risk of transmitting bovine spongiform encephalopathy through bone grafts derived from bovine bone. Biomaterials 2001; 22: 1599–1606.
45. Schwartz Z, Weesner T, van Dijk S, et al. Ability of deproteinized cancellous bovine bone to induce new bone formation. J Periodontol 2007; 71: 1258–1269.
46. Araújo M, Linder E, Wennström J, Lindhe J. The influence of Bio-Oss collagen on healing of an extraction socket: an experimental study in the dog. Int J Periodontics Restorative Dent 2008; 28: 123–135.
47. Araújo M, Linder E, Lindhe J. Effect of a xenograft on early bone formation in extraction sockets: an experimental study in dog. Clin Oral Implants Res 2009; 20: 1–6.
48. Piattelli M, Favero GA, Scarano A, et al. Bone reactions to anorganic bovine bone (Bio-Oss) used in sinus augmentation procedures: a histologic long-term report of 20 cases in humans. Int J Oral Maxillofac Implants 1999; 14: 835–840.
49. Froum S, Cho S, Elian N, et al. Extraction sockets and implantation of hydroxyapatites with membrane barriers: a histologic study. Implant Dent 2004; 13: 153–164.
50. Molly L, Vandromme H, Quirynen M, et al. Bone formation following implantation of bone biomaterials into extraction sites. J Periodontol 2008; 79: 1108–1115.
51. Hardwick R, Scantlebury T, Sanchez R, et al. Membrane design criteria for guided bone regeneration of the alveolar ridge. In: Guided Bone Regeneration in Implant Dentistry, Buser D, Dahlin C, Schenk RK, eds. Quintessence, 1994, pp. 101–136.
52. Hellem S, Astrand P, Stenstrom B, et al. Implant treatment in combination with lateral augmentation of the alveolar process: a 3-year prospective study. Clin Implant Dent Relat Res 2003; 5: 233–240.
53. Llambes F, Silvestre F, Caffesse R. Vertical guided bone regeneration with bioabsorbable barriers. J Periodontol 2007; 78: 2036–2042.
54. Louis P, Gutta R, Said-Al-Naief N, et al. Reconstruction of the maxilla and mandible with particulate bone graft and titanium mesh for implant placement. J Oral Maxillofac Surg 2008; 66: 235–245.
55. Simion M, Scarano A, Gionso L, et al. Guided bone regeneration using resorbable and non-resorbable membranes: a comparative histologic study in humans. Int J Oral Maxillofac Implants 1996; 11: 735–742.
56. Simion M, Fontana F, Rasperini G, et al. Vertical ridge augmentation by expanded polytetrafluoroethylene membrane and a combination of intraoral autogenous bone graft and deproteinized anorganic bovine bone (Bio Oss). Clin Oral Implants Res 2007; 18: 620–629.
57. Gielkens P, Bos R, Raghoebar G, et al. Is there evidence that barrier membranes prevent bone resorption in autologous bone grafts during the healing period? A systemic review. Int J Oral Maxillofac Implants 2007; 22: 390–398.

58. Becker W, Becker B, Mellonig J, et al. A prospective multi-center study evaluating periodontal regeneration for class II furcation invasions and intrabony defects after treatment with bioabsorbable barrier membrane: 1 year results. J Periodontol 1996; 67: 641–649.
59. Laurell L, Falk H, Fornell J, et al. Clinical use of bioabsorbable matrix barrier in guided tissue regeneration therapy. J Periodontol 1994; 65: 967–975.
60. Christgau M, Bader N, Schmalz G, et al. GTR therapy of intrabony defects using 2 different bioabsorbable membranes: 12 month results. J Clin Periodontol 1998; 25: 499–509.
61. Schallhorn RG, McClain PK. Combined osseous composite grafting, root conditioning, and guided tissue regeneration. Int J Periodontics Restorative Dent 1988; 8: 8–31.
62. Machtei E. The effect of membrane exposure on the outcome of regenerative procedures in humans: a meta-analysis. J Periodontol 2001; 72: 512–516.
63. Murphy K. Post-operative healing complications associated with Gore-tex periodontal material. Part II. Effect of complications on regeneration. Int J Periodontics Restorative Dent 1995; 15: 548–561.
64. Bunyaratavej P, Wang HL. Collagen membranes: a review. J Periodontol 2001; 72: 215–229.
65. Kois J. Predictable single tooth peri-implant esthetics: five diagnostic keys. Compend Contin Educ Dent 2001; 22: 199–206.
66. Goaslind D, Robertson B, Mahan J, et al. Thickness of facial gingiva. J Periodontol 1977; 48: 768–771.
67. Linkevicius T, Apse P, Grybauskas S, et al. The influence of soft tissue thickness on crestal bone changes around implants: a 1-year prospective controlled clinical trial. Int J Oral Maxillofac Implants 2009; 24: 712–719.
68. Jung R, Sailer I, Hämmerle C, et al. *In vitro* color changes of soft tissues caused by restorative materials. Int J Periodontics Restorative Dent 2007; 27: 251–257.
69. Ngom P, Diagne F, Benoist H, et al. Intra-arch and inter-arch relationships of the anterior teeth and periodontal conditions. Angle Orthod 2006; 76: 236–242.
70. Fuhrmann R. Three-dimensional evaluation of periodontal remodeling during orthodontic treatment. Semin Orthod 2002; 8: 23–28.
71. Wennstrom J. Mucogingival therapy. Ann Periodontol 1996; 1: 671–701.
72. Kassab M, Cohen R. The etiology and prevalence of gingival recession. J Am Dent Assoc 2003; 134: 220–225.
73. Patel M, Nixon P, Chan M. Gingival recession: part 1. Aetiology and non-surgical management. Brit Dent J 2011; 211: 251–254.
74. Richman C. Is gingival recession a consequence of an orthodontic tooth size and/or tooth position discrepancy? A paradigm shift. Compend Cont Educ Dent 2011; 32: 62–69.
75. Esposito M, Maghaireh H, Grusovin M, et al. Interventions for replacing missing teeth: management of soft tissues for dental implants. Cochrane Database Syst Rev 2012; (2): CD006697.
76. Chen S, Darby I, Reynolds E. A prospective clinical study of non-submerged immediate implants: clinical outcomes and esthetic results. Clin Oral Implants Res 2007; 18: 552–562.
77. Le B, Borzabadi-Farahani A. Labial bone thickness in area of anterior maxillary implants associated with crestal labial soft tissue thickness. Implant Dent 2012; 21: 406–410.
78. Bengazi F, Wennstrom J, Lekholm U. Recession of the soft tissue margin at oral implants. A 2-year longitudinal prospective study. Clin Oral Implants Res 1996; 7: 303–310.
79. Wennstrom J, Bengazi F, Lekholm U. The influence of the masticatory mucosa on the peri-implant soft tissue condition. Clin Oral Implants Res 1994; 5: 1–8.
80. Chung D, Oh T, Shotwell J, et al. Significance of keratinized mucosa in maintenance of dental implants with different surfaces. J Periodontol 2006; 77: 1410–1420.
81. Schrott A, Jimenez M, Hwang J, et al. Five-year evaluation of the influence of keratinized mucosa on peri-implant soft tissue health and stability around implants supporting full-arch mandibular fixed prostheses. Clin Oral Implants Res 2009; 20: 1170–1177.
82. Bouri A, Bissada N, Al-Zahrani M, et al. Width of keratinized gingiva and the health status of the supporting tissues around dental implants. Int J Oral Maxillofac Implants 2008; 23: 323–326.
83. Kim B, Kim Y, Yun P, et al. Evaluation of peri-implant tissue response according to the presence of keratinized mucosa. Oral Surg Oral Med Oral Path Oral Rad Endo 2009; 107: 24–28.
84. Cairo F, Pagliaro U, Nieri M. Soft tissue management at implant sites. J Clin Periodontol 2008; 35: 163–167.
85. Wennstrom J, Derks J. Is there a need for keratinized mucosa around implants to maintain health and tissue stability? Clin Oral Implants Res 2012; 23: 136–146.
86. Pluemsakunthai W, Le BT, Kasugai S. Alveolar ridge alteration following immediate implant placement in different implant-buccal gap plate distance: a micro-computed tomography analysis in dogs. J Oral Maxillofac Surg 2013; 71(9 Suppl): e54–e55.
87. Le B, Borzabadi-Farahani A, Pluemsakunthai W. Is buccolingual angulation of maxillary anterior implants associated with the crestal labial soft tissue thickness? Int J Oral Maxillofac Surg 2014; 43: 874–878.

CHAPTER 15

Trans-Alveolar Sinus Elevation and Contiguous Sinus Floor Elevation

Daniel R. Cullum[1] & Douglas Deporter[2]
[1]Private Practice, Coeur d'Alene, ID; Loma Linda University Department of OMS, Loma Linda, CA; UCLA Department of OMS, Los Angeles, CA, USA
[2]Discipline of Periodontics, Faculty of Dentistry, University of Toronto, Toronto, ON, Canada

Introduction

Management of the edentulous posterior maxilla can be challenging due to pneumatization of the maxillary sinus, reduced alveolar dimensions, and poor bone quality.[1] When first introduced, endosseous dental implants had a threaded geometry and machined surface finish, and were recommended for use in lengths ≥10 mm in mandible and ≥13 mm in maxilla.[2] Initial attempts to use short dental implants as a less invasive approach had unacceptable failure rates in 7 mm lengths, reported at 18.5–26%.[3–6] These implants were minimally rough and the resulting bone–implant interfaces with short implant lengths were thought to be inadequate to resist tensile components of off-axis loads.[7] Dental implant reconstruction with conventional length implants often required a lateral window sinus grafting procedure, also known as the Caldwell–Luc approach.[8–10] Successful implant outcomes in grafted sinus sites include the amount of native subantral bone[11,12] and implant surface design, with moderately rough surfaces performing better than machined.[13,14] Implant design modifications with rougher surface textures, enhanced threads, and tapered designs have enabled broader application in shorter lengths[15,16] (see also Chapter 10). Lateral window sinus grafting carries potential morbidity and risks such as encountering sinus septa,[17] sinus membrane perforation,[18] acute or chronic reactive sinusitis, graft infection with sequestration and oro-antral fistula formation,[19,20] arterial damage with risk of bleeding,[21] or implant displacement into the sinus.[22,23] However, for many surgeons, the lateral window sinus graft remains a predictable and common procedure to treat vertical bone deficiencies in the posterior maxilla in spite of the treatment cost, post-operative pain and edema, and an extended graft healing time of up to 9 months.

Tatum[9] also described a crestal or trans-alveolar approach and combined crestal and lateral techniques along with his description of the open lateral window graft. Summers introduced the "osteotome sinus floor elevation" (OSFE) procedure, a closed, indirect, localized crestal sinus floor up-fracture with minimal elevation and simultaneous implant placement.[24] Summers also described a "bone-added osteotome sinus floor elevation" (BAOSFE) with particulate bone "added" to the sinus floor fracture to achieve larger elevations.[25] This was accomplished using concave-tipped, end-cutting hand osteotomes and a surgical mallet. Saadoun and Le Gall suggested the use of tapered blunt-nose osteotomes for this procedure.[26] Recent systematic literature reviews support the conclusion that implants placed using BAOSFE can show comparable outcomes to those for implants placed in native bone.[27–29] With proper case selection, BAOSFE is equally successful as open window sinus grafting with either simultaneous or delayed implant placement.[30–32]

Modifications of the trans-alveolar sinus elevation (TASE) concept have been proposed, including endoscopic and Piezosurgery®-assisted sinus floor up-fracture,[33–35] use with guided surgery technology,[36] as part of tooth extraction,[37,38] and as a staged approach to increase residual bone height.[39,40] Newer TASE methods that have been introduced to expose and directly raise the sinus membrane include hydraulic pressure,[41] Piezosurgery-assisted hydraulic pressure,[42,43] nasal suction,[44] and inflatable balloons.[45] Other TASE techniques have been advocated to elevate larger segments of sinus floor, including joined adjacent sites,[39] localized management of the sinus floor (LMSF),[46] sinus alveolar crest tenting (SACT),[47] and contiguous sinus floor elevation (CSFE).[48,49] Still others have promoted TASE without the addition of particulate graft materials (OSFE).[50,51] This chapter will discuss clinical applications of the various TASE procedures to advance a minimally invasive approach to sinus elevation.

Anatomic considerations

The maxillary sinus is an inverted pyramidal-shaped cavity lined with a thin Schneiderian membrane, and having a mean volume of 14.9 mL (9.5–20 mL).[52,53] After tooth loss, maxillary alveolar resorption and sinus pneumatization can reduce the bone height available for dental implants. The relative slope or steepness of the sinus floor (Figure 15.1) and the presence of Underwood's septa (see Figure 15.19a) also influence the potential difficulty of implant placement and the risk of sinus membrane tearing during the the lateral window sinus grafting procedure.[54,55] With limited atrophy and the presence of adjacent teeth, a sloping sinus floor is often present. In the anterior region of the maxillary sinus, the bucco-palatal dimension is narrower and the anterior sinus floor slope can be steep (Figure 15.1a). In such cases, the use of osteotomes for lateral and vertical manipulation of bone can help to "evert" the membrane as it is released and elevated. Severe sinus pneumatization can result in a broad flat sinus floor requiring a broad base of elevation, limiting the amount of vertical elevation achievable and increasing the risk of membrane perforation using the BAOSFE technique[56] (Figure 15.1b). Narrower,

Minimally Invasive Dental Implant Surgery, First Edition. Edited by Daniel R. Cullum and Douglas Deporter.

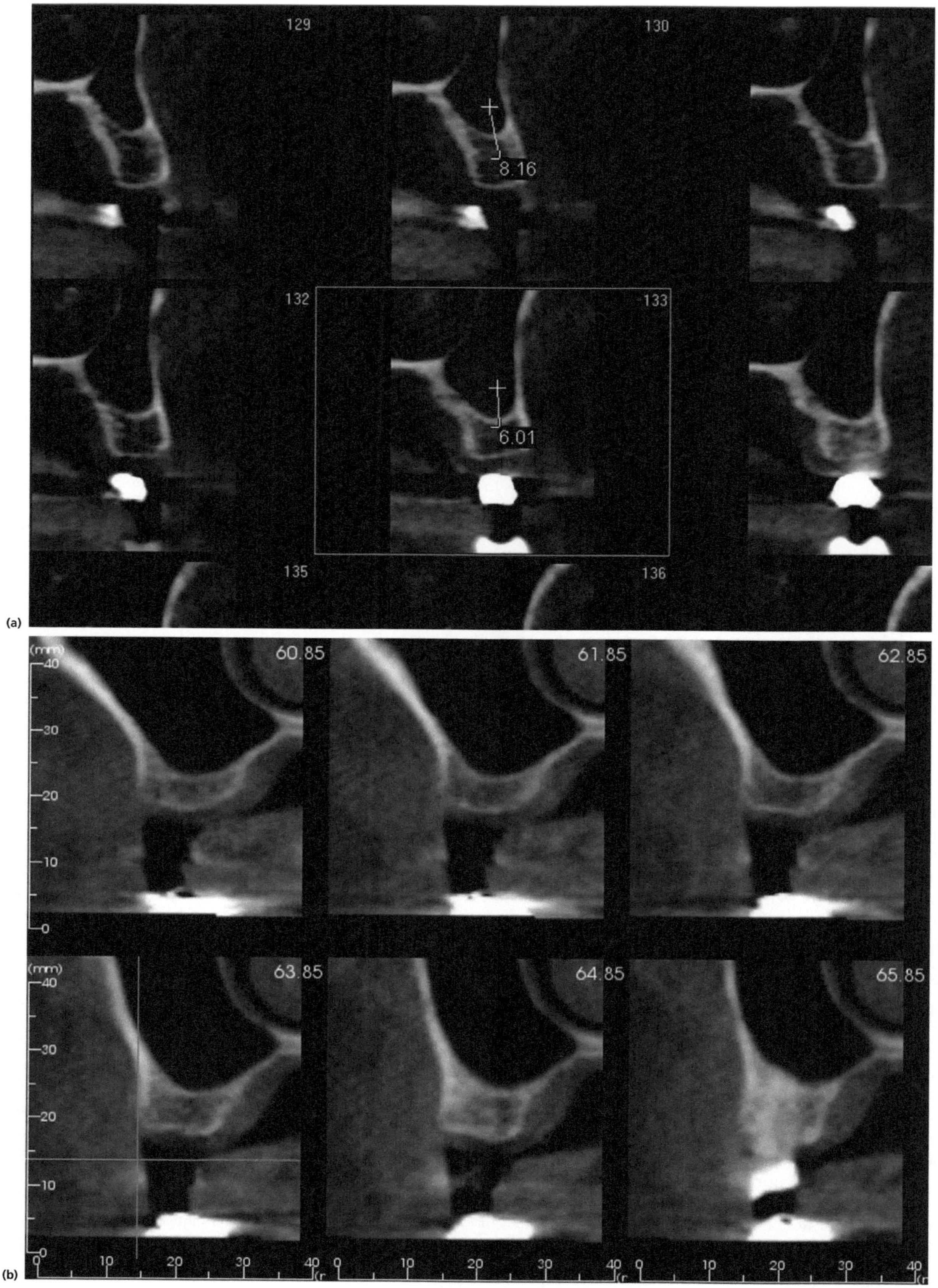

Figure 15.1 Cone beam computed tomography (CBCT) images of sinus anatomy. (a) The anterior region of the maxillary sinus typically has a narrower bucco-palatal dimension, and the anterior sinus floor slope can be steep. (b) In the posterior sinus regions, or with increasing pneumatization and atrophy, the sinus anatomy becomes broader and flatter. © Daniel R. Cullum.

steeper sinus floor angle cases are more amenable to a TASE procedure than a lateral wall approach, while the reverse is true with an atrophic broader flat anatomy.

Preoperative CBCT scanning is invaluable to evaluate alveolar and sinus dimensions for treatment planning, and also can confirm the presence of an intact sinus ostio-meatal complex, chronic sinusitis or other soft tissue pathology, such as membrane thickening, pseudo-cyst, retention cyst, or mucocele (see Chapter 2). In such situations, some clinicians have advocated preoperative medical evaluation or endoscopic assessment, avoiding treatment altogether, or direct excision and repair of a lesion at the time of open sinus grafting.[57] However, the sinus seems to recover nicely after TASE grafting procedures in patients with asymptomatic membrane thickening or limited soft tissue pathology.[58,59]

TASE bone manipulation procedures require an adequate buccopalatal ridge width and with threaded implants 5–7 mm of subantral bone height.[25] With less than this minimal bone height, a classic BAOSFE approach requires greater elevation, which increases the risk of sinus membrane perforation[60,61] or mandates the use of a shorter implant.[62,63] A residual bone height of ≤4 mm has been associated with increased implant failure rate following TASE using threaded dental implants.[64,65] Healed grafted sites or osteoporotic bone may reduce compliance with an increased risk of buccal or palatal wall fracture, altered resistance of the sinus floor to TASE, reduced vascular supply, and/or reduced primary stability.

Surgical considerations

Minimally invasive application of TASE preserves the vascular supply of the periosteum and sinus membrane, and develops adequate but limited localized sinus elevation with less pain and edema while allowing a shorter overall healing interval compared with a lateral sinus graft. Understanding and experience with the classic OSFE and BAOSFE techniques are critical in TASE as other more recent technique modifications build on these skills, and circumstances may require their use in spite of an initial plan to use a modified technique.

Preoperative patient preparation with chlorhexidine rinses and a loading dose of antibiotic (e.g. amoxicillin) are recommended. Intravenous sedation can be beneficial, and the patient should be seated in a semi-reclined position. Control of the osteotome is by the dominant hand of the surgeon, while the other hand is used to palpate and support the ridge for continuous feedback at the developing osteotomy. A light malleting force is used with short repeated taps on the osteotome by the surgeon or the assistant under direction from the surgeon. Palpating the ridge along with visual, and auditory cues will help avoid sudden fracture of buccal bone or loss of vertical reference causing sinus breach. The initial sharp clear ringing sound softens and dulls as bone begins to respond. Slow, progressive, and repetitive manipulations are necessary to produce the desired result. Careful force application and control are necessary with these techniques. Support for the patient's head by a second assistant can help non-sedated patients better tolerate the percussive forces and minimize the risk of paroxysmal vertigo[66–69] (see later discussion in "Avoiding and managing complications" section).

If the local bone is primarily cancellous (types III or IV), surgical burs may not be needed and the site treated solely with osteotomes compacting bone both laterally and apically, and resulting in faster implant site healing.[70] This technique also has been advocated to improve initial implant stability,[71,72] although not all investigators agree.[73] Initial site preparation in denser bone may require the use of pilot burs[74] and/or piezoelectric surgical tips[75–77] to minimize forces needed to advance the osteotomes with the mallet. Summers described the "ridge expansion osteotomy" at ridges with slightly reduced horizontal dimension using an osteotome condensation and expansion technique.[78] In this application, limited crestal drilling with a 1.4–2 mm diameter pilot drill is followed with increasing diameter osteotomes for progressive bone compression, slight crestal expansion, and/or implant "axis re-orientation."[48] Bone compression and expansion of 1–1.5 mm is fairly straightforward, but beyond this can exceed bone compliance and result in uncontrolled buccal fracture without employing more advanced expansion techniques (see Chapters 16 and 17).[79]

In the classic OSFE approach, once the initial site has been defined with a pilot bur, further site development is accomplished with increasing diameter osteotomes and progressive bone condensation (Figure 15.2). The surgeon must avoid the tendency to tip the osteotome instruments distally during site preparation. With initial osteotome trial length determination, the tip should stop short of the sinus floor by about 1 mm[24] (Figure 15.2a). Confirmation of the trial length and fracture of the floor without any elevation allows the clinician to feel more confident with further site development using increasing diameter osteotomes (Figure 15.2b). Periapical radiographs and intermittent nose blow testing are helpful to confirm position, trial length, and membrane integrity. Sinus floor elevation or "up-fracture" is generally best attempted after the surgeon has reached the largest diameter osteotome corresponding to the final implant diameter (Figure 15.2c). Up-fracture is achieved with a slow gentle release of the apical bone/sinus floor, often with a discernable dulling sound with percussion of the mallet. If resistance is significant, greater force can result in a sudden loss of purchase of the osteotome and sinus membrane breach. It is often necessary to return to a size smaller osteotome or Piezosurgery tip to reduce the apical bone thickness and force needed to fracture the floor. Developing apical mobilization is important before continuing with the final diameter osteotome and final site development (Figure 15.2c). Once the sinus floor has been up-fractured, the implant is placed with a typical sinus floor elevation of 1–2 mm (and often 3 mm with good apical mobilization) with OSFE (see Figure 15.2d).

Boyne[80] concluded from a study in monkeys that implants with rounded apices placed with 2–3 mm of sinus membrane elevation and no added graft developed substantial bone around their apices, provided the sinus membrane remained intact. At 5 mm of elevation, however, the amount of apically formed bone without added graft decreased by 50%, and at around 6 mm of elevation the incidence of membrane perforation and implant failure increased significantly. These animal data have been confirmed in patients treated using the osteotome approach without added graft. Thus, generally the treatment will lead to 1–3 mm of increased bone height.[49,81,82] Application of short implants (7 mm × 4.1 mm sintered porous-surfaced (SPS) implants) using OSFE without graft material is demonstrated in Figure 15.3a. The implants were restored with individual crowns and had been in function for >7 years and show substantial bone around the implant apices above the original sinus floor level (Figure 15.3b). Placement of short implants (7–8 mm) in ≥5 mm subantral bone without any graft may be the least invasive TASE approach.

The BAOSFE technique described by Summers[25] used pressure from compaction of bone gathered from the concave cutting tip of the osteotome and/added graft particles mixed with blood to elevate

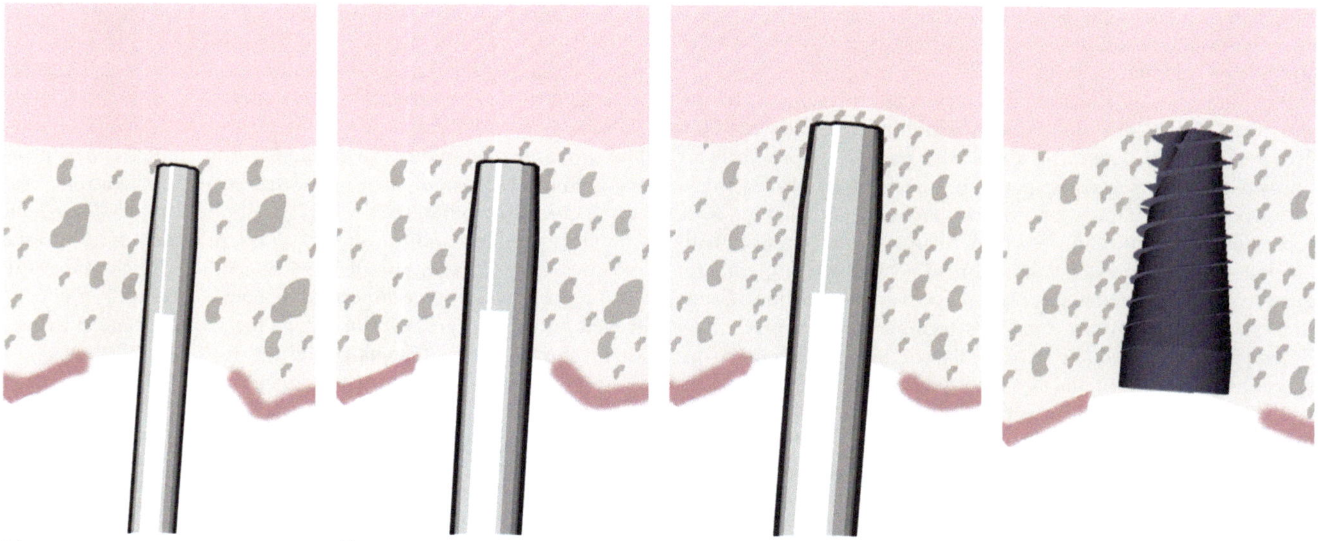

(a) (b) (c) (d)

Figure 15.2 Bone manipulation with OSFE/floor up-fracture. (a) Limited crestal drilling with a 1.4–2 mm diameter pilot drill, or in D4 bone, placement of a 2 mm concave-tipped osteotome is completed 1–2 mm short of the sinus floor for trial length determination. Confirmation of the trial length is completed with osteotome advancement to the level of the floor and then fracture of the floor without any elevation. (b) The next larger size osteotome is advanced to the sinus floor with fracture. (c) The procedure is repeated with increasing diameter osteotomes to the final diameter with floor fracture and elevation of 2–3 mm. (d) The implant is inserted into the OSFE site. © Daniel R. Cullum.

the membrane. The osteotome tip was not advanced beyond the trial length depth of the original sinus floor (Figure 15.4). Repeated addition of small increments of graft particles with each increasing diameter osteotome was used to achieve incremental elevations of the sinus membrane of 0.5–1 mm (Figure 15.4d–f). Osteotomes with depth stops can be useful to ensure that the instruments do not advance uncontrollably and breach the sinus membrane.[83] Successive periapical radiographs can be used to confirm membrane integrity with particulate graft containment showing as an enlarging spherical density beyond the point of up-fracture. After 3–4 mm of sinus elevation has been achieved with addition of graft particles, a self-threading implant can be placed to optimize initial stability[25] (Figure 15.4h; see further discussion below in the "Procedures" section).

During site development the surgeon should confirm visually the persistence of an intact socket "ceiling" of compressed bone[49] and an intact membrane. Having the patient blow gently through the nose with intermittent pinching of the nostrils should detect any sinus membrane perforation. A small perforation without apical displacement will often close spontaneously if no implant is placed or it can usually be sealed with a resorbable collagen sponge,[84] recombinant platelet-derived growth factor (PDGF) or platelet-rich autogenous fibrin clots or gel. (See further discussion in the "Avoiding and Managing Complications" section.) If a small perforation

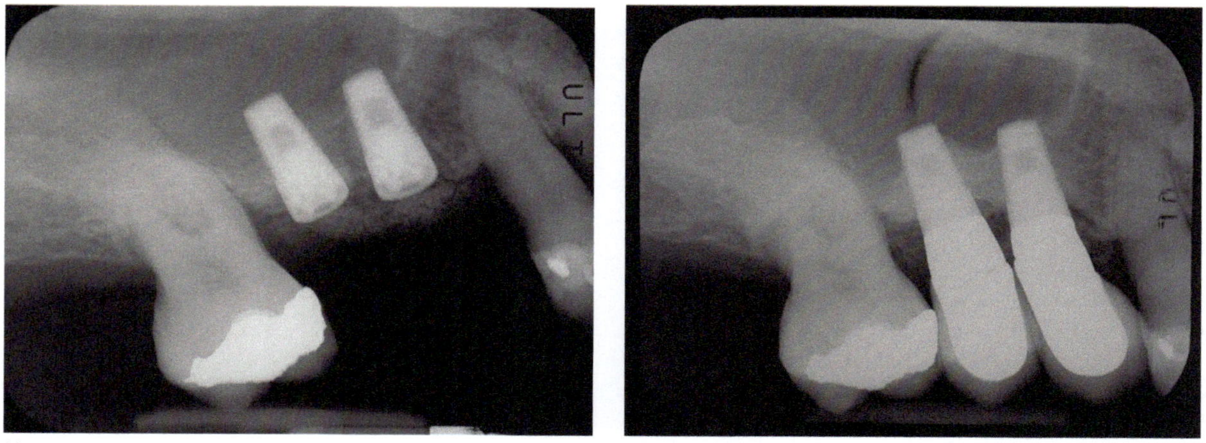

(a) (b)

Figure 15.3 OSFE and short implants. (a) Application of short implants is demonstrated with placement of two (7 mm × 4.1 mm) SPS implants using OSFE without graft material. (b) The implants were restored with individual crowns (in function for >7 years); substantial bone can be seen around the implant apices above the original sinus floor level. Restorations provided by Dr Reynaldo Todescan, Toronto, ON, Canada. Reproduced with permission from Dr Todescan.

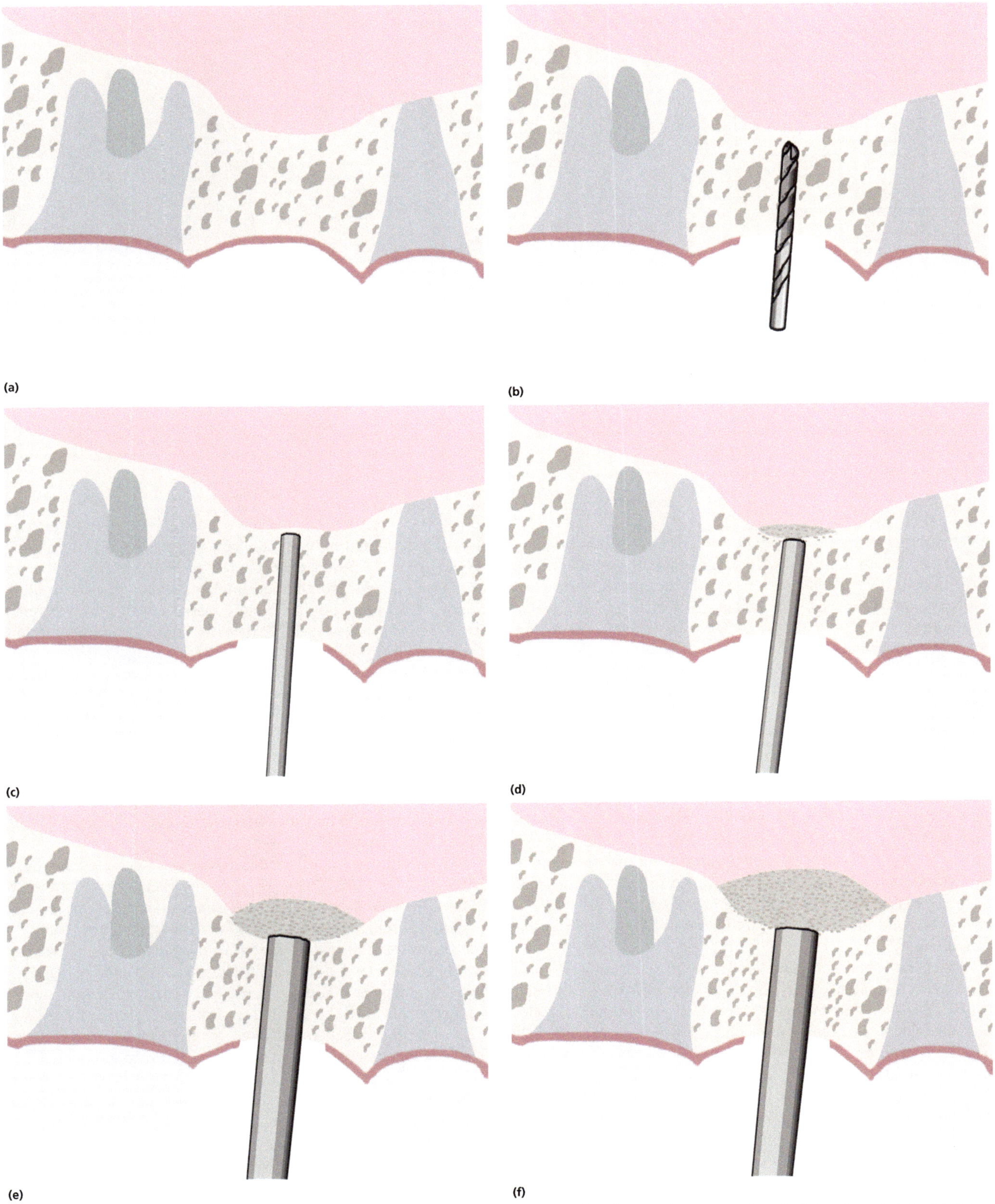

Figure 15.4 Bone manipulation with BAOSFE. (a) Preoperative cancellous posterior maxillary bone with 7–9 mm of residual sinus bone height. (b) Using a 2 mm diameter pilot drill (or osteotome in type IV bone), initial site development should stop 1–2 mm short of the sinus floor. (c) After trial length is confirmed, a 2 mm diameter osteotome is advanced to approach but not breach the sinus floor. (d–f) Small portions of particulate graft material are added to the site for each increasing diameter osteotome, while maintaining the osteotome within the alveolus or with limited (0.5–1 mm) advancement of the osteotome tip into the sinus. Periapical radiographs should demonstrate an advancing intact spherical density.

(*Continued*)

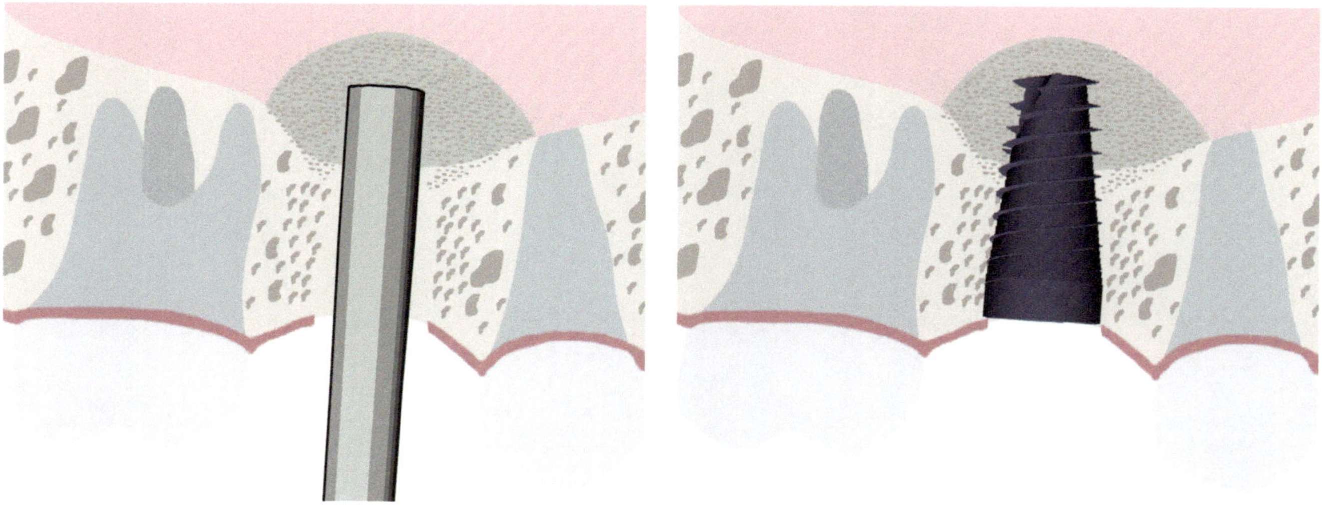

(g) (h)

Figure 15.4 (Continued)

(g) The final osteotome is advanced incrementally with the addition of further graft material to the final height plus 1 mm. (h) The implant is inserted incrementally to the desired position, not to exceed the confirmed height of the osteotome elevation. This avoids the potential risk of membrane tear on implant insertion. © Daniel R. Cullum.

of the sinus membrane is suspected with OSFE, the procedure may be completed with limited elevation as membrane perforation less than 2 mm during OSFE appears to have limited impact on implant success.[50] BAOSFE (i.e. with added particulate graft material) membrane perforation is more of a concern owing to the risk of loss of graft containment. In the healthy sinus, ciliary function would likely clear small particulate material via the ostium. However, if the ostium is not patent or the volume or particle size too large, sinus infection could develop.[85]

An implant placed using TASE techniques gains primary stability from the existing native subantral bone. Techniques to gain primary stability with a threaded parallel wall implant include finishing with an osteotome or bur slightly smaller in diameter than the implant being placed,[75,86] avoiding countersinking in crestal bone, and using self-threading implants. However, using a tapered implant design may offer the most predictable primary stability in limited residual alveolus bone.[87] Submerged implant healing may be considered in sites where the original subantral bone height is <4 mm to avoid the risk of implant micromotion or displacement into the sinus.[22,23]

Post-operatively for the first 7–10 days, patients are advised to avoid heavy physical activity, nose blowing or sucking through straws, and asked only to sneeze through an open mouth. As with lateral window sinus grafting procedures, post-operative antibiotics are a consideration for BAOSFE techniques that have substantial graft volume. Healing time before implant site re-entry and/or prosthesis fabrication will vary from 4 to 6 months. This will depend on the amount of original native bone and the degree of sinus elevation as sufficient time is needed to allow the apical grafted site to mature. Testing implants with resonance frequency analysis (implant stability quotient (ISQ), Ostell®, Gothenburg, Sweden) at surgery and before undertaking prosthetic procedures has been suggested to confirm adequate site healing.[88,89]

Tapered implants with lengths of ≤7 mm can offer an advantage when used with BAOSFE as they can be placed in as little as 3–4 mm residual height of subantral bone,[87] requiring limited sinus elevation and reducing the risk of membrane perforation[60] (Figure 15.5). Deporter et al.[62] reported 98% survival at 3 years for 7 mm tapered, press-fit SPS implants placed in a mean bone height of 4.2 mm. Similar results were achieved by Corrente et al.,[90] while Pjetursson et al.[91] reported good outcomes for 8 mm long threaded implants placed using BAOSFE. Del Fabbro et al.[29] concluded that length was less important than previously thought, with similar survival rates being reported for implants of <8.5 mm (97.16%), 8.5–10 mm (97.66%), and >10 mm (98.11%) lengths. However, this application still requires further study as some data showed a survival rate of only 47.6% when 6 mm long ITI implants were used in 3–4 mm of native bone without grafting.[92] Generally, short implants (≤8 mm)[93] are finding a wider application following improvements in implant surface technology and surgical techniques (see Chapter 10).

Many technique modifications have been suggested for both OSFE and BAOSFE. Deporter and coworkers[62,87] and others[49] allowed their implant-specific osteotomes to advance beyond the level of the original sinus floor in order to assist with graft compaction and to shape the osteotomy to fit a tapered implant. Advancing each larger diameter osteotome to the trial length and completing floor fracture prior to adding the particulate graft is a helpful modification of the BAOSFE technique. This pre-fracture of the floor reduces the force needed and increases predictability of the elevation.[49] Some clinicians have avoided adding any graft material,[91,94] and others have proposed using autogenous platelet-rich fibrin clots (see Figure 15.9d) rather than particulate graft to facilitate the elevation and eliminate the potential for loss of graft containment into the sinus cavity.[93,95]

A significant advance in technique with dense bone quality includes the use of specialized side-cutting reamer burs (e.g. Crestal Lift Control®, Meisinger USA, Golden, CO) to access the sinus floor with minimal risk of membrane damage (Figure 15.6). Reamer burs with a modified cutting surface and a drill stop system have been used to advance bone chips to reach the sinus floor. Ahn et al.[96] described this approach mainly at molar sites with a sinus

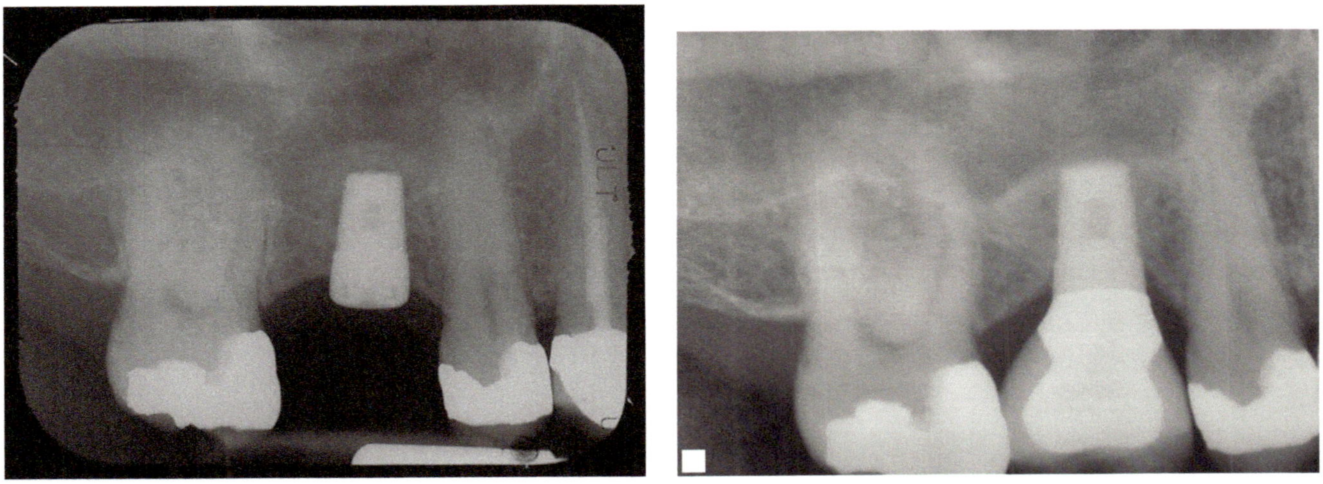

(a) (b)

Figure 15.5 BAOSFE and short implants. (a) Placement of a short implant (7 mm) with BAOSFE is demonstrated on the immediate post-implantation radiograph. Sinus floor elevation of 3 mm from the cortical margins of the original sinus floor is visible. (b) A radiograph of the restored implant after 6 years in function shows bone remodeling and remnants of the cortical outline of the original sinus floor.

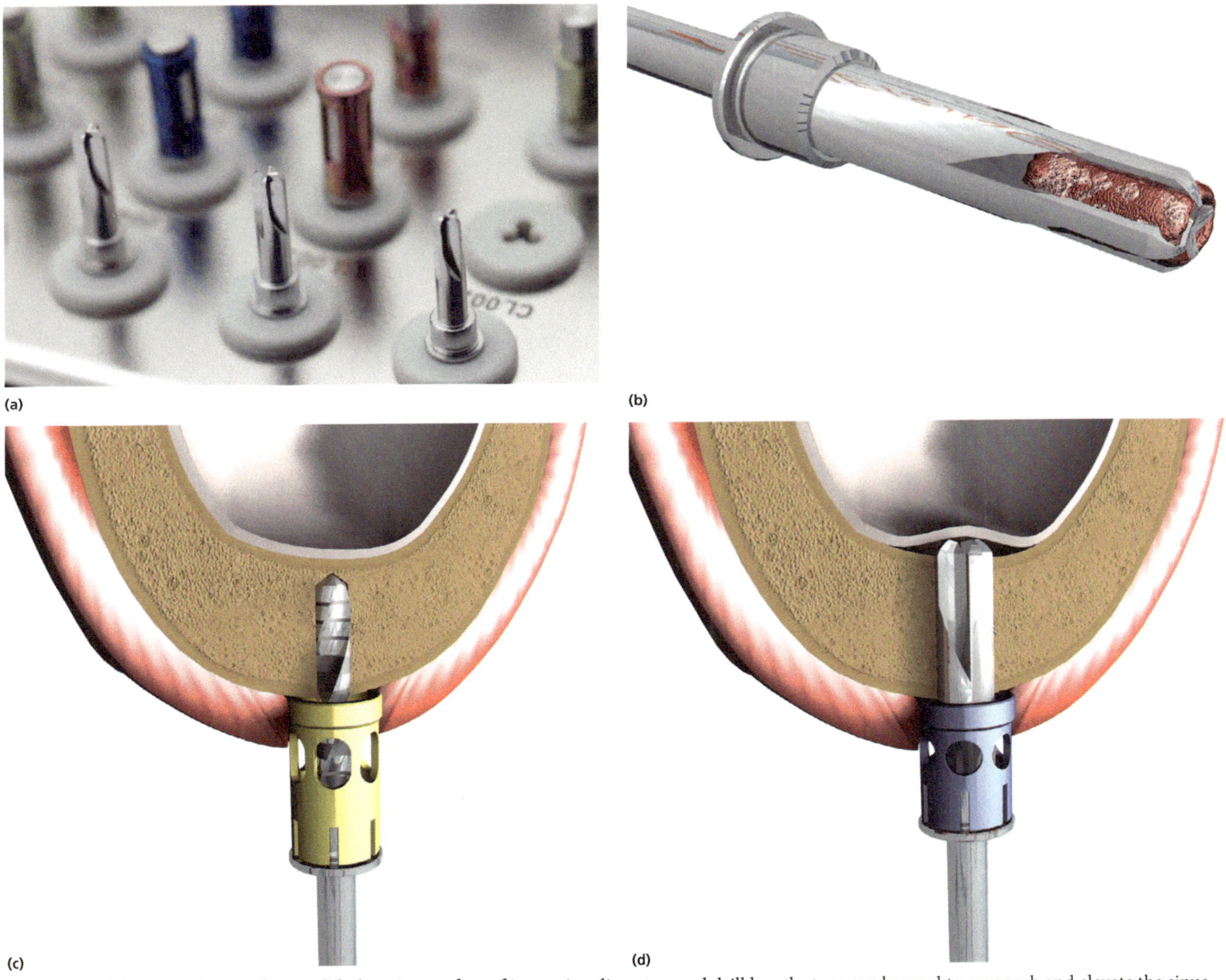

(a) (b) (c) (d)

Figure 15.6 (a) Reamer burs with a modified cutting surface of increasing diameters and drill length stops can be used to approach and elevate the sinus floor (Crestal Lift Control®, Meisinger USA, Golden CO). *Source:* Meisinger USA, Golden CO. (b) The tip of the reamer bur collects bone as it advances and mobilizes the bone apically, acting as a buffer to protect and mobilize the sinus membrane. (c) Trial length determination is completed with the drill stop system. (d) Sequential reamer bur diameters are used to advance bone chips to reach the sinus floor. The burs are designed to thin and displace apically the sinus cortical bone while maintaining membrane integrity.

membrane perforation rate of 5% and outcomes similar to those achieved using BAOSFE via osteotomes. Drill speed is at 50 rpm or less with final reamer diameter 0.5–1.5 mm smaller than the planned implant. The burs are designed to thin and displace apically the sinus floor cortical bone without making direct contact with the membrane. Autogenous bone also can be collected and retrieved for later use using the reamer. After access to the sinus floor is achieved, various methods of adding graft for membrane elevation can be used, including traditional osteotomes (as with BAOSFE) or rotary bone spreaders to lateralize and expand the volume of the added graft.

For sites with ≤4–5 mm of remaining subantral bone, Summers[39] and others[40] suggested that trephines and BAOSFE be used for preparatory site grafting or *future site development* followed by delayed implant placement after graft site healing. This approach has also been called the "crestal core elevation technique" and advanced as a minimally invasive option to avoid an open window sinus graft.[82] A trephine can be used to free a core of subantral bone for up-fracture with an osteotome of corresponding diameter (Figure 15.7) and the site back-filled with exogenous graft material. After adequate site healing, implants then can be placed using a combination of burs and osteotomes. A further modification has been described[97] using a trephine with a minimum 4–5 mm of subantral bone. Apical movement of the trephined plug was completed to permit simultaneous placement of 9 or 10 mm length implants without the addition of graft material.

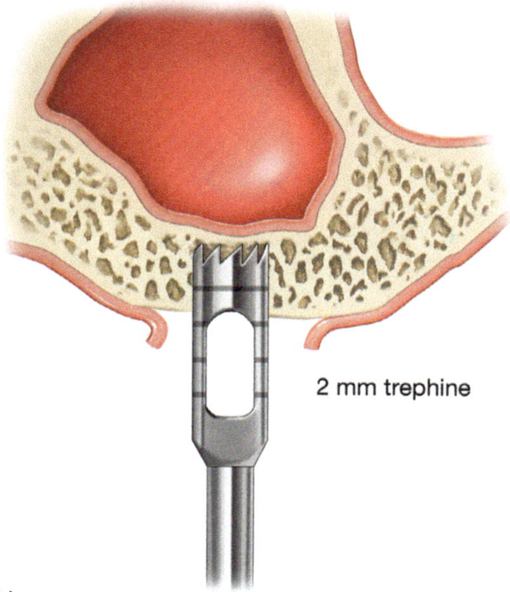

(a)

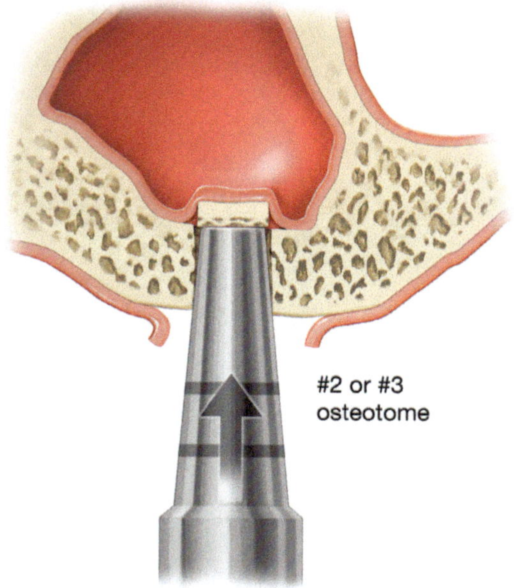

(b)

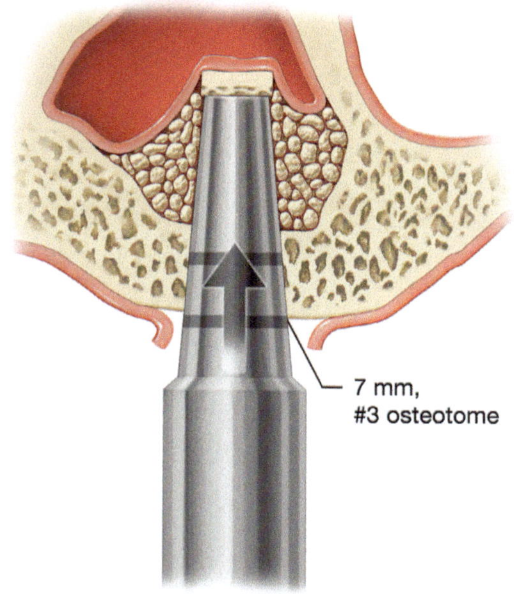

(c)

Figure 15.7 "Future site development." (a) "Future site development" begins with a surgical trephine of 2 mm internal diameter. It is necessary to leave some bone beneath the sinus floor so as to avoid tearing the sinus membrane with the trephine. (b) The sinus floor up-fracture is done with an osteotome diameter corresponding to that of the trephine. (c) Osteotome elevation and grafting is completed and the site is allowed to heal with delayed implant placement.

Advanced trans-alveolar sinus elevation techniques

With successful application of the basic TASE approaches described above, clinicians may choose to use more advanced techniques, such as Piezosurgery-assisted elevations,[42,43,76,77] inflatable balloons,[98,99] hydraulic pressure using saline[41,100] or pressure from a radiopaque gel,[101] and other advanced osteotome-mediated crestal techniques, to loosen and elevate the membrane with or without the addition of graft material. The premise of these techniques is to reduce local tension (elasticity, adhesion force, and influence of local anatomy) that may cause membrane tear at >5 mm of elevation at a single site by elevating a larger section of membrane.[102] The most straightforward example is the use of implants at adjacent sites. The ability to join sites together[39] by merging the individual apical elevations, enlarges the apical footprint, and reduces the risk of membrane tears.

Techniques using ultrasonic bone-cutting surgical tips[42,43,76,77] have been advanced to expose the sinus floor with minimal risk of membrane damage (Figure 15.8a and b). Piezosurgery inserts can be used to expose the membrane with insertion of a hydraulic adapter into the osteotomy to allow sinus elevation by gentle hydraulic pressure.[43] Significant elevations of 5–8 mm have been reported with these tips (Figure 15.8c).

Alternatively, the hydrodynamic piezoelectric internal sinus elevation (HPISE) technique[42] can be completed after initial osteotomy preparation with a reamer bur or Piezosurgery tip. HPISE uses a specially designed 2 mm internally irrigated carbide tip (tip S028E®, Bukbu Dental Co., Daegu, S. Korea and HPISE tip, S0281®, S-Dental Co., Daegu, South Korea) to cut through the sinus floor and elevate the sinus membrane with hydraulic and ultrasonic forces[42] (Figure 15.9a–c). The HPISE tip can be seen on activation, as it enters a first molar osteotomy site to elevate the membrane (Figure 15.9b). Final osteotomy site preparation is completed with burs or osteotomes. Exogenous graft material is then delivered into the membrane-contained space before implant placement. Alternatively, concentrated growth factor (CGF) or platelet-rich fibrin can be prepared from the patient's centrifuged venous blood (Figure 15.9d) and used as the graft material[103] (Figure 15.9e). After graft delivery, the implant is fully seated into the elevated site (Figure 15.9f). It should be noted, however, that these modifications can be technique-sensitive and require specialized equipment and experience. Nevertheless, they may be helpful where extensive membrane elevations, sloping sinus floor, or septa are risks.

Other advanced osteotome-mediated techniques including LMSF,[46] SACT,[47] CSFE,[48] and/or a combined approach with simultaneous ridge expansion and implant placement[49] (see Chapter 17) also have been advocated as alternatives to open lateral sinus grafting procedures. Bruschi et al.[46] described LMSF for vertical site development with simultaneous implant placement without added graft material. After surgical exposure of the ridge crest (see Chapter 17), a bone incision was completed into the palatal bone strut parallel to the sinus wall. A blunted chisel was malleted into the osteotomy to effect an "in-fracture" of the palatal bone to the medial, and then osteotomes were used for elevation of the antral floor and osteotomy development in continuity with the mobilized palatal wall.

The SACT approach was described by Winter et al.[47] for adjacent implant sites and later modified for use with Piezosurgery.[104] A rectangular section of bone was cut within the bucco-palatal ridge width approaching the sinus floor and 2 mm narrower than

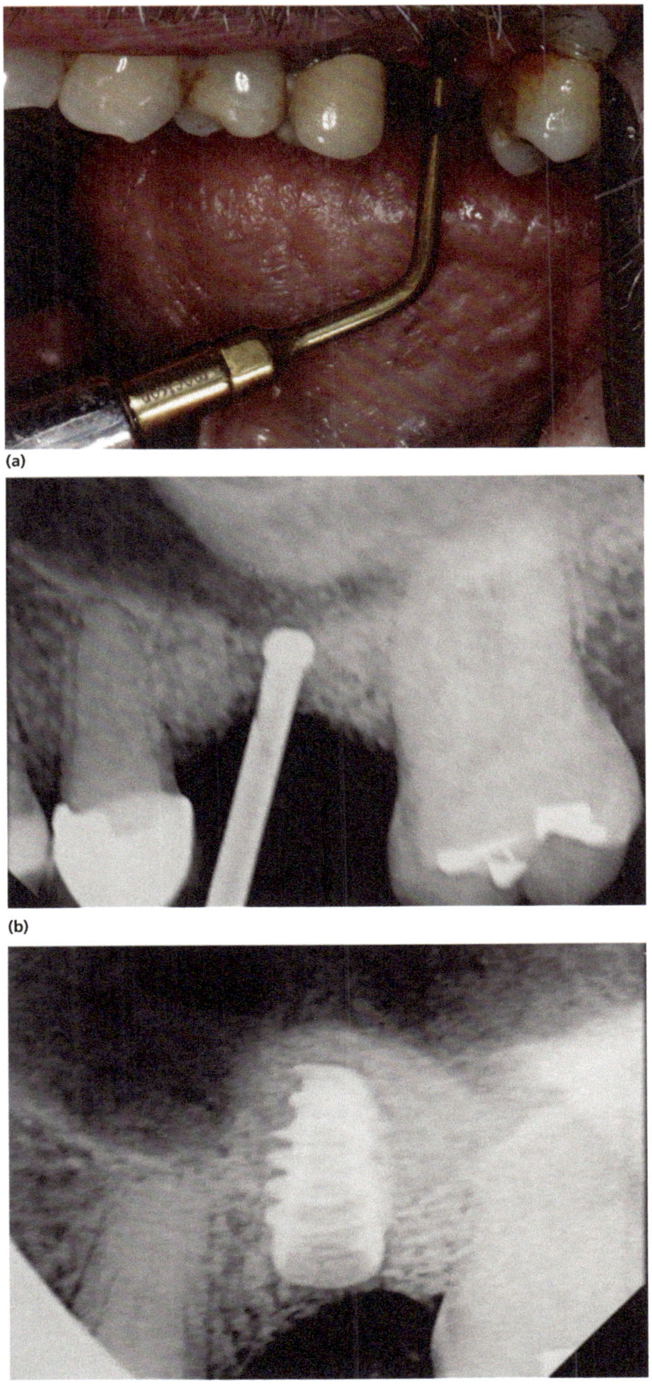

Figure 15.8 Piezosurgery-assisted and hydraulic techniques. (a) Piezosurgery inserts are used to approach the sinus floor and uncover the sinus membrane. (b) A radiograph demonstrated the relationship between the sinus floor and instrument tip. (c) After implant placement, the apical deposit of particulate graft material placed with an osteotome can be seen to have resulted in significant membrane elevation. © Daniel R. Cullum.

the planned implant diameters to ensure initial implant stability. Gentle apical manipulation and elevation of the bone segment was achieved with a combination of osteotomes to mobilize the bone floor followed by sinus curettes to elevate the sinus membrane. The elevated sinus cavity defect was filled with absorbable

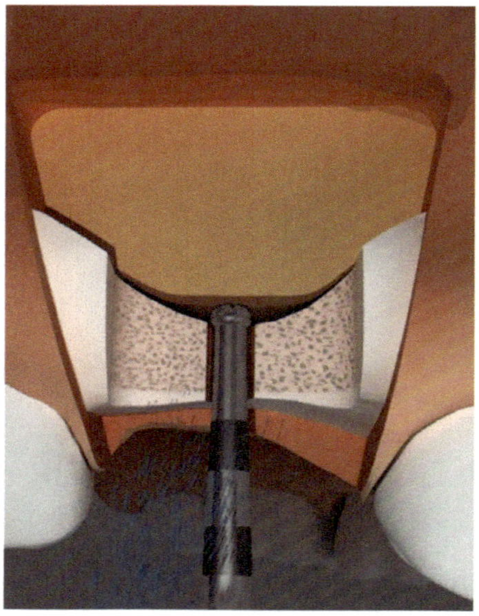
(a)

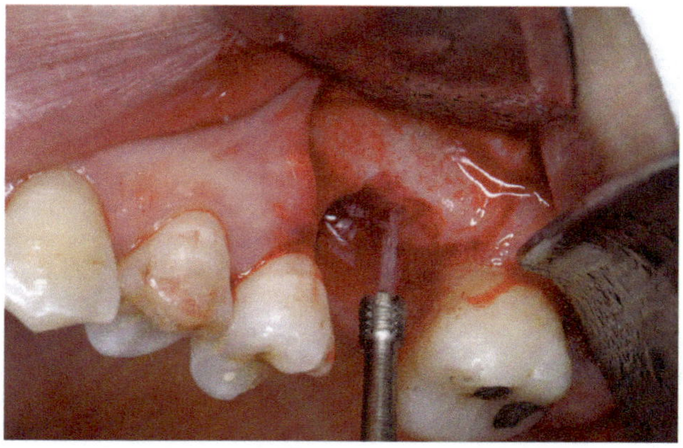
(b)

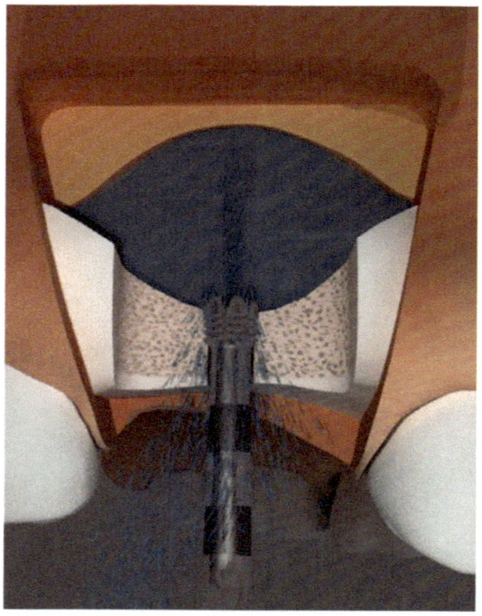
(c)

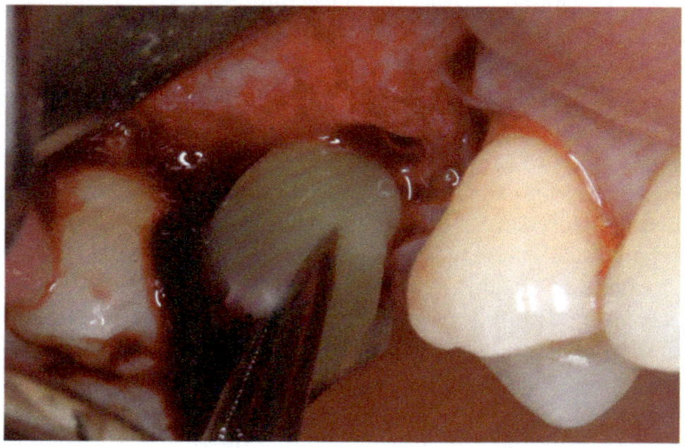
(d)

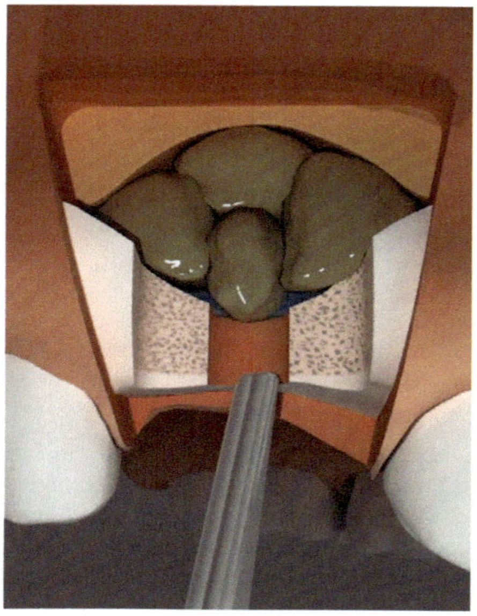
(e)

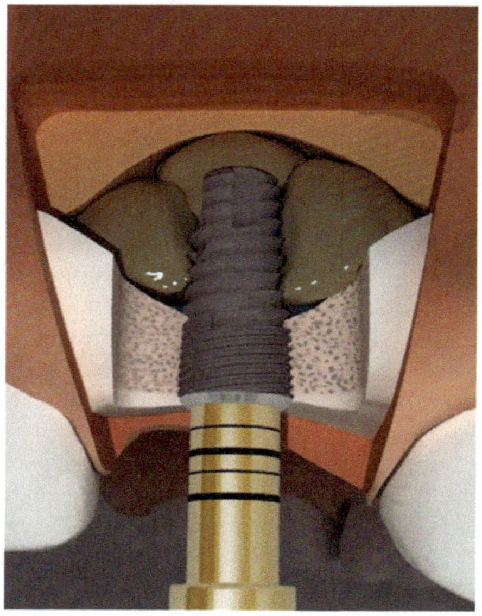
(f)

Figure 15.9 (a) Piezoelectric® surgery inserts can be used to approach the sinus floor and uncover the membrane. (b) After initial osteotomy preparation, a specially designed 2 mm, internally irrigated carbide HPISE tip (#S0281®, Bukbu Dental Co., Daegu, South Korea) is activated with irrigation spray as it enters a first molar osteotomy site. (c) The HPISE tip can be used to cut through the sinus floor, and the hydraulic and ultrasonic forces then can be used to elevate the sinus membrane. Final osteotomy site preparation is then completed with burs or osteotomes. (d) Platelet-rich fibrin can be inserted and manipulated into the site to support the apical advancement of the membrane achieved with the hydraulic forces. (e) The graphic demonstrates CGF (prepared from the patient) delivered into the membrane-contained space as the graft material in lieu of particulate bone graft. (f) The implant is placed into the elevated sinus cavity. *Source:* Dr Dong-Seok Sohn. Reproduced with permission of Dr Sohn.

collagen (Collatape®, Zimmer Dental, Carlsbad, CA) and tapered, wide-diameter implants placed (length 11.99 mm and diameter 5.94 mm) with stabilization against the buccal and palatal bony walls. The mean preoperative native bone height was 2.87 mm, with mean membrane elevation of 9.12 mm. The implant survival rate was 91.4%, which is comparable to similar higher risk atrophic cases treated using open window sinus grafting. Bruschi et al.[105] also described a similar "transcrestal sinus floor elevation" using chisels and reported 95.5% survival of 66 implants placed in 46 patients after up to 16 years' follow-up.

Cullum introduced another advanced TASE approach termed contiguous sinus floor elevation (CSFE).[48,49] This involves using the sequential (side-by-side) overlapping application of osteotomes, Piezosurgery, and/or reamer drills to create a trough in the crestal bone followed by elevation of the associated segment of sinus floor using a "floor fracture" only or a combined "bone-added" technique. Fracture of the sinus floor is completed using small and medium-sized concave-tipped osteotomes. (Figures 15.10a–c and 15.11a). This is followed by floor elevation (without added graft) and/or membrane elevation (with added graft) using contiguous sinus floor elevators (Figure 15.10d and e). Tapered implants typically are placed simultaneously, with adequate initial stability achieved via contact with the buccal and palatal walls of the bony trough (Figure 15.10f). This technique has the advantage of partially "up-fracturing" the surrounding bone walls, increasing their vertical height (i.e. "delamination"), and therefore increasing the native bone contact on the implant surfaces. It is discussed in greater detail in the "Procedures" section.

Implants inserted using these advanced TASE techniques can have minimal initial alveolar support and will require the longer healing intervals more typical of guided bone regeneration wounds. However, the time required is generally less than that needed with lateral sinus grafting, as there is comparatively limited detachment of the membrane and a smaller graft volume. There is, theoretically,

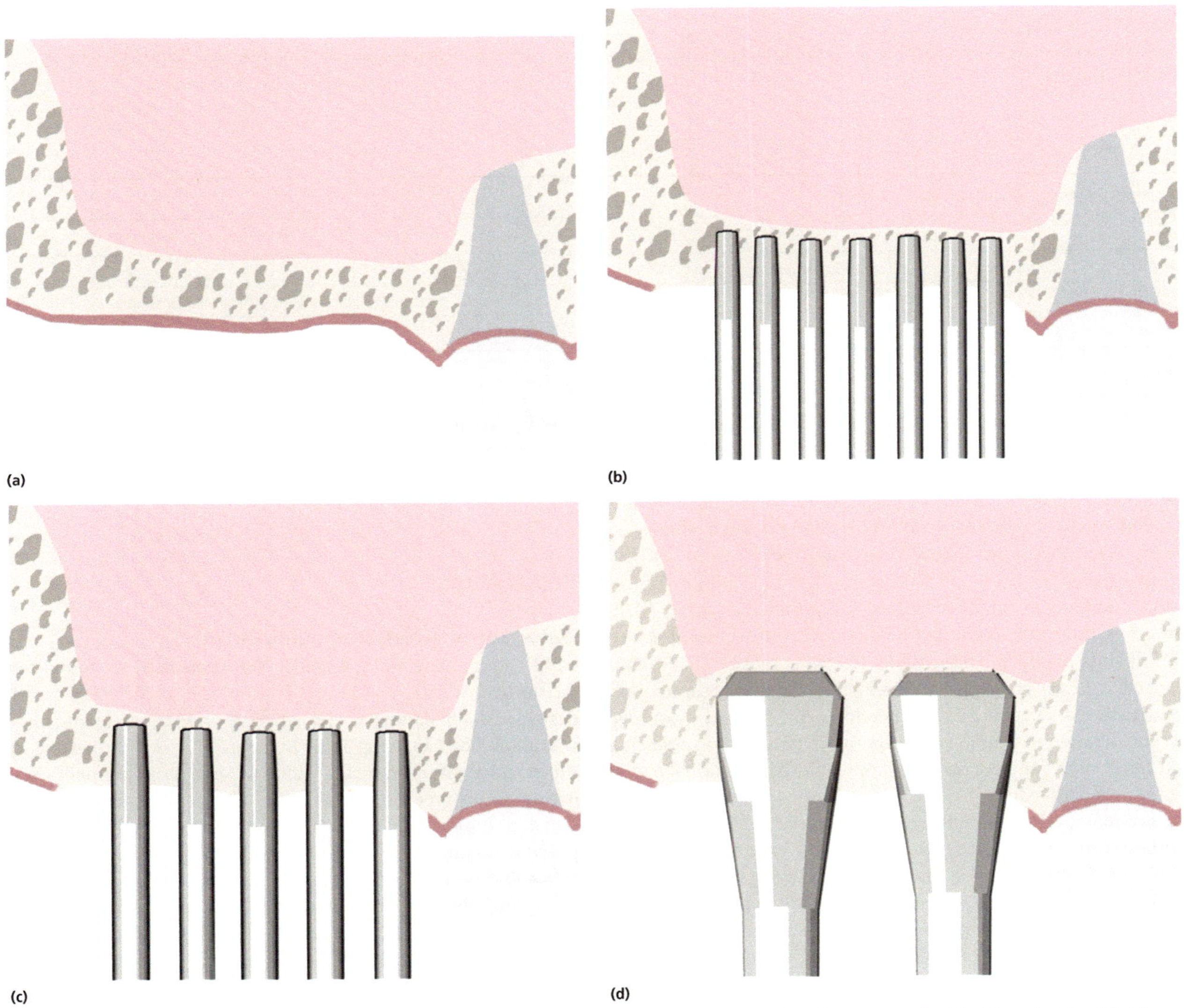

Figure 15.10 Graphic of CSFE at the edentulous posterior maxilla. (a) An edentulous posterior maxilla with 3–4 mm of residual bone height. (b) A bone trough was completed to the level of the sinus floor. Concave-tipped osteotomes were used to sequentially fracture the sinus floor with a stepped or slightly overlapping (mesio-distally) placement of the instruments. (c) Larger diameter concave-tipped osteotomes were used to widen and sequentially fracture the sinus floor with a stepped or slightly overlapping placement of the instruments. (d, e) CSFE was completed with progressive apical advancement using contiguous elevators (3 and 4 mm widths) with the addition of particulate graft material.

(Continued)

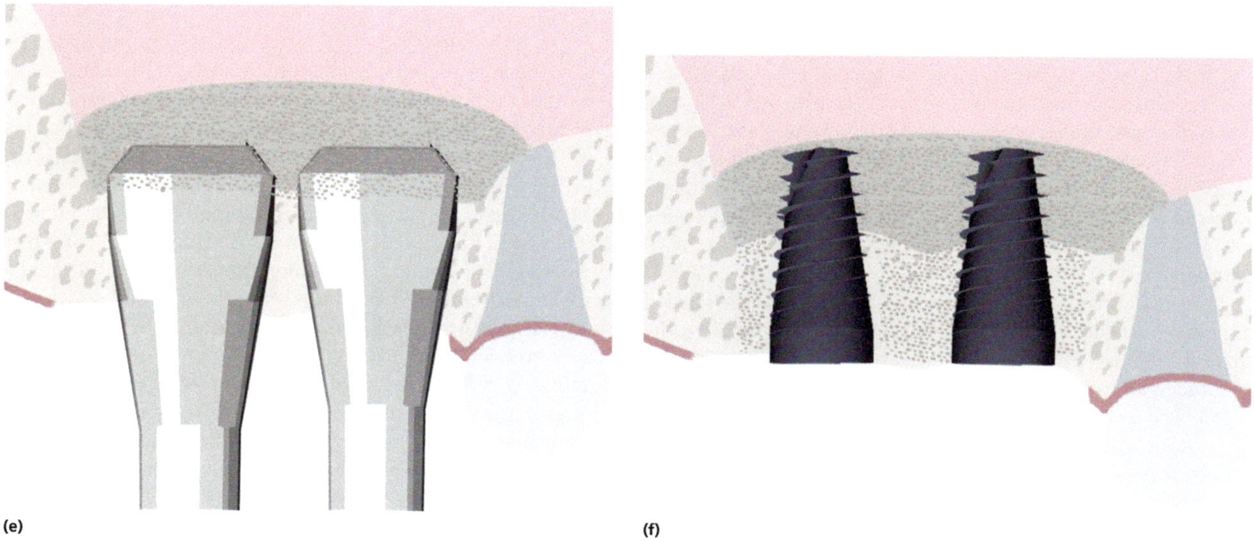

Figure 15.10 (Continued)
(f) Final site development was completed with the implant-specific osteotome followed by placement of tapered wide-diameter fixtures (5–6 mm). © Daniel R. Cullum.

Table 15.1 Indications for TASE techniques based on height of sinus elevation and minimum 3–4 mm residual bone volume

Sinus elevation (mm)	Indicated TASE technique
1–3	OSFE (no added graft material)[24,49,50,107–110]
2–4	BAOSFE[25–28,62] and bone core elevation without graft[96]
4 to >5	"Future site development" with delayed implant placement,[39,40] bone cores,[96] joined adjacent sites, Piezosurgery-assisted/hydraulic elevation,[42,48] and CSFE[49]
6 to >8	Piezosurgery-assisted/hydraulic elevation,[42,48] CSFE,[49] and SACT[47] or consider lateral sinus graft

an increased risk of implant displacement into the sinus during the early healing interval; however, this has not been our clinical experience. With sites that originally had <3 mm of subantral bone height and were treated by preparatory open window grafting, moderately rough threaded implants have been shown to have significantly higher failure rates than those placed entirely in native maxillary bone (13.9% versus. 3.4%).[106] While success seems favorable with implants placed using these advanced TASE approaches, there are no published data to allow direct comparison with implants placed in native bone. Access is more difficult with advanced TASE techniques, and developing proficiency can require considerable patience and skill. Therefore, the surgeon must give due consideration to training and experience necessary in assessing the surgical risks and benefits compared with the traditional lateral sinus grafting procedure.

In summary, classic, modified, and advanced TASE techniques, including short implants (see also Chapter 10) have been discussed for managing the posterior maxilla with varying residual levels of subantral bone. Table 15.1 outlines indications for use of these techniques. Patient selection includes assessment of risk factors such as smoking, a history of chronic sinusitis, poorly controlled diabetes, uncontrolled periodontal disease, and/or a long history of anti-resorptive drug therapy for management of osteoporosis. Any factors that impair bone vascularity or sinus function can impair sinus graft healing and implant integration. Edentulous sites should have adequate bucco-palatal ridge width to ensure at least 2 mm of buccal bone thickness will remain after osteotomy preparation to avoid post-surgical buccal bone loss.[111–113] With larger elevations and/or severe atophic sites with a broad flat sinus floor anatomy, a traditional lateral sinus graft may be more appropriate based on surgeon preference and experience.

Procedures

Osteotome sinus floor elevation

OSFE site preparation can utilize flat-, concave-, or round-tipped instruments. Figure 15.11a and b show two of the most useful tip designs. Manipulation of the sinus floor with these instruments will allow bone bending into the sinus of 1–2 mm or sinus floor "up-fracture" of up to 3 mm. Using a 2 mm diameter pilot drill (or osteotome in type IV bone), initial site development should stop 1–2 mm short of the sinus floor. A trial length radiograph can be completed to confirm this vertical reference. Thereafter, a 2 mm diameter osteotome is advanced gently with repeated mallet strikes in order to approach but not breach the sinus floor (percussion note dulls as the floor fractures) (Figure 15.3a). This step is repeated with increasing-diameter osteotomes at the desired 3-D position, taking care to avoid angulation errors or creation of an irregularly shaped osteotomy that could compromise primary implant stability (Figure 15.3b and c). If strong resistance is encountered, changing the osteotome to a different design (round, concave, flat, or cutting) or using a Piezosurgery insert or reamer bur to reduce floor thickness may be necessary. Alternatively, a return to a smaller size osteotome with limited force

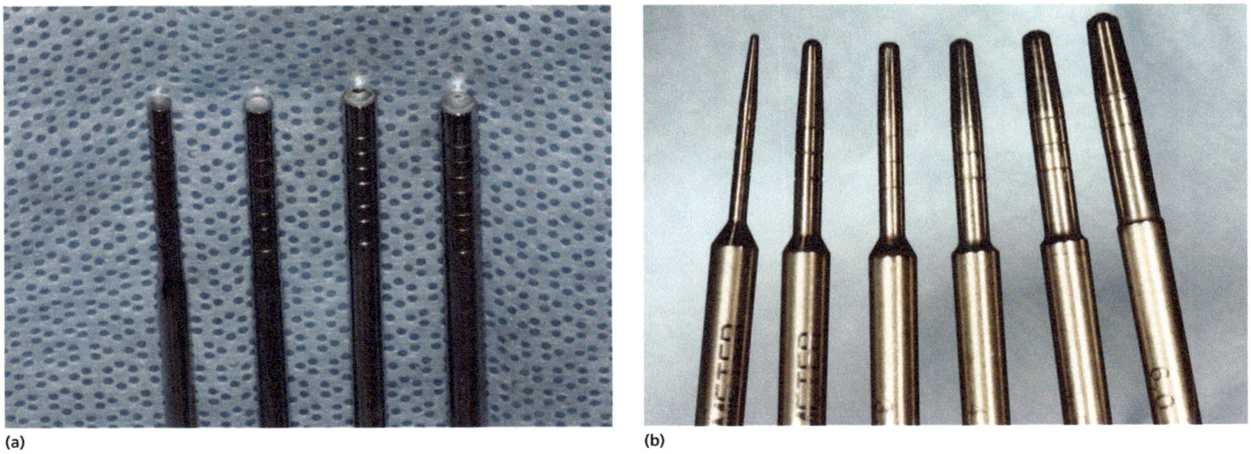

Figure 15.11 Osteotomes designs. (a) Parallel-walled osteotomes with a concave cutting tip design (H&H Co., Ontario, CA). (b) Rounded, tapered osteotome design (Nobel Biocare, Yorba Linda, CA). *Source:* (a) © Daniel R. Cullum (b) Cullum DR, Ridge Expansion and Piezoelecric Bone Surgery. In: The Piezoelectric Bone Surgery. A New Paradigm, Vercellotti T, ed. Quintessenza Edizioni, 2015. Reproduced with permission of Quintessence Publishing Co., Inc..

can allow progressive floor bending or fracture of 1–3 mm. Mobilization of the sinus floor slightly beyond the anticipated implant length is desirable to avoid the final vertical implant position being more apical than the OSFE height achieved (Figure 15.3d) which carries the risk of membrane damage as the implant in being inserted. An example is shown in Figure 15.12a. Extraction of the maxillary right second premolar root was followed by OSFE site preparation of 2–3 mm with implant placement and provisional restoration (Figure 15.12b). The sinus floor (at the horizontal level of the adjacent root apices) was manipulated with an intact roof using concave-tipped osteotomes. Bone levels are demonstrated 18 months and 8 years after treatment in Figure 15.12c and d.

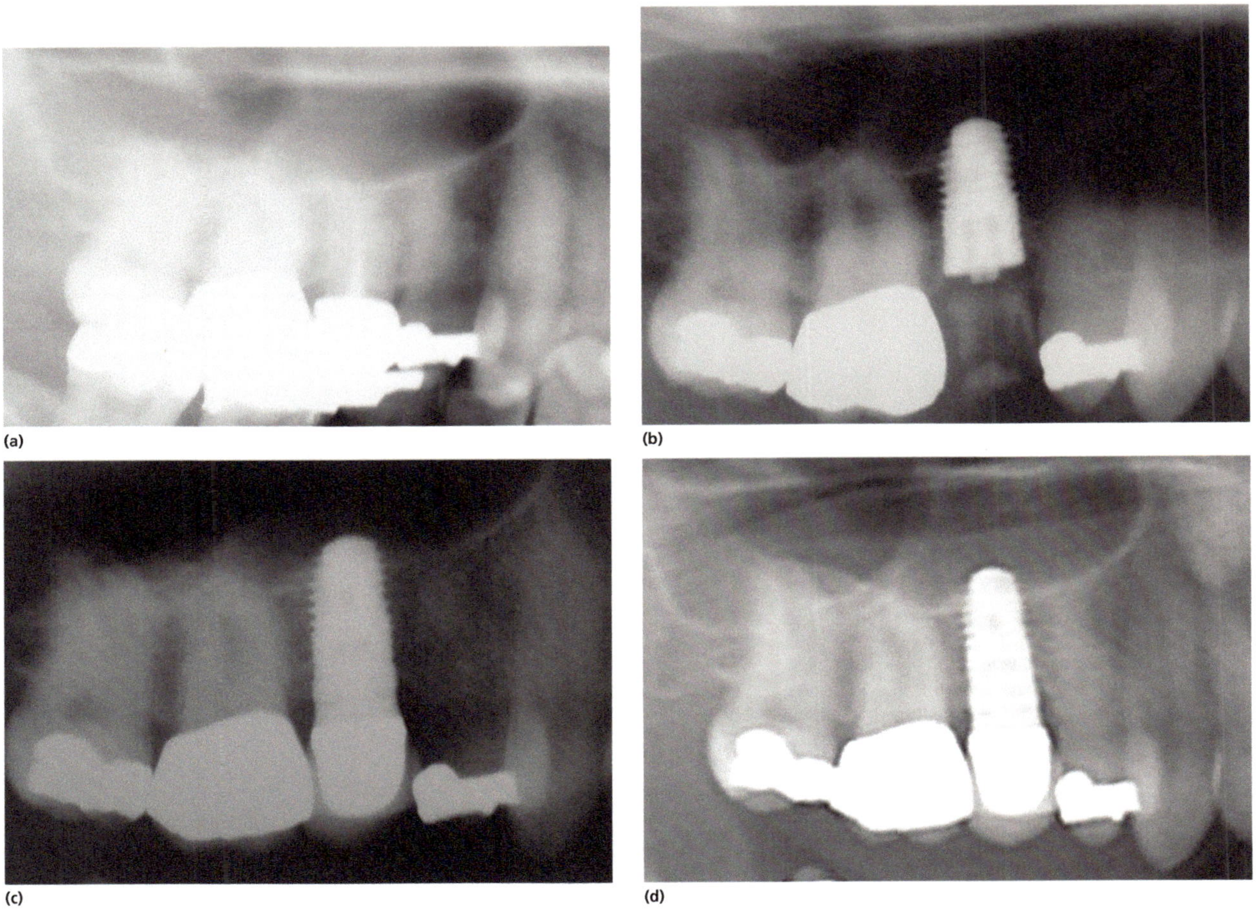

Figure 15.12 Radiographic series of an osteotome sinus floor elevation with immediate implant placement. (a) A preoperative radiograph of a fractured tooth #4 and associated sinus pneumatization. (b) The immediate post-op image of an immediate implant placement using TASE with OSFE/floor fracture with an immediate provisional restoration. (c, d) The 18-month and 8-year post-treatment radiographs demonstrating stable bone levels at the TASE site. © Daniel R. Cullum.

Bone-added osteotome sinus floor elevation

BAOSFE site preparation utilizes similar technique to OSFE, but includes the use of added particulate graft material (Figure 15.4). Once the sinus floor trial length has been determined (Figure 15.4a–c), small portions of particulate graft material are added to the site for each 0.5–1 mm advancement of the osteotome tip (Figure 15.4d). Dense xenograft material can be readily viewed in intraoperative periapical radiographs to verify the growing, intact, apical spherical dome of graft particles. Intraoperative "nose blow" testing can be used to confirm an intact membrane. The advancing "plug" of graft material mixed with blood exerts hydraulic force at the implant apex and lifts the sinus membrane outwardly over a larger circumferential area to achieve sinus elevations of 3–5 mm.

Preoperative clinical and radiographic images in Figure 15.13a and b demonstrate an edentulous maxillary left first molar site with 7–8 mm of alveolar bone height to the sinus floor. A 2 mm twist

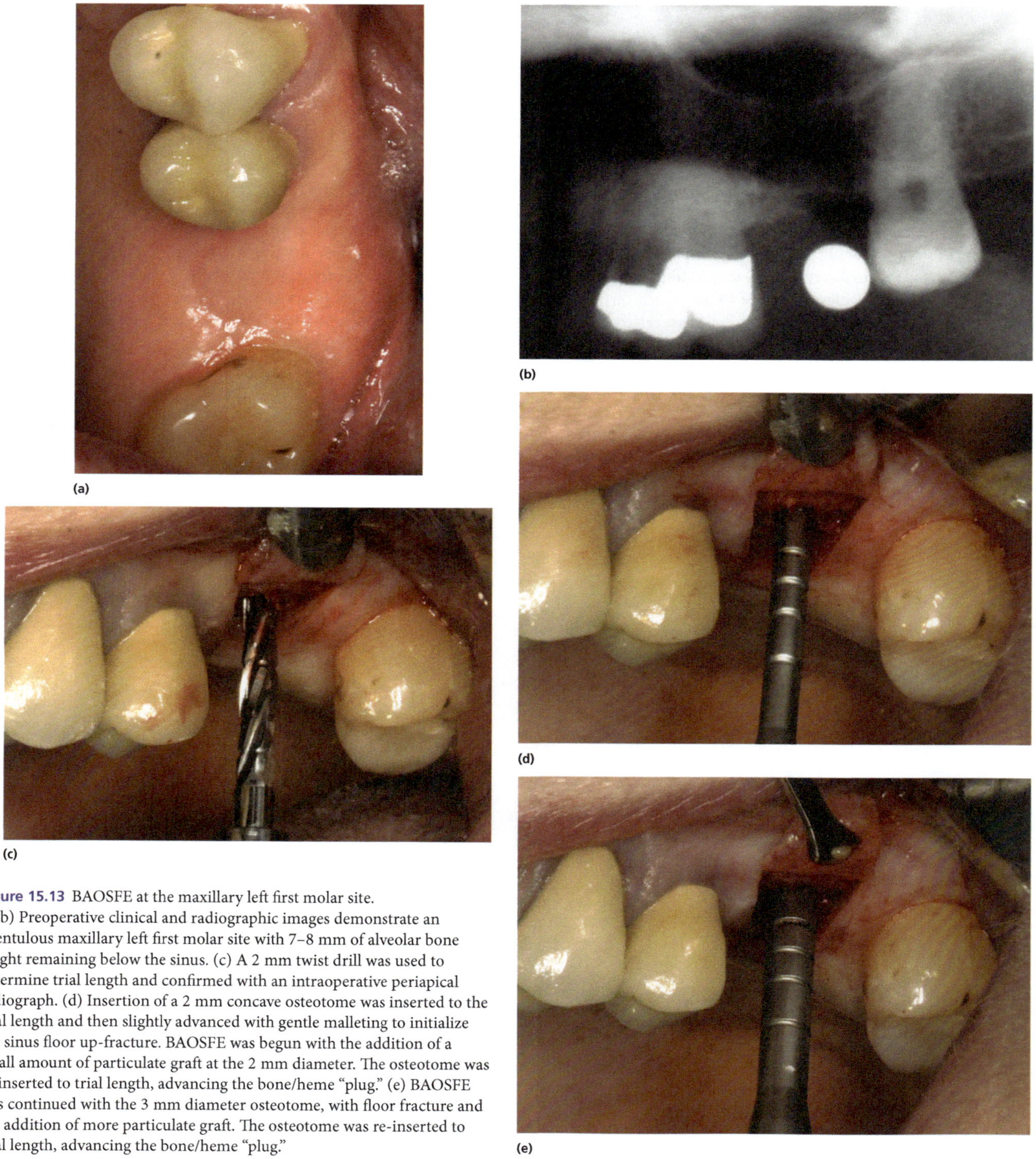

Figure 15.13 BAOSFE at the maxillary left first molar site. (a, b) Preoperative clinical and radiographic images demonstrate an edentulous maxillary left first molar site with 7–8 mm of alveolar bone height remaining below the sinus. (c) A 2 mm twist drill was used to determine trial length and confirmed with an intraoperative periapical radiograph. (d) Insertion of a 2 mm concave osteotome was inserted to the trial length and then slightly advanced with gentle malleting to initialize the sinus floor up-fracture. BAOSFE was begun with the addition of a small amount of particulate graft at the 2 mm diameter. The osteotome was re-inserted to trial length, advancing the bone/heme "plug." (e) BAOSFE was continued with the 3 mm diameter osteotome, with floor fracture and the addition of more particulate graft. The osteotome was re-inserted to trial length, advancing the bone/heme "plug."

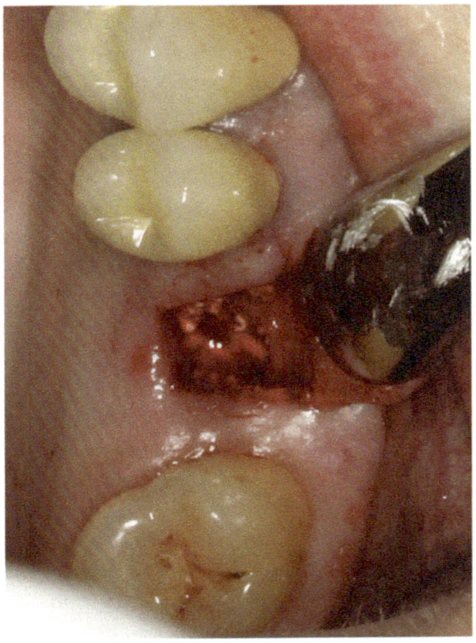

(f)

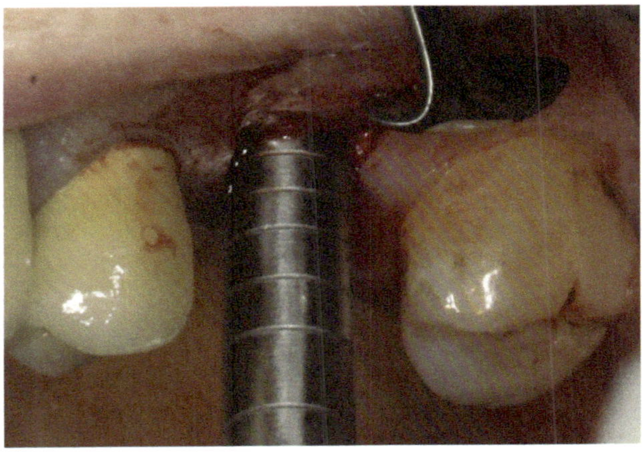

(g)

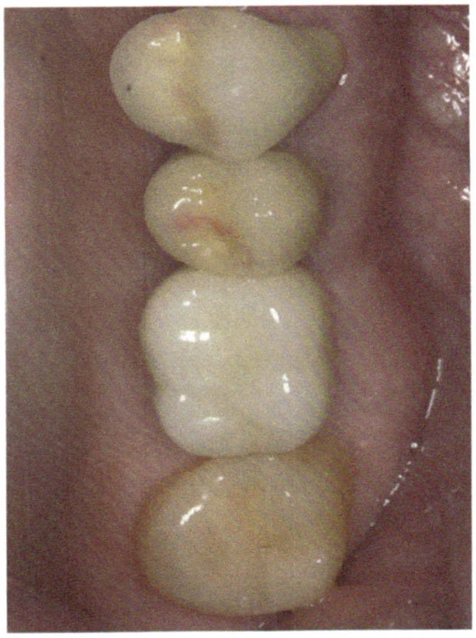

(i)

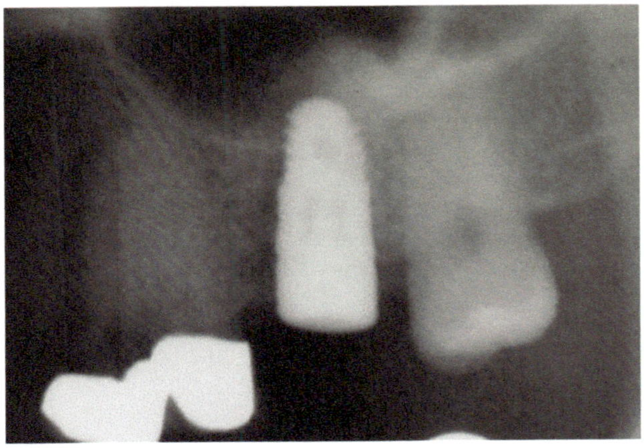

(h)

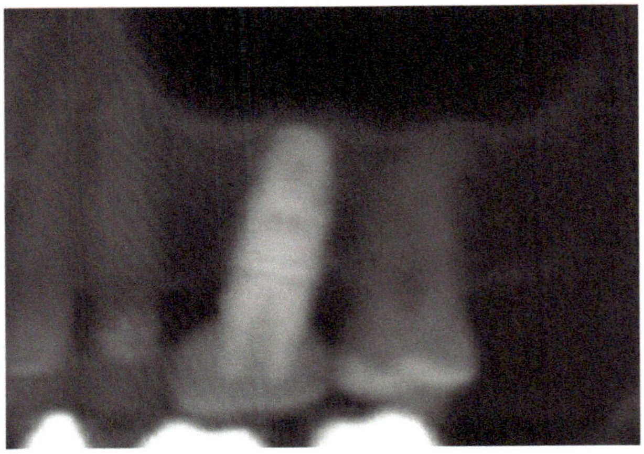

(j)

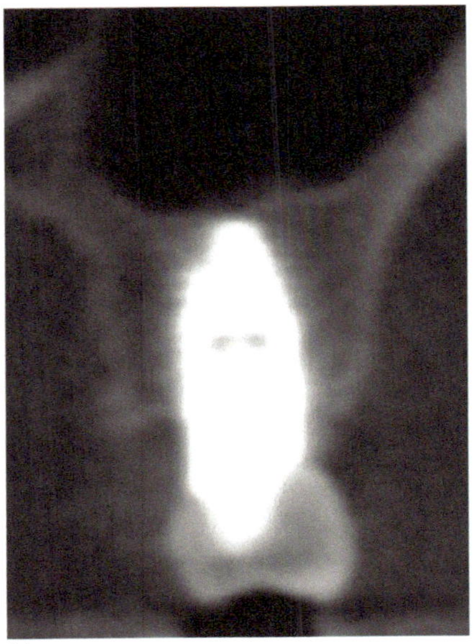

(k)

Figure 15.13 (Continued)
(f) Increasing diameter osteotomes were used following the same steps (initial floor fracture followed by re-insertion of the same diameter osteotome to trial length and advancing the bone/heme "plug"). (g) Final site development was completed with the largest diameter osteotome corresponding to the planned implant (5.5 mm diameter). Floor fracture was followed with addition of particulate graft and re-insertion to trial length and 1 mm beyond. Further graft material was added incrementally to advance the osteotome 3–4 mm to the final height of 12 mm. Direct tactile evaluation and nose blow testing was completed to confirm an intact sinus membrane prior to inserting the implant. (h) The post-operative radiograph demonstrates implant insertion and an overlying spherical density consistent with graft containment of the 5.5 mm × 11 mm implant. A transgingival initial healing protocol was used. (i–k) The 42-month post-op clinical and CBCT images demonstrating the new bone contours of the elevated sinus floor. © Daniel R. Cullum.

drill was used to determine trial length, which was confirmed with a periapical radiograph (Figure 15.13c). Insertion of a 2 mm concave-tipped osteotome was then completed to the trial length and advanced 0.5 mm with gentle malleting to initiate floor fracture (Figure 15.13d). A small amount of particulate graft was added and the osteotome re-inserted to trial length to advance the bone/heme "plug" and begin BAOSFE. A 3 mm diameter osteotome was then inserted to trial length, continuing the BAOSFE with floor fracture of a slightly larger concentric ring. This was followed by the addition of more graft and re-insertion of the osteotome to the trial length. At this point, periapical radiographs should demonstrate floor mobilization and the initiation of a small dome of graft material. Nose-blow testing should be applied intermittently throughout this process (Figure 15.13e). BAOSFE was continued with increasing-diameter osteotomes following the same process with initial floor fracture followed by re-insertion of the same osteotome to trial length and advancement of the bone/blood "plug" (Figure 15.13f). For final site development, the diameter of osteotome (or slightly undersized) corresponding to the planned implant is used (5.5 mm for this patient). The floor fracture is completed (Figure 15.13g) and repeated additions made of particulate graft with osteotomes. The goal is to develop a final osteotomy height of the intended implant length plus 1 mm of additional elevation. Confirming an intact elevated ceiling prior to inserting the implant will reduce the possibility of undiagnosed perforation and loss of containment of graft material. A post-operative radiograph following implant insertion shows an apical dome consistent with graft containment (Figure 15.13h). Figure 15.13i–k shows the clinical and radiographic status after 42 months' clinical function.

Bone-added osteotome sinus floor elevation at a sloping floor and in adjacent sites

In higher density bone, it may be necessary to use Piezosurgery or rotary instruments for preparation of the intra-alveolar osteotomy, followed by the same diameter osteotome for floor up-fracture and the BAOSFE steps. In the case of an ascending anterior sinus floor, the use of smaller diameter blunt-tipped/tapered osteotomes and the addition of graft material before sinus floor up-fracture will reduce the risk of membrane damage in the sloped region. Sinus septa will increase the risk of membrane perforation using the open, lateral wall approach but, like the sloping sinus floor, can be safely managed with BAOSFE using blunt-tipped osteotomes. BAOSFE also can be used where two or more adjacent implants are planned. In the patient demonstrated in Figure 15.14a and b, the right maxilla had a retained primary molar and an edentulous site at the congenitally missing first premolar location. CBCT cross-sectional images demonstrated limited residual bone height (Figure 15.14c). Pilot drilling was completed for trial length determination (Figure 15.14d). A tapered osteotome was used for apical floor fracture at the sloped region of the sinus floor (Figure 15.14e). Progressive addition and advancement of particulate xenograft using BAOSFE at both implant sites was used to join and expand the elevations. Radiographs demonstrated the membrane-contained graft material at the joined sites (Figure 15.14f and g) with one final tapered osteotome inserted to depth (Figure 15.14h). Figure 15.14i–k shows the immediate post-operative clinical and radiographic conditions. An elevation of >8 mm was achieved at the joined adjacent sites.

Bone-added osteotome sinus floor elevation with the use of reamer burs

Reamer burs represent a significant advancement in sinus floor manipulation techniques as they can be used with minimal risk of membrane damage and reduce or avoid the use of osteotomes in sites with denser bone.[95] Figure 15.6 demonstrates some of these specialized side-cutting reamer burs which are designed to thin

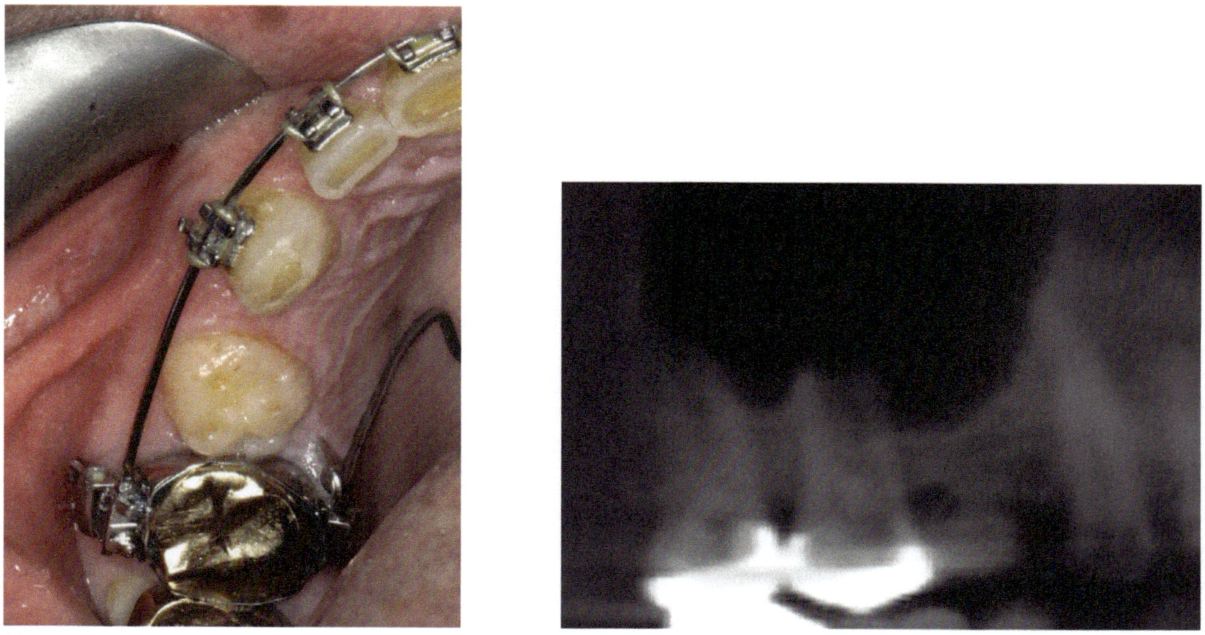

(a) (b)

Figure 15.14 Adjacent-site BAOSFE at a site with an anterior sloped sinus wall. (a, b) Preoperative clinical and radiographic images of the right maxilla with a retained primary molar and an edentulous site at the first premolar. Both premolars were congenitally missing.

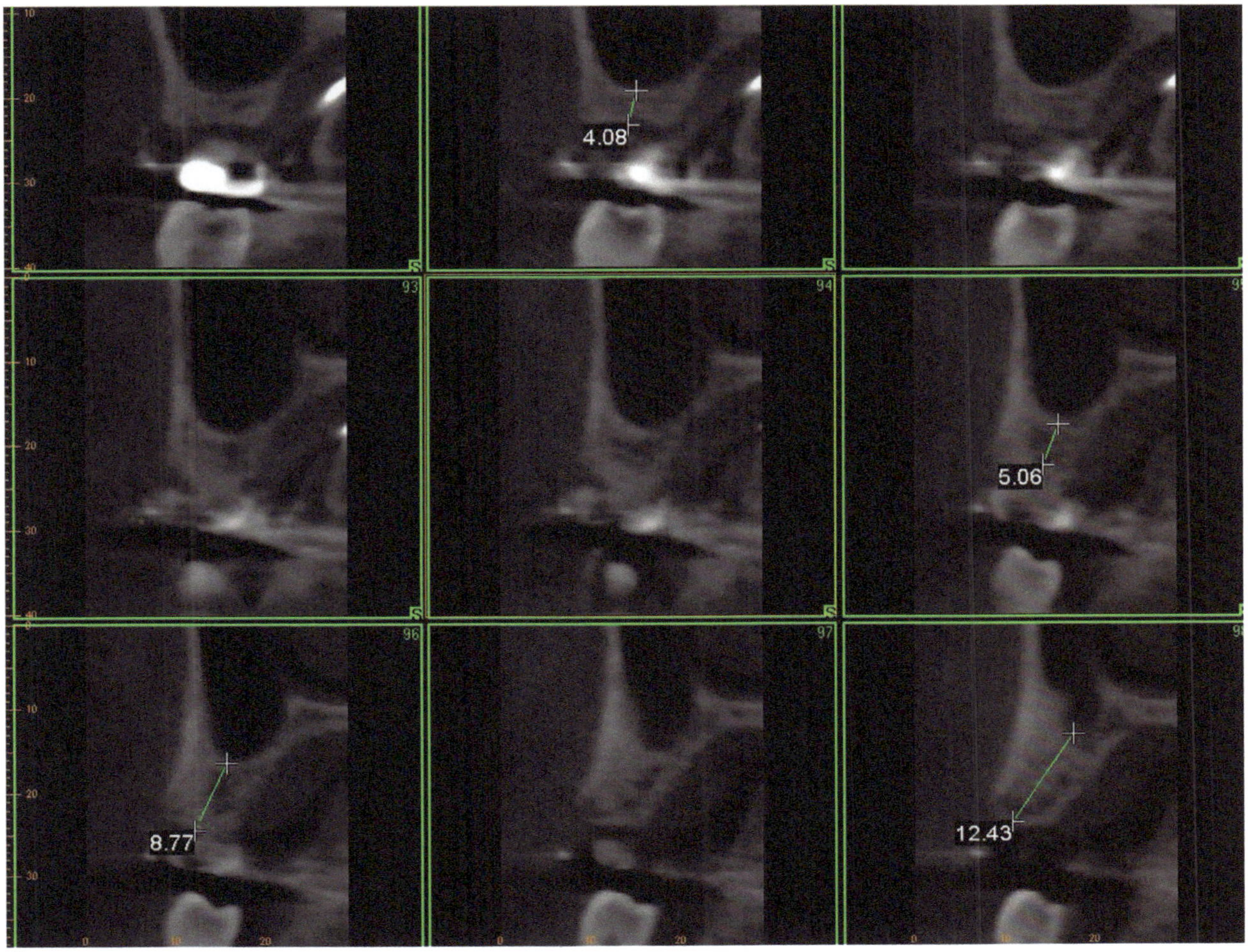

(c)

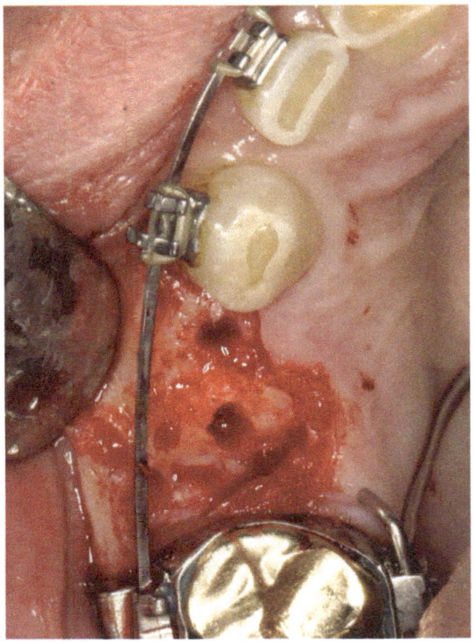

(d)

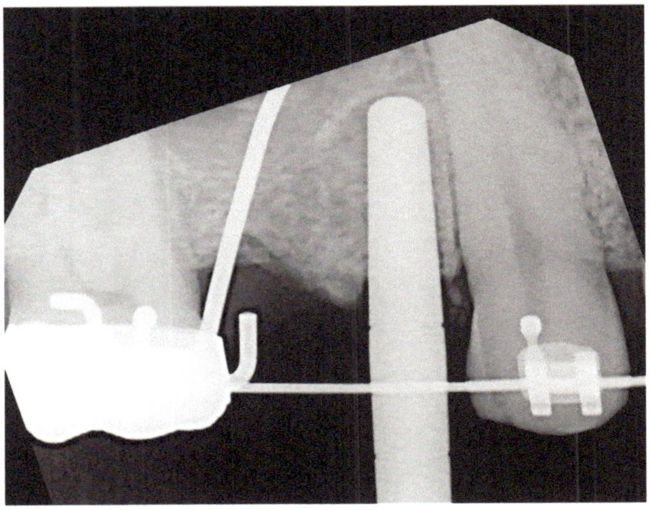

(e)

Figure 15.14 (Continued)
(c) CBCT images demonstrate limited residual bone height. (d) The pilot drill was used to prepare the sites for trial length determination. (e) A radiograph of the sinus floor up-fracture showing a tapered osteotome on the sloped region of the sinus floor.

(Continued)

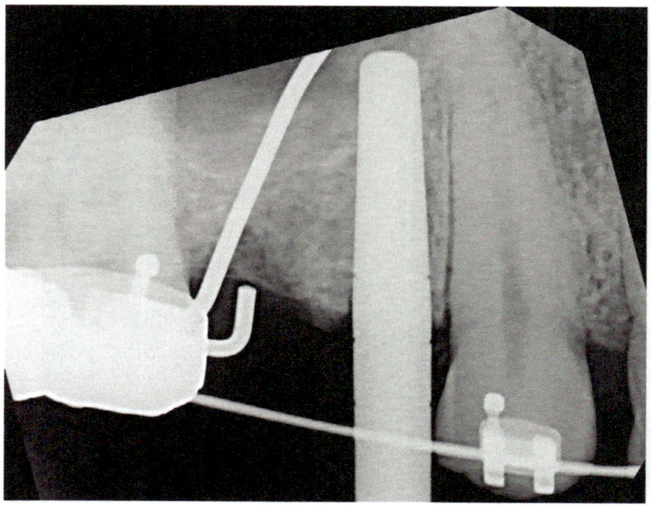

(f)

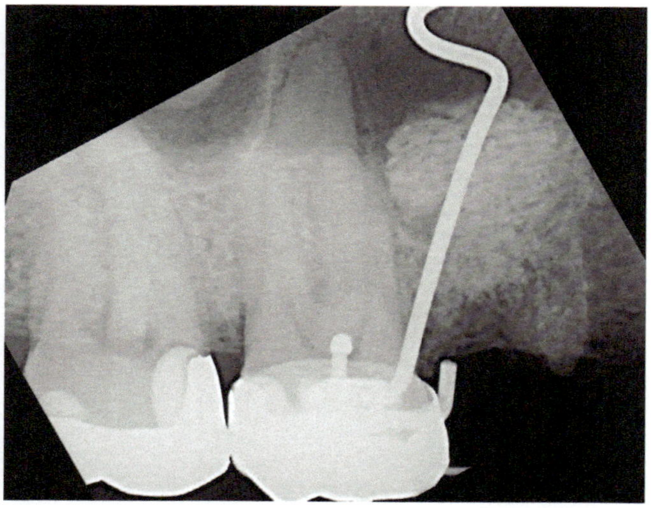

(g)

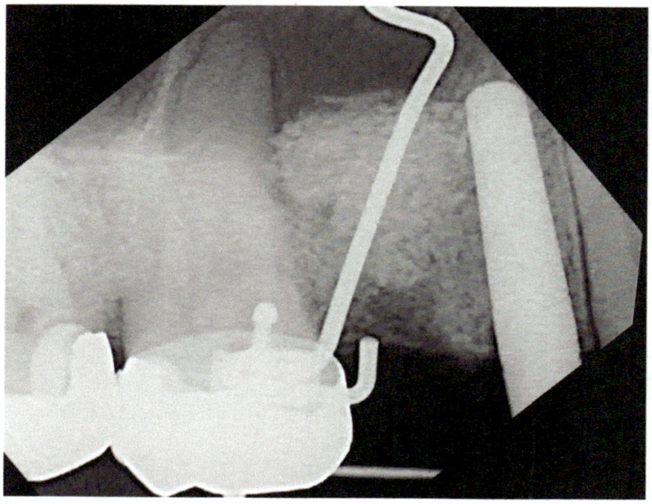

(h)

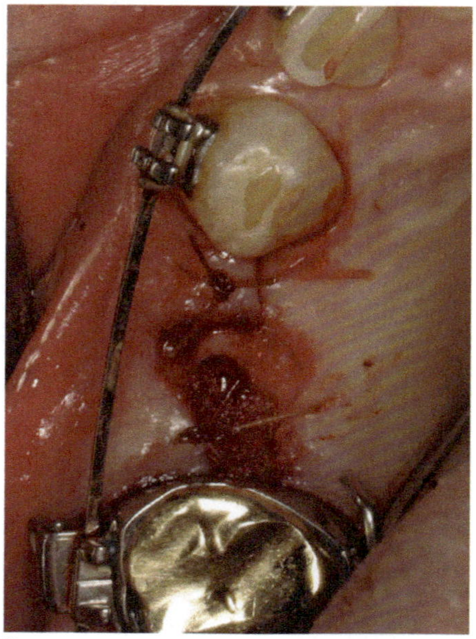

(i)

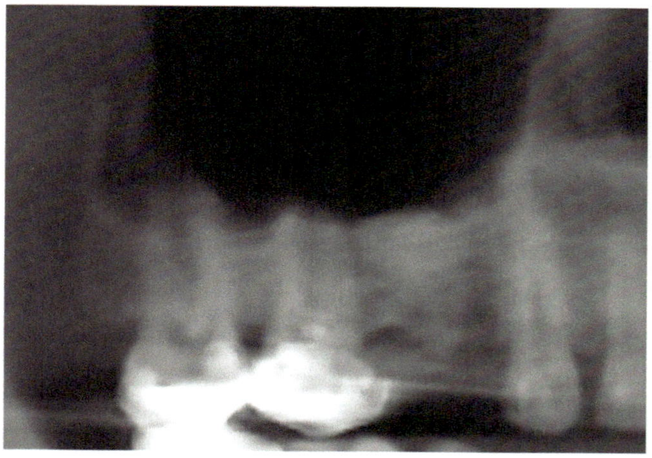

(j)

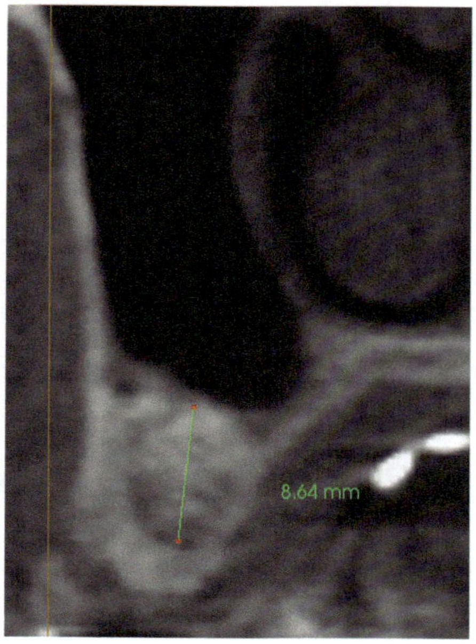

(k)

Figure 15.14 (Continued)
(f) A radiograph of the initial apical advancement with BAOSFE using a tapered osteotome. (g) A radiograph of the membrane-contained graft material at two joined adjacent sites with BAOSFE. (h) A radiograph of the membrane-contained graft at the joined adjacent sites at the point of final apical and lateral graft insertion using a tapered osteotome. (i) The immediate post-operative clinical picture after grafting. A crestal soft tissue void was filled with dense collagen saturated with heme. (j, k) The post-operative CBCT images demonstrated 8 mm of sinus elevation for future site development at the joined sites using BAOSFE. © Daniel R. Cullum.

and displace apically the sinus cortical bone floor without making direct contact with the membrane. Preoperative clinical and radiographic images can be seen in Figure 15.15a–c for a patient treated with a modified reamer drill approach for an edentulous site at the maxillary right first molar. The failing adjacent second molar tooth also was to be removed. CBCT cross-sectional imaging showed a residual bone height of 4.56 mm (Figure 15.15c). The edentulous site was exposed first (Figure 15.15d). The trial length for the first molar site was determined using a 2 mm twist drill with a stop feature. This was followed by site development using reamer drills of increasing diameter to the sinus floor and then beyond by 1 mm (Figure 15.15e). Drill speed was at 50 rpm or less, with the final

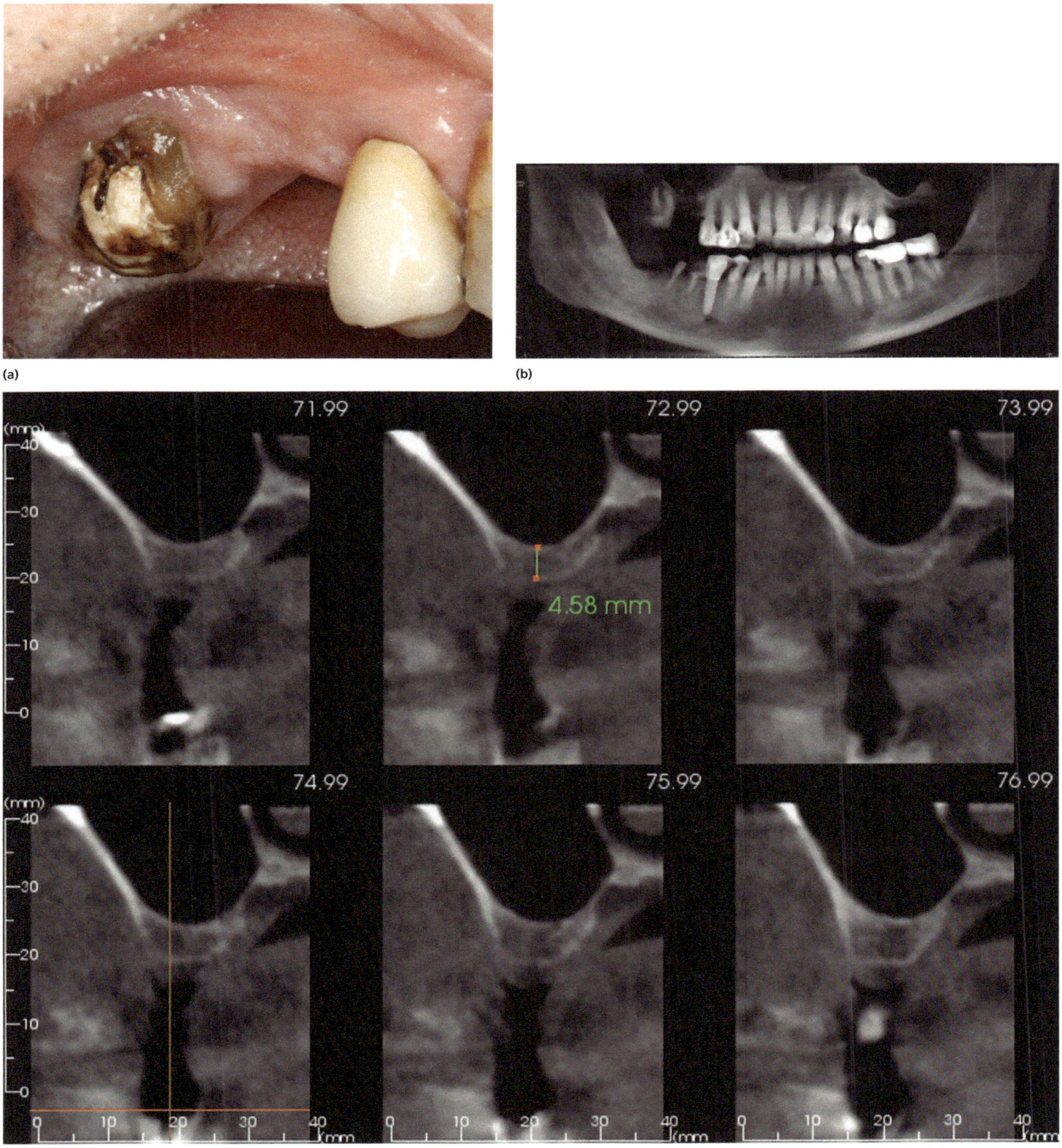

(a) (b) (c)

Figure 15.15 BAOSFE with reamer burs at a maxillary right first molar site. (a, b) The preoperative clinical and radiographic images of an edentulous site at the maxillary right first molar. The failing adjacent second molar was to be removed and grafted. (c) The CBCT cross-sectional image showed a residual bone height of 4.56 mm.

(Continued)

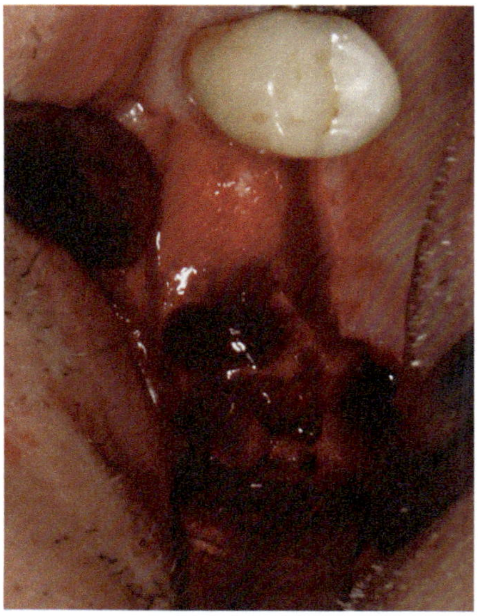

(d)

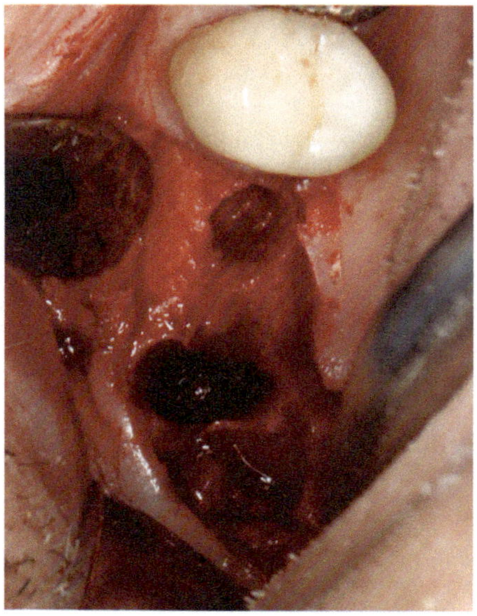

(e)

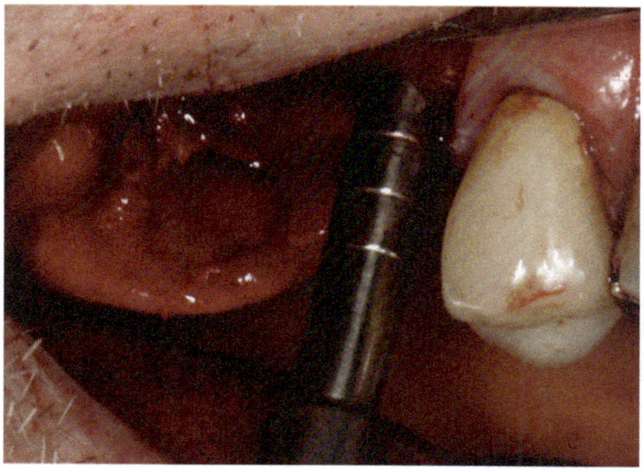

(f)

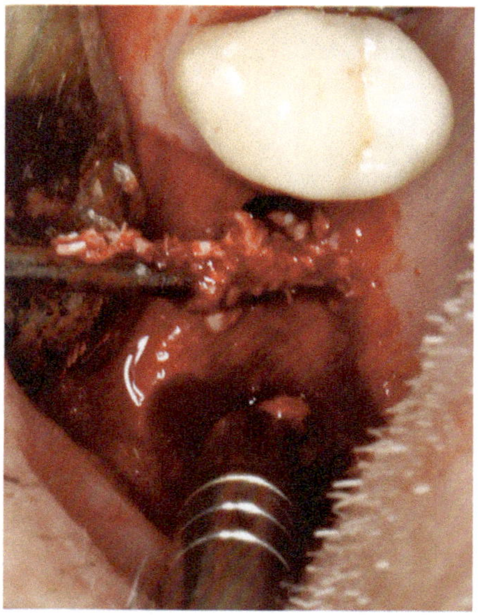

(g)

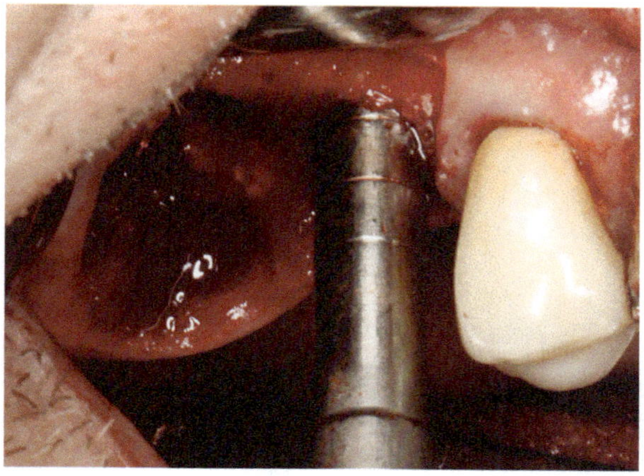

(h)

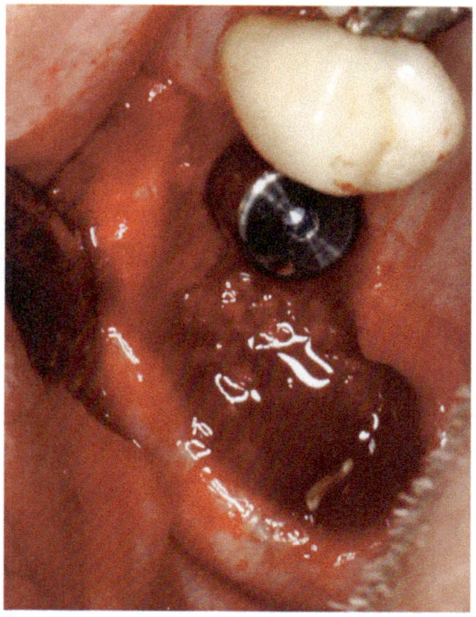

(i)

Figure 15.15 (Continued)

(d) The edentulous site has been exposed. (e) The trial length was determined with a 2 mm twist drill and stop, followed by site development with reamer drills of increasing diameter and with drill stops to the sinus floor. The sinus floor was then intruded with a 1 mm longer reamer drill. (f) Confirmation of sinus floor proximity and an intact membrane was confirmed with a periapical radiograph, nose blow test, and osteotome sounding. (g) Bone graft material was added progressively with the osteotomes, using lateral and vertical displacement following the same process as for BAOSFE. (h) Addition of particulate bone was completed with final osteotome insertion to a depth of 10 mm. (i) Implant placement (5.0 mm × 10 mm) was achieved with adequate buccal bone volume.

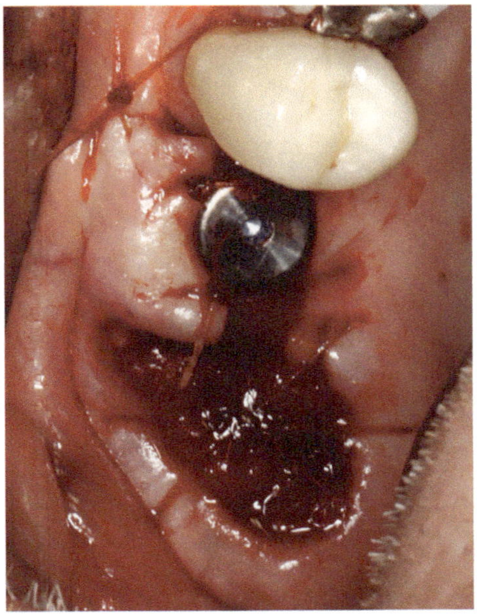

(j)

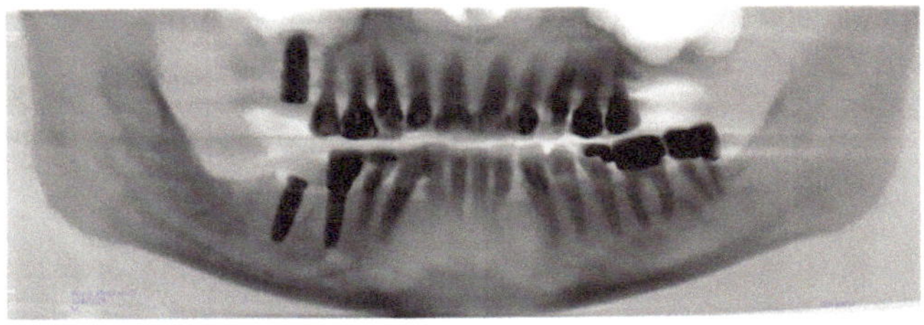

(k)

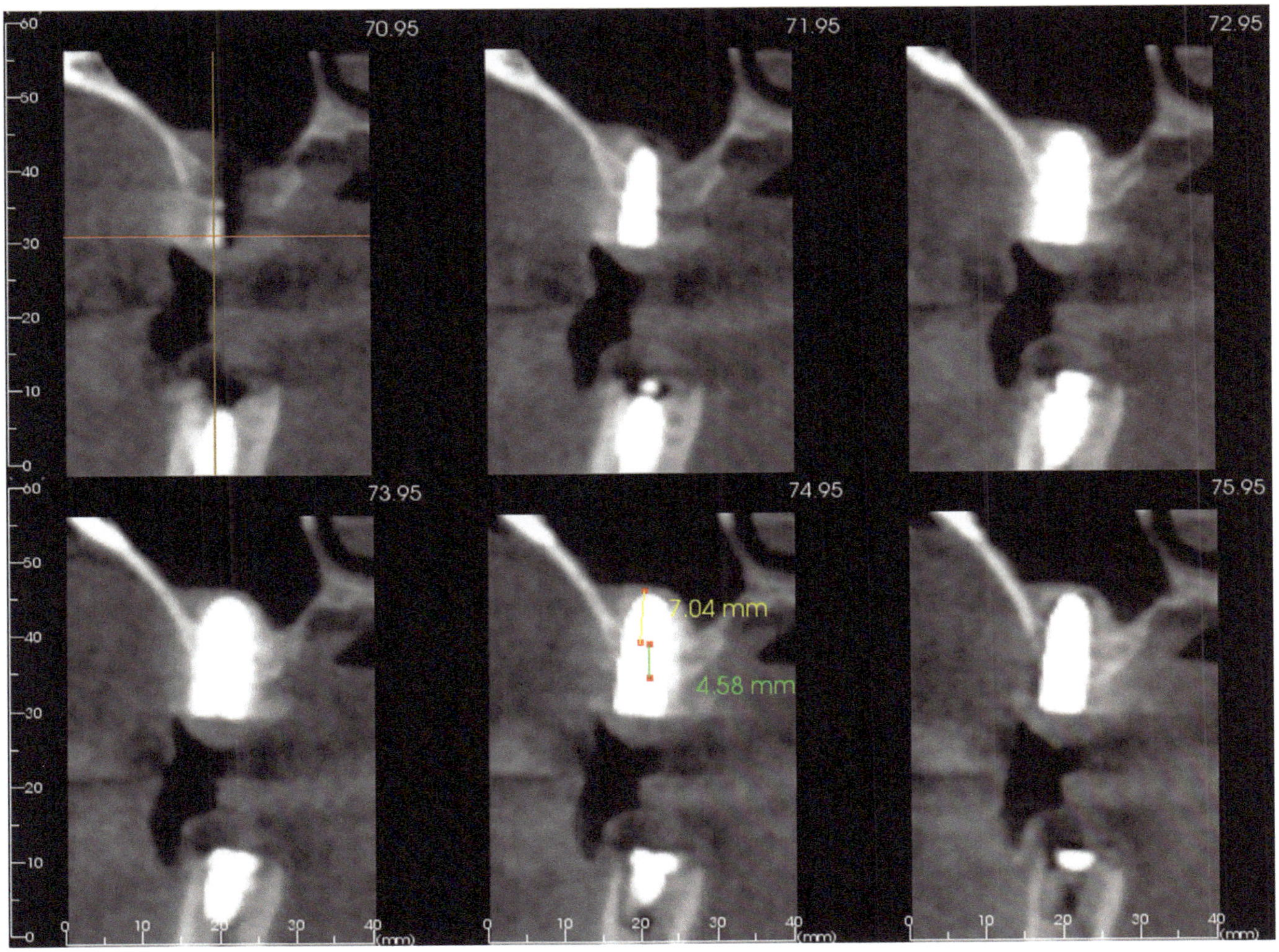

(l)

Figure 15.15 (Continued)
(j) Implant in position with a healing cap for a single-stage protocol. The distal extraction site was grafted with an open technique, allowing the soft tissue flap to be apically positioned (k, l) Post-operative CBCT images showed a contained particulate graft elevation following implant positioning.

(Continued)

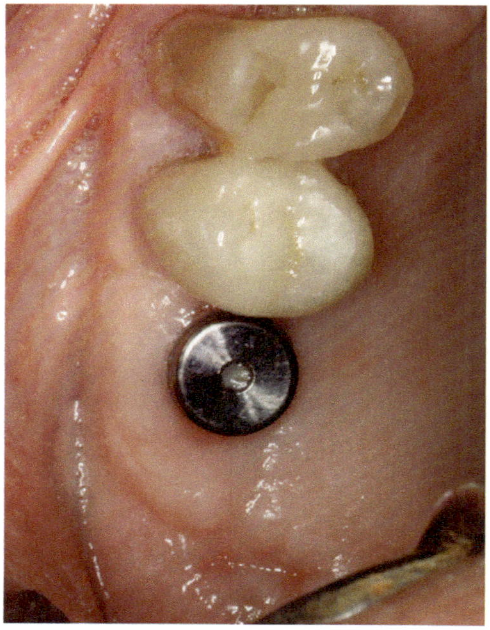

(m)

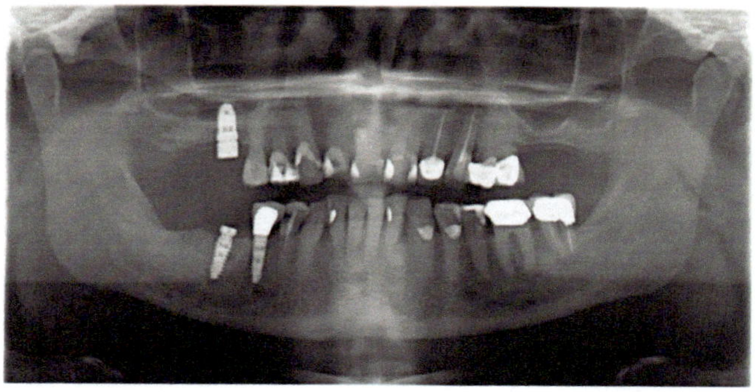

(n)

Figure 15.15 (Continued)
(m, n) Clinical and radiographic 4-month follow-up images demonstrate good healing and tissue contours. © Daniel R. Cullum.

reamer diameter 0.5–1.5 mm smaller than the planned implant. Confirmation of sinus floor proximity and an intact membrane was completed with osteotome sounding, a nose blow test, and a periapical radiograph (Figure 15.15f). Bone graft material was added incrementally using osteotomes with both lateral and vertical graft displacement, and the implant inserted (Figure 15.15g–i). The extraction site was grafted with an open modified BioCol® technique (Figure 15.15j). Post-operative CBCT images showed contained particulate graft elevation and the final implant position (Figure 15.15k and l). Clinical and radiographic 4-month follow-up images demonstrated good healing and tissue contours (Figure 15.15m and n).

Hydrodynamic piezoelectric sinus floor elevation

A preoperative CBCT scan of an edentulous maxillary first molar site displayed minimal residual bone height beneath the sinus, but good bucco-palatal ridge width (Figure 15.16a). After site exposure, initial osteotomy preparation was completed with a specially designed piezoelectric 2 mm diameter carbide tip (HPISE tip; S0281, Bukbu Dental Co., Daegu, South Korea) to approach the sinus floor and remove bone to uncover and elevate the membrane using hydraulic and ultrasonic forces[42] (Figure 15.16b). Final osteotomy site preparation then was completed with burs and osteotomes (Figure 15.16c). Graft material, in this case CGF prepared by centrifuging the patient's blood, was delivered into the elevated membrane-contained space[103] (Figure 15.16d). The implant was placed with a healing cap and left for single-stage healing (Figure 15.16e and f). Post-operative CBCT images demonstrated an intact sinus elevation and substantial vertical height gain (Figure 15.16g). Figure 15.16h and i show the restored implant with excellent hard and soft tissue contours and peri-implant bone levels.

Contiguous sinus floor elevation

CSFE site preparation is completed using a trans-alveolar approach with the sinus being elevated along an intra-bony trough created using a "stepped" and "overlapping" osteotome technique[49] (Figure 15.10a–f). Fracture of the floor is completed along the entire length of the defect to the largest diameter osteotome that the ridge will allow while maintaining appropriate buccal and palatal cortical wall thicknesses. Sinus floor elevations of 8 mm or more can be completed with grafting of the elevated sinus portion. This elevation of a larger portion of the sinus floor as one contiguous segment reduces the potential for breach complications.

Figure 15.17a and b demonstrate preoperative panoramic and CBCT images for a patient with limited alveolar height and bone density. A palatal incision was used to expose the edentulous segment. Concave-tipped osteotomes were used to fracture the residual sinus floor, progressing to the largest diameter osteotome that the ridge width would allow. Malleting the osteotomes was completed gently at each site until the note dulled, indicating fracture, but without elevating the sinus floor (Figure 15.17c). As each site was completed in this manner, the osteotome was sequentially stepped with slight overlaps across the entire antero-posterior dimension of the intended implant sites. In denser bone or if a localized area has more residual bone height, the surgeon can create a trough to thin the overlying bone with a Piezosurgery tip or a rongeur, which also allows bone to be saved for subsequent grafting of the defect. Adjusting the anterior–posterior angle of the osteotomes to keep the apical surface perpendicular to the sinus floor can prevent uneven fracture or perforation. After the bone roof was fractured but intact, CSFE instruments (Figure 15.17d and e) in 2, 3, and 4 mm widths (H&H Co. Ontario, CA) were used progressively to advance added graft material and raise the floor by 8 mm at the #14 site (Figure 15.17f). The tapered osteotome corresponding to the

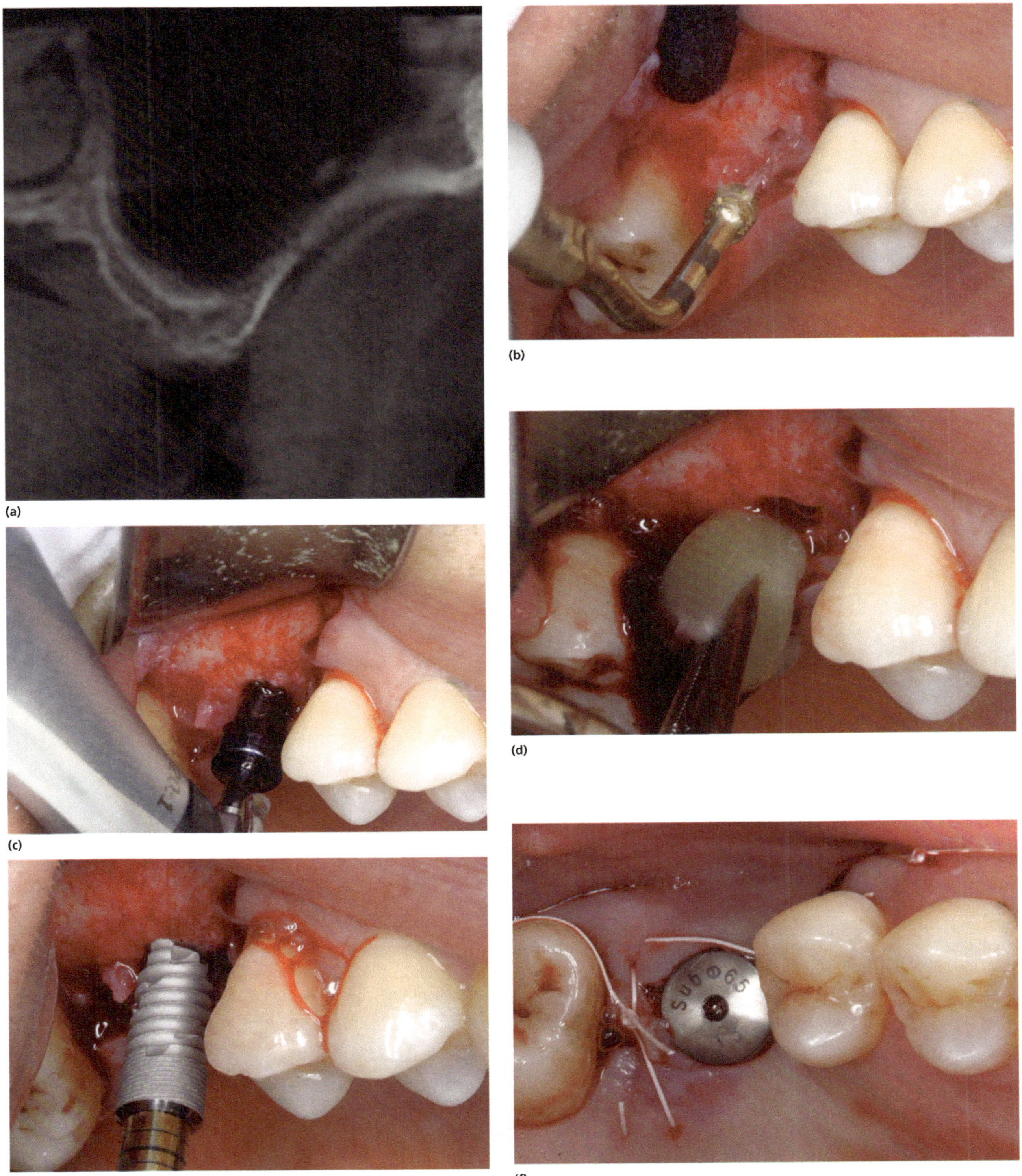

(a) (b) (c) (d) (e) (f)

Figure 15.16 HPISE case. *Source:* Dr Dong-Seok Sohn. Reproduced with permission of Dr Sohn. (a) The CBCT scan of an edentulous maxillary first molar site with minimal bone beneath the sinus but good bucco-palatal ridge width. (b) After initial osteotomy preparation with a pilot bur, osteotome, or Piezosurgery® tip, a specially designed 2 mm diameter carbide tip (HPISE® tip; S0281, Bukbu Dental Co., Daegu, South Korea) was used to cut through the sinus floor. The tip is internally irrigated and uses a jet of saline to elevate the sinus membrane. (c) After the membrane was elevated with the HPISE tip, final osteotomy site preparation was completed with implant drills. (d) CGF (platelet-rich fibrin clots) was prepared from the patient's centrifuged venous blood and placed into the elevated sinus as the graft material. (e) After graft delivery, the implant was placed. (f) The soft tissue was closed around the healing cap for single-stage healing.

(Continued)

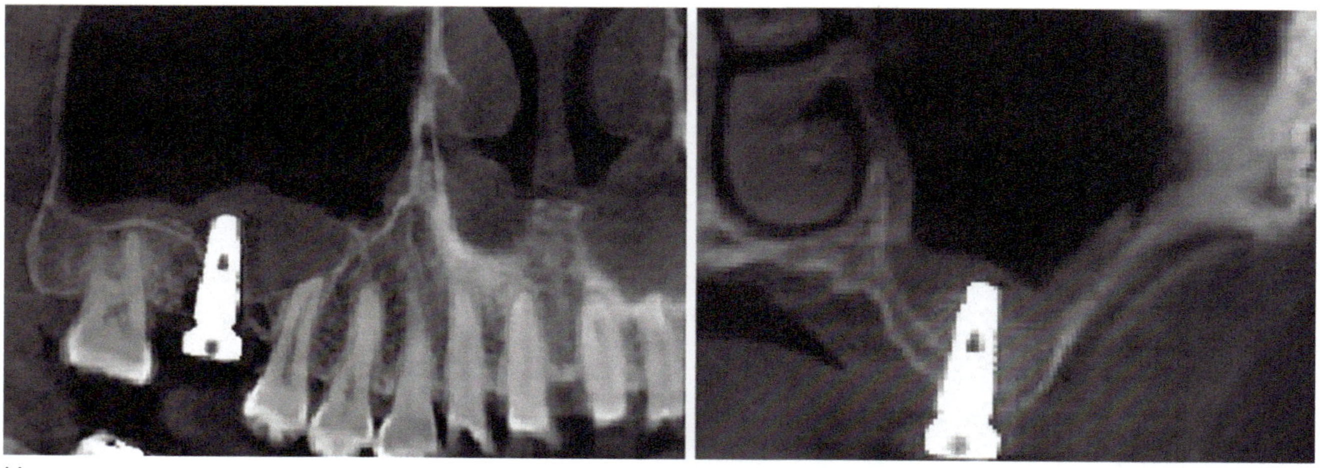

(g)

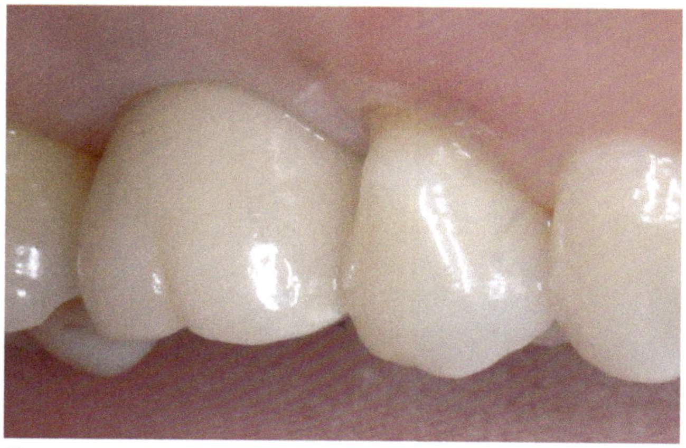

(h)

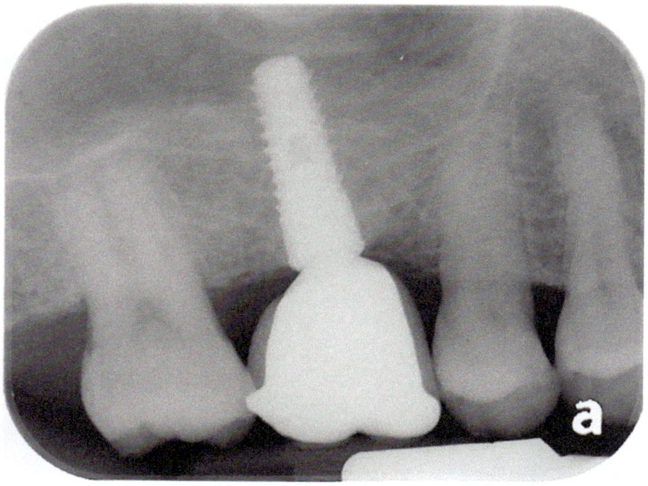

(i)

Figure 15.16 (Continued)
(g) The post-operative CBCT images demonstrate the intact sinus elevation and significant vertical height gain. (h) The clinical image of the restored implant showing excellent hard and soft tissue contours. (i) The post-restoration periapical radiograph shows maturing apical bone and good interproximal bone maintenance.

final implant diameter was inserted with elevation to allow placement of a 6.0 mm × 10 mm long implant with 1 mm of undisturbed graft apically (Figure 15.17g). Immediate and 4-year post-operative radiographs demonstrate the treatment outcome (Figure 15.17h and i).

Progressive mobilization with the largest instrument possible will spread the forces and tension from elevation over a larger area, reducing the risk of membrane tear and allowing greater elevation. If implant insertion is not feasible, grafting without implant placement can be completed for a staged implant approach. Closure over

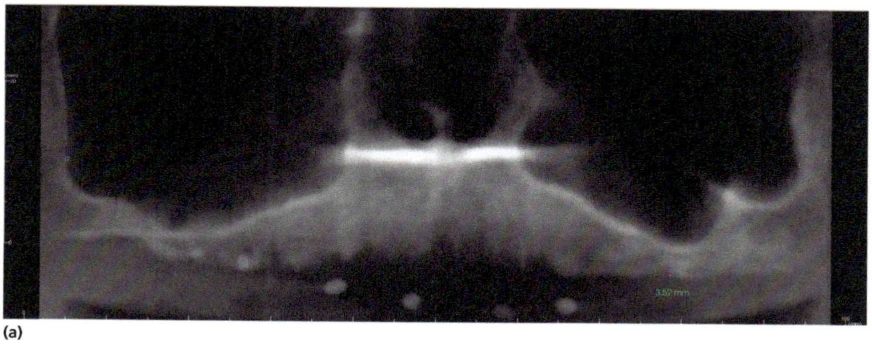

(a)

Figure 15.17 CSFE at the edentulous left posterior maxilla. (a, b) The preoperative panoramic and CBCT images of a patient with limited alveolar height and bone density.

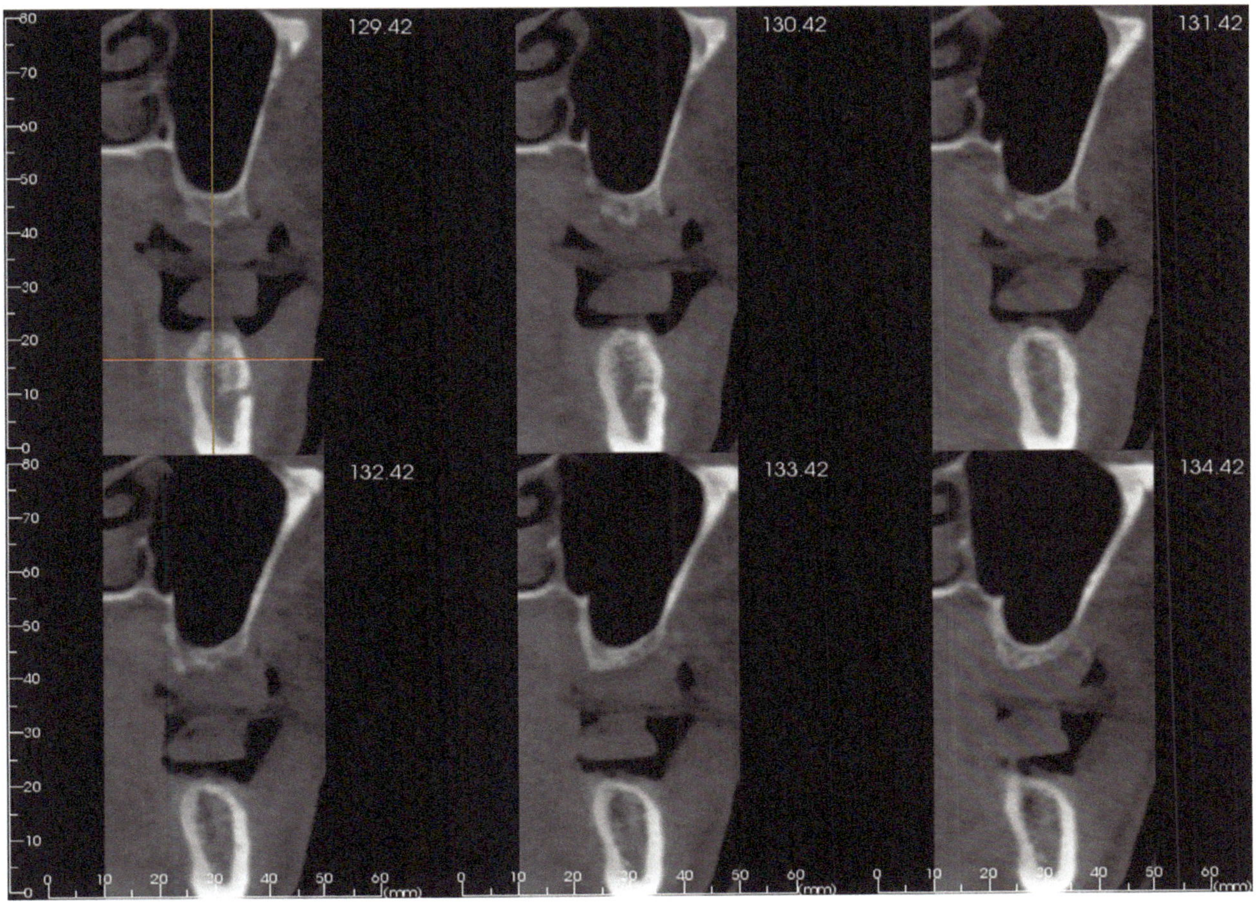

(b)

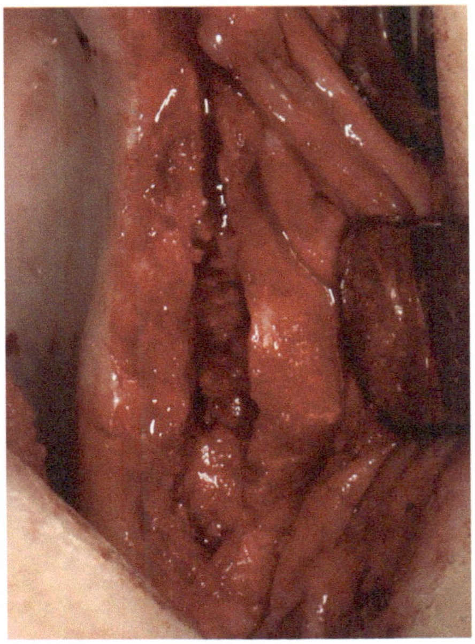

(c)

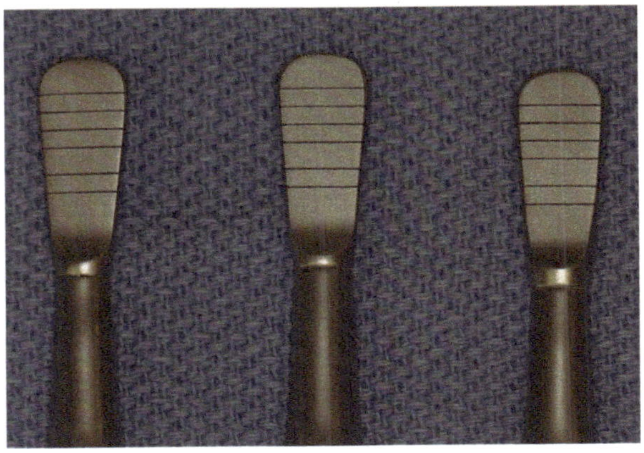

(d)

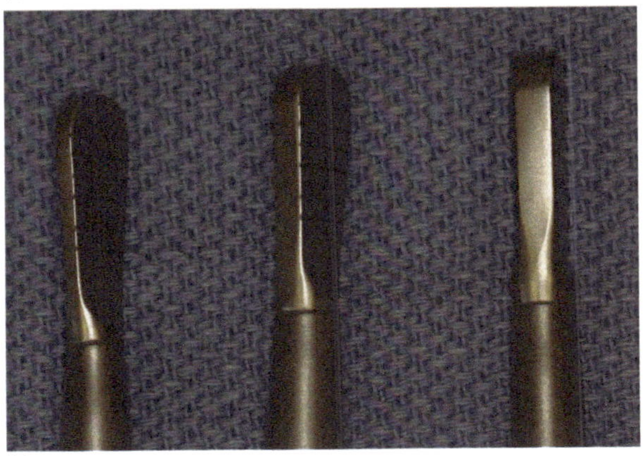

(e)

Figure 15.17 (Continued)
(c) A bone trough with stepped floor fracturing was completed using concave osteotomes. The osteotome was malleted gently until the note dulled, indicating fracture without any elevation of the sinus floor. The osteotomes were sequentially stepped across the antero-posterior dimension with slight overlaps. (d, e) CSFE instruments. CSF elevators 2, 3, and 4 mm widths (H&H Co., Ontario, CA).

(Continued)

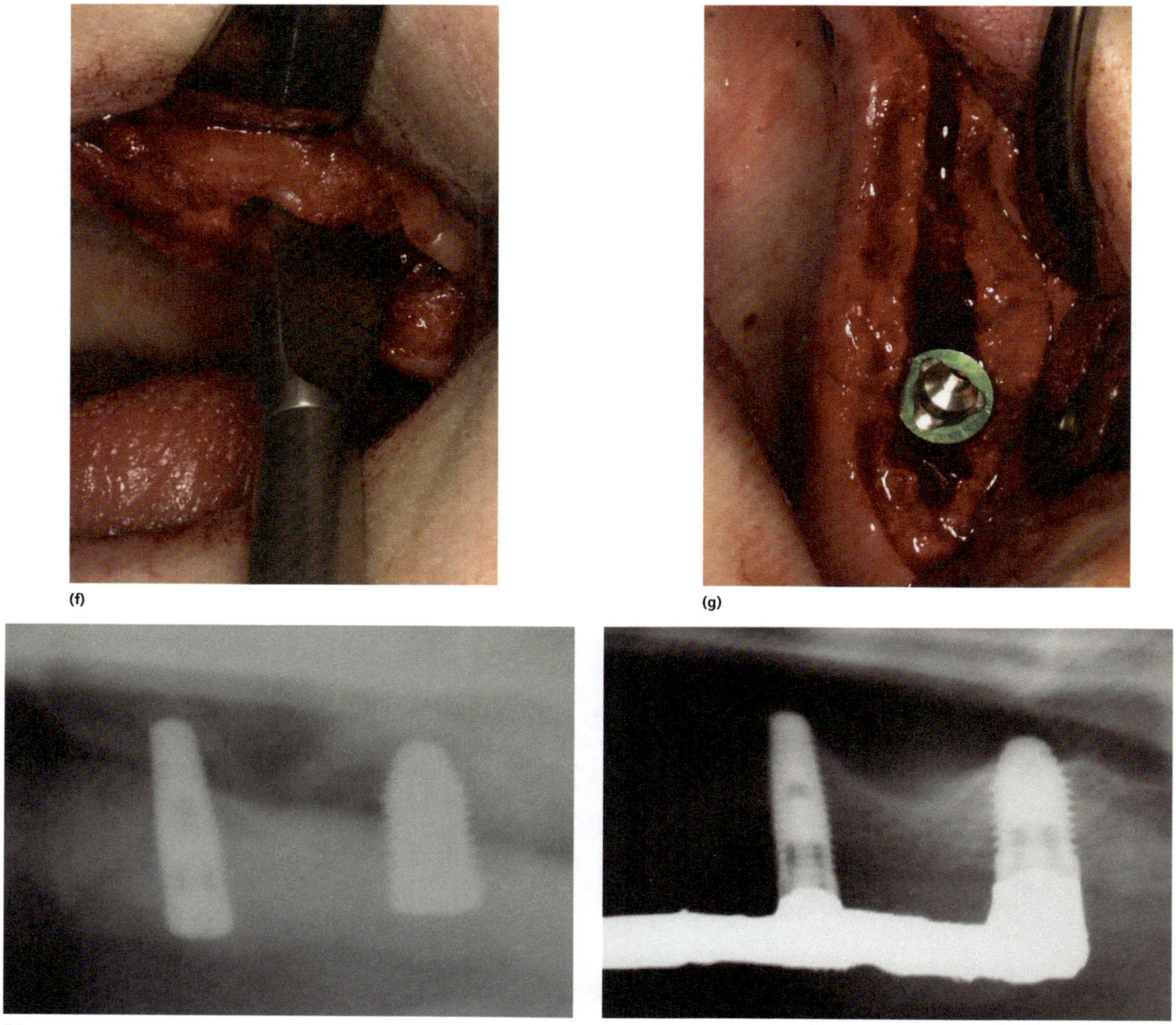

(f) (g) (h) (i)

Figure 15.17 (Continued)

(f) CSFE can be completed with progressive apical advancements using the CSFE instruments with or without the addition of particulate graft material. (g) A 6.0 mm × 10 mm implant was placed after 8 mm of CSFE. (h, i) The immediate and 4-year post-operative radiographs demonstrate the outcome with the CSFE procedure. a–h © Daniel R. Cullum.

implants can be primary for a two-stage protocol or near primary for single-stage cases. Alternatively, periodontal plastic procedures (subepithelial connective tissue grafts, or apically repositioned, lateral, finger, or pedicle flaps) can be utilized for primary and soft tissue augmented closure. A common application of this technique is for single-stage restoration of a maxillary first molar site with 3–5 mm of residual bone height (Figure 15.18).

The patient in Figure 15.19 shows CSFE being used at a single molar edentulous site. Preoperative CBCT and clinical images demonstrated an anterior sinus floor slope with 3–4 mm of residual bone height and a medial sinus septa (Figure 15.19a and b). A palatal papilla-sparing incision gave access to the ridge for preparation of a mesial to distal bone trough using rotary and Piezosurgery instrumentation. The CSFE trough and sinus floor fracture were completed using concave-tipped osteotomes (Figure 15.19c). The 3 mm contiguous sinus floor elevator (Figure 15.17d and e) and particulate graft material then were used to elevate the floor and membrane by 5–6 mm (Figure 15.19d). The final osteotome corresponding to the final implant diameter was inserted to 10 mm (Figure 15.19e), followed by insertion of a 10 mm × 6.0 mm diameter implant (Figure 15.19f). A healing cap was placed for single-stage healing, and the soft tissue flap was apically positioned. The wound was covered with light-cured periodontal dressing. A similar CSFE procedure was completed at the right first molar site (Figure 15.19b and c). The 4-month clinical and panoramic radiographs demonstrate excellent wound healing at both implant sites (Figure 15.19g and h). Figure 15.19i–k shows 1 year post-restoration images with good tissue contours, and interproximal and apical bone.

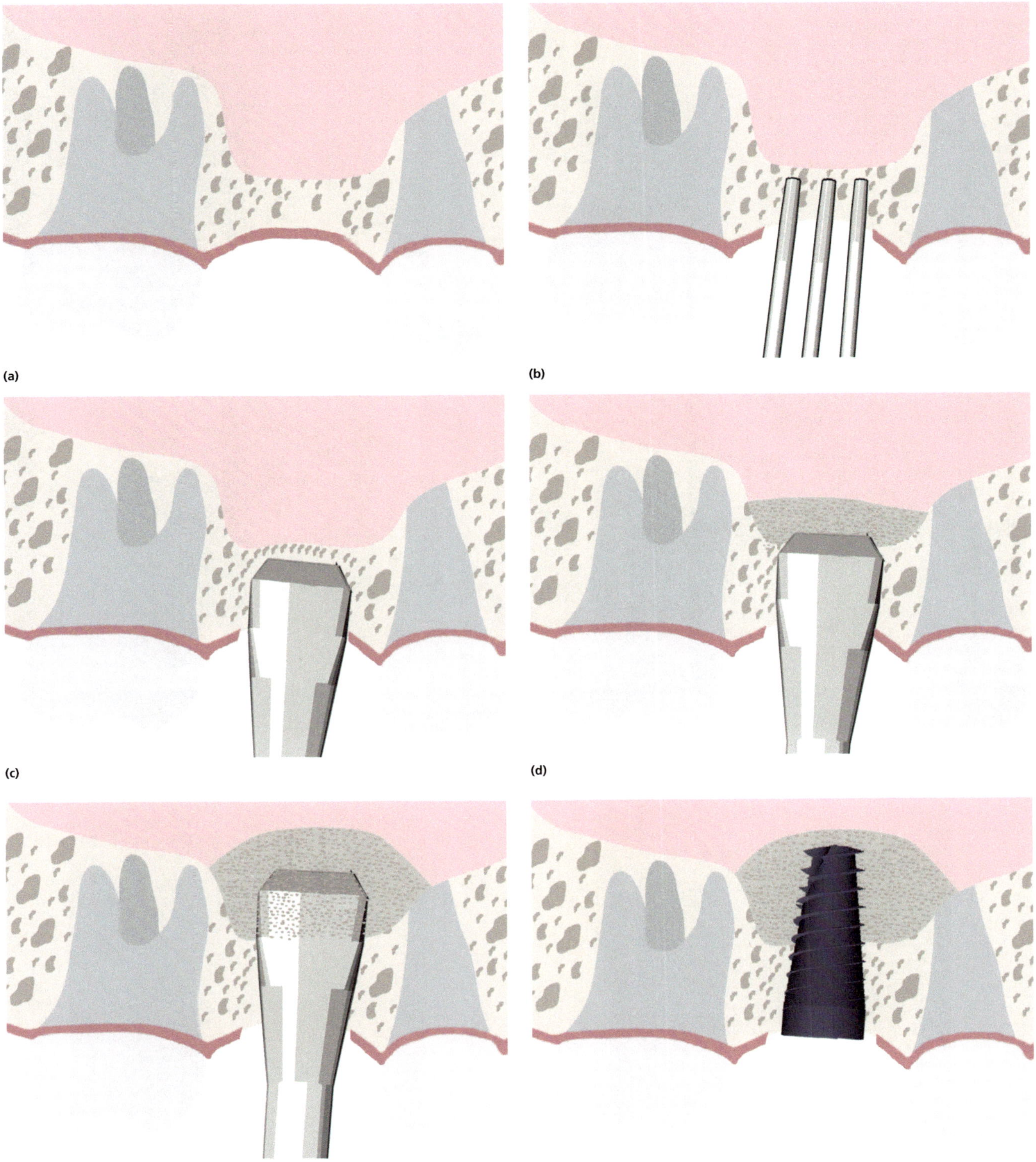

(a) (b) (c) (d) (e) (f)

Figure 15.18 A CSFE graphic for a single molar site. (a) An edentulous first molar site is depicted with 3–4 mm of residual bone height and a medial sinus septa. b) A bone trough is completed to the sinus floor. Concave-tipped osteotomes are used to sequentially fracture the sinus floor using a stepped or slightly overlapping placement of the instruments. (c–e) CSFE is completed with progressive apical advancement with contiguous osteotomes (3 and 4 mm widths) and addition of particulate graft material. (f) Final site development is completed with the implant-specific osteotome followed by placement of a tapered wide-diameter (5–6 mm) fixture. © Daniel R. Cullum.

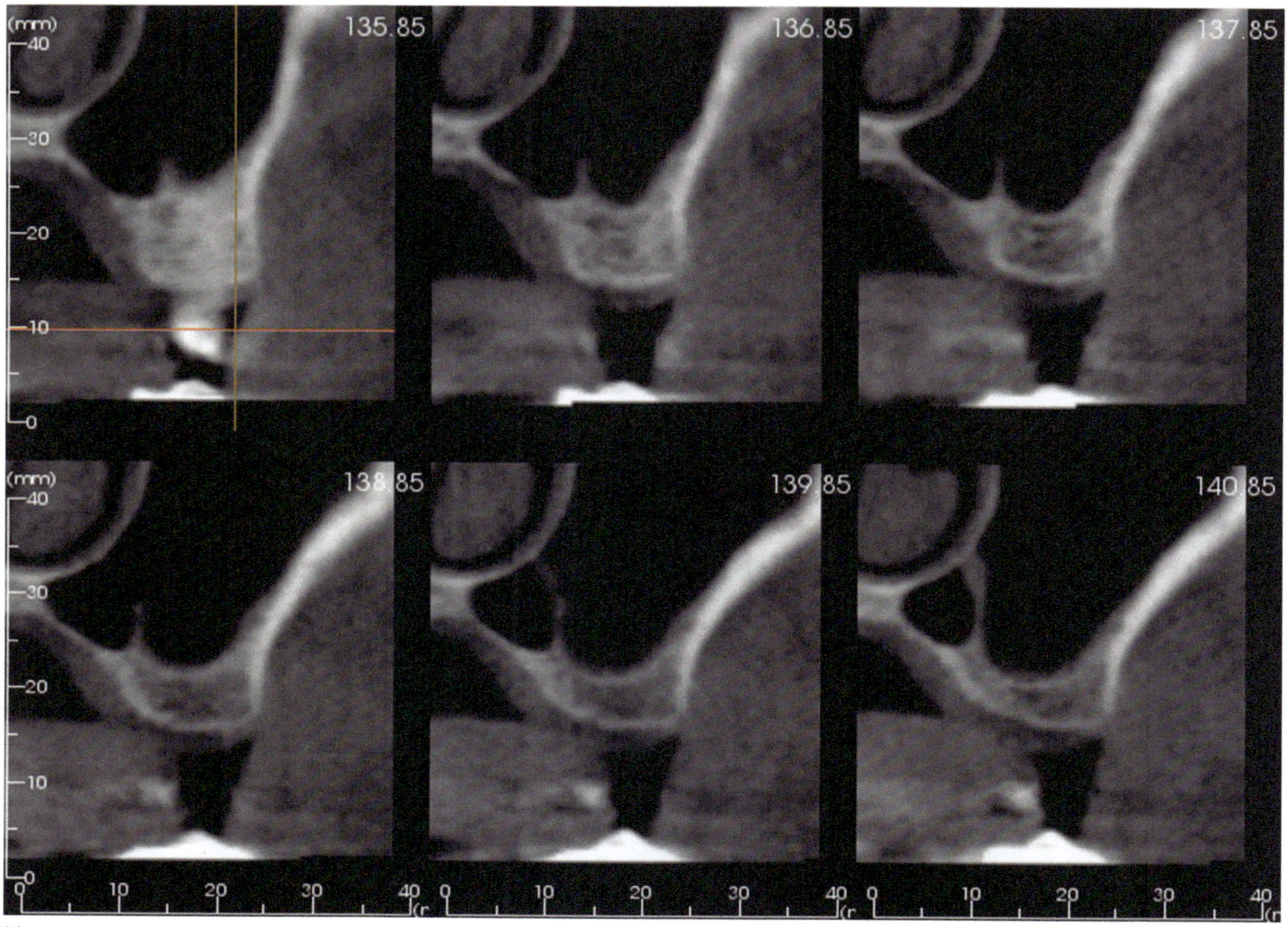

(a)

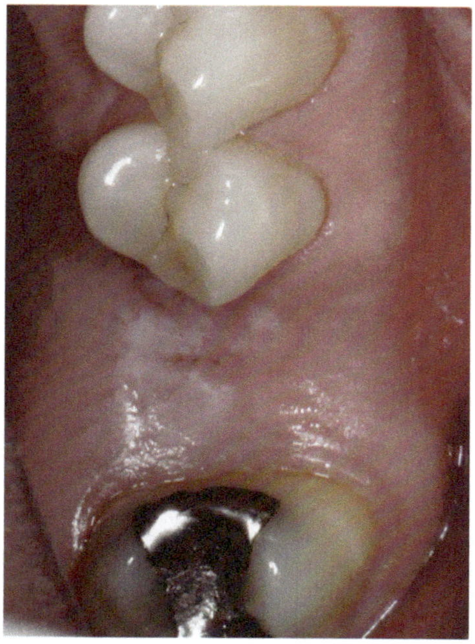

(b)

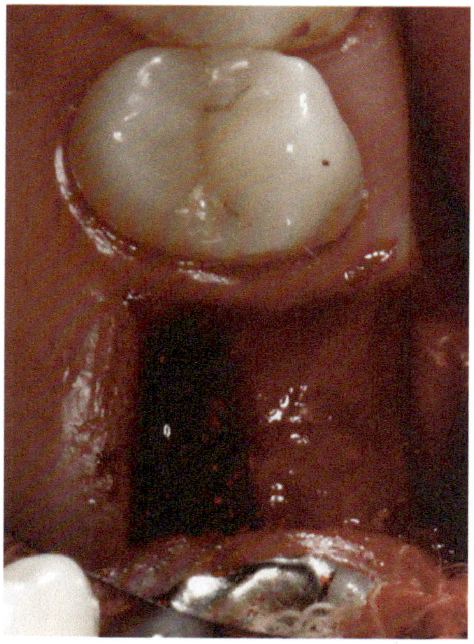

(c)

Figure 15.19 CSFE at a single molar site. (a) Preoperative CBCT images demonstrate 4 mm of residual bone height and a medial sinus septa. (b) A preoperative clinical image of the edentulous first molar site. (c) The CSFE trough after concave-tipped osteotome site development and sinus floor up-fracture.

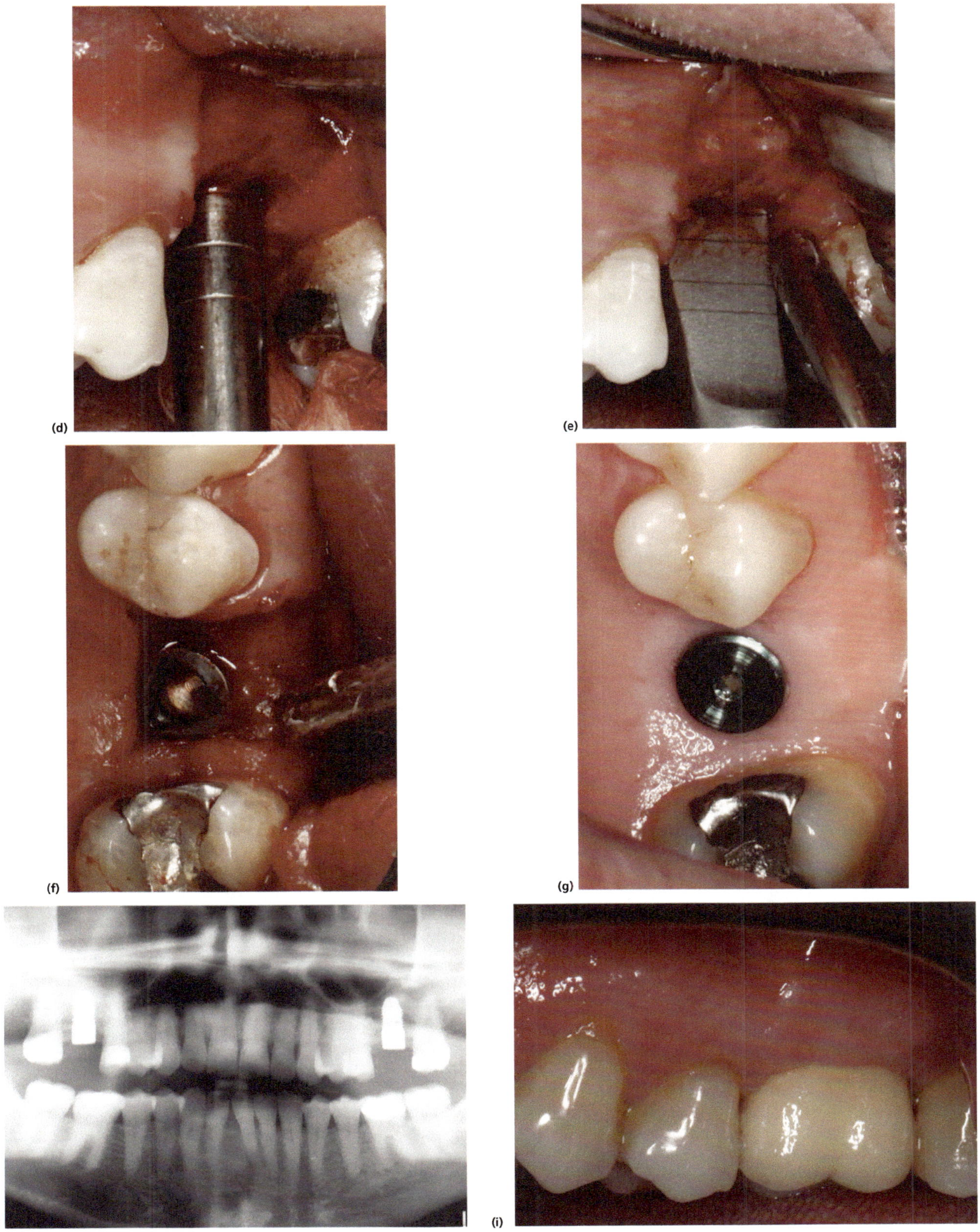

Figure 15.19 (Continued)

(d) Contiguous elevators were used to elevate the sinus floor and membrane 5–6 mm with added particulate graft. (e) The osteotome corresponding to the final implant diameter was inserted with elevation to 7 mm to allow placement of a 10 mm long × 6.0 mm diameter implant and leaving 1 mm minimum of undisturbed graft apically. (f) The implant (6.0 mm diameter) had good primary stability. A healing cap was placed for single-stage site healing and the soft tissue flap apically positioned. A similar procedure also was completed at the right first molar site. (g, h) The 4-month clinical and panoramic radiographs demonstrate excellent wound healing, tissue contours, and bone apical to the implants. (i–k) The 1-year post-restoration images demonstrate good tissue contours and interproximal bone heights. © Daniel R. Cullum.

(Continued)

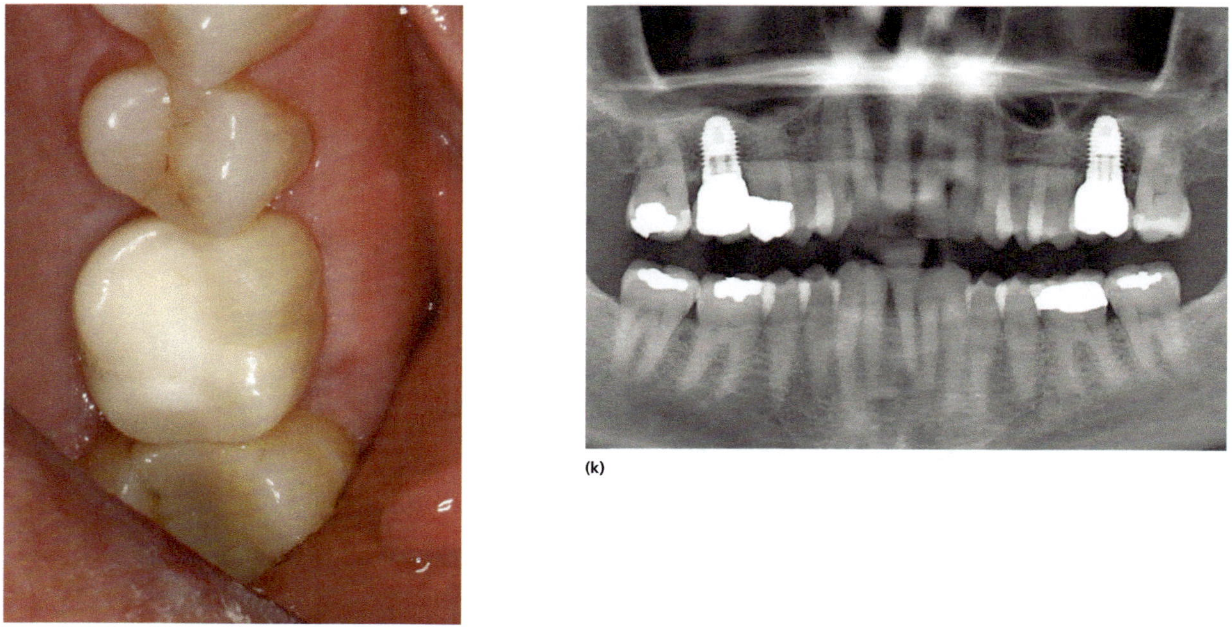

(j)

(k)

Figure 15.19 (Continued)

Avoiding and managing complications

TASE techniques can be minimally invasive, require specialized instruments, and are more technique-sensitive than guided bone regeneration or the Caldwell–Luc approach to sinus grafting. Site anatomy can limit the amount of elevation and affect choice of TASE technique, mandating care in case selection. Patient tolerance is greatly improved with the use of intravenous sedation and modifications using side-cutting drills or Piezosurgery tips. Benign paroxysmal vertigo is a rare self-limiting finding, and can be avoided by using light force, supporting the patient's head and avoiding Trendelenburg positioning during the procedure.[66–69] If site development appears to have reached the tactile limit of an osteotome technique, consideration should be given to placing a shorter implant, using site grafting with delayed implant placement, joining adjacent BAOSFE sites, using contiguous sinus floor elevation for broader membrane mobilization, or converting the procedure to a lateral wall approach.

Other complications with TASE procedures include those common to all traditional implant surgery, including improper implant positioning, inadequate primary stability, infection, and failure of osseointegration. Preoperative CBCT assessment and planning are critical to a full understanding of the 3-D bony topography of the residual crest, sinus floor, and membrane thickness/pathology (see Chapter 2). Potential complications increase with residual bone heights less than 4–5 mm, in part from limited implant support and primary stability and due to the amount of elevation required for implant placement.[107] Manipulation of the sinus from a trans-alveolar approach gives limited visibility and requires judicious use of tactile and auditory skills as well as surgical judgment and intuition. Challenges with sinus floor manipulation and elevation can occur intraoperatively or during the early or post-operative periods. These include sinus membrane perforation, tears, complete sinus breach and displacement of graft or implant into the sinus proper, acute infection, and chronic sinusitis. Any gross loss of graft containment or implant displacement requires immediate surgical intervention and/or specialist referral.

Perforation of the sinus membrane with site preparation can occur even prior to trial length determination with rotary or osteotome instrumentation. This is often due to bone volume buccally or palatally to the pneumatized sinus giving the appearance of greater bone height in traditional 2-D radiographic images (Figure 15.20). The diagnosis of membrane perforation during an OSFE procedure is straightforward. with loss of apical resistance and a positive nose blow test. Application of drill stop guides and reamer drills (Figure 15.6) can be helpful in avoiding this problem.

Diagnosis and management of sinus breach can be more challenging with a "bone-added" technique than with OSFE. A positive nose blow test can be more difficult to discern as a membrane tear can be masked by partially contained graft particles. Confirmation of a progressively increasing discrete, spherical dome of mineralized graft material at the implant apex on a periapical radiograph is a reliable indication of containment. Loss of rebound resistance of the sinus membrane with osteotome advancement usually indicates a larger tear. While loss of graft containment can typically be seen with an intraoperative periapical radiograph, CBCT imaging may be needed for accurate diagnosis. Using the implant to complete the final elevation gives the operator no tactile feedback, as the rotational torque resistance of the implant insertion has no relationship to the continuity of the sinus membrane. Caution also is necessary with vertical adjustment for final implant platform height (especially with a flapless approach). Apical advancement may be more than the surgeon realizes and cause sinus breach with internal bleeding or loss of graft containment. Figure 15.20 demonstrates a sinus membrane tear and intra-sinus bleeding without loss of graft containment after a TASE procedure. Post-operative CBCT views (Figure 15.21) suggested a partial membrane tear with a horizontal radiodensity consistent with bleeding and clot formation. There did not appear to be loss of graft containment manifested by the apical peri-implant graft density. The intraoperative periapical images appeared to demonstrate an intact sinus membrane and graft containment prior to the final vertical height platform adjustment. The patient was asymptomatic and made routine post-operative progress, as seen in Figure 15.19g–j.

Treatment options with sinus breach include the following:

1 Aborting the procedure and patching the perforation with collagen or autogenous platelet-rich fibrin with or without particulate grafting of the alveolar portion.
2 Mobilizing the sinus membrane around the periphery of the osteotomy to elevate a larger portion followed by patching with

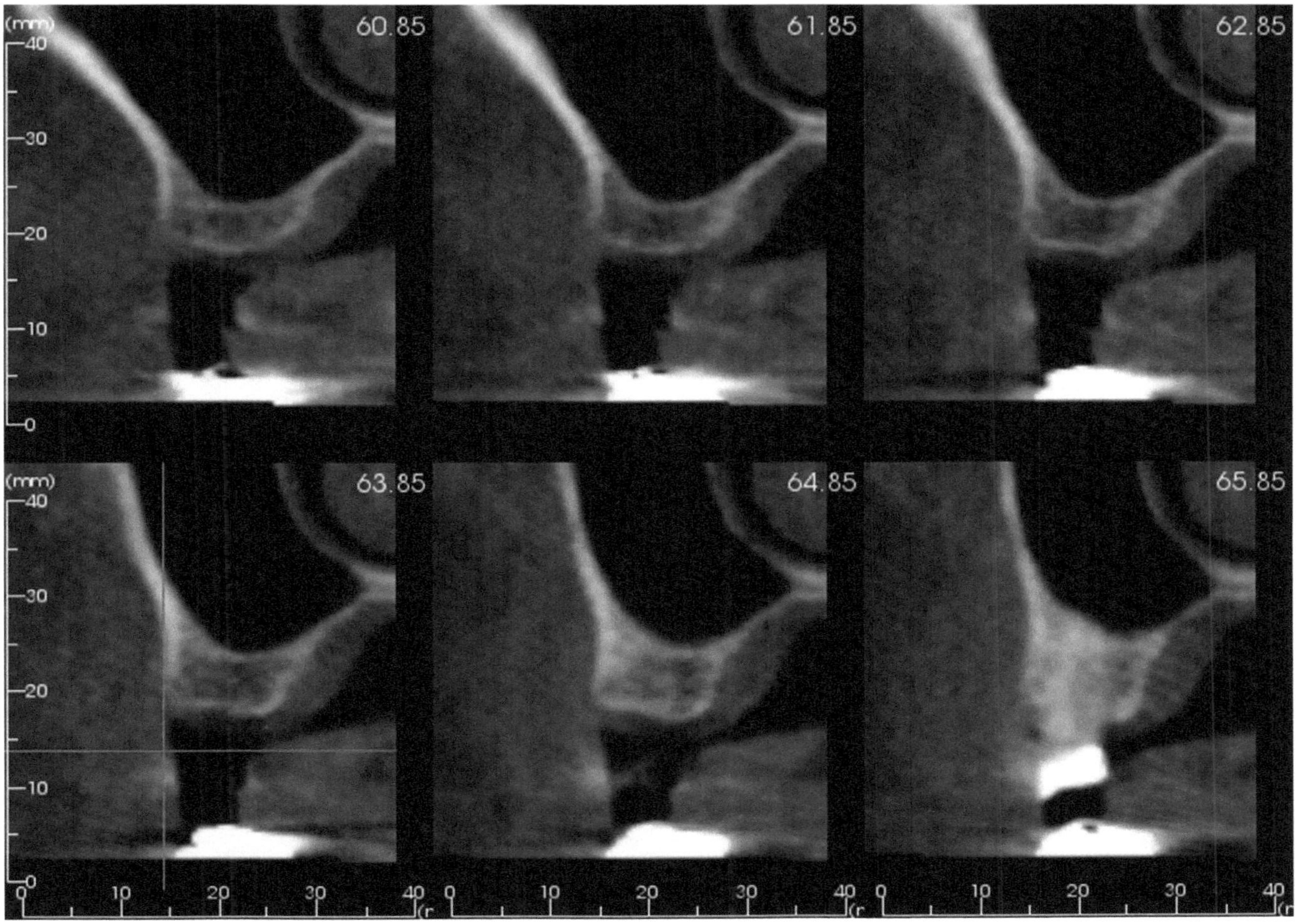

Figure 15.20 A CBCT images demonstrating bone volume buccally and palatally to the pneumatized sinus. A thicker palatal alveolar height can give the impression of greater bone height in traditional 2-D radiographic images. The CBCT image demonstrate an anterior to posterior slope from 8 mm to 4 mm of the residual bone height. © Daniel R. Cullum.

collagen or autogenous platelet-rich fibrin clots and/or placing a shorter implant (with adequate diameter and height) below the tear height.

3 Converting to a CSFE with mobilization of a larger portion of the membrane anterior and posterior to the tear followed by patching with collagen or autogenous platelet-rich fibrin and grafting for a staged procedure or with simultaneous implant placement if adequate repair and containment has been achieved.
4 Converting the procedure to a lateral wall approach and collagen or platelet-rich fibrin patching, sinus grafting, and possible implant placement.

If the breach is noted early and has a small diameter, it is often possible to place a small pledget of collagen saturated with blood, platelet-rich fibrin or recombinant human PDGF (rhPGDF; off-label use of GEM 21S®, Osteohealth, Shirley, NY), and then to enlarge site diameter with Piezosurgery or rotary instruments. If the added collagen has sealed the small tear and adequate sinus floor can be gathered with a concave-tipped osteotome, the procedure can often be completed with implant placement. In this case, it is prudent to place the implant without undue apical pressure. If the loss in sinus membrane continuity results in dispersal of graft material, suction evacuation of the osteotomy is indicated to remove accessible graft material. The intra-sinus portion can be evacuated using a Fraser suction tip (as for retrieval of a displaced tooth root fragment), followed by sinus irrigation with saline for complete debridement. This should be accomplished with the patient placed in a more upright position. The residual sinus membrane defect then can be sealed at the apex with collagen or collagen impregnated with xenograft (BioOss Collagen™, Geistlitch Pharma, Princeton, NJ) saturated with blood, platelet-rich autogenous plasma, or rhPDGF (off-label use of GEM 21S growth factor; Osteohealth, Shirley, NY). Grafting of the defect avoiding any apical pressure or displacement of the graft particles and primary soft tissue closure would be recommended to ensure containment of graft particles during the healing interval.

Displacement of an implant into the sinus is also a concern, as even partial overseating of a cylindrical implant can result in complete displacement with attempts to remove the fixture. Engagement of a fixture mount or implant abutment can aid in maintaining an occlusal force while reverse-turning the implant. A Caldwell–Luc approach or functional endoscopic sinus surgery can give access for debridement or implant removal, which should not be delayed.[22] If the patient develops acute post-operative sinusitis symptoms, evaluation for delayed endoscopic debridement may be indicted. Preoperative assessment of sinus health and patency of the sinus ostium would influence management. If the patient has had any significant sinusitis history or issues with patency of the ostium,[85] more aggressive treatment may be indicated in concert with medical specialist evaluation. Appropriate post-operative

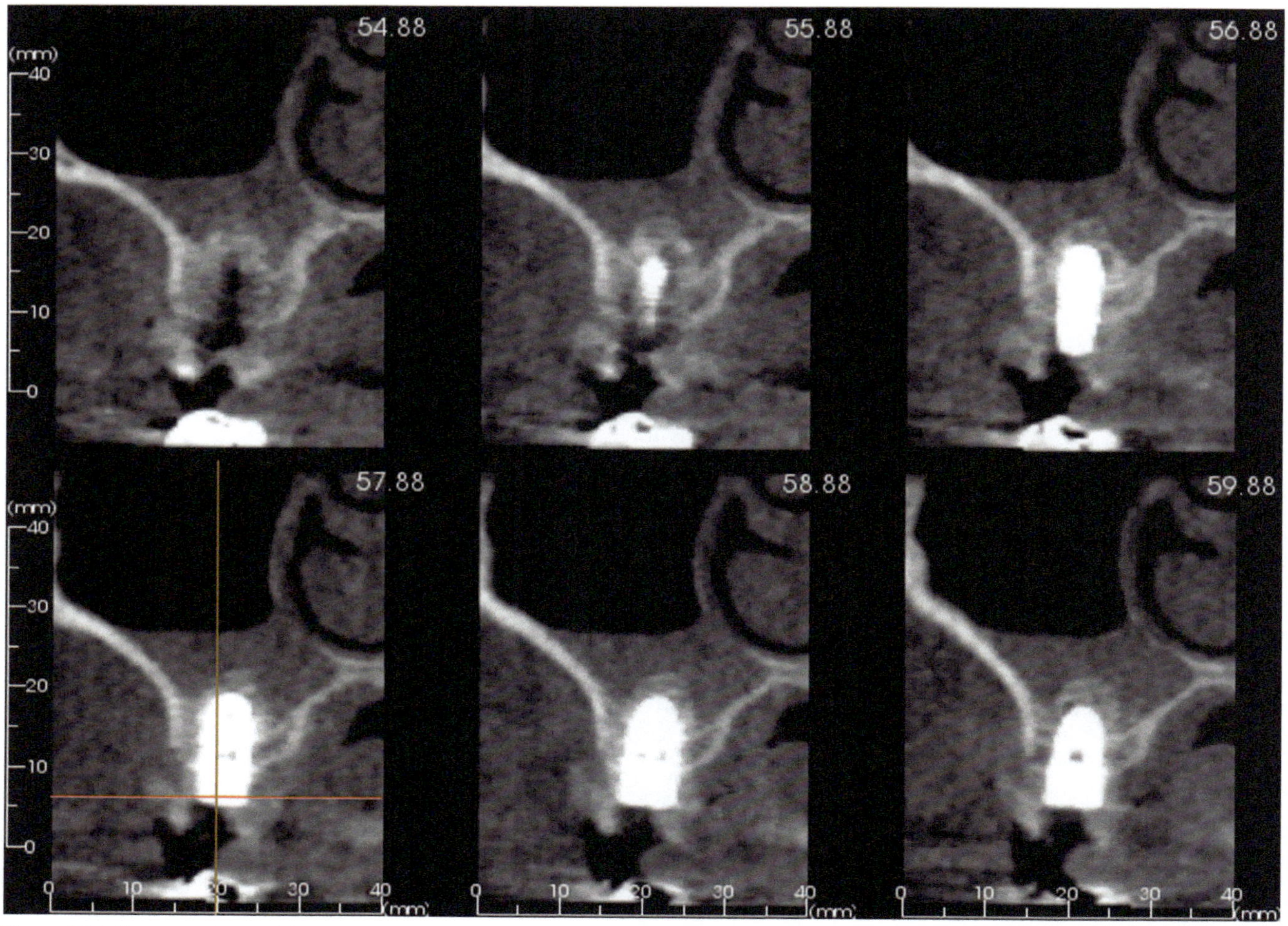

Figure 15.21 Post-operative CBCT views suggest a partial membrane tear with a horizontal radiodensity consistent with bleeding within the sinus. There appears to be graft containment manifested by the spherical apical peri-implant graft density.© Daniel R. Cullum.

sinus precautions, sinus spectrum antibiotics, and post-operative convalescence also would be indicated.

Conclusions

TASE procedures are an effective and minimally invasive approach for placing dental implants in the resorbed posterior maxilla, but require advanced training and recognition of the indications and limitations of the various approaches. Planning for OSFE (i.e. with no graft material used), the appropriate implant length can be 1–2(3) mm longer than the available subantral bone height, whereas with BAOSFE the planned implant length can be 3–4(5) mm longer than the available subantral bone height. The vertical height elevation achievable with OSFE or BAOSFE will be reduced for sites with broad and flat sinus floor anatomy. Therefore, to safely place a 10 mm long implant with these techniques, 6–8 mm of original subantral bone height is required; otherwise a more advanced technique may be needed. Many implant sites requiring sinus elevation have <7 mm of bone; in this situation, short, tapered implants (≤8 mm) in combination with TASE may be an appealing option. However, little data exist on outcomes with short, threaded implants in sites with ≤4 mm of subantral bone height. Use of reamer drills and Piezosurgery tips to approach the sinus floor are both significant technical advances that can reduce the need for osteotomes and malleting. However, a sloping sinus floor or sinus septa are best managed with the classic BAOSFE or the hydraulic technique. Application of advanced techniques, including joined adjacent sites and CSFE, offer potential for significantly greater sinus elevation. However, they also present greater technical demands for the surgeon. Careful treatment planning for selection of a TASE or open lateral sinus grafting technique will ensure that patients with edentulous posterior maxillae are treated successfully with the least invasive and most predictable approach.

References

1. Atwood D. Reduction of residual ridges: A major oral disease entity. J Prosthetic Dent 1971; 26: 266–279.
2. Van Steenberghe D, Lekholm U, Bolender C, et al. The applicability of osseointegrated oral implants in the rehabilitation of partial edentulism: a prospective multicenter study on 558 fixtures. Int J Oral Maxillofac Implants 1990; 5: 272–282.
3. Wyatt C, Zarb G. Treatment outcomes of patients with implant-supported fixed partial prostheses. J Oral Maxillofac Implants 1998; 13: 204–211.
4. Tawil G, Younan R. Clinical evaluation of short machined surface implants followed for 12 to 96 months. Int J Oral Maxillofac Implants 2003; 18: 894–901.
5. Weng D, Jacobson Z, Tarnow D, et al. A prospective multicenter clinical of 3i machined-surface implants. Results after 6 years of follow-up. Int J Oral Maxillofac Implants 2003; 18: 417–423.
6. Herrmann I, Lekholm U, Holm S, Kultje C. Evaluation of patient and implant characteristics as potential prognostic factors for oral implant failures. Int J Oral Maxillofac Implants 2005; 20: 220–230.

7. Pilliar R, Sagals G, Meguid S, et al. Threaded versus porous-surfaced implants as anchorage units for orthodontic treatment. Three-dimensional fine element analysis of peri-implant bone tissue stresses. Int J Oral Maxillofac Implants 2006; 21: 879–889.
8. Boyne PJ, James RA. Grafting of the maxillary sinus floor with bone and marrow. J Oral Surg 1980; 38: 613–616.
9. Tatum H Jr. Maxillary and sinus implant reconstructions. Dent Clin North Am 1986; 30: 207–229.
10. Smiler D, Johnson P, Lozada J. Sinus lift grafts and endosseous implants: treatment of the atrophic posterior maxilla. Dent Clin North Am 1992; 36: 151–186.
11. Geurs N, Wang I-C, Shulman L, Jeffcoat M. Retrospective radiographic analysis of sinus graft and implant placement procedures from the Academy of Osseointegration Consensus Conference on Sinus Grafts. Int J Periodontics Restorative Dent 2001; 21: 517–523.
12. Chao Y-L, Chen H-H, Mei C-C, et al. Meta-regression analysis of the initial bone height for predicting implant survival rates of two sinus elevation procedures. J Clin Periodontol 2010; 37: 456–465.
13. Wallace S, Froum S. Effect of maxillary sinus augmentation on the survival of endosseous dental implants. A systematic review. Ann Periodontol 2003; 8: 328–343.
14. Del Fabbro M, Testori T, Francetti L, Weinstein R. Systematic review of survival rates for implants placed in the grafted maxillary sinus. Int J Periodontics Restorative Dent 2004; 24: 565–577.
15. Albrektsson T, Wennerberg A. Oral implant surfaces: part I: review focusing on topographic and chemical properties of different surfaces and *in vivo* responses to them. Int J Prosthodont 2004; 17: 536–543.
16. Bernard J, Szmukler-Moncler S, Pessotto S, et al. The anchorage of Brånemark and ITI implants of different lengths. I. An experimental study in the canine mandible. Clin Oral Implants Res 2003; 14: 593–600.
17. Velasquez-Plata D, Hovey L, Peach C, Alder M. Maxillary sinus septa: a 3-dimensional computerized tomographic scan analysis. Int J Oral Maxillofac Implants 2002; 17: 854–860.
18. Becker S, Terheyden H, Steinriede A, et al. Prospective observation of 41 perforations of the Schneiderian membrane during sinus floor elevation. Clin Oral Implants Res 2008; 19: 1285–1289.
19. Misch CM. The pharmacological management of maxillary sinus elevation surgery. J Oral Implantol 1992; 18: 15–23.
20. Schwartz-Arad D, Herzberg R, Dolev E. The prevalence of surgical complications of the sinus graft procedure and their impact on implant survival. J Periodontol 2004; 75: 511–516.
21. Hong Y-H, Mun S-K. A case of massive maxillary sinus bleeding after dental implant. Int J Oral Maxillofac Surg 2011; 40: 758–760.
22. Chiapasco M, Felisati G, Maccari A, et al. The management of complications following displacement of oral implants in the paranasal sinuses: a multicenter clinical report and proposed treatment protocols. Int J Oral Maxillofac Surg 2009; 38: 1273–1278.
23. Ridaura-Ruiz L, Figueiredo R, Guinot-Moya R, et al. Accidental displacement of dental implants into the maxillary sinus: a report of nine cases. Clin Implant Dent Relat Res 2009; 11(Suppl 1) e38–e45.
24. Summers R. A new concept in maxillary implant surgery: the osteotome technique. Compend Contin Educ Dent 1994; 15: 152–160.
25. Summers R. The osteotome technique: part 3: less invasive methods of elevating the sinus floor. Compend Contin Educ Dent 1994; 15: 698–708.
26. Saadoun AP, Le Gall MG. Implant site preparation with osteotomes: principles and clinical application. Pract Periodontics Aesthet Dent 1996; 8:453–463.
27. Shalabi M, Manders P, Mulder J, et al. A meta-analysis of clinical studies to estimate the 4.5-year survival rate of implants placed with the osteotome technique. Int J Oral Maxillofac Implants 2007; 22: 110–116.
28. Tan W, Lang N, Zwahlen M, Pjetursson B. A systematic review of the success of sinus floor elevation and survival of implants inserted in combination with sinus floor elevation. Part II: transalveolar technique. J Clin Periodontol 2008; 35(Suppl 8): 241–254.
29. Del Fabbro M, Corbella S, Weinstein T, et al. Implant survival rates after osteotome-mediated sinus augmentation: a systematic review. Clin Implant Dent Relat Res 2012; 14(Suppl 1): e159–e168.
30. Jurisic M, Markovic A, Radulovic M, et al. Maxillary sinus floor augmentation: comparing osteotome with lateral window immediate and delayed implant placements. An interim report. Oral Surg Oral Med Oral Pathol Oral Radiol Endod 2008; 106: 820–827.
31. Kim S-M, Park J-W, Suh J-Y, et al. Bone-added osteotome technique versus lateral approach for sinus floor elevation: a comparative radiographic study. Implant Dent 2011; 20: 465–470.
32. Uckan S, Tamer Y, Deniz K. Survival rates of implants inserted in the maxillary sinus area by internal or external approach. Implant Dent 2011; 20: 476–479.
33. Nkenke E, Schelegel A, Schultze-Mosgau S, et al. The endoscopically controlled osteotome sinus floor elevation: a preliminary prospective study. Int J Oral Maxillofac Implants 2002; 17: 557–566.
34. Engelke W, Schwarzwaller W, Behnsen A, Jacobs HG. Subantroscopic laterobasal sinus floor augmentation (SALSA): an up-to-5-year clinical study. Int J Oral Maxillofac Implants 2002; 17: 135–143.
35. Vercellotti T, Nevins M, Jensen OT. Piezoelectric bone surgery for sinus bone grafting. In: The Sinus Graft, 2 ed., JensenOT, ed. Chicago, IL: Quintessence, 2006, pp. 273–279.
36. Leziy S, Miller B. Guided implant surgery and the use of osteotomes for rehabilitation of the maxilla. Pract Proced Aesthet Dent 2006; 18: 293–295.
37. Fugazzotto PA. Sinus floor augmentation at the time of maxillary molar extraction: technique and report of preliminary results. Int J Oral Maxillofac Implants 1999; 14: 536–542.
38. Barone A, Cornelinin R, Ciaglia R, Covani U. Implant placement in fresh extraction sockets and simultaneous osteotome sinus floor elevation: a case series. Int J Periodontics Restorative Dent 2008; 28: 283–289.
39. Summers RB. The osteotome technique: part 4 – future site development. Compend Contin Educ Dent 1995; 16: 1080–1092.
40. Kang T. Sinus elevation using a staged osteotome technique for site development prior to implant placement in sites with less than 5 mm of native bone. Int J Periodontics Restorative Dent 2008; 28: 73–81.
41. Sotirakis EG, Gonshor A. Elevation of the maxillary sinus floor with hydraulic pressure. J Oral Implantol 2005; 31: 197–204.
42. Sohn DS, Lee JS, An KM, Choi BJ. Piezoelectric internal sinus elevation (PISE) technique: a new method for internal sinus elevation. Implant Dent 2009; 18: 458–463.
43. Sentineri R, Dagnino G. Sinus physiolift: a new technique for a less invasive great sinus augmentation with crestal approach. J Osteol Biomater 2011; 2: 69–75.
44. Ucer C. Nasal suction technique for maxillary sinus floor elevation: a report of 24 consecutive patients. Int J Oral Maxillofac Implants 2009; 24: 1138–1143.
45. Kfir E, Kfir V, Mijiritsky E, et al. Minimally invasive antral membrane balloon elevation followed by maxillary bone augmentation and implant fixation. J Oral Implantol 2006; 32: 26–33.
46. Bruschi G, Scipioni A, Calesini G. Localized management of the sinus floor with simultaneous implant placement. Int J Oral Maxillofac Implants 1998; 13: 219–226.
47. Winter A, Pollack AS, Odrich RB. Sinus/alveolar crest tenting (SACT): a new technique for implant placement in atrophic maxillary ridges without bone grafts or membranes. Int J Periodontics Restorative Dent 2003; 23: 557–565.
48. Cullum DR, Jensen OT. Trans-alveolar sinus elevation combined with ridge expansion. In: The Sinus Graft, 2nd ed., Jensen OT, ed. Chicago, IL: Quintessence, 2006, pp. 251–262.
49. Cullum DR. Advances in Bone Manipulation Techniques: Part 1. Osteotome Site Development and Minimally Invasive Sinus Elevation. Selected Readings in Oral and Maxillofacial Surgery. San Francisco, CA: Guild for Scientific Advancement in Oral and Maxillofacial Surgery, 2010, vol. 18, no. 4.
50. Schmidlin P, Muller J, Bindl A, Imfeld T. Sinus floor elevation using an osteotome technique without grafting materials or membranes. Int J Periodontics Restorative Dent 2008; 28: 401–409.
51. Gabbert O, Koob A, Schmitter M, Rammelsberg P. Implants placed in combination with internal sinus lift without graft material: an analysis of short-term failure. J Clin Periodontol 2009; 36: 177–183.
52. Gray H. Anatomy of the Human Body, 28th ed. Philadelphia, PA: Lea & Febiger, 1966.
53. Uchida Y, Masaaki G, Katsuki T, Soejima Y. Measurement of maxillary sinus volume using computerized tomographic images. Int J Oral Maxillofac Implants 1998; 13: 811–818.
54. Cho S, Wallace S, Froum S, Tarnow D. Influence of anatomy on Schneiderian membrane perforations during sinus elevation surgery: three-dimensional analysis. Pract Proced Aesthet Dent 2001; 13: 160–163.
55. Katranji A, Fotek P, Wang H. Sinus augmentation complications: etiology and treatment. Implant Dent 2008; 17: 339–346.
56. Garbacea A. Lozada JL, Church CA, et al. The incidence of maxillary sinus membrane perforation during endoscopically assessed crestal sinus floor elevation: a pilot study. J Oral Implantol 2012; 38: 345–359.
57. Pikos M. Maxillary sinus membrane repair: update on technique for large and complete perforations simultaneous excision and repair of sinus lesions. Implant Dent 2008; 17: 24–29.
58. Timmenga NM, Raghobar GM, Boering G, Van Weissenbruch R. Maxillary sinus function after sinus lifts for insertion of dental implants. J Oral Maxillofac Surg 1997; 55: 936–939.
59. Ferringo N, Laureti M, Fanali S. Dental implant placement in conjunction with osteotome sinus floor elevation: a 12-year life-table analysis from a prospective study on 588 ITI implants. Clin Oral Implants Res 2006; 17: 194–205.
60. Reiser G, Rabinovitz Z, Bruno J, et al. The evaluation of maxillary sinus membrane response following elevation with the crestal osteotome technique in human cadavers. Int J Oral Maxillofac Implants 2001; 16: 833–840.

61. Barengo M, Sivolella Z, Majzoub G, Cordioli G. Endoscopic evaluation of the bone added osteotome sinus floor elevation procedure. Int J Oral Maxillofac Surg 2004; 35: 185–194.
62. Deporter DA, Caudry S, Kermalli J, Adegbembo A. Further data on the predictability of the indirect sinus elevation procedure using with short, porous-surfaced dental implants. Int J Periodontics Rest Dent 2005; 25: 585–593.
63. Toffler M. Treating the atrophic maxilla by combining short implants with minimally invasive osteotome procedures. Pract Proced Aesthet Dent 2006; 18: 301–308.
64. Rosen P, Summers R, Mellado J, et al. The bone-added osteotome sinus floor elevation technique. Multicenter retrospective report of consecutively treated patients. Int J Oral Maxillofac Implants 1999; 14: 853–858.
65. Toffler M. Osteotome-mediated sinus floor elevation: a clinical report. Int J Oral Maxillofac Implants 2004; 19: 266–273.
66. Penarrocha-Diago M, Perez H, Garcia A, Guarinos J. Benign paroxysmal positional vertigo as a complication of osteotome expansion of the maxillary alveolar ridge. Int J Oral Maxillofac Surg 2001; 59: 106–107.
67. Simmons J, Triplett R, Schow S. Benign paroxysmal positional vertigo as a complication associated with osteotome use in the maxillofacial region. Int J Oral Maxillofac Implants 2005; 20: 477 (abstract).
68. Sammartino G, Mariniello M, Scaravilli M. Benign paroxysmal positional vertigo following closed sinus floor elevation procedure: mallet osteotomes vs. screwable osteotomes. A triple blind randomized controlled trial. Clin Oral Implants Res 2011; 22: 669–672.
69. Vernamonte S, Mauro V, Vernamonte S, Messina A. An unusual complication of osteotome sinus floor elevation: benign paroxysmal positional vertigo. Int J Oral Maxillofac Surg 2011; 40: 216–218.
70. Nkenke E, Kloss F, Schultze-Mosgau S, et al. Histomorphometric and fluorescence microscopic analysis of bone remodeling after installation of implants using an osteotome technique. Clin Oral Implants Res 2002; 13: 595–602.
71. Shayesteh Y, Khojasteh A, Siadat H, et al. A comparative study of crestal bone loss and implant stability between osteotome and conventional implant insertion techniques: a randomized controlled clinical trial study. Clin Implant Dent Relat Res 2013; 15: 350–357.
72. Nevins M, Nevins ML, Schupbach P, et al. The impact of bone compression on bone-to-implant contact of an osseointegrated implant: a canine study. Int J Periodontics Restorative Dent 2012; 32: 637–645.
73. Nobrega A, Norton A, Silva J, et al. The osteotome versus conventional drilling technique for implant site preparation: a comparative study in the rabbit. Int J Periodontics Restorative Dent 2012; 32: e109–e115.
74. Buchter A, Kleinheinz J, Wiesmann H, et al. Interface reaction at dental implants inserted in condensed bone. Clin Oral Implants Res 2005; 16: 509–517.
75. Sforza N, Marzadori M, Zucchelli G. Simplified osteotome sinus augmentation technique with simultaneous implant placement: a clinical study. Int J Periodontics Restorative Dent 2008; 28: 291–299.
76. Fu P-Y. Piezoelectric-assisted osteotome-mediated sinus floor elevation: an innovative approach. Implant Dent 2010; 19: 299–303.
77. Kim J-M, Sohn D-S, Heo J-U, et al. Minimally invasive sinus augmentation using ultrasonic piezoelectric vibration and hydraulic pressure: a multicenter retrospective study. Implant Dent 2012; 21: 536–542.
78. Summers RB. The osteotome technique: part 2 – the ridge expansion osteotomy (REO) procedure. Compend Contin Educ Dent 1994; 15: 422–436.
79. Cullum D. Advances in Bone Manipulation Techniques. Part 2: Osteo-Mobilization for Horizontal and Vertical Implant Site Development. Selected Readings in Oral and Maxillofacial Surgery. San Francisco, CA: Guild for Scientific Advancement in Oral and Maxillofacial Surgery, 2010, vol. 18, no. 5.
80. Boyne P. Analysis of performance of root-form endosseous implants placed in the maxillary sinus. J Long Term Eff Med Implants 1993; 3: 143–159.
81. Leblebicioglu B, Ersanli S, Karabuda C, et al. Radiographic evaluation of dental implants placed using an osteotome technique. J Periodontol 2005; 76: 385–390.
82. Kolerman R, Moses O, Artzi Z, et al. Maxillary sinus augmentation by the crestal core elevation technique. J Periodontol 2011; 82: 41–51.
83. Tilotta F, Lazaroo B, Gaudy JF. Gradual and safe technique for sinus floor elevation using trephines and osteotomes with stops. A cadaveric anatomic study. Oral Surg Oral Med Oral Pathol Oral Radiol Endod 2008; 106: 210–216.
84. Yamada J, Park H-J. Internal sinus manipulation (ISM) procedures: a technical report. Clin Implant Dent Relat Res 2007; 9: 128–135.
85. Hunter W, Bradick J, Houser S, et al. Maxillary sinusitis resulting from ostium plugging by dislodged bone graft: case report. J Oral Maxillofac Surg 2009; 67: 1495–1498.
86. Bragger U, Gerber C, Joss A, et al. Patterns of tissue remodeling after placement of ITI dental implants using an osteotome technique: a longitudinal radiographic case cohort study. Clin Oral Implants Res 2004; 15: 158–166.
87. Deporter D, Todescan R, Caudry S. Simplifying management of the posterior maxilla using short porous-surfaced dental implants and simultaneous indirect sinus elevation. Int J Periodontics Restorative Dent 2000; 20: 477–485.
88. Lai H-C, Zhang Z-Y, Wang F, et al. Resonance frequency analysis of stability on ITI implants with osteotome sinus floor elevation technique without grafting: a 5-month prospective study. Clin Oral Implants Res 2008; 19: 469–475.
89. Markovic A, Colic S, Drazic R, et al. Resonance frequency analysis as a reliable criterion for early loading of sandblasted/acid-etched active surface implants placed by the osteotome sinus floor elevation technique. Int J Oral Maxillofac Implants 2011; 26: 718–724.
90. Corrente G, Abundo R, Bermond des Ambrois A, et al. Short porous implants in the posterior maxilla: a 3-year report of a prospective study. Int J Periodontics Restorative Dent 2009; 29: 23–29.
91. Pjetursson B, Ignjatovic D, Matuliene G, et al. Transalveolar maxillary floor elevation using osteotomes with or without grafting material. Part I: implant survival and patients' perception. Clin Oral Implants Res 2009; 20: 667–676.
92. Renouard F, Nisand D. Impact of implant length and diameter on survival rates. Clin Oral Implants Res 2006; 17(Suppl 2): 35–51.
93. Pjetursson B, Ignjatovic D, Matuliene G, et al. Transalveolar maxillary floor elevation using osteotomes with or without grafting material. Part II: radiographic tissue remodeling. Clin Oral Implants Res 2009; 20: 677–683.
94. Taschieri S, Del Fabbro M. Post-extraction osteotome sinus floor elevation technique using plasma-rich growth factors. Implant Dent 2011; 20: 418–424.
95. Toffler M, Toscano N, Holtzclaw D. Osteotome-mediated sinus floor elevation using only platelet-rich fibrin: an early report on 110 patients. Implant Dent 2010; 19: 447–453.
96. Ahn S-H, Park E-J, Kim E-S. Reamer-mediated transalveolar sinus floor elevation without osteotome and simultaneous implant placement in the maxillary molar area: clinical outcomes of 391 implants in 380 patients. Clin Oral Implants Res 2012; 23: 866–872.
97. Fugazzotto P. Immediate implant placement following a modified trephine trephine/osteotome approach: success rates of 116 implants up to 4 years in function. Int J Oral Maxillofac Implants 2002; 17: 113–120.
98. Mazur Z. The use of minimally invasive antral membrane balloon elevation (MIAMBE) to treat posterior maxilla: a clinical presentation. J Implant Reconstr Dent 2010; 2: 26–31.
99. Peñarrocha-Diago M, Galán-Gil S, Carrillo-García C, et al. Transcrestal sinus lift and implant placement using the sinus balloon technique. Med Oral Patol Oral Cir Bucal 2012; 17: e122–e128.
100. Bensaha T. Outcomes of flapless crestal maxillary sinus elevation under hydraulic pressure. Int J Oral Maxillofac Implants 2012; 27: 1223–1229.
101. Pommer B, Watzek G. Gel-pressure technique for flapless transcrestal maxillary sinus floor elevation: a preliminary cadaveric study of a new surgical technique. Int J Oral Maxillofac Implants 2009; 24: 817–822.
102. Stelzle F, Benner K-U. Evaluation of different methods of indirect sinus floor elevation for elevation heights of 10 mm: an experimental ex vivo study. Clin Implant Dent Relat Res 2011; 13: 124–133.
103. Kim J-M, Sohn D-S, Bae M-S, et al. Flapless transcrestal sinus augmentation using hydrodynamic piezoelectric internal sinus elevation with autologous concentrated growth factors alone. Implant Dent 2014; 23: 168–174.
104. Soardi C, Wang H-L. New crestal approach for lifting sinus in the extremely atrophic upper maxillae. Clin Adv Periodontics 2012; 2: 179–185.
105. Bruschi G, Crespi R, Cappare P, Gherlone E. Transcrestal sinus floor elevation: a retrospective study of 46 patients up to 16 years. Clin Implant Dent Relat Res 2012; 14(5): 759–767.
106. Barone A, Orlando B, Tonelli P, Covani U. Survival rate for implants placed in the posterior maxilla with and without sinus augmentation: a comparative cohort study. J Periodontol 2011; 82: 219–226.
107. Spray J, Black C, Morris H, Ochi S. The influence of bone thickness on facial marginal bone response: stage 1 placement through stage 2 uncovering. Ann Periodontol 2000; 5: 119–128.
108. Qahash M, Susin C, Polimeni G, et al. Bone healing dynamics at buccal peri-implant sites. Clin Oral Implants Res 2008; 19: 166–172.
109. Takuma T, Oishi K, Manabe T, et al. Buccal bone resorption around posterior implants after surgery: a 1-year prospective study. Int J Oral Maxillofac Implants 2014; 29: 634–641.
110. Calin C, Petre A, Drafta S. Osteotome-mediated sinus floor elevation: a systematic review and meta-analysis. Int J Oral Maxillfac Implants 2014; 29: 558–576.
111. Nedir R, Bischof M, Vazquez L, et al. Osteotome sinus floor elevation without grafting material: a 1-year prospective pilot study with ITI implants. Clin Oral Implants Res 2006; 17: 679–686.
112. He L, Chang X, Liu Y. Sinus floor elevation using osteotome technique without grafting materials: a 2-year retrospective study. Clin Oral Implants Res 2013; 24: 63–67.
113. Fermergard R, Astrand P. Osteotome sinus floor elevation without bone grafts – a 3-year retrospective study with Astra Tech implants. Clin Implant Dent Relat Res 2012; 14: 198–205.

CHAPTER 16

Ridge Expansion

Daniel R. Cullum
Private Practice, Coeur d'Alene, ID; Loma Linda University Department of OMS, Loma Linda, CA; UCLA Department of OMS, Los Angeles, CA, USA

Introduction

When teeth are extracted without simultaneous socket preservation grafting, predictable loss in alveolar ridge width and height occurs (Figure 16.1a and b).[1,2] While osseointegrated implants have greatly advanced dental reconstruction,[3–5] adequate bone quality and quantity are required for long-term implant success.[6] Various approaches have been introduced to manage vertical and horizontal alveolar dimension loss, including: (i) guided bone regeneration (GBR),[7] (ii) block and particulate grafting,[8–11] (iii) "ridge splitting,"[12–16] (iv) distraction osteogenesis,[17,18] (v) composite microvascular free flaps,[19] and (vi) the use of biologics and biomimetics.[20–23] These methods as originally proposed often required multiple or staged procedures with prolonged healing intervals, increased cost, and post-operative discomfort. Refinements in techniques and indications have led to faster, less invasive, and predictable treatment options being available, many of which are discussed in this textbook.[24–31]

Alternatives to conventional implant site development procedures include a group of bone manipulation techniques including ridge expansion (RE) or "bone spreading" that can be used to mobilize vital bone via plastic bending, shaping, or condensation of tissue as a "bone flap" or "bone–periosteal flap."[12,15,32–37] These approaches result in contour or dimensional changes while preserving bone integrity and viability. The concept is to manipulate the residual bone to create an intrabony cavity with a wider base or taller roof (i.e. a "four-wall bony defect") that heals like an extraction site by allowing access for mesenchymal stem cells and normal wound healing mechanisms[35] (Figure 16.1c and d).

These RE techniques can be broadly categorized as *osteo-condensation*[32,33] and *osteo-mobilization*,[37] and are commonly used in maxilla where bone is spongy and malleable. Overcoming sinus pneumatization with trans-alveolar sinus elevation[38–41] has been discussed in Chapter 15, and can be used as a combined procedure with RE to achieve simultaneous increases in horizontal and vertical ridge dimensions of the deficient posterior maxilla[16,41,42] (see Chapter 17). Other bone manipulation techniques have application in the mandible with the technological advances of office-based cone beam computed tomography (CBCT) to facilitate treatment planning, piezoelectric bone surgery, rotary expanders, and tapered implant designs.[34,37,43] The advantages of these techniques include a reduced need for graft materials, simultaneous implant placement, reduced discomfort, and faster native bone healing. This chapter will review the scientific basis, clinical indications, and applications for bone manipulation to achieve RE in a minimally invasive manner, including appropriate flap designs and soft tissue enhancement techniques for esthetic dental implant reconstruction.

Literature review

Tatum first described RE techniques in the maxilla using partial-thickness flaps to preserve blood supply to the alveolus.[12] His rationale was that the preservation of blood supply via periosteal retention would minimize post-operative bone resorption. Summers later described a number of "osteotome" techniques for implant site development using full thickness flaps, hand end-cutting osteotomes and a surgical mallet to develop implant osteotomies.[32,33] His "RE osteotomy" advanced the principle of avoiding bone removal during implant site development by using limited or no drilling. Osteotomes of increasing diameter were used to achieve lateral compression/condensation of spongy maxillary bone, and in so doing to increase peri-implant bone density and bone-to-implant contact, and in some instances to increase ridge width at the osteotomy site (Figure 16.2a). *Osteo-condensation* best describes these minimally invasive osteotome techniques. A modification of the technique uses rotary mechanical expanders instead of hand osteotomes to accomplish the osteo-condensation, reducing surgical manipulation and patient awareness[37,43] (Figure 16.2b).

Osteo-mobilization involves the use of precise bone osteotomies of the residual alveolus to allow progressive intraoperative manipulation and outward mobilization of buccal bone, thereby increasing alveolar horizontal dimension.[37] The outcome is an expansion defect that opens crestally, like a book at its binding. The defect created has its widest dimension crestally and tapers apically, and the procedure often restores the alveolar volume and contour to near-normal dimensions (Figure 16.1c and d). The technique in its most basic form has been described as "ridge-splitting," achieving widening with a "greenstick" fracture or "out-fracture" of the buccal cortical plate using osteotomes, bone chisels, and/or rotary mechanical instruments.[13,14] Grafting and/or fixation of the fractured buccal segment can be completed using GBR principles with or without

Minimally Invasive Dental Implant Surgery, First Edition. Edited by Daniel R. Cullum and Douglas Deporter.

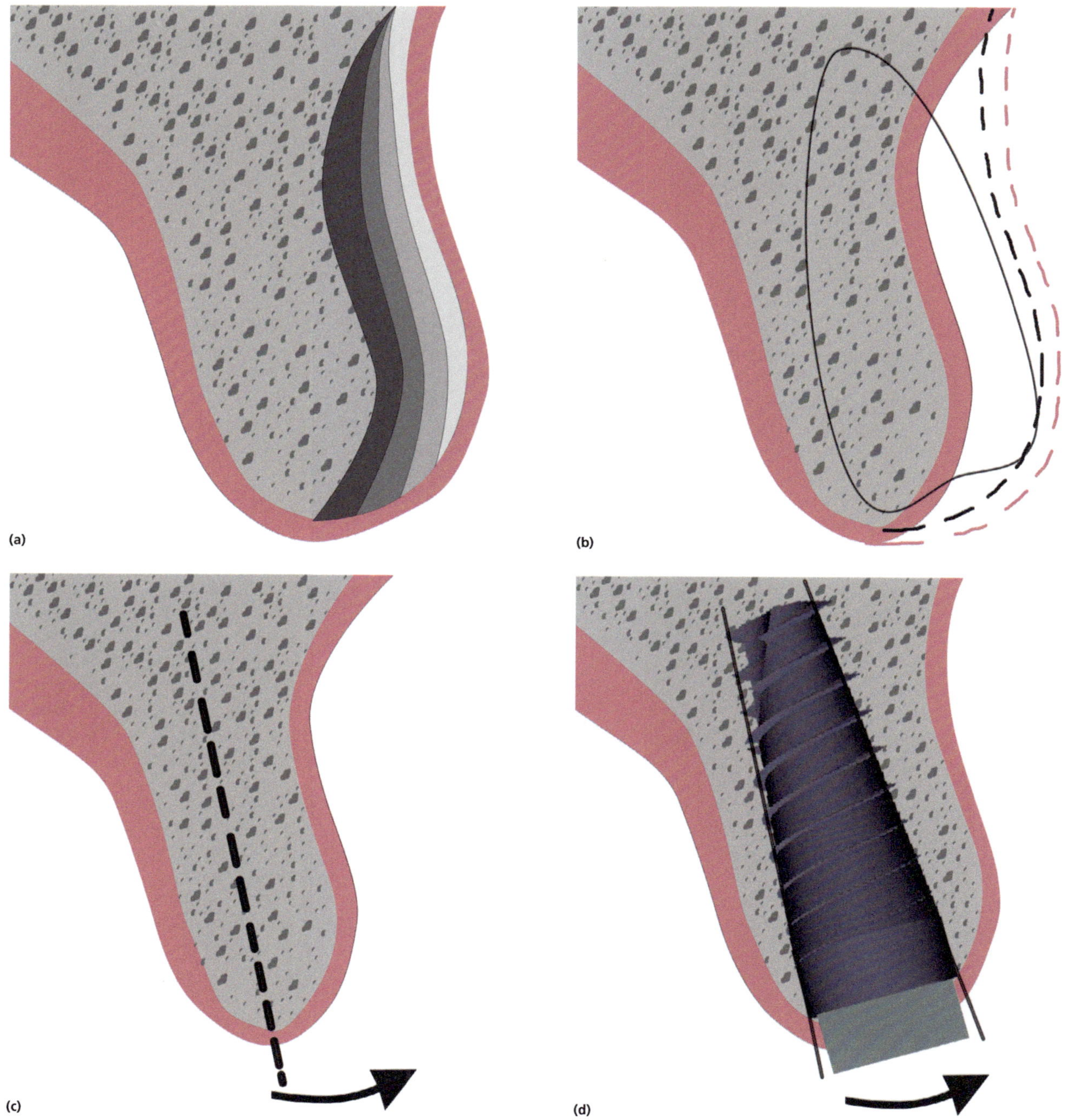

Figure 16.1 Progressive horizontal bone loss resulting in reduced bone volume and bone incision design for ridge expansion. (a) Progressive horizontal bone loss. (b) Progressive horizontal bone loss resulting in reduced bone volume and challenges for "restorative-driven" implant positioning. (c) Bone incision design for osteo-mobilization. (d) Osteo-mobilization with buccal bone manipulation to the facial for site development to allow a "restorative-driven" implant position. *Source:* (a–c) © Daniel R. Cullum. (d) Cullum DR, Ridge Expansion and Piezoelecric Bone Surgery. In: The Piezoelectric Bone Surgery. A New Paradigm, Vercellotti T, ed. Quintessenza Edizioni, 2015. Reproduced with permission of Quintessence Publishing Co., Inc.

simultaneous implant placement and primary soft tissue closure.[44–46] However, the buccal segment often ends up with a limited or complete compromise of blood supply, acting as a free graft with a high risk of resorption. Another variation of RE (also referred to as "bone spreading") mobilizes the buccal cortical plate from the stable palatal cortex, maintaining the continuity of the expanded buccal segment as a viable "bone flap" or "bone–periosteal flap."[12,15,16] RE techniques include the use of mechanical expanders of rotary "screw" design (Figure 16.2b) and/or hand osteotomes of several modified designs (Figure 16.3).[12,15,37,43]

RE in the maxilla is best approached using a partial-thickness flap or a limited crestal access with a "flapless" approach

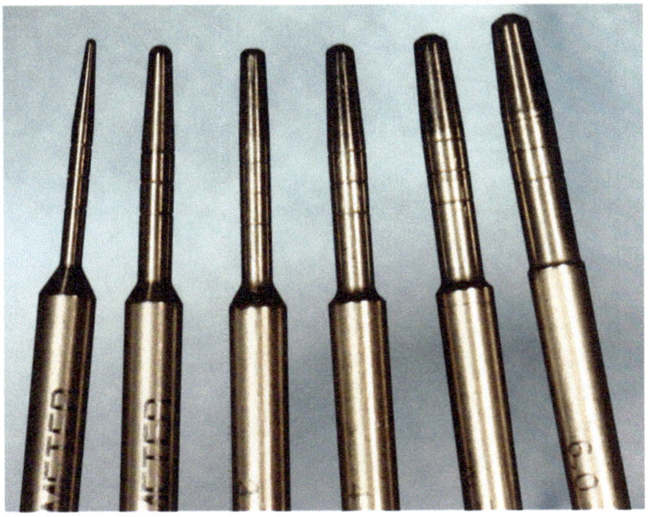
(a)

Figure 16.2 (a) Tapered osteotomes (NobelBiocare USA, Yorba Linda, CA). (b) Rotary "screw" expanders (Meisinger USA, Centennial, CO) for osteo-condensation. *Source*: (a) Cullum DR, Ridge Expansion and Piezoelectric Bone Surgery. In: The Piezoelectric Bone Surgery. A New Paradigm, Vercellotti T, ed. Quintessenza Edizioni, 2015. Reproduced with permission of Quintessence Publishing Co., Inc. (b) © Daniel R. Cullum

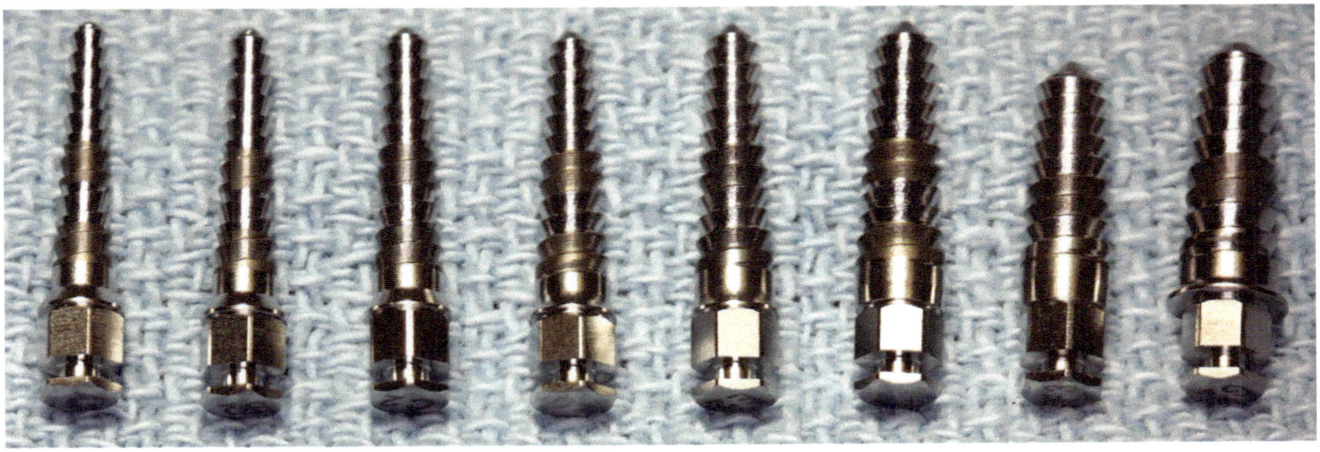
(b)

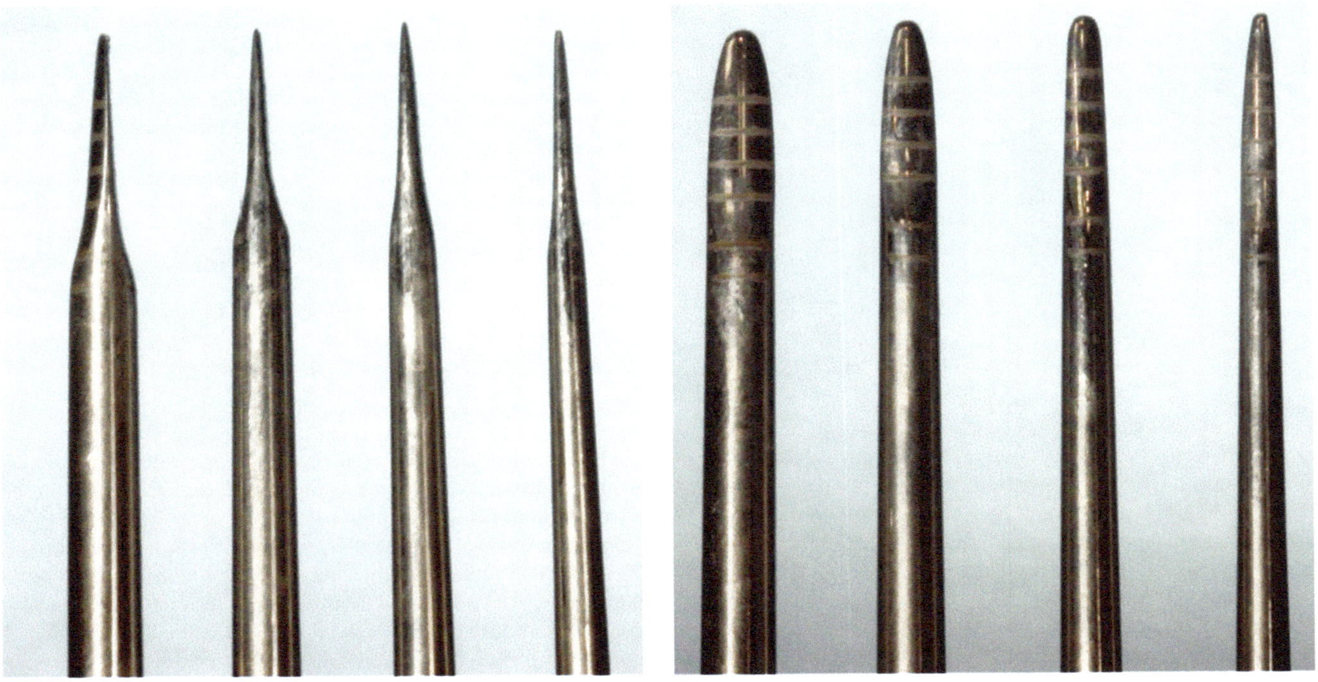
(a) (b)

Figure 16.3 Modified osteotomes for RE (H&H Co, Ontario, CA): (a, b) "spade" osteotomes;

(Continued)

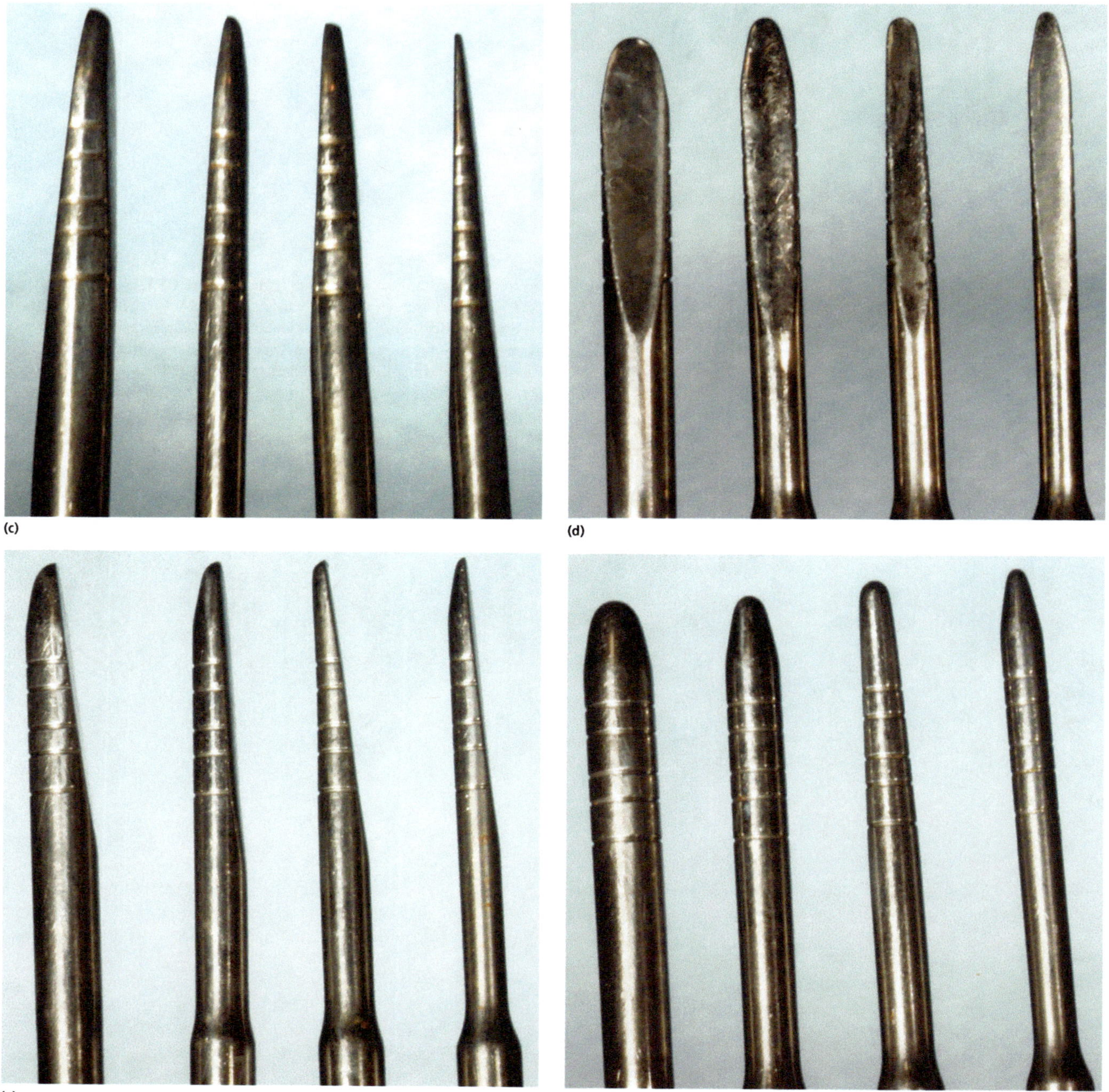

(c) (d) (e) (f)

Figure 16.3 (Continued)
(c, d) "bi-bevel" osteotomes; (e, f) "D" osteotomes. *Source:* Cullum DR, Ridge Expansion and Piezoelecric Bone Surgery. In: The Piezoelectric Bone Surgery. A New Paradigm, Vercellotti T, ed. Quintessenza Edizioni, 2015. Reproduced with permission of Quintessence Publishing Co., Inc.

to preserve the vascular supply[35,47,48] (Figure 16.4). Osteomobilization techniques utilizing substantial bone flap mobilization require maintenance of a thick supraperiosteal dissection to preserve vascular supply[49] or a planned full-thickness flap to permit over-grafting of the expanded segment using GBR and primary closure. The "split graft" with "greenstick" out-fracture and the "island flap" described by Jensen[50] are "osteo-periosteal" bone flaps with osteotomies designed to maintain continuity of the overlying soft tissue flap, the latter with complete mobilization of the bone as an "island." The intervening bone gap is grafted and requires primary closure with implant placement delayed after adequate graft healing.

Preservation of the vascular supply using an intact bone–periosteal flap (minimum thickness of 2 mm) allows normal healing of the inter-bone gap without the need for grafting.[35] In order for this procedure to be successful, the soft tissue flap design (full thickness, partial thickness, or flapless), including its thickness, mobilization, and stability is critical to avoid unwanted resorption

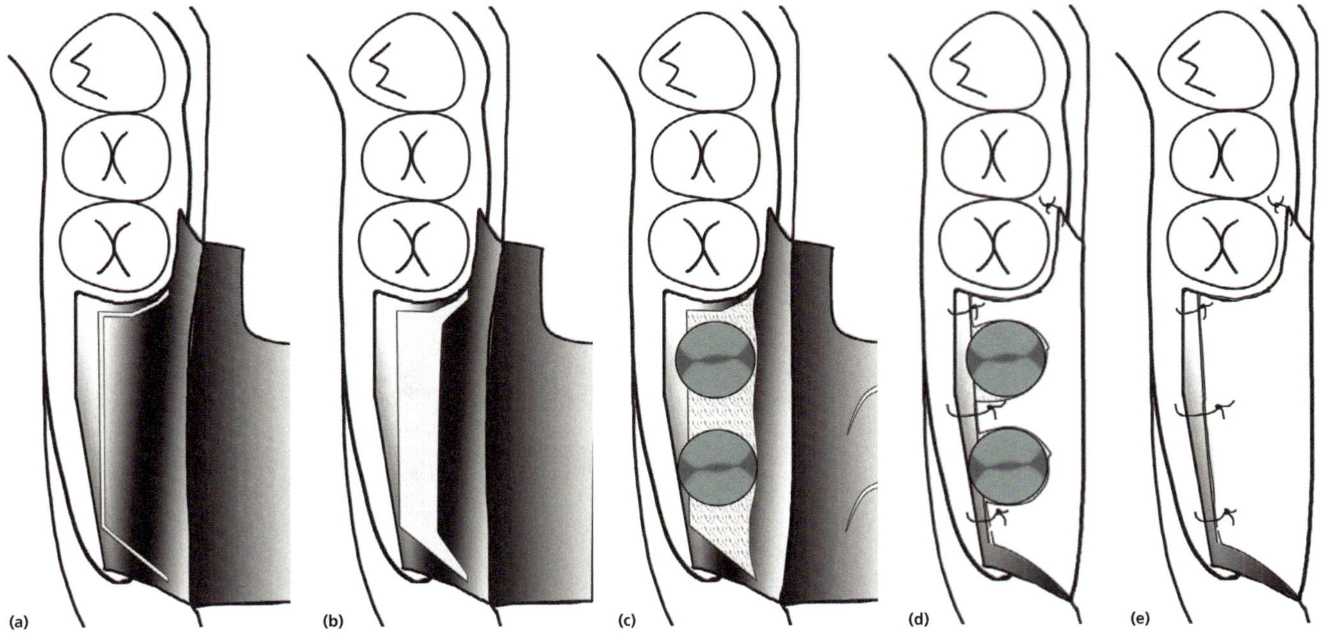

Figure 16.4 Posterior maxilla – split-thickness RE with intrabony osteotomy, internal lateral beveled bone incisions, transgingival tapered implant placement with apical repositioned flap. (a) Palatal incised, buccal-based, split-thickness flap design with completion of Piezosurgery intrabony incisions. (b) The buccal bone–periosteal flap is progressively mobilized to the facial with chisels and "D" expanders. Care is taken to maintain flap continuity and preserve the overlying periosteum. (c) Implants placed with expansion gap filled with heme-saturated collagen and particulate grafting of the anterior and posterior vertical buccal defects. (d) With an abundance of attached tissue, anterior-based "finger" flaps are developed and the flap is anterior and apically repositioned. (e) Alternate closure for a staged approach, showing near primary closure with periosteal margins exposed for secondary intention healing. © Daniel R. Cullum.

of the expanded segment.[47] Ultrasonic bone-cutting instrumentation has increased bone cutting efficiency and reduced lateral thermal damage to bone, thus increasing predictability of the procedure.[34,51,52] Significant differences in terminology and technical difficulty with the broad group of procedures described as "RE" may account for the varied reports of success and complications.

Anatomic considerations

Evaluation of facial, dento-facial, and dento-gingival parameters and esthetics must be completed prior to initiating an RE procedure.[53–55] Treatment planning considerations should include smile assessment, quality and quantity of keratinized gingival tissue (width and biotype), vestibular depth, muscle or frenal tissue attachments and adjacent teeth or implants at the intended surgical site (see Chapters 1 to 8).[55–58] Enhancement of soft tissues may be necessary to prevent wound dehiscence during initial healing or later recession of the soft tissues surrounding the final implant-supported restoration. Preparatory or simultaneous soft tissue procedures, such as laser frenoplasty, vestibuloplasty, and/or augmentation with connective tissue grafting, are often needed.[30,59–61]

In the anterior maxilla flapless or split-thickness exposure will preserve crestal blood supply to the alveolus, providing more predictable hard and soft tissue outcomes after healing. In the posterior maxilla, split-thickness flap development is clinically more challenging than a full-thickness flap, but allows retention of the periosteal blood supply to the bone flap.[12] In posterior mandible it is not practical to use split-thickness dissections since the periosteum here is thinner and more friable. Final soft tissue levels also are esthetically less critical; therefore, in posterior mandible, a full-thickness flap approach is preferred.[37] In all cases, the viability and thickness of the cortical buccal bone flap after its mobilization will determine if additional bone augmentation with over-grafting is necessary.

Bone quantity and quality can vary greatly, and will require careful preoperative clinical and radiographic analysis.[62] Office-based CBCT technology allows preoperative analysis of ridge dimensions, sinus anatomy, and relative indication of bone density (see Chapter 2).[63] With recently grafted sites or osteoporotic bone there can be altered or inconsistent bone quality and compliance. This can result in increased risk of buccal or palatal bone wall fracture, reduced vascular supply, and/or reduced primary implant stability and load-bearing capacity.[64,65] Examples of anatomical variances showing sites with progressively more complex expansion sites are demonstrated on CBCT analysis in Figure 16.5.

Anatomic factors that will influence risk with RE include:[37]

1 Significant cortical bone thickness and density, making it less flexible.
2 Volume of the medullary component of bone. The procedure becomes more difficult with progressive atrophy; that is, "bi-cortical" bone.
3 Varying degrees of undercut (vertical dimension) and/or a steep slope up to adjacent tooth roots (horizontal dimension). Increased undercut or convexity will act as a "buttress" for the buccal plate, reducing its mobility and increasing the risk of fracture or apical one-third buccal perforation.
4 Mesio-distal dimension of the bone flap. The longer this dimension, the greater area over which the bending moment is spread.

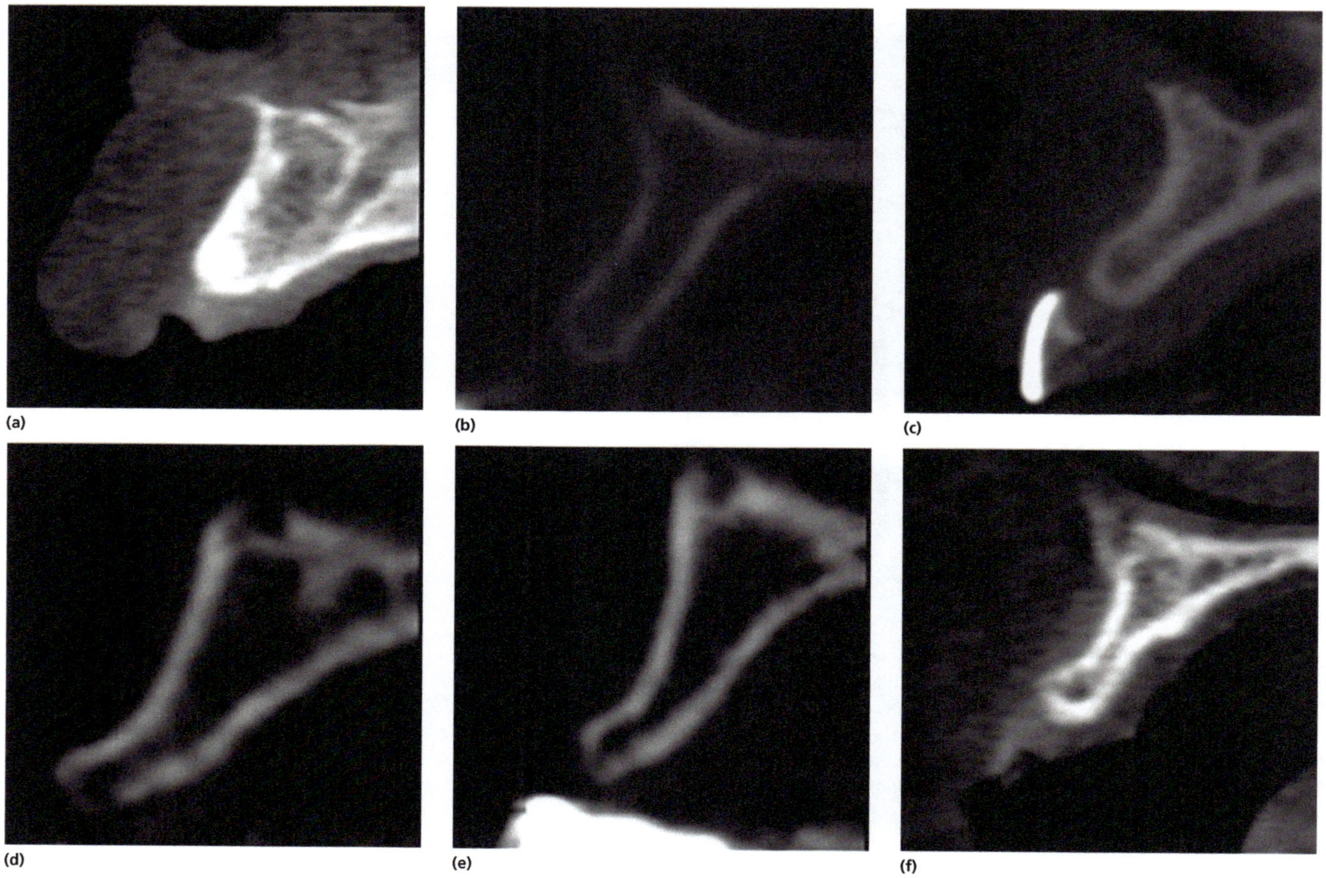

Figure 16.5 CBCT images of increasing degrees of horizontal bone loss, labial undercut, reduced marrow volume, and cortical bone margin thickness. (a) Mild horizontal dimensional loss after grafting for site preservation. (b) Mild horizontal loss with minimal undercut and good marrow–cortical bone anatomy. (c) Mild horizontal bone loss with increasing undercut and reduced marrow space. (d) Moderate horizontal bone loss with moderate undercut and reduced marrow space. (e) Moderate to severe horizontal bone loss with moderate undercut and reduced marrow space. (f) Severe horizontal bone loss with severe undercut and reduced marrow space with thick "bi-cortical" bone. *Source*: (a) Cullum DR, Ridge Expansion and Piezoelectric Bone Surgery. In: The Piezoelectric Bone Surgery. A New Paradigm, Vercellotti T, ed. Quintessenza Edizioni, 2015. Reproduced with permission of Quintessence Publishing Co., Inc. (b–f) © Daniel R. Cullum.

5 Too large an implant diameter. An implant with diameter >4.3 mm significantly increases risk of fracture.
6 Implant design with an aggressive tapered macrogeometry and a non-expanded collar. A tapered implant will fit the "v"-shaped expansion defect, while a non-expanded collar design will maintain maximum buccal bone thickness and avoid excess pressure on the coronal bone flap margin (Figure 16.6; optimal implant design).

The location of the RE also can affect the outcome. Expansion at an isolated maxillary canine location can be predictable with moderate bone volume and compliance. Management of a multi-tooth segment with osteo-mobilization can be completed anteriorly from the maxillary canine to the central incisor or posteriorly toward the molar region. However, the canine position will often act as a "buttress" around the corner of the arch, increasing the risk of uncontrolled fracture. Designing the bone flap through the canine site, therefore, typically requires a planned vertical bone release at the mesial or distal of the canine to avoid a vertical fracture usually at the height of contour of the implant site.[37] The list of anatomic factors that reduce bone compliance also increase the difficulty. Defects with severe atrophy, undercut, "bi-cortical" bone, and small mesio-distal dimension are best managed with other augmentation techniques.

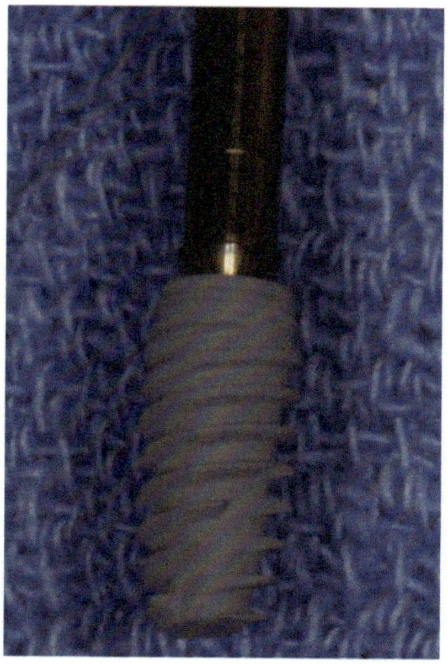

Figure 16.6 Tapered implant design features. © Daniel R. Cullum.

Surgical considerations

The advantages of RE techniques can include simultaneous implant placement, shorter treatment time, less discomfort, and the restoration of the buccal arch dimension for restorative-driven implant positioning. For patients with potential wound healing compromise, such as those with diabetes, the vascular bone flap may be less susceptible to overlying soft tissue dehiscence following RE than following block or particulate grafting procedures. In patients with a history of stroke or peripheral vascular disease, there may be a risk of traumatic displacement of a vascular plaque, making preoperative medical consultation advisable. Post-operative vertigo is a rare and usually self-limiting complication of osteotome techniques, and may require management with an Epley maneuver.[66,67]

Osteo-condensation is indicated for limited expansion of 1–2 mm in ridges already having 6–7 mm width. Application is straightforward with favorable ridge anatomic features such as a thin buccal cortical plate of mild to moderate density, an adequate marrow volume, and a rectangular cross-sectional shape with minimal undercut and moderate mesio-distal dimension. Osteo-mobilization is indicated for patients with mild to moderate horizontal bone loss with ridge widths of 4–5 mm requiring expansion of 3–4 mm. Adequate vertical alveolar height above the inferior alveolar nerve or sinus and favorable anatomy also need consideration. Progressive implementation of RE techniques for horizontal site development would require surgical competence with GBR procedures and should begin with less demanding bone manipulation procedures such as osteo-condensation with rotary screw expansion[43] or osteo-mobilization with "split grafting."[50] "Ridge splitting" and osteo-mobilization of a bone flap are more demanding techniques, and expansion with a flapless approach or use of a bone–periosteal flap are even more complex.[15,37] Risk increases as the amount of required expansion increases, and sites with a need for >4 mm of expansion will be at great risk of fracture. Both osteo-condensation and osteo-mobilization can be completed as a staged approach, but their primary advantage is with simultaneous implant placement.

Routine preoperative patient preparation is completed, including chlorhexidine mouth rinses and preoperative oral antibiotics. The patient is seated in a semi-reclined position with head support. In using osteotomes, the surgeon must pay continuous attention to tactile, visual, and auditory cues in order to avoid sudden fracture of the buccal bone or loss of vertical reference. Slow, progressive, and repetitive bending and relaxation of the buccal bone is necessary to produce the desired expansion result.

Precise osteotomies require the use of Piezosurgery® inserts (Figure 16.7a) and gentle malleting with a #64 mini "Beaver" blade (Figure 16.7b). Intermittent insertion of a surgical template can be helpful for determining initial site development dimensions, inter-implant positioning, and vertical position referencing during the procedure. However, drilling pilot holes should not be undertaken until after expansion of the bone flap has been accomplished in order to preserve as much bone as possible. As the buccal bone is manipulated facially, the expansion defect can be opened further with apical and 3-D position adjustments using Piezosurgery inserts (Figure 16.7c) and/or rotary instruments.

A tapered implant design is preferable so as to enhance and support the expansion yet avoid fracture of the buccal plate either at the height of contour or at the apical one-third (area of greatest undercut) (Figure 16.8). Implant primary stability and bone flap stability are required for maintenance of vascularity, viability, and implant integration.[35]

RE in the esthetic zone can avoid open flap and particulate grafting procedures; however, periosteal preservation is critical to reduce the degree of bone and soft tissue remodeling and the risk of soft tissue recession. A "flapless" access offers maximal

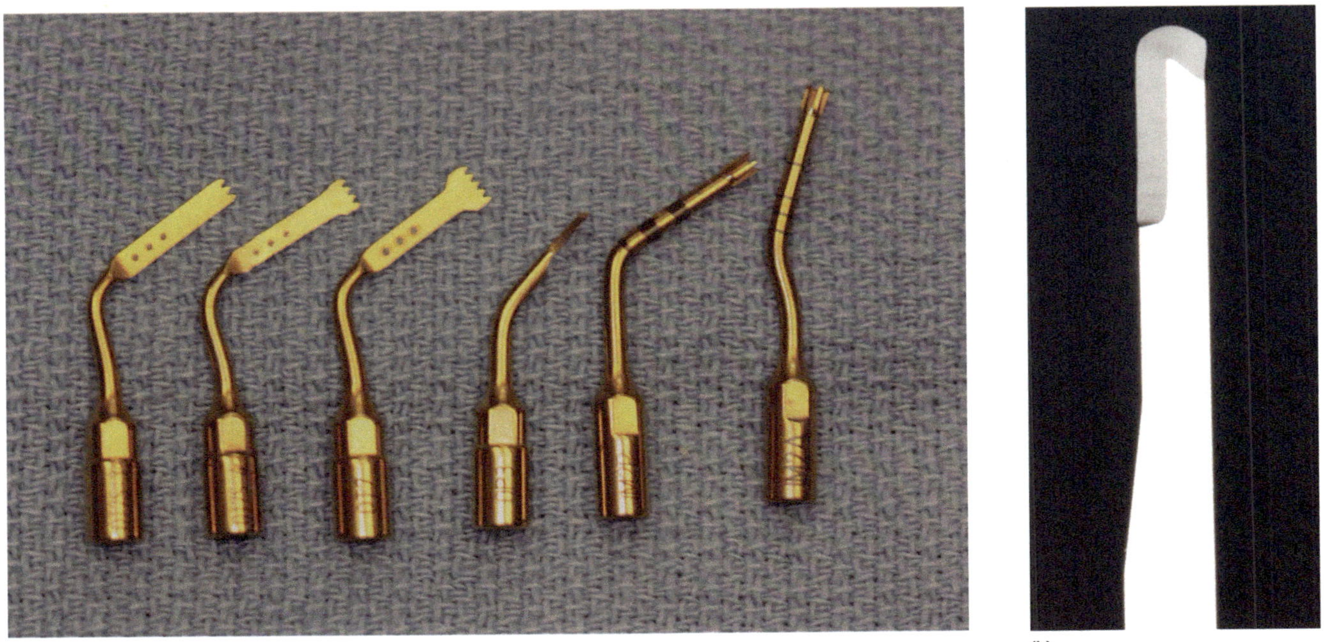

(a) (b)

Figure 16.7 Bone sectioning instruments. Piezosurgery inserts: (a) Piezosurgery inserts from left to right: OT7S3, OT7S4, OT7, OP3, and Implant site preparatiion inserts IM2P and IM2A (Piezosurgery USA, Columbus, OH). (b) #64 "mini" Beaver blade (#S6400, Sable Industries, Vista, CA).

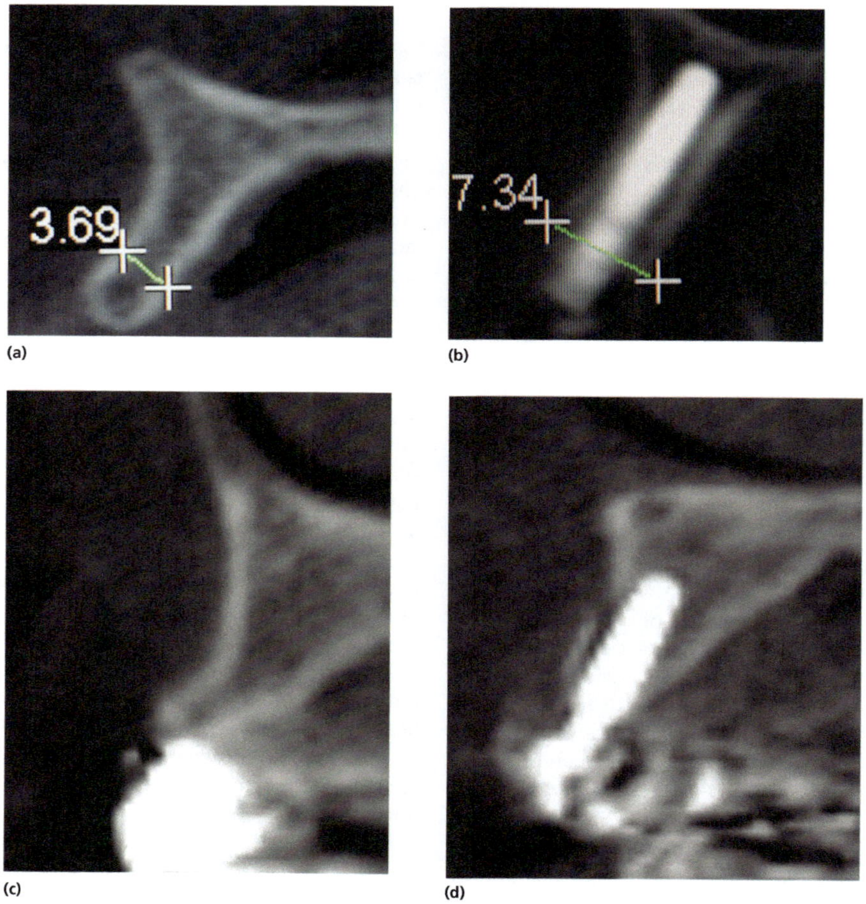

Figure 16.8 (a, b) Preoperative and post-operative CBCT of RE demonstrating horizontal dimensional change. (c, d) Preoperative and post-operative CBCT of RE demonstrating severe facial undercut and fracture at the apical one-third of the buccal plate. *Source*: (a, b) Cullum DR, Ridge Expansion and Piezoelecric Bone Surgery. In: The Piezoelectric Bone Surgery. A New Paradigm, Vercellotti T, ed. Quintessenza Edizioni, 2015. Reproduced with permission of Quintessence Publishing Co., Inc. (c, d) © Daniel R. Cullum.

vascular preservation, but with obvious restricted visibility. A palatal split-thickness incision will allow repositioning of keratinized tissue to the buccal in order to maintain or improve vestibular depth and the width of keratinized tissue around the implant (Figure 16.9a–h). Both partial-thickness flaps and a "flapless" approach demand more technical care and time at surgery. Challenges in implant positioning most often occur in the mesiodistal and facial dimensions. Maintaining adequate distance from adjacent teeth or implants is essential. Facial angulation and/or facial positioning often result in a compromise of buccal bone thickness and increase the risk of crestal bone loss and soft tissue recession. In cases requiring minimal expansion (existing ridge width of 6–7 mm), it is often necessary to complete additional palatal purchase to avoid the implant being too buccal (Figure 16.9i). If the buccal bone thickness is compromised during the procedure, grafting the expansion gap with particulate bone and even shimming the defect open as a "split graft" can be used for site development and delayed implant placement.[48] A modification of the split graft can be completed with an intentional out-fracture as an osteo-periosteal island flap; however, an extended healing interval may be needed as a greater remodeling of final bone dimensions is likely.[50]

Mechanical rotary expanders have the advantage of reduced patient manipulation compared with osteotomes and a mallet (Figure 16.2b). Like osteotomes, mechanical expanders can be used with osteo-condensation in the maxilla limited to smaller expansions of 1–2 mm. Mechanical expanders, however, are the most practical approach in mandible, where access and bone density typically prevent the use of osteotomes. The technique maintains native bone on the implant surface, and horizontal augmentation can be enhanced by use of a slow turnover graft material and resorbable barrier. Osteo-condensation with rotary mechanical expanders and over-grafting should be straightforward for surgeons experienced with GBR procedures.

Rotary expanders also can be used with osteo-mobilization at horizontal multi-tooth defects in the mandible (Figure 16.10). Following full-thickness flap exposure, bone incisions/osteotomies using ultrasonic bone surgery and rotary expansion can allow correction of mandibular horizontal deficiencies often without a GBR over-graft provided that a viable buccal bone flap of 2 mm minimum thickness can be maintained (Figure 16.10g, h). Additionally, an implant design with an aggressive cutting thread and tapered body design (Figure 16.6) can function like a rotary expander, reducing the amount of initial osteo-mobilization needed (see also Figure 16.11).

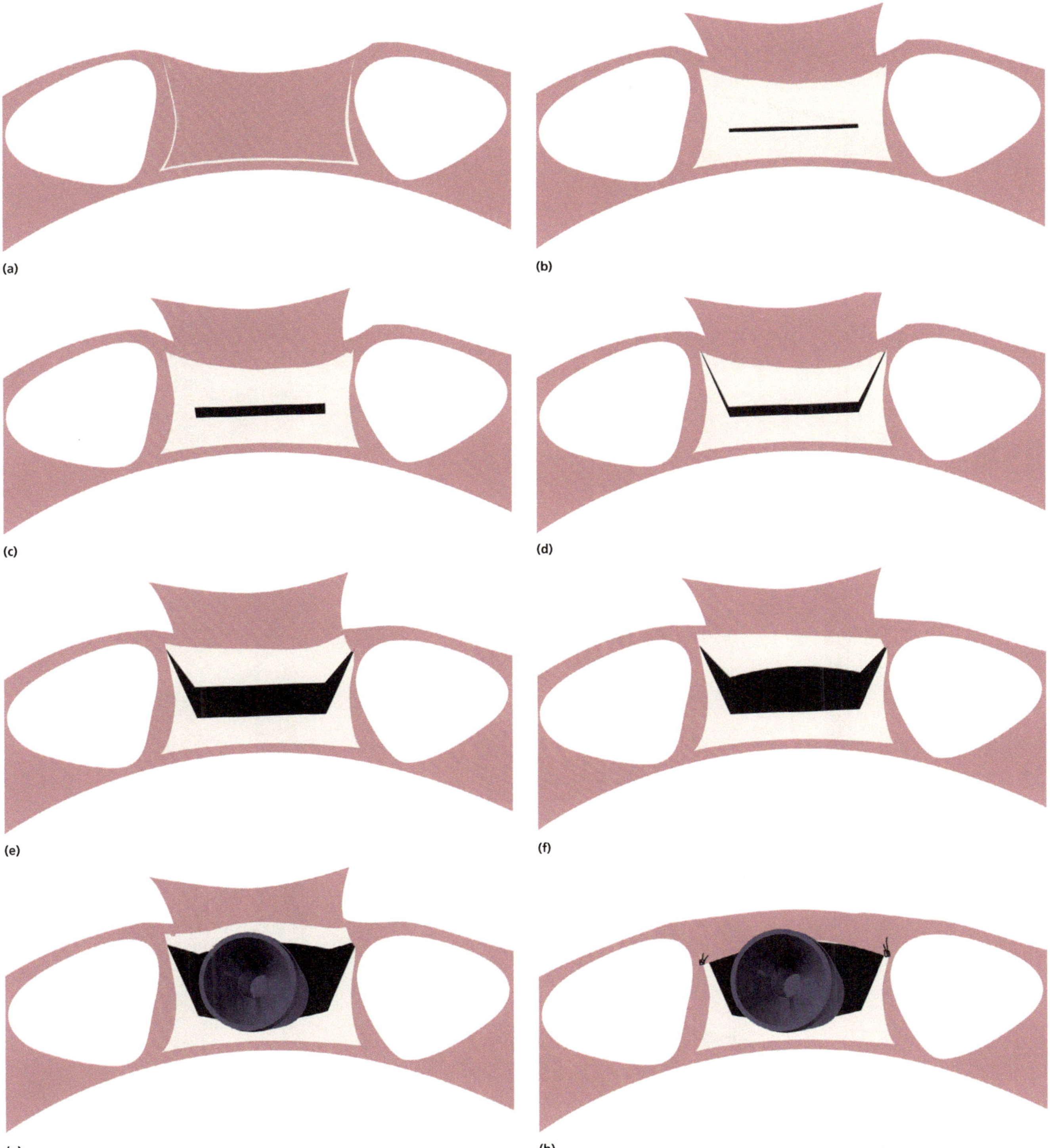

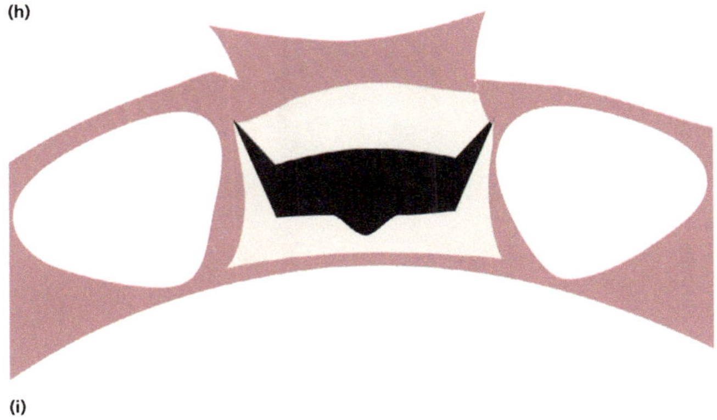

Figure 16.9 Anterior maxilla – split-thickness RE with intrabony osteotomy, internal lateral-beveled bone incisions, transgingival tapered implant placement with apical repositioned flap. (a) Palatal incised, buccal-based, split-thickness flap design. (b) Horizontal Piezosurgery bone incision. (c) Osteo-mobilization with "spade" expanders. (d) Internal beveled bone incision with #64 "Beaver" blade. (e) Osteo-mobilization with "spade" and "bi-bevel" expanders. (f) Osteo-mobilization with "D" and tapered osteotomes. (g) Tapered implant placed with collagen in the intact intrabony gap. (h) Apical repositioning of the facial flap with lateral beveled soft tissue releasing incisions. (i) In cases requiring minimal expansion (ridge width of 6–7 mm) it is often necessary to complete additional palatal purchase to avoid the implant being too buccal or flared to the facial. © Daniel R. Cullum.

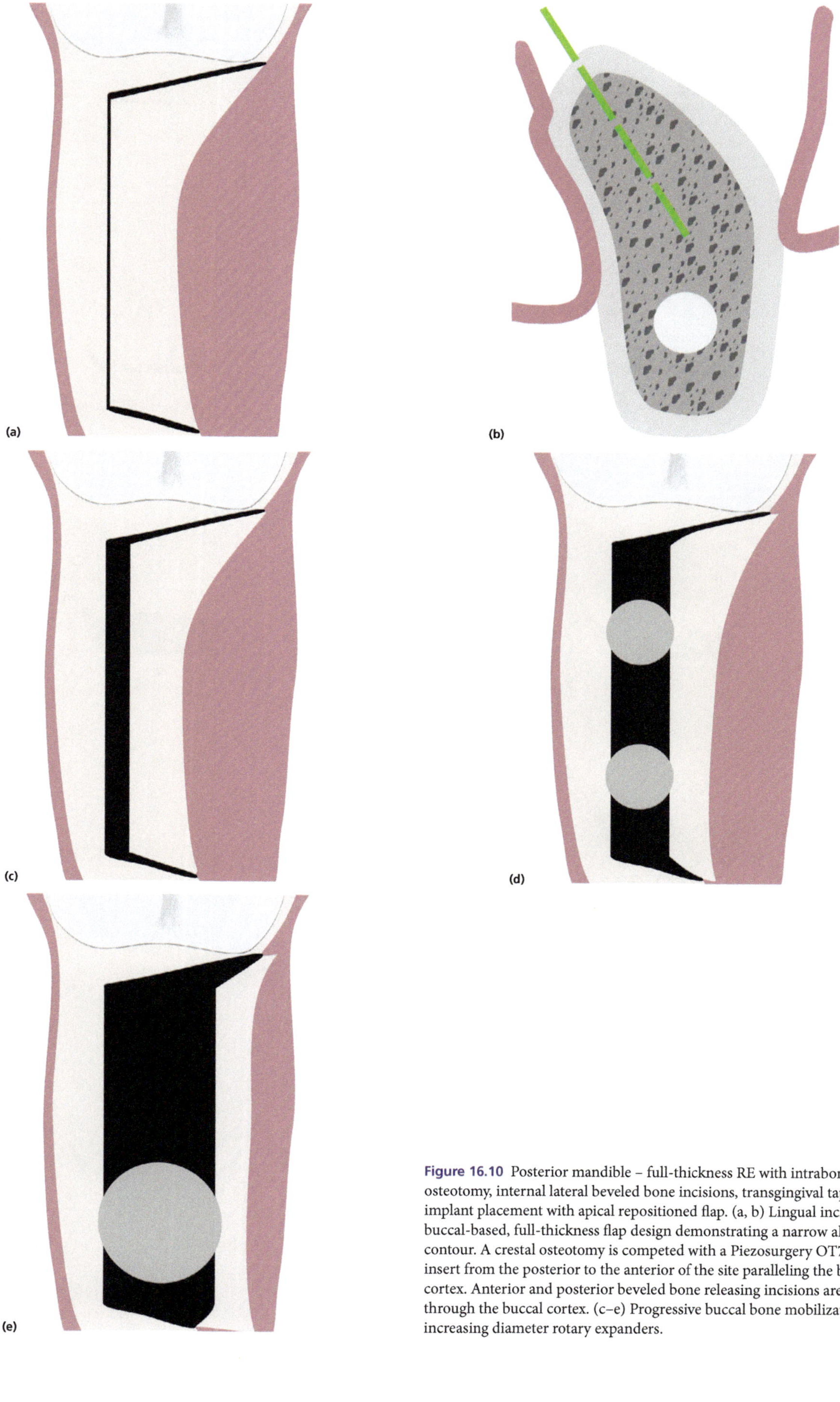

Figure 16.10 Posterior mandible – full-thickness RE with intrabony osteotomy, internal lateral beveled bone incisions, transgingival tapered implant placement with apical repositioned flap. (a, b) Lingual incised, buccal-based, full-thickness flap design demonstrating a narrow alveolar contour. A crestal osteotomy is competed with a Piezosurgery OT7S4 insert from the posterior to the anterior of the site paralleling the buccal cortex. Anterior and posterior beveled bone releasing incisions are made through the buccal cortex. (c–e) Progressive buccal bone mobilization with increasing diameter rotary expanders.

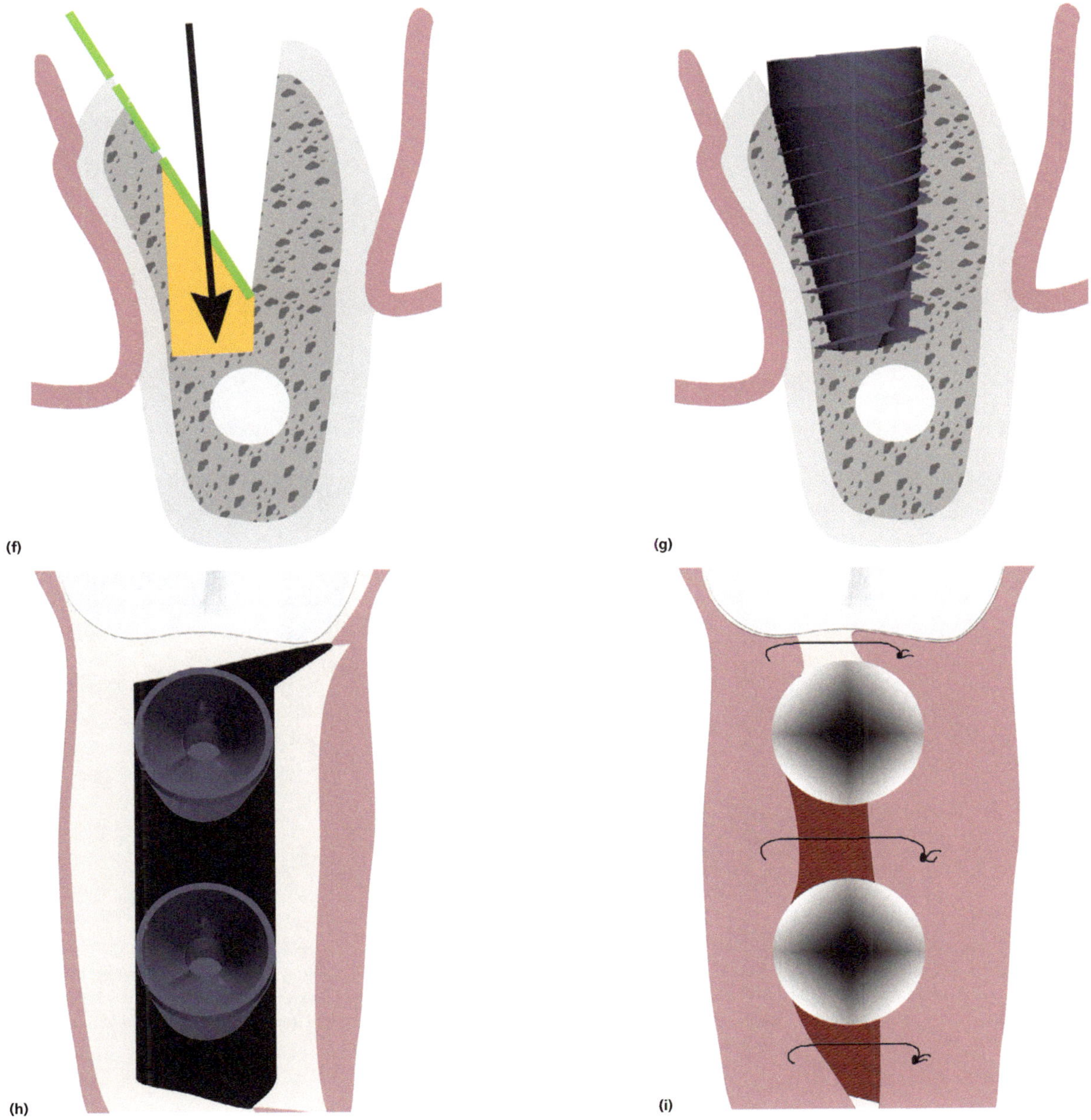

Figure 16.10 (Continued)
(f) With the anterior expander removed (Figure 16.10e, f), lingual apical preparation is completed with the Piezosurgery IM2P insert and twist drills to "upright" the long axis of the implant site preparation. (g, h) Tapered implant insertion. (i) Apical repositioning of the facial flap with lateral beveled soft tissue releasing incisions. *Source*: (a, h) Cullum DR, Ridge Expansion and Piezoelectric Bone Surgery. In: The Piezoelectric Bone Surgery. A New Paradigm, Vercellotti T, ed. Quintessenza Edizioni, 2015. Reproduced with permission of Quintessence Publishing Co., Inc. (b–g, i) © Daniel R. Cullum.

Should a residual buccal plate be thin or fracture occur, the flapless design, unlike the partial-thickness approach, allows for progression to a full-thickness design as needed to permit over-grafting and primary closure. Typically primary soft tissue closure and delayed healing would be indicated, although limited graft volumes can be treated with careful closure to a healing abutment with a transgingival healing protocol. This "over-grafting" technique cannot be utilized over periosteum of a split-thickness flap. Therefore, a strategic choice is necessary based on preoperative assessment for the appropriate treatment pathway[37] (Table 16.1).

Single-stage implant placement at the time of RE often is possible provided that an intact bone flap of optimal thickness remains. Soft tissue management with apical positioning and selective use of finger flaps and/or connective tissue grafting can allow wound closure to a gingival or periosteal margin.[68,69] Additionally, with a thin gingival biotype or the esthetic need for additional soft tissue thickness, such as to simulate a "root eminence," subepithelial connective tissue grafting can be completed through a closed tunnel with crestal access[37,61] (see Chapter 8). A light-cured periodontal dressing (e.g. Barricaide™, Densply-Caulk, Milford,

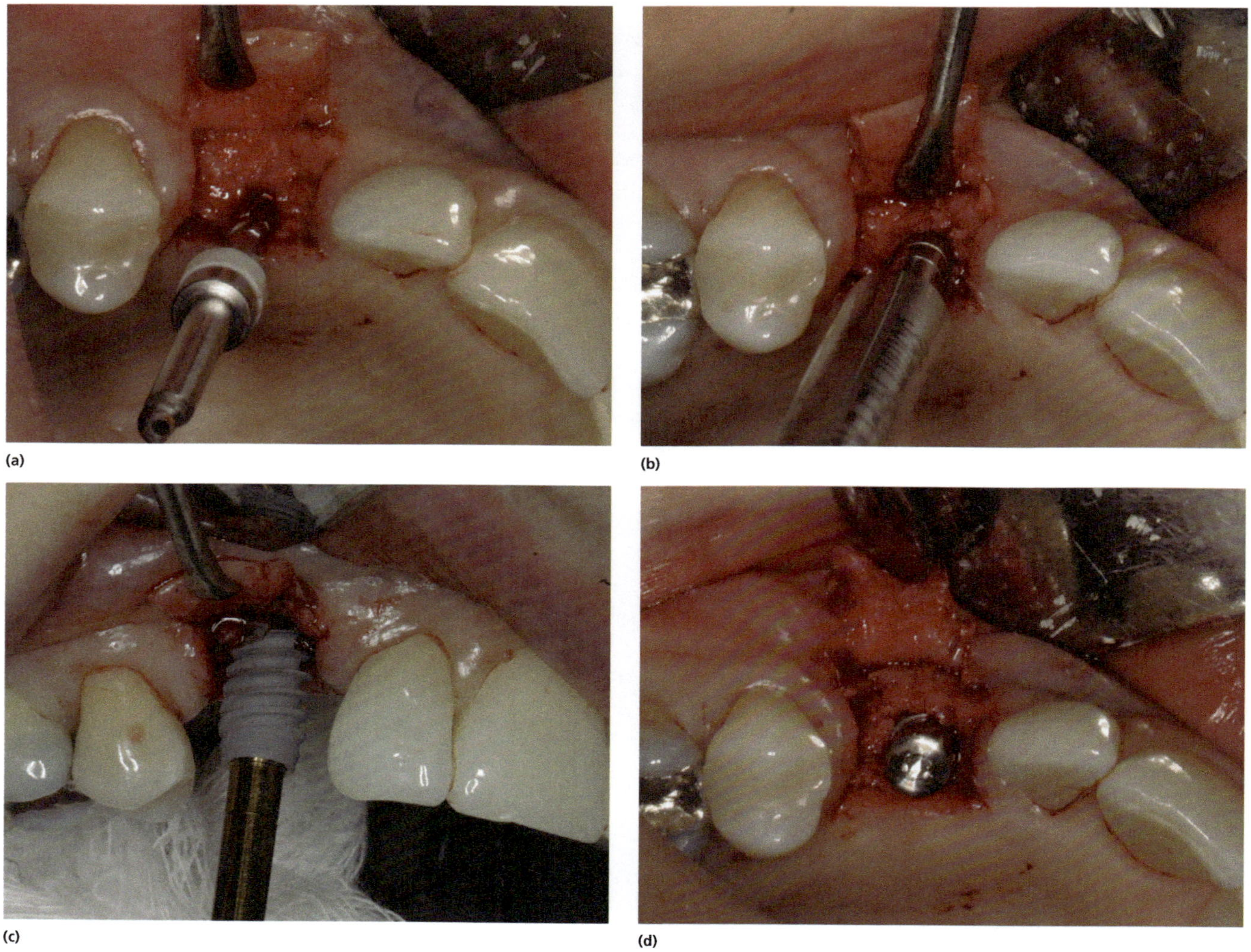

Figure 16.11 Full-thickness flap exposure osteo-condensation/axis re-orientation (RE osteotomy) with buccal bone manipulation for "restorative-driven" implant position. (a) A palatal incised full-thickness flap design is completed for planned apical positioning. A 2 mm twist drill is used for the initial osteotomy in a palatal position at the anticipated location of the final palatal implant margin. (b) Osteo-condensation and buccal bone manipulation with progressive tapered osteotomes. (c) Implant insertion with axis re-orientation to ideal position. (d) Implant and healing cap placed with expanded crestal bone intact with adequate volume for healing with single-stage placement. © Daniel R. Cullum.

DE) can aid in protection of transgingival wounds during the initial post-operative period.[16] When a two-stage healing protocol is utilized, uncovering (i.e. re-entry) with apical soft tissue flap positioning or additional soft tissue augmentation can be completed to enhance the transgingival interface. With increasing operator experience, management of narrower ridge widths, smaller flaps, and reduced wound exposure will further enhance the minimally invasive benefits of these procedures.

Table 16.1 Summary of RE procedure selection

Site	Flap design	Wound healing	MGMT of fracture
Mandible/maxilla	Full thickness	GBR principles	"Over-graft"
Maxilla	Partial thickness	Local regeneration	"Split graft"
Maxilla	Mini-flap/flapless	Local regeneration	Either[a]

[a]A procedure with a "mini-flap" or "flapless" approach can be converted to an open flap exposure if required to manage a complication.

Procedures

Osteo-condensation in the maxilla: full-thickness flap

Use of a full-thickness flap design in the maxilla in combination with osteo-condensation can be completed with osteotomes (Figure 16.11) or with rotary expansion screws.[43] In Figure 16.11a, a 2 mm drill was used to start the osteotomy at the desired palatal margin of the future implant site. An RE osteotomy was completed using tapered osteotomes with asymmetric "axis re-orientation" site development toward the facial.[33] Adequate buccal bone thickness (>2 mm) was maintained (Figure 16.11d), and the case was managed with apical soft tissue flap positioning and single-stage implant placement. In many cases, however, buccal bone thickness will end up <2 mm, necessitating over-grafting using GBR principles, primary wound closure, and a staged healing interval.

Osteo-condensation in the mandible: full-thickness flap

In mandible, osteo-condensation with full-thickness flap exposure and rotary screw expanders offers a similar minimally invasive approach. A 1.4 mm pilot drill is followed with increasing diameter screw expanders for progressive bone condensation (Figure 16.12). Screw manipulation will result in lateral forces causing an asymmetric expansion of the buccal cortical bone (less dense than its lingual counterpart), partially restoring the lost buccal dimension. With screw expansion of greater than 1.5 mm, the potential for vertical fractures of the buccal plate is increased (Figure 16.12c). If the residual buccal plate thickness after expansion is <2 mm, overgrafting with particulate xenograft and a collagen barrier should be completed (Figure 16.12d and e). The goal is to have a healed buccal bone dimension of 2 mm or greater. Often, this can be accomplished with a single-stage implant healing protocol (Figure 16.12f). Preoperative and 1-year post-restoration images demonstrate the clinical changes in dimension. (Figure 16.12g and h). The advantage with RE is that the implant has native bone and its cells, rather than graft material, on its surface. However, the surgeon must avoid the tendency to try to over-utilize this technique, since mandibular cortical bone does have limited compliance. With the need for more than 1.5 mm expansion in mandible, osteo-mobilization should be considered since the rotary screw technique will increase risk of cortical fractures and/or horizontal fractures into the periodontal ligament space of adjacent teeth.

Osteo-mobilization in the mandible: full-thickness flap exposure

For this procedure, a full-thickness flap incision is designed for maximal soft tissue mobilization and its apical positioning for a transgingival healing protocol. A crestal incision is completed on the lingual

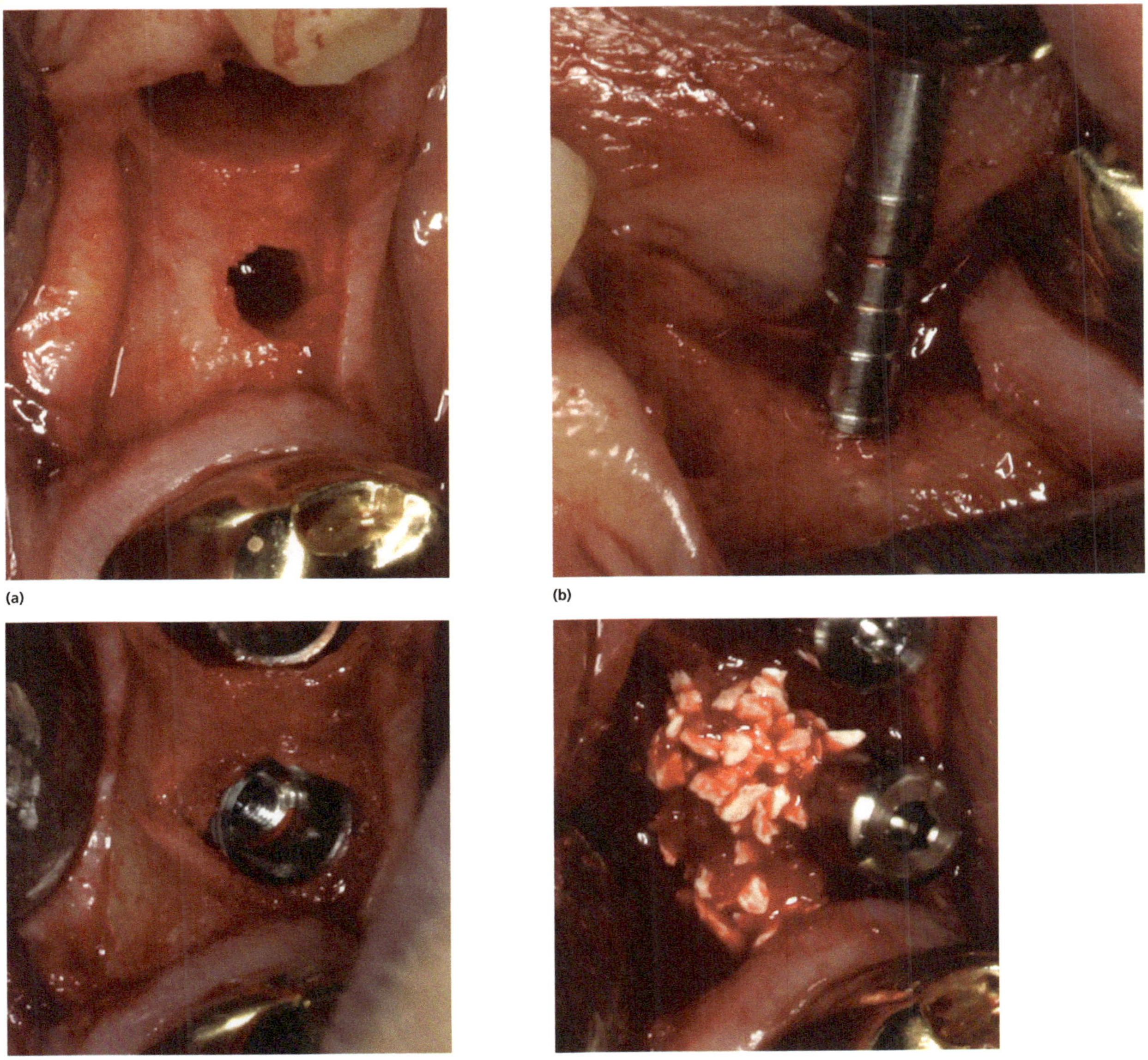

(a) (b) (c) (d)

Figure 16.12 Expansion by osteo-condensation in the mandible. (a) Bucally-based, lingual crestal soft tissue incision for full-thickness flap and 2 mm drill preparation. (b) Rotary screw expansion was completed to a maximum of 4mm. (c) Self-tapping, aggressive thread pattern, tapered implant design in position with expanded and partially fractured buccal cortex at the mid-implant height of contour. (d) Particulate xenograft for lateral augmentation.

(Continued)

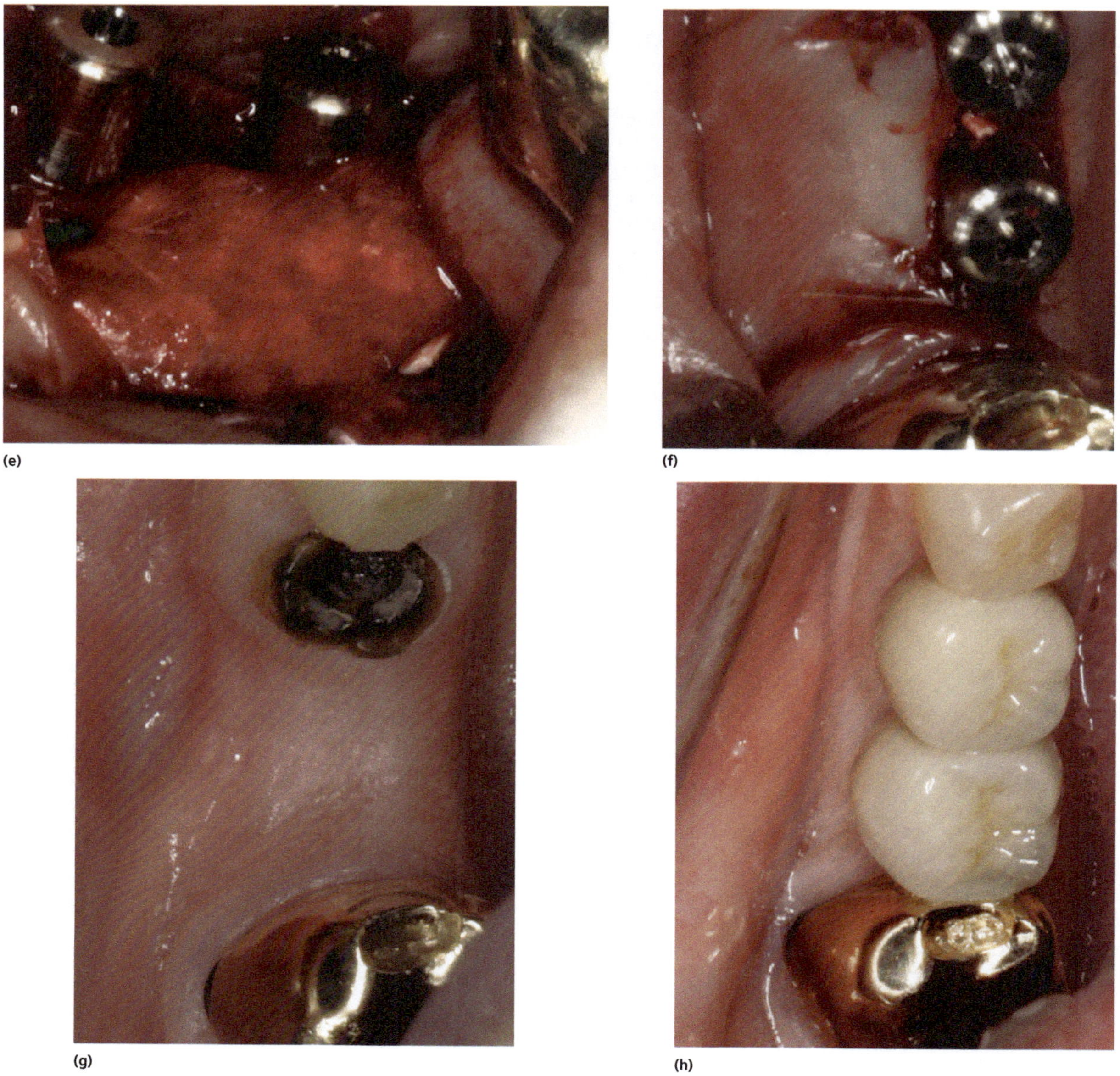

Figure 16.12 (Continued)
(e) Collagen barrier (Cytoplast RTM®, Osteogenics, Lubbock, TX) with transgingival healing caps in position. (f) Closure with apical repositioned flap with transgingival healing. (g, h) Preoperative and 1-year post-restoration views demonstrating contour enhancement and stable soft tissue. © Daniel R. Cullum.

aspect to maximize the amount of keratinized gingival tissue in the flap. The mesial and distal corners are extended to increase the flap length for optimal fit with apical positioning (Figure 16.10a–f). Using Piezosurgery inserts OT7 or OT7S4 for the osteotomies will minimize the time required and local trauma to section the bone (Figure 16.7a). The narrower OT7S4 insert allows the surgeon to make a fine cut of only 0.35 mm width with minimal lateral thermal injury to the bone. The initial ridge width should be at least 4.0–5.0 mm in order to leave the expanded bone flaps with adequate thickness for regeneration. The bone is first sectioned at the crest, paralleling the buccal cortex and maintaining a minimum 2 mm buccal thickness, to a depth of 8–9 mm (Figure 16.10b). In a posterior edentulous segment, the osteotomy should extend well past the last implant site at the posterior aspect, then gently angle out laterally through the buccal cortex and an anterior vertical beveled bone incision completed (Figure 16.10a). At an interdental expansion site, vertical beveled bone incisions are completed at both ends. These incisions are completed with Piezosurgery insert OT7S4 (Figure 16.7a) starting from the internal aspect of the alveolus and cutting vertical through the buccal cortex at a 45° angle toward the facial and parallel to any adjacent tooth root. This sectioning allows the bone flap to bend open at the vertical releases, and the bevels reduce the discontinuity defects after expansion. Care should be taken when sectioning through the buccal cortex to place the vertical defect 3 mm away from the final implant site while avoiding any adjacent tooth root.

Once the bone incisions have been completed, threaded rotary expanders (e.g. Meisinger USA, Centenial, CO) (Figure 16.2b) with progressively increasing diameter can be used to create the expansion defect.[37] Alveolar purchase at the desired implant site(s) is initiated with a 1.4 mm twist drill. Developing more than one site together can assist in bone flap mobilization. Expansion screws of progressively increasing diameter are inserted at the sites using a handpiece at low speed (30–50 rpm) and maximum torque (50 N cm), or a hand-racheting device to expand the intrabony gap (Figure 16.10c–e). In the example shown, the posterior expansion screw was left in position, while the anterior implant site was developed with rotary instrumentation and Piezosurgery insert IM2P (Figure 16.7a). The implant site was uprighted to the buccal from its initial lingual orientation (Figure 16.10b, f, and g), and the implant was then inserted at the anterior site (Figure 16.10g) with apical development and "uprighting" with insertion of the implant at the posterior site (Figure 16.10h).

Adequate apical preparation of the osteotomy with implant drills or Piezosurgery is required as inadequate apical lingual bone removal can result in a wedging effect on the bone flap with fracture of the buccal segment and/or lingual inclination of the implant. This usually will occur at the greatest depth of contour change (undercut) at about two-thirds the vertical height of the buccal bone flap. Should the crestal buccal bone thickness end up being <2 mm, placement of the implant more apically may help to increase the crestal buccal bone thickness, provided that there are no proximity risks to the inferior alveolar nerve. Also, if the crestal buccal bone thickness is <2 mm or has any vertical microfractures, then over-grafting following GBR principles is recommended. Loss of continuity of the buccal segment or a complete "ridge split" is discussed further on in the "Avoiding complications" section.

Wound closure after a successful expansion with adequate buccal bone thickness allows for single-stage implant placement. Bovine collagen (e.g. CollaTape®, Zimmer Dental, Carlsbad, CA) can be placed in the RE defect between the buccal and lingual cortices to assist with clot retention. Particulate bone graft material is placed at the vertical releases of the buccal bone flap to avoid potential cortical defects. The flap design allows for apical repositioning often with a beveled releasing incision at the anterior margin for mobilization. Apical flap positioning is completed to the implant margin with interproximal sutures, minimizing the exposed wound. Primary closure can be obtained around the healing caps by developing finger flaps incised from the flap if there is adequate keratinized tissue width (Figure 16.10i), and the wound can be protected with a light-cured periodontal dressing.

Figure 16.13 demonstrates a patient treated with osteomobilization for replacement of an edentulous mandibular left first molar adjacent to an extraction site. This case is an example of maintaining the buccal soft tissues in the mandible to preserve blood supply. The clinical images show a significant horizontal bone defect and minimal attached tissue (Figure 16.13a). A buccally-based, lingual full-thickness crestal incision was created with limited dissection exposing only the ridge crest

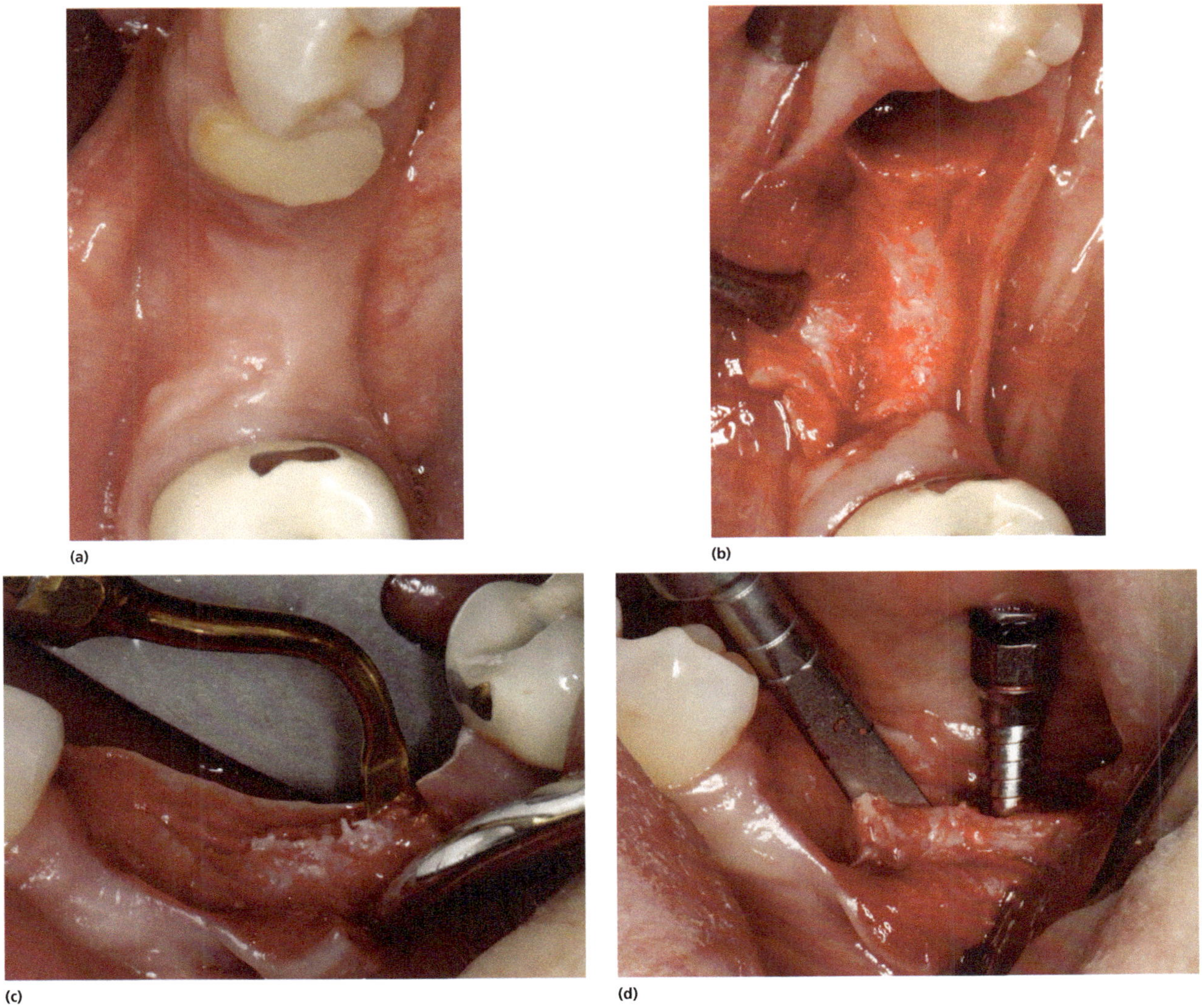

Figure 16.13 Osteo-mobilization in the mandible adjacent to an extraction site. (a) Preoperative clinical image demonstrating horizontal dimensional loss at the lower left first molar site. (b) Buccally-based lingual crestal full-thickness incision exposing only the ridge crest. Incision design allows for possible apical positioning. (c) Piezosurgery bone osteotomy is completed from anterior to posterior of the site followed by beveled lateral cortical releasing incisions. (d) Increasing diameter rotary expanders are inserted at the first molar site with anterior osteotomy expansion assisted with a flat chisel. *(Continued)*

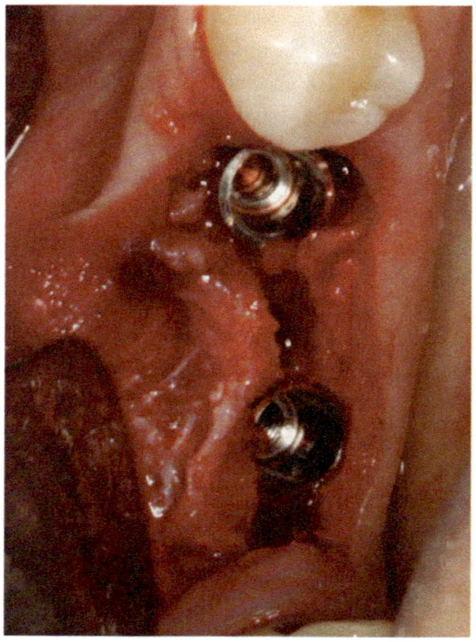
(e)

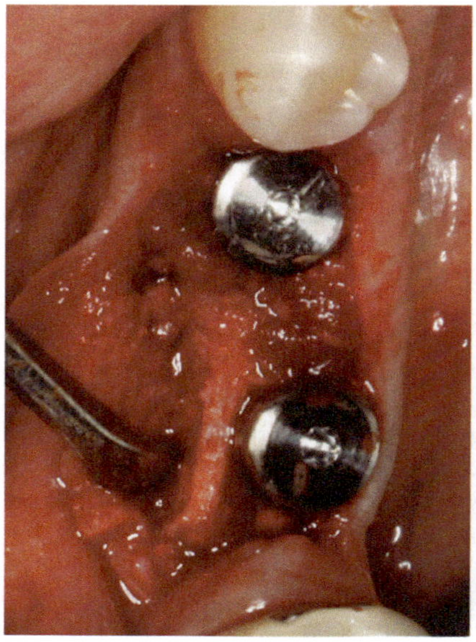
(f)

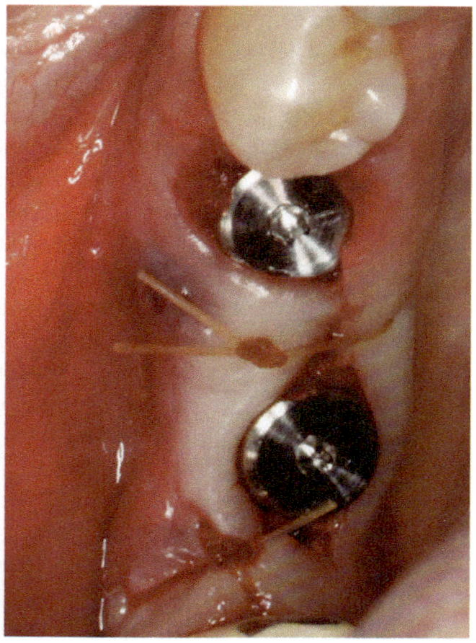
(g)

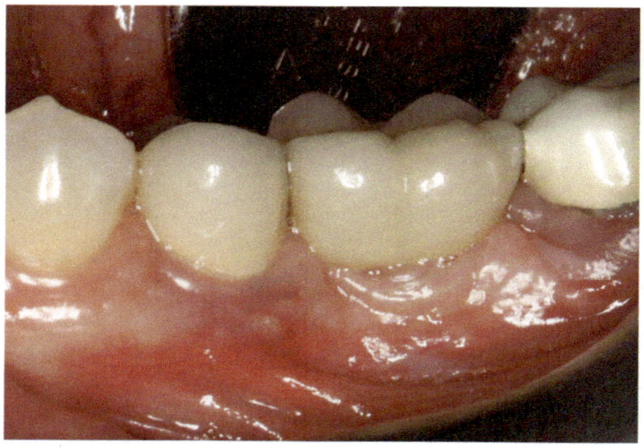
(h)

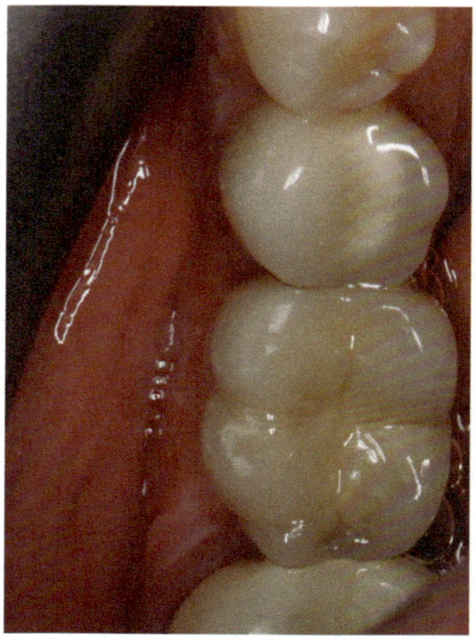
(i)

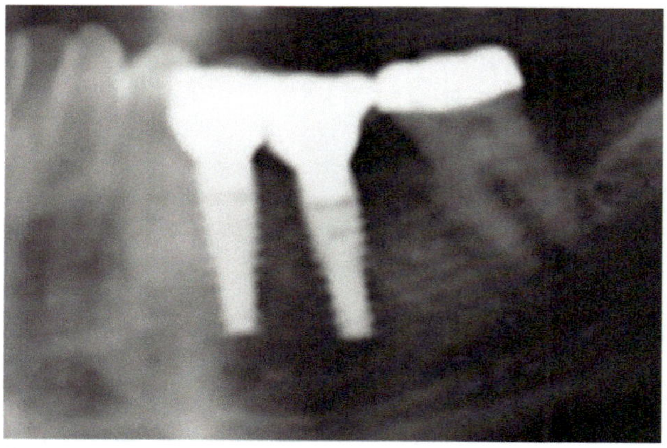
(j)

Figure 16.13 (Continued)
(e) After immediate site development at the adjacent premolar, 4.3 mm diameter implants are placed with the expansion gap. (f) Healing caps (5 mm × 5 mm) were inserted and particulate graft was placed in the adjacent immediate site and the expansion gap and covered with collagen (CollaTape®, Zimmer, Carlsbad, CA). (g) Transgingival healing was facilitated with apical flap positioning around the healing cap. (h–j) Post-restoration clinical images and radiograph after 19 months. © Daniel R. Cullum.

(Figure 16.13b). The antero-posterior osteotomy (Figure 16.13c) and the posterior beveled vertical release were completed with a Piezosurgery OT7S4 insert. Rotary expanders of increasing diameter assisted by a flat chisel were used to complete development of the anterior osteotomy expansion (Figure 16.13d). Implants were placed into the expanded segment after osteo-mobilization and immediate implant site preparation at the adjacent premolar (Figure 16.13e). Healing caps (5 mm × 5 mm) were inserted and particulate graft was placed in the adjacent immediate site and the expansion gap and covered with collagen (CollaTape) (Figure 16.13f). Single-stage healing was allowed after flap positioning around the healing caps (Figure 16.13g). Images 19 months after restoration demonstrate the enhanced and stable bone and tissue contours (Figure 16.13h–j).

Osteo-mobilization for horizontal deficiency in the maxilla: flap designs for periosteal retention (split thickness, mini-flap, or flapless)

RE in maxilla uses osteo-mobilization of the buccal cortical plate away from the stable palatal cortex while maintaining the continuity of the expanded buccal segment as a viable "bone flap" or "bone–periosteal flap."[15,16] Ideally, the procedure can be approached using a partial-thickness dissection or a limited crestal access with a "flapless" approach,[47] and the actual expansion done with hand instrumentation, including expanders, chisels, and osteotomes of several modified designs[37] (Figure 16.3a–f).

For a split-thickness flap, a buccally-based palatal incision is developed to just above the level of the periosteum using the #64 "mini" Beaver blade. The incision can be extended one to two teeth anteriorly and/or posteriorly with a marginal release at the mucogingival junction (Figure 16.4a). The flap can be further extended with a beveled vertical release to gain access, visibility or soft tissue mobilization for repositioning. Beveling the vertical incision 45° away from the periosteal base will limit significantly the potential for visible scar formation. Incision design for apical flap positioning improves soft tissue vestibular depth and quantity of keratinized tissue, with the residual soft tissue defect remote from the implant site (Figure 16.4d and e). With posterior edentulous spans, the flap should extend well distal to the site or to the tuberosity with lateral/vertical release. Larger expansion sites require greater soft tissue mobilization with a periosteal release incision at the distal and/or superior margins to enhance mobility of the flap. Care is necessary to avoid flap perforation, particularly at the mucogingival junction. The palatal aspect of the ridge may be exposed with split-thickness dissection or be assessed with bone sounding to determine the inclination of the palatal vault.[15] Often, with experience, the procedure can be completed with minimal flap development,[37] unless a larger flap is required for soft tissue management. Alternately, a limited palatal crestal incision can be completed for a "flapless" or mini-flap exposure in anterior regions or for single-tooth posterior sites (Figure 16.9a).

The patient seen in Figure 16.14a shows a moderate horizontal bone defect planned for split-thickness flap RE at the left central incisor site. The bone incisions should be done using Piezosurgery

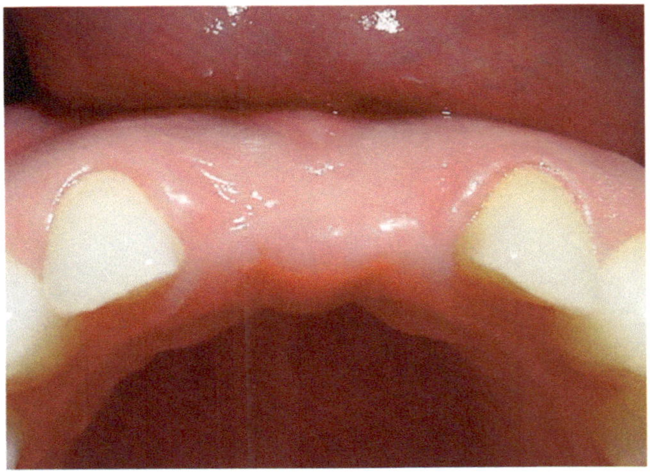

(a)

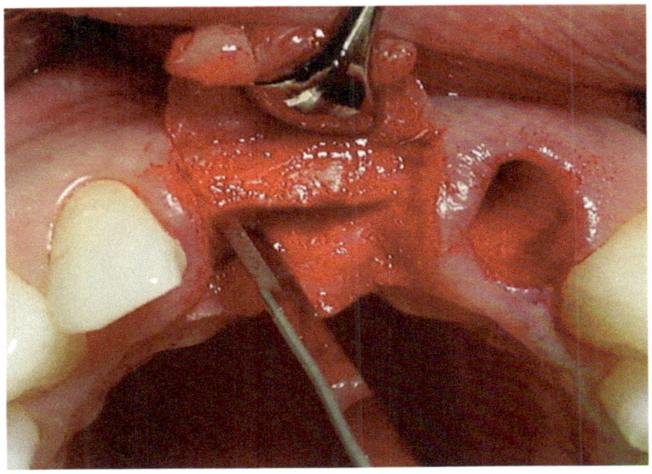

(b)

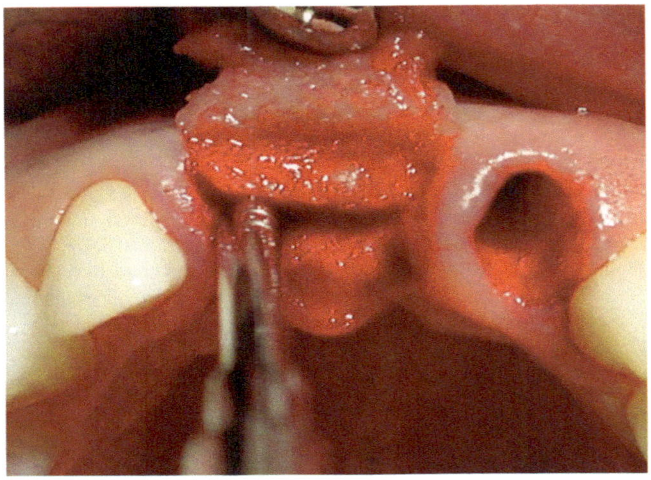

(c)

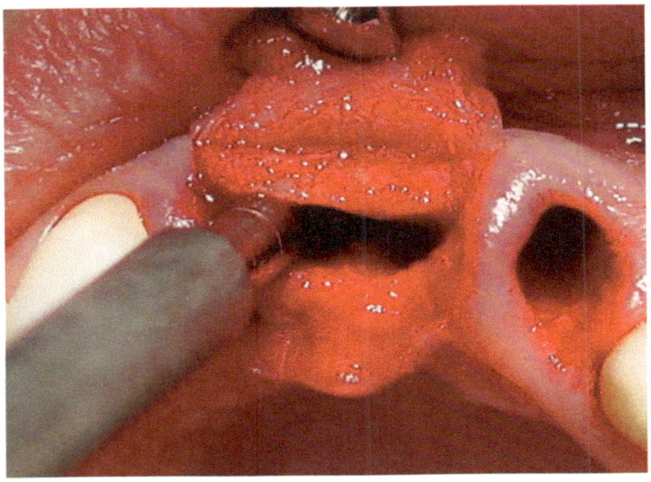

(d)

Figure 16.14 Split-thickness flap esthetic zone RE. (a) Preop horizontal ridge defect at the maxillary central incisors. (b) Split-thickness flap dissection is completed with bone incision and initial osteo-mobilization ("spade" expanders); beveled intrabony incision is completed with a #64 "mini" Beaver blade. (c) Horizontal osteo-mobilization with "D" osteotome with developing expansion gap. (d) Progressive expansion with tapered osteotomes and expansion gap. (e) After 4.3 mm diameter implant placement, surgical guide evaluation of the implant position shows vertical height reduction of labial plate is required.

(Continued)

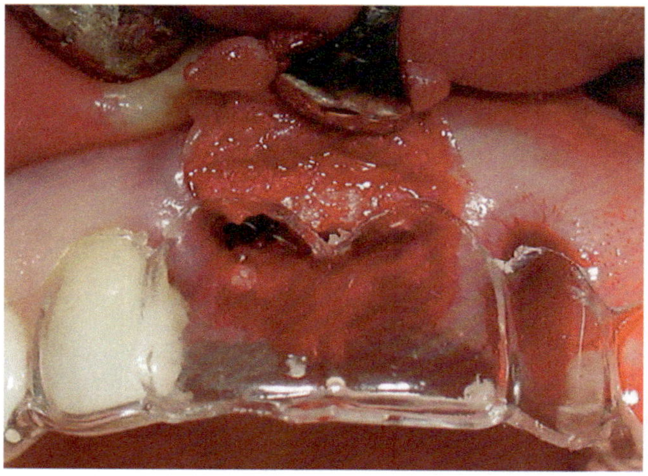

(e)

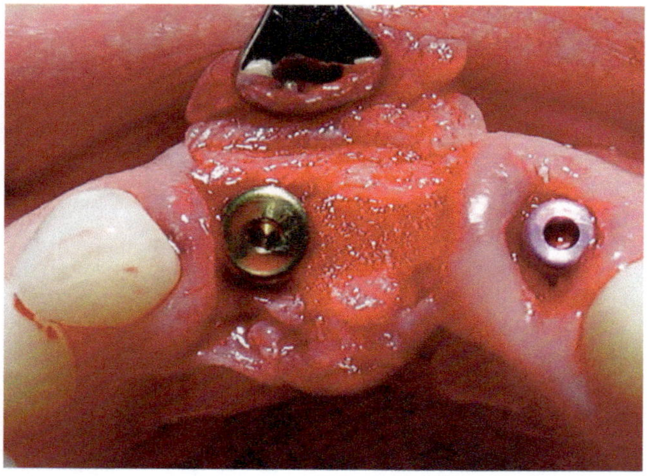

(f)

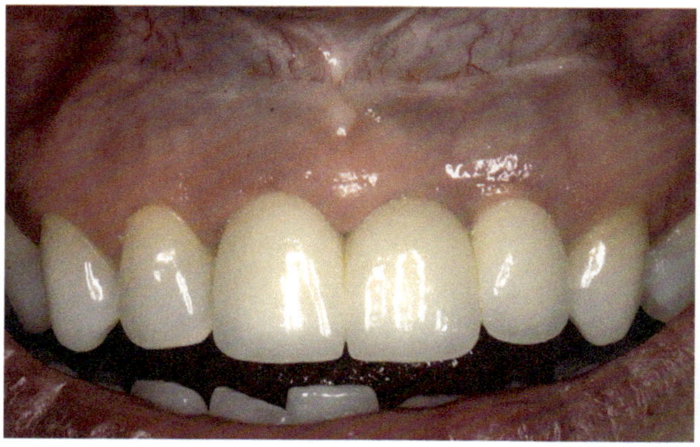

(g)

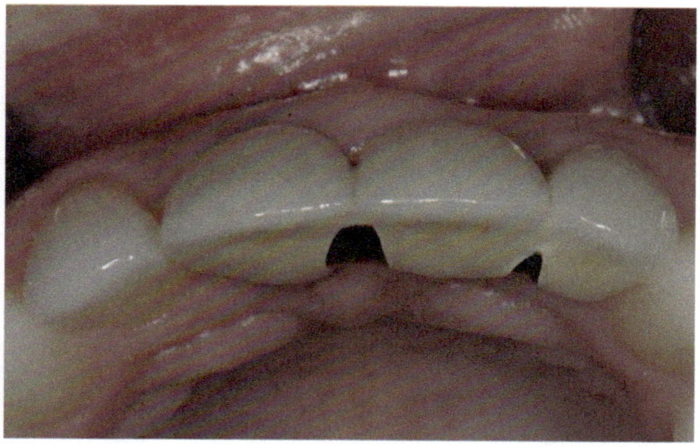

(h)

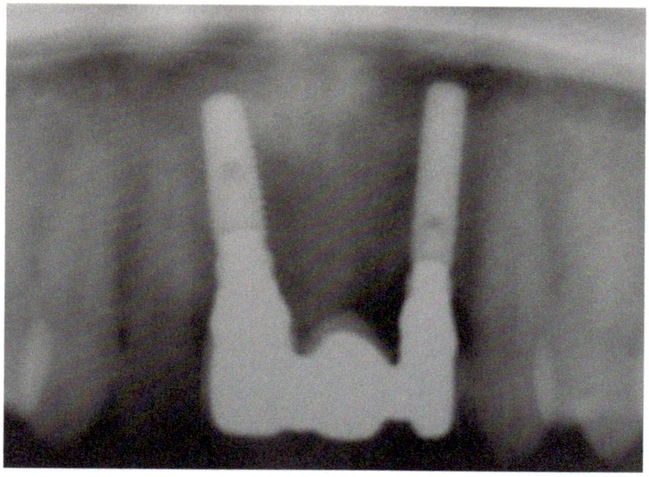

(i)

Figure 16.14 (Continued)

(f) Implants with healing caps in position and collagen placed in the intrabony gap. (g–i) The 43-month post-op results and radiograph demonstrate good bone maintenance. (Restorations: Earl Ness, DDS, MSD.) *Source*: (a, h, i) Cullum DR, Ridge Expansion and Piezoelecric Bone Surgery. In: The Piezoelectric Bone Surgery. A New Paradigm, Vercellotti T, ed. Quintessenza Edizioni, 2015. Reproduced with permission of Quintessence Publishing Co., Inc. (b–g) © Daniel R. Cullum.

insert OT7S3 or -4 as this allows a fine cut (0.35 mm in width). A #64 "mini" Beaver blade (Figure 16.7d) also can be used to section the residual alveolar ridge with a gentle malleting action[15] (Figure 16.14b). The #64 "mini" blade should be progressively advanced and then mobilized in a mesio-distal direction for removal from the site (buccal–palatal manipulation risks blade fracture). The ridge should have a minimal initial thickness of 4.0 mm in order to leave the expanded bone flaps with adequate thickness for regeneration. Initial osteo-mobilization can be completed (Figure 16.9c) with "spade" expanders[37] (Figure 16.3a and b) to about 10 mm depth. A lateral buccal bending moment can then be used to manipulate and begin the expansion process. Beveled vertical intrabony incisions are then made at the mesial and distal aspects of the site (Figure 16.9d). These should be completed at a 45° angle (away from the site) parallel to any adjacent tooth roots (Figure 16.14b). The incisions are made in the medullary space only, preserving continuity of the buccal cortex while releasing stress and allowing bending of the intact cortex (i.e. like opening a book with the buccal cortex as the binding) (Figure 16 9f and g). Occasionally, however, it is necessary to section through the buccal cortex for adequate mobilization of the bone flap.

Osteo-mobilization at single tooth edentulous sites can be assisted with the use of a mallet and progressively thicker instruments designed for RE, such as "bi-beveled" expanders and "D" expanders[37] (Figure 16.3c–f). The narrowest tips are used for lateral incisors, while the mid and widest tips are used for central incisors, canines, and premolars (based on the mesial–distal dimension of the edentulous site). Simultaneous palpation with the non-dominant hand gives the surgeon a feel for the bone mobilization as it occurs. The apical bone also can be mobilized with sequential use of "spade" osteotomes or chisels using an elevation force and twisting action of the instruments (see further discussion in "Avoiding complications" section).

Site development was continued using "D"-shaped expanders[37] (Figure 16.14c). The "D" is first placed with the flat surface against the palatal bone and advanced to the desired depth, shaping the buccal plate. Then, the instrument is turned 180° so that the flat surface faces buccally and reinserted to depth, and the apical corners of the buccal bone are manipulated to the facial. Attention to 3-D positioning is important as the instruments follow the path of least resistance, and can be displaced or deflected by internal variations in bone density. Adjustment of positioning must be active with each step. This includes use of Piezosurgery or rotary instruments. A 2 mm twist drill is inserted after crestal expansion to complete apical preparation and to confirm orientation with an intraoperative periapical radiograph. To complete site development, implant-specific tapered osteotomes are used progressively to the final site diameter (Figure 16.14d). The buccal plate often displays significant rebound of 20–30% with instrument removal. Implant insertion usually will display moderate to significant torque resistance with excellent primary stability. After placement of a 4.3 mm diameter implant, surgical guide evaluation of the implant position showed vertical height reduction of the labial plate was needed (Figure 16.14e). The implants are seen with healing caps in position and collagen placed in the intrabony gap in Figure 16.14f. Clinical and radiographic results can be seen in Figure 16.14g–i after 43 months demonstrating good bone and soft tissue maintenance.

Micro-flap access and subepithelial tunnel connective tissue grafting have been described with RE to address additional soft tissue demands in the esthetic zone.[37,61] Micro-flap access can be used to expose the ridge crest with expansion following the described protocol but without direct visualization (Figure 16.15a–d). If further soft tissue enhancement is desired, a crestally accessed supraperiosteal tunnel can be developed with a #64 "mini" Beaver blade after bone expansion and implant placement (Figure 16.15e) for insertion of a connective tissue graft harvested from the palate or tuberosity (see Chapter 8). The graft is trimmed to fit the desired dimensions and guided into the closed pocket with a 6-0 horizontal mattress suture (Figure 16.15f and g). Preoperative CBCT images of an edentulous left maxillary lateral incisor site demonstrated a severe undercut as well as significant cortical plate thickness and moderate dimensional loss (Figure 16.15h and i). The apical one-third required careful management because of the undercut.[37] In such situations, crestal bone can usually be mobilized, but the undercut can offer strong resistance or risk sudden perforation due to the geometric curvature. Wider spade expanders or a standard tapered chisel (Figure 16.16a and b) can be used to mobilize the broadest apical portion of the undercut (Figure 16.16c and d) using gentle progressive lifting of the instrument tip at the site apex. Additionally, turning the instrument like tightening and loosening with a screwdriver will mobilize the apical buccal cortex in continuity with the periosteum.[37] The immediate post-operative CBCT image demonstrated osteo-mobilization and adequate remaining thickness of the facial bone plate (Figure 16.15j). At 42 months post-restoration, clinical images demonstrated excellent tissue contours and health (Figure 16.15k–m).

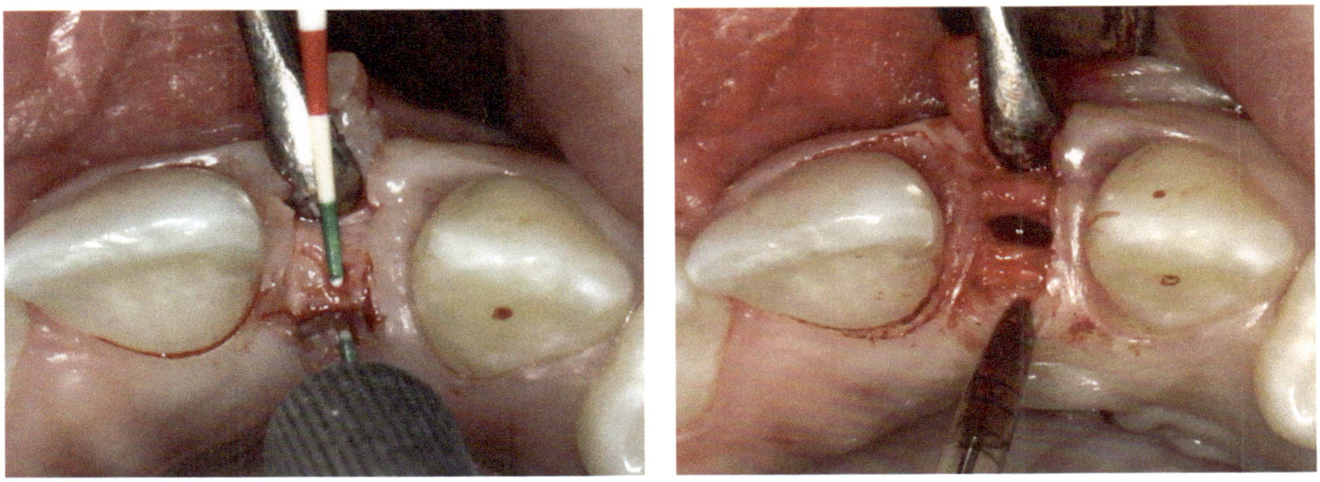

(a) (b)

Figure 16.15 Esthetic mini-flap RE with subepithelial connective tissue eminence graft. (a) Buccal-based "mini-flap" exposure. (b) Expansion gap after Piezosurgery bone incision and initial osteo-mobilization with "spade" expanders.

(Continued)

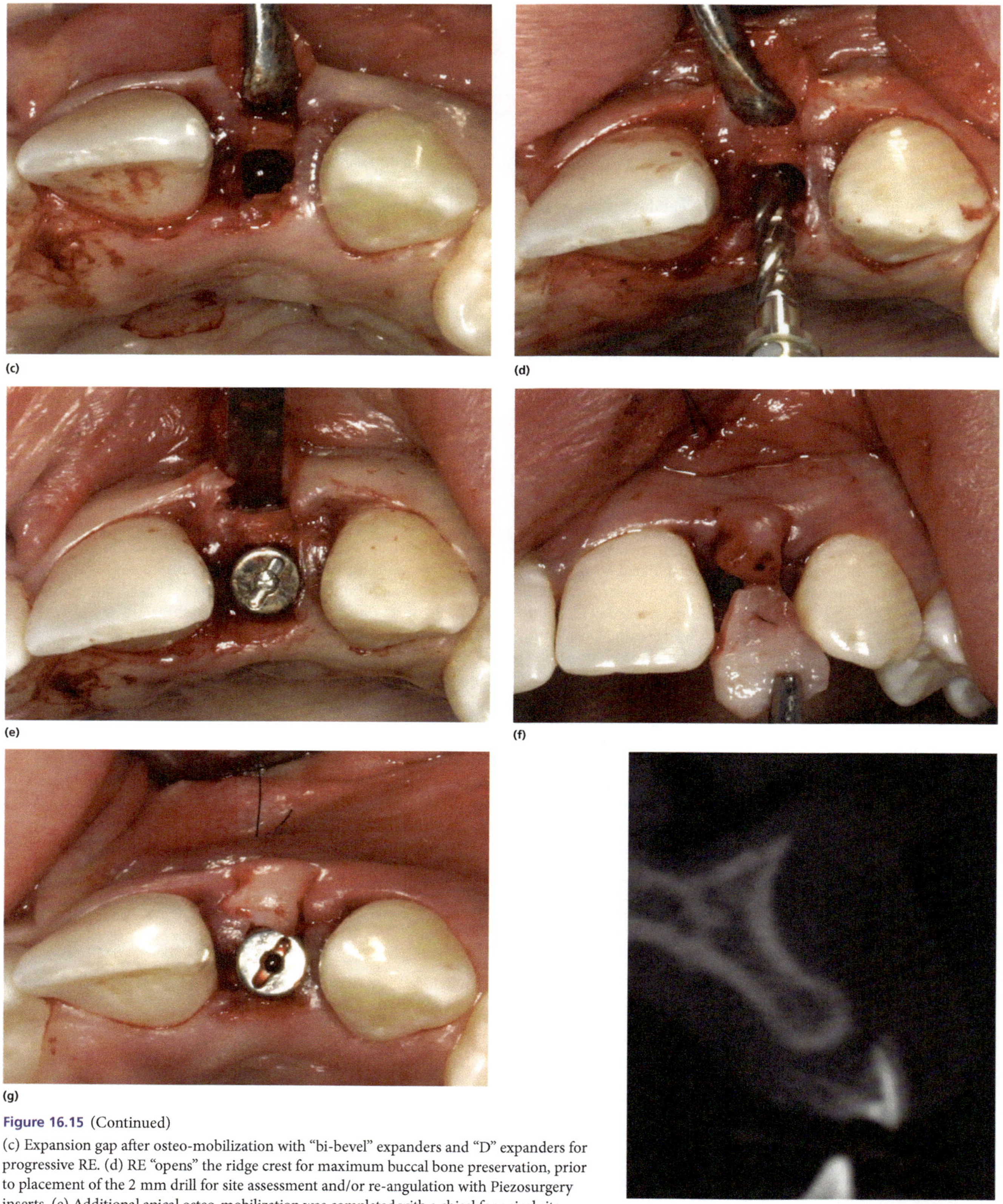

(c) (d) (e) (f) (g) (h)

Figure 16.15 (Continued)

(c) Expansion gap after osteo-mobilization with "bi-bevel" expanders and "D" expanders for progressive RE. (d) RE "opens" the ridge crest for maximum buccal bone preservation, prior to placement of the 2 mm drill for site assessment and/or re-angulation with Piezosurgery inserts. (e) Additional apical osteo-mobilization was completed with a chisel for apical site development to prevent perforation of the undercut. Final osteotome site development and implant placement. Closed supraperiosteal pocket was developed, allowing visualization of the intact expanded crest. (f, g) Connective tissue graft harvested from the tuberosity was trimmed and shaped to the defect with insertion and fixation with a 6-0 nylon horizontal mattress suture for single-stage healing. (h, i) Preop edentulous #10 CBCT images with severe undercut, cortical plate thickness, and moderate dimensional loss.

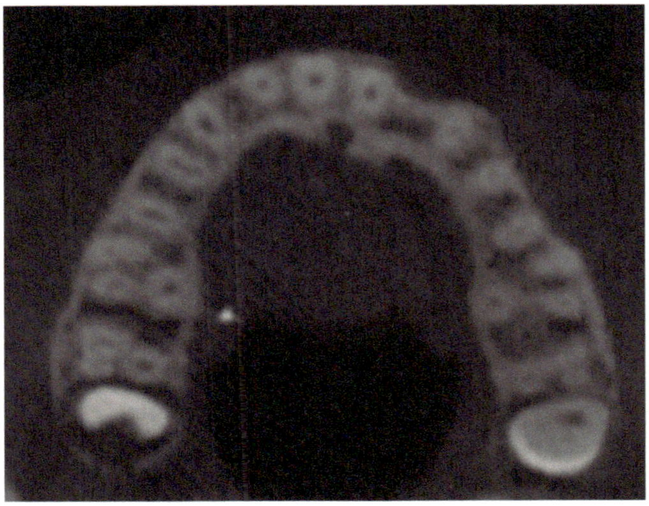

(i)

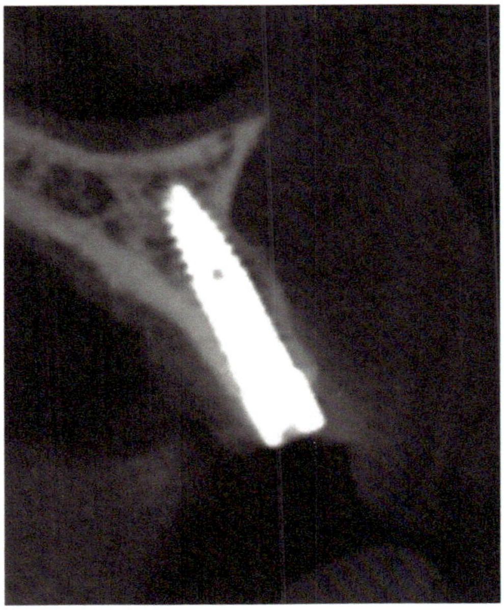

(j)

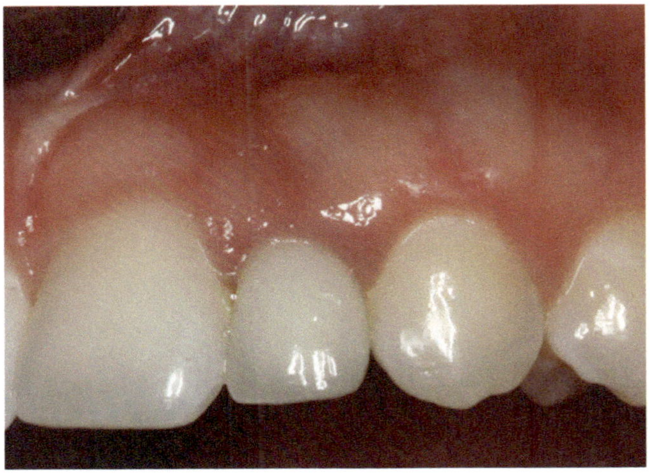

(k)

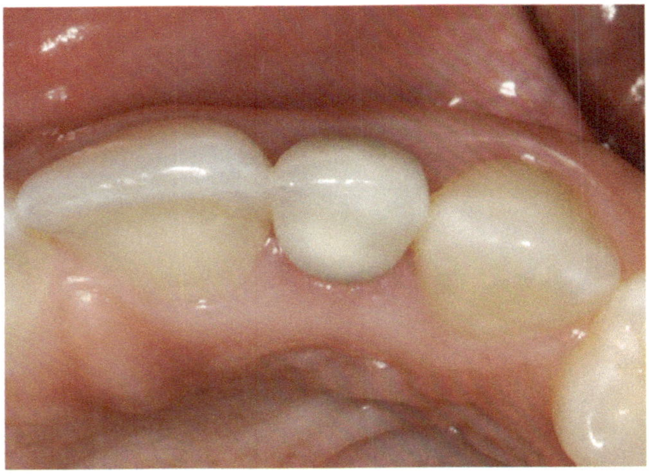

(l)

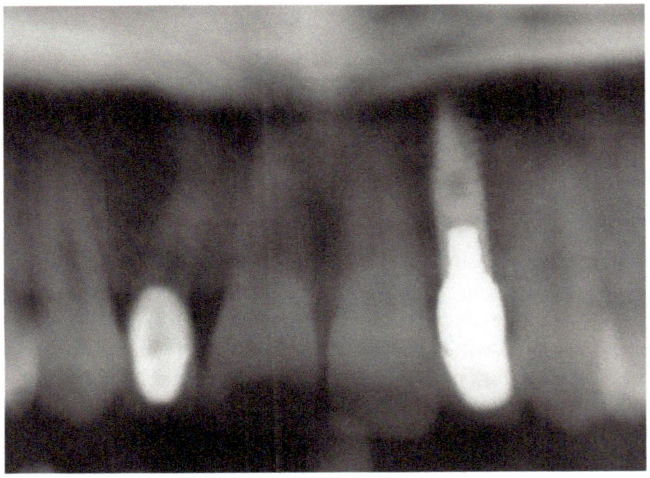

(m)

Figure 16.15 (Continued)
(j) Immediate post-op CBCT image demonstrating osteo-mobilization and adequate thickness of the facial bone plate. (k, l) The 42-month post-restoration clinical images with excellent tissue contours and health. (m) The 42-month post-restoration radiographic image with stable bone levels. *Source*: (a-c, e-h, j, k, m) Cullum DR, Ridge Expansion and Piezoelectric Bone Surgery. In: The Piezoelectric Bone Surgery. A New Paradigm, Vercellotti T, ed. Quintessenza Edizioni, 2015. Reproduced with permission of Quintessence Publishing Co., Inc. (d, i, l) © Daniel R. Cullum.

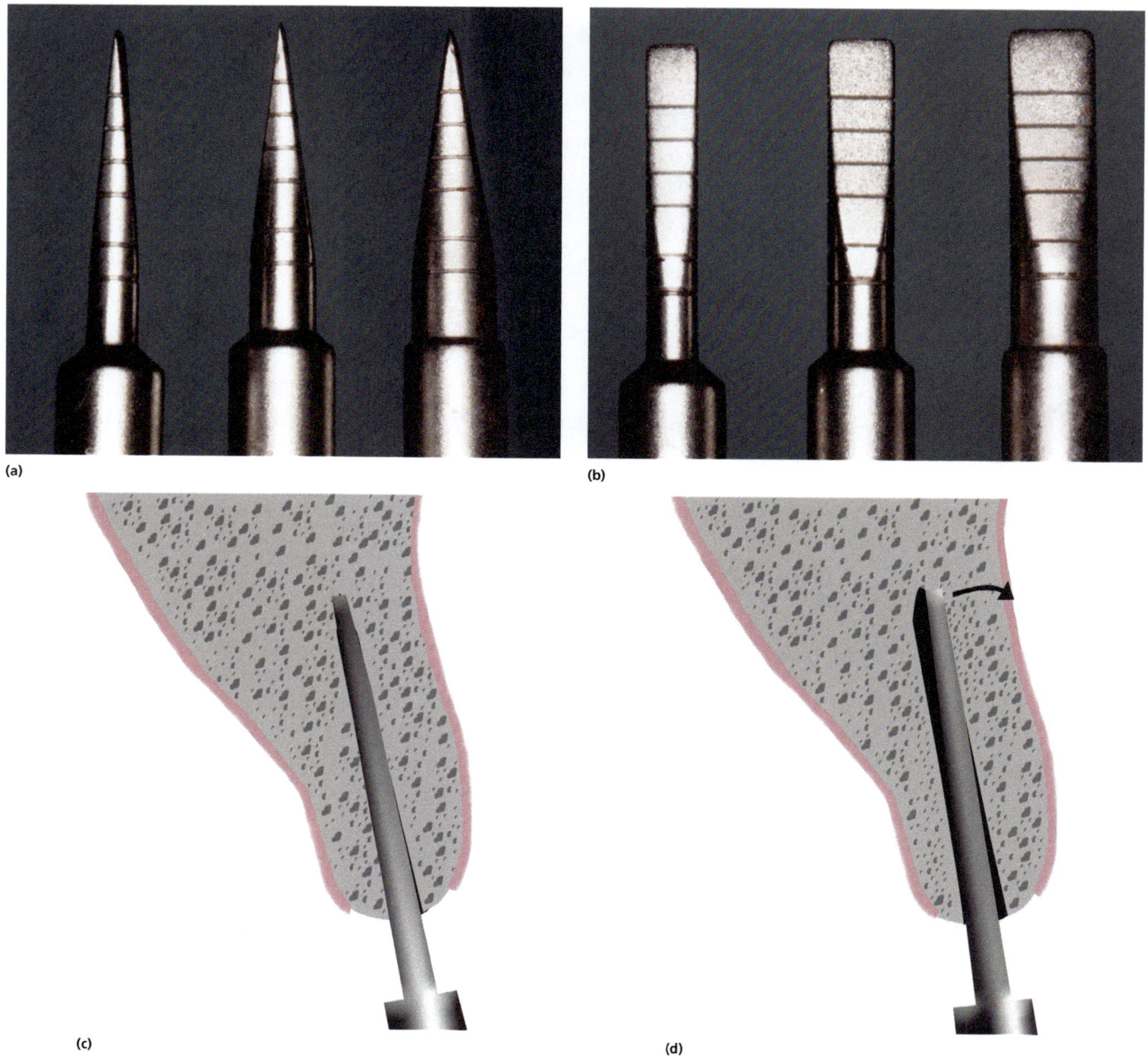

Figure 16.16 Apical implant site modification to correct/reduce labial inclination. (a, b) Bi-beveled chisels (H&H Co, Ontario, CA). (c, d) Apical buccal cortical manipulation with chisels to reduce facial angulation or risk of apical perforation. *Source*: (a, b) Cullum DR, Ridge Expansion and Piezoelectric Bone Surgery. In: The Piezoelectric Bone Surgery. A New Paradigm, Vercellotti T, ed. Quintessenza Edizioni, 2015. Reproduced with permission of Quintessence Publishing Co., Inc.

Avoiding complications

The most common challenges with RE are the same 3-D positioning issues seen with traditional implant placement, although new users of the technique are most concerned with buccal plate fractures. Buccal plate fractures can vary from small vertical fracture lines to a complete "split" creating a free bone graft (Figure 16.17a). With a full-thickness flap approach, management of these situations can be completed with a GBR over-graft (see Figure 16.12c–e); however, a larger "split" defect may need to be managed with screw fixation of the fracture segment, a barrier membrane, and primary wound closure (Figure 16.17b and c). Preoperative and post-operative CBCT images demonstrate the ridge dimensions and screw fixation of the buccal cortex (Figure 16.17d and e) The patient went on to have uneventful healing, with the final restoration radiographic image demonstrating stable bone dimensions (Figure 16.17f).

Another risk with facial manipulation of a bone flap is excessive buccal inclination of the implant. To avoid this problem, after the bone expansion gap is opened, modification of its apical portion can be completed with Piezosurgery inserts or rotary instrumentation to reduce excess facial inclination unless apical perforation or fracture of the labial plate might result. Alternatively, an increased crestal purchase of the lingual/palatal bone using the same instruments can improve final implant angulation and position (Figure 16.9i). Rarely, if the position or the angle of the osteotomy

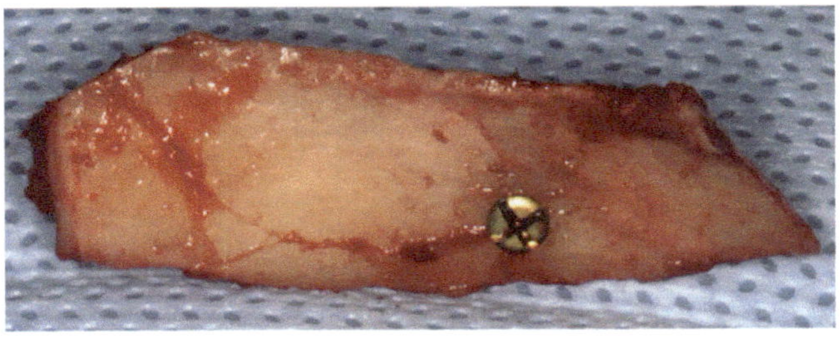

(a)

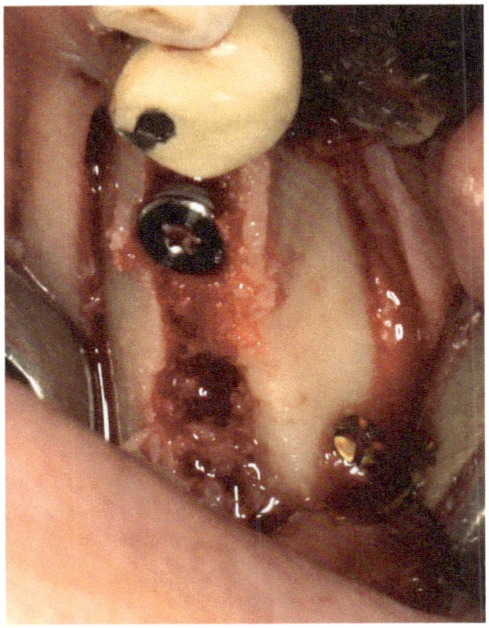

(b)

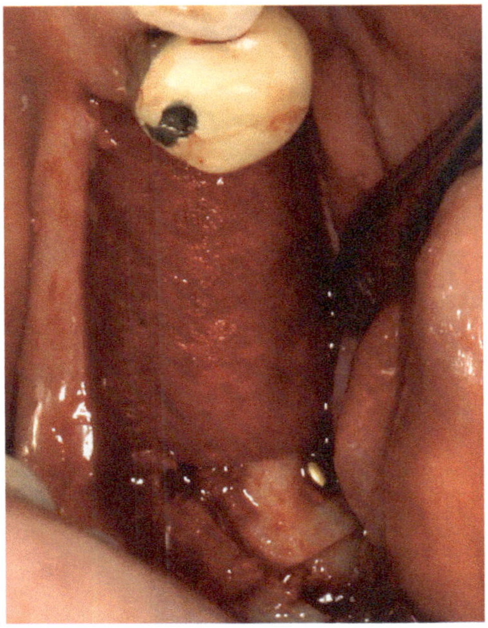

(c)

Figure 16.17 “Ridge split” with re-graft and screw fixation of buccal segment. (a) Mechanical rotary expanders are sequentially placed in bone gap for osteo-mobilization. After implant placement there was partial loss of anterior bone flap continuity, which resulted in a complete “split” with a free autograft. The implants had adequate primary stability and position. (b) Reconstruction of the complete “ridge split” defect was with screw fixation of the free buccal segment and particulate grafting of the intrabony gap. (c) Collagen barrier (Cytoplast RTM, Osteogenics, Lubbock, TX) was placed followed with primary closure. (d) Preoperative CBCT scan demonstrating ridge dimensions in the #29–30 region.

(*Continued*)

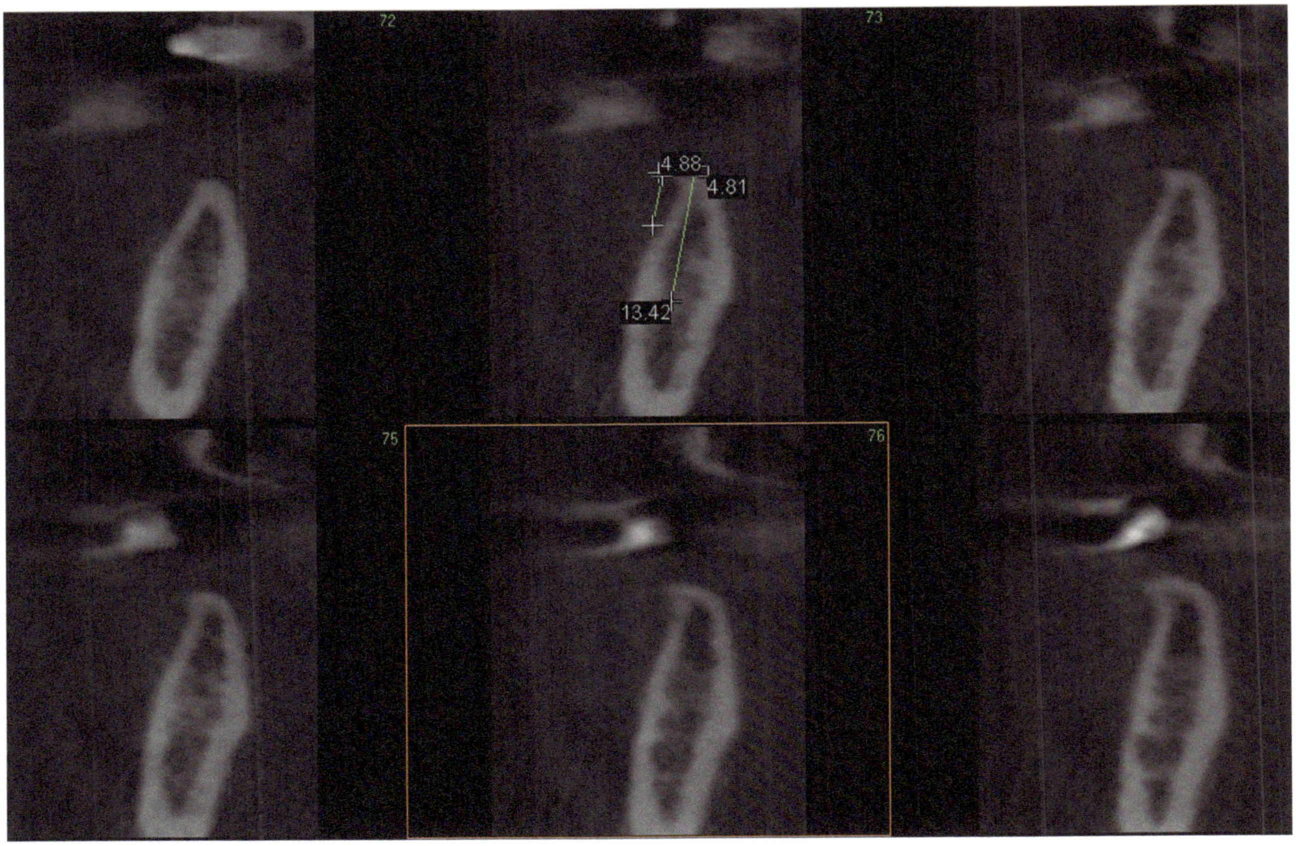

(d)

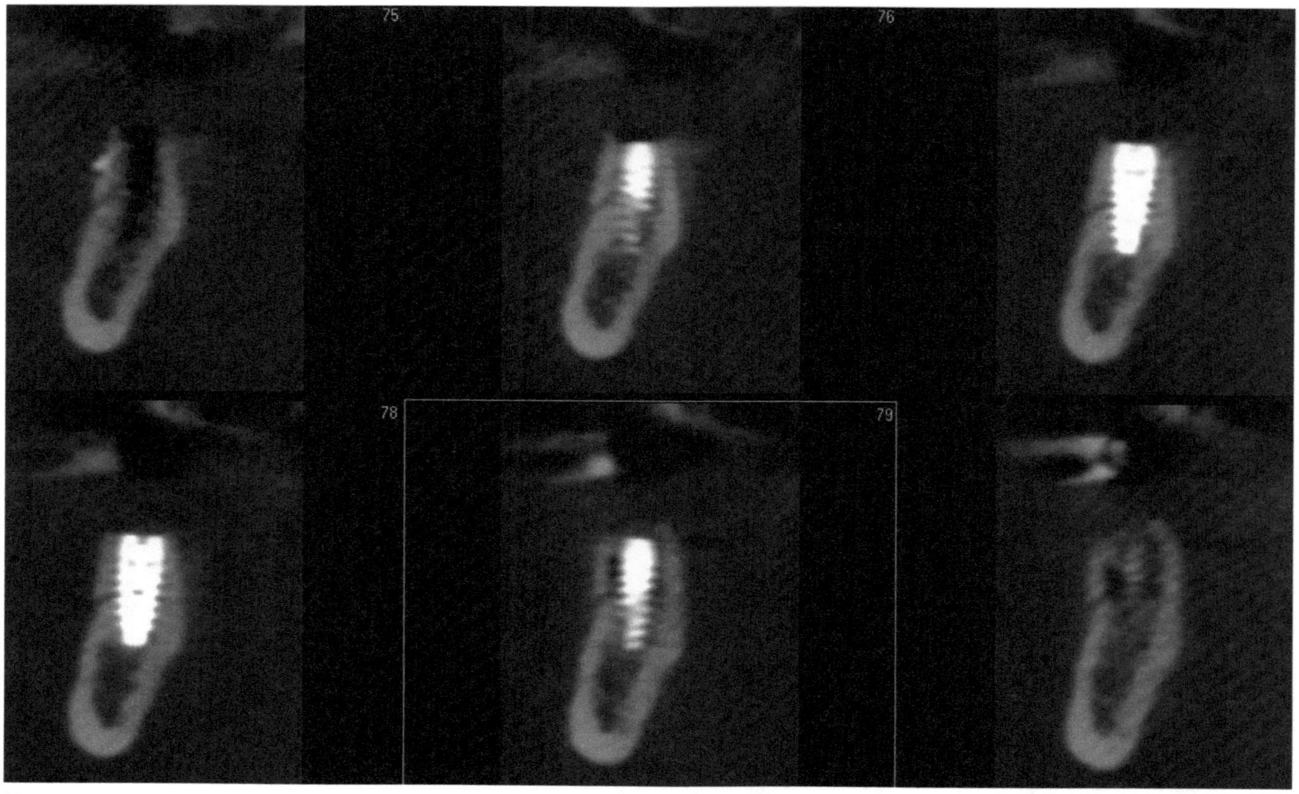

(e)

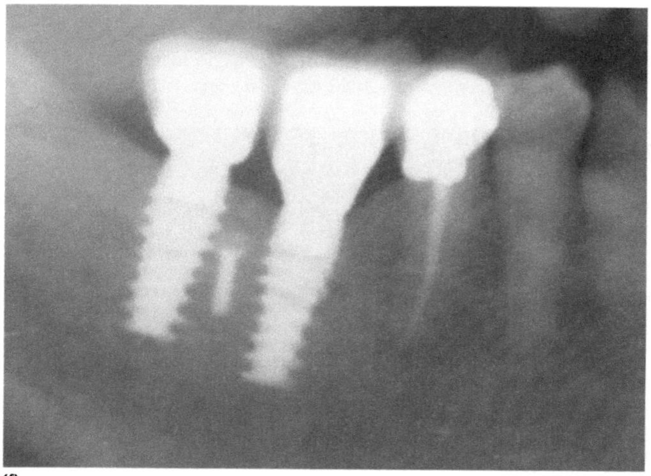

(f)

Figure 16.17 (Continued)
(e) Post-operative CBCT demonstrating screw fixation of buccal segment.
(f) Post-restoration panoramic demonstrating good implant position and bone levels. © Daniel R. Cullum.

cannot be optimized, a site with split-thickness dissection may require interpositional grafting as a "split graft" followed by delayed implant placement. If a full-thickness flap has been used, the site also could be managed with conventional GBR.

Another risk is the presence of a significant labial alveolar undercut.[37] To avoid apical perforation or buccal fracture in such sites, factors to be considered include: (i) amount of labial undercut; (ii) ridge width, bone quality, and compliance; (iii) bone incision design with partial or complete intrabony release; (iv) anatomy of the maxilla or mandible; and (v) position in the arch. It may be necessary to use a standard tapered chisel design for lateral mobilization of the apical bone at the undercut in continuity with the periosteum using gentle progressive lifting and turning of the instrument (Figure 16.16). Alternative techniques to manage a significant labial undercut include sectioning the alveolar/nasal base with a curved chisel for out-fracture.[49,70]

The use of a tapered implant design that conforms to the shape of the expansion defect and a non-flared implant collar design can reduce the risk of fracture of the expanded bone flap. Grafting of the expansion gap can be completed if there is fracture or vascular compromise. Grafting of vertical bone release incisions is recommended to prevent a contour deficiency. Post-operative vertigo is a rare complication of osteotome techniques, and advising patients in advance as part of the informed consent process is necessary. A careful history to rule out any prior episodes, avoiding even moderate mallet strikes and proper patient positioning can be preventative. Rare cases may require management with an Epley maneuver to allow repositioning of the otoliths in the inner ear apparatus.[66,67]

Summary

A group of minimally invasive bone manipulation techniques using RE have been described. These approaches can offer patients a less invasive treatment option than traditional preparatory block grafting or GBR procedures, while maintaining native bone on the implant surface. Careful design of the soft tissue incision is essential, as this will determine the bone manipulation approach to be undertaken. Full-thickness flap exposure offers good vision, but comes with the disadvantage of a compromised vascular supply to the manipulated buccal bone segment. Partial-thickness flaps offer more favorable vascular support to the healing wound, but are more challenging to perform and are not useful in the posterior mandible. A variety of instruments, including various hand osteotomes and chisels used with a mallet, mechanical rotary screw expanders, and specialized Piezosurgery tips, are used to expand individual implant sites (osteo-condensation) or alveolar segments (osteo-mobilization), and can be used with or without particulate over-grafting in a single- or two-stage implant placement protocol. The key for success in RE procedures is ensuring that the thickness of the expanded buccal bone flap is ≥2 mm to minimize the risk of post-surgical crestal bone loss and soft tissue recession. RE is an elegant procedure to restore lost alveolar dimensions, retain adequate buccal bone and soft tissue thickness, and allow implants to be placed in restoratively driven positions.

References

1. Atwood D. Reduction of residual ridges: a major oral disease entity. J Prosthetic Dent 1971; 26: 266–279.
2. Tallgren A. Alveolar bone loss in denture wearers as related to facial morphology. Acta Odontol Scand 1970; 28: 251–270.
3. Brånemark P, Hanson B, Adell R, et al. Osseointegrated implants in the treatment of the edentulous jaw. Experience from a 10-year period. Scand J Plast Reconstr Surg Suppl 1977; 16: 1–132.
4. Adell R, Leckholm U, Rockler B, et al. A 15-year study of osseointegrated implants in the treatment of the edentulous jaw. Int J Oral Surg 1981; 10: 387–416.
5. Leckholm U, Zarb G. Patient selection and preparation. In: Tissue Integrated Prosthesis: Osseointegration in Clinical Dentistry, Brånemark PI, Zarb G, Albrektsson T, eds. Chicago, IL: Quintessence, 1985, pp. 199–210.
6. Truhlar R, Orenstein I, Morris H, et al. Distribution of bone quality in patients receiving endosseous dental implants. J Oral Maxillofac Surg 1997; 11: 38–45.
7. Hammerle C, Jung R, Feloutzis A. A systematic review of the survival of implants in bone sites augmented with barrier membranes (guided bone regeneration) in partially edentulous patients. J Clin Periodontol 2002; 29(Suppl 3): 226–231.
8. Misch CM. Comparison of intra-oral donor sites for onlay grafting prior to implant placement. Int J Oral Maxillofac Implants 1997; 12: 767–776.
9. Boyne P, Cole M, Strolinger D, et al. A technique for osseous reconstruction of deficient edentulous maxillary ridges. J Oral Maxillofac Surg 1985; 43:87–91.
10. Boyne P, James R. Grafting of the maxillary sinus floor with bone and marrow. J Oral Surg 1980; 38: 613–616.
11. Khoury F. Augmentation osseuse et chirugie implantare. Implant 1999; 5: 221–237.
12. Tatum OH Jr. Maxillary and sinus implant reconstructions. Dent Clin North Am 1986; 30: 207–229.
13. Khoury F. Die modifizierte Alveolar-Extensionsplastik. Z Zahnärztl Implantol 1987; 3: 174–178.
14. Simion M, Baldoni M, Zaffe D. Jawbone enlargement using immediate implant placement associated with a split-crest technique and guided bone regeneration. Int J Periodontics Restorative Dent 1992; 2: 462–473.
15. Scipioni A, Brushi G, Calesini G. The edentulous ridge expansion technique: a five-year study on 123 implants with 1–5 year follow-up. Int J Periodontics Restorative Dent 1994; 14: 451–459.
16. Cullum D, Jensen O. Trans-alveolar sinus elevation combined with ridge expansion. In: The Sinus Bone Graft, 2nd ed., Jensen O, ed. Chicago, IL: Quintessence, 2006, pp. 251–262.
17. Chin M, Toth B. Distraction osteogenesis in maxillofacial surgery using internal devices. J Oral Maxillofac Surg 1996; 54: 45–53.
18. Jensen O, Cockrell R, Kuhlke L, et al. Anterior maxillary alveolar distraction osteogenesis: a prospective 5-year clinical study. Int J Oral Maxillofac Implants 2002; 17: 52–68.
19. Roummanas E, Markowitz B, Lorant J, et al. Reconstructed mandibular defects: fibula-free flaps and osseointegrated implants. Plast Reconstr Surg 1997; 99: 356–365.
20. Boyne P, Marx R, Nevins M, et al. A feasibility study evaluating rhBMP-2/absorbable collagen sponge for maxillary sinus floor augmentation. Int J Periodontics Restorative Dent 1997; 17: 11–25.
21. Marx R, Carlson E, Schimmele S, et al. Platelet-rich plasma: growth factor enhancement for bone grafts. Oral Surg Oral Med Oral Pathol Oral Radiol Endod 1998; 85: 638–646.
22. Boyan B, Weesner T, Lohmann C, et al. Porcine fetal enamel matrix derivative enhances bone formation induced by demineralized freeze-dried bone allograft *in vitro*. J Periodontol 2000; 71: 1278–1286.
23. Simion M, Rocchietta I, Dellavia C. Three-dimensional ridge augmentation with xenograft and recombinant human derived growth factor-BB in humans: report of two cases. Int J Periodontics Restorative Dent 2007; 27: 109–115.
24. Lang N, Bragger U, Hammerle C, et al. Immediate trans-mucosal implants using the principle of guided tissue regeneration. I. Rationale, clinical procedures and 30-month results. Clin Oral Implants Res 1994; 5: 154–163.
25. Bartee B. The use of high-density polytetrafluoroethylene membranes to treat osseous defects: clinical reports. Implant Dent 1995; 4: 21–26.
26. Garber D, Belser U. Restoration-driven implant placement with restoration-generated site development. Compend Contin Educ Dent 1995; 16: 798–802.
27. Buser D, Mericske-Stern R, Bernard JP, et al. Long-term evaluation of non-submerged ITI implants. Part I: 8-year life table analysis of a prospective multi-center study with 2359 implants. Clin Oral Implants Res 1997; 8: 161–172.
28. Whorle P. Single tooth replacement in the esthetic zone with immediate provisionalization: fourteen consecutive case reports. Pract Periodontics Aesthet Dent 1998; 9: 1107–1114.
29. Covani U, Crespi R, Cornelini R, et al. Immediate implants supporting single crown restorations: a 4-year prospective study. J Periodontol 2004; 75: 982–988.
30. Kan J, Rungcharassaeng K, Morimoto T, Lozada J. Facial gingival tissue stability after connective tissue graft with single immediate tooth replacement in the esthetic zone: consecutive case report. J Oral Maxillofac Surg 2009; 67: 40–48.
31. Chiapasco M, Casentini P. Implant-supported dental restorations in compromised sites: optimization of results with a multidisciplinary integrated approach. In: Bone Augmentation in Oral Implantology, Khoury F, Antoun H, Missika P, eds. Chicago, IL: Quintessence, 2007, pp. 29–52.
32. Summers R. A new concept in maxillary implant surgery: the osteotome technique. Compend Contin Educ Dent 1994; 15: 152–160.
33. Summers R. The osteotome technique: part 2 – the ridge expansion osteotomy (REO) procedure. Compend Contin Educ Dent 1994; 15: 422–436.
34. Vercellotti T. Piezoelectric bone surgery in implantology: a case report – a new piezoelectric ridge expansion technique. Int J Periodontics Restorative Dent 2000; 20: 358–365.
35. Scipioni A. Bone regeneration in the edentulous ridge expansion technique: histologic and ultrastructural study of 20 clinical cases. Int J Periodontics Restorative Dent 1999; 19: 269–277.
36. Bravi F, Bruschi G, Ferrini F. A 10-year multicenter retrospective clinical study of 1715 implants placed with the edentulous ridge expansion technique. Int J Periodontics Restorative Dent 2007; 27: 557–565.
37. Cullum D. Advances in Bone Manipulation Techniques: Part 2. Osteo-mobilization for Horizontal and Vertical Implant Site Development. Selected Readings in Oral and Maxillofacial Surgery. San Francisco, CA: Guild for Scientific Advancement in Oral and Maxillofacial Surgery, 2010, vol. 18, no. 5.
38. Summers R. The osteotome technique: part 3 – less invasive methods of elevating the sinus floor. Compend Contin Educ Dent 1994; 15: 698–710.
39. Horowitz R. Clinical uses of osteotomes for sinus augmentation at the time of implant placement. Compend Contin Educ Dent 1997; 18: 441–454.
40. Saadoun A, Le Gall M. Implant site preparation with osteotomes: principles and clinical application. Pract Periodontics Aesthet Dent 1996; 8: 453–463.
41. Cullum D. Advances in Bone Manipulation Techniques: Part 1. Osteome Site Development and Minimally Invasive Sinus Elevation. Selected Readings in Oral and Maxillofacial Surgery. San Francisco, CA: Guild for Scientific Advancement in Oral and Maxillofacial Surgery, 2010; vol. 18, no. 4.
42. Bruschi G, Scipioni A, Calesini G. Localized management of the sinus floor with simultaneous implant placement. Int J Oral Maxillofac Implants 1998; 13: 219–226.
43. Cortes A, Cortes D. Non-traumatic bone expansion for immediate implant placement: an analysis of 21 cases. Implant Dent 2010; 19: 92–97.
44. Engelke W, Diederichs C, Jacobs H, Dwecker I. Alveolar reconstruction with splitting and osteotomy and micro-fixation of implants. Int J Oral Maxillofac Implants 1997; 12: 462–473.

45. Malchodi L, Scarano A, Quaranta M, et al. Rigid fixation by means of titanium mesh in edentulous ridge expansion for horizontal ridge expansion in the maxilla. Int J Oral Maxillofac Implants 1998; 13: 701–705.
46. Coatam G, Marrotti A. The segmental ridge-split procedure. J Periodontol 2003; 74: 757–770.
47. Jensen O, Cullum D, Baer D. Marginal bone stability using 3 different flap approaches for alveolar split expansion for dental implants – a 1-year clinical study. J Oral Maxillofac Surg 2009; 67: 1921–1930.
48. Jensen O. The book bone flap: sequential alveolar crest expansion. In: The Osteoperiosteal Flap, Jensen O, ed. Chicago, IL: Quintessence, 2010, pp. 96–99.
49. Horrocks G. The controlled assisted ridge expansion technique for implant placement in the anterior maxilla: a technical note. Int J Periodontics Restorative Dent 2010; 30: 495–501.
50. Jensen O. The book bone flap: the island flap. In: The Osteoperiosteal Flap, O, ed. Chicago, IL: Quintessence, 2010, pp. 101–114.
51. Blus C, Szmukler-Montcler S. Split-crest and immediate implant placement with ultrasonic bone surgery: a 3-year life-table analysis with 230 treated sites. Clin Oral Implants Res 2006; 17: 700–707.
52. Danza M, Guidi R, Carinci F. Comparison between implants inserted into piezo split and unsplit alveolar crests. J Oral Maxillofac Surg 2009; 67: 2460–2465.
53. Chiche G, Pinault A. Artistic and scientific principles applied to esthetic dentistry. In: Esthetics of Anterior Fixed Prosthodontics, Chiche G, Pinault A, eds. Chicago, IL:Quintessence, 1994, pp. 13–32.
54. Kois J. Predictable single-tooth peri-implant esthetics: five diagnostic keys. Compend Contin Educ Dent 2004; 25: 895–906.
55. Sclar A. Systematic evaluation of the esthetic implant patient. In: Soft Tissue and Esthetic Considerations in Implant Therapy. Chicago, IL: Quintessence, 2003, pp. 13–41.
56. Tarnow D, Magner A, Fletcher P. The effect of the distance from the contact point to the crest of bone on the presence or absence of the inter-proximal dental papilla. J Periodontol 1992; 63: 995–996.
57. Tarnow D, Cho S, Wallace S. The effect of inter-implant distance on the height of inter-implant bone crest. J Periodontol 2000; 71: 546–549.
58. Goodacre J, Bernal G, Rerengcharassaeng K, et al. Clinical complications with implants and implant prostheses. J Prosthetic Dent 2003; 90: 121–132.
59. Palacci P, Ericsson I, Engstrand P, Rangert B. Optimal Implant Positioning and Soft Tissue Management for the Brånemark System. Chicago, IL: Quintessence, 1995, pp. 59–70.
60. Sclar A. Surgical techniques for management of peri-implant soft tissues. In: Soft Tissue and Esthetic Considerations in Implant Therapy. Chicago, IL: Quintessence, 2003, pp. 52–56.
61. Cullum D. Esthetic reconstruction of lateral incisors using micro-flap ridge expansion. Clinical Innovation Abstract, Academy of Osseointegration, Annual Meeting Program, 2003, CI-10, p. 58.
62. Ulm C, Solar P, Gsellmann, B, et al. The edentulous maxillary alveolar process in the region of the maxillary sinus – a study of physical dimension. Int J Oral Maxillofac Surg 1995; 24: 279–282.
63. Worthington P, Rubenstein J, Hatcher D. The role of cone-beam computed tomography in the planning and placement of implants. J Am Dent Assoc 2010; 141(Suppl 3): 19s–24s.
64. Agaloo T, Moy P. Which hard tissue augmentation techniques are the most successful in furnishing bony support for implant placement? Int J Oral Maxillofac Implants 2007; 22(Suppl): 49–70.
65. Misch CE. Bone character: second vital implant criterion. Dent Today 1988; 7: 39.
66. Peñarrocha M, Pérez H, García A, Guarinos J. Benign paroxysmal positional vertigo as a complication of osteotome expansion of the maxillary alveolar ridge. J Oral Maxillofac Surg 2001; 59: 106–107.
67. Saker M, Ogle O. Benign paroxysmal vertigo subsequent to sinus lift via closed technique. J Oral Maxillofac Surg 2005; 63: 1385–1387.
68. Khoury F, Tunkel J. Bone augmentation and soft tissue management. In: Bone Augmentation in Oral Implantology, Khoury F, Antoun H, Missika P, eds. Chicago, IL: Quintessence, 2007, pp. 75–114.
69. Palacci P, Nowzari H. Soft tissue enhancement around dental implants. Periodontol 2000 2008; 47: 113–132.
70. Scipioni A, Calesini G, Micarelli C, et al. Morphogenic bone splitting: description of an original technique and its application in esthetically significant areas. Int J Prosthodont 2008; 21: 389–397.

CHAPTER 17

Ridge Expansion Combined with Trans-Alveolar Sinus Elevation

Daniel R. Cullum
Private Practice, Coeur d'Alene, ID; Loma Linda University Department of OMS, Loma Linda, CA; UCLA Department of OMS, Los Angeles, CA, USA

Introduction

Management of the posterior edentulous maxilla can be challenging for patients with significant bone loss and sinus pneumatization. Restoration of lost alveolar dimensions allows for a "restorative-driven" implant position with long-term stability, optimal esthetics, and function. This chapter will discuss ridge expansion (RE) with osteo-mobilization combined with trans-alveolar sinus elevation (TASE) procedures for simultaneous restoration of posterior maxillary alveolar ridge width and height. The rationale, clinical indications, and applications for these procedures, including flap design and soft tissue enhancement techniques, will be reviewed. While combining RE and indirect sinus elevation techniques in a single sitting has a steep learning curve, the benefit is a minimally invasive, transgingival, single intervention with limited use of grafting materials and a shorter healing interval.

Literature review

Alveolar atrophy follows tooth extraction with progressive bone loss (horizontally, vertically, or both) and altered bone quality[1–3] (Figure 17.1a) Vertical and horizontal alveolar dimension losses have been managed with various modifications of guided bone regeneration,[4–7] block and particulate grafting,[7–11] RE,[12–18] distraction osteogenesis,[19,20] composite microvascular free flaps,[21] and/or the use of biologics and biomemetics[22–27] to restore height and contour. These methods often require multiple, staged procedures with prolonged healing intervals, increased cost, and post-operative discomfort.

In addition to horizontal and vertical bone loss, the edentulous posterior maxilla often poses the challenge of progressive sinus pneumatization and poor bone quality[2,22,28] (Figure 17.1b–e). The reconstruction of alveolar height within the pneumatized sinus has been addressed with a variety of procedures including grafting via a Caldwell–Luc/lateral wall approach using autogenous inlay, onlay, and interpositional grafts,[9 10] particulate grafting,[12] and biologics/growth factor enhanced regeneration.[22,26] Another strategy is to use short or tilted implant placement (see Chapters 10 and 12) to avoid the need for involving the sinus.[29,30]

An alternative to these conventional implant site development procedures is to use one or more of a group of bone manipulation techniques to mobilize vital bone with plastic bending, shaping, and condensation as a buccal "bone flap" or "bone–periosteal flap."[12,13,16] Tatum[12] was the first to describe bone manipulation techniques in the maxilla and the use of partial-thickness flaps for RE to preserve blood supply to the alveolus. His rationale was that preservation of the blood supply with periosteal retention would minimize or prevent bone resorption. Summers later described a series of "osteotome" techniques for implant site development in maxilla using full-thickness flaps, hand instruments, and a surgical mallet.[31–33] He advanced the principle of bone preservation (i.e. avoiding bone removal) and "osteo-condensation" using minimally invasive osteotome techniques. These approaches result in contour or dimensional changes while preserving bone integrity and viability. The concept is to manipulate the residual bone to create an intrabony cavity with a wider base or taller roof (i.e. a "four-wall bony defect") that heals like an extraction socket, with access for mesenchymal stem cells and normal wound healing mechanisms.[34] Bone manipulation techniques are most commonly utilized in maxilla owing to its cancellous bone nature. Traditional TASE procedures have a limit to the amount of sinus elevation possible without risk of a sinus membrane tear.[31,35–38] TASE procedures generally require a residual height of 7 mm subantral bone with adequate horizontal (bucco-palatal) bone dimension for insertion of a 10 mm implant.[35–41] Several modified TASE techniques have been shown to allow successful placement of implants in posterior maxilla in combination with RE.[16,42,43]

RE techniques can be broadly categorized as *osteo-condensation* and *osteo-mobilization*, as discussed in Chapter 16.[44] Osteo-mobilization describes a group of bone manipulation techniques that rely on precise bone osteotomies of the residual alveolus to allow progressive intraoperative expansion and mobilization of buccal bone to increase the alveolar horizontal (bucco-palatal) dimension (see Chapter 16). The edentulous RE (ERE) technique described by Scipioni et al.[13] (also referred to as "bone spreading") utilized a split-thickness flap design for retention of periosteum and its blood supply. The technique mobilizes the buccal cortical plate from the stable palatal cortex with an expansion defect opening like a book at its binding and maintaining continuity of the expanded buccal segment as a viable bone flap or bone–periosteal flap.[13,16,42–44] The defect created is tapered with its widest dimension at the ridge crest (Figure 17.2), and the result can be restoration of alveolar volume and arch contour to near-normal dimensions. Preservation of the vascular supply with an intact buccal bone–periosteal flap of 2 mm or greater thickness allows for healing of the inter-bone gap without the need for grafting.[34]

In its most aggressive form, RE has been described as "ridge splitting." Using a full-thickness mucoperiosteal flap for access, the ridge widening ultimately can result in an "out-fracture" of the buccal cortex that then acts as a free graft with limited or no blood supply.[15] In this scenario, fixation of the buccal segment with

Minimally Invasive Dental Implant Surgery, First Edition. Edited by Daniel R. Cullum and Douglas Deporter.

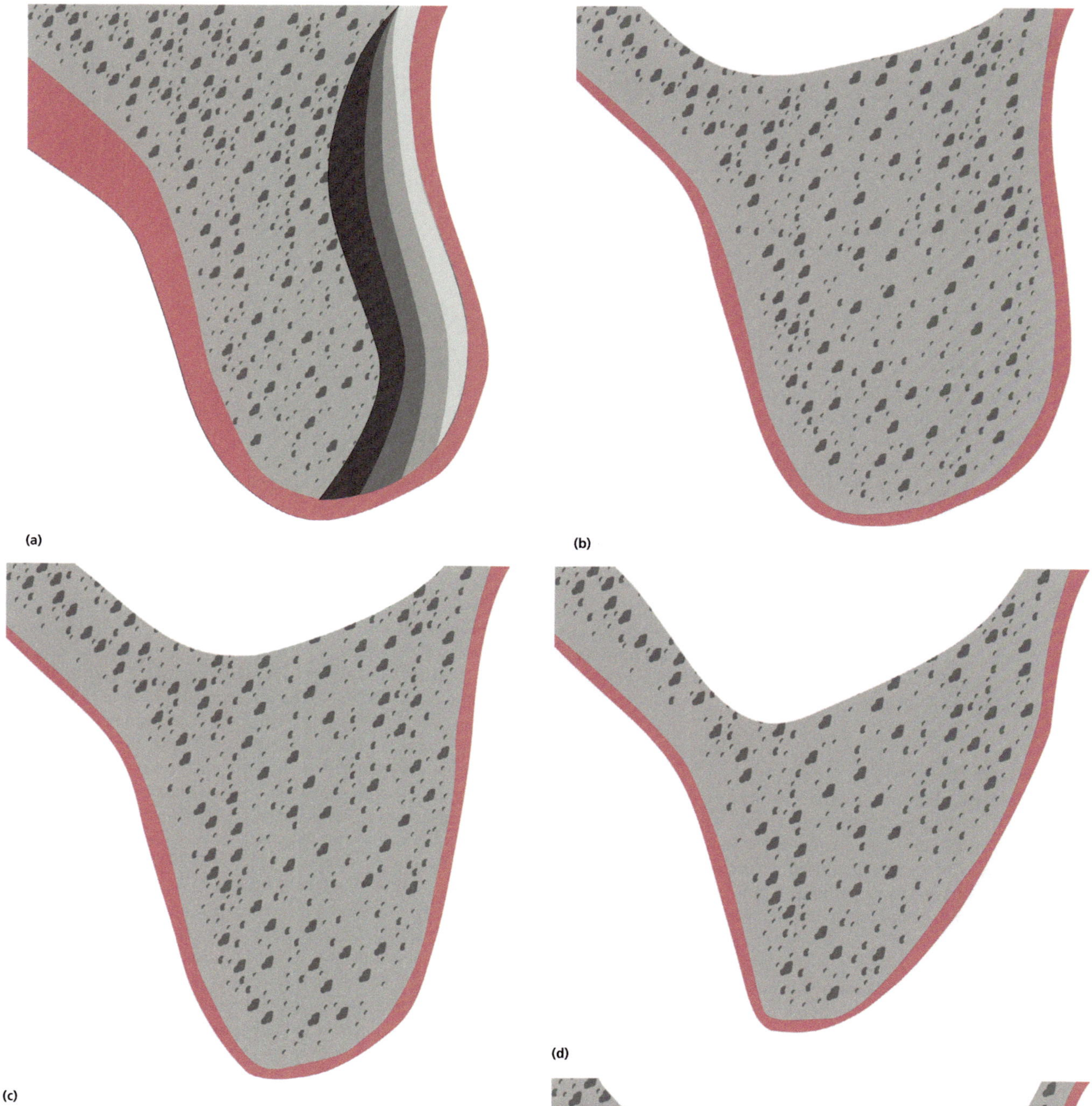

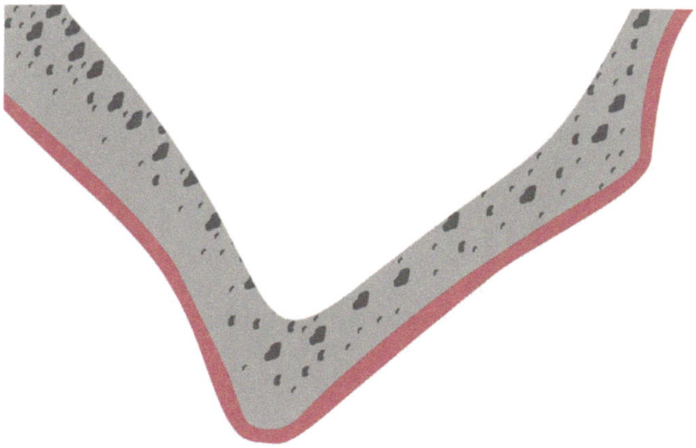

Figure 17.1 An example of progressive bone loss and sinus pneumatization. (a) A healed edentulous site in posterior maxilla. (b) Horizontal buccal dimensional bone loss with slight increase in vertical sinus height. (c–e) Progressive patterns of combined horizontal buccal and vertical alveolar bone loss are demonstrated with increasing pneumatization of the sinus. This can result in a severe bone volume deficiency and present positioning challenges for implant reconstruction. (a–d) © Daniel R. Cullum.

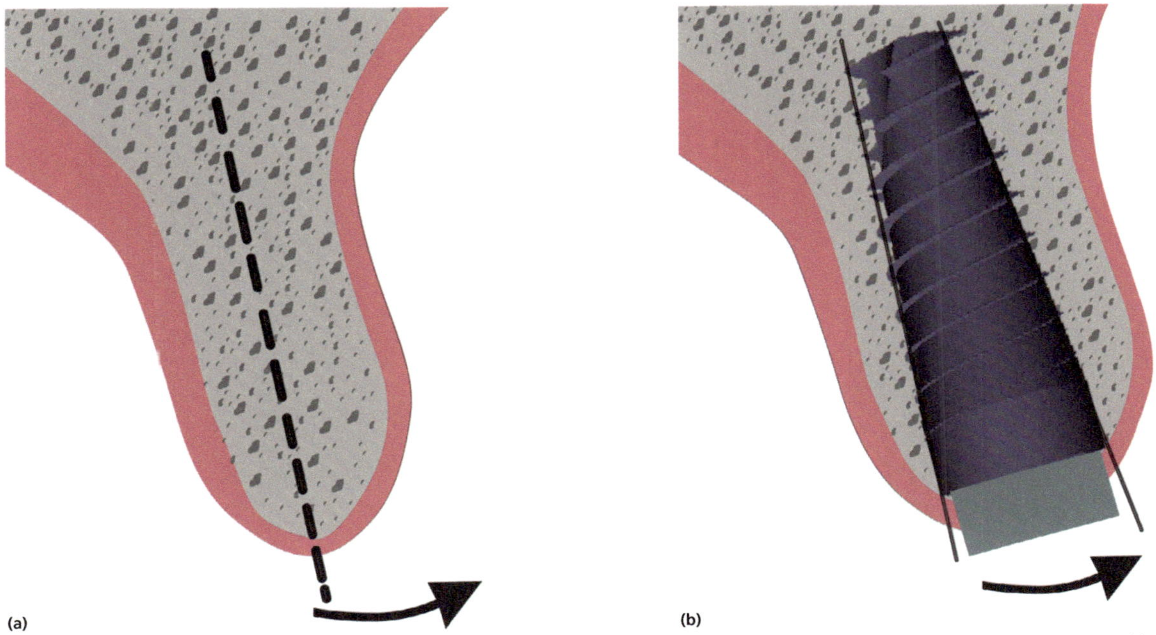

Figure 17.2 Reduced horizontal dimension with restored alveolar contours following ridge sectioning, RE, and implant insertion. (a) Reduced horizontal dimensions resulted from alveolar remodeling. The vertical line represents the position for bone sectioning and RE by osteo-mobilization of the buccal plate. (b) The alveolar contours were restored by sectioning, RE, and implant insertion. *Source:* (a) © Daniel R. Cullum. (b) Cullum DR, Ridge Expansion and Piezoelectric Bone Surgery. In: The Piezoelectric Bone Surgery. A New Paradigm, Vercellotti T, ed. Quintessenza Edizioni, 2015. Reproduced with permission of Quintessence Publishing Co., Inc.

screws and over-grafting (particulate graft and a barrier), whether or not implant placement is included, along with primary soft tissue closure, will be central to a successful outcome.[15] Factors influencing the residual blood supply to the bone flap include use of piezoelectric bone surgery, flap design and management, and bone flap thickness/viability. These variables may account for the varied reports of success and complications with the technique.[12–14,41–51]

RE with osteo-mobilization can be combined simultaneously with TASE techniques to increase the horizontal and vertical dimensions of the deficient posterior maxilla for implant site development. Use of osteotome-mediated sinus floor elevation (OSFE) and bone-added, osteotome-mediated sinus floor elevation (BAOSFE) can result in combined elevations of 1–3 mm and 2–4 mm respectively[33] (see Chapter 15). Bruschi et al.[41] described localized management of the sinus floor (LMSF) with simultaneous implant placement. They advocated a palatally angled bone incision for fracture medially and superiorly to gain width and height when combined with the RE technique (Figure 17.3). A

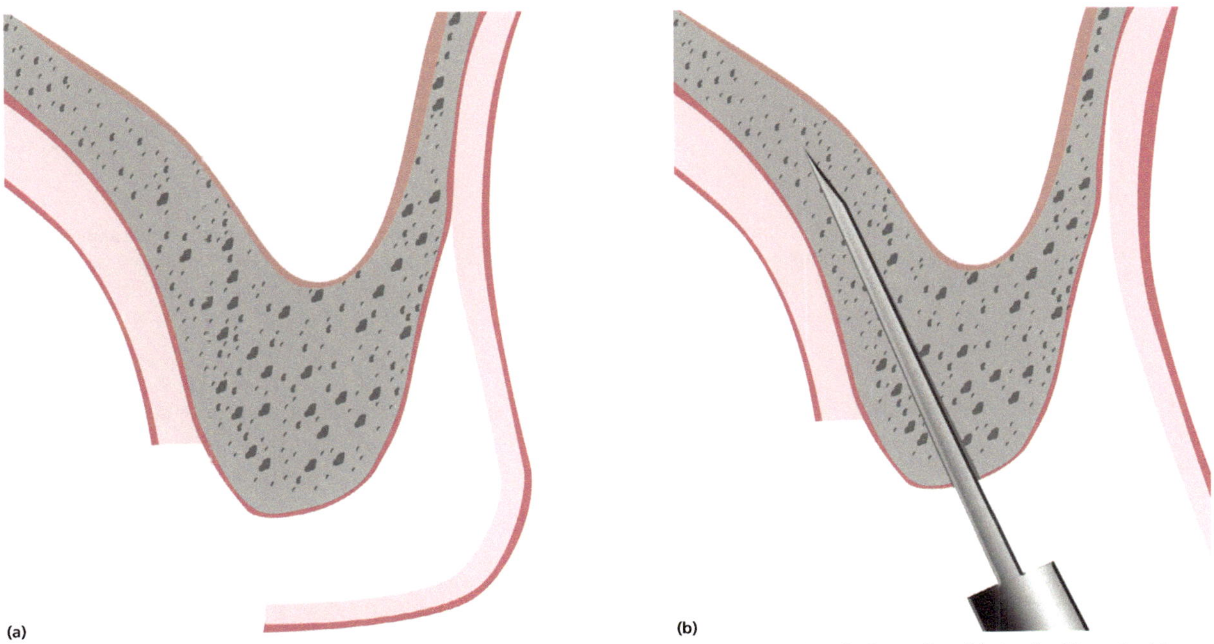

Figure 17.3 ERE combined with LMSF. (a) A palatal incision allows elevation of a buccally-based, split- thickness flap. (b) A palatal bone incision can be initiated using a #64 "Beaver" blade and surgical mallet.

(Continued)

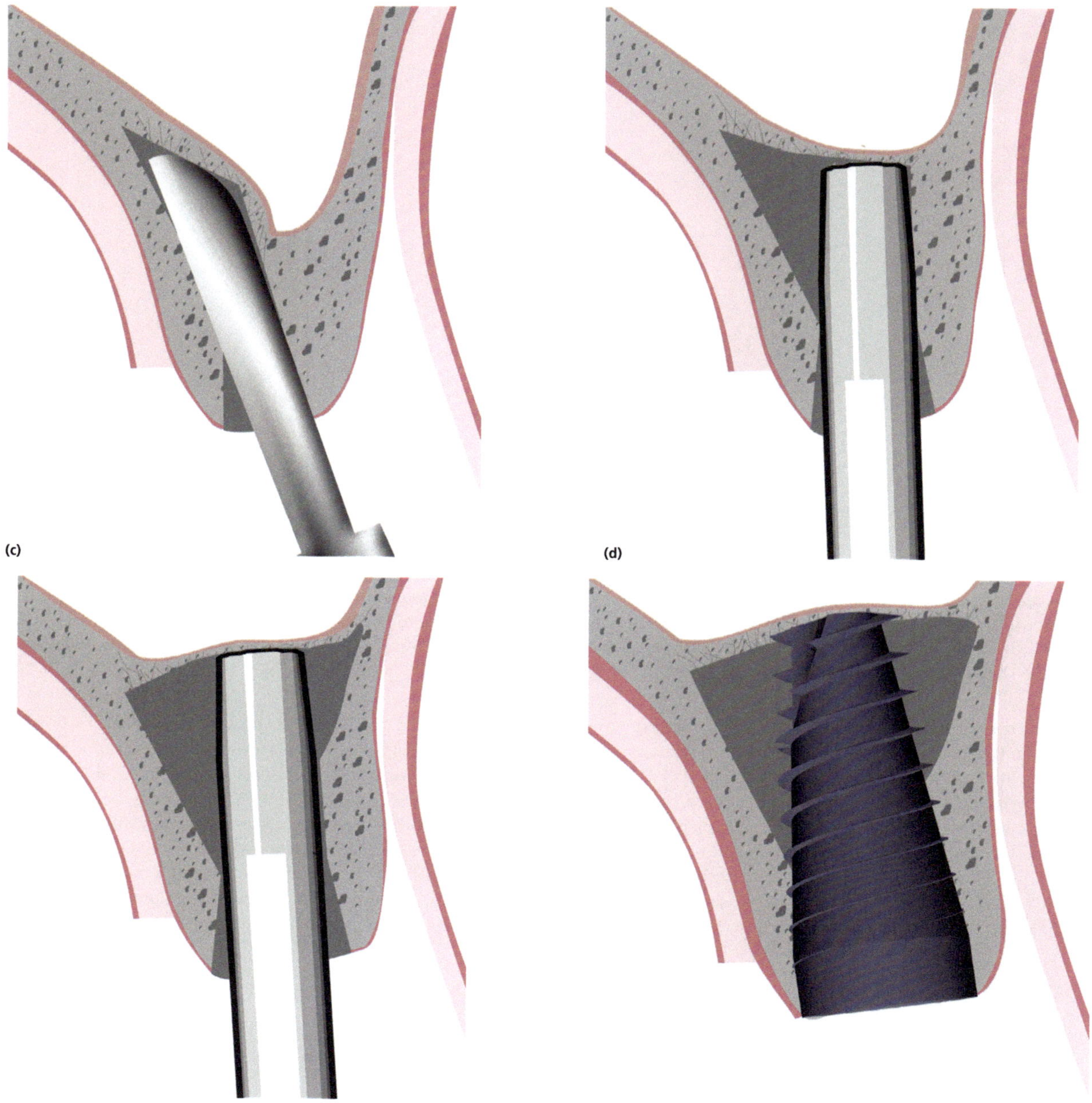

Figure 17.3 (Continued)
(c) A medial bony "in-fracture" of the sinus floor. (d) A concave-tipped osteotome can be used to intrude and elevate the apical region and medialize the sinus floor. (e) Further elevation and expansion is completed to the desired implant dimension using osteotomes. (f) A tapered implant is placed at the RE and LMSF site. (a–f) © Daniel R. Cullum.

patient with 10-year follow-up treated with this technique is demonstrated in Figure 17.4.

Contiguous sinus floor elevation (CSFE) has been advanced as another TASE technique to safely gain additional intra-sinus elevation[51] (see Chapter 15) and can be combined with RE to gain additional ridge width[16] (Figure 17.5).

This involves fracture and elevation of a larger mesio-distal segment of the sinus floor to allow increased elevations with reduced risk of sinus membrane tear or complications (see further discussion in "Ridge expansion and contiguous sinus floor elevation" section).

Anatomic considerations

Preoperative clinical evaluation and treatment planning considerations should include smile assessment, attached gingival tissue (width and biotype), vestibular depth, and muscle or frenal tissue attachments.[52–54] Appropriate 3-D implant placement

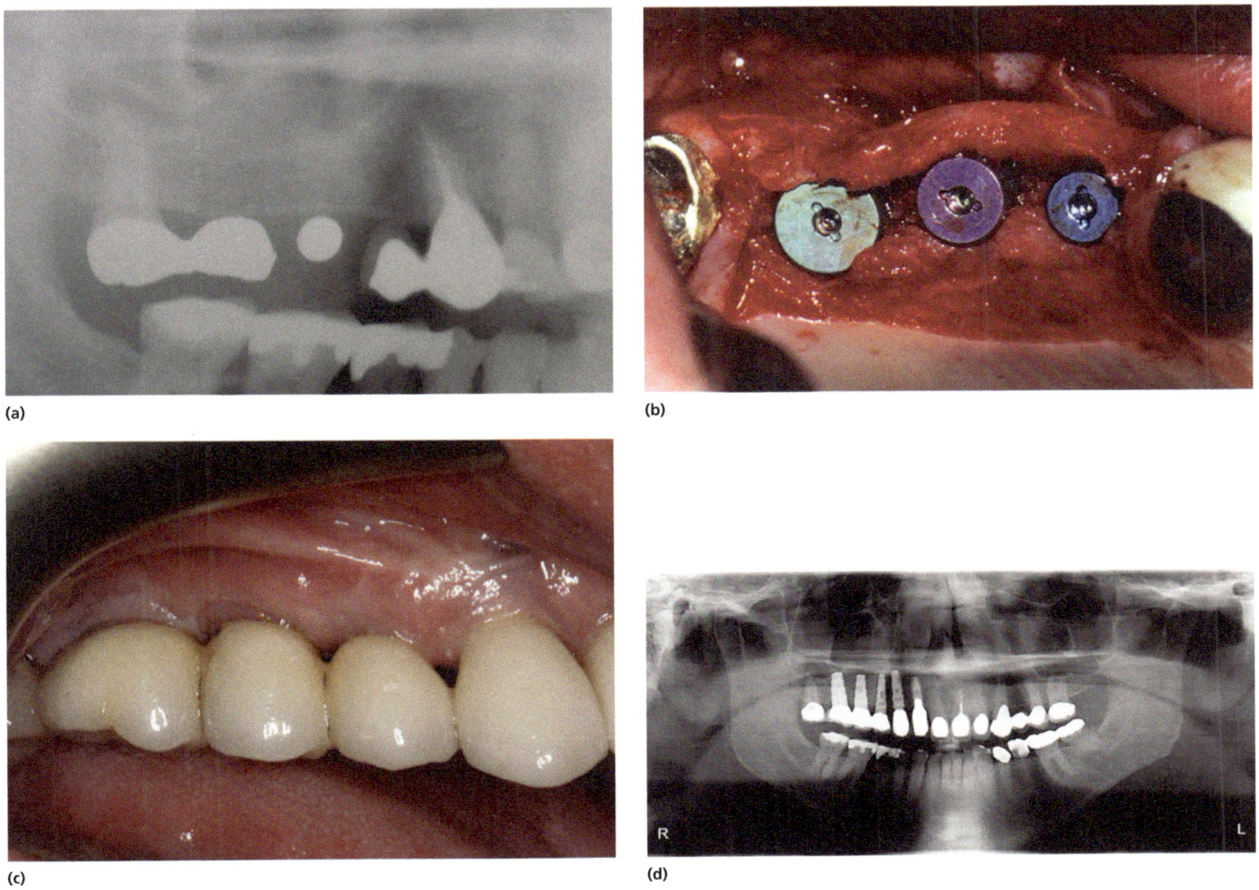

Figure 17.4 Clinical images of a patient treated with the ERE–LMSF technique: (a) preoperative radiograph; (b) intra-operative ERE–LMSF with intact periosteal–bone flap; (c) clinical and (d) radiographic images at 10 years follow-up. *Source*: (a, b) Cullum DR, Trans-Alveolar Sinus Elevation Combined with Ridge Expansion. In: The Sinus Bone Graft, 2nd ed., Jensen OT, ed. Chicago, IL: Quintessence, 2006.[16] Reproduced with permission of Quintessence Publishing Co., Inc. (c, d) © Daniel R. Cullum.

and management of any esthetic or soft tissue compromises are necessary to prevent problems during initial healing or long-term stability of the prosthetic reconstruction.[55–58] Preparatory or simultaneous soft tissue procedures, such as laser frenoplasty, vestibuloplasty, and/or augmentation with connective tissue grafting may be necessary[59–61] (see Chapter 8). In the maxilla, split-thickness flap development is more challenging than a full-thickness flap, but will allow retention of the periosteal blood supply to the buccal bone.

Bone quantity and quality vary greatly in the edentulous maxilla and require careful preoperative clinical and radiographic analyses.[62,63] Office-based cone-beam computed tomography (CBCT) technology allows preoperative analysis of sinus anatomy and pathology, ridge dimensions, and relative indication of bone density[64] (see Chapter 2). Sinus anatomy will influence the suitability of the TASE procedure and the amount of elevation possible with it, a broader and flatter sinus floor requiring a larger floor "footprint" to elevate compared with a narrower and steeper form (see Chapter 15). With recently grafted extraction sites or osteoporotic bone there can be altered or inconsistent bone compliance, with increased risk of buccal or palatal wall fracture, reduced vascular supply, or reduced implant primary stability and load-bearing capacity.[16,51] Cortical bone thickness, increasing ridge undercuts, marrow density, bone height to sinus, and proximity of zygoma or nasal floor will all influence bone compliance and the ease of bone flap expansion[44] (see Chapter 16).

Osteo-mobilization procedures generally require a residual ridge bucco-palatal widths of 4–5 mm and when used in combination with TASE procedures, residual ridge heights of 4–5 mm. If the ridge has significant cortical buccal bone thickness, a significant undercut, or lacks a medullary component, there is a greater risk of fracture during its expansion and elevation. Additionally, with greater mobilization of the bone flap, partial fracture or loss of continuity, there is increased risk of bone resorption during healing, and all of these possibilities are a concern with narrower ridges. Likewise, with reduced alveolar vertical bone height mobility of the buccal bone flap is reduced, as is the potential for adequate implant primary stability. With advanced degrees of resorption, the alveolar crest approaches the base of the zygoma, where the bone is more cortical with less compliance.[16]

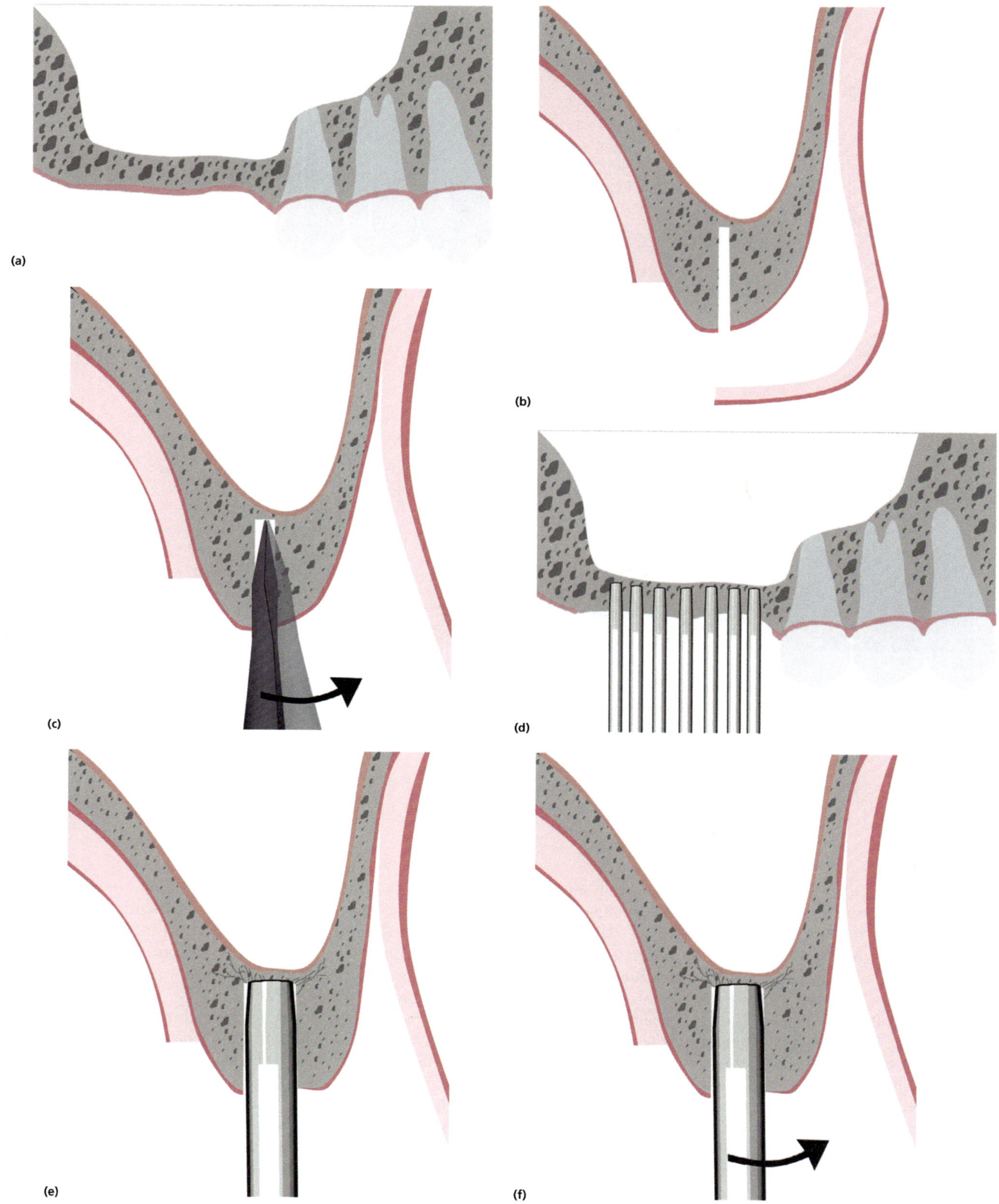

Figure 17.5 RE combined with CSFE and a split-thickness flap dissection. (a, b) A palatal incision is used to create a buccally-based, split-thickness flap design. With moderate sinus pneumatization Piezosurgery bone incisions are completed to a depth 1–2 mm below the sinus floor. (c) Osteo-mobilization are achieved using chisels to produce horizontal RE. (d, e) Sequential floor fractures are developed by walking a 2 mm diameter concave-tipped osteotome across the sinus floor (fracture without elevation). (f) RE with the 2 mm CSFE instrument or chisels.

(*Continued*)

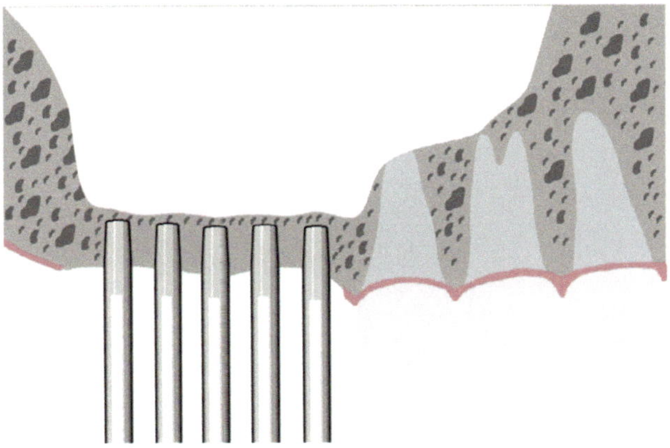

(g)

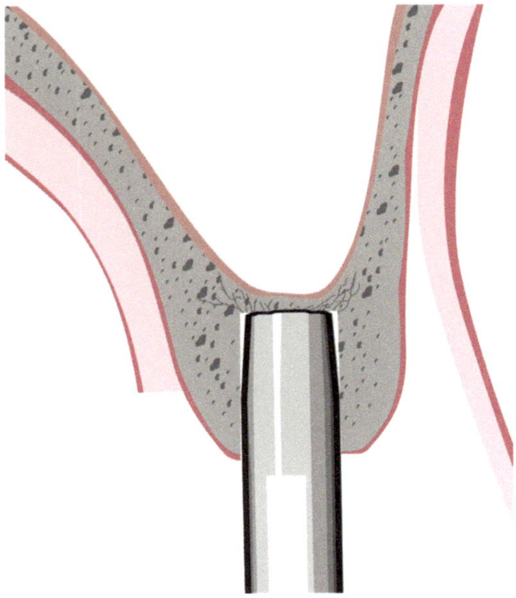

(h)

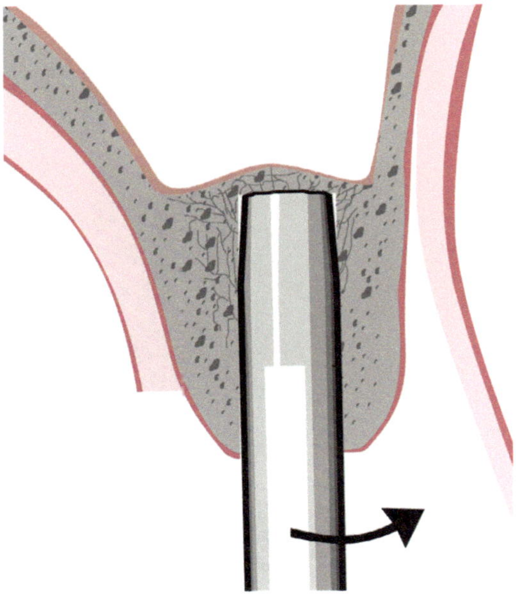

(i)

Figure 17.5 (Continued)

(g, h) Floor fracture is produced by walking a 3 mm diameter concave-tipped osteotome across the sinus floor (fracture ± elevation). (i) RE is continued with the 3 mm diameter CSFE instrument with elevation and expansion. Steps g–i are repeated with 4 mm diameter instruments with initial 0.5 mm sinus floor elevation to widen the contiguous sinus floor fracture to 4 mm. (j, k) Contiguous sinus floor elevators can be used to mobilize and elevate the sinus floor 1–3 mm and to continue osteo-mobilization of the buccal bone-periosteal flap.

(Continued)

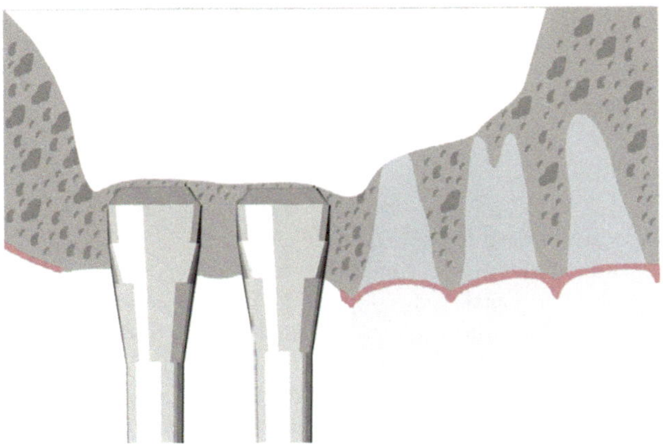

(j)

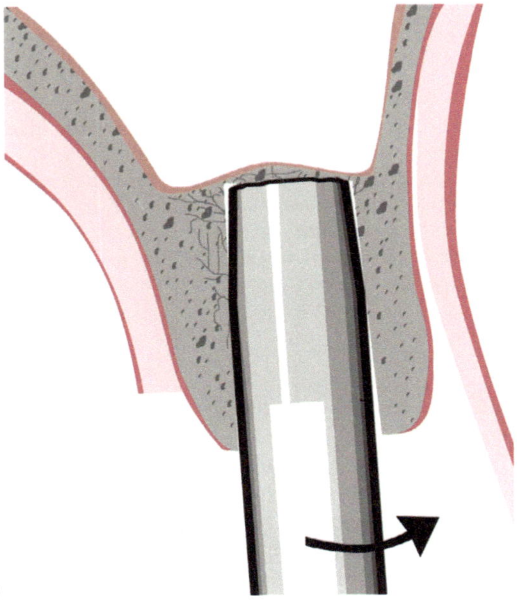

(k)

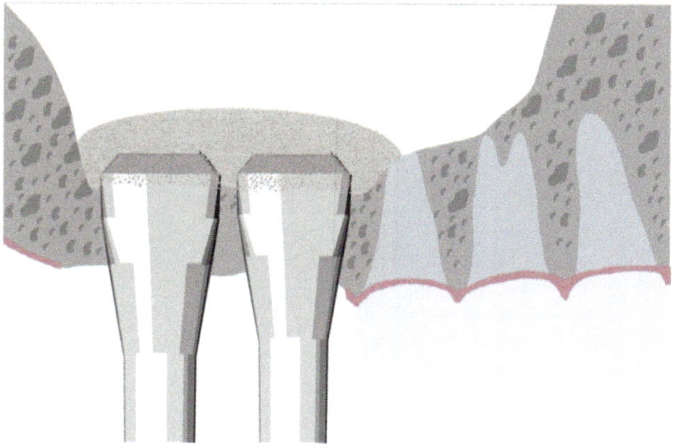

(l)

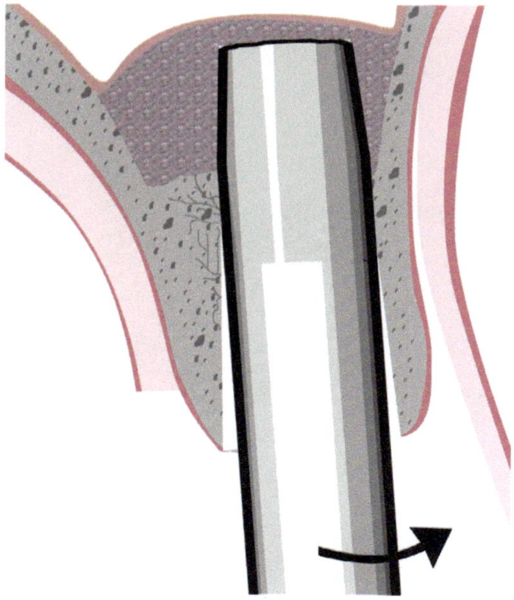

(m)

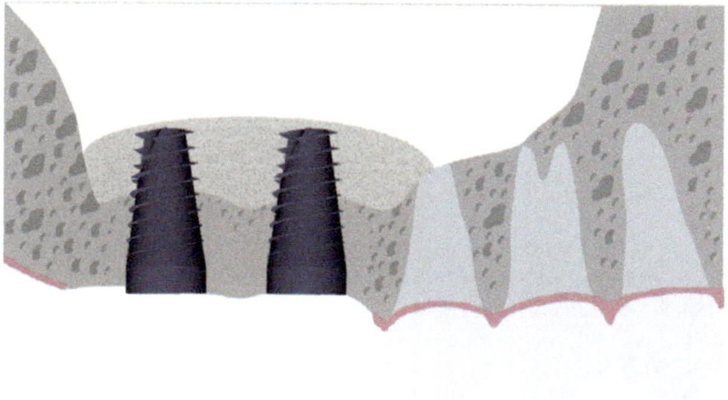

(n)

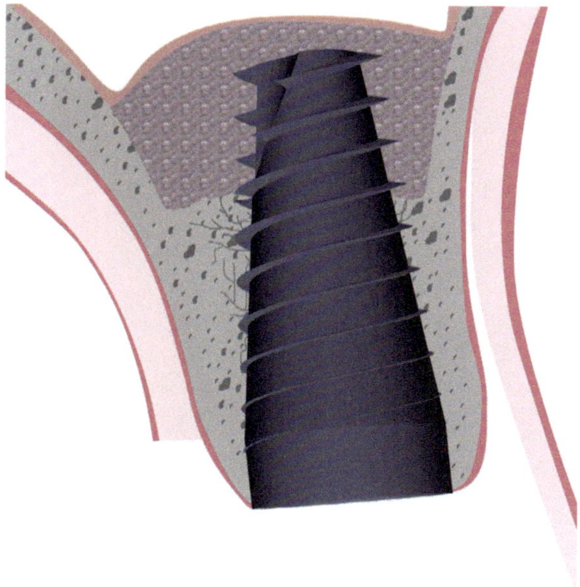

(o)

Figure 17.5 (Continued)
(l) Contiguous sinus floor elevators can be used to continue mobilization and elevation to 3–5 mm with the addition of particulate graft, and to continue osteo-mobilization of the bone–periosteal flap. (m) The final osteotome for a 5–6 mm implant diameter is shown here to complete the expansion; an intact membrane should be confirmed prior to implant placement and ensuring its primary stability. (n, o) Implant in position following RE and CSFE. (a–o) © Daniel R. Cullum.

Surgical considerations

Combined TASE and RE with osteo-condensation and osteo-mobilization in maxilla requires surgical proficiency with each component procedure (see Chapters 15 and 16). Combining these techniques can be challenging, and the surgeon is strongly cautioned to have mastered each technique separately and use a progressive implementation strategy, including live surgery observation and case mentoring. The combined procedures can be completed as a staged approach, but the primary advantage is with simultaneous implant placement.

Preoperative patient preparation is with chlorhexidine mouth rinse and a loading dose of an oral antibiotic. Intravenous sedation and local anesthesia are administered with the patient in a semi-reclined position. Operating from a sitting position, an arm-rest offers a stable base to control force application. Support of the patient's head is important for all osteotome procedures. The expander or osteotome is guided by the surgeon's right hand while the left hand palpates the ridge and palate for continuous tactile feedback. The surgeon directs repeated tapping of the instrument by the assistant. Tactile, visual, and auditory cues require careful attention to avoid sudden fracture of the buccal bone or loss of vertical reference with regard to the sinus floor.

Expansion techniques make use of piezoelectric surgery with specialized cutting inserts[65] (Figure 17.6), hand instrumentation, including a #64 mini Beaver blade (Sable Industries, Vista, CA) (Figure 17.7), bone chisels with several modified designs, and tapered osteotomes (Figure 17.8). Mechanical expanders of rotary "screw" design have limited use due to poor bone quality in the posterior maxilla and limited residual bone height to the sinus.[44]

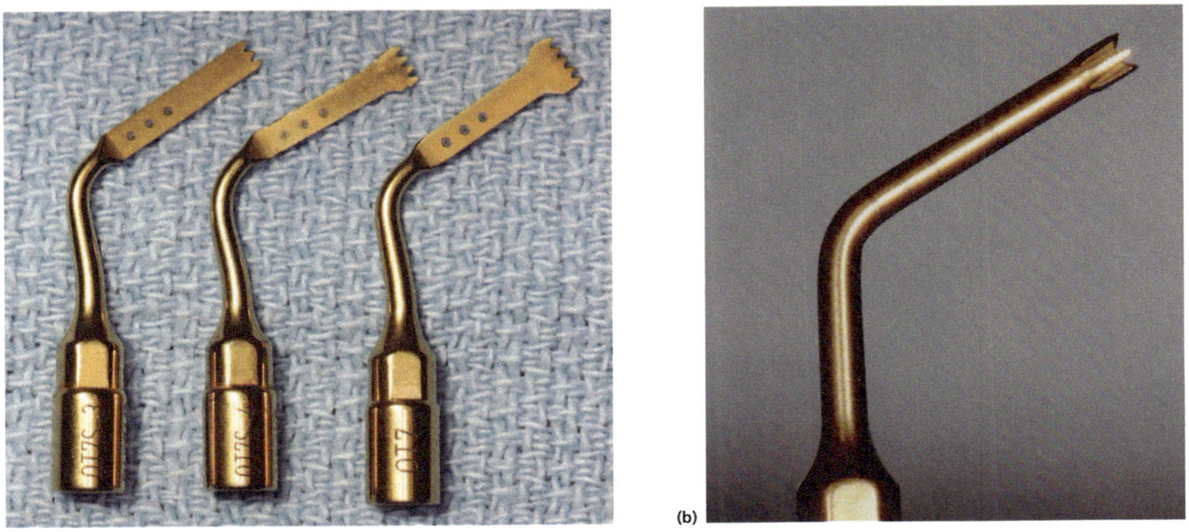

Figure 17.6 Piezosurgery inserts (Piezosurgery® USA, Columbus, OH): (a) OT7S3, OT7S4, and OT7; (b) IM2P. (a) © Daniel R. Cullum.

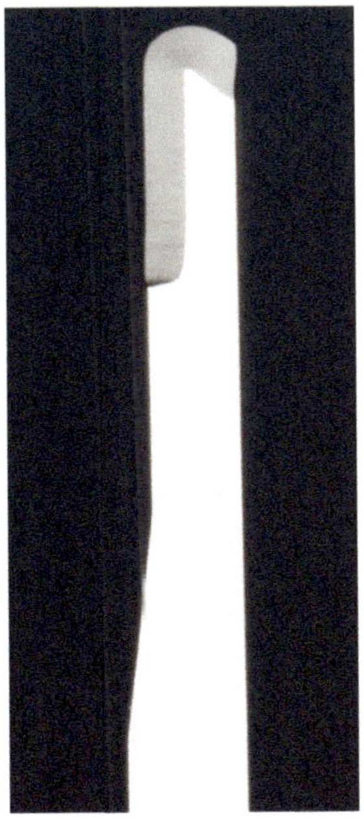

Figure 17.7 A #64 mini blade (#S6400, Sable Industries, Vista, CA). © Daniel R. Cullum.

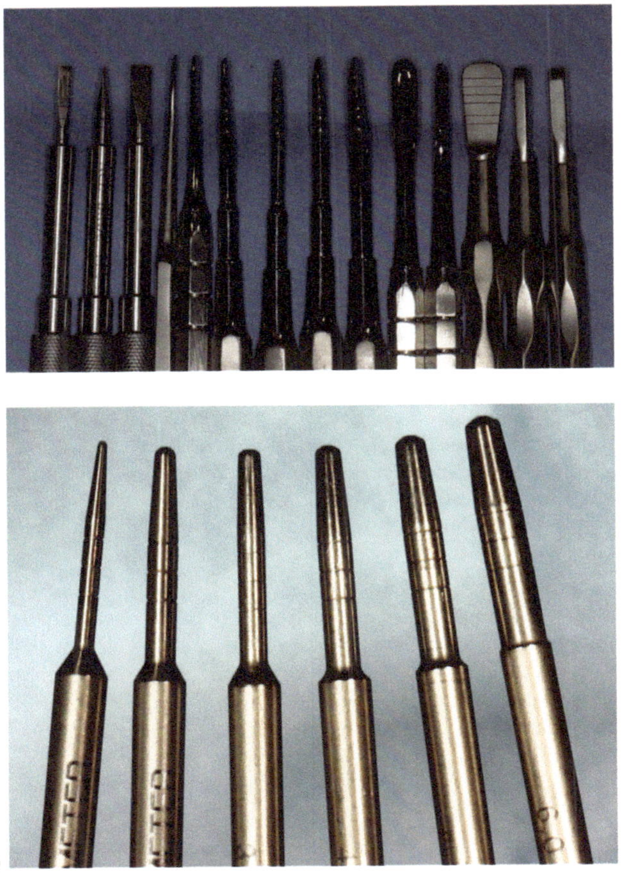

Figure 17.8 RE and osteo-condensation instruments. (a) Surgical mono-bevel and bi-bevel chisels, D-expanders, and contiguous sinus floor elevators. (b) Tapered osteotomes (Nobel Biocare, Yorba Linda, CA). *Source:* (a) Cullum DR, Trans-Alveolar Sinus Elevation Combined with Ridge Expansion. In: The Sinus Bone Graft, 2nd ed., Jensen OT, ed. Chicago, IL: Quintessence, 2006.[16] Reproduced with permission of Quintessence Publishing Co., Inc. (b) © Daniel R. Cullum.

A palatal incision allows for a full-thickness or split-thickness flap design and apical positioning of attached gingival tissue to the buccal, helping to maintain or improve vestibular depth and width of attached gingiva around the implant (Figure 17.9). The palatal incision design also allows development of a mesially- or distally-based rotational flap to aid primary closure around an implant healing cap[66] (Figure 17.9d). A split-thickness design can allow for a more palatal incision and a wider zone of attached tissue than does a full-thickness flap design. The residual palatal partial thickness periosteal layer with a split-thickness flap approach can be left exposed for healing by secondary intention. Split-thickness flaps

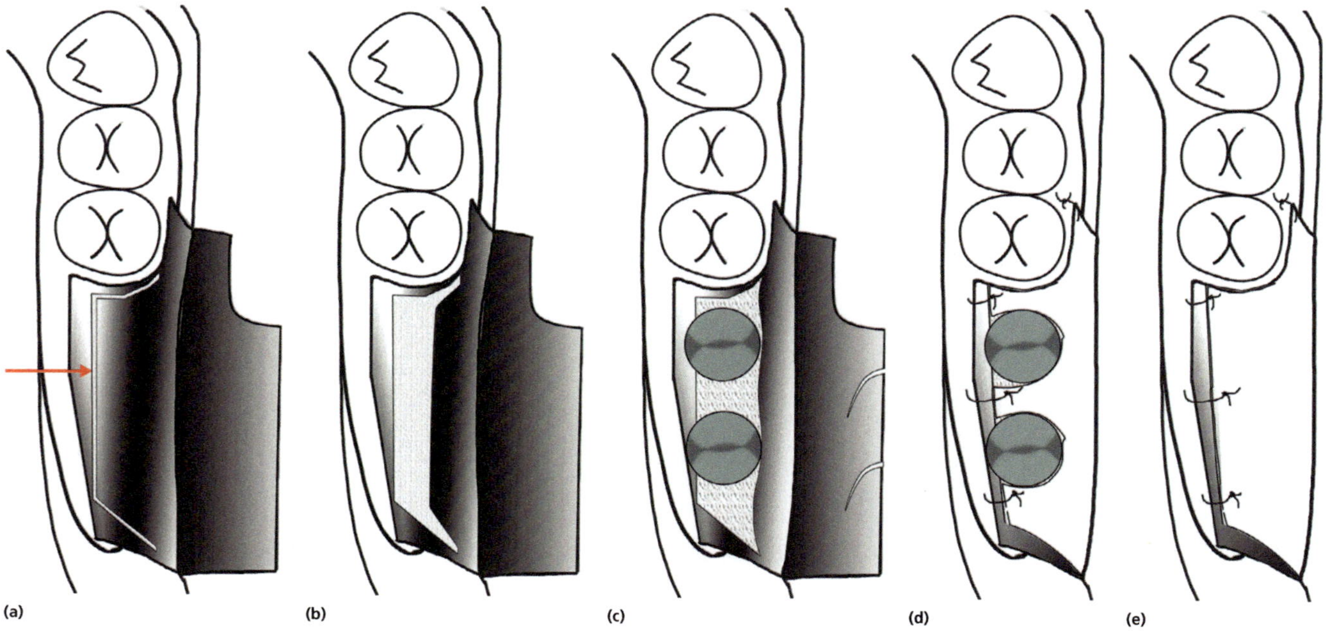

Figure 17.9 Demonstration of a split-thickness RE in posterior maxilla with intrabony osteotomy, internal lateral beveled bone incisions, transgingival tapered implant placement, and apical-positioned flap. (a) A palatal incision is used to create a buccally-based, split-thickness flap allowing completion of Piezosurgery intrabony incisions (arrow). (b) A buccal bone–periosteal flap is progressively mobilized to the facial using chisels and "D" expanders. Care is needed to maintain flap continuity and preserve the overlying periosteum. (c) Implants are placed and the remaining expansion gap filled with heme-saturated collagen and particulate grafting of the anterior and posterior vertical buccal defects. (d, e) With an abundance of attached gingival tissue, anteriorly based rotational "finger" flaps can be developed and positioned anteriorly and apically. Or (e), near-primary closure with periosteal margins exposed for secondary intention healing. (a–e) © Daniel R. Cullum.

will demand more technical care at surgery, and while dissection time is reduced with experience, the demand remains.

RE is completed with slow and repetitive bending and relaxation with progressively larger "D"-shaped instruments (Figure 17.8a) to produce the desired expansion result (Figure 17.9b) As the buccal bone is manipulated facially, the expansion defect is opened and trial length radiographs can be completed (as described for the TASE procedures – see Chapter 15). Expansion of 2 to 3 mm is completed with bone chisels gently malleted to a point just short of the sinus floor. A surgical guide can be inserted for intermittent reference of the inter-implant and vertical positions, and to give a dento-gingival reference for the desired final vertical and bucco-palatal implant position. Apical and 3-D position adjustments can be accomplished with the use of Piezosurgery and/or rotary instruments. With a low sinus the expanded buccal segment must have adequate elasticity and compressive rebound to achieve primary implant stability. Implant selection must include a design shaped to fit the final defect of the alveolar crest expansion. A tapered implant design with a non-expanded collar (see Figure 16.6) can support the expansion yet avoid stress on the crestal buccal margin, reducing the risk of vertical fracture at the height of contour or excessive post-operative crestal bone loss. Also, a non-cutting implant apex can support any added graft material used with the TASE component with less risk of cutting through the elevated sinus membrane.

Challenges in implant positioning most often occur in the mesio-distal and facial directions. It is essential to maintain adequate distances to adjacent teeth or implants and to avoid excessive facial implant angulation. Use of Piezosurgery with tip insert IM2P can facilitate "differential implant site preparation" for asymmetric osteotomy shaping (Figure 17.6b) with selective removal of bone to adjust the position or inclination of the implant.[65] Excessive facial angulation and/or facial positioning often will result in a compromise of the buccal hard and soft tissue volumes, leading to resorption and recession. If the implant position is not acceptable, the implant should be removed and the site grafted for delayed implant placement.[44] Delayed implant placement also can be beneficial when the buccal plate ends up too thin or develops a fracture during the procedure. Transgingival (i.e. non-submerged) implant placement can be used when good initial implant stability is achieved and an intact buccal bone flap of optimal thickness (>2 mm) remains (Figure 17.9d). With increasing operator experience, narrower ridge widths, smaller flaps, and reduced wound exposure can be utilized, enhancing the minimally invasive benefits of these procedures. A light-cured periodontal dressing (Barricaide™, Densply-Caulk, Milford, DE) can aid in protection of transgingival wounds during the initial post-operative period.[16] RE combined with LMSF or CSFE in situations with a residual alveolar height of 4–5 mm may require a healing interval of up to 6 months.[16,41] Transitional loading on a reduced occlusal platform and/or a splinted provisional prosthesis can be considered to incorporate progressive implant loading.

Use of a full-thickness flap with "ridge splitting" is simpler for access. With thinner ridge widths (less than 4 mm), anatomic concerns for increased fracture potential, or limited surgical experience, a splitting technique using a full-thickness flap with over-grafting, submerged healing (following a bone graft/guided bone regeneration protocol), and primary closure may be preferred. This "over-grafting" technique cannot be applied over the intact periosteum with a split-thickness flap. Therefore a strategic choice is necessary beforehand based on preoperative clinical and CBCT assessment.

Ridge expansion and trans-alveolar sinus elevation procedures for maxillary horizontal and vertical deficiency

After the surgeon has developed experience with RE and TASE procedures separately, their combined application has great potential as a minimally invasive procedure. RE combined with TASE procedures is indicated for elevations of 1–2 mm with OSFE, 2–4 mm with BAOSFE, and 4–7 mm with CSFE.

Soft tissue flap design

Full-thickness

A palatal incision is developed through the periosteum to bone at the planned palatal margin of the final implant position. It should be extended anteriorly and posteriorly to the adjacent teeth with a marginal release to preserve the papillae, or with an edentulous posterior segment distally to the tuberosity with a lateral release. At the anterior buccal margin, the incision can be extended one tooth horizontally at the level of the mucogingival junction with a vertical release for additional access.

Split-thickness

The same buccally-based palatal incision is developed with sharp dissection just above the level of the periosteum using the #64 "mini" Beaver blade (Figure 17.7). The split-thickness flap can be extended to the anterior or posterior, one to two teeth, with a marginal release at the mucogingival junction (Figure 17.9a). The flap can be further extended with a beveled vertical release to gain access, visibility, or soft tissue mobilization for repositioning. Beveling the vertical incision 45° away from the periosteal base significantly reduces or eliminates vertical scar formation. With edentulous spans that extend anteriorly to the esthetic zone or in patients with esthetic display to the molar region, the flap should extend one to two teeth distal to the site or to the tuberosity with lateral/vertical release. The release of the periosteum at the distal and superior margins with a "cut-back" incision greatly enhances mobility of the soft tissue flap. Apical flap positioning improves soft tissue vestibular depth and quantity of attached tissue, with the residual soft tissue defect remote from the expansion and implant site (Figure 17.9d). Care is necessary to avoid perforation on dissection of the flap by using a sharp blade and slightly increasing the blade angle (more vertically) as the mucogingival junction is approached.[16] The palatal aspect of the ridge may be exposed with split-thickness dissection, or bone sounding can be used to determine the clinical anatomic dimensions of the ridge and inclination of the palatal vault. Often with experience, the procedure can be completed with minimal flap development.[49] Larger expansion sites may require greater soft tissue mobilization to allow movement of the bone flap and apical soft tissue repositioning.

Bone incision design

After soft tissue dissection, the bone incisions are made (arrow Figure 17.9a) utilizing Piezosurgery OT7 or OT7S4 inserts (Figure 17.6a) to section the residual alveolus from anterior to posterior with a distal lateral release at the tuberosity or the end of the edentulous span. An anterior beveled intrabony release is then completed with the Piezosurgery OT7S4 insert as described for RE (see Chapter 16) (Figure 17.9a). The bone incisions are completed to a level 1–2 mm below the sinus floor and following the floor contour. Trial length radiographs are completed as described for the TASE procedures (see Chapter 15), after which bone chisels (H&H Co., Ontario, CA) are gently malleted to this depth to begin initial osteomobilization for ridge width expansion of 2–3 mm (Figures 17.7a and 17.9b). After the initial RE has been completed, the appropriate TASE technique is selected based on the residual bone height and the required amount of elevation.

Ridge expansion and trans-alveolar sinus elevation procedures

Ridge expansion combined with osteotome sinus floor elevation

RE combined with OSFE for elevation of 1–3 mm can be used with either a partial- or full-thickness flap. An example with a full-thickness flap is shown in Figure 17.10. The edentulous right maxillary first molar site was treated with a limited full-thickness flap exposure (Figure 17.10a–c). RE with intrabony osteotomy development was completed to a level 1–2 mm below the sinus floor. Internal laterally-beveled bone incisions were completed

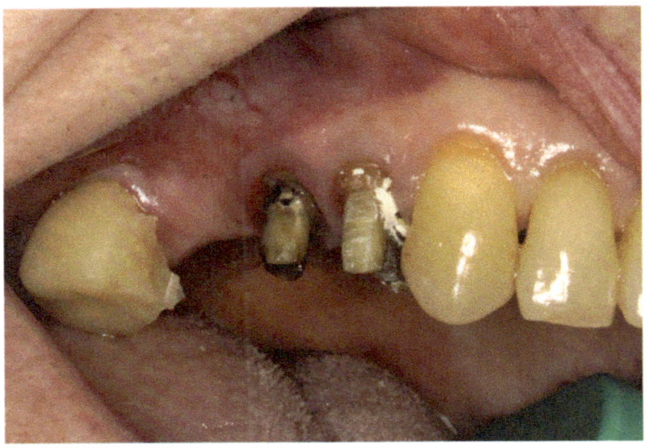

(a)

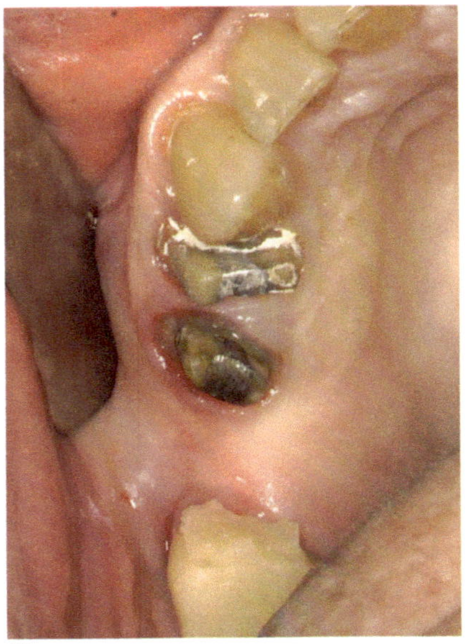

(b)

Figure 17.10 An edentulous right maxillary first molar site was accessed using limited full-thickness flap exposure. RE used an intrabony osteotomy and internally laterally-beveled bone incisions to allow laterally-beveled placement of a tapered implant. Over-grafting and apical repositioned flap/rotational finger flaps also were used. Simultaneous extraction of the first and second premolar teeth and immediate implant placement with OSFE and connective tissue grafting also were completed. (a, b) The preoperative clinical view of the edentulous right maxillary first molar site.

(Continued)

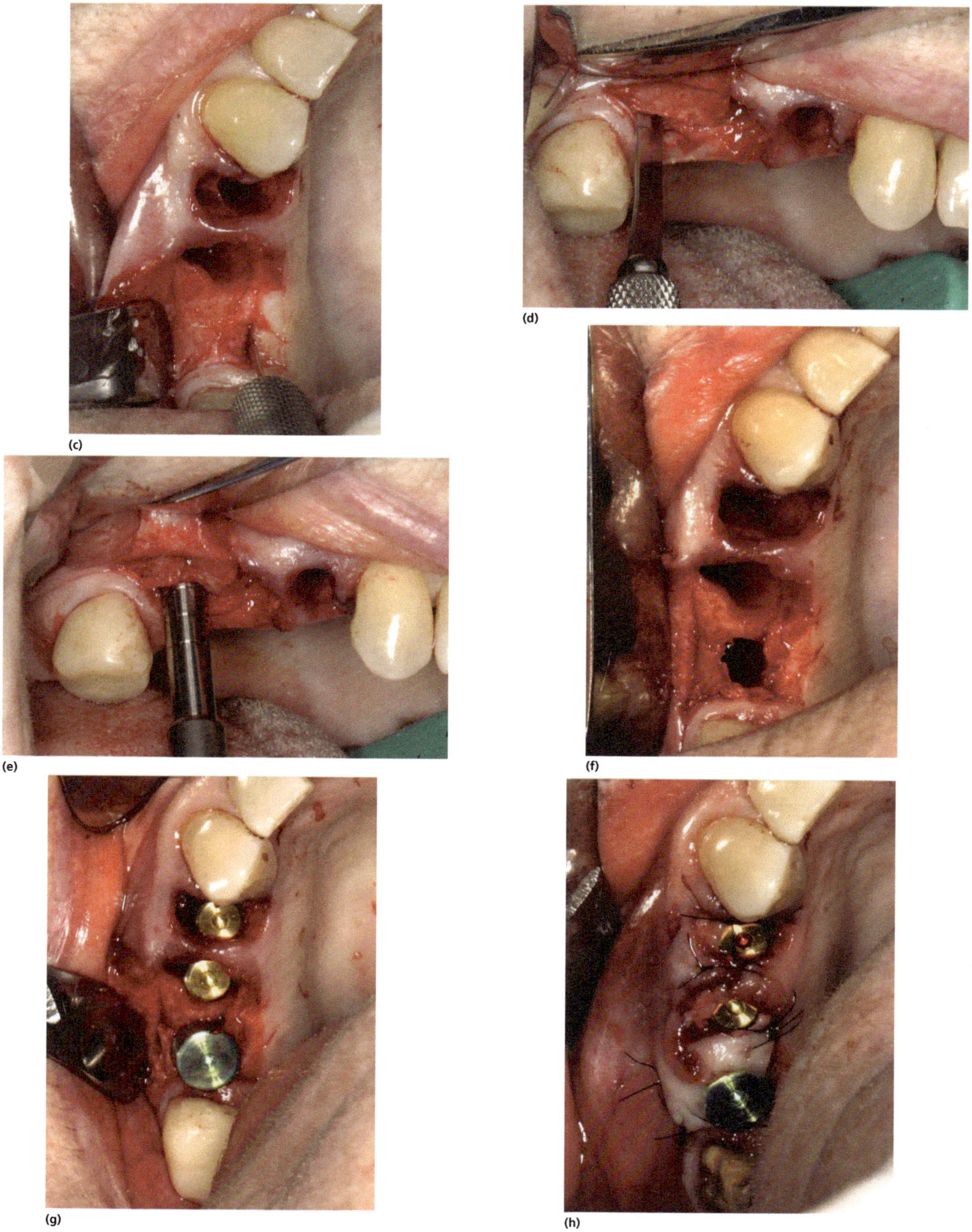

Figure 17.10 (Continued)
(c) Limited site exposure was achieved with a buccally-based, full-thickness flap design with reduced horizontal dimension. (d) A horizontal (anterior to posterior) bone incision was completed below the sinus floor. The posteriorly-beveled lateral/vertical bone incision using a #64 mini blade is demonstrated. (e) The tapered 6 mm diameter osteotome in position after achieving RE to the final diameter required and an apical sinus floor fracture (OSFE) of 2 mm. Note the small vertical crestal fracture. (f–h) Occlusal views of the site after osteotome removal demonstrating the dimensional changes: (f) implant placement was finished with an intact crestal fracture of the buccal plate; the fracture was over-grafted using particulate xenograft; (g) an apically positioned/anterior pedicle rotation flap was used to allow transgingival healing. A buccal connective tissue graft was placed at the premolar sites.

(*Continued*)

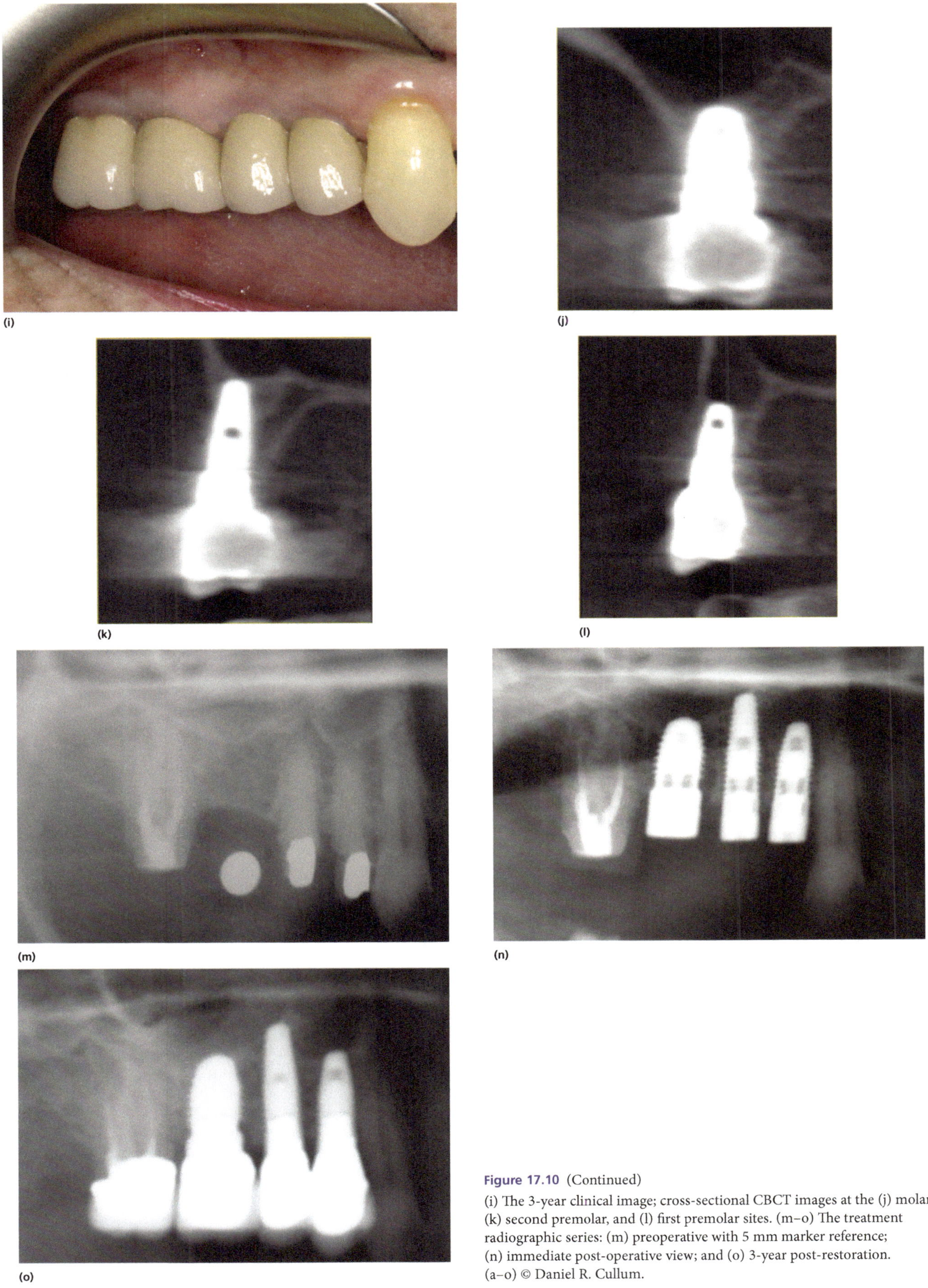

Figure 17.10 (Continued)
(i) The 3-year clinical image; cross-sectional CBCT images at the (j) molar, (k) second premolar, and (l) first premolar sites. (m–o) The treatment radiographic series: (m) preoperative with 5 mm marker reference; (n) immediate post-operative view; and (o) 3-year post-restoration. (a–o) © Daniel R. Cullum.

with the #64 mini blade (Figure 17.10d). The final tapered osteotome (6.0 mm diameter) can be seen in Figure 17.10e in position after completion of RE and apical sinus floor fracture (OSFE) of 2 mm. There is a small vertical crestal fracture, which was overgrafted after tapered implant placement. Closure was via an apical positioned flap/rotational finger flap around the healing cap for a transgingival protocol (Figure 17.10g). Simultaneous extraction of the first and second premolar teeth was also completed with immediate implant placement using OSFE and connective tissue grafting at the facial aspect (Figure 17.10h). The patient can be seen 3 years after restoration in Figure 17.10i, and cross-sectional CBCT images are seen at the molar, second premolar, and first premolar (Figure 17.10j–l). Figure 17.10m–o demonstrates the radiographic series with a preoperative view (with 5 mm marker reference), an immediate post-operative view, and 3 years post-restoration.

Ridge expansion and bone-added osteotome sinus floor elevation

RE and BAOSFE of 2–4 mm can be completed as described in Chapter 15 with either a partial- or full-thickness flap. A partial-thickness flap exposure is demonstrated for the patient in Figure 17.11. Clinical and CBCT images show a failing left maxillary bridge and edentulous premolar sites (Figure 17.11a–d). The failing bridge and molar were removed (Figure 17.11e). A palatally incised, buccally-based partial-thickness flap exposure and Piezosurgery were used to complete the bone incisions, including an anterior beveled bone vertical releasing incision (in the figure) (Figure 17.11f). RE was completed with increasing size "D" expanders and chisels across the expansion site (Figure 17.11g–i and n). RE was continued with tapered osteotomes, which also were used with particulate xenograft for a "bone-added" sinus floor fracture and elevation of 3–4 mm (BAOSFE) at the distal site (Figure 17.11j–m). Tapered implants and healing caps were inserted with good primary stability and an intact periosteal-bone flap (Figure 17.11o). The posterior extraction defect was grafted using particulate xenograft and a modified BioCol® technique (as described in Chapter 5). Primary wound closure was completed with apical positioning of the buccal flap at the anterior region and with an anterior-based rotational "Palacci" flap[66] at the molar implant site. A buccal flap of keratinized tissue from the tuberosity was advanced anteriorly for closure over the extraction defect (Figures 17.11p and q). The 18-month post-restoration clinical result and radiographs are shown in Figure 17.11r–v.

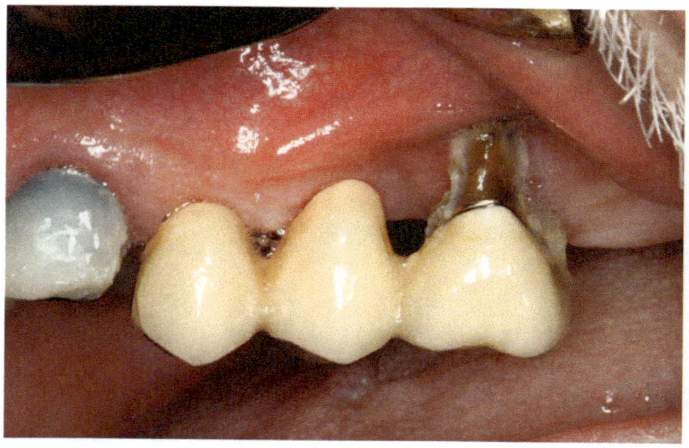

(a)

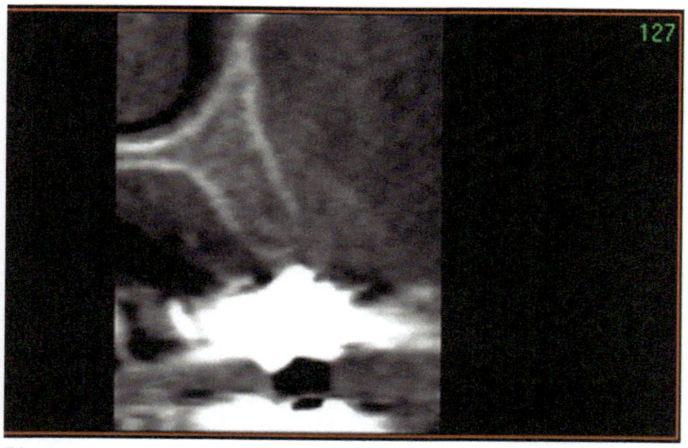

(b)

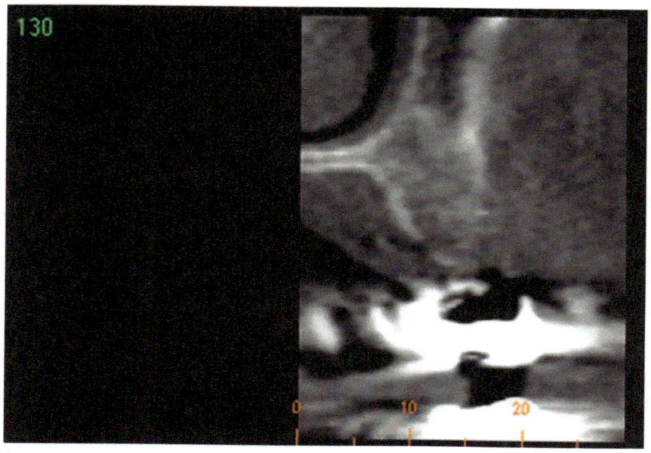

(c)

Figure 17.11 A failing left maxillary bridge with edentulous premolar sites. (a–d) Preoperative images: (a) clinical view; cross-sectional CBCT images for (b) the first premolar, (c) second premolar, and

(Continued)

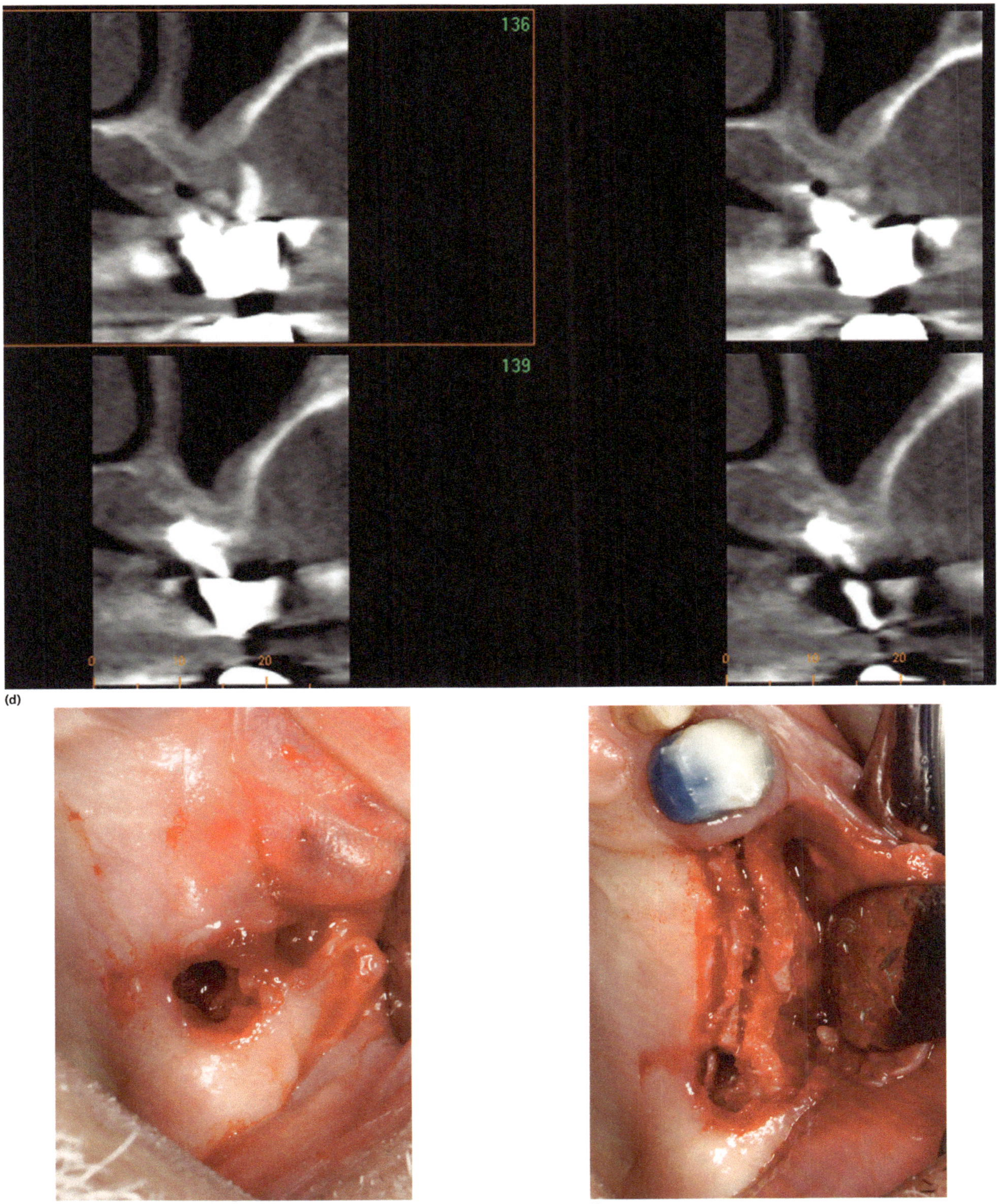

(d) (e) (f)

Figure 17.11 (Continued)

(d) mesial of the first molar sites. (e) The post-extraction occlusal view of the residual ridge and defect. (f) A palatal incision was used to create a buccally-based partial-thickness flap exposure and demonstrated a narrow alveolar contour; bone incisions are completed short of the sinus floor and the anteriorly-beveled vertical incision (not visible) were done using Piezosurgery. RE was completed using increasing size "D" expanders

(*Continued*)

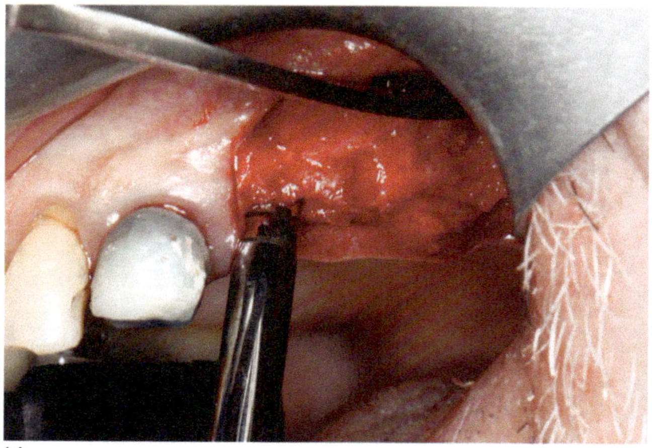

(g)

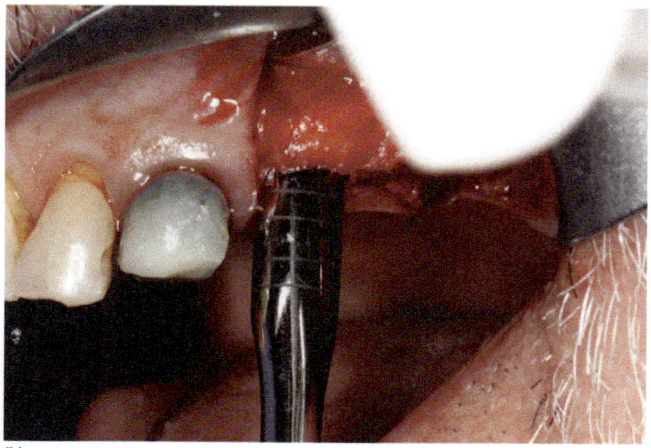

(h)

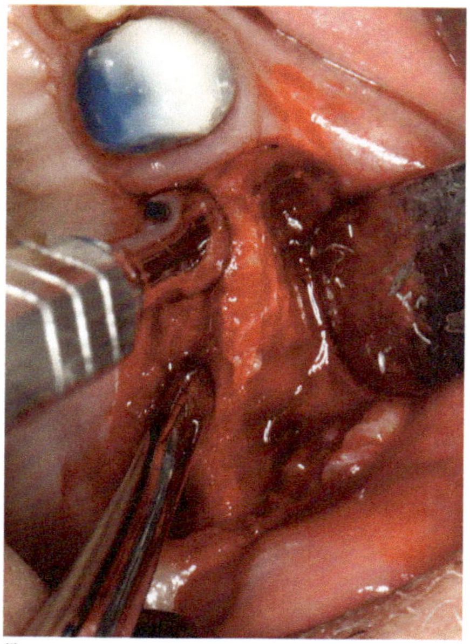

(i)

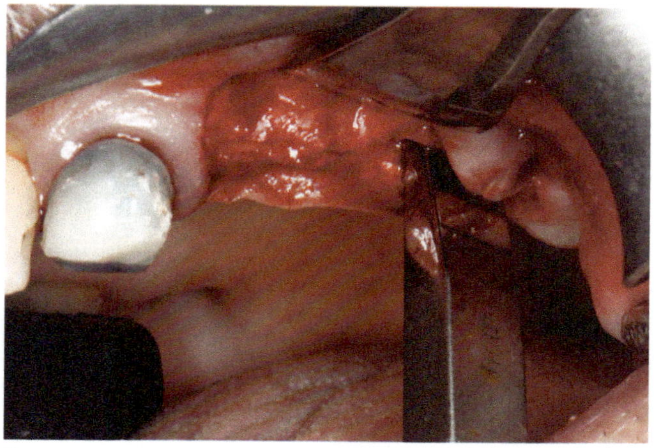

(j)

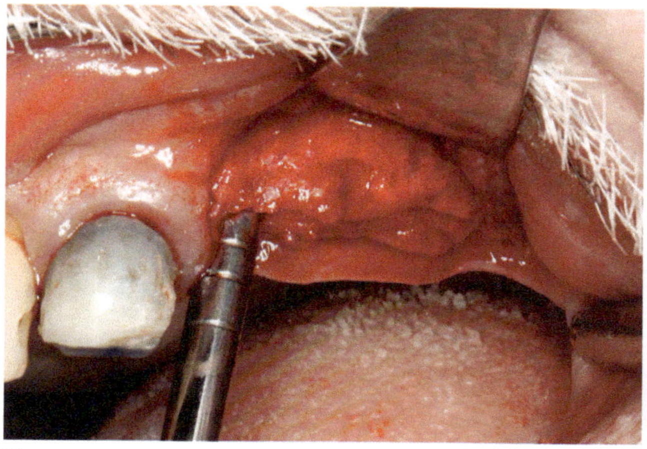

(k)

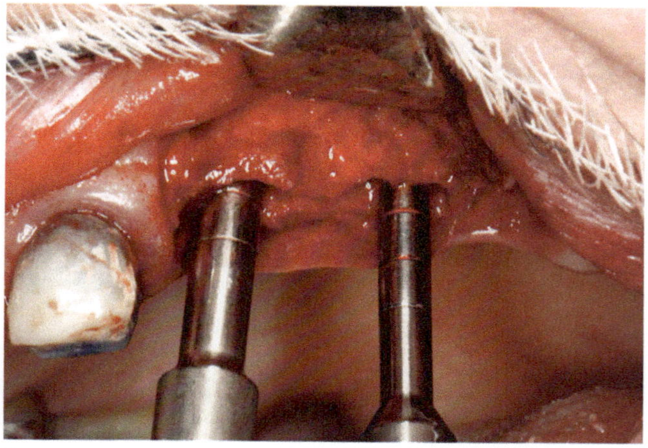

(l)

Figure 17.11 (Continued)
(g, h, i) and chisels (j) across the expansion site. (k) Tapered ostetomes continued the RE. (l–n) RE was continued using increasing diameter tapered osteotomes and included sinus floor up-fracture and BAOSFE at the distal site resulting in elevation of 3–4 mm. (o–q) Occlusal views demonstrating "D" expanders for initial expansion

(*Continued*)

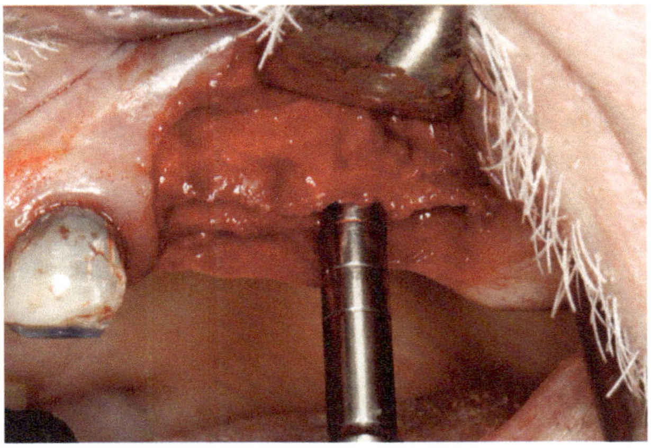

(m)

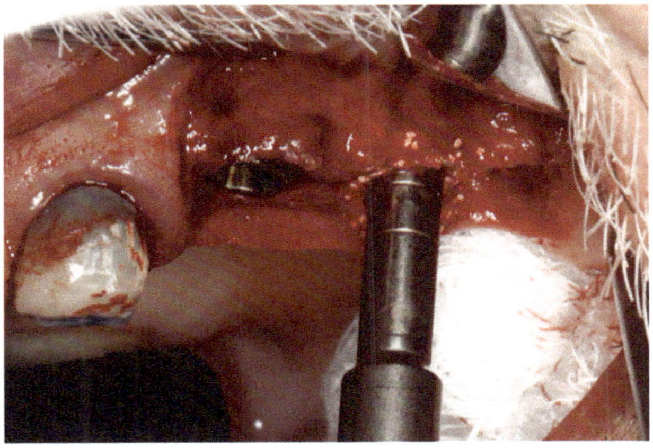

(n)

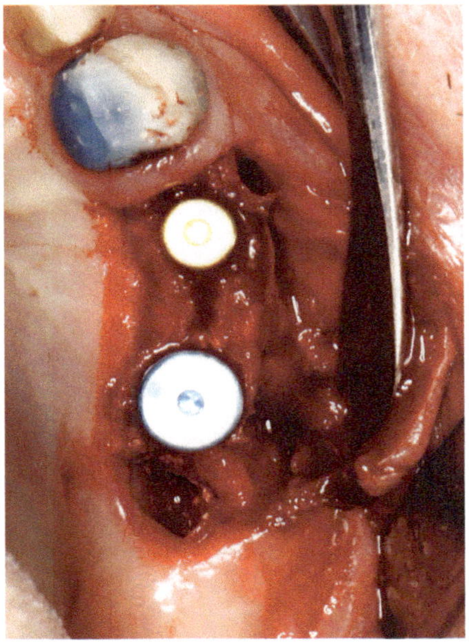

(o)

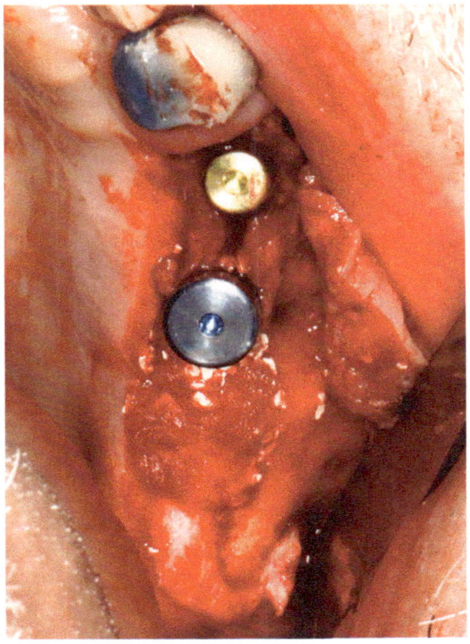

(p)

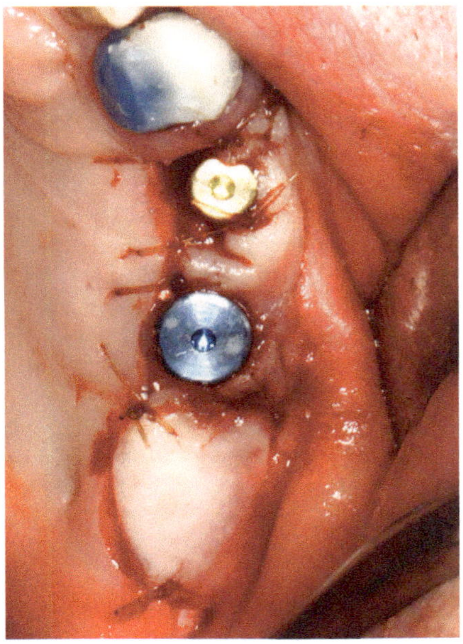

(q)

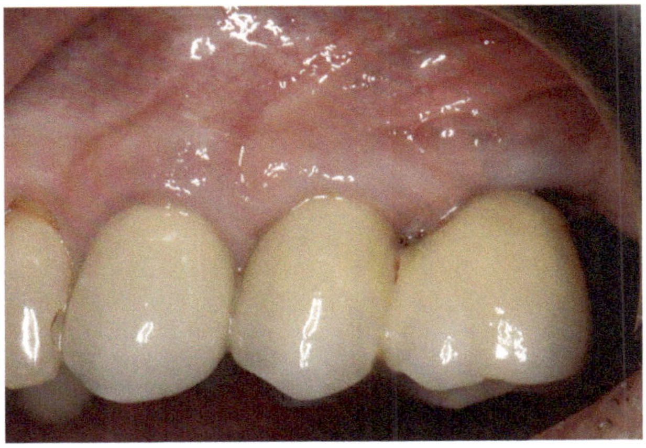

(r)

Figure 17.11 (Continued)

(o), and healing caps in position with an intact bone/periosteal flap; (p) the posterior extraction defect was grafted and covered with a single layer of collagen (q), and primary closure achieved using apical positioning of the buccal flap around the implants and an anteriorly advanced buccal flap for distal closure. (r) The 18-month post-restoration clinical result.

(Continued)

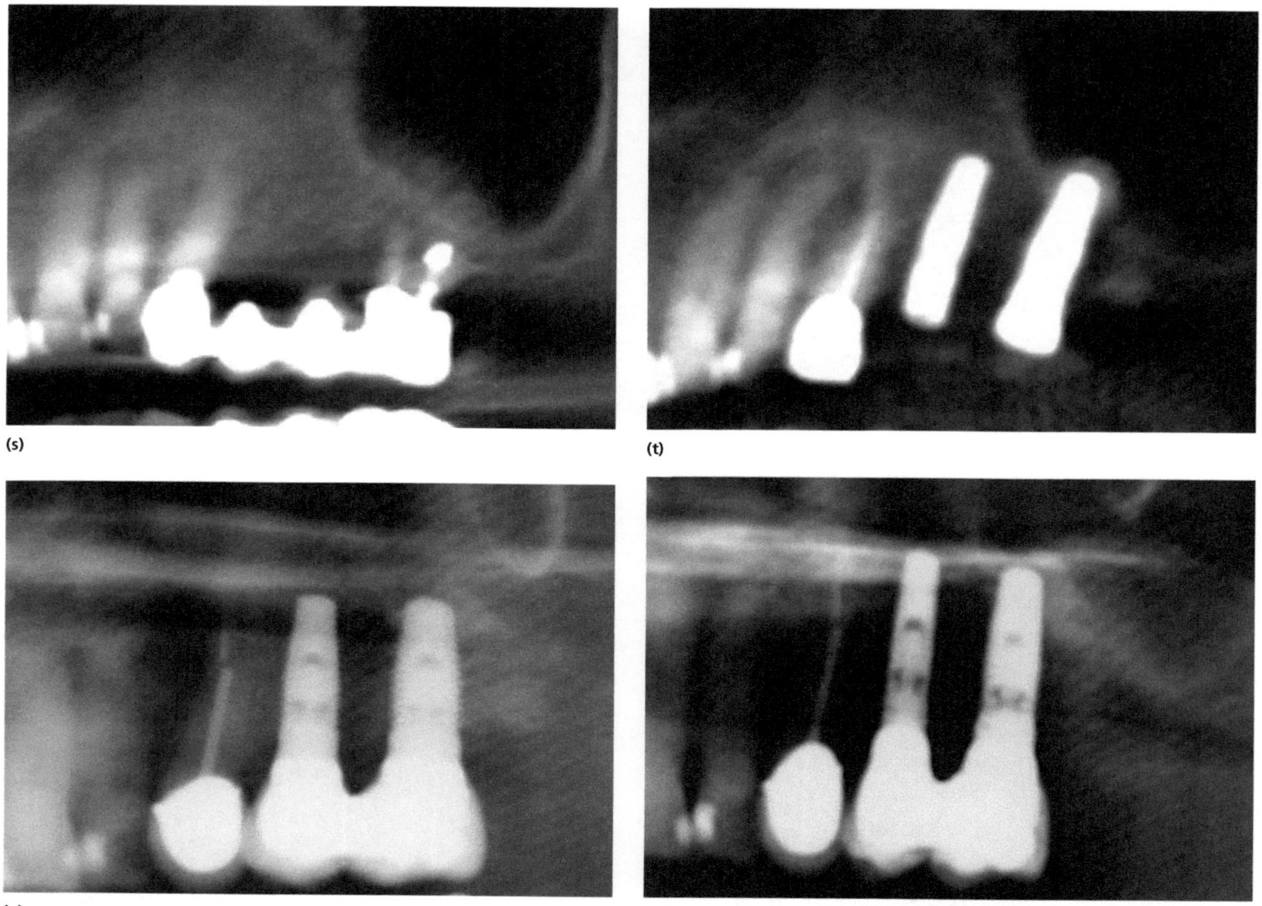

(s) (t) (u) (v)

Figure 17.11 (Continued)
The treatment radiographic series: (s) preoperative; (t) immediate post-op; (u) restored; (v) 18-month post-restoration condition. (a–v) © Daniel R. Cullum.

Ridge expansion and contiguous sinus floor elevation

An example of CSFE with RE is shown in Figure 17.12. A palatally-based incision at the right maxillary edentulous site was completed (Figure 17.12a). A split-thickness flap was elevated and bone incisions completed as described previously (Figures 17.5a and b and 17.12b). RE to a width of 2 mm was completed and the sinus floor fractured from the anterior to the posterior of the defect by overlapping use of a standard 2 mm concave-tipped osteotome (Figures 17.5d and e and 17.12c). The sinus floor bone will bend and/or fracture depending on its compliance, but at this point no attempt should be made to elevate the floor. The RE was continued with larger bone chisels and "D" expanders, with lateral bending creating a 3 mm bone gap (Figure 17.5f). The floor manipulation was changed at the new expanded width of 3 mm with a 3 mm diameter concave-tipped osteotome (Figure 17.5g and h). Expansion up to 4 mm can often be completed if needed, followed by a contiguous floor fracture with 4 mm diameter osteotomes with a concave cutting tip design. Contiguous sinus floor elevators (Figure 17.12d and e) can be used to start vertical elevation and for horizontal manipulation for expansion at the 3–4 mm width (Figure 17.5i and j). These instruments are designed to achieve the sinus floor elevation of 6–8 mm by spreading the forces over a large area (2, 3, 4 mm × 10 mm sizes). A surgical guide can be placed to determine implant positions, and to assist with the development of a palatal purchase for the implant(s) using Piezosurgery or rotary instruments. A tapered osteotome (Figure 17.8b) then was used to complete implant site development (Figure 17.5m). Tapered implant (6.5 mm diameter) placement was completed with good rotational stability and an intact bone–periosteal flap (Figure 17.12f). Collagen was placed in the expansion gap and a cover screw on the implant (Figure 17.12g). Without adequate primary stability the implant should be removed and the defect grafted for delayed implant placement. Figure 17.12h shows passive flap closure with slight apical positioning. The radiographs in Figure 17.12i–k demonstrate preoperative (with 5 mm marker), immediate post-op, and 4-year post-restoration panoramic images. The 4-year restored clinical view can be seen in Figure 17.12l. Long-term follow-up after 10 years 8 months is seen in clinical and cross-sectional CBCT images in Figure 17.12m and n.

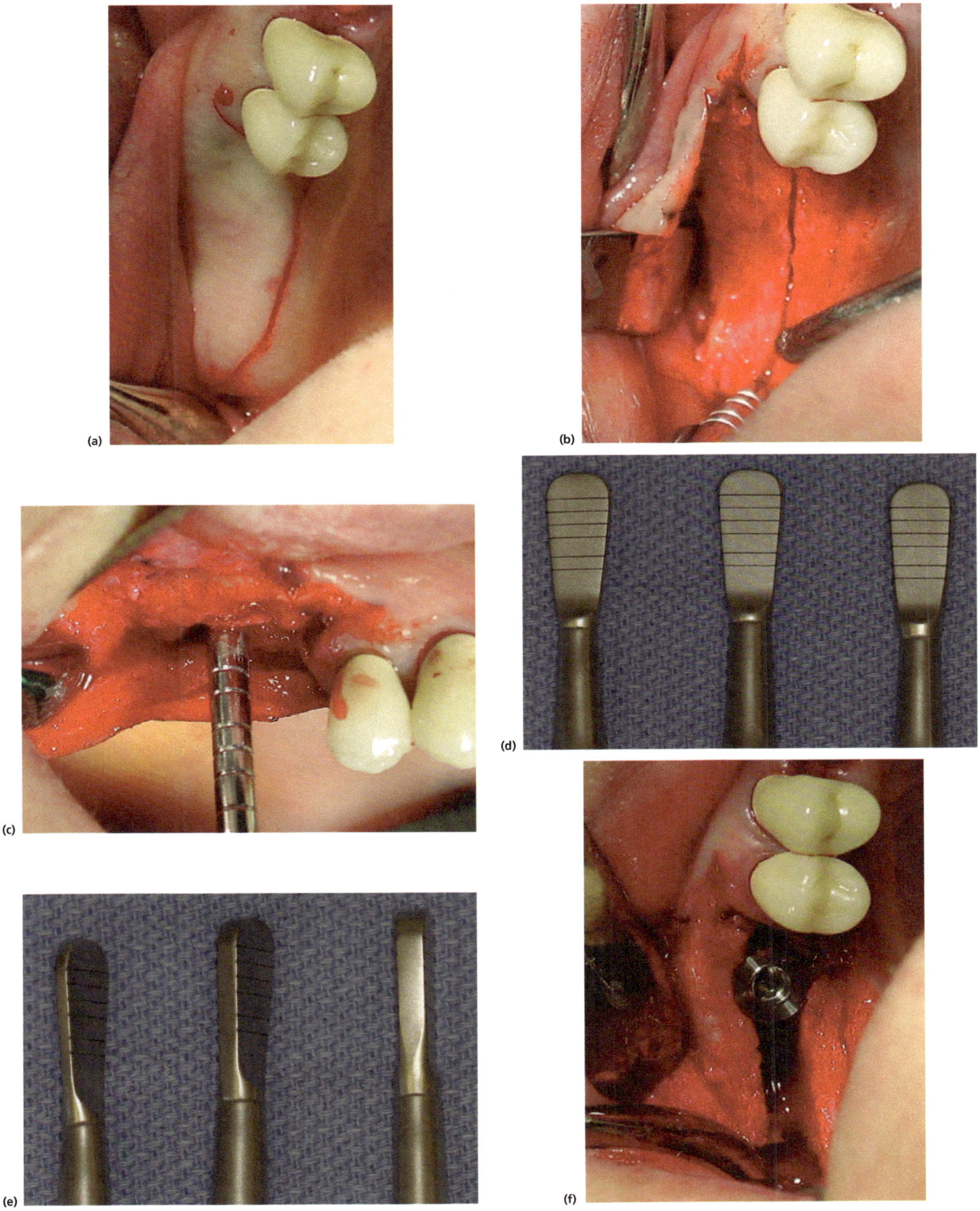

Figure 17.12 This edentulous right posterior maxillary site was managed with RE and CSFE including a split-thickness flap dissection for replacement of the first molar. (a) The incision design at the edentulous right posterior maxillary site. (b) The spit-thickness flap dissection is seen. The bone incision was completed and extended posteriorly to the tuberosity with an anterior vertical beveled bone-releasing incision. (c) After horizontal RE by osteo-mobilization creating a 2 mm bone expansion gap, sequential stepped overlapping floor fracture was completed using a 2 mm concave-tipped osteotome. After further expansion, sinus floor up-fracture was completed with both 3 and 4 mm diameter-concave tipped osteotomes. (d, e) Contiguous sinus floor elevators 2, 3, and 4 mm diameter × 10 mm (H&H Co., Ontario, CA) were used to up-fracture the sinus floor and achieve horizontal bending with osteo-mobilization and sinus floor elevation. (f) Final site development was completed with the appropriate tapered osteotome to allow placement of a 6.5 mm diameter implant; an intact bone–periosteal flap was maintained and good primary stability achieved. *(Continued)*

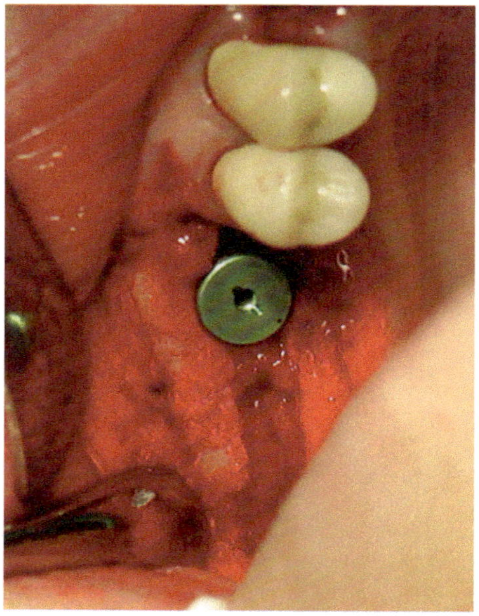
(g)

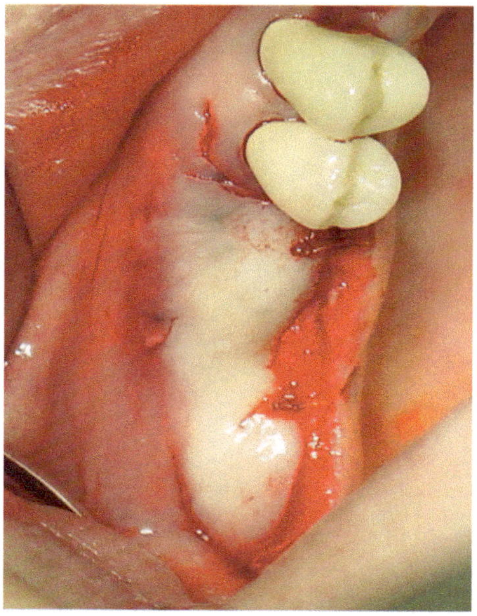
(h)

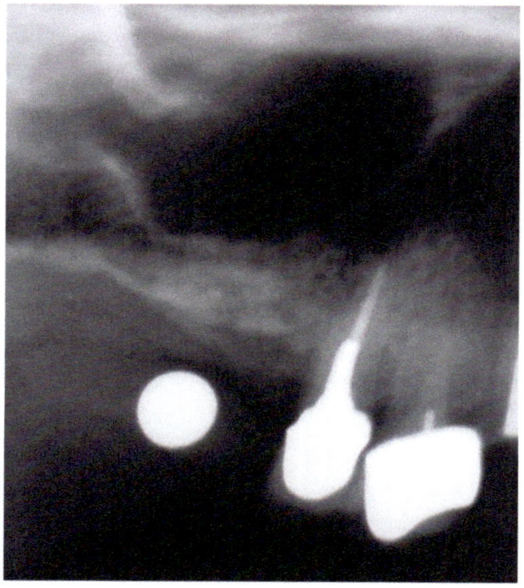
(i)

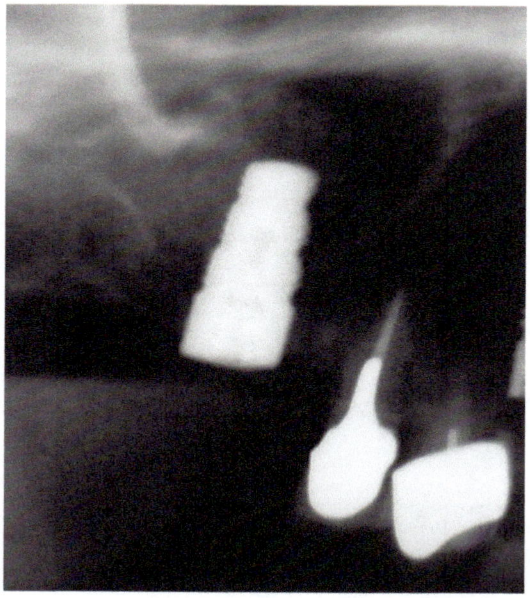
(j)

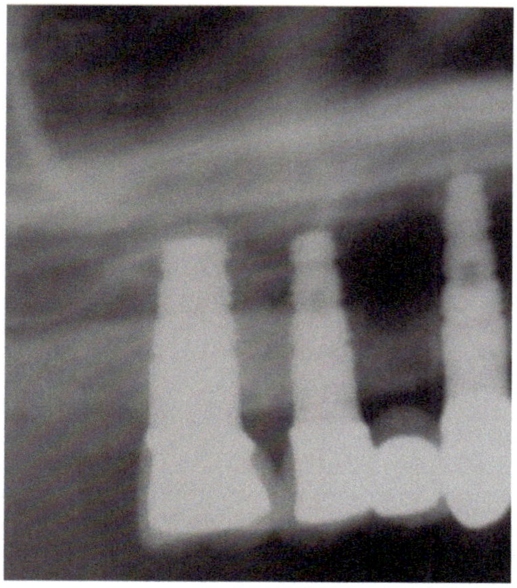
(k)

Figure 17.12 (Continued)

(g) Collagen (Collatape®, Zimmer Dental, Carlsbad, CA) was placed in the intrabony expansion gap and particulate xenograft graft used at the anterior vertical bone incision. (h) Passive flap closure was achieved with slight apical positioning. Treatment radiographic series: (i) at preop, (j) immediate post-op, and (k) 4-year post-restoration time intervals.

(Continued)

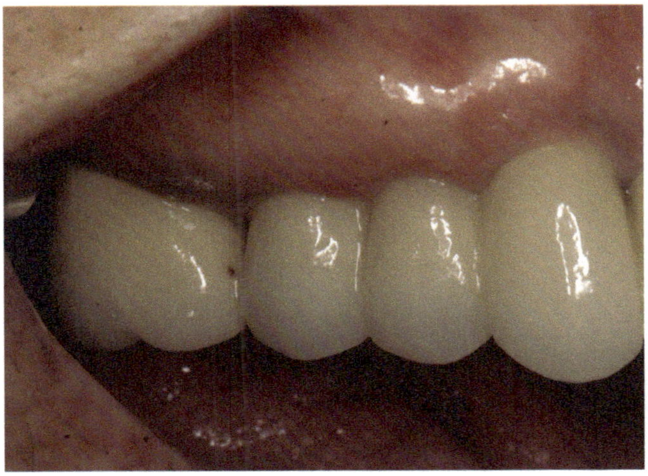

(l)

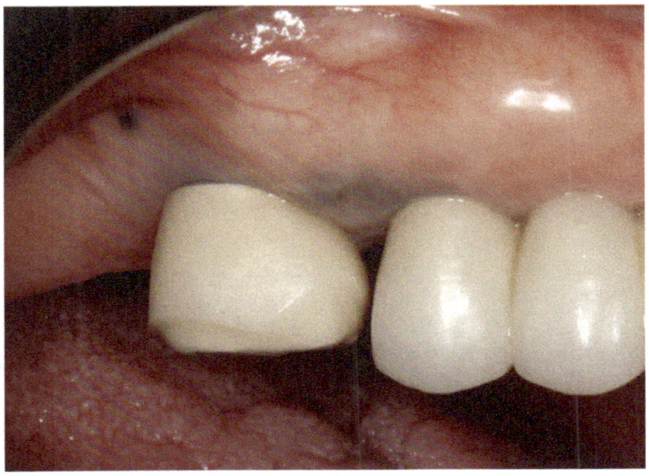

(m)

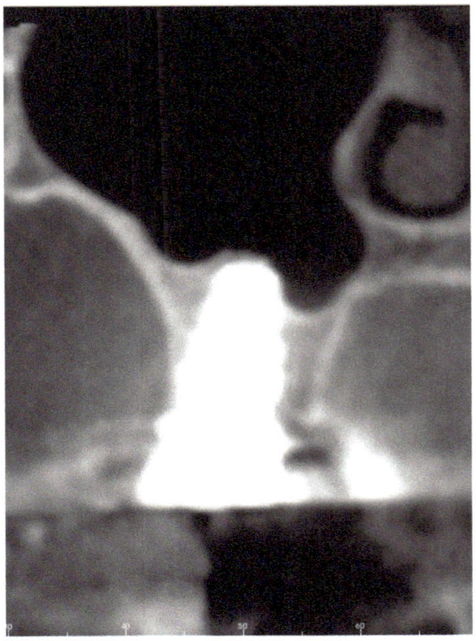

(n)

Figure 17.12 (Continued)
(l) The clinical presentation at 48 months showed stable soft tissue contours. (m) Clinical and (n) CBCT images at 10 years 8 months post-op demonstrating excellent maintenance of the bony reconstruction. *Source*: (a–c, f–i) Cullum DR, Trans-Alveolar Sinus Elevation Combined with Ridge Expansion. In: The Sinus Bone Graft, 2nd ed., Jensen OT, ed. Chicago, IL: Quintessence, 2006.[16] Reproduced with permission of Quintessence Publishing Co., Inc. (d, e, j–n) © Daniel R. Cullum.

Avoiding complications

Simultaneous use of RE and TASE techniques offers patients and clinicians the ability to manipulate the residual atrophic maxilla to restore adequate dimensions for implant placement without the need for extensive use of grafting materials. Complications as described in Chapters 15 and 16 can occur; however, combined use of the techniques can significantly increase their incidence during the learning process. It is strongly recommended that the surgeon become proficient with each technique separately first before applying the combined approach and to start in patients with moderate bone volumes.

With RE, manipulation of the bone flap (Figure 17.2b) can result in excessive buccal inclination of the implant(s). After the bone expansion gap is opened, modification of the implant osteotomy can be completed with Piezosurgery implant site preparation inserts. Often, an increased crestal purchase of the palatal bone margin can reduce unwanted facial angulation. Rarely, if the position or the angle of the osteotomy cannot be optimized, the site may require inter-positional or grafting with split-thickness flap design and delayed implant placement. Grafting of the expansion gap should be completed if the buccal plate has any fracture or vascular compromise. Grafting of the buccal vertical bone release incisions is recommended to prevent a contour deficiency. Buccal plate fracture can range from small vertical fracture lines to a complete "split." With a full-thickness flap approach, management is of moderate to advanced complexity with guided bone regeneration over-grafting needed to augment a thin or fractured buccal plate. A larger "split" defect can be managed with screw fixation of the fracture segment, grafting, and a barrier membrane. (see Chapter 16).

A number of factors are important to consider to avoid apical perforation or buccal fracture, including the amount of buccal alveolar ridge undercut, ridge width, bone quality and compliance, bone incision design with partial or complete intrabony release, and anatomic location in the arch (e.g. proximity to zygoma or a multi-tooth defect with osteo-mobilization around the corner of the arch at the canine site). The use of a tapered implant design that conforms to the shape of the expansion defect increases primary stability and can reduce the risk of fracture of the bone–periosteal flap (Figure 17.2b). Undue apical force during the procedure should be avoided as it may result in apical displacement of an implant into the sinus. Also, with a single-stage approach, any significant biting force during the early healing period could displace the implant. Consideration of a staged approach would be appropriate if there are any concerns with patient compliance in the post-operative period. Management of sinus complications, including small tears or breach, are discussed in detail in Chapter 15. Prior to treatment, discussion with patients of the potential complications with osteotome techniques should include post-operative vertigo. This rare complication is usually self-limiting; however, it may require management with an Epley maneuver.[67,68]

Summary

Bone manipulation techniques for combined RE and TASE procedures offer patients a combined treatment option for site development. The soft tissue incision design determines the bone manipulation approach to be used. Full-thickness flap exposure can be used in conjunction with osteotome techniques and particulate over-grafting for a single- or two-stage implant placement protocol. Partial-thickness flaps help preserve the vascular supply to the buccal bone flap, helping to limit bone resorption of the expanded segment. The exposed marrow on the internal aspect of the bone flap is a source of pleuripotent mesenchymal stem cells for regeneration. The need for grafting materials is significantly reduced, and shorter healing intervals are generally required. Buccal expansion and TASE restores lost alveolar dimensions and allows simultaneous reconstruction of horizontal and vertical defects with implant placement in a restorative-driven position.

References

1. Atwood D. Reduction of residual ridges: a major oral disease entity. J Prosthetic Dent 1971; 26: 266–279.
2. Atwood D. Bone loss of the edentulous ridges. J Periodontol 1979; 50: 11–21.
3. Tallgren A. Alveolar bone loss in denture wearers as related to facial morphology. Acta Odontol Scand 1970; 28: 251–270.
4. Hammerle C, Jung R, Feloutzis A. A systematic review of the survival of implants in bone sites augmented with barrier membranes (guided bone regeneration) in partially edentulous patients. J Clin Periodontol 2002; 29(Suppl 3): 226–231.
5. Lang N, Bragger U, Hammerle C, et al. Immediate trans-mucosal implants using the principle of guided tissue regeneration. I. Rationale, clinical procedures and 30-month results. Clin Oral Implants Res 1994; 5: 154–163.
6. Bartee B. The use of high-density polytetrafluoroethylene membranes to treat osseous defects: clinical report. Implant Dent 1995; 4: 21–26.
7. Misch CM. Comparison of intra-oral donor sites for onlay grafting prior to implant placement. Int J Oral Maxillofac Implants 1997; 12: 767–776.
8. Keller E, van Rockel N, Desjardins R, et al. Prosthetic–surgical reconstruction of the severely resorbed maxilla with iliac bone grafting and tissue-integrated prostheses. Int J Oral Maxillofac Implants 1987; 2: 155–165.
9. Boyne P, Cole M, Strolinger D, et al. A technique for osseous reconstruction of deficient edentulous maxillary ridges. J Oral Maxillofac Surg 1985; 43: 87–91.
10. Boyne P, James R. Grafting of the maxillary sinus floor with bone and marrow. J Oral Surg 1980; 38: 613–616.
11. Khoury F. Augmentation osseuse et chirugie implantare. Implant 1999; 5: 221–237.
12. Tatum OH Jr. Maxillary and sinus implant reconstructions. Dent Clin North Am 1986; 30: 207–229.
13. Scipioni A, Brushi G, Calesini G. The edentulous ridge expansion technique: a 5-year study on 123 implants with 1 to 5 year follow-up. Int J Periodontics Restorative Dent 1994; 14: 451–459.
14. Vercellotti T. Piezoelectric bone surgery in implantology: a case report – a new piezoelectric ridge expansion technique. Int J Periodontics Restorative Dent 2000; 20: 358–365.
15. Simion M, Baldoni M, Zaffe D. Jawbone enlargement using immediate implant placement associated with a split-crest technique and guided bone regeneration. Int J Periodontics Restorative Dent 1992; 12: 462–473.
16. Cullum D, Jensen OT. Trans-alveolar sinus elevation combined with ridge expansion. In: The Sinus Bone Graft, 2nd ed., JensenOT, ed. Chicago, IL: Quintessence, 2006, pp. 251–262.
17. Chiapasco M, Ferrini F, Casentini P, et al. Dental implants placed in expanded narrow edentulous ridges with the Extensio-Crest® device; a 1 to 3-year multicenter study. Clin Oral Implants Res 2006; 17: 265–272.
18. Cortes AR, Cortes DN. Non-traumatic bone expansion for immediate implant placement: an analysis of 21 cases. Implant Dent 2010; 19: 92–97.
19. Chin M, Toth B. Distraction osteogenesis in maxillofacial surgery using internal devices. J Oral Maxillofac Surg 1996; 54: 45–53.
20. Jensen OT, Cockrell R, Kuhlke L, et al. Anterior maxillary alveolar distraction osteogenesis: a prospective 5-year clinical study. Int J Oral Maxillofac Implants 2002; 17: 52–68.
21. Roummanas E, Markowitz B, Lorant J, et al. Reconstructed mandibular defects: fibula free flaps and osseointegrated implants. Plastic Reconstr Surg 1997; 99: 356–365.
22. Boyne P, Marx R, Nevins M, et al. A feasibility study evaluating rhBMP-2/absorbable collagen sponge for maxillary sinus floor augmentation. Int J Periodontics Restorative Dent 1997; 17: 11–25.
23. Howell T, Fiorellini J, Jones A, et al. A feasibility study evaluating rhBMP-2/absorbable collagen sponge for alveolar ridge preservation or augmentation. Int J Periodontics Restorative Dent 1997; 17: 124–139.
24. Boyan B, Weesner T, Lohmann C, et al. Porcine fetal enamel matrix derivative enhances bone formation induced by demineralized freeze-dried bone allograft *in vitro*. J Periodontol 2000; 71: 1278–1286.
25. Simion M, Rocchietta I, Dellavia C. Three-dimensional ridge augmentation with xenograft and recombinant human derived growth factor-BB in humans: report of two cases. Int J Periodontics Restorative Dent 2007; 27: 109–115.
26. Marx R, Carlson E, Schimmele S, et al. Platelet-rich plasma: growth factor enhancement for bone grafts. Oral Surg Oral Med Oral Pathol Oral Radiol Endod 1998; 85: 638–646.
27. Simion M, Rocchietta I, Montforte M, Maschera E. Three-dimensional alveolar bone reconstruction with a combination of recombinant human platelet-derived growth factor-BB and guided bone regeneration. A case report. Int J Periodontics Restorative Dent 2008; 28: 239–243.
28. Buser D, Mericske-Stern R, Bernard J, et al. Long-term evaluation of non-submerged ITI implants. Part I: 8-year life table analysis of a prospective multicenter study with 2359 implants. Clin Oral Implants Res 1997; 8: 161–172.
29. Deporter D, Caudry S, Kermalli J, et al. Further data on the predictability of the indirect sinus elevation procedure used with short, porous-surfaced dental implants. Int J Periodontics Restorative Dent 2005; 25: 585–593.
30. Krekmanov L, Kahn M, Rangert B, Lindstrom H. Tilting of posterior mandibular and maxillary implants for improved prosthesis support. Int J Oral Maxillofac Implants 2000; 15: 405–414.
31. Summers RB. A new concept in maxillary implant surgery: the osteotome technique. Compend Contin Educ Dent 1994; 15: 152–160.
32. Summers RB. The osteotome technique: part 2 – the ridge expansion osteotomy (REO) procedure. Compend Contin Educ Dent 1994; 15: 422–436.
33. Summers RB. The osteotome technique: part 3 – less invasive methods of elevating the sinus floor. Compend Contin Educ Dent 1994; 15: 698–710.
34. Scipioni A. Bone regeneration in the edentulous ridge expansion technique: histologic and ultrastructural study of 20 clinical cases. Int J Periodontics Restorative Dent 1999; 19: 269–277.
35. Rosen P, Summers R, Mellado J, et al. The bone-added osteotome sinus floor elevation technique: multi-center retrospective report of consecutively treated patients. Int J Oral Maxillofac Implants 1999; 14: 853–858.
36. Toffler M. Site development in the posterior maxilla using osteocompression and apical alveolar displacement. Compend Contin Educ Dent 2001; 22: 775–780.
37. Toffler M. Treating the atrophic maxilla by combining short implants with minimally-invasive osteotome procedures. Pract Proced Aesthet Dent 2006; 18: 301–308.
38. Ferringo N, Lauureti M, Fanali S. Dental implant placement in conjunction with osteotome sinus floor elevation: a 12-year life-table analysis from a prospective study on 588 ITI implants. Clin Oral Implants Res 2006; 17: 194–205.
39. Pjetursson B, Ignjatovic D, Matuliene G, et al. Trans-alveolar maxillary floor elevation using osteotomes with or without grafting material. Part I: implant survival and patients' perception. Clin Oral Implants Res 2009; 20: 667–676.
40. Pjetursson B, Ignjatovic D, Matuliene G, et al. Trans-alveolar maxillary floor elevation using osteotomes with or without grafting material. Part II: radiographic tissue remodeling. Clin Oral Implants Res 2009; 20: 677–683.
41. Bruschi G, Scipioni A, Calesini G. Localized management of the sinus floor with simultaneous implant placement. Int J Oral Maxillofac Implants 1998; 13: 219–226.

42. Bravi F, Bruschi G, Ferrini F. A 10-year multicenter retrospective clinical study of 1715 implants placed with the edentulous ridge expansion technique. Int J Periodontics Restorative Dent 2007; 27: 557–565.
43. Jensen OT. The book bone flap: sequential alveolar crest expansion. In: The Osteoperiosteal Flap, Jensen OT, ed. Chicago, IL: Quintessence, 2010, pp. 96–99.
44. Cullum D. Advances in Bone Manipulation Techniques: Part 2. Osteo-mobilization for Horizontal and Vertical Implant Site Development. Selected Readings in Oral and Maxillofacial Surgery. San Francisco, CA: Guild for Scientific Advancement in Oral and Maxillofacial Surgery, 2010, vol. 18, no. 5.
45. Coatam G, Marrotti A. The segmental ridge-split procedure. J Periodontol 2003; 74: 757–770.
46. Malchodi L, Scarano A, Quaranta M, et al. Ridge fixation by means of titanium mesh in edentulous ridge expansion for horizontal ridge expansion in the maxilla. Int J Oral Maxillofac Implants 1998; 13: 701–705.
47. Blus C, Szmukler-Montcler S. Split-crest and immediate implant placement with ultrasonic bone surgery: a 3-year life-table analysis with 230 treated cases. Clin Oral Implants Res 2006; 17: 700–707.
48. Danza M, Guidi R, Carinci F. Comparison between implants inserted into piezo split and unsplit alveolar crests. J Oral Maxillofac Surg 2009; 67: 2460–2465.
49. Jensen OT, Cullum D, Baer D. Marginal bone stability using 3 different flap approaches for alveolar split expansion for dental implants – a 1-year clinical study. J Oral Maxillofac Surg 2009; 67: 1921–1930.
50. Horrocks G. The controlled assisted ridge expansion technique for implant placement in the anterior maxilla: a technical note. Int J Periodontics Restorative Dent 2010; 30: 495–501.
51. Cullum D. Advances in Bone Manipulation Techniques: Part 1. Osteome Site Development and Minimally Invasive Sinus Elevation. Selected Reviews in Oral and Maxillofacial Surgery. San Francisco, CA: Guild for Scientific Advancement in Oral and Maxillofacial Surgery, 2010, vol. 18; no. 4.
52. Sclar A. Systematic evaluation of the esthetic implant patient. In: Soft Tissue and Esthetic Considerations in Implant Dentistry. Chicago, IL: Quintessence, 2003, pp. 13–41.
53. Kois J, Kan J. Predictable peri-implant gingival aesthetics: surgical and prosthodontic rationales. Pract Proced Aesthet Dent 2001; 13: 691–698.
54. Kois J. Predictable single-tooth peri-implant esthetics: five diagnostic keys. Compend Contin Educ Dent 2004; 25: 895–906.
55. Tarnow D, Magner A, Fletcher P. The effect of the distance from the contact point to the crest of bone on the presence or absence of the inter-proximal dental papilla. J Periodontol 1992; 63: 995–996.
56. Salama H, Salama M, Garber D, et al. Developing optimal peri-implant papillae within the esthetic zone: guided soft tissue augmentation. J Esthet Dent 1995; 7: 125–129.
57. Tarnow D, Cho S, Wallace S. The effect of inter-implant distance on the height of inter-implant bone crest. J Periodontol 2000; 71: 546–549.
58. Goodacre J, Bernal G, Rerengcharassaeng K, et al. Clinical complications with implants and implant prostheses. J Prosthetic Dent 2003; 90: 121–132.
59. Khoury F, Tunkel J. Bone augmentation and soft tissue management. In: Bone Augmentation in Oral Implantology, KhouryF, AntounH, MissikaP, eds. Chicago, IL: Quintessence, 2007, pp. 75–114.
60. Palaci P, Ericsson I, Engstrand P, Rangert B. Optimal Implant Positioning and Soft Tissue Management for the Brånemark System. Chicago, IL: Quintessence, 1995, pp. 59–70.
61. Sclar A. Surgical techniques for management of peri-implant soft tissues. In: Soft Tissue and Esthetic Considerations in Implant Dentistry. Chicago, IL: Quintessence, 2003, pp. 52–56.
62. Ulm C, Solar P, Gsellmann B, et al. The edentulous maxillary alveolar process in the region of the maxillary sinus – a study of physical dimension. Int J Oral Maxillofac Surg 1995; 24: 279–282.
63. Uchida Y, Goto M, Katsuki T, Soejima Y. Measurement of maxillary sinus volume using computerized tomographic images. Int J Oral Maxillofac Implants 1998; 13: 811–818.
64. Worthington P, Rubenstein J, Hatcher D. The role of cone-beam computed tomography in the planning and placement of implants. J Am Dent Assoc 2010; 141(Suppl 3): 19s–24s.
65. Vercellotti T, Stacchi C, Russo C, et al. Ultrasonic implant site preparation using Piezosurgery: a multicenter case series study analyzing 3579 implants with a 1- to 3-year follow-up. Int J Periodontics Restorative Dent 2014; 34: 11–18.
66. Palacci P, Nowzari H. Soft tissue enhancement around dental implants. Periodontol 2000 2008; 47: 113–132.
67. Peñarrocha M, Pérez H, García A, et al. Benign paroxysmal vertigo as a complication of osteotome expansion of the maxillary alveolar ridge. J Oral Maxillofac Surg 2001; 59: 106–107.
68. Saker M, Ogle O. Benign paroxysmal vertigo subsequent to sinus lift via closed technique. J Oral Maxillofac Surg 2005; 63: 1385–1387.

SECTION V

Immediate Implant Reconstruction

CHAPTER 18

Immediate Implant Placement for Single- and Multi-Rooted Teeth

Daniel R. Cullum[1] & Douglas Deporter[2]

[1]Private Practice, Coeur d'Alene, ID; Loma Linda University Department of OMS, Loma Linda, CA; UCLA Department of OMS, Los Angeles, CA, USA

[2]Discipline of Periodontics, Faculty of Dentistry, University of Toronto, Toronto, ON, Canada

Introduction

Management of extraction sites with immediate placement of endosseous dental implants was first advanced by Schulte et al.[1] Early treatment used open flap exposure and advancement for primary closure at the immediate site. More recent technological advances, including dental implant design and cone beam computed tomography (CBCT) diagnosis and planning, have enabled the routine use of immediate implants for replacement of single- and multi-rooted teeth with minimally invasive methods. Also, complementary techniques with bone and/or soft tissue grafting and application of biomimetic and biologic agents allow simultaneous reconstruction of confounding hard and soft tissue defects (see also Chapters 7, 8, and 19). Applications in single- and multi-rooted teeth come with varying demands on implant design, instrumentation, and surgical skills, including an understanding of implant positioning and peri-implant gap management for long-term bone volume maintenance. Simultaneous application of trans-alveolar sinus elevation (TASE) procedures can allow minimally invasive vertical sinus augmentation with immediate maxillary posterior implant placement. Minimally invasive treatment principles will be presented for immediate implant placement of single- and multi-rooted teeth offering significant advantages of reduced treatment time, cost, and often a single surgical procedure.

Literature review

The placement of immediate implants at fresh extraction sites was originally conceived for single-rooted teeth[1] and shown in both animal[2] and human[3,4] studies to be feasible provided that good initial implant stability was achievable.[5,6] Figure 18.1 demonstrates a patient treated in Dr Schulte's clinic with an immediate aluminum oxide endosseous dental implant (Frialit-1®, Friadent, Mannheim, Germany) at the maxillary right lateral incisor position, after more than 35 years follow-up.

Chen et al.[7] published a review of early studies using immediate implants for single-rooted teeth. Most reports in the review used submerged implant site healing and had similar short-term survival rates to implants placed in healed sites, provided that implants were placed well within the confines of the socket to ensure a maximum number of bone walls. Experiments in dogs showed that when the gaps ("jumping distances") between socket walls and implant surface were in the region of 1 mm, grafting appeared unnecessary to achieve fill with new bone, although only mesio-distal sections were examined.[8] As the gap widened, the amount of bone-to-implant contact that formed during healing decreased and the point of highest bone-to-implant contact shifted apically.[9] When buccal and lingual gaps were assessed in dogs, placement of an immediate dental implant without grafting had the same loss in buccal bone height seen at control, non-implanted extraction sockets.[10,11] Conversely, in a similar dog model, when circumferential gaps (1.35 mm wide) around implants were grafted with a bone autograft or xenograft, the loss in buccal bone height was prevented.[12,13] This would suggest that the presence of a buccal gap at the time of implant placement with grafting may be desirable. Clinically, >3 mm wide, well-contained peri-implant defects can fill without grafting, but substantial horizontal resorption (thinning ~56%) of the buccal bone surface results.[14] After implant insertion, grafting of buccal bone defects with xenograft[12] or an allograft[15] could be of benefit in retaining buccal bone contour and height over the implant, minimizing the risk of late soft tissue recession. Grafting the gap with a xenograft also has been shown to increase amounts of bone and bone-to-implant contact at the entrance of the previous tooth socket.[13] Some clinicians have proposed that placement of xenograft[16] or connective tissue into a buccal, subperiosteal pouch over an implant can help to stabilize local ridge anatomy;[17] whether this approach can maintain buccal bone volume over time has yet to be studied.

From early experience, investigators suggested that immediate implants be routinely overseated by 1 mm to compensate for inevitable loss in buccal bone and soft tissue height.[2,18] Others advocated seating the implant 2 mm apical to the coronal bone margins to aid primary soft tissue closure over an expanded polytetrafluoroethylene barrier.[5] Other early users of immediate implants followed a similar approach with or without added graft material for treatment of sites without four intact bone walls using guided bone regeneration (GBR) principles.[19–21] Immediate implant placement using non-submerged healing and collagen barriers was completed with openings made to slip the barrier over and around the implant neck.[22–24] Ferrus et al.[25] studied clinical outcomes following immediate implant placement in maxillary incisor, cuspid, or bicuspid sites. No graft materials or barriers were used to manage peri-implant gaps; rather, the soft tissues were repositioned and sutured to achieve a semi-submerged outcome. The peri-implant gap fill was greater and vertical bone loss less in bicuspid compared with anterior tooth implant locations. In bicuspid sites where the buccal

Minimally Invasive Dental Implant Surgery, First Edition. Edited by Daniel R. Cullum and Douglas Deporter.

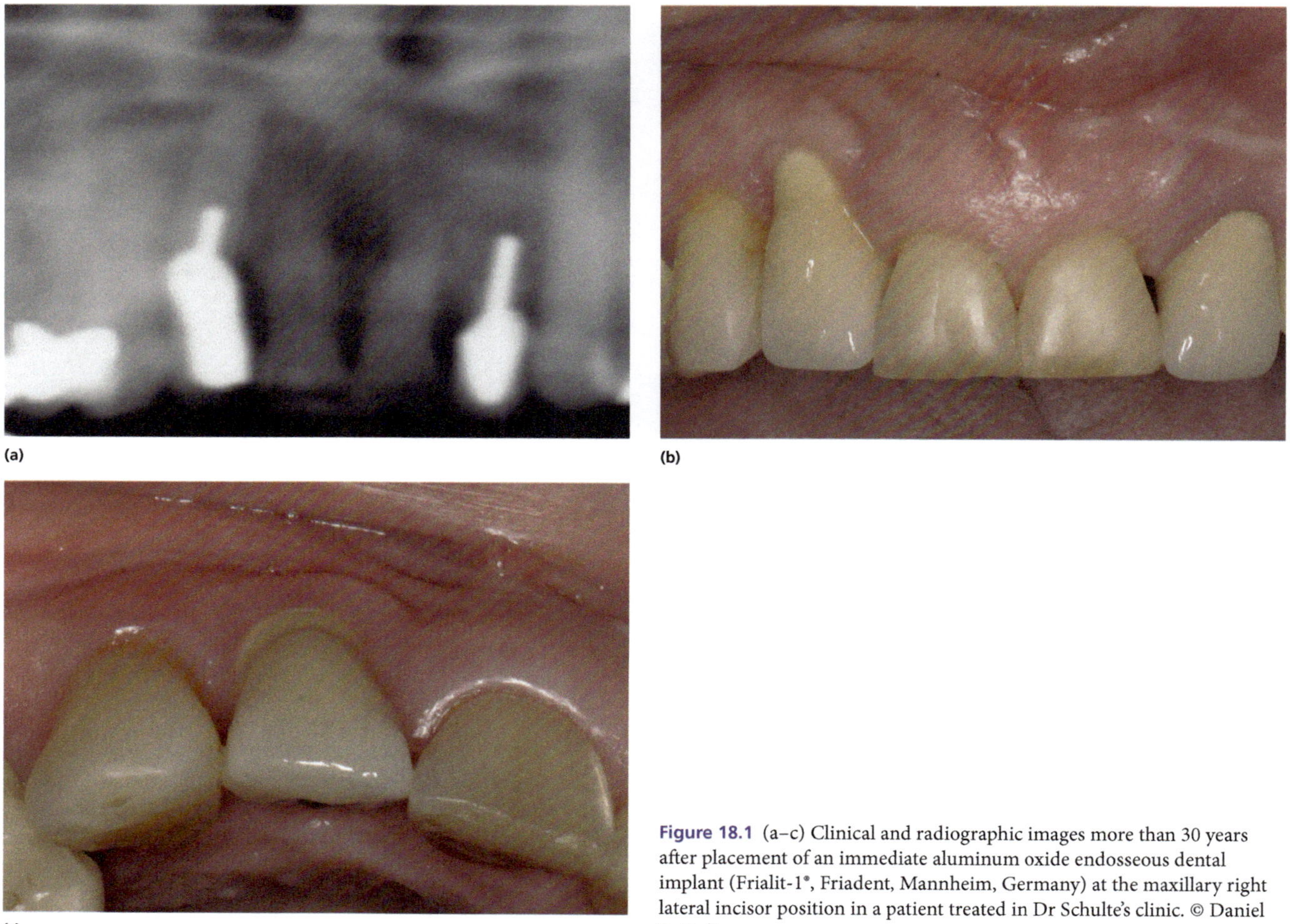

(a) (b) (c)

Figure 18.1 (a–c) Clinical and radiographic images more than 30 years after placement of an immediate aluminum oxide endosseous dental implant (Frialit-1®, Friadent, Mannheim, Germany) at the maxillary right lateral incisor position in a patient treated in Dr Schulte's clinic. © Daniel R. Cullum.

bone was initially thick (>1 mm) and the buccal jumping distance large (>1 mm), substantial bone fill occurred. This would suggest that bicuspid sites are the most favorable maxillary sites for immediate implant placement.

Schnitman et al.[26] reported survival of immediate implants with immediate loading using provisional restorations for full-arch segments. The immediately loaded implants were placed to support provisional prostheses and were not expected to integrate, but rather to shield additional implants placed using a two-stage healing protocol. Initial unanticipated success with the immediate load implants opened a new understanding of principles in use today. A flapless approach can now be advocated both to preserve the periosteum and its blood supply to the extraction site and to allow immediate provisional restoration to fulfill patient esthetic demands[27–29] (see Chapter 19). Implant positioning in maxillary anterior tooth sites is more critical since buccal bone and soft tissue dimensions can be thin and subject to vertical resorption without augmentation grafting.[15,30–35] Use of soft tissue grafting in maxillary anterior sites may be appropriate to reduce the risk of recession that accompanies buccal horizontal and vertical bone resorption.[17,36]

Immediate implantation into molar extraction sockets is challenging as the standard implant shapes and sizes are markedly different from the anatomical sites that they are to replace. This results in the technical challenge of developing the osteotomy in the desired 3-D position leaving larger residual defects between the implant and socket walls.[37,38] Further considerations include the reason for tooth loss, since implants intended to replace teeth lost for periodontal reasons, especially at maxillary molar sites, may be at greater risk of failure[39]. Indeed, most clinicians would hesitate to place immediate implants in patients with chronic or refractory periodontal disease. Other risk factors include smoking and the existence of an acute infection at the extraction site.[40]

Prosthetic considerations

Planning for immediate placement includes consideration of 3-D implant positioning for the final prosthesis design for possible screw retention[35,41,42] (Figure 18.2a–c). Palatal positioning has been determined to be a key factor in the long-term stability of crestal bone volume and subsequent soft tissue stability.[43,44,45] Screw retention often requires implant placement to be completed in a more upright position than the original tooth root (Figure 18.2c–e). This is required to allow the screw access opening to exit far enough away from the incisal edge for adequate material thickness to remain for strength and esthetics of the prosthesis[35] (see Chapters 1 and 2). This is also a significant consideration with immediate provisional restoration (see Chapter 19) and for long-term soft tissue maintenance.[29] A significant alveolar undercut can restrict the desired position, forcing

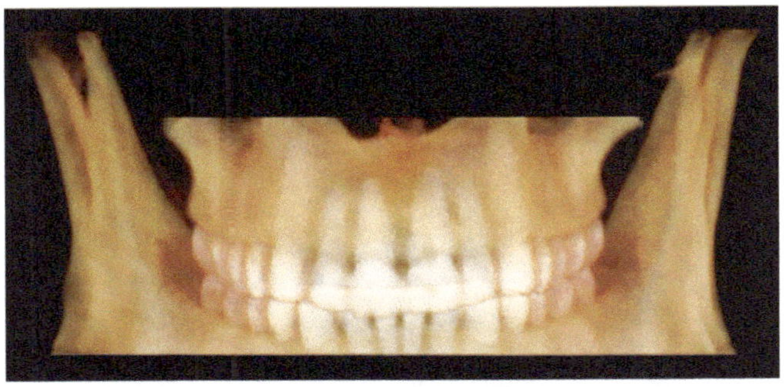
(a)

Figure 18.2 (a) Preoperative 3-D reconstruction of failing maxillary central incisors. (b) CBCT cross-sectional images showing the root proximity to the facial bone in the apical one-third region. (c) Implant positioning and angulation for screw retention, with the screw access positioned for emergence through the cingulum area and an anticipated facial bone gap of >2 mm (arrow).

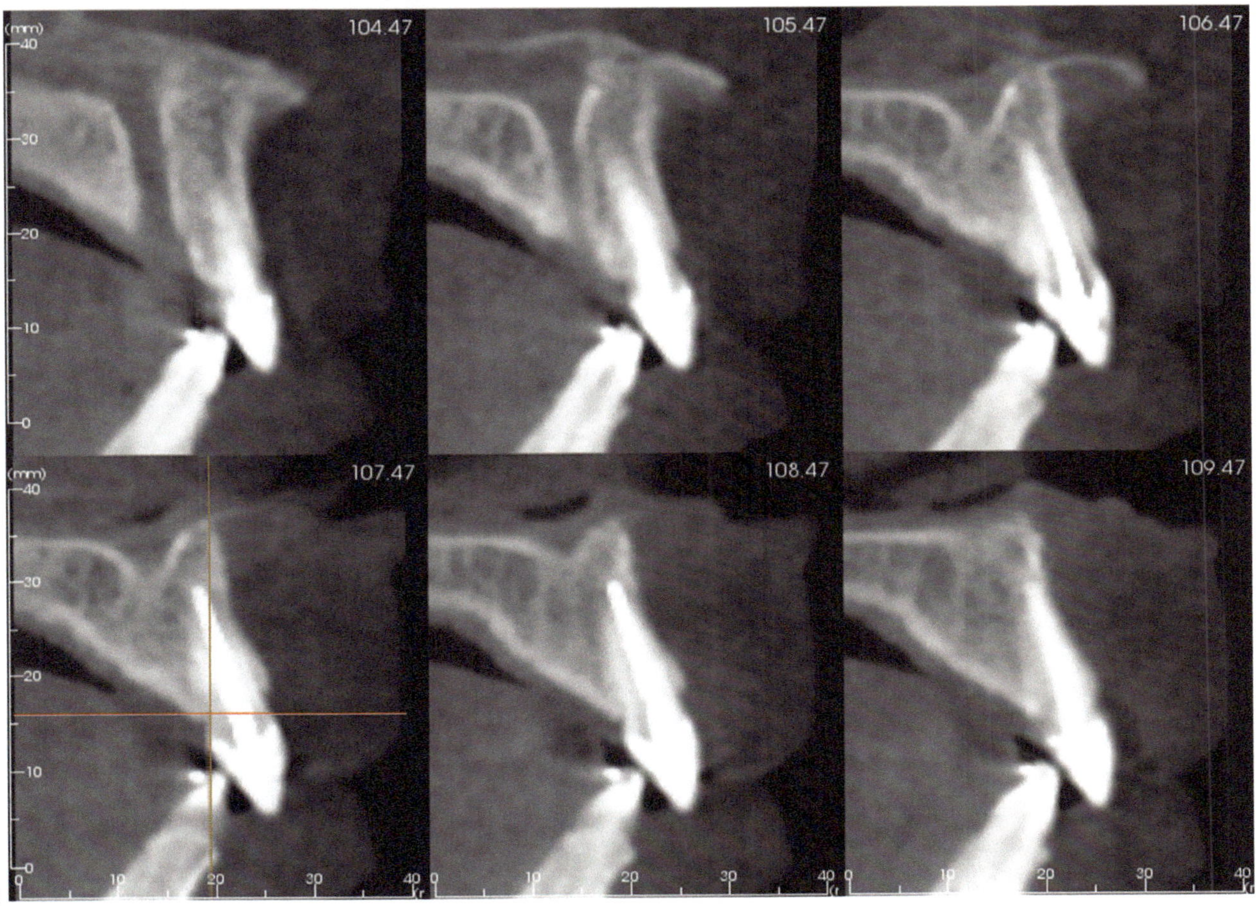

(b)

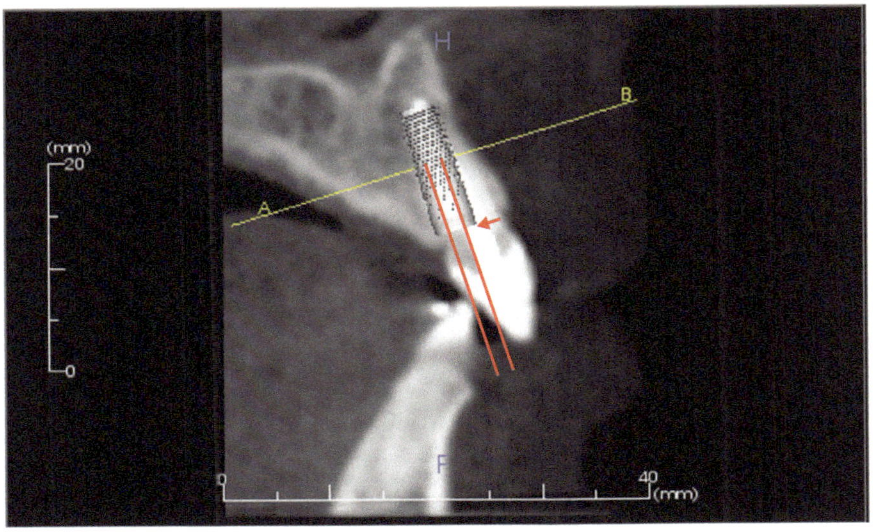

(c)

(Continued)

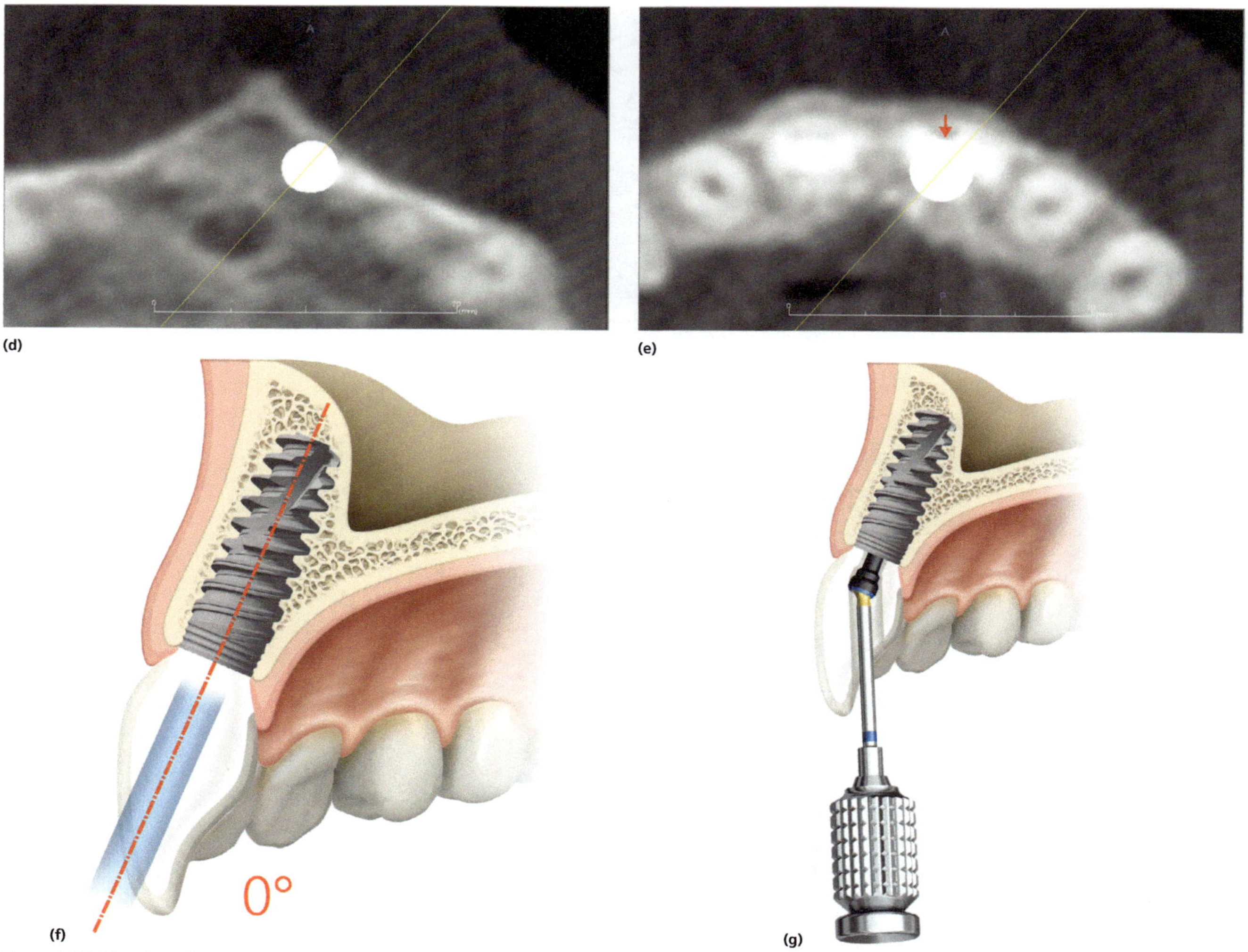

Figure 18.2 (Continued)
(d, e) Axial views of the planning with the apical view (d) close to the facial plate and the crestal view (e) demonstrating the planned facial gap (arrow). (f, g) Graphic representation of the problem with implant screw access through the facial of the potential implant crown. A modified abutment screw and driver design, Angulated Screw Channel® (Nobel Biocare, Yorba Linda, CA) allows off-axis placement and removal of the retention screw when positioning does not allow direct cingulum access. *Source*: (a–e) © Daniel R. Cullum. (f, g) Nobel Biocare. Reproduced with permission of Nobel Biocare.

implant placement with a more facial angulation to avoid the risk of protrusion of the implant body through the undercut[41] (Figure 18.2c and d). Implant placement with increased facial angulation typically requires use of an angled abutment and cement retention, influencing the prosthesis design and the potential for immediate provisional restoration. A recent modified angulated screw channel abutment allows "off-axis" access to the retention screw when implant positioning does not allow direct cingulum access (Angulated Screw Channel®, Nobel Biocare, Yorba Linda, CA) (Figure 18.2f and g). Limiting the facial angulation will also reduce the risk of recession[45] (see later discussion and Chapter 2). Further considerations include use of a narrower diameter or shorter implant to allow a more optimal position and reducing anatomic risk.[46,47]

A reduced inter-arch dimension will influence the planned restoration and desired implant placement. Short crown heights may mandate screw retention in order to have adequate material thickness for prosthetic strength, esthetics, and durability (see Chapters 1 and 3). Screw retention is indicated if the implant site is determined at preoperative planning to have a restricted vertical dimension (<6 mm), if findings at surgery restrict further apical implant positioning due to anatomy (e.g. inferior alveolar nerve proximity) or would result in the implant position being too deep relative to the interproximal bone height of an adjacent tooth, or if the prosthesis design must be retrievable (for hygiene and long-term maintenance).[42]

Anatomic considerations

Clinical and radiographic assessment with 3-D imaging allows accurate diagnosis and planning (see Chapter 2). Pretreatment diagnosis of extraction site defects that can limit immediate placement, such as missing bone walls or apical defects, will allow the clinician to plan for treatment alternatives.[31,37,48] For single-rooted teeth, the extraction defect must be evaluated for the relative position of the root defect compared with the desired implant position. Assessment of facial and palatal bone thickness, root prominence, labial undercut, adjacent teeth or implants, and other anatomical structures (nerve, blood vessels, sinus, nasal cavity, etc.) must also be completed[41] (Figure 18.3). Bone density

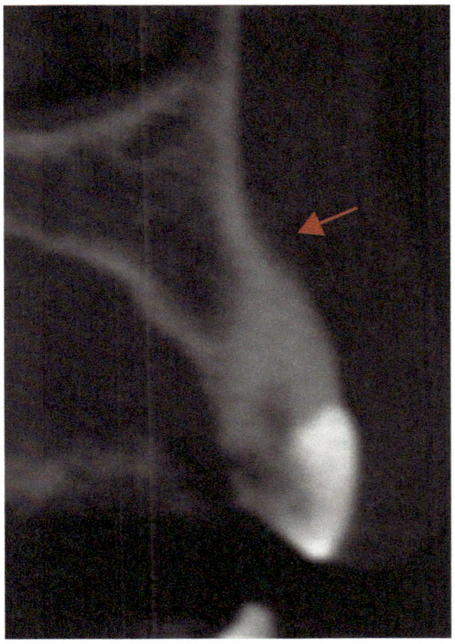

(a)

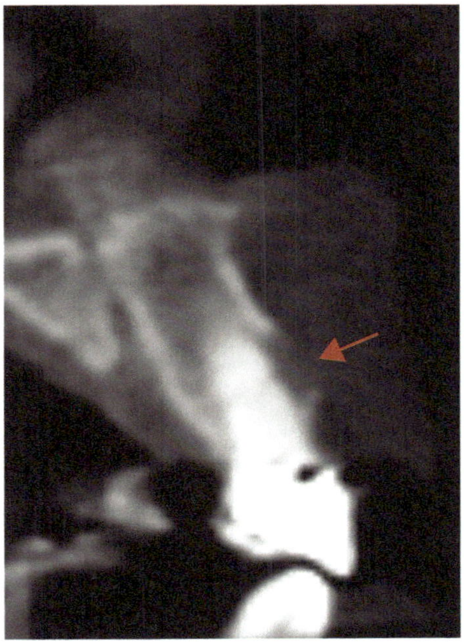

(b)

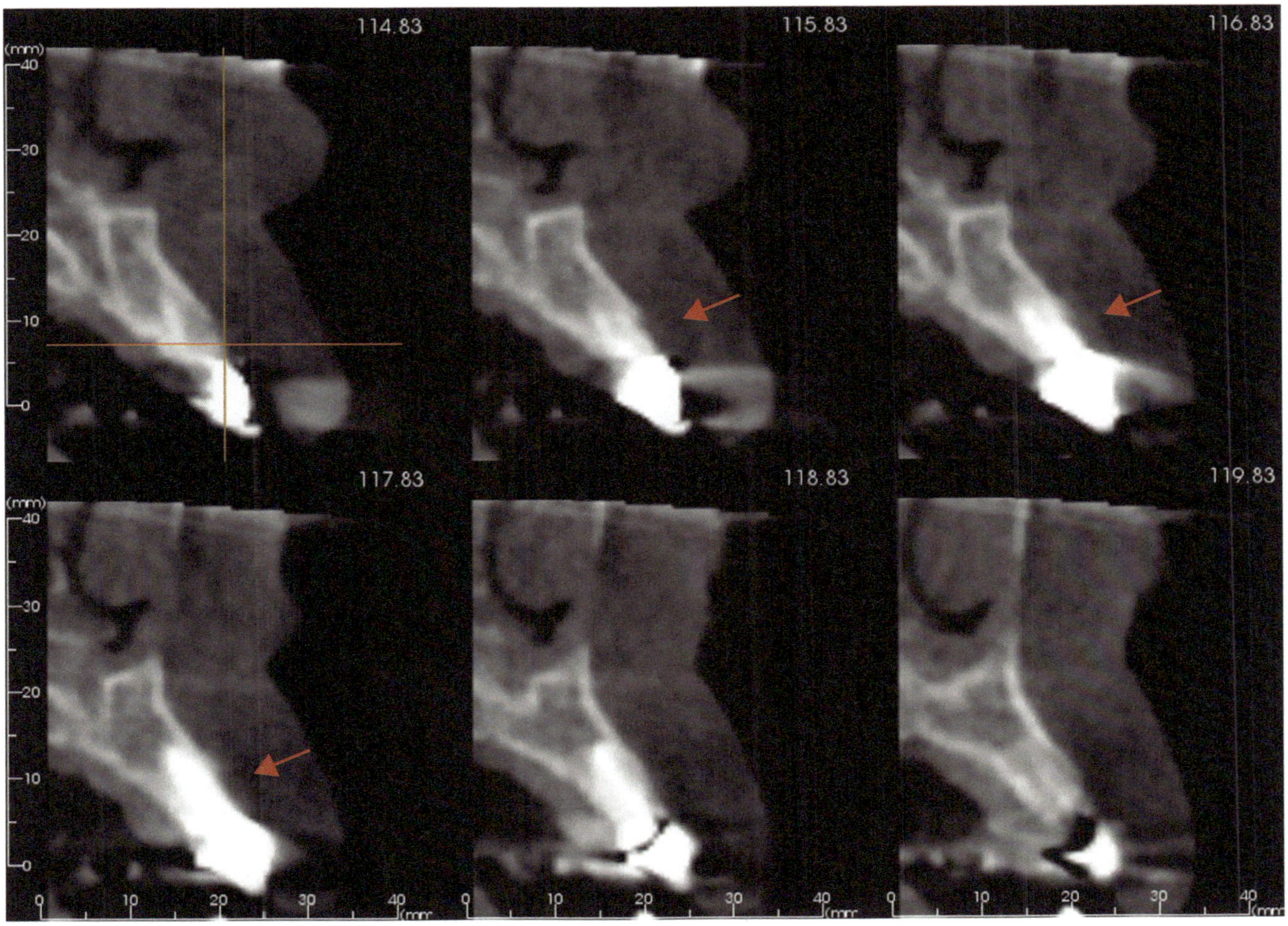

(c)

Figure 18.3 CBCT anterior site evaluation. (a) Maxillary canine demonstrating apical root perforation at the alveolar undercut (arrow). (b) Facial bone plate defect/fenestration (arrow). (c) Buccal crestal bone defect (arrow).

(Continued)

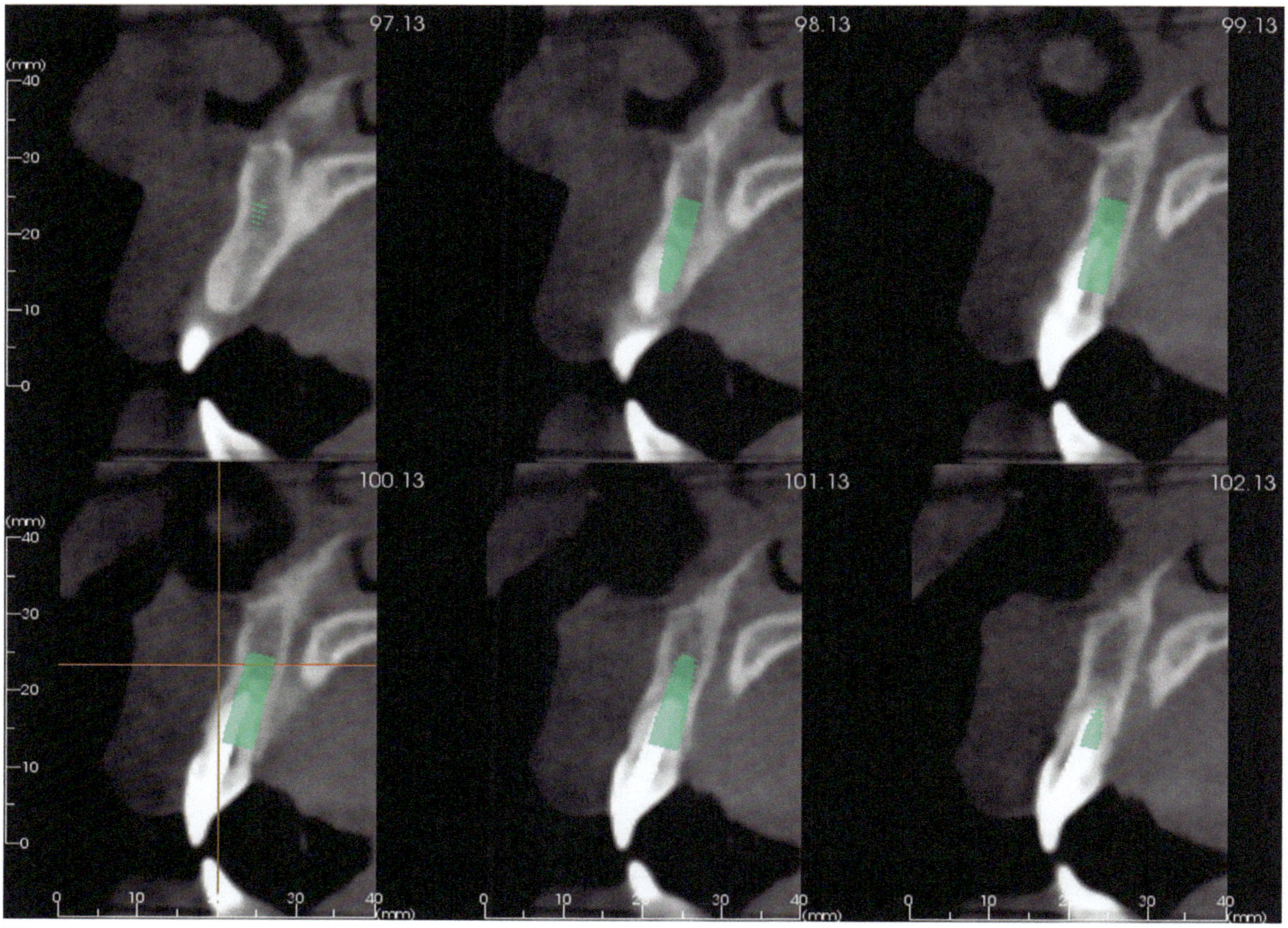

(d)

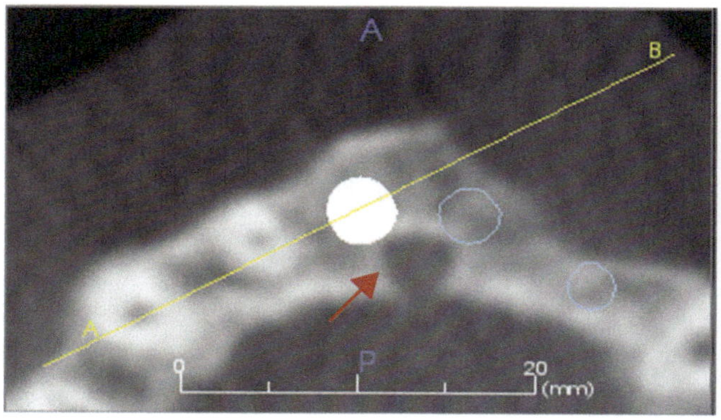

(e)

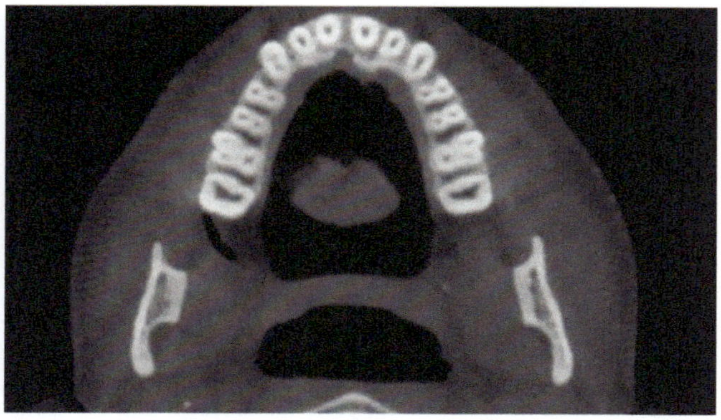

(f)

Figure 18.3 (Continued)
(d, e) Proximity to the naso-palatine canal (arrow). (f) Bucccal root prominence and dehiscence demonstrated here at the maxillary canine and first molars sites.

can vary at specific locations within the arch and between the maxilla and mandible, potentially influencing primary stability of immediate implants.[6] Immediate sites have the added challenge of developing an implant osteotomy within a sloped or "off-axis" residual defect, or between adjacent roots of multi-rooted teeth resulting in variable gap dimensions as discussed earlier.[43] The anterior mandible displays narrow mesio-distal dimensions of the incisor teeth, often with inadequate interproximal dimension to avoid interproximal bone loss, even with the use of 3 mm diameter implant designs. Consideration of removal of an adjacent incisor with a cantilever pontic or management of the four incisors with a two implant-supported four-unit bridge often

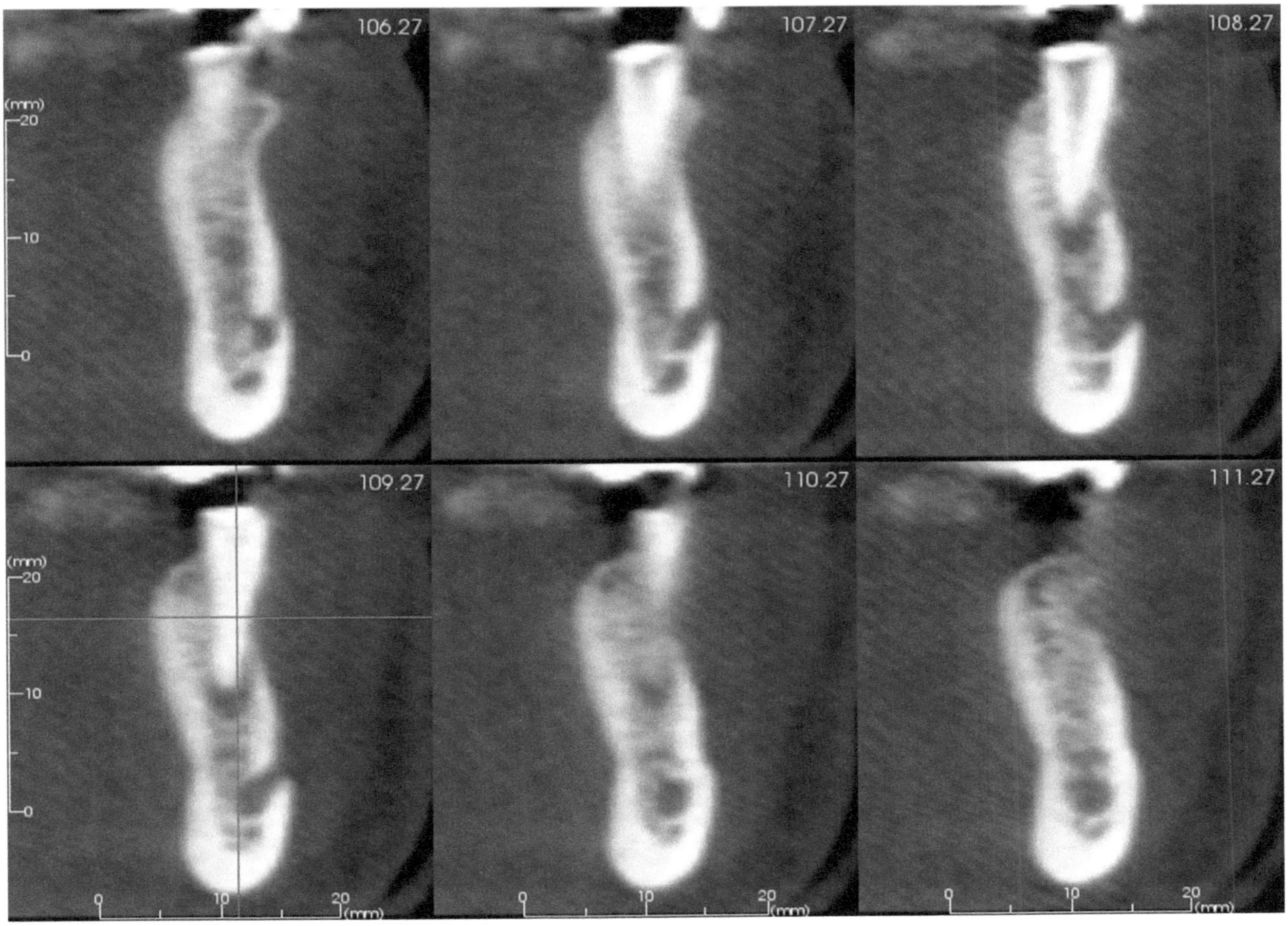

(g)

Figure 18.3 (Continued)

(g) Apical inflammation and proximity to the inferior alveolar nerve. (a–g) © Daniel R. Cullum.

may be more practical solutions to inadequate mesio-distal space dimensions.

Atieh et al.[38] published a systematic review of outcomes with over 1000 immediate maxillary and mandibular molar implants after 1–11 years in function. Survival rates were consistent with molar implants placed in healed extraction sites (93.9–100%). Many of the early molar implants had been placed in one or more of the individual molar root sockets, resulting in eccentric placement with poor emergence profiles and anatomically compromised crowns. Placing immediate molar implants centrally in the mesio-distal dimension of the inter-radicular bone is technically more challenging, but facilitates a more ideal crown anatomy and better access for home care. The depth of osteotomy preparation should engage approximately 4 mm of apical bone or require the use of wider diameter implants to gain adequate primary stability.[6] In the mandible this increases the risk of perforating the lingual bone or encroaching upon the mandibular canal. Froum et al.[37] reported data from a series of CT scan assessments showing that 53% of mandibular first molar and 73% of mandibular second molar sites were considered at high risk of complication with immediate implant placement. At posterior maxillary sites, sinus pneumatization can be extensive and may require simultaneous TASE procedures (see Chapter 15) for immediate implant placement.[49]

The anatomy of the inter-radicular septum can be a factor in achieving good immediate molar implant positioning and stability.[42,50,51] (Figure 18.4a–c). At molar sites in the mandible, the septum may be too narrow to allow stable and congruent use of surgical burs (see later discussion). Maxillary molars often present with trifurcation of the roots and a furcal bone plateau (Figure 18.4d–f). Softer bone densities typical of these sites may be amenable to development with, concave-tipped osteotomes, avoiding bur chatter or fracture of poorer quality furcal bone. Denser bone site preparation follows that described in the "Surgical considerations" section.

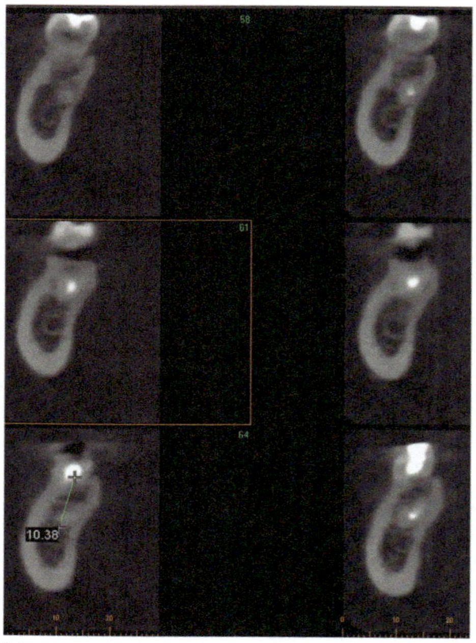

(a)

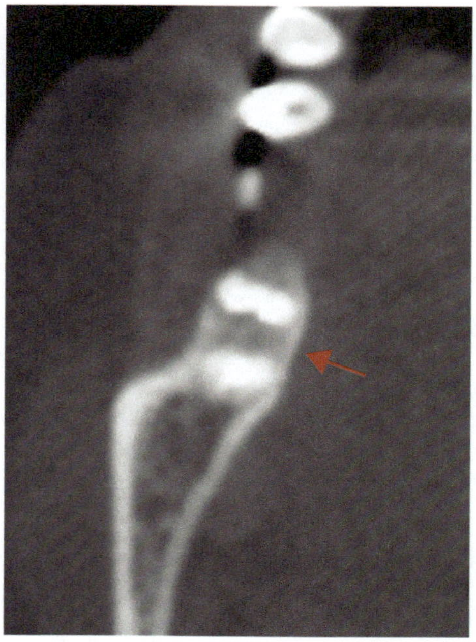

(c)

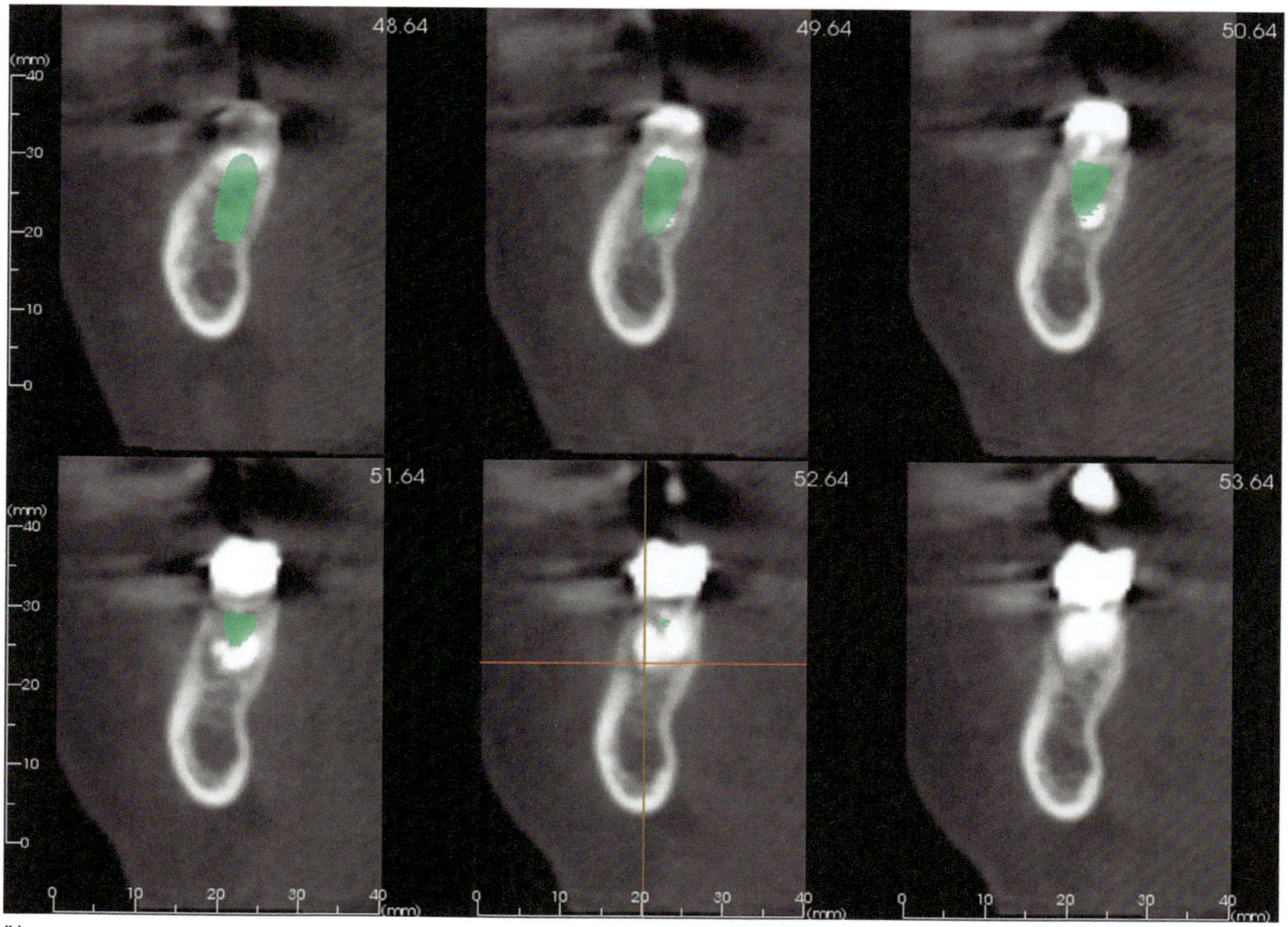

(b)

Figure 18.4 CBCT evaluation of inter-radicular molar anatomy. (a) Cross-sectional view demonstrating minimal distance from the root apex to the inferior alveolar nerve. (b, c) Mandible CBCT axial and cross-sectional images showing adequate height above the nerve and inter-radicular bone dimension at the right mandibular second molar (arrow).

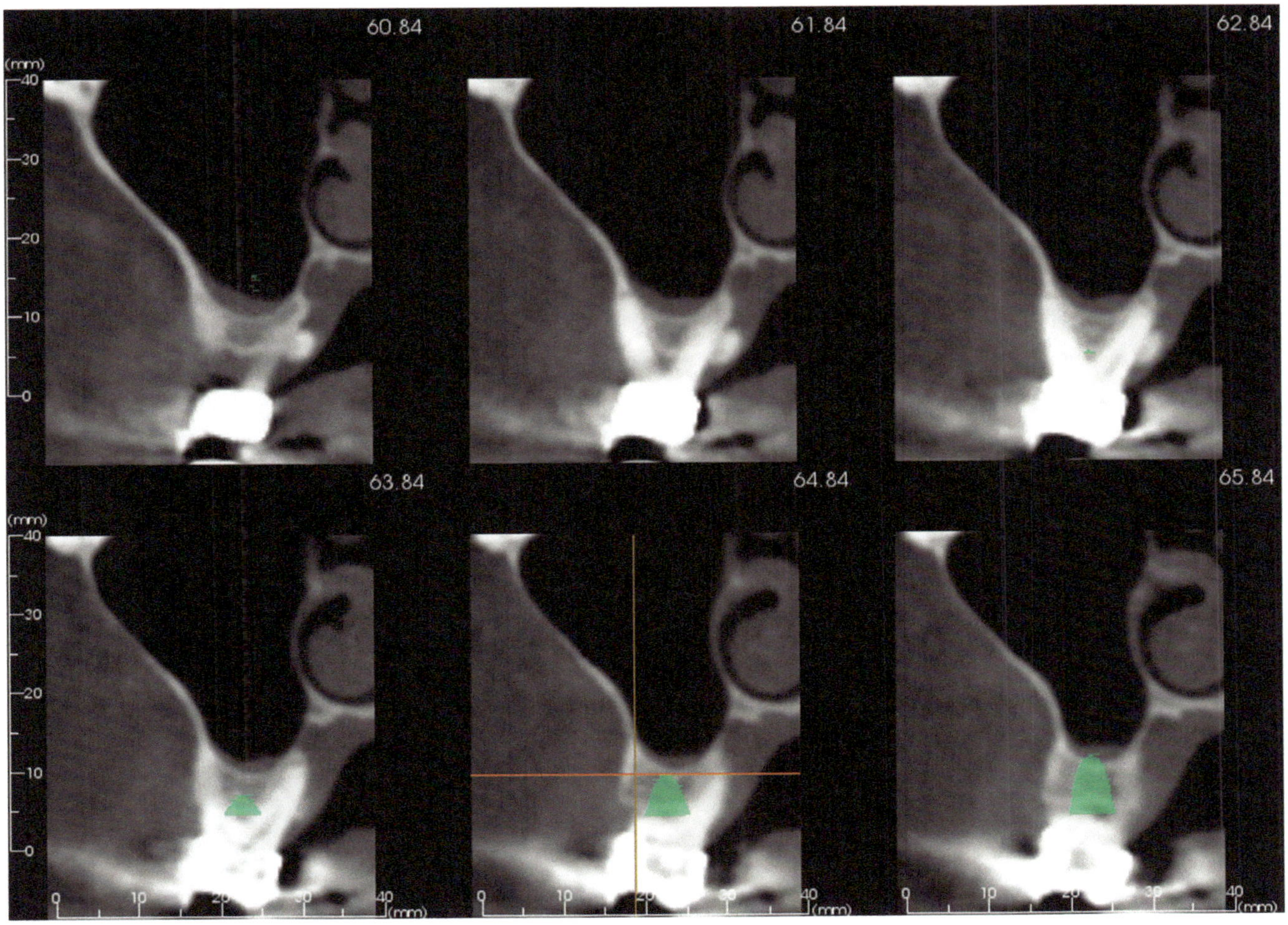

(d)

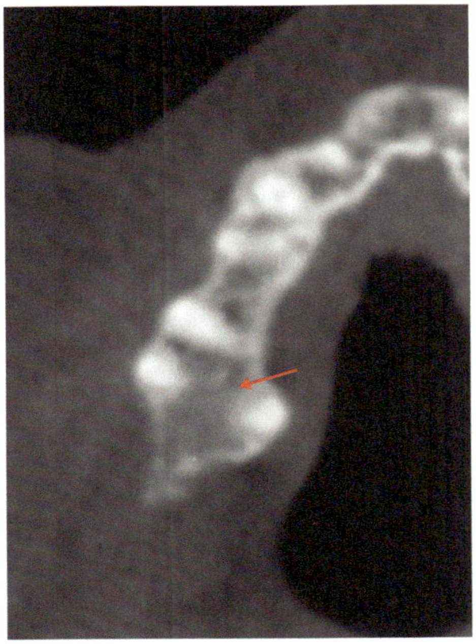

(e)

Figure 18.4 (Continued)
(d, e) Maxillary molar CBCT axial and cross-sectional images demonstrating a broad inter-radicular plateau of bone (arrow) (e), with 3–4 mm of residual subantral bone height (d).

(Continued)

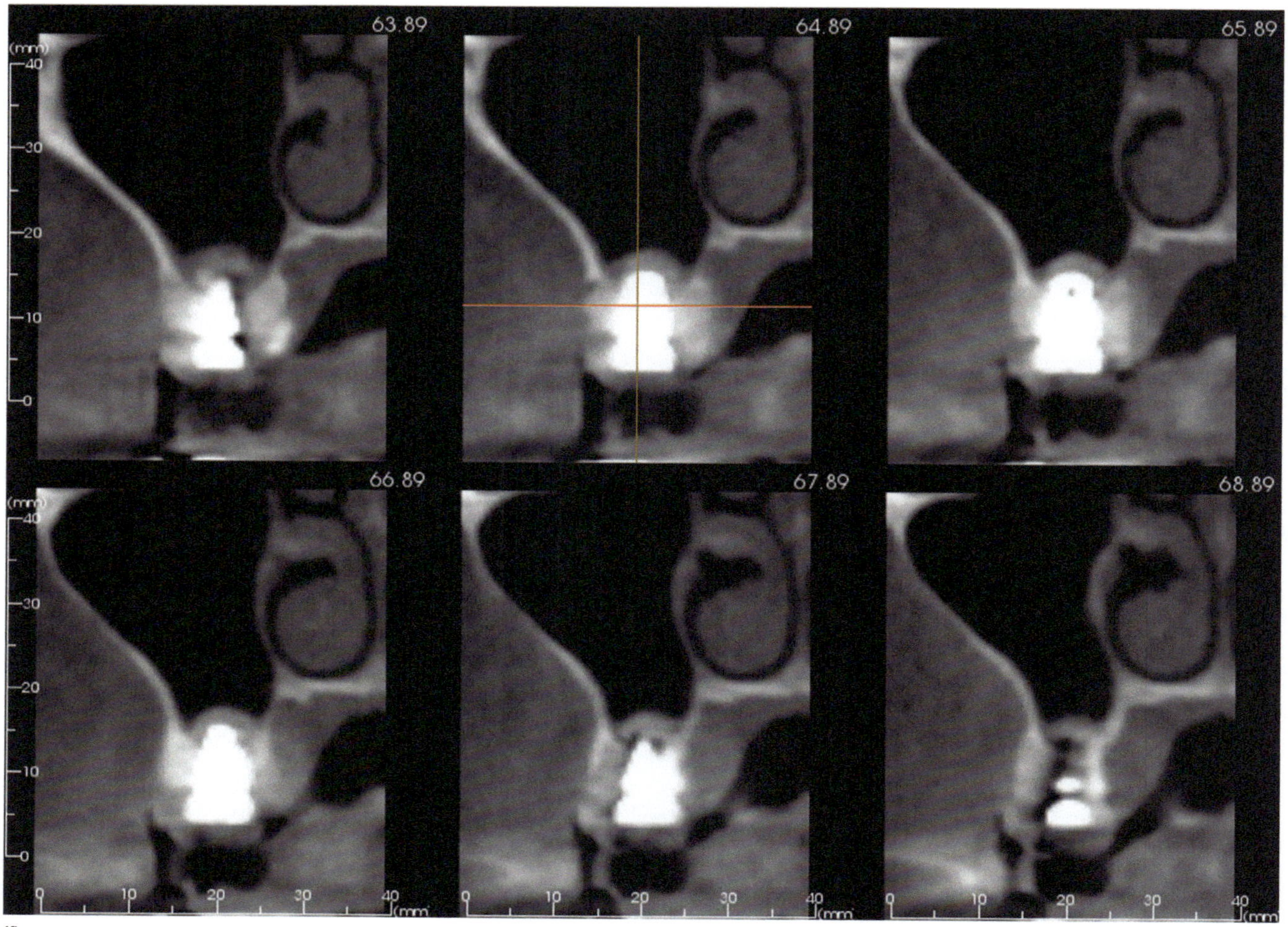

(f)

Figure 18.4 (Continued)

(f) Post-operative images showing immediate 7.5 mm × 5.8 mm diameter implant with combined TASE (see Chapter 15) for immediate molar replacement. (a–f) © Daniel R. Cullum.

Surgical considerations

The recommended protocol for immediate implant placement includes atraumatic tooth removal (discussed in Chapter 5), minimal or no flap elevation, and sectioning for multi-rooted or ankylotic teeth. Using adjunctive techniques such as Piezosurgery®, root extractor devices (Benex®, Meisinger USA, Centennial, CO), and electric periotome devices (Powertome®, Bridgeport, OR) can be helpful. Meticulous debridement and apical socket curettage are necessary to ensure complete removal of pathology and periodontal remnants (Figure 18.5a). Site evaluation with periodontal probing is necessary to determine the residual crestal bone height and the support of the surrounding bone walls and/or defects. With larger defects, open access may be necessary to ensure complete debridement or access for grafting. Implant site development can then proceed, keeping in mind the limitations of the extraction site anatomy and desired final 3-D implant position.

Techniques to obtain an initial purchase at an "off-axis" or sloping extraction site include the use of twist drills or pointed drills to obtain purchase followed by "up-righting" of the osteotomy with standard drill preparation[51,52] (Figure 18.5b and c) or the use of Piezosurgery inserts (Figure 18.5d) for "differential" or asymmetric implant site preparation.[53] Care is needed to maintain adequate adjacent tooth or implant distances and avoiding facial malpositioning or misangulation[49,52] (Figure 18.5e).

The remaining peri-implant bone gap/defect of the extraction socket is grafted with any harvested autogenous bone mixed with mineralized allograft[15] or xenograft material[27,54,55] (Figure 18.5f). An open flap approach may be necessary if there has been loss of buccal or interproximal bone requiring GBR.[29,55] Typically, with the implant placed against the palatal or lingual wall of the extraction site, particulate graft material is packed with moderate pressure into the buccal defect to ensure that no voids remain. The remaining crestal soft tissue defect can be sealed with dense collagen (CollaPlug®, Zimmer Dental, Carlsbad, CA) sectioned to the desired shape and saturated with blood or recombinant human platelet-derived growth factor (rhPDGF – "off-label" use) and stabilized with a "figure-of-eight" chromic suture as a modified BioCol® technique[56] (Figure 18.5g; see further description in Chapter 5). The site can be protected from salivary enzymes, gross food particles, and tongue manipulation with light-cured periodontal dressing (Barricaid®, Dentsply-Caulk, Milford, DE). The site can be seen after 16 days' healing in Figure 18.5i and on radiographs after more than 4 years

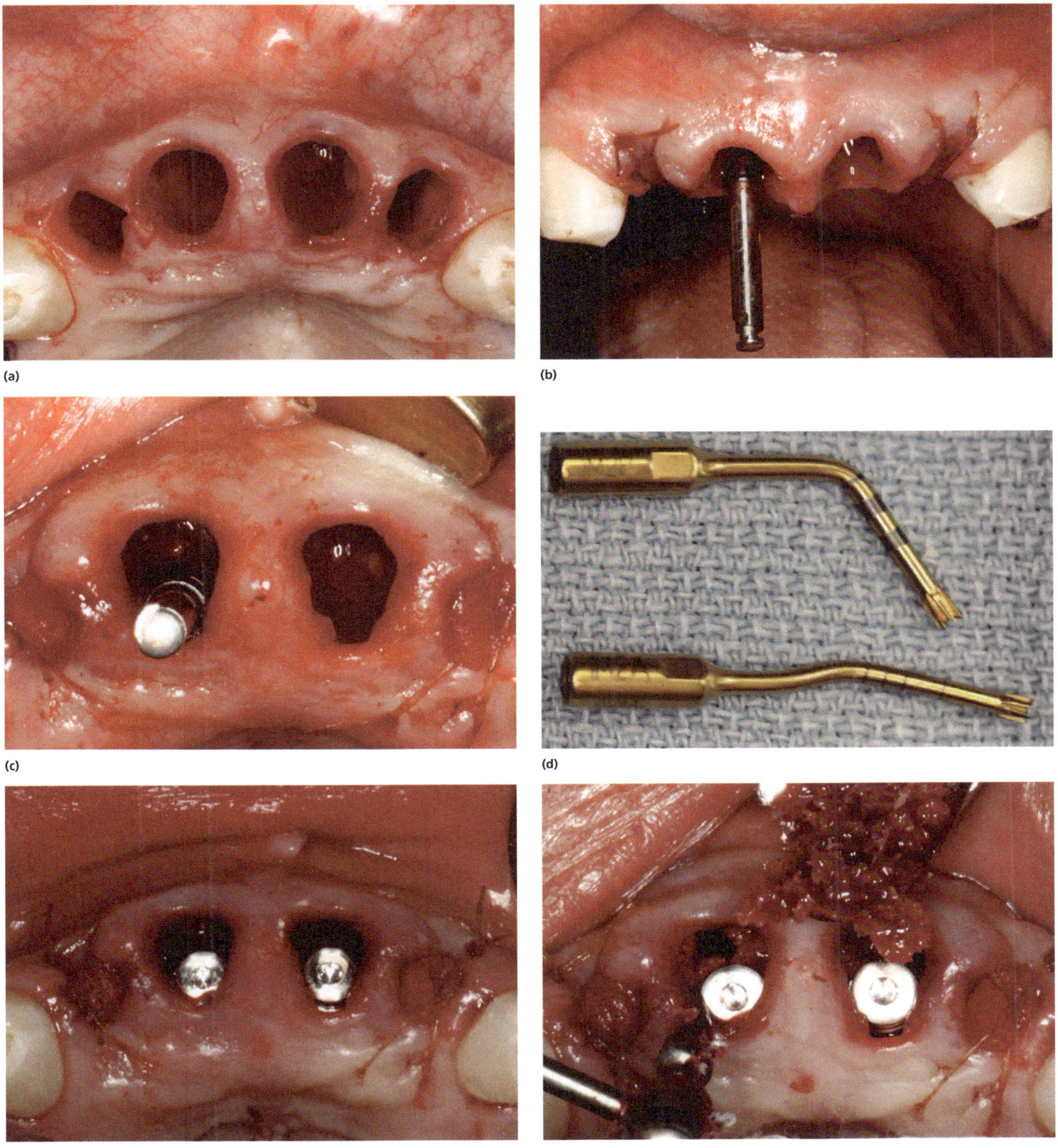

(a) (b) (c) (d) (e) (f)

Figure 18.5 (a) Complete debridment and site evaluation with periodontal probing is necessary to determine the residual crestal bone height and the existence of surrounding bone walls and/or defects. (b, c) A 2 mm drill in position after obtaining an initial purchase at the "off-axis" sloping extraction site. (d) Piezosurgery inserts IM2A and IM2P. (e) Re-angulation and 3-D position adjustment of the osteotomy can be completed intraoperatively to attain implant placement in the palatal aspect of the tooth socket maintaining adequate adjacent tooth or implant distances and avoiding facial malpositioning or misangulation. (f) The facial bone gaps were grafted (mineralized particulate allograft), as were the two adjacent lateral incisor extraction sites.

(Continued)

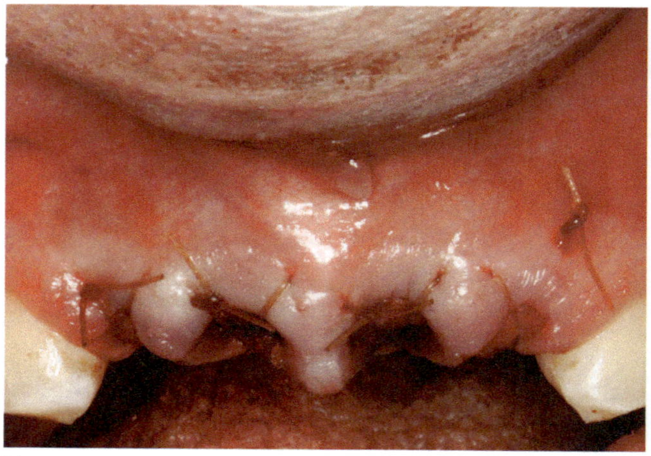

(g)

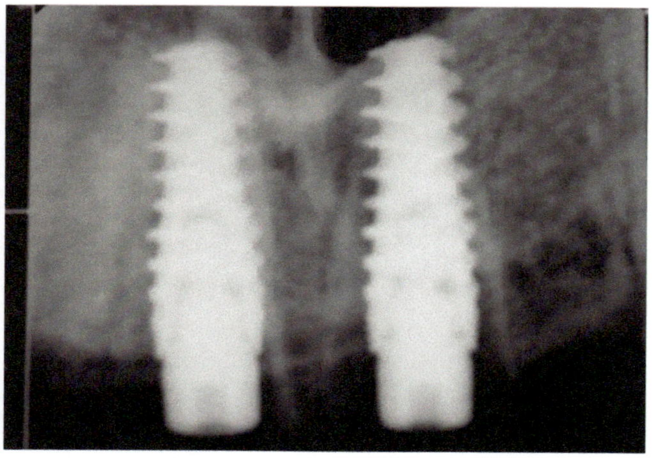

(h)

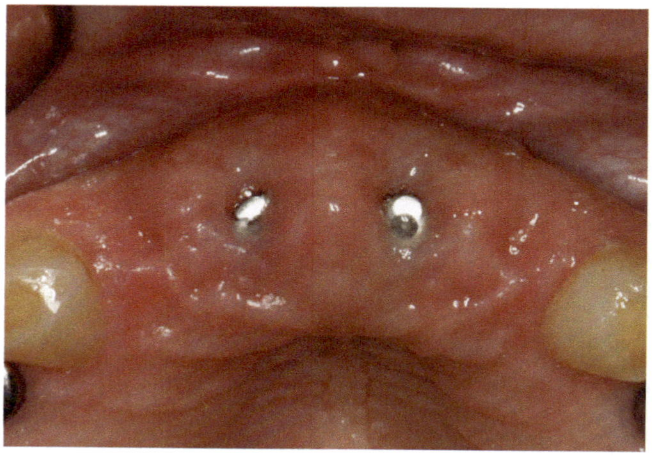

(i)

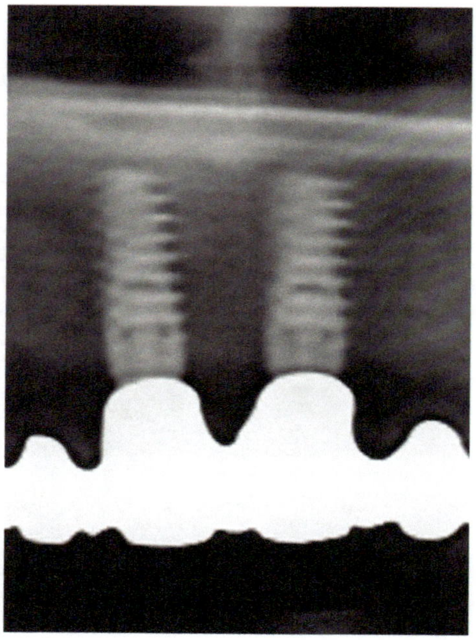

(j)

Figure 18.5 (Continued)
(g) The crestal soft tissue gap was sealed with rhPDGF ("off-label" use, GEM 21S®, Osteohealth, Shirley, NY) saturated collagen (CollaPlug®, Zimmer Dental, Carlsbad, CA) and secured with 4-0 chromic gut suture and with light-cured periodontal dressing. (h) Final intraoperative periapical radiograph. (i) Clinical healing after 16 days. (j) Post-treatment restored radiograph after 4 years and 8 months. (a–j) © Daniel R. Cullum.

in Figure 18.5j. An immediate non-loaded provisional restoration can be considered with adequate implant primary stability and positioning (see Chapter 19). Immediate placement with partial or significant bone wall defects can be completed with GBR, flap advancement for primary closure, and submerged healing. If need be, a free connective tissue graft or palatal pedicle connective tissue flap can be used to augment tissue thickness and/or wound closure[57,58] (see Chapter 8).

The role of 3-D imaging is significant for planning immediate implant surgery. However, computer-guided surgery must be used with caution in immediate sites. The presence of an anatomical defect with a significant slope can cause the drill to deflect from the intended guided path, altering the direction/inclination of the osteotomy and/or causing binding within the guide sleeve. Extraction sites at retained primary teeth offer the best anatomic locations to use this technology, as they have a greater volume of apical bone for implant stability and a shorter extraction site defect (see Chapters 2 and 9). Low-dose CBCT imaging can be a helpful tool for post-treatment assessment of implant positioning and on rare occasions for intraoperative evaluation when adjacent anatomy cannot be clearly defined on periapical radiographs.

Design features that facilitate immediate implant placement include tapered macrodesigns that produce primary stability and facilitate optimal 3-D positioning. With maxillary anterior immediate implant placement, implant designs without cutting threads tend to be displaced to the facial by resistance of the dense palatal bone, as would attempts to use a tap or thread former without an opposing buccal bone wall for stability and cutting pressure. This can result in the implant following the path of least resistance with buccal displacement of the crestal aspect of the implant body, reducing the dimension of the facial bone gap and increasing facial angulation. A reduced coronal implant diameter will reduce this tendency for buccal displacement and allow for an adequate buccal gap dimension to remain for hard and soft tissue grafting and minimal risk of soft and hard tissue loss. Examples of implant designs well-suited for immediate placement for single-rooted teeth can be seen in Figure 18.6.

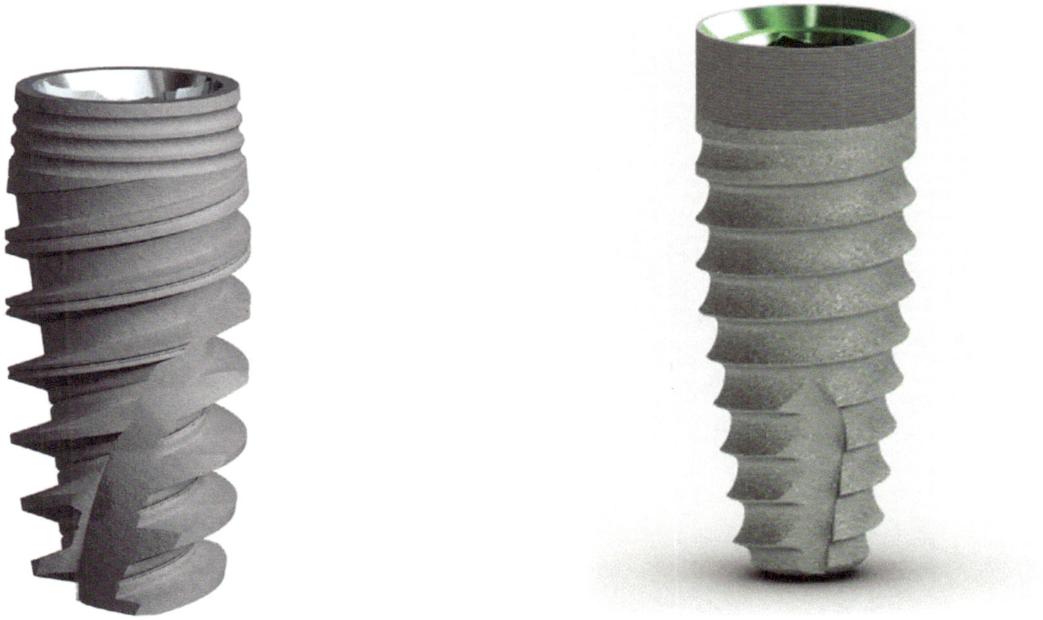

(a) (b)

Figure 18.6 (a, b) Implant design features for regular platform immediate applications include significant taper with aggressive thread design (Nobel Active®, Nobel Biocare, Yorba Linda, CA, and Tapered Internal®, BioHorizons, Birmingham, AL). *Source*: (a) Nobel Biocare. Reproduced with permission of Nobel Biocare. (b) BioHorizons. Reproduced with permission from BioHorizons.

Molar implant procedures can be more technique-sensitive, particularly in mandible where larger diameter drills can bind at the osteotomy walls. With a narrow (<3 mm in width) inter-radicular septum in the mandible the pilot drill can be started on an angle near its base to gain a stable starting point and then be slowly "uprighted" to reduce bur chatter and drifting for optimal implant positioning[51] (Figure 18.7). Some clinicians have suggested the use of trephines[43] or beginning and/or completing the osteotomy before tooth removal to help with obtaining a purchase while drilling,[59,60] although this increases the challenge of final root removal.

For molar replacement, a minimum implant diameter of 4 mm is recommended for biomechanical considerations.[46,47] Many

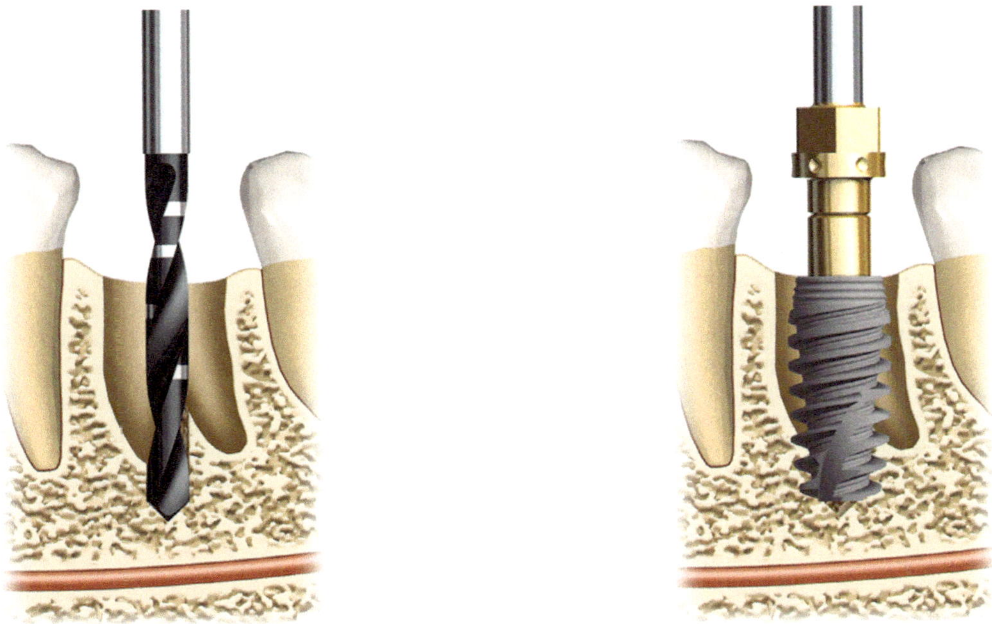

(a) (b)

Figure 18.7 (a, b) Drill location for a mandibular molar after apical purchase and drill "uprighting" for desired final implant position. Nobel Biocare, Yorba Linda, CA. Reproduced with permission of Nobel Biocare.

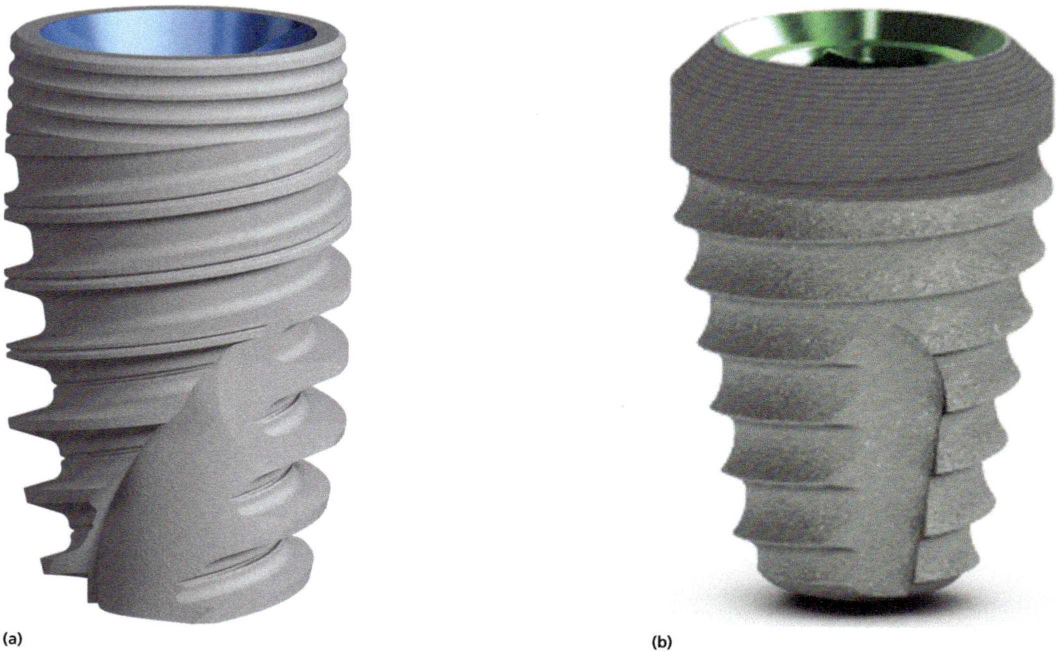

Figure 18.8 (a–c) Posterior immediate implant designs with wider diameter and platform-switching features (Nobel Active®, Nobel Biocare, Yorba Linda, CA, and Tapered Internal Plus®, BioHorizons, Birmingham, AL). *Source:* (a) Nobel Biocare. Reproduced with permission of Nobel Biocare. (b) BioHorizons. Reproduced with permission from BioHorizons.

clinicians prefer to use wider diameter implants to increase the possibility of having a larger emergence profile for the final restoration and reducing potential food retention[35] (Figure 18.8). 3-D finite element analyses and retrospective clinical data have shown wide-diameter implants (6 mm versus 3.7 mm or 4.7 mm diameter) with a minimum of 1.8 mm buccal bone thickness after osteotomy preparation can reduce peri-implant stress and associated crestal bone loss in first molar locations.[47] Implants with a coronal diameter of 6.5 mm for immediate molar sites demonstrated success rates in the maxilla[50] and mandible[51] of 99.5% and 99% respectively.

Wider diameter implants may achieve greater primary stability by bone contact where the inter-radicular septum fuses with the buccal and lingual cortices.[61] A tapered "ultrawide" implant design has been proposed for use as an immediate replacement for molar teeth (Figure 18.9a–e). Survival rates were reported to be 95.8% at healed extraction sites and 95.7% at immediate extraction sites after a mean follow-up of 14 months. Minimal crestal bone loss with a non-submerged initial healing period was reported and attributed to the implant diameter (with reduced crestal bone stresses) and the built-in platform-switch feature. However, during osteotomy preparation, ultrawide implant sites must maintain adequate buccal bone thickness (>2 mm) or risk long-term buccal bone loss and dehiscence. A clinical example of this ultrawide design can be seen at a maxillary molar site in Figure 18.9b–g. Regardless of implant diameter, 3-D positioning at surgery to maintain an adequate buccal bone gap to receive grafting should not be compromised in order to ensure long-term bone stability.

Immediate provisionalization has been well-documented as a treatment option for single-rooted teeth and with straight and angled implants as part of multiple-unit splinted restorations[26,38,40,62] (see Chapters 12 and 19). Several groups of investigators have looked at the effect of immediate loading of wide-diameter implants placed immediately into molar extraction sockets and have shown similar success results when compared with conventional staged treatment.[38,40,43,61]

Classification of extraction socket defects to determine the appropriate management requires evaluation of gingival biotype, number of intact socket walls, and existence of horizontal bone and soft tissue loss.[48] It has been suggested that the decision to undertake immediate treatment should be made based on how much damage is present after tooth extraction. Surgical exposure for immediate implant placement can be limited to a flapless approach with completion of grafting of the intrabony defect when less than one-third of the buccal plate is partially dehisced or missing in the mid-buccal region only.[15] With increasing defect size, however, further conservative surgical exposure may require an intrasulcular incision design, an envelope flap with extension to adjacent teeth, and even one or more vertical releasing incisions. For small buccal ridge defects (<2 mm width), a flapless or sulcular incision only may be adequate, but for larger defects an open-book flap design (see Chapter 14) may be needed to enhance visualization and access to the site needing augmentation grafting.[15,55,63] A distal, curvilinear, vertical incision that follows the gingival margin of the distal tooth with elevation of the papilla on the mesial side of the edentulous site will allow a wide subperiosteal reflection to be completed exposing two to three times the treatment area.[55]

Immediate reconstruction in the maxilla can offer the advantage of development of a vascular pedicle flap to attain tension-free primary closure at larger defect sites[57] (see Chapter 8). Using the palatal tissue in a free or vascular design provides increased tissue volume for graft containment with limited facial dissection,

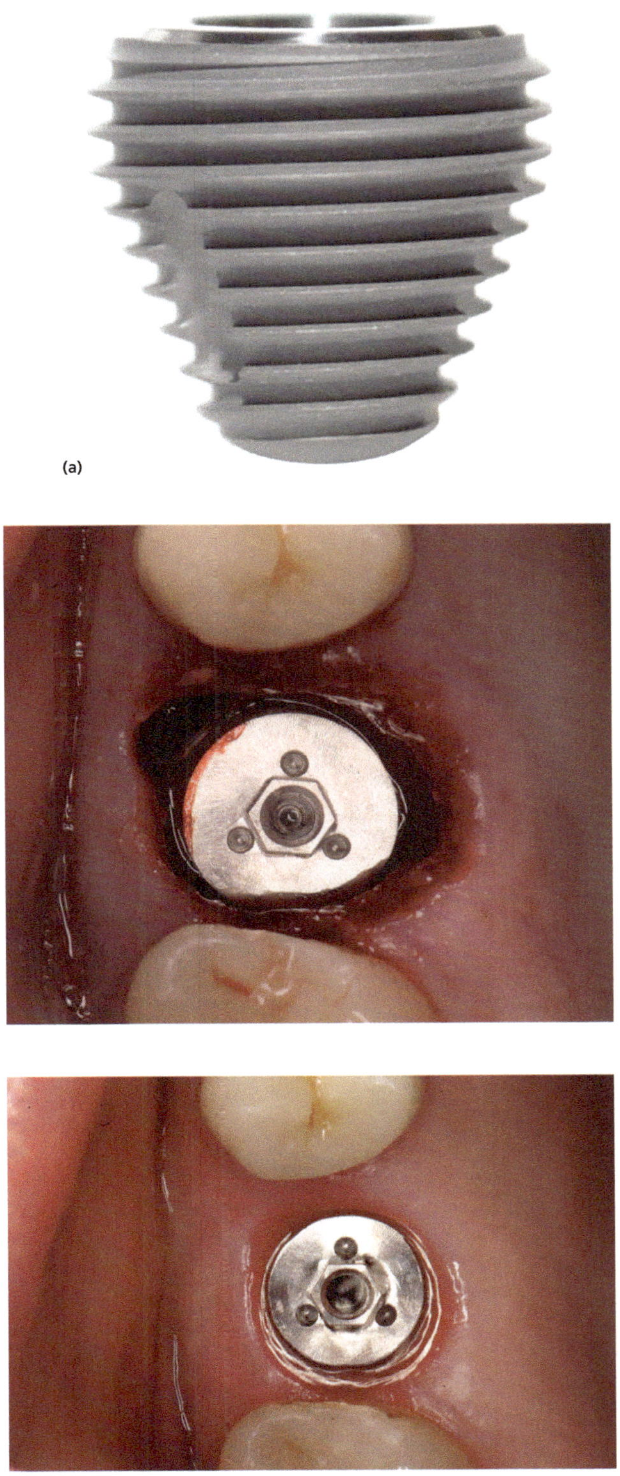

(a)

(c)

(e)

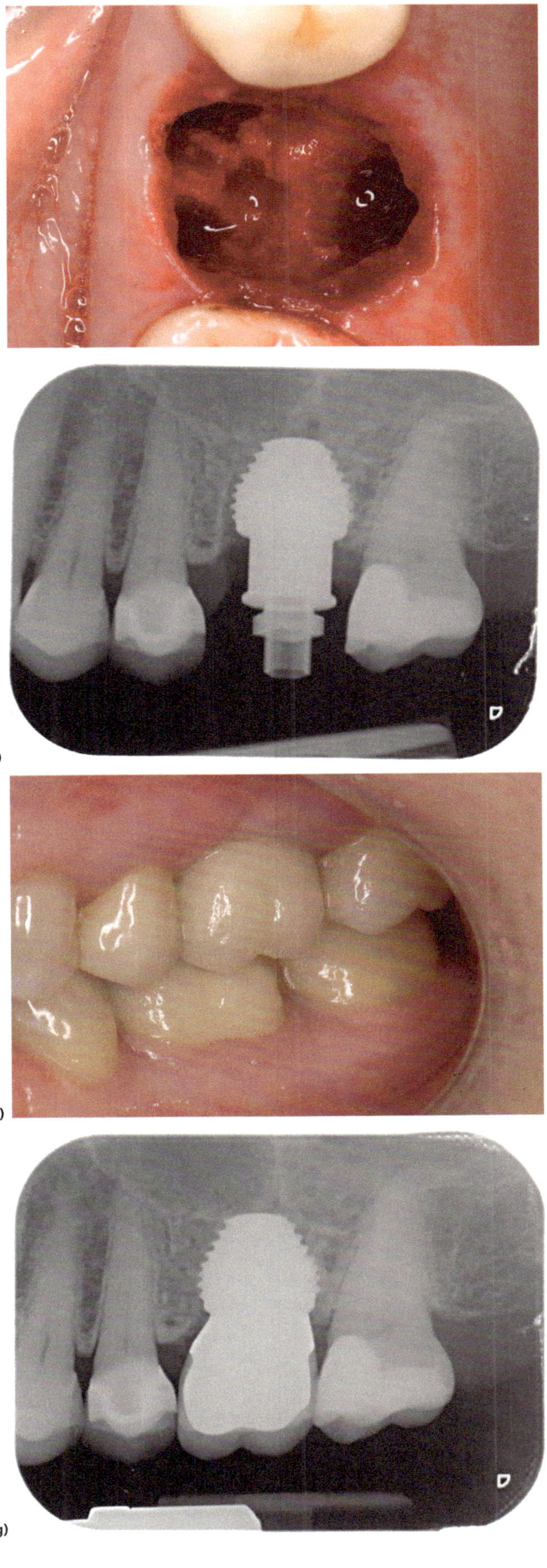

(b)

(d)

(f)

(g)

Figure 18.9 "Ultrawide" immediate implants. (a) "Ultrawide" immediate implant design in 7, 8, and 9 mm diameters (Max®, Keystone Dental, Burlington, MA). (b–g) Clinical and radiographic images of a patient with placement of an immediate "ultrawide" implant and after restoration. *Source:* Andrew Ackermann. Reproduced with permission of Andrew Ackermann.

thereby maintaining vascular supply, avoiding loss of vestibular height, and increasing the keratinized tissue margin. These advantages apply to larger volume defects or thin tissue biotypes with high esthetic demand.

In a retrospective analysis of 42 single-tooth implants placed in the esthetic zone, Evans and Chen[64] reported a significant increase in crown length after immediate implant placement as a result of a mean marginal tissue recession of 0.9 mm. They also found that a thin tissue biotype showed greater recession than a thick biotype (1 mm versus 0.7 mm respectively). In contrast, in a randomized control study, Block et al.[65] found no statistically significant differences in crestal or interproximal bone levels in the anterior maxilla when comparing immediate or delayed implant placement with immediate provisionalization. The authors concluded that immediate implant placement with immediate provisional restoration resulted in approximately 1 mm less facial gingival recession compared with that in the delayed control group. When overall treatment outcomes were compared, immediate implants were preferred over a staged approach by patients.[66,67]

Factors influencing the stability of the facial gingival margin position include:

1 Adequate buccal, crestal bone volume/level.[15,33,68–72] <2 mm buccal thickness is prone to resorption. This is especially true if full-thickness flap elevation is utilized without bone augmentation. There is also increased risk with volume shrinkage following particulate graft procedures with larger defects (multiple tooth sites or greater than a three-walled defect)[25] or in cases with significant root prominence.[73]
2 Soft tissue quality and quantity[58,59,64,74–76] (biotype/thickness, keratinized tissue width, and translucency of prosthetic material; see also Chapter 8). Adequate tissue thickness (thick biotype) with underlying bone support are key factors to esthetic implant success.
3 Palatal positioning[44,68] with anterior implants to maintain adequate crestal/buccal bone volume.
4 Implant angulation. Soft tissue recession is greater with implant angulation to the facial, and this often presents as a late finding after the prosthetic phase.[29,30,44,45]
5 Depth of implant placement.[14,33,64,69] A high, scalloped, thin biotype and triangular tooth form may require deeper positioning relative to the interproximal and/or palatal bone margin and is at higher risk of facial and interproximal adverse tissue level changes.
6 Implant diameter. Smaller diameter implants require less bone volume within the alveolar housing but also less facial inclination to avoid perforation of an undercut.[69]
7 Abutment connection design. An internal "Morse" taper design reduces abutment mobility, microgap dimension, and bacterial colonization compared with flat or parallel-walled connections.[77,78,79]
8 Platform shifting medializes the abutment–implant microgap and helps maintain a higher crestal bone level.[78,80–83]
9 Crestal implant surface/macrogeometry. Microthreads and laser microgroves seem to enhance tissue stability of the biologic width.[84–86]
10 Prosthetic restoration. Screw-retained restorations or avoiding excess cement with cemented restorations are a consideration,[87,88] especially with anterior restorations, where a deeper interdental col and/or high gingival scalloped anatomy[33] may increase the risk of subgingival cement retention.[72,87,88]

Procedures with single-rooted teeth

Flapless procedures are indicated for intact maxillary anterior extraction sites with moderate labial bone thickness after atraumatic tooth removal. The advantage of a flapless approach is in minimizing facial bone resorption by preservation of the periosteal blood supply. Figure 18.10a–c demonstrates a patient with caries affecting the maxillary canine teeth after an extended provisional phase. Panoramic and CBCT cross-sectional images also demonstrated atypical anatomic findings with thin facial bone and root apices perforating the alveolus (Figure 18.10e and f). After extraction, site evaluation was completed with a periodontal probe, including assessment of tissue thickness (Figure 18.10g). Moderate vertical bony defects of less than one-third of the mesio-distal dimension may be managed with this approach provided that an adequate facial gap dimension (>2–3 mm) will remain for grafting. Implant placement requires obtaining adequate apical initial drill purchase, proper 3-D orientation following sequential site enlargement and the use of a tapered implant design. 3-D positioning typically offers the greatest challenges with immediate placement. Correct positioning of the implant osteotomy at an internally sloped extraction defect and maintaining this orientation while drilling with increasing diameter drills can cause drill chatter and slippage or prevent apical purchase at implant insertion. Implant position in the site shown in Figure 18.10h was mid-cingulum toward the incisal due to an alveolar undercut. Implant placement can be seen on the post-operative low-dose cross-sectional CBCT images (Figure 18.10j and k). After 4 months, the patient was restored and the definitive restorations with preservation of the soft tissue contours are seen in Figure 18.10l and m. Follow-up after 6 years with stable bone and soft tissue contours can be seen in the clinical and panoramic radiographic images in Figure 18.10n and o.

Limited exposure and grafting of partial defects with otherwise intact bony walls is common; for example, with the buccal defect displayed in Figure 18.11a. Alternately, a vestibular semi-lunar or vertical access incision can be used to manage fenestration defects at the time of immediate implant placement to preserve the crestal soft tissue and periosteum. Bone grafting of the dehiscence is completed with GBR principles (Figure 18.11b and c; see complete case in Figure 18.14). Open flap procedures can allow greater visibility, but typically will result in greater bone resorption and remodeling because of the interruption of the periosteal blood supply. When a flap is elevated, strong consideration should be given to buccal augmentation or "esthetic contour" grafting. Open flap exposure for management of smaller buccal wall defects can be combined with GBR as a single or staged procedure or with primary closure and submerged healing. Patients with more challenging extractions and/or a greater bone wall defect (especially if the defect involves the interproximal region) should be managed with a staged procedure using GBR and delayed implant placement.

Simultaneous soft tissue augmentation using autogenous connective tissue, vascular pedicle flaps, or porcine dermal matrix grafting material can be considered for patients with thin gingival biotype at esthetic zone sites or with excessive gingival display (a high smile line). This will reduce the risk of recession or translucency of implant components through the thin tissue. Using palatal tissue in a free or vascular pedicle design will allow an increase in tissue volume for graft containment and increase the zone of

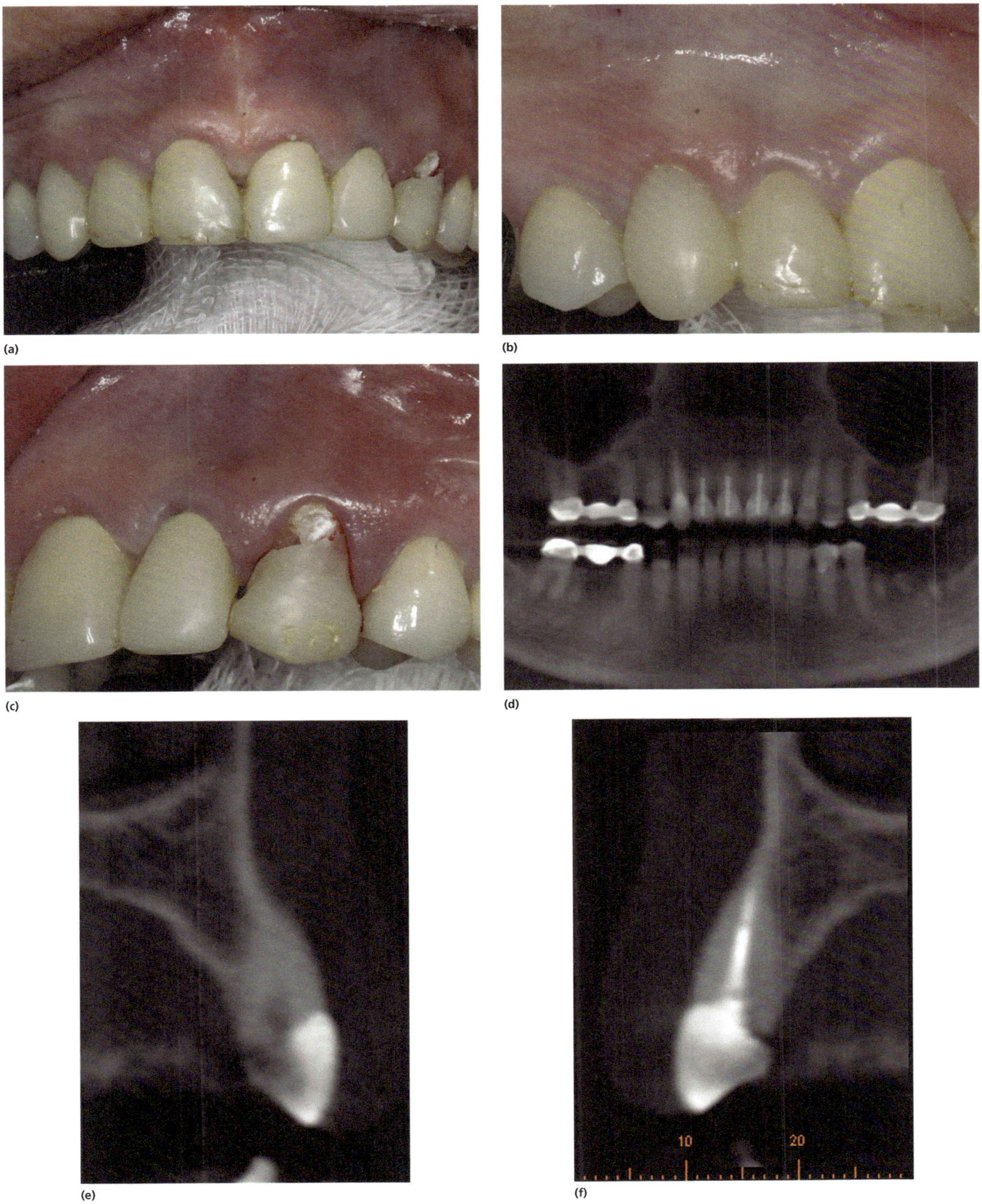

Figure 18.10 Flapless single-stage implants (anterior maxilla). (a–c) After an extended provisional phase, the patient presented with caries involving the maxillary canine teeth and failing anterior maxillary provisional restorations. (d–f) Panoramic and CBCT cross-sectional images demonstrated anatomic finding with thin facial bone and the root apices at or perforating the undercut of the alveolus. *(Continued)*

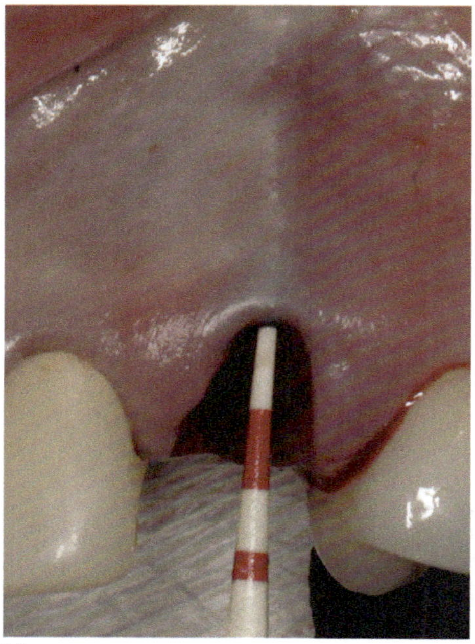

(g)

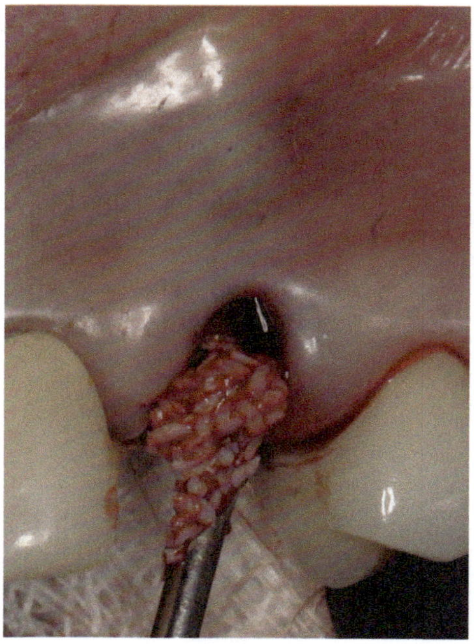

(h)

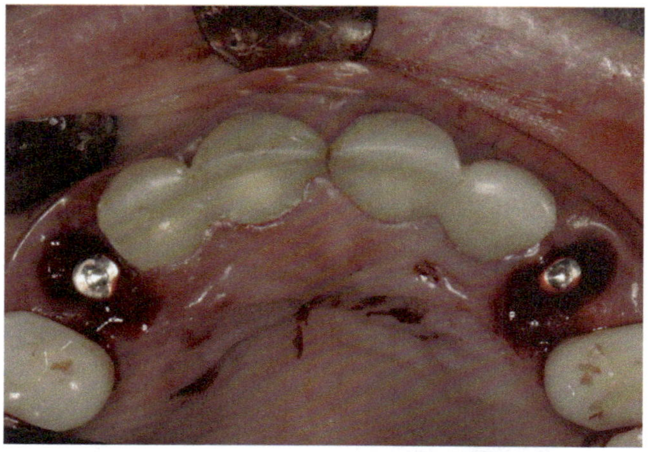

(i)

Figure 18.10 (Continued)

(g) Extraction site evaluation is completed and the soft tissue thickness is assessed with a periodontal probe. (h) Implant placement required obtaining adequate apical initial drill purchase, proper 3-D orientation following sequential site enlargement, and an adequate facial bone volume/facial gap dimension (>2–3 mm) for grafting. After grafting, the crestal soft tissue void can be filled with collagen or connective tissue. (i) Implant positioning with healing caps in place. Position is mid-cingulum toward the incisal due to the challenge of the alvelolar undercut. (j, k) CBCT immediate post-operative cross-sectional images demonstrate adequate palatal position, facial gap/graft, and implant angulation.

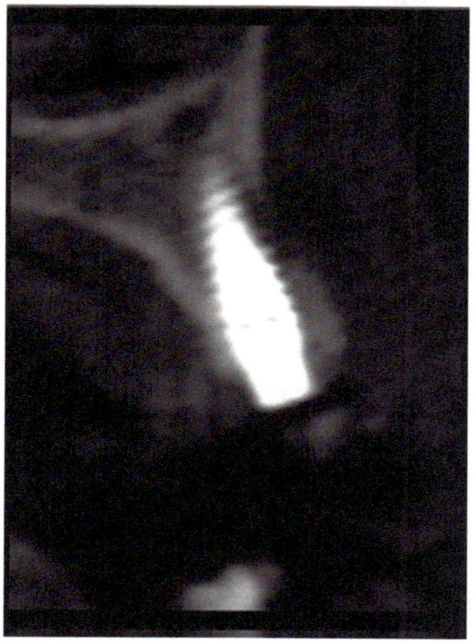

(j)

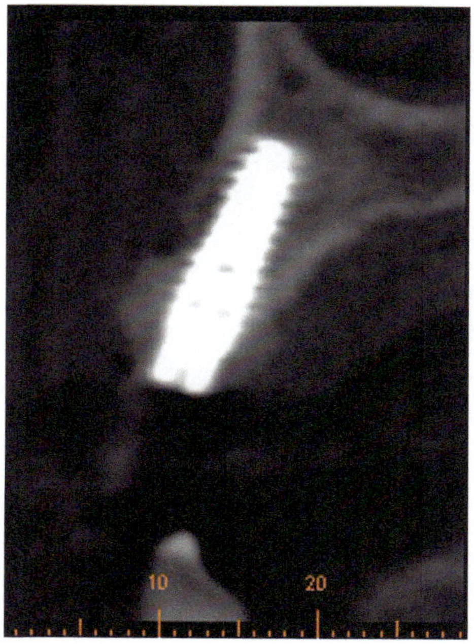

(k)

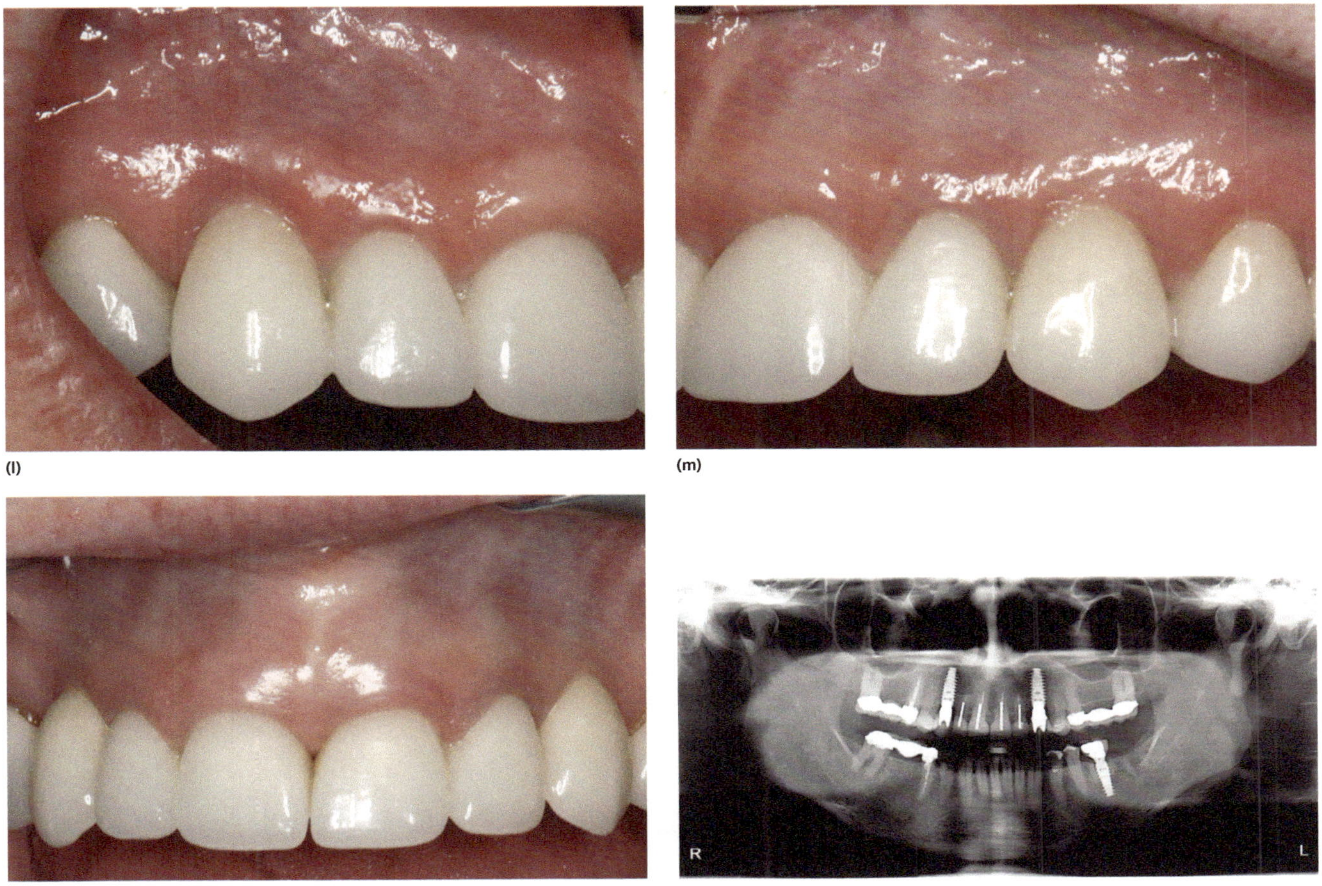

(n) (o)

Figure 18.10 (Continued)
(l, m) After 4 months' healing the patient was restored, and clinical images of the definitive restorations show excellent bone and soft tissue contours. (n, o) Follow-up clinical and panoramic radiographic images after 6 years demonstrate stable bone and soft tissue contours. (a–o) © Daniel R. Cullum.

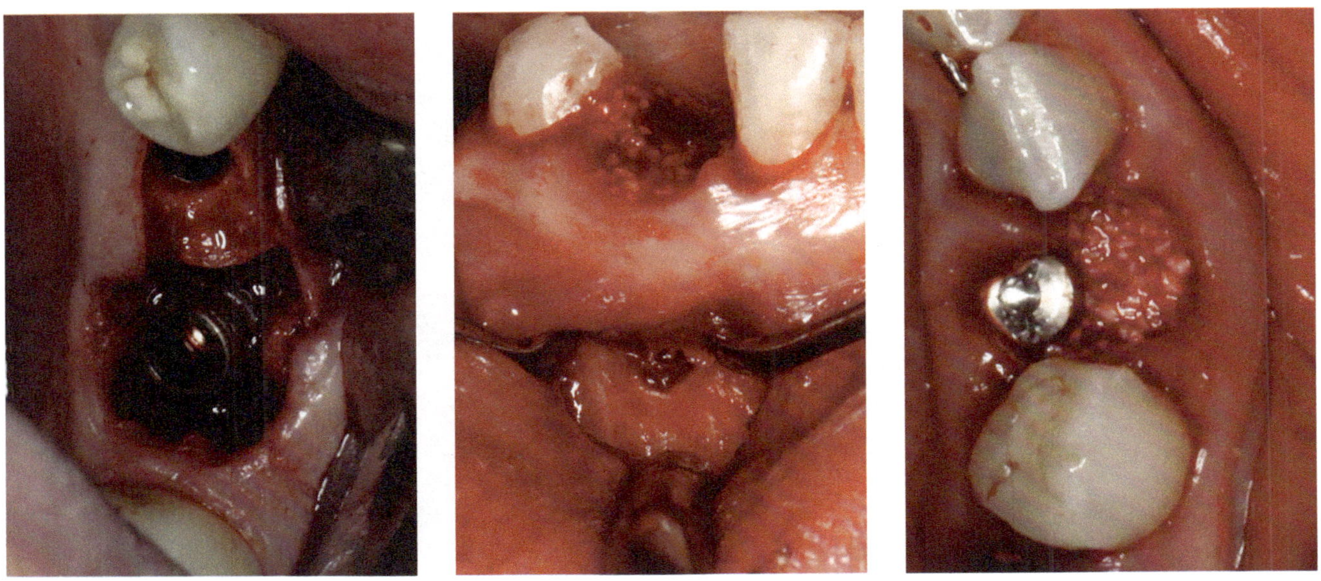

(a) (b) (c)

Figure 18.11 (a) Limited flap exposure demonstrating a buccal defect at a mandibular first molar site. (b, c) A mandibular canine site shows a limited vertical incision with tunnel vestibular access can be used with a fenestration defect for access and GBR, while preserving the crestal soft tissue and periosteum for particulate gap grafting. (a–c) © Daniel R. Cullum.

marginal keratinized tissue. Figure 18.12a and b shows a patient after extraction of the maxillary right first premolar, canine, and lateral incisor teeth. Immediate implants were placed in the premolar and canine positions and grafting done with particulate xenograft at the bone gaps and socket of the lateral incisor. On the facial view (Figure 18.12b), the greater portion of a 5 mm tall healing abutment is visualized with a reduced tissue volume and deficient coronal height. Connective tissue was harvested from the maxillary tuberosity and a split-thickness tunnel developed on the facial aspect to allow graft insertion and stabilization using 6-0 nylon horizontal mattress sutures (Figure 18.12c–e). The connective tissue graft can be seen augmenting the vertical and horizontal soft tissue dimension after an additional "figure-of-eight" suture and modified BioCol treatment of the adjacent sites (Figure 18.12f and g). The soft tissue contours and minimal inflammation typical of this type of minimally invasive procedure can be seen after 12 days in Figure 18.12h and i.

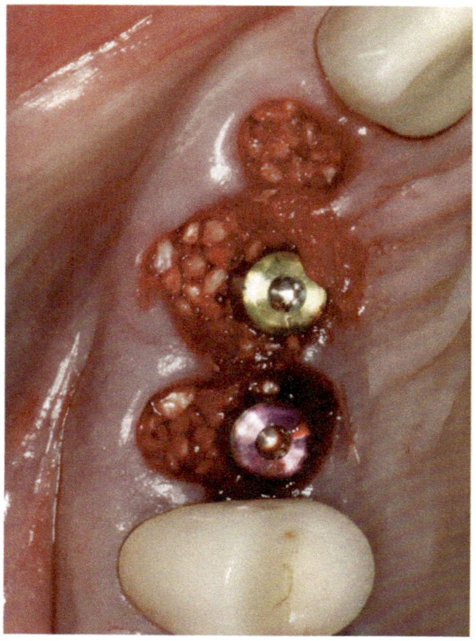
(a)

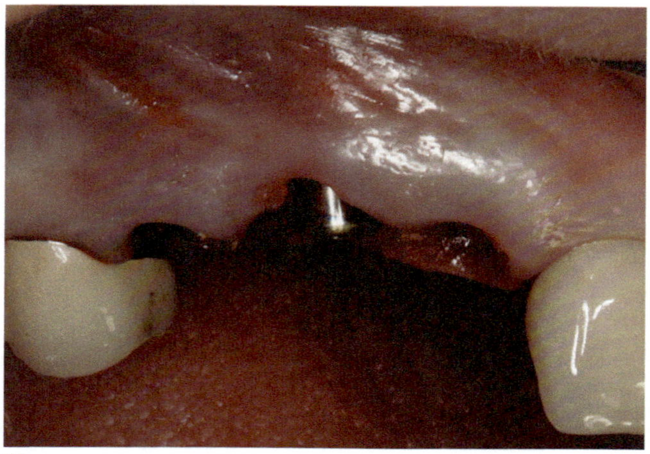
(b)

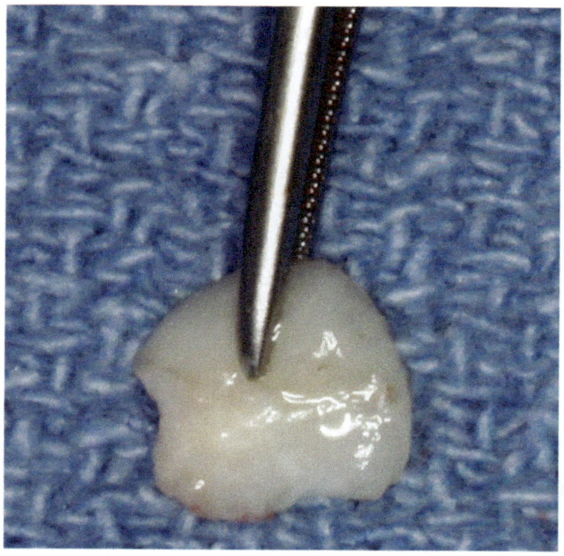
(c)

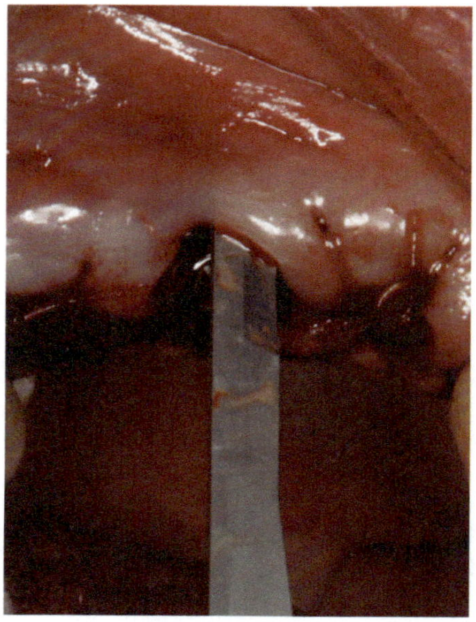
(d)

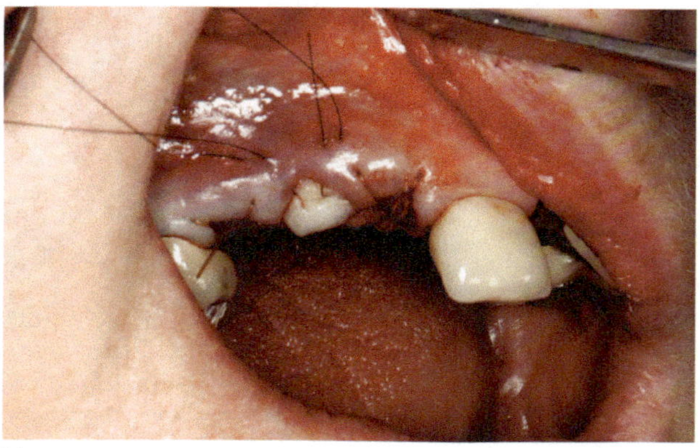
(e)

Figure 18.12 Immediate implant with simultaneous soft tissue enhancement. (a) Immediate implants have been placed in the right maxillary premolar and canine positions with particulate xenograft placed at the bone gaps and socket of the adjacent lateral incisor. (b) On facial view the greater portion of a 5 mm tall healing cap is visualized with a reduced tissue volume and deficient coronal height. (c) Connective tissue was harvested from the maxillary tuberosity. (d) A split-thickness tunnel was developed on the facial aspect of the canine site. (e) The connective tissue graft insertion was completed using 6-0 nylon horizontal mattress sutures for positioning.

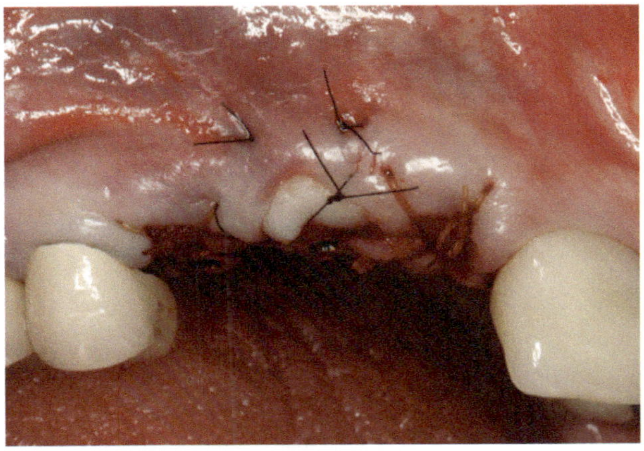

(f)

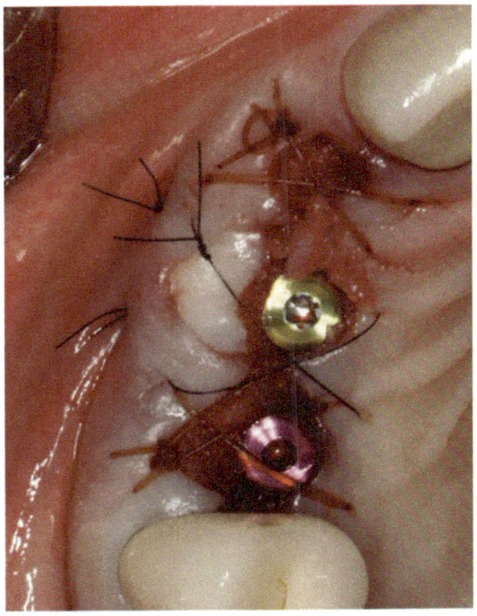

(g)

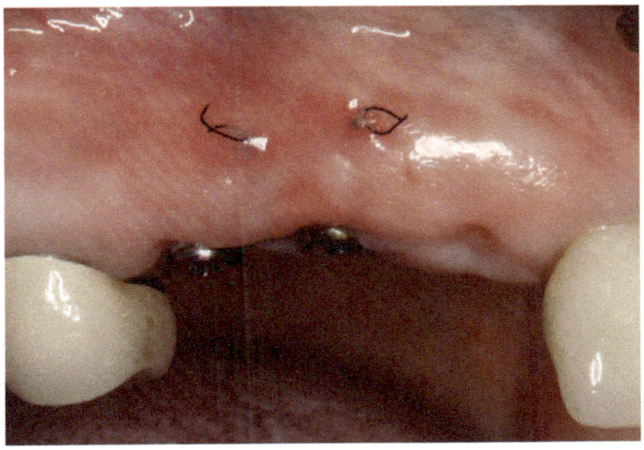

(h)

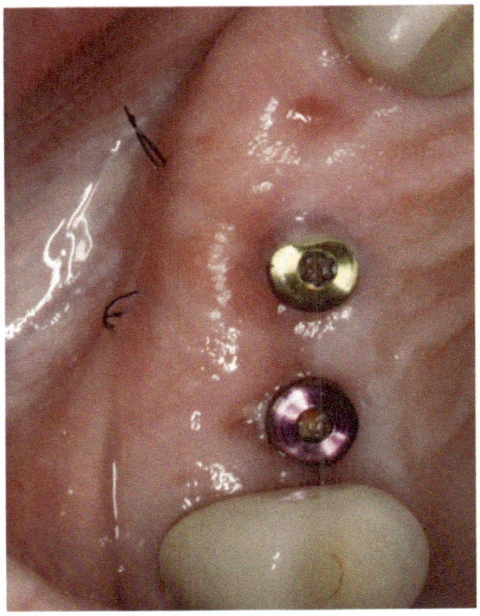

(i)

Figure 18.12 (Continued)
(f, g) The CT graft in position after an additional "figure-of-eight" suture, augmenting the vertical and horizontal soft tissue dimension. Modified BioCol® treatment of the adjacent sites was also completed. (h, i) After 12 days, soft tissue contours and minimal inflammation are seen typical of this type of minimally invasive procedure. (a–i) © Daniel R. Cullum.

Immediate procedures for multi-rooted teeth

Mandibular molars

Immediate management of mandibular molars is a predictable treatment requiring adequate interfurcal bone height above the inferior alveolar nerve and a tapered implant macrodesign with adequate apical thread engagement. Figure 18.13a and b shows a patient who presented with symptomatic apical involvement of the mandibular right canine and first and second molar teeth. CBCT analysis confirmed apical pathology but anatomic suitability for immediate implant placement (Figure 18.13c–f). The patient declined endodontic treatment for philosophical reasons and requested immediate implant therapy. After molar extraction and site debridement, the interfurcal bone was removed with Piezosurgery to obtain an adequate bone plateau for a 2 mm drill purchase. The osteotomy sites were developed with periapical radiographic guidance and copious irrigation (Figure 18.13g and h) to a drill diameter one size smaller than the planned implant. The implants were initially inserted slightly short of the intended depth and seated fully only after length confirmation on radiograph (Figure 18.13i). With an anatomic lingual to buccal ridge slope, often implants placed level with the buccal bone can end up submerged as much as 5 mm below the lingual soft tissue margin. Ideally, the implant should be placed toward the lingual aspect of the socket and result in a large buccal gap of 3–5 mm (Figure 18.13i). Using this approach, adequate primary stability can be attained with implant stability quotient readings in the 60–70 range. If necessary to allow complete seating of a flared healing abutment, the lingual and interproximal bone levels can be contoured to within 1 mm height of the implant platform. The buccal bone gap should be packed with a mineralized particulate graft (Figure 18.13j). Any crestal soft tissue defect can be sealed with dense collagen saturated with the patient's blood, rhPDGF, or a connective tissue graft shaped to the gap dimensions and secured with a "figure-of-eight" chromic suture (Figure 18.13k and l). With this open grafting technique it is recommended that the site be covered with a protective

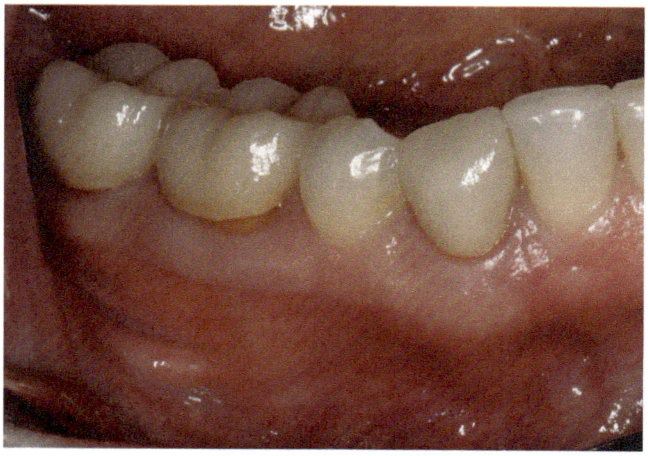

(a)

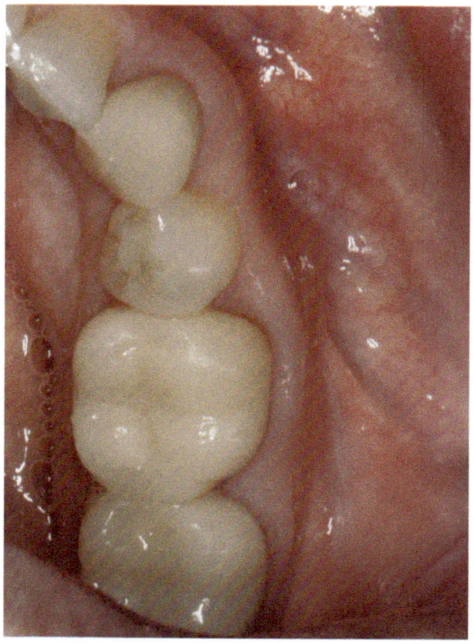

(b)

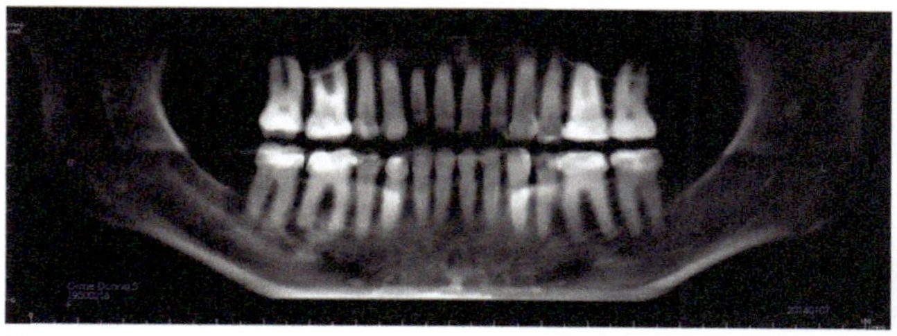

(c)

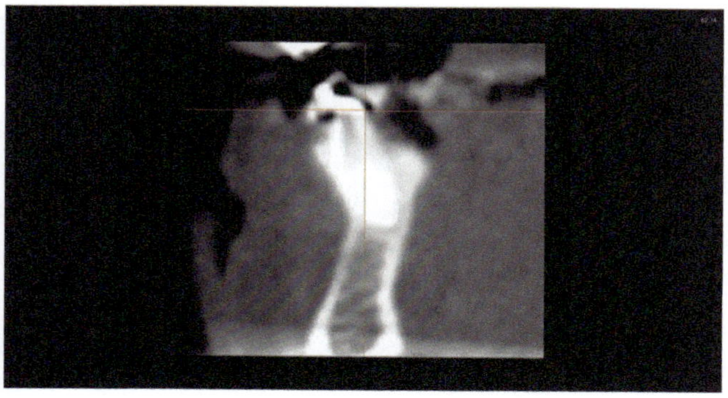

(d)

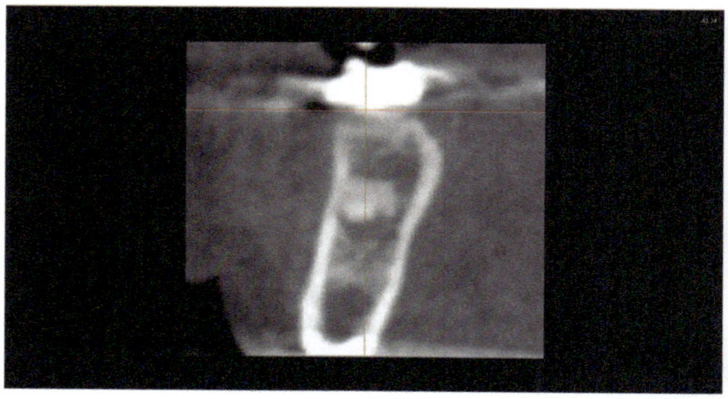

(e)

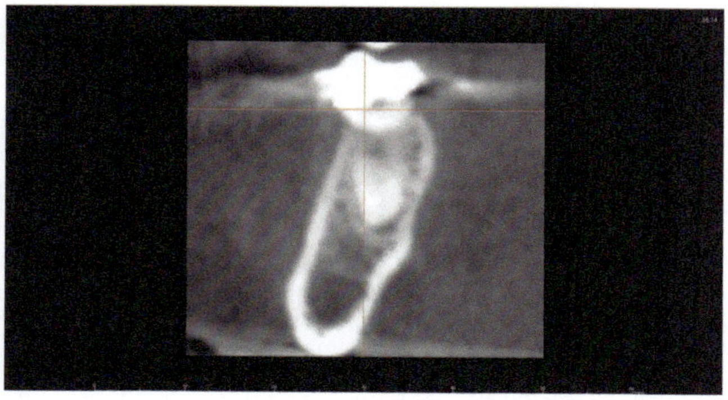

(f)

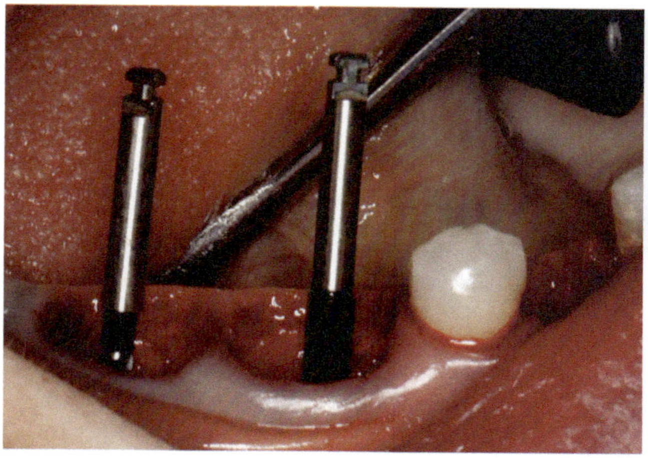

(g)

Figure 18.13 (a, b) A patient presented with symptomatic apical involvement of the right canine and first and second molar teeth and declined endodontic treatment. (c–f) CBCT analysis confirmed the apical pathology and necessary anatomic requirements for immediate implant placement. (g, h) After a 2 mm drill purchase, the osteotomy sites were developed with periapical radiographic guidance.

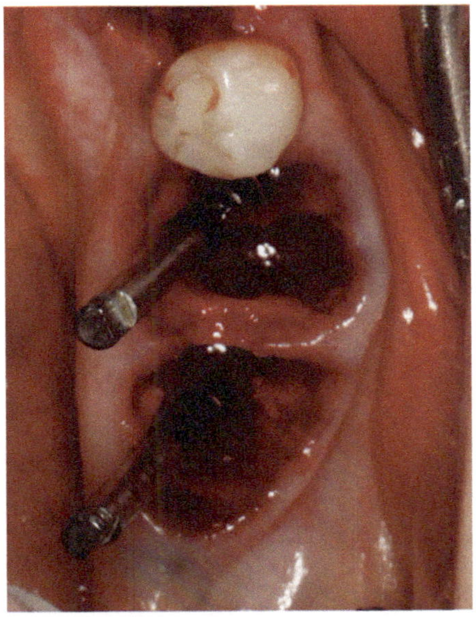

(h)

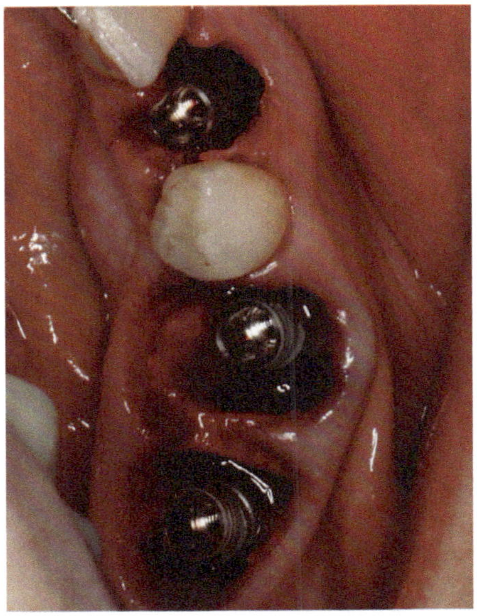

(i)

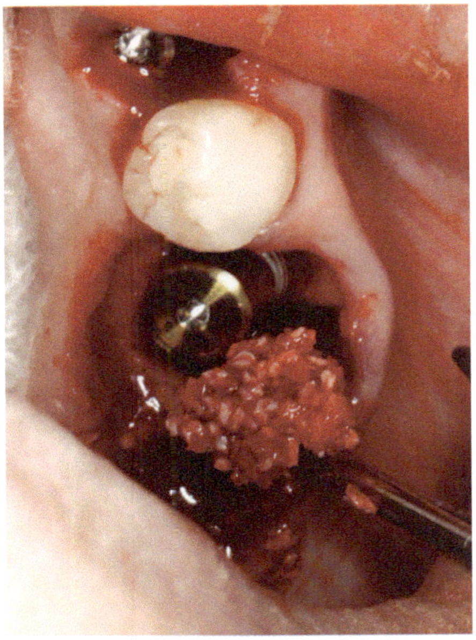

(j)

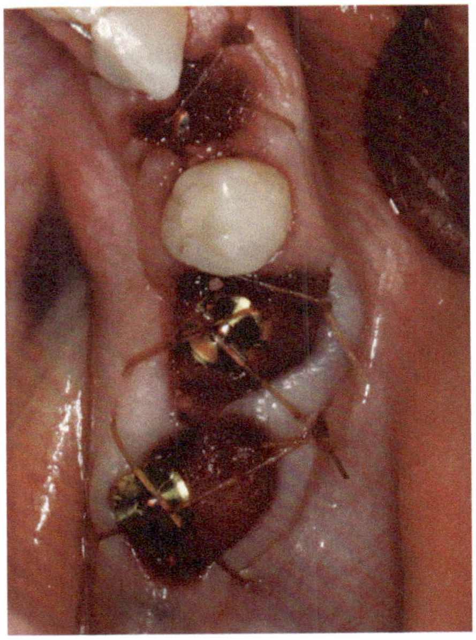

(k)

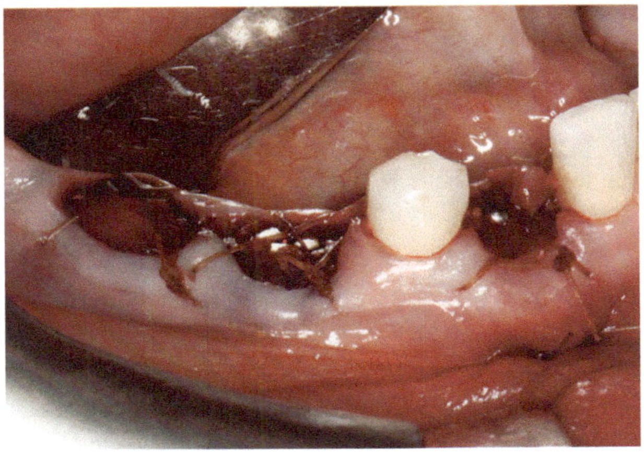

(l)

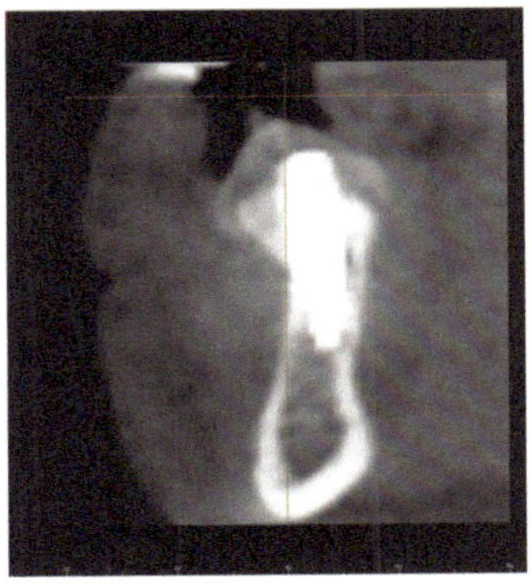

(m)

Figure 18.13 (Continued)

(i) The 5.0 mm diameter implants (Noble Active®, Nobel Biocare, Yorba Linda, CA) were placed in the inter-radicular bone of the molar sites and a 4.3 mm diameter implant at the canine. The implants should be placed toward the lingual aspect of the socket and level with the intact buccal bone plate. (j) The buccal bone gap was packed with a mineralized particulate graft. (k, l) The crestal soft tissue defect was sealed with dense collagen saturated with the patient's blood and secured with a "figure-of-eight" chromic suture. (m, o) Post-operative cross-sectional CBCT images demonstrate implant positioning, and in (n), a common challenge with immediate placement. The implant preparation and seating was displaced by the dense lingual bone plate. The site maintained an intact buccal apical wall and good crestal buccal dimension that was grafted as shown in (j). *(Continued)*

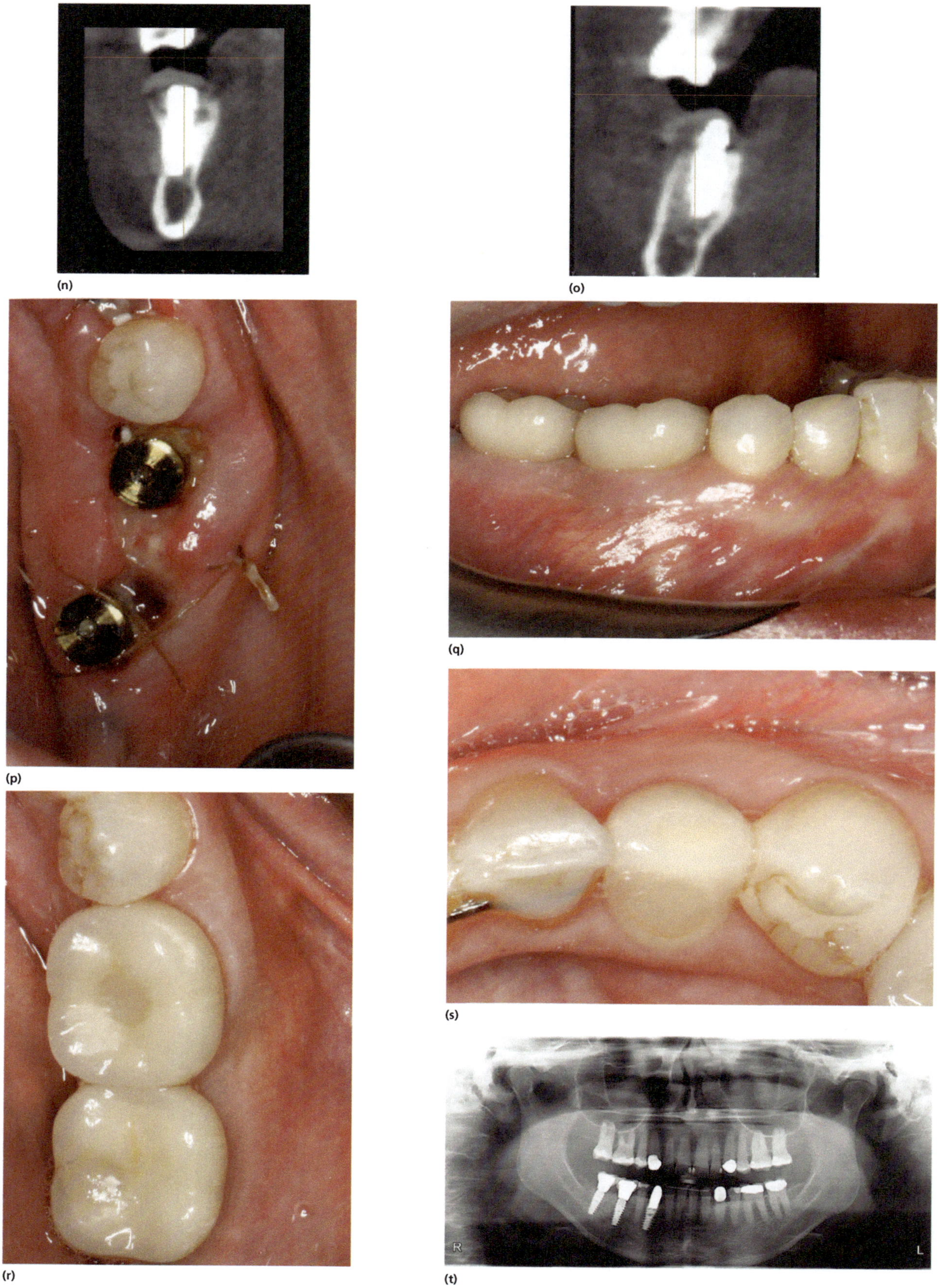

Figure 18.13 (Continued)
(p) On removal of the dressing after 10 days, the site shows fibrin formation and early wound healing with minimal inflammation. (q–s) Six months after surgery the final restorations and radiograph are seen demonstrating excellent bone and soft tissue contours. (a–t) © Daniel R. Cullum.

periodontal dressing (Barricaid). Figure 18.13n demonstrates a common challenge with immediate placement. The implant preparation and seating was displaced by the dense lingual bone plate. The site maintained an intact buccal apical wall and good crestal buccal dimension that was grafted as shown in figure 18.13j. Postoperative cross-sectional CBCT images demonstrate the three implants in the canine, first molar, and second molar sites (Figures 18.13m–o). On removal of the dressing after 10 days, the site showed fibrin formation and early wound healing with minimal inflammation (Figure 18.13p). Six months after surgery, the final restorations and radiograph demonstrating excellent bone and soft tissue contours can be seen in Figure 18.13q–s.

Maxillary molars and trans-alveolar sinus elevation

In the posterior maxilla with minimal vertical alveolar height, a 10 mm × 5.0 mm diameter or 8 mm × 5.5 mm (or greater) diameter implant can be placed in the inter-radicular region biased toward the palatal. However, a failing maxillary molar is often associated with significant sinus pneumatization. Immediate implant placement in these situations often can be managed with elevation of the bone using osteotome sinus floor elevation (OSFE), bone-added osteotome sinus floor elevation (BAOSFE), or contiguous sinus floor elevation (CSFE) techniques[49] (see Chapter 15) (Figure 18.14). After tooth sectioning, extraction, and thorough socket debridement, the inter-radical bone is evaluated. After drill purchase and trial

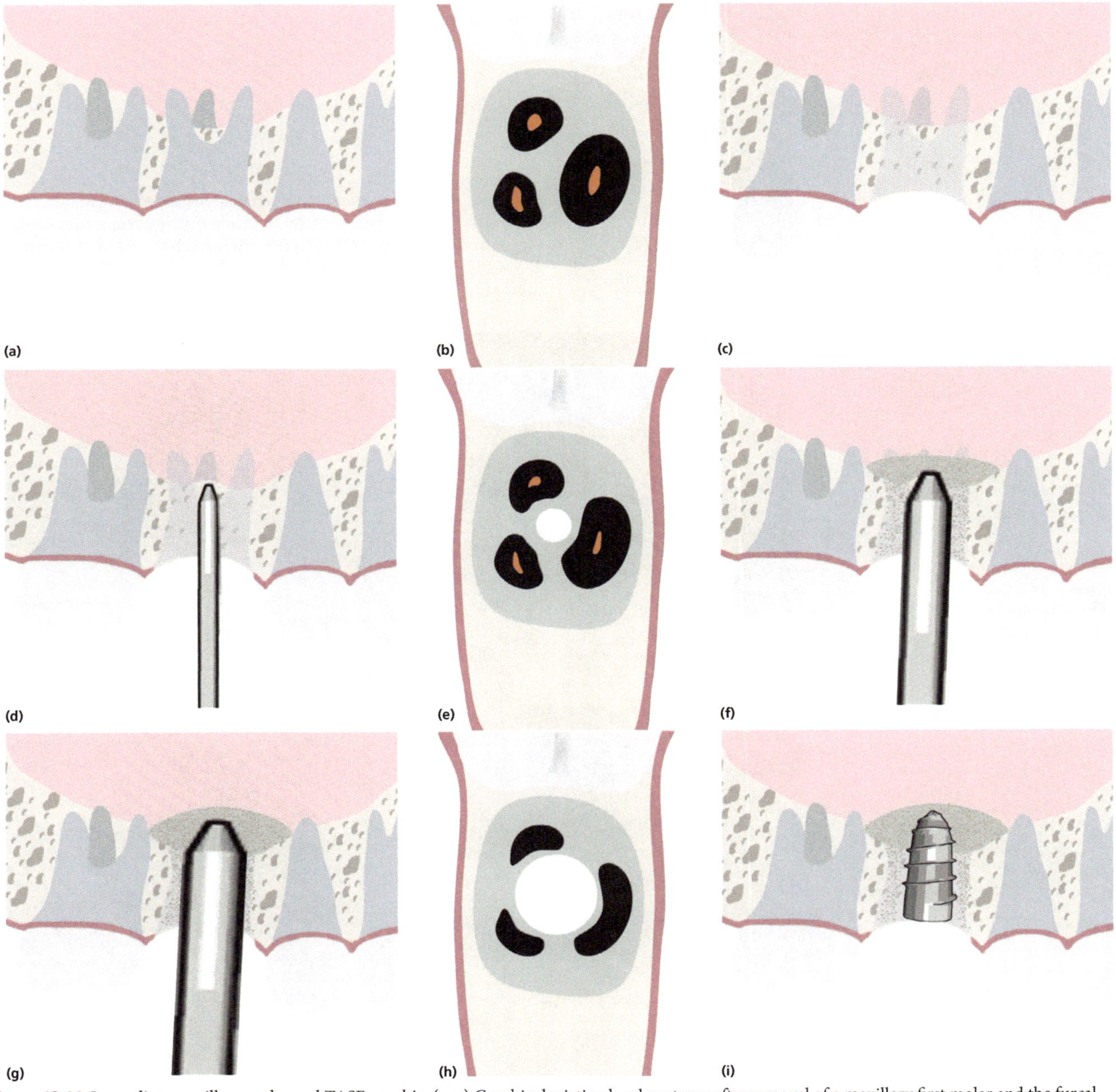

Figure 18.14 Immediate maxillary molar and TASE graphic. (a–c) Graphic depicting local anatomy after removal of a maxillary first molar and the furcal plateau of bone. (d, e) A 2 mm drill or osteotome (less dense bone) is used to complete initial site evaluation and trial length determination. (f–h) Osteotomes are used here demonstrating progressive addition of particulate graft for BAOSFE to the anticipated implant height with manipulation of the bone into the palatal edge of the socket. (i) Final implant insertion is completed with grafting of the implant crestal bone gap. (a–i) © Daniel R. Cullum.

length determination, the osteotomy can be enlarged and elevated using osteotomes (Figure 18.14d–h). The surgeon must take care to develop the osteotomy to the desired final implant position toward the palatal. With adequate vertical ridge dimension, simultaneous insertion of a tapered implant can be completed with good primary stability (Figure 18.14i).

A clinical example of this procedure after removal of the left maxillary first molar is shown in Figure 18.15. Preoperative CBCT diagnosis demonstrated the presence of a furcal bone plateau with a height of 3–4 mm and divergent roots, a scenario expected to give a good prognosis for this combined minimally invasive approach (Figure 18.15a and b). If the inter-radicular bone is less than 3 mm in width on evaluation, vertical height reduction can be completed with a rongeur for adequate width to allow a 2 mm drill purchase. A trial length radiograph is completed with a 2 mm drill or, in soft bone, a concave cutting osteotome tip *in situ*. The osteotomy "footprint" is

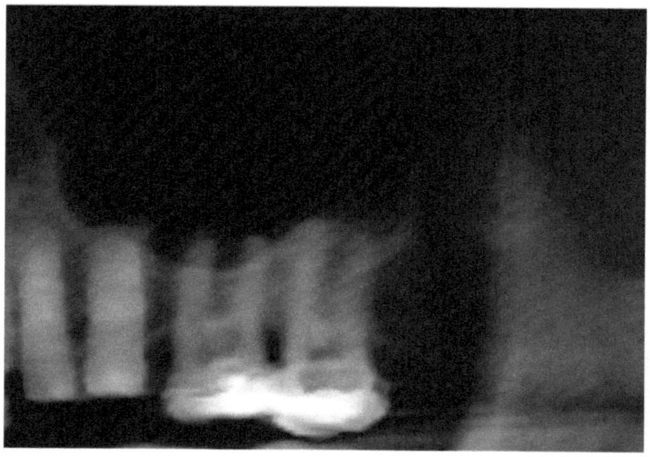

(a)

Figure 18.15 (a, b) Preoperative representation of moderate sinus pneumatization into the first molar furcation region. Preoperative CBCT diagnosis demonstrating the presence of a furcal bone plateau with a height of 3–4 mm and divergent roots gives a good prognosis for this combined minimally invasive approach.

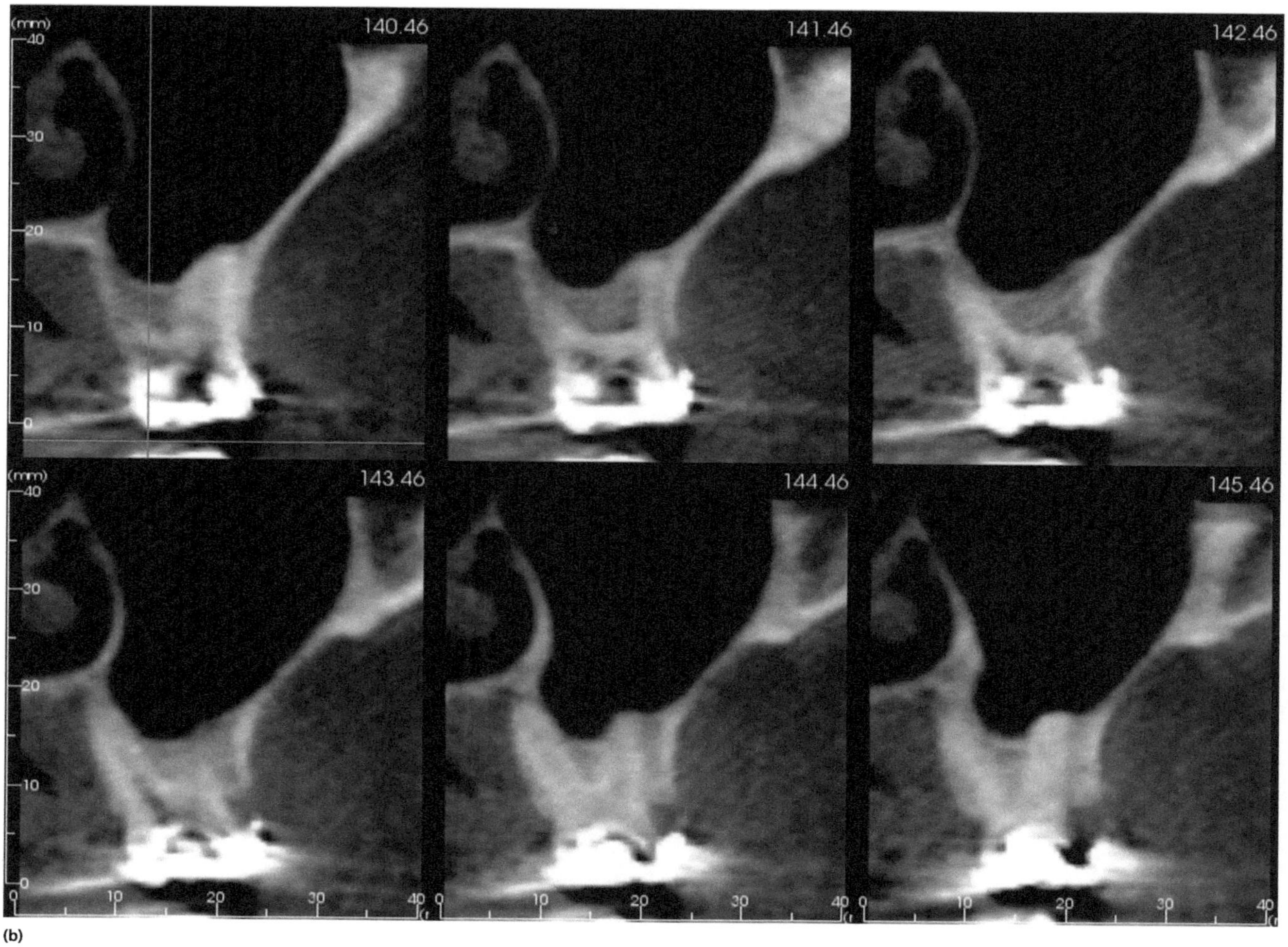

(b)

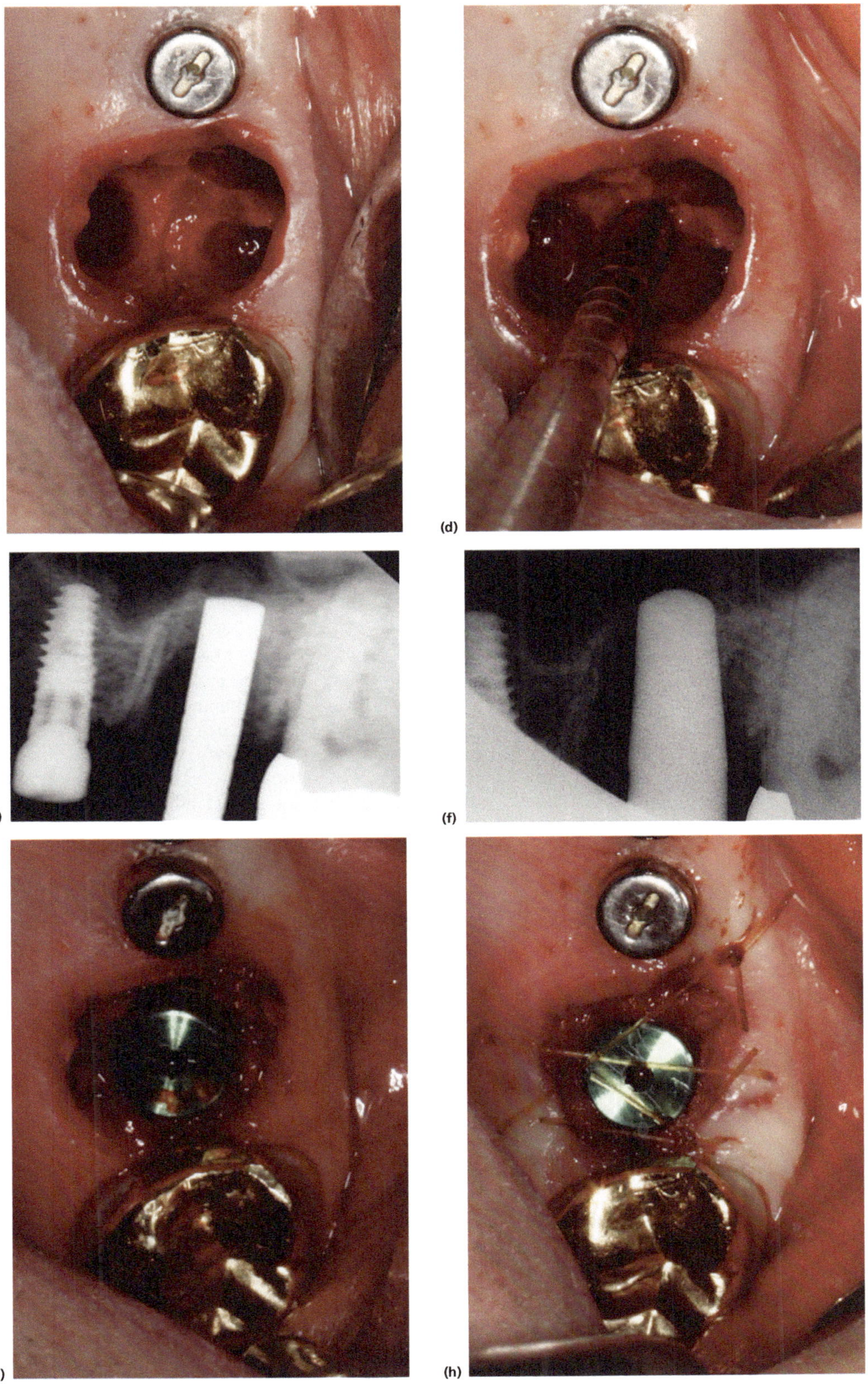

(c) (d) (e) (f) (g) (h)

Figure 18.15 (Continued)
(c) After tooth extraction and thorough socket debridement the furcal region was assessed to be too narrow and removed with a rongeur to gain adequate width to allow a 2 mm drill purchase. (d, e) A trial length radiograph was completed with the 2 mm drill and the osteotomy enlarged and elevated using concave cutting-tipped osteotomes to a diameter of 4 mm with added particulate graft as a BAOSFE procedure. (f) For continued BAOSFE 5 and 6 mm diameter tapered osteotomes were used to mobilize the sinus floor and membrane to final elevation at 11 mm. (g) Placement of a 6.0 mm × 10 mm length tapered implant (Nobel Replace®, Nobel Biocare, Yorba Linda, CA) was completed with a healing cap The crestal bone gap was grafted with moderate packing of the graft material to the surrounding bone crest height. (h) The crestal soft tissue gap was sealed with collagen and secured with a "figure-of-eight" suture and covered with periodontal dressing. *(Continued)*

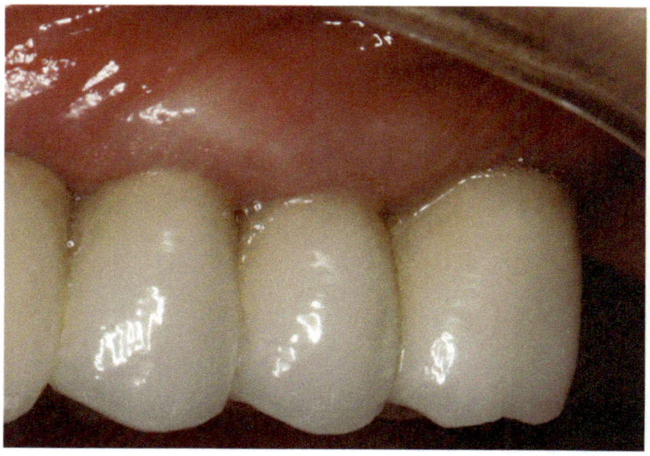

(i)

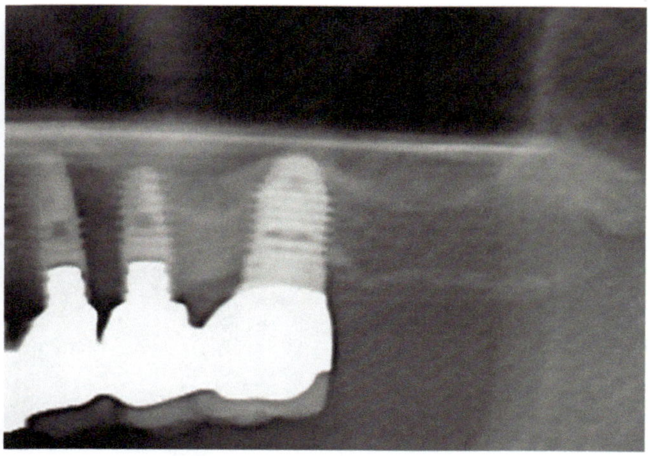

(j)

Figure 18.15 (Continued)
(i) Final implant-supported restoration can be seen clinically after 3 years. (j) Radiograph of restoration showing bone heights after more than 4 years. The original sinus floor cortical bone is still visible, along with the vertical augmented bone above the apex. (a–j) © Daniel R. Cullum.

enlarged using increasing diameter osteotomes re-inserted to the trial length with added particulate graft material (Figure 18.15d and e). Tapered osteotomes of 5 and 6 mm diameters and further additions of graft material can be used to finish site development and mobilize the sinus floor/membrane aiming for a final elevation slightly greater than the final planned implant length (Figure 18.15f). Placement of a 6.0 mm × 10 mm length tapered implant was completed, followed by addition of a healing abutment. The remaining implant bone gaps around the extraction socket were packed using moderate pressure with any harvested autogenous bone mixed with mineralized allogenic or xenograft material (Figure 18.15g). The crestal soft tissue defect can then be sealed with dense collagen saturated with heme or rhPDGF as a modified BioCol technique, and stabilized with a "figure-of-eight" chromic suture (Figure 18.15h). The site was protected with light-cured Barricaid periodontal dressing. Figure 18.15i and j demonstrate the final restoration clinically after 3 years and radiographically after more than 4 years. The original sinus cortical floor is still visible, blending with the vertical augmented bone above the apex.

Conclusions

Placing immediate implants is an efficient, minimally-invasive and evidence-based treatment option to offer patients. There are significant clinical demands on the surgeon, including considerations of suitable implant design, implant positioning, and grafting. A "flapless" approach can preserve the alveolar blood supply and help maintain soft tissue and bone levels when combined with palatal implant positioning, facial bone gap grafting and screw-retained restorations. A key factor in any immediate site development is ensuring that the buccal bone thickness remains around 2 mm or that an adequate buccal gap remains for grafting with a slow-resorbing particulate material. Failing to fulfill these requirements will almost invariably lead to buccal bone loss, soft tissue recession and exposure of implant components. Implant positioning also must allow for a proper emergence profile for provisional and final restorations to achieve optimal esthetics and function and to avoid food impaction. Molar sites often are not addressed in this fashion, and can result in maintenance challenges. Larger diameter implants can be useful in molar sites by offering greater surface contact with bone and better emergence profiles, but must not be so large in diameter as to obliterate the necessary buccal gap and prevent its required grafting. Whether standard or wide-diameter implants are planned, they must obtain adequate primary stability apically in virgin bone and/or by contact with the lingual/palatal bone plates. Maxillary molars often require simultaneous TASE procedures, which can be completed with high predictability. Clinical application of immediate implant therapy offers both clinicians and patients rewarding and gratifying minimally invasive treatment options.

References

1. Schulte W, Kleinekenscheidt H, Lindner K, et al. The Tübingen immediate implant in clinical studies. Dtsch Zahnarztl Z 1978; 33: 348–359 (in German).
2. Barzilay I, Graser G, Iranpour B, Proskin H. Immediate implantation of pure titanium implants into extraction sockets of *Macaca fascicularis*. Part I: clinical and radiographic assessment. Int J Oral Maxillofac Implants 1996; 11: 299–310.
3. Gelb D. Immediate implant surgery: three-year retrospective evaluation of 50 consecutive cases. Int J Oral Maxillofac Implants 1993; 8: 388–399.
4. Gomez-Roman G, Kruppenbacher M, Weber H, Schulte W. Immediate post-extraction implant placement with root-analog stepped implants: surgical procedure and statistical outcome after 6 years. Int J Oral Maxillofac Implants 2001; 16: 503–513.
5. Lazzara R. Immediate implant placement into extraction sites: surgical and restorative advantages. Int J Periodontics Restorative Dent 1989; 9: 333–343.
6. Lioubavina-Hack N, Lang N, Karring T. Significance of primary stability for osseointegration of dental implants. Clin Oral Implants Res 2006; 17: 244–250.
7. Chen S, Wilson T, Hammerle C. Immediate or early placement of implants following tooth extraction: review of biologic basis, clinical procedures and outcomes. Int J Oral Maxillofac Implants 2004; 19(Suppl): 12–25.
8. Botticelli D, Berglundh T, Buser D, Lindhe J. The jumping distance revisited. An experimental study in the dog. Clin Oral Implants Res 2003; 14: 35–42.
9. Akimoto K, Becker W, Persson R, et al. Evaluation of titanium implants placed into simulated extraction sockets: a study in dogs. Int J Oral Maxillofac Implants 1999; 14: 351–360.
10. Araujo M, Sukekava F, Wennstrom J, Lindhe J. Ridge alterations following implant placement in fresh extraction sockets: an experimental study in the dog. J Clin Periodontol 2005; 32: 645–652.
11. Araujo M, Sukekvava F, Wennstrom J, Lindhe J. Tissue modeling following implant placement in fresh extraction sockets. Clin Oral Implants Res 2006; 17: 615–624.

12. Abushahba F, Renvert S, Polyzois I, Claffey N. Effect of grafting materials on osseointegration of dental implants surrounded by circumferential bone defects. An experimental study in the dog. Clin Oral Implants Res 2008; 19: 329–334.
13. Araujo M, Linder E, Lindhe J. Bio-Oss® collagen in the buccal gap at immediate implants: a 6-month study in the dog. Clin Oral Implants Res 2011; 22: 1–8.
14. Botticelli D, Berglundh T, Lindhe J. Hard-tissue alterations following immediate implant placement in extraction sites. J Clin Periodontol 2004; 31: 820–828.
15. Le BT, Borzabadi-Farahani A. Simultaneous implant placement and bone grafting with particulate mineralized allograft in sites with buccal wall defects, a three-year follow-up and review of literature. J Craniomaxillofac Surg 2014; 42: 552–559.
16. Caiazzo A, Brugnami F, Mehra P. Buccal plate preservation with immediate post-extraction implant placement and provisionalization: preliminary results of a new technique. Int J Oral Maxillofac Surg 2013; 42: 666–670.
17. Yoshino S, Kan J, Rungcharassaeng K, et al. Effects of connective tissue grafting on the facial gingival level following single immediate implant placement and provisionalization in the esthetic zone: a 1-year randomized controlled prospective study. Int J Oral Maxillofac Implants 2014; 29(2): 432–440.
18. Small P, Tarnow D. Gingival recession around implants: a 1-year longitudinal prospective study. Int J Oral Maxillofac Implants 2000; 15: 527–532.
19. Becker W, Becker B. Guided tissue regeneration for implants placed into extraction sockets and for dehiscences: surgical techniques and case reports. Int J Periodontics Restorative Dent 1990; 10: 376–391.
20. Nyman S, Lang N, Buser D, Bragger U. Bone regeneration adjacent to titanium dental implants using guided tissue regeneration: a report of two cases. Int J Oral Maxillofac Implants 1990; 5: 9–14.
21. Wilson T. Guided tissue regeneration around dental implants in immediate and recent extraction sites: initial observations. Int J Periodontics Restorative Dent 1992; 12: 185–193.
22. Lang N, Bragger U, Hammerle C, Sutter F. Immediate transmucosal implants using the principle of guided tissue regeneration. I. Rationale, clinical procedures and 30-month results. Clin Oral Implants Res 1994; 5: 154–163.
23. Hammerle C, Bragger U, Schmid B, Lang N. Successful bone formation at immediate transmucosal implants: a clinical report. Int J Oral Maxillofac Implants 1998; 13: 522–530.
24. Lang N, Tonetti M, Suvan J, et al. Immediate implant placement with transmucosal healing in areas of aesthetic priority. A multicenter randomized-controlled clinical trial. I. Surgical outcomes. Clin Oral Implants Res 2007; 18: 188–196.
25. Ferrus J, Cecchinato D, Pjetursson E, et al. Factors influencing ridge alterations following immediate implant placement into extraction sockets. Clin Oral Implants Res 2010; 21: 22–29.
26. Schnitman P, Wöhrle P, Rubenstein J. Immediate fixed interim prostheses supported by two-stage threaded implants: methodology and results. J Oral Implantol 1990; 16: 96–105.
27. Covani U, Cornelini R, Barone A. Buccal bone augmentation around immediate implants with and without flap elevation: a modified approach. Int J Oral Maxillofac Implants 2008; 23: 841–846.
28. Wöhrle P. Single-tooth replacement in the aesthetic zone with immediate provisionalization: fourteen consecutive cases report. Pract Periodontics Aesthet Dent 1998; 10: 1107–1114.
29. De Carvalho B, de Carvalho E, Consani R. Flapless single-tooth immediate implant placement. Int J Oral Maxillofac Implants 2013; 28: 783–789.
30. Caneva M, Salata L, de Souza S et al. Influence of implant positioning in extraction sockets on osseointegration: histomorphometric analyses in dogs. Clin Oral Implants Res 2010; 21: 43–49.
31. Huynh-Ba G, Pjetursson B, Sanz M, et al. Analysis of the socket wall dimensions in the upper maxilla in relation to immediate implant placement. Clin Oral Implants Res 2010; 21: 37–42.
32. Benic G, Mokti M, Chen C, et al. Dimensions of buccal bone and mucosa at immediately placed implants after 7 years: a clinical and cone beam computed tomography study. Clin Oral Implants Res 2012; 23: 560–566.
33. Kois J. Predictable single tooth peri-implant esthetics. Five diagnostic keys. Compend Contin Educ Dent 2001; 22: 199–208.
34. Grunder U. Crestal ridge width changes when placing implants at the time of tooth extraction with and without soft tissue augmentation after a healing period of 6 months: report of 24 consecutive cases. Int J Periodontics Restorative Dent 2011; 31: 9–17.
35. Chen S, Buser D. Esthetic complications due to implant malpositions: etiology, prevention and treatment. In: Dental Implant Complications: Etiology, Prevention and Treatment, FroumS, ed. Ames, IA: Wiley-Blackwell, 2010, chapter 8, pp. 134–155.
36. Rungcharassaeng K, Kan J, Yoshino S, et al. Immediate implant placement and provisionalization with and without a connective tissue graft: an analysis of facial gingival tissue thickness. Int J Periodontics Restorative Dent 2012; 32: 657–663.
37. Froum S, Casanova L, Byrne S, Cho S. Risk assessment before extraction for immediate implant placement in the posterior mandible: a computerized tomographic scan study. J Periodontol 2011; 82: 395–402.
38. Atieh M, Payne A, Duncan W, et al. Immediate placement or immediate restoration/loading of single implants for molar replacement: a systematic review and meta-analysis. Int J Oral Maxillofac Implants 2010; 25: 401–415.
39. Deng F, Zhang H, Zhang H, et al. A comparison of clinical outcomes for implants placed in fresh extraction sockets versus healed sites in periodontally compromised patients: a 1-year follow-up report. Int J Oral Maxillofac Implants 2010; 25: 1036–1040.
40. Urban T, Kostopoulos L, Wenzel A. Immediate implant placement in molar regions: risk factors for early failure. Clin Oral Implants Res 2012; 23: 220–227.
41. Greenstein G, Cavallaro J, Tarnow D. Practical application of anatomy for the dental implant surgeon. J Periodontol 2008; 79: 1833–1846.
42. Pjetursson BE, Thoma D, Jung R, et al. A systematic review of the survival and complication rates of implant-supported fixed dental prostheses (FDPs) after a mean observation period of at least 5 years. Clin Oral Implants Res 2012; 23: 22–38.
43. Prosper L, Crespi R, Valenti E, et al. Five-year follow-up of wide-diameter implants placed in fresh molar extraction sockets in the mandible: immediate versus delayed loading. Int J Oral Maxillofac Implants 2010; 25: 607–612.
44. Lee E, Gonzalez-Martin O, Fiorellini J. Lingualized flapless implant placement into fresh extraction sockets preserves buccal alveolar bone: a cone beam computed tomography study. Int J Periodontics Restorative Dent 2014; 34: 61–68.
45. Le BT, Borzabadi-Farahani A, Pluemsakunthai W, et al. Is buccolingual angulation of maxillary anterior implants associated with the crestal labial soft tissue thickness? Int J Oral Maxillofac Surg 2014; 43(7): 874–878.
46. Renouard F, Nisand D. Impact of implant length and diameter on survival rates. Clin Oral Implants Res 2006; 17(Suppl 2): 35–51.
47. Ormianer Z, Palti A, Demiralp B, et al. Implant-supported first molar restorations: correlation of finite element analysis with clinical outcomes. Int J Oral Maxillofac Implants 2012; 27: e1–e12.
48. Caplanis N, Lozada J, Kan J. Extraction defect assessment, classification and management. J Calif Dent Assoc 2005; 33: 853–863.
49. Cullum, DR. Advances in Bone Manipulation Techniques: Part 1. Osteome Site Development and Minimally Invasive Sinus Elevation. Selected Readings in Oral and Maxillofacial Surgery. San Francisco, CA: Guild for Scientific Advancement in Oral and Maxillofacial Surgery, 2010, vol. 18, no. 4.
50. Fugazzotto P. Implant placement at the time of maxillary molar extraction: treatment protocols and report of results. J Periodontol 2008; 79: 216–223.
51. Fugazzotto P. Implant placement at the time of mandibular molar extraction: description of technique and preliminary results of 341 cases. J Periodontol 2008; 79: 737–747.
52. Park HH. A Chair-side Technique for Immediate Implant Placement with Provisionalization to Optimize Esthetic Outcome. Selected Readings in Oral and Maxillofacial Surgery. San Francisco, CA: Guild for Scientific Advancement in Oral and Maxillofacial Surgery, 2011, vol. 19, no. 2.
53. Vercellotti T, Stacchi C, Russo C, et al. Ultrasonic implant site preparation using piezosurgery: a multicenter case series study analyzing 3579 implants with a 1 to 3-year follow-up. Int J Periodontics Restorative Dent 2014; 34: 11–18.
54. Albiero AM, Benato R, Degidi M. Buccal plate regeneration with immediate post-extraction implant placement and restoration: case reports. Int J Periodontics Restorative Dent 2014; 34: e67–e72.
55. Le B, Burstein J. Esthetic grafting for small volume hard and soft tissue contour defects for implant site development. Implant Dent 2008; 17: 136–141.
56. Sclar AG. Strategies for management of single tooth extraction sites in aesthetic implant therapy. J Oral Maxillofac Surg 2004; 62(Suppl 2): 90–105.
57. Khori F, Happe A. The palatal subepithelial connective tissue flap method for soft tissue management to cover maxillary defects: a clinical report. Int J Oral Maxillofac Implants 2000; 15: 415–418.
58. Zuhr O, Hurzeler M. Plastic-Esthetic Periodontal and Implant Surgery. A Microsurgical Approach. Quintessence, 2012.
59. Rebele S, Zuhr O, Hurzeler M. Pre-extractive interradicular implant bed preparation: case presentations of a novel approach to immediate implant placement at multirooted molar sites. Int J Periodontics Restorative Dent 2013; 33: 88–95.
60. Hamouda NI, Mourad SI, El-Kenawy MH, Maria OM. Immediate implant placement into fresh extraction socket in the mandibular molar sites: a preliminary study of a modified insertion technique. Clin Implant Dent Rel Res 2015; 17(Suppl S1): e107–e116.
61. Vandeweghe S, Ackermann A, Bronner J, et al. A retrospective, multicenter study on a novo wide-body implant for posterior regions. Clin Implant Dent Relat Res 2012; 14: 281–292.
62. Krekmanov L, Kahn M, Rangert B, Lindström H. Tilting of posterior mandibular and maxillary implants for improved prosthesis support. Int J Oral Maxillofac Implants 2000; 15: 405–414.
63. Hellem S, Astrand P, Stenström B, et al. Implant treatment in combination with lateral augmentation of the alveolar process: a 3-year prospective study. Clin Implant Dent Relat Res 2003; 5: 233–240.

64. Evans C, Chen S. Esthetic outcomes of immediate implant placements. Clin Oral Implants Res 2008; 19: 73–80.
65. Block M, Mercante D, Lirette D, et al. Prospective evaluation of immediate and delayed provisional single tooth restorations. J Oral Maxillofac Surg 2009; 67: 89–107.
66. Schropp L, Isidor F, Kostopoulos L, et al. Patient experience of, and satisfaction with, delayed-immediate vs delayed single-tooth implant placement. Clin Oral Implants Res 2004; 15: 498–503.
67. Hof M, Pommer B, Ambros H, et al. Does timing of implant placement affect implant therapy outcome in the aesthetic zone? A clinical, radiological, aesthetic, and patient-based evaluation. Clin Implant Dent Relat Res. Article first published online: 20 Feb 2014. DOI: 10.1111/cid.12212.
68. Le BT, Borzabadi-Farahani A. Labial bone thickness in area of anterior maxillary implants associated with crestal labial soft tissue thickness. Implant Dent 2012; 21: 406–410.
69. Qahash M, Susin C, Polimeni G, et al. Bone healing dynamics at buccal peri-implant sites. Clin Oral Implants Res 2008; 19: 166–172.
70. Grunder U, Gracis S, Capelli M. Influence of the 3-D bone-to-implant relationship on esthetics. Int J Periodontics Restorative Dent 2005; 25: 113–119.
71. Covani U, Bortolaia C, Barone A, et al. Bucco-lingual crestal changes after immediate and delayed implant placement. J Periodontol 2004; 75: 1605–1612.
72. Nisapakultorn K, Suphanantachat S, Silkosessak O, Rattanamongkolgul S. Factors affecting soft tissue level around anterior maxillary single-tooth implants. Clin Oral Implants Res 2010; 21: 662–670.
73. Nevins M, Cameo M, DePaoli S, et al. A study of the fate of the buccal wall of extraction sockets of teeth with prominent roots. Int J Periodontics Restorative Dent 2006; 26: 19–29.
74. Jung R, Holderegger C, Sailer I, et al. The effect of all-ceramic and porcelain-fused-to-metal restorations on marginal peri-implant soft tissue color: a randomized controlled clinical trial. Int J Periodontics Restorative Dent 2008; 28: 357–365.
75. Jung R, Sailer I, Hämmerle C, et al. *In vitro* color changes of soft tissues caused by restorative materials. Int J Periodontics Restorative Dent 2007; 27: 251–257.
76. Linkevicius T, Apse P, Grybauskas S, et al. The influence of soft tissue thickness on crestal bone changes around implants: a 1-year prospective controlled clinical trial. Int J Oral Maxillofac Implants 2009; 24: 712–719.
77. Morris HF, Ochi S, Creum P, et al. AICRG Part I: a 6-year multi-centered, multidisciplinary clinical study of a new and innovative implant design. J Oral Implantol 2004; 30: 125–133.
78. Pozzi A, Tallarico M, Moy P. Three-year post-loading results of a randomized, controlled, split-mouth trial comparing implants with different prosthetic interfaces and design in partially posterior edentulous mandibles. Eur J Oral Implantol 2014; 7: 47–61.
79. Gracis S, Michalakis K, Vigolo P. Internal vs. external connections for abutments/reconstructions: a systematic review. Clin Oral Implants Res 2012; 23(Suppl 6): 202–216.
80. Vandeweghe S, DeBruyn H. A within-implant comparison to evaluate the concept of platform-switching. A randomized controlled trial. Eur J Oral Implantol 2012; 5: 253–262.
81. Rodriquez-Ciurana X, Vela-Nebot X, Segala-Torres M, et al. The effect of inter-implant distance on the height of inter-implant bone crest when using platform-switched implants. Int J Periodontics Restorative Dent 2009; 29: 141–151.
82. Elian N, Bloom M, Dard M, et al. Effect of inter-implant distance (2 and 3 mm) on the height of inter-implant bone crest: a histomorphometric evaluation. J Periodontol 2011; 82: 1749–1756.
83. Elian N, Bloom M, Dard M, et al. Radiological and micro-computed tomography analysis of the bone at dental implants inserted 2, 3 and 4 mm apart in a minipig model with platform switching incorporated. Clin Oral Implants Res 2014; 25: e22–e29.
84. Iorio-Siciliano V, Marzo G, Blasi A, et al. Soft and hard tissue modifications at immediate transmucosal implants (with Laser-Lok microtextured collar) placed into fresh extraction sites: a 6-month prospective study with surgical re-entry. Int J Periodontics Restorative Dent 2014; 34: 541–549.
85. Lee D-W, Choi Y-S, Park K-H, et al. Effect of microthread on the maintenance of marginal bone level: a 3-year prospective study. Clin Oral Implants Res 2007; 18: 465–470.
86. Nevins M, Kim M, Jun S, Guze K. Histologic evidence of connective tissue attachment to laser micro-grooved abutments: a canine study. Int J Periodontics Restorative Dent 2010; 30: 245–255.
87. Wilson T. The positive relationship between excess cement and peri-implant disease: a prospective clinical endoscopic study. J Periodontol 2009; 80: 1388–1392.
88. Sailer I, Mühlemann S, Zwahlen M, et al. Cemented and screw-retained implant reconstructions: a systematic review of the survival and complication rates. Clin Oral Implants Res. 2012; 23(Suppl 6): 163–201.

CHAPTER 19

Immediate Esthetic Zone Tooth Replacement

Daniel R. Cullum[1] & Howard Park[2]

[1]Private Practice, Coeur d'Alene, ID; Loma Linda University Department of OMS, Loma Linda, CA; UCLA Department of OMS, Los Angeles, CA, USA
[2]Private Practice, Santa Monica, CA; UCLA Department Department of OMS, Los Angeles, CA, USA

Introduction

Management of extraction sites with simultaneous endosseous implant placement was first advanced by Schulte et al.[1] Immediate implant placement offers patients the significant advantages of fewer surgical procedures and shorter overall treatment times. In selected cases, treatment can be further accelerated by the use of a fixed, appropriately prepared and contoured, provisional implant crown that can help maintain peri-implant soft tissue architecture. This approach eliminates the need to wear a removable prosthesis. However, the literature has many reports of esthetic complications following these procedures, including recession of the facial gingiva and loss of papilla height.[2–8] Small and Tarnow suggested that, regardless of the technique used, approximately 1 mm of apical migration of the free gingival margin can be expected following abutment connection.[8] While there are several possible etiological factors for gingival recession, a compromised buccal plate is thought to be the most significant.[9,10] Many clinicians believe immediate implants with or without immediate provisional restoration should not be attempted in the esthetic zone, especially if the buccal plate is compromised.[9,11] Valentini et al. have challenged this guideline by reporting cases in which immediate implants with immediate provisional restorations were restored definitively with good esthetic results when followed up to 1 year.[12] Evaluation of intact buccal plates with direct measurements following extraction of anterior maxillary teeth showed less than 1 mm thickness near the crest in 81 of 93 consecutive patients.[13] These findings were consistent with several recent cone beam computed tomography (CBCT) scan studies which showed that fewer than 5–10% of teeth in studied individuals have an intact buccal plate with thickness greater than 1 mm in the maxillary anterior area.[14–16] Many other factors need to be considered before employing immediate provisional restorations in the anterior maxilla. Considerations in obtaining an optimal esthetic outcome include individual anatomy, preservation of vascular supply, implant size and design, primary stability, implant positioning, dimensions of the buccal bone gap, whether the restoration is screw- or cement-retained, design of the provisional restoration, and post-healing emergence profile development. Further anatomic concerns include the role of a thin gingival biotype and the pre-treatment gingival margin position. This chapter describes a practical and predictable integrated surgical and prosthetic approach, independently developed over 14 years, for immediate esthetic zone implant placement with immediate provisional restoration.[17]

Literature review

Since the original Brånemark protocol was presented in 1981,[18] the use of dental implants has expanded from edentulous arches to include partially edentulous segments and single tooth replacements in the esthetic zone.[2–4] With excellent survival rates, dental implants have become the preferred method to replace single teeth,[5] with increasing demand for reduced treatment time, patient comfort, and expense. Schulte et al.[1] are credited with being the first clinicians to attempt immediate implant placement into fresh extraction sockets. However, their report of 95 cases with up to 2½ year follow-up was published in German and had limited exposure and impact at the time. Schnitman et al.[19] were the first to report on immediate loading of dental implants placed in healed extraction sites. These clinicians followed seven full-arch cases in which immediate loading had been applied to three implants while additional implants were left unloaded for traditional healing. The loaded implants were planned as transitional implants and were not expected to develop osseointegration; however, 18 of these 21 implants became fully integrated. Ericsson et al.[20] confirmed that implants placed using non-submerged healing in edentulous sites with immediate (loaded) provisional restorations performed similarly to control implants placed using submerged healing. Subsequently, Wöhrle[21] reported on 14 consecutively treated cases of immediate provisional restoration of immediately placed implants. Kan et al.[22] and others[12,23–26] also reported favorable outcomes with the potential for preserving gingival architecture using immediate implants and immediate provisional restoration of maxillary anterior single-tooth implants. However, these reports also identified challenges, including facial gingival recession and shortened papilla height, as restorations were evaluated over longer time intervals.[11,12,27,28] As these esthetic complications became more apparent, investigators began examining possible etiological factors, including the integrity of buccal plate,[10] grafting versus non-grafting of the buccal gap in extraction sockets,[29–31] implant diameter, macrodesign and surface treatment, palatal implant positioning,[32] abutment design and emergence, flap versus flapless surgery,[33–35] gingival biotype,[36] and the effect of simultaneous connective tissue grafting.[37,38]

The phenomenon of bone volume loss following tooth removal was recognized as early as 1960 by Lam,[39] who reported vertical bone loss of 2.0–4.5 mm. Johnson[40] reported 50% ridge width loss following extraction. Interest in extraction socket remodeling was renewed more recently when the concept of preserving bone volume by placing implants immediately into fresh extraction sockets

Minimally Invasive Dental Implant Surgery, First Edition. Edited by Daniel R. Cullum and Douglas Deporter.

was proposed.[41–45] These studies affirmed the reports by Lam and Johnson, and also refuted the concept that bone could be preserved with immediate dental implant placement alone. Araújo et al.[43,44] reported data from a canine study with full-thickness flap exposure and complete elevation of the periosteum suggesting that the buccal plate continued to remodel and resulted in a net loss of 1.3–1.4 mm in horizontal dimension.

The majority of the studies evaluating the effect of a compromised buccal plate on facial gingival margin position involved raising a full-thickness flap to visually confirm the buccal defect and perform subsequent hard and soft tissue grafting.[10,11,27,42,46–50] However, elevation of a full-thickness flap compromises blood supply to the residual alveolar bone and increases subsequent resorption.[51–54] This has raised enough concern regarding the esthetics of peri-implant tissues that flapless procedures are often preferred over flap procedures.[33,34] Management of the gap space between the buccal plate and the implant in fresh extraction sockets has been studied extensively.[29–31,55] While new bone will regenerate spontaneously without the need for grafting, studies have shown that grafting the gap will minimize horizontal bone loss.[56–58]

Advancement of CBCT has allowed visualization of bone volume not previously possible with conventional radiographs (see Chapter 2). Several CBCT studies have shown that the thickness of buccal plate near the crest with natural teeth is less than 1.0 mm in the majority of patients.[14,15,17] This thickness has been independently verified by others who took direct measurements following extractions.[13] Most of the crestal buccal bone consists of bundle bone (lamina dura) providing the attachment surface for Sharpey's fibers of the periodontal ligament. The thickness of this bone layer varies from anterior to posterior teeth, ranging from 0.22 to 0.54 mm, and resorbs completely following tooth extraction.[59,60] These studies essentially confirm that even the intact crestal buccal plate will disappear following extraction even with socket preservation grafting (see Chapter 5). Owing to the beam hardening effect of CBCT technologies, bone thickness of less than 1.0 mm next to the implant body is difficult to visualize, making buccal plate evaluation a challenge preoperatively.[61–63] Roe et al.[64] studied the buccal plate thickness of 21 patients who received immediate implants with immediate provisional restorations. Only those with intact buccal plates at the time of implant placement were selected for the study. CBCT evaluation 1 year after the implant placement showed the greatest bone loss occurred at the crestal level, averaging 1.23 mm in horizontal dimension and 0.82 mm in vertical dimension. However, this study did not measure any concomitant soft tissue changes. Another CBCT study followed 14 patients for 7 years and noted that five patients did not show any detectable remaining buccal bone but had mid-buccal free gingival margins only 1 mm more apical compared with their contralateral tooth.[65]

While the challenges of a thin gingival biotype include a higher risk for soft tissue recession, Kan et al.[36] demonstrated that it is often difficult to assess the situation preoperatively using visual inspection and probing techniques. This suggests that, when contemplating immediate implants with immediate provisional restoration in the esthetic zone, consideration should be given to treat every patient as if they display a thin biotype (see Chapter 8).

For successful immediate implant placement, macrodesigns must produce primary stability and facilitate optimal 3-D positioning (see Chapter 18). Implant designs without adequate taper and cutting thread pattern tend to push to the facial due to resistance from the dense palatal bone. This can result in additional risk of facial displacement of the crestal aspect of the implant body, increasing facial angulation and reducing the dimension of the facial bone gap. An additional implant design feature of benefit in the esthetic zone is a reduced coronal diameter, which reduces the tendency of the crestal portion of the implant to be displaced facially. This feature also allows for increased facial gap dimension and the subsequent formation of increased volumes of hard and soft tissues, thus reducing short- and long-term risks of gingival recession. Implant designs most suitable for immediate placement in the maxillary anterior include an internal and tapered abutment connection to minimize the microgap and micromotion and a reduced abutment diameter relative to the crestal platform of the implant body ("platform switching") to reduce dimensional changes required for biological width formation around the implant–abutment junction (see discussion in Chapters 3, 4, and 18).

Based on these findings, it has become generally accepted that immediate implant placement in the maxillary anterior region should be against the palatal bone wall leaving approximately a 2–3 mm horizontal gap between the facial aspect of the implant body and the buccal plate.[29,32,42,46,47] Simultaneous bone grafting of the facial gap will then ensure long-term stability of the labial plate of bone over the implant body.

Provisional abutment design

Many abutment options are available for clinical application with provisional restorations, including several forms of "plastic," ceramic, titanium, zirconia, and other hybrid designs. For immediate provisional restoration as outlined later, "plastic" abutments and "direct" and screw-retained pick-up technique are demonstrated where the advantages of resiliency and simple modification in the surgical setting outweigh the potential for delamination, fracture, and fatigue. For delayed application at a healed site, an "indirect" screw-retained titanium abutment has the advantage of allowing laboratory fabrication. In any case, the provisional abutment must be strong enough to last through the implant integration period without risk of screw loosening, delamination, or fracture. The immediate provisional restoration is developed to avoid soft tissue recession using a flat or concave tissue emergence for initial healing and implant osseointegration, shock dampening, and resiliency. However, it must also have sufficient longevity and facilitate delayed abutment modifications of the emergence profile for soft tissue sculpting. Perhaps future developments in the digital world will soon produce immediate fabrication or milling of an abutment, and allow later re-design and fabrication in incremental sizes and/or shape modifications in a cost-effective manner.

Immediate placement of the final abutment has been advanced to reduce tissue recession associated with repeated removal/re-insertion of abutments. The same biologic and clinical principles apply, and would require selection of a narrower buccal emergence profile with an "immediate" final abutment placement to minimize risk of soft tissue recession during the healing interval. However, while maintaining a narrow emergence profile is an option, we find that the resulting crown is often clinically unacceptable both esthetically and functionally, and the result can be compromised due to food impaction and retention. Additionally, prosthetic compensation for eccentric or palatal positioning cannot be completed without customization as a secondary process. There is currently no system that allows immediate custom final abutment fabrication. Fabrication of an under-contoured immediate provisional healing abutment or provisional restoration and delayed emergence profile development have been applied with excellent esthetic and functional results (see Chapter 4). The time invested in these types of cases can produce outstanding results and gratification.

A screw-retained provisional restoration is preferred to eliminate potential cement entrapment in the immediate extraction wound. Screw retention with a plastic or titanium abutment (see Chapter 4) can allow for direct custom fabrication of an immediate provisional at surgery and prevent the need for a removable appliance. Perhaps the most important challenge of the screw-retained provisional is the requirement for the surgeon to place the implant palatally and with an angulation allowing the screw access opening to come out through the cingulum.

A "platform-switched" feature facilitates fabrication of the immediate provisional restoration by reducing the potential for interproximal or palatal tissue contact preventing complete seating or deflection of the crown contour. Plastic abutments are not radiodense; therefore, if used, their complete seating must be confirmed clinically.

Preoperative evaluation and planning

The following checklist may be helpful for preoperative clinical and radiographic evaluation.

1 Soft tissue evaluation:
   i. free gingival margin level compared with contralateral tooth;
   ii. gingival biotype: thin versus thick;
   iii. papilla shape: high scalloping versus broad and blunted;
   iv. high frenum attachment;
   v. pre-existing mucogingival defect.
2 Hard tissue evaluation:
   i. alveolar bone levels on adjacent teeth;
   ii. integrity of buccal plate via probing and/or CBCT;
   iii. palatal bone volume assessment via CBCT.
3 Occlusion:
   i. open bite versus deep bite (class II div II).
4 Infection:
   i. apical pathology;
   ii. fistular tracts;
   iii. acute infection with buccal abscess.
5 Pre-existing restorations on adjacent teeth:
   i. full coverage crowns;
   ii. veneers;
   iii. class IV or V composite restorations.
6 Smoking/tobacco use.

With the broad application of CBCT technologies, 3-D imaging and planning software have become cost-effective with minimal radiation exposure (see Chapters 2, 9, and 18). These are powerful tools in combination with the preoperative history and clinical examination to allow formulation of a comprehensive diagnosis and treatment plan (see Chapters 1–3). For an immediate implant and provisional restoration, the most critical information is the quantity of facial soft tissue, the height of interproximal bone, and the volume of palatal bone available. Integrity of buccal bone is helpful, but does not change treatment planning significantly when utilizing palatal implant positioning with a flapless approach. From our clinical experience, adequate palatal bone can be readily available despite any compromise at the buccal plate. This has been confirmed by a recent CBCT study demonstrating 98% of maxillary central incisors to have adequate palatal bone for immediate implant placement.[66] Periapical radiographs also can be used to estimate the appropriate length of implant needed, and to evaluate the interseptal bone at adjacent teeth. If the bone level on adjacent teeth is compromised, it is important to identify and recognize the limitation for papillary regeneration and to have a frank discussion with the patient before proceeding or choosing another technique.[67–70]

The presence of apical pathology and/or a facial fistula are not necessarily contraindications for immediate implant placement as protocols have been developed for these situations.[71] Immediate implant survival rates have recently been studied looking at various factors, including the presence of infection, vertical root fracture, failing endodontic treatment, and antibiotic therapy. The only statistically significant factor seen to increase the survival rate was post-operative antibiotic therapy.[72] Further risk factors include patients with a high smile line, class II division II "deep bite," or thin gingival biotype with triangular tooth shapes and "high scalloped" papillae.[73] These latter situations should be avoided or treated only following significant experiences with and mastery of the technique. The presence of restorations or future restorative procedures on adjacent teeth can present increased risk for gingival marginal recession at an implant restoration exposing finishing margins, and again should be discussed with patients preoperatively. The heights of interdental papillae around the implant restoration will be determined by the level of alveolar bone on the adjacent teeth (see discussion in Chapters 3 and 18).

Surgical techniques

The extraction technique should follow a minimally invasive protocol (as outlined in Chapter 5). A surgical guide is typically not mandatory for a single implant site, but is most helpful for multiple teeth, or if the preoperative work-up demonstrates the need for an altered vertical or palatal position for the implant relative to the native tooth root position. The guide should be designed to allow the implant retaining screw to emerge through the cingulum and away from the incisal edge of the future implant crown. This will help to ensure that the implant shoulder will not be too close to the buccal plate, and leave a larger buccal bone gap. A larger gap (>2 mm) is more favorable for placement of a sufficient volume of bone graft material to ensure long-term tissue stability. The extraction should be completed without flap elevation using only an intra-sulcular incision to prevent "pulling" of the interdental papillae from the adjacent teeth. It is often necessary to use Proximator® instruments or Piezosurgery® root extraction inserts to mobilize the root fragments. Alternatively, a rotary instrument may be needed to section the root and minimize injury to surrounding bone (see Chapter 5). Following tooth removal, the socket is aggressively curetted and debrided to remove completely any granulation tissue. Decortication of the socket wall is not performed; however, irrigation with a clindamycin solution for 5 seconds or povodine iodine solution for 30 seconds can be completed following the debridement. Site assessment is completed with a periodontal probe used to confirm interproximal, facial, and palatal bone levels.

With an adequate volume of palatal bone (confirmed via visualization and bone sounding, if CBCT was not taken preoperatively), a small round bur or sharp-pointed precision drill (Figure 19.1a) on a drill extender is used to gain a purchase point about halfway from the palatal crest to the root apex and along the palatal socket wall. Subsequent development using sequentially larger diameter drills is completed at reduced drill speed of <700 rpm with intermittent drill force and copious saline irrigation. A challenge with this technique is the tendency for the increasing diameter drills to be displaced off the palatal wall, as this can result in the final osteotomy being

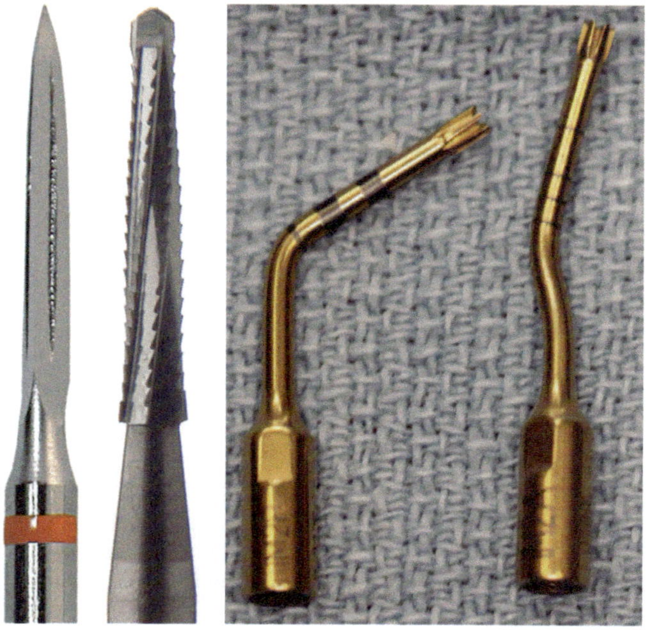

(a) (b) (c)

Figure 19.1 (a) Pointed precision drill and (b) "latch type" Lindemann bur (Meisinger USA, Golden, CO). (c) Piezosurgery® IM1 and IM2a inserts (Piezosurgery USA, Columbus, OH).

too close to the buccal plate. Judicious application of a Lindemann (side-cutting) bur or Piezosurgery IM2P insert (Figure 19.1b and c) is often necessary to prepare the palatal wall so as to prevent facial displacement of the osteotomy.

Depending on tactile feedback during osteotomy preparation, it is often necessary to slightly "under-prepare" the site. This allows the implant to be placed with high insertion torque, typically in the range of ≥35 to 50 N cm depending on the implant design. Upon seating the implant, there should be at least a 2 mm gap present between the buccal plate and the facial aspect of the implant (Figure 19.2). Many implant designs do not have a cutting thread, and tend to push away from resistance provided by the dense palatal bone. This can result in additional risk of facial displacement of the crestal aspect of the implant body, increasing the facial angulation and reducing the dimension of the facial bone gap. An additional implant design feature of benefit in the esthetic zone is a reduced coronal diameter. This feature allows for the formation of increased volumes of hard and soft tissues.

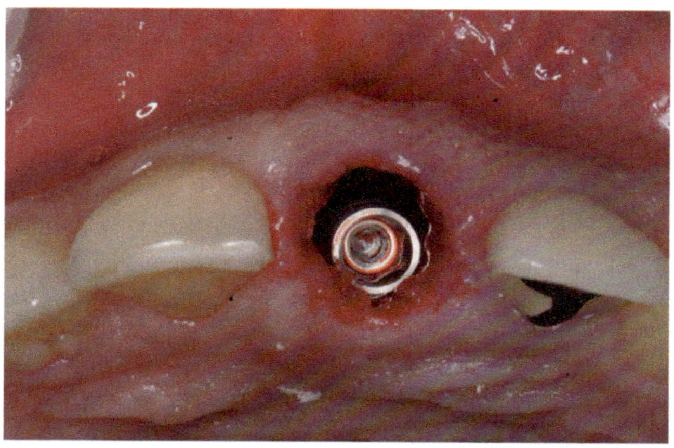

Figure 19.2 A minimum 2 mm buccal gap is visually confirmed following the seating of the implant in the extraction socket. Exposed threads are visible on the facial aspect of the implant. Placement was 3 mm apical from the desired gingival margin of the final restoration.

Proper apico-coronal positioning of the implant is dictated by the desired final position of the "ideal" free gingival margin. Seating the implant approximately 3 mm apical to the ideal free gingival margin is recommended to allow a proper emergence profile and biologic width development (see Chapters 1, 4, and 18). When an implant is placed following these principles, it is common at this point to visualize exposed facial threads of the coronal two-thirds of the implant within the buccal bone gap (Figure 19.2). If the buccal plate is missing, a greater volume of bone graft material should be used to over-correct the defect. A thickness of graft material of at least 3 mm should be present between the overlying mucosa and the implant shoulder. If the buccal plate is intact and the gap is less than 2 mm, the implant should be removed and replaced with a narrower diameter or the osteotomy repositioned further to the palatal to create more gap space. This often requires removing additional palatal bone and/or possibly using a longer implant. Using wide-diameter implants to gain primary stability should be avoided.

As we have stressed, grafting of the facial bone gap is critical for long-term maintenance of facial bone volume and soft tissue support. The use of various graft materials has been advanced; however, there are no definitive data that one is superior. Over the past 14 years, we have used particulate autogenous cancellous, mineralized cancellous and cortico-cancellous allografts, as well as equine and bovine mineralized xenografts. Our clinical experience demonstrates that all lead to clinical osseointegration of the immediate implant, and that all are superior in contour maintenance compared with not grafting the facial bone gap. Addition of a graft material will not be an adequate substitute for a minimal gap dimension (<2 mm), from improper implant placement towards the facial, or with excessive facial angulation. It is our clinical observation that contour maintenance is less predictable with particulate autogenous bone and is greatest with xenografts. Our combined experience is a preference for small (0.25–1.0 mm range) particle equine mineralized xenograft (Equimatrix®, Osteohealth, Shirley, NY) or a 1 : 1 equal volume mixture of mineralized allograft (Miner-Oss®, BioHorizons, Birmingham, AL) and mineralized bovine xenograft (Bio-Oss®, Geistlich, Geistlich Pharma North America Inc., Princeton, NJ). We prefer to saturate the graft either in venous autologous blood or in a clindamycin solution. Placement of a layer of sectioned fibrillar collagen (e.g. Collaplug®, Zimmer Dental, Carlsbad, CA) saturated in recombinant human platelet-derived growth factor (off-label use of GEM 21S®, Osteohealth, Shirley, NY) can be added to the protocol to seal the crestal graft at the interface of the provisional; however, a barrier is not needed as a properly contoured immediate provisional protects the site nicely.

The provisional restoration

Considerations for immediate provisional restoration include atraumatic tooth removal, ideal implant position, and adequate primary implant stability (rotational torque values >30 N cm and implant stability quotient reading >65). A screw-retained provisional restoration is preferred to eliminate potential cement entrapment and/or frequent dislodging of the provisional crown. Another advantage of the screw-retained provisional is that it forces the surgeon to place the implant in an adequately palatal position to allow the screw access to come out through the cingulum. In our experience, this has been the single most important factor in producing acceptable esthetic outcomes.

Materials needed include: (i) a pre-fabricated plastic or titanium engaging abutment and abutment screw (Figure 19.3a and b); (ii) a pre-fabricated methyl methacrylate shell crown (Figure 19.3c) or hollowed-out plastic denture tooth of appropriate size and shade (Figure 19.3d); (iii) an implant analog (Figure 19.3d); (iv) a long-shafted driver (Figure 19.3a and d); (v) a lab handle (Figure 19.3e); (vi) acrylic or flowable composite and shade guide (Figure 19.3f–h); and (vii) various acrylic burs (Figure 19.3i), polishing discs, and pumice/wheel.

The provisional restoration is indexed by a direct intraoral "pick-up" technique. The crown and abutment are adjusted for height and interproximal dimension and the crestal aspect of the provisional is luted to the abutment with a bonding agent and flowable composite or jet acrylic of matching shade (Figure 19.4a and b). The access opening is maintained with placement of a

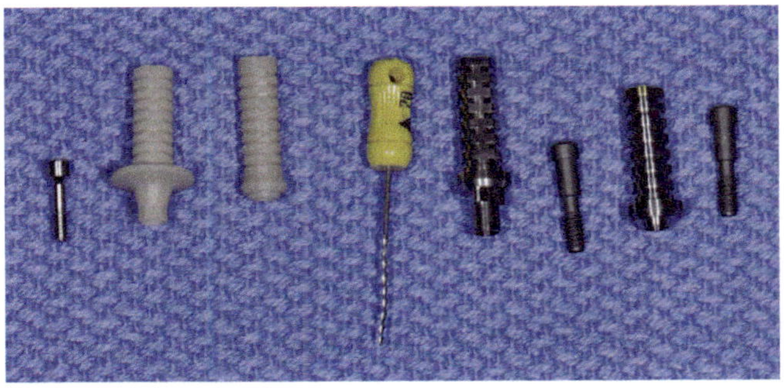

(a)

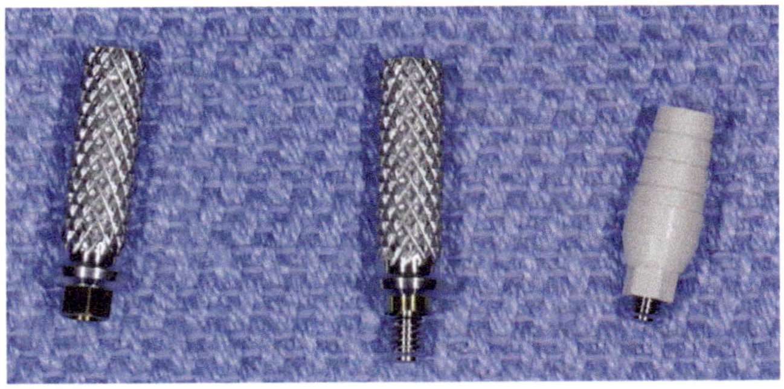

(b)

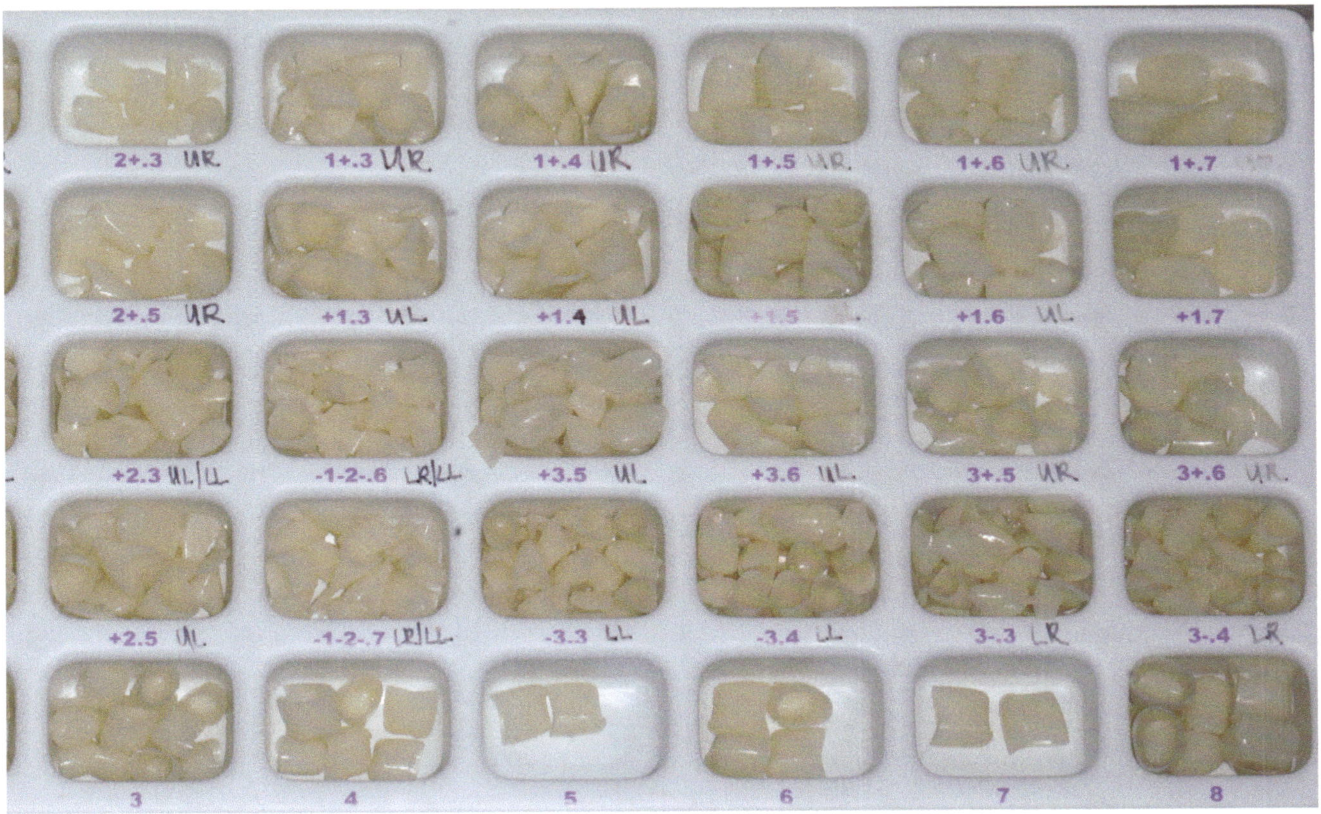

(c)

Figure 19.3 (a) An assortment of engaging and non-engaging plastic and titanium temporary abutments (Nobel Biocare, Yorba Linda, CA). Non-engaging abutments are used with multiple-unit provisionals to avoid any insertion draw conflict. An endodontic file or an explorer can be used to remove cotton pellets from the temporary abutments while the acrylic is curing in the mouth. Alternatively, the screw access can be maintained by leaving the driver in position during curing. An extra-long driver is often needed to engage screws due to the anatomic crown height. (b) Another assortment of engaging and non-engaging plastic and titanium temporary abutments (BioHorizons, Birmingham, AL). (c) An assortment of anterior crown forms. *(Continued)*

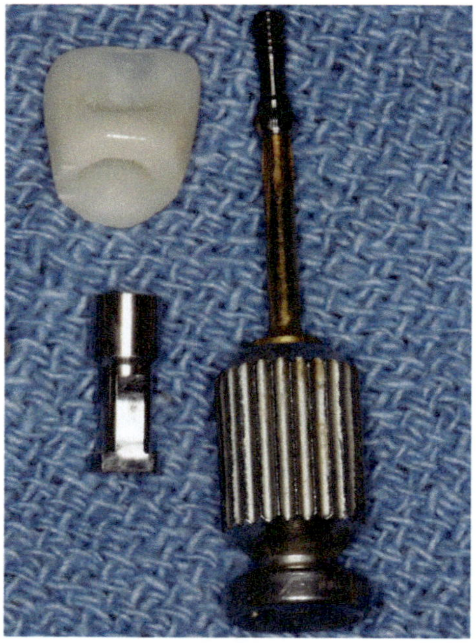

(d)

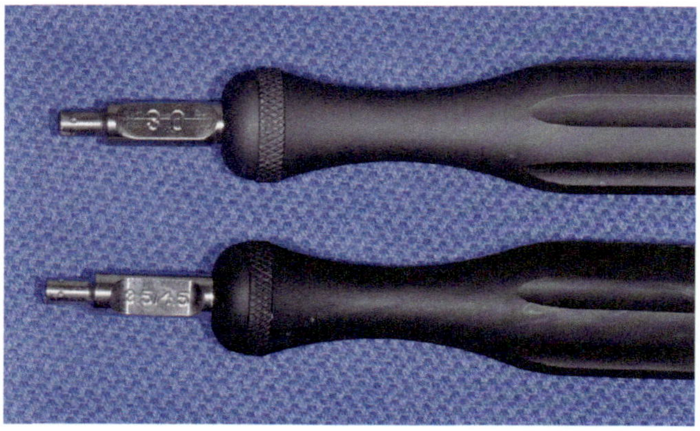

(e)

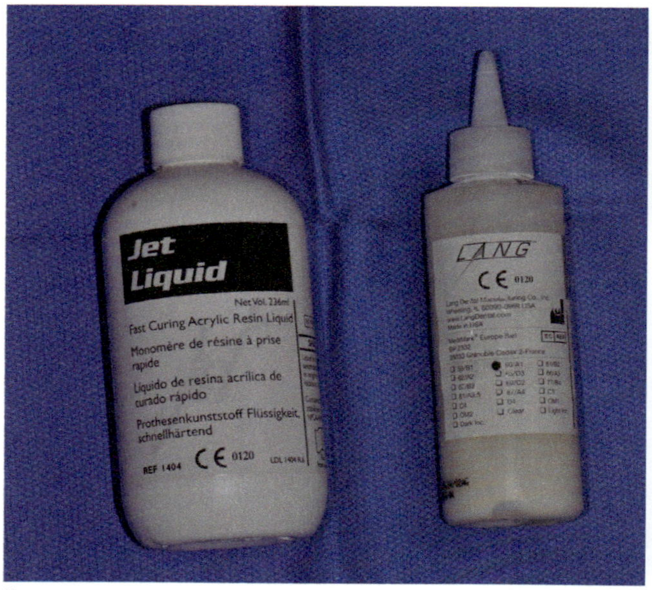

(f)

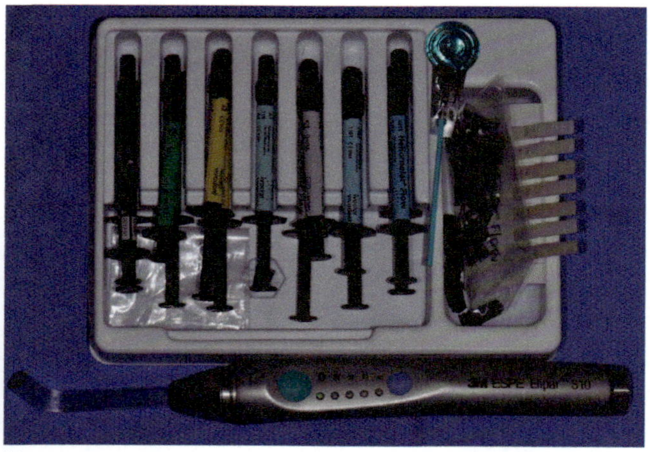

(g)

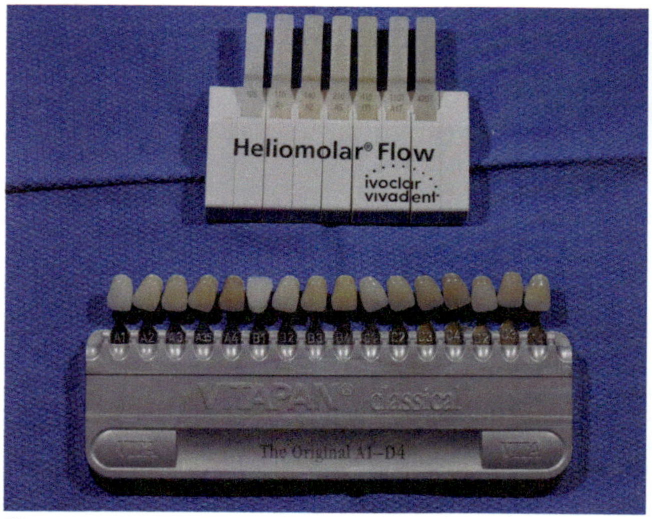

(h)

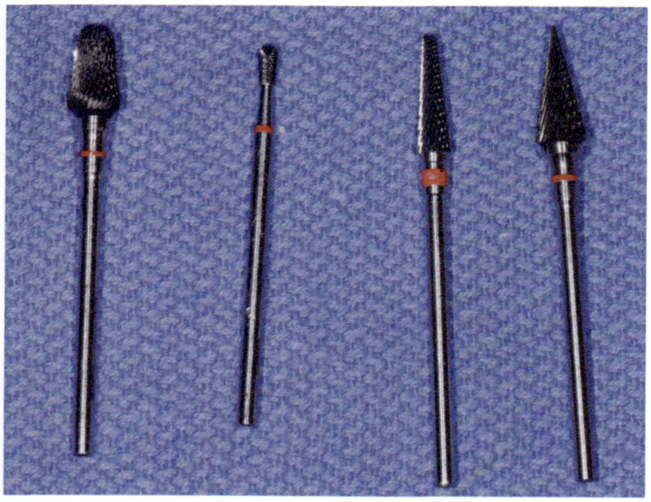

(i)

Figure 19.3 (Continued)

(d) A hollowed-out plastic denture tooth of appropriate size and shade, an implant analog, a long-shafted driver, and an abutment screw. (e) Laboratory handles used to hold implant analogs during fabrication of a provisional restoration. (f, g) Acrylics and flowable composites of various shades. (h) Shade guides. (i) Various acrylic burs. *Source:* (d) © Daniel R. Cullum

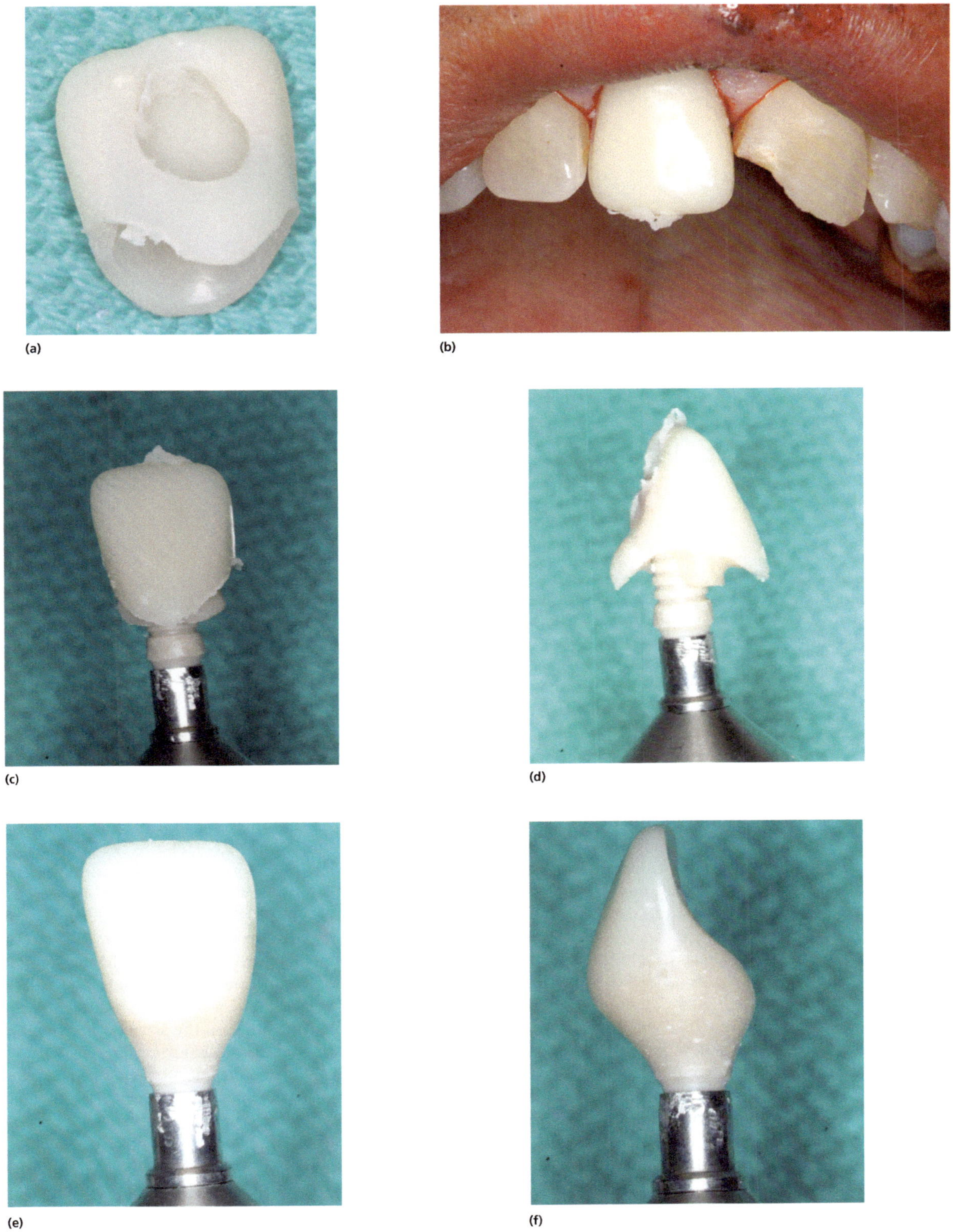

Figure 19.4 (a) The selected temporary crown is trimmed and a screw access created. (b) The temporary crown is delivered with acrylic in its coronal portion over the temporary abutment with the screw access cleared by removing the cotton pellet before the acrylic sets. (c, d) The temporary crown–abutment is unscrewed and removed from the mouth with the occlusal pick-up intact. Voids at the gingival aspect are visible. (e–g) The abutment surface is cleansed and dried, and the subgingival portion of the temporary crown back-filled with acrylic or flowable composite, shaped, and polished.

(Continued)

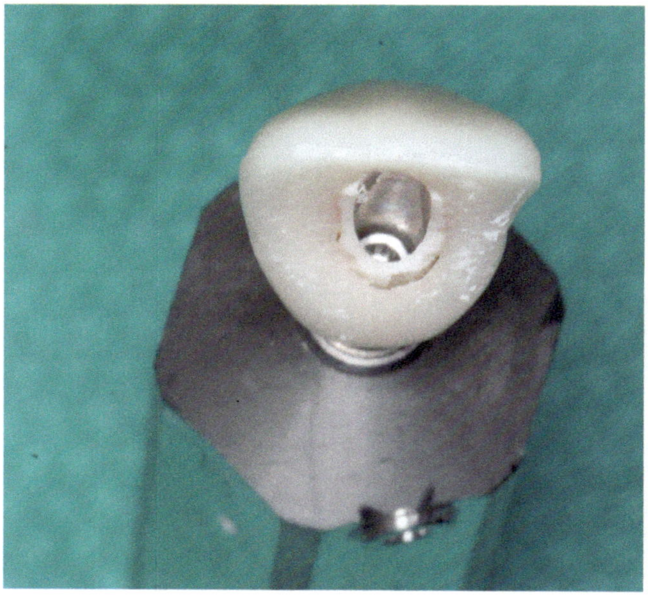

(g)

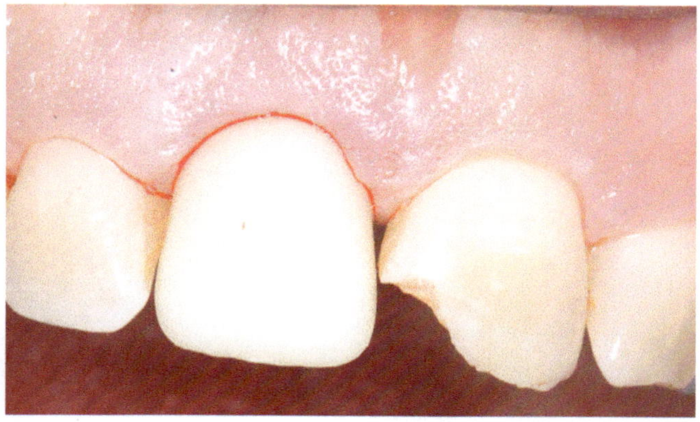

(h)

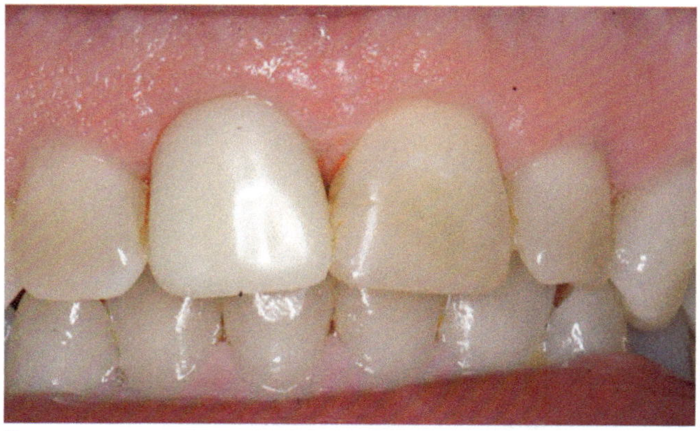

(i)

Figure 19.4 (Continued)
(h) The immediate post-op view of the right maxillary central incisor in Figure 19.2 after immediate provisional restoration. The provisional restoration can be seen after 4 months (i) and the final restoration after 18 months (j), demonstrating harmonious soft tissue levels and an esthetically pleasing result.

cotton pellet, which is then removed before the composite is light-cured or the acrylic is set (Figure 19.4b). An alternate technique to maintain the access opening is to place the long-shafted abutment screwdriver in position while the composite is light cured (Figure 19.5a). The temporary crown–abutment combination then is unscrewed and removed from the mouth with the occlusal pick-up intact. Voids at the gingival aspect of the abutment are visible and the abutment surface is cleansed and dried (Figures 19.4c and d and 19.5b). The subgingival "emergence" or cervical portion of the provisional restoration is then back-filled out of the mouth (Figures 19.4e–g and 19.5c). The facial subgingival aspect is intentionally under-contoured (Figure 19.4f and g) as any convexity in this area will result in pressure on the healing soft tissues and increase risk of recession of the free gingival margin. Shaping the crown form is completed using acrylic burs (Figure 19.3i). The provisional is re-inserted to confirm the desired facial under-contour and the resulting coronal facial soft tissue level (Figure 19.3h). Fine articulating ribbon and "film strips" are used to ensure no direct occlusal contact in centric, lateral, and protrusive movements. The provisional abutment and crown are polished with pumice and glazed with Palaseal® (Heraeus-Kulzer Dental, LLC). The screw access is filled with cotton pellet and sealed with flowable composite or Fermit® (Inovar Vivadent Inc.). The provisional restoration after 4 months and the final restoration after 18 months can be seen in Figure 19.4i and j.

The patient's own tooth can be used, as demonstrated for the case shown in Figure 19.6a–h. The patient presented with internal resorption at the left mandibular central incisor (Figure 19.6a and i). The tooth was removed with immediate implant reconstruction using the modified tooth crown as the provisional (Figure 19.6b–d) restoration. The outcomes can be seen immediately post-op (Figure 19.6e), at 2 weeks (Figure 19.6f), and after 3 months just prior to the definitive restorative treatment (Figure 19.6g). The definitive restoration can be seen after 2 years in function in Figure 19.6h and j. The challenge with this approach is to achieve adequate strength of the crown form since the palatal access opening leaves a minimal thickness of tooth substance. Often, a modified natural tooth crown is too fragile and will fracture, leaving a facial veneer of dentin and enamel that can still be adequate depending on the size and positioning. Having the provisional restoration fracture or present with screw loosening during the osseointegration period can require undesirable manipulation of the implant, increasing risk of failed integration. The use of a ceramic or metal-ceramic crown removed from a failing tooth is limited as its modification and customization are difficult, if not impossible.

If there is adequate time before the procedure, a pre-fabricated custom crown can be made in the laboratory, as demonstrated in Figure 19.7. The maxillary right canine had a hopeless prognosis (Figure 19.7a and g). After minimally invasive tooth root removal, an immediate implant was placed in a palatal position and the laboratory-processed provisional crown form (Figure 19.7b) modified and luted to the abutment as described previously (Figure 19.7c). After grafting of the buccal gap, the provisional restoration was placed (Figure 19.7d). Figure 19.7e

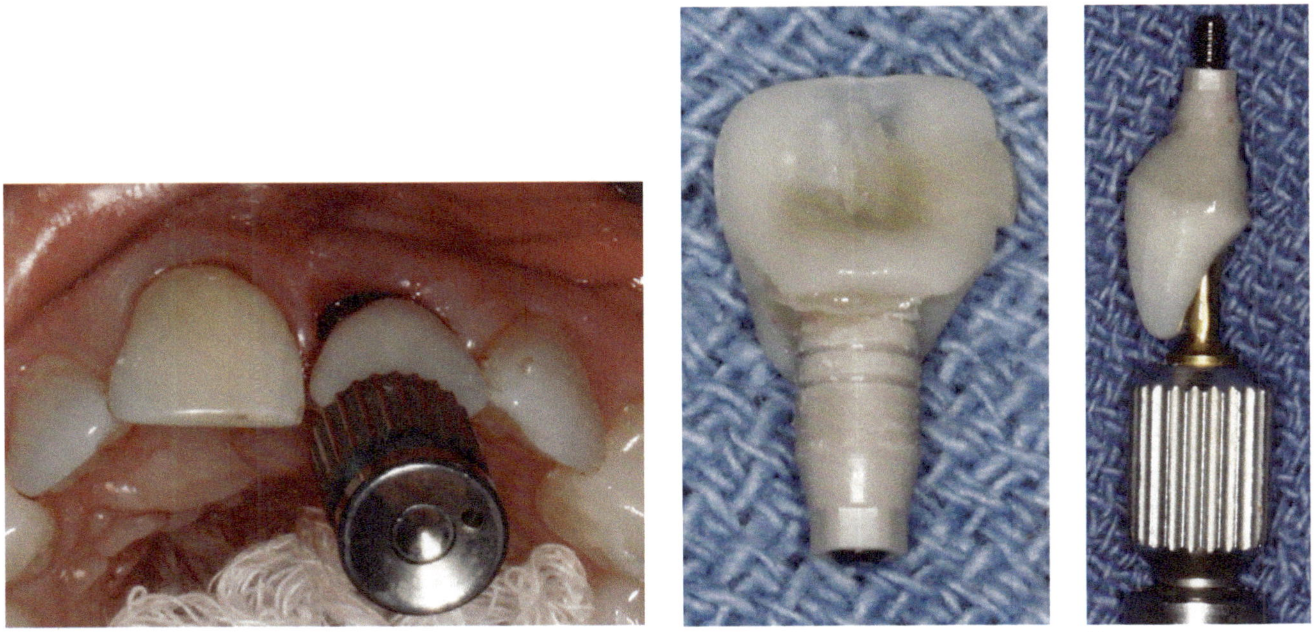

(a) (b) (c)

Figure 19.5 (a) Alternatively, after seating the crown form over the abutment and with the long-shafted driver in position (to block out the screw access opening), flowable composite can be placed in the occlusal aspect. (b) The abutment is removed from the mouth with the crestal "pick-up" intact. These direct techniques purposefully avoid the soft tissue–bone interface to prevent wound contamination and moisture. (c) The abutment surface is cleansed and dried, and the voids and subgingival portion of the abutment–temporary crown back-filled using flowable composite, shaped, and polished. *Source:* © Daniel R. Cullum

shows the patient after 1 week. The definitive restoration can be seen clinically and on a periapical radiograph after 2 years in Figure 19.7f and h.

Immediate provisional restoration with simultaneous connective tissue grafting is often considered with patients displaying a thin tissue biotype or minor gingival height discrepancies. Connective tissue and tunnel grafting (see Chapter 8) can be completed to augment the soft tissue to reduce the risk of recession during initial healing or after restorative contours are incorporated into the final restoration. After fabrication of the provisional restoration, particulate grafting of the bone gap is completed with the provisional removed from the wound. Connective tissue grafting if used is completed as the last step, requiring the surgeon to complete and place the provisional restoration. It is most uncommon for a restorative team member to be able to accomplish this process after completion of the surgical phase and grafting without damage or loss of the precisely positioned graft.

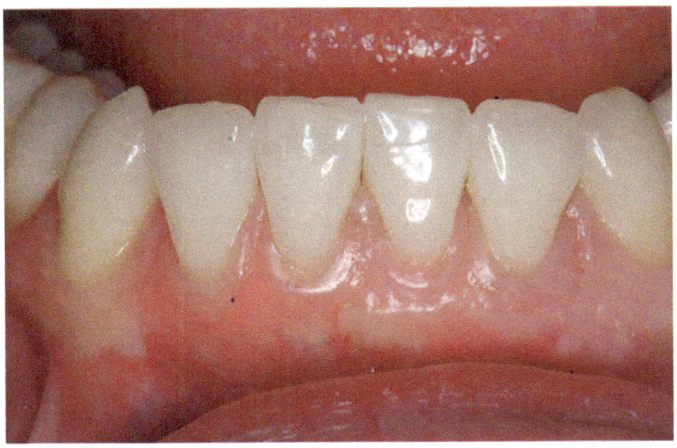

(a)

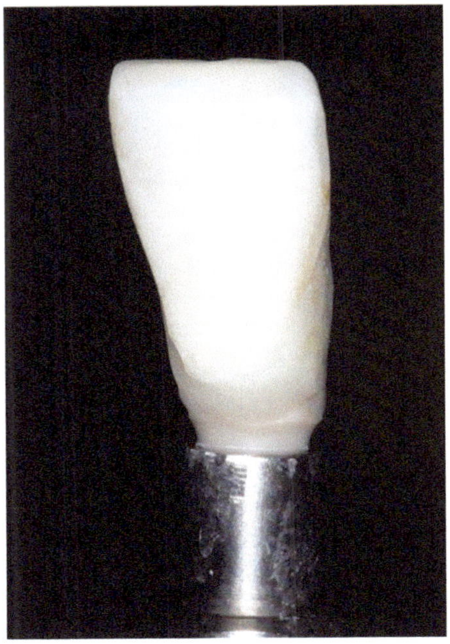

(b)

Figure 19.6 (a) A failing mandibular left central incisor. (b–d) After extraction and implant placement, the patient's tooth was used as a veneer and bonded to the temporary abutment with composite.

(Continued)

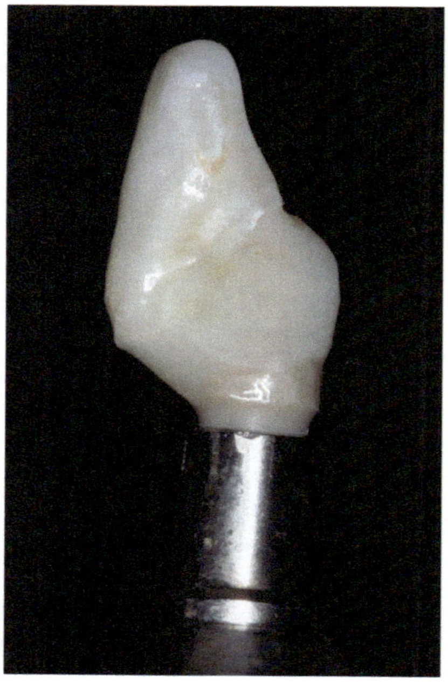

(c)

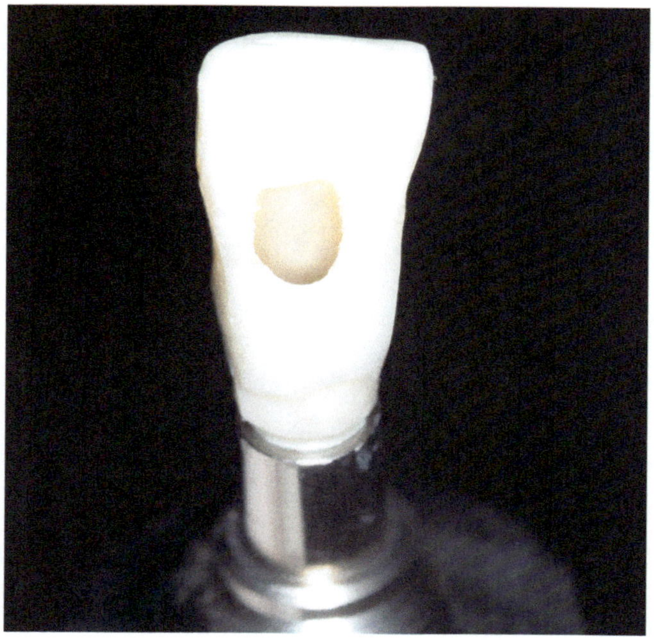

(d)

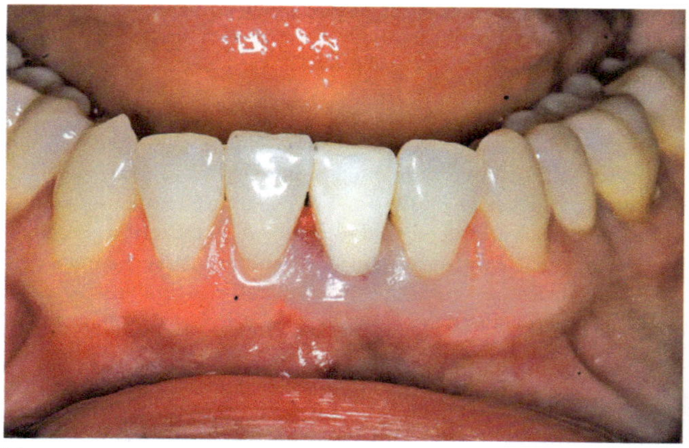

(e)

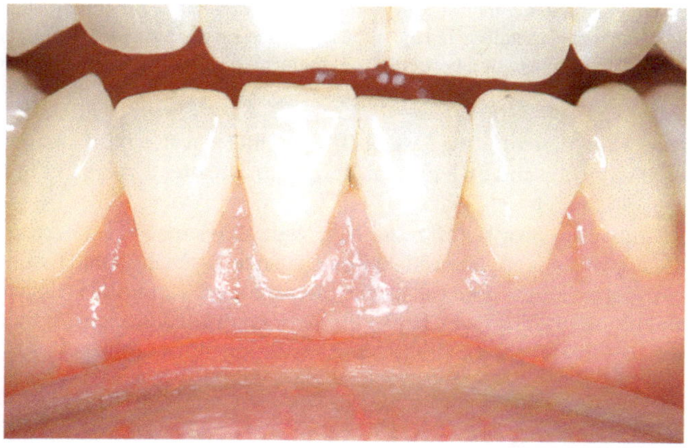

(f)

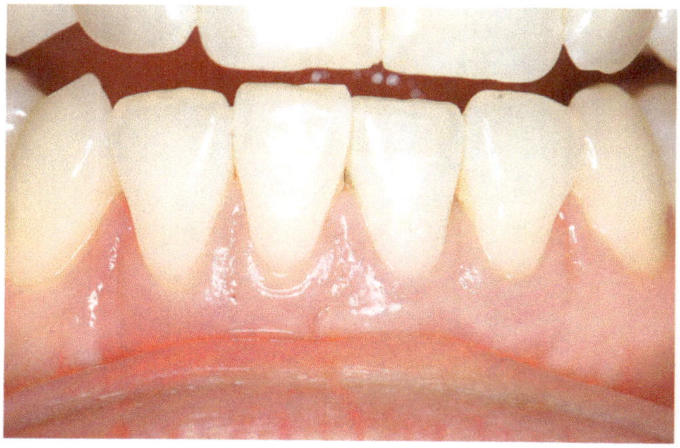

(g)

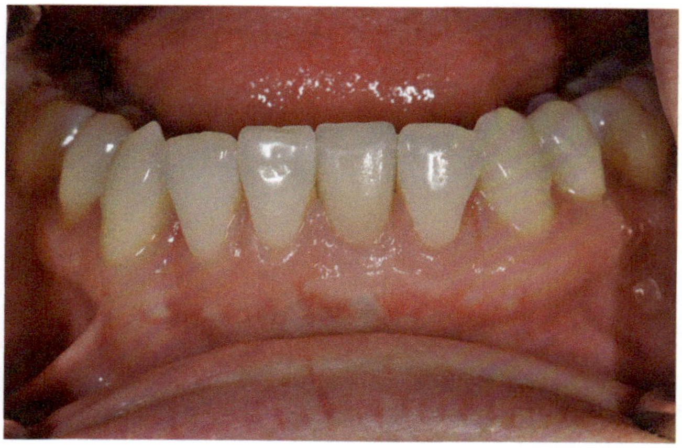

(h)

Figure 19.6 (Continued)
(e) The immediate post-operative image with the temporary crown in place. (f) The 2-week post-op situation. (g) The 3-month post-op situation. (h) The definite restoration is seen here after 2 years in function.

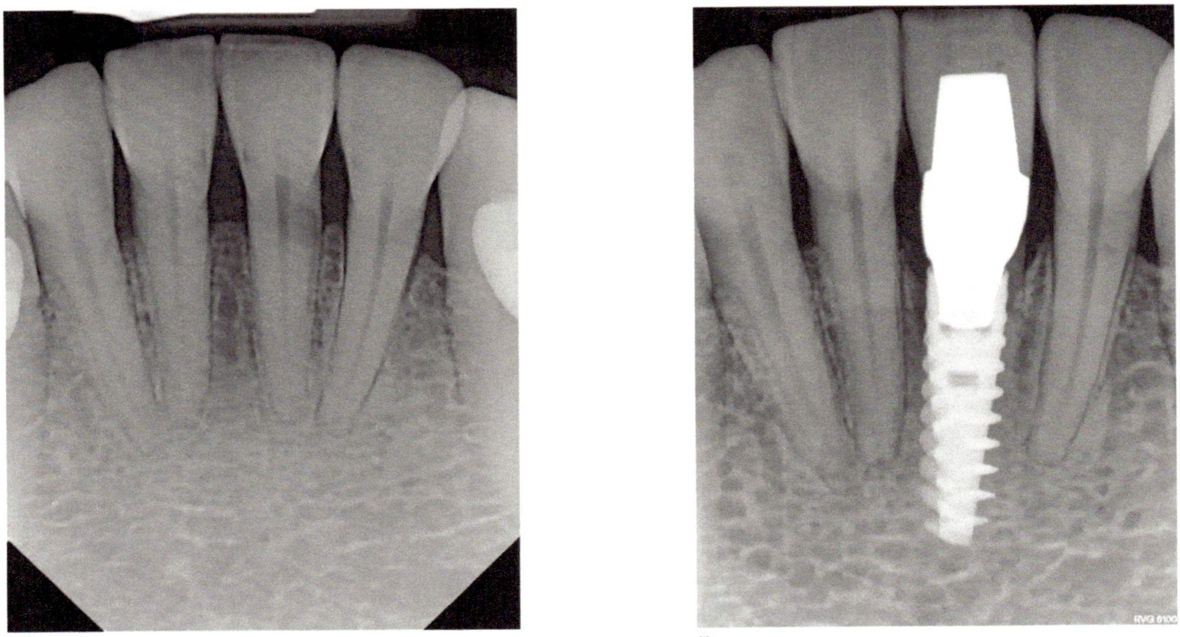

(i) (j)

Figure 19.6 (Continued)
(i) The pre-treatment periapical radiograph of the lower left central incisor with internal resorption. (j) The post-treatment periapical radiograph of the definitive restoration after 2 years in function.

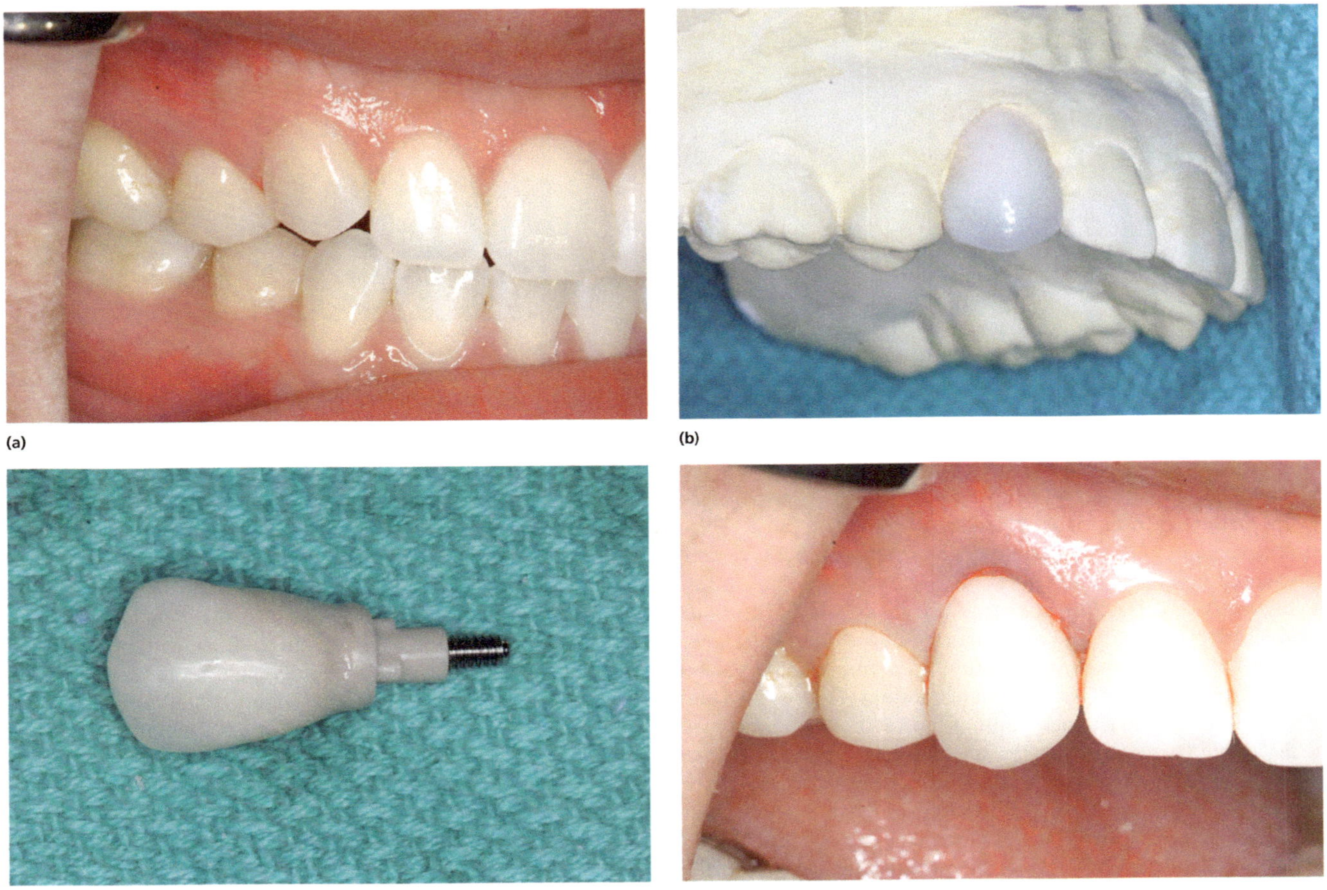

(a) (b) (c) (d)

Figure 19.7 (a) A maxillary right canine with internal root resorption. (b) A laboratory-processed acrylic crown. (c) The temporary crown converted to a screw-retained provisional. (d) The immediate post-op situation with the inserted temporary crown.

(Continued)

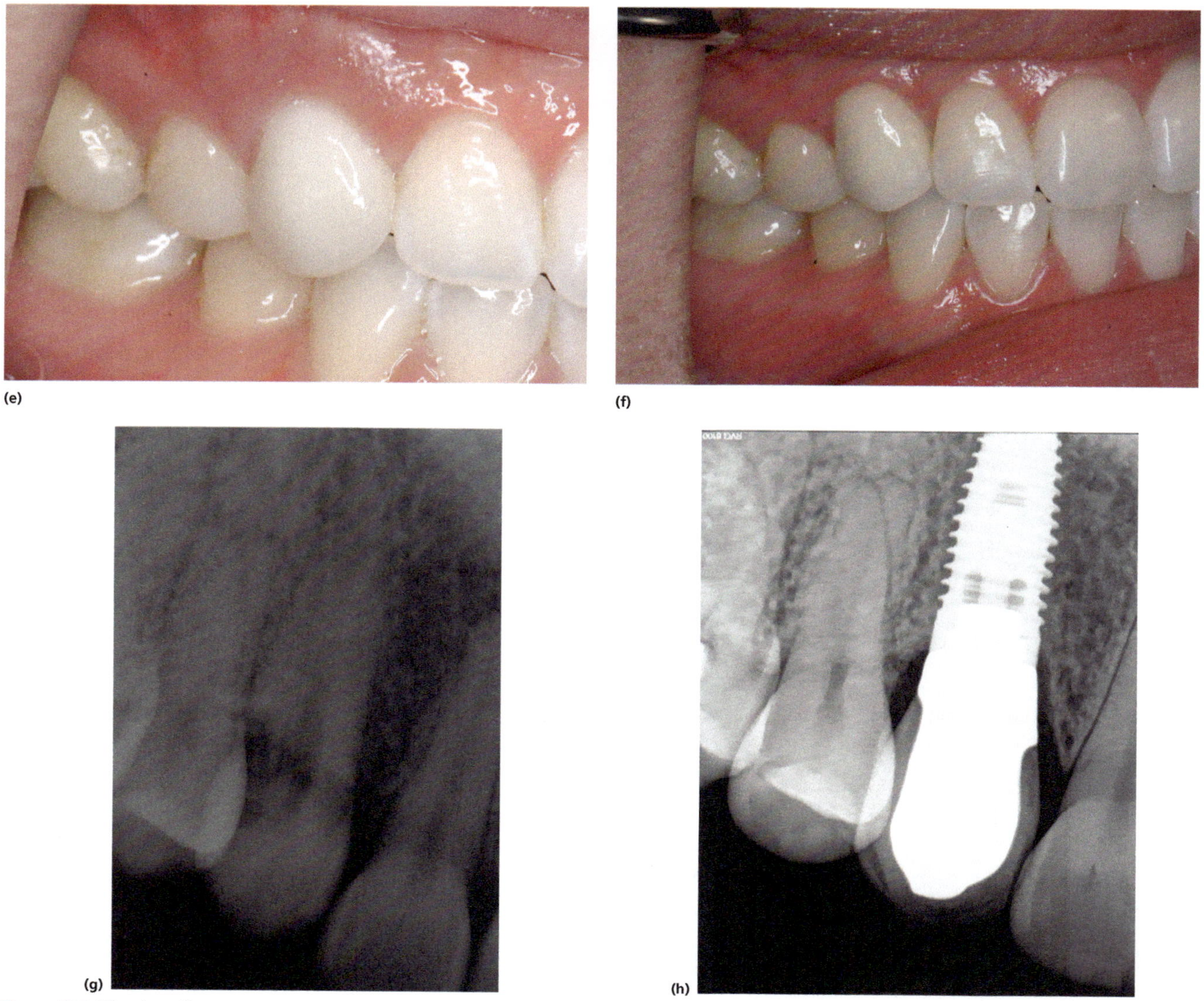

Figure 19.7 (Continued)
(e) The 1-week post-op situation. (f) The definitive restoration after 2 years in function. (g) The pre-treatment periapical radiograph showing the internal root resorption. (h) The post-restoration periapical radiograph with the definitive restoration after 2 years in function.

The patient seen in Figure 19.8a shows a 1.5 mm facial recession defect and interproximal papilla loss. Minimal bone volume was noted on cross-sectional CBCT (Figure 19.8b). After minimally invasive extraction, the facial bone was intact with bone probing depths of 2.5–3.0 mm to the gingival margin (Figure 19.8c). The initial 2 mm drill position was completed for palatal implant placement and provisional restoration (Figure 19.8d and e). Facial soft tissue augmentation, if indicated, can be achieved using tissue harvested from the maxillary tuberosity or palate. Two strategies are followed, depending on the facial soft tissue thickness encountered and the desired gingival margin position. For augmentation of a thin biotype or to enhance the root eminence, a supraperiosteal pouch can be dissected within the buccal sulcus over the root eminence region (Figure 19.8f). The dissection must be precise to maintain subsequent graft positioning. The suitably contoured graft is inserted using a horizontal mattress suture of 6-0 nylon or 4-0 polytetrafluoroethylene. The suture traverses from the vestibule through the sulcus where it is passed through the graft and back through the sulcus to the vestibule. The graft then is pulled into the pouch, increasing the overlying tissue thickness. In the case shown, the graft also was used to augment vertical tissue height with 2.5 mm of tissue exposed on the facial aspect (Figure 19.8g). There is typically adequate vascular supply from the submerged portion to support a satisfactory vertical height gain in soft tissue when used with an under-contoured provisional crown (Figure 19.8h). The immediate post-op cross-sectional CBCT demonstrates the facial bone volume after grafting of the buccal gap (Figure 19.8i), while Figure 19.8j shows the maturing soft tissue graft and under-contoured non-functional restoration at 18 days. Final clinical and radiographic images show the pleasing coronal gingival position and bone levels (Figure 19.8k and l).

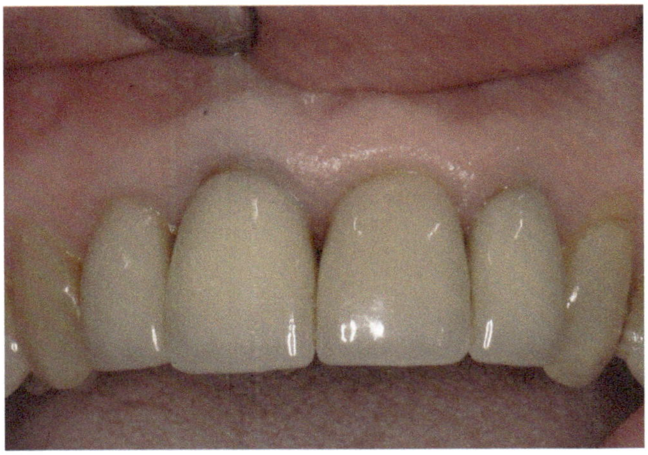

(a)

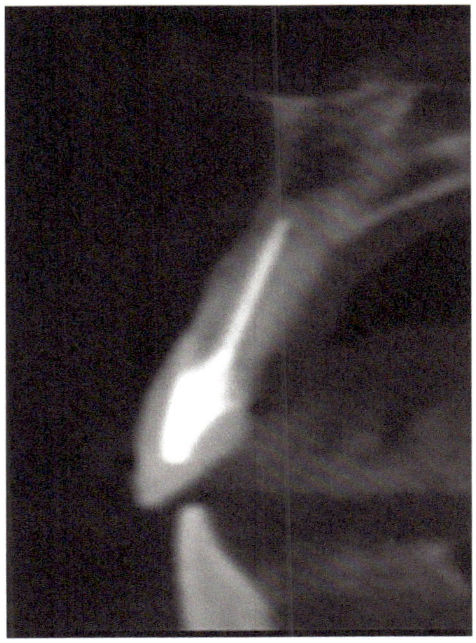

(b)

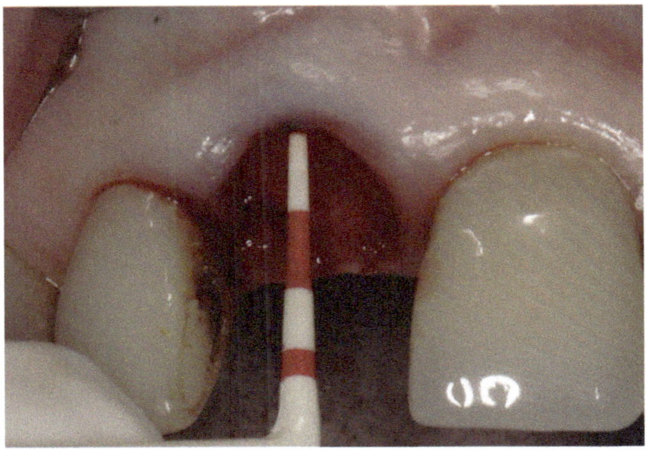

(c)

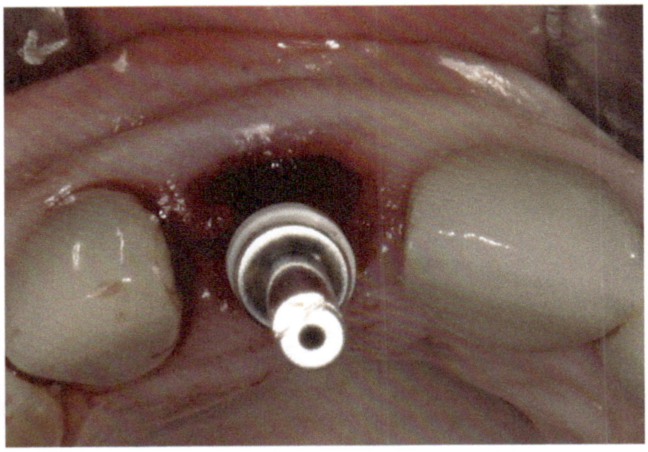

(d)

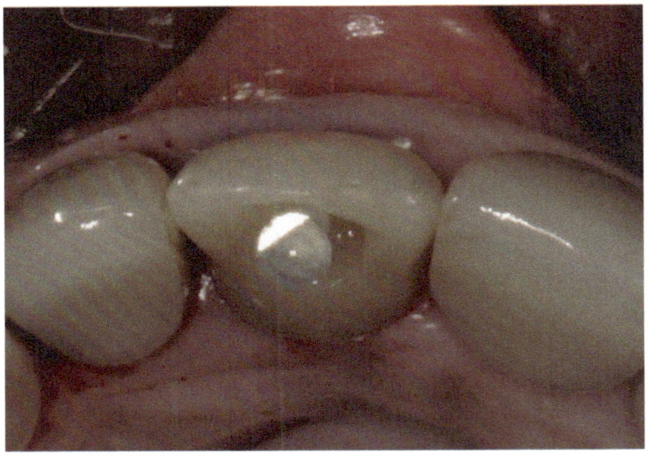

(e)

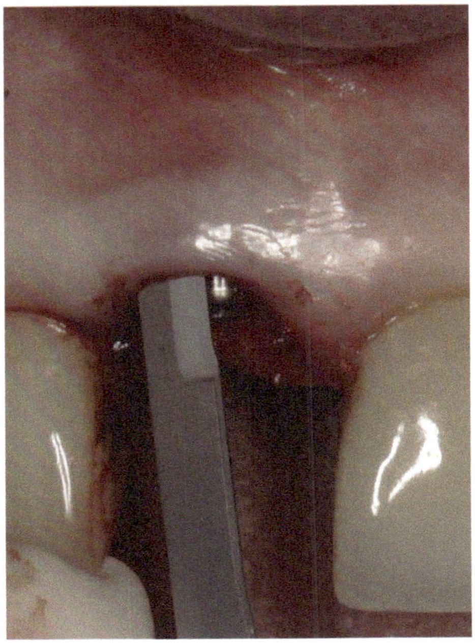

(f)

Figure 19.8 (a) This female patient presented with a 1.5 mm gingival recession at the right maxillary central incisor relative to the contralateral tooth. (b) CBCT cross-sectional images of the tooth revealed limited buccal and palatal bone volumes. (c) After minimally invasive extraction, the facial bone remained intact with bone probing depths of 2.5–3.0 mm to the gingival margin. (d) The initial 2 mm drill position was completed for palatal implant placement. (e) Provisional fabrication was completed by the "direct technique" with an under-contoured facial aspect. The provisional was removed to facilitate access for bone and soft tissue grafting. (f) A precise supraperiosteal pouch was dissected from within the buccal sulcus over the root eminence region in order to contain the grafted connective tissue in position.

(Continued)

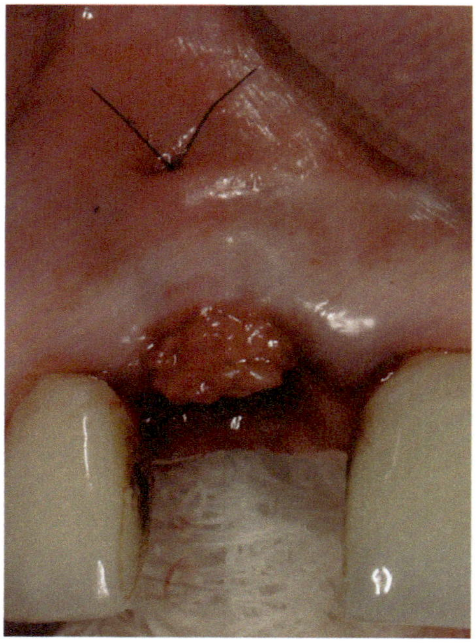
(g)

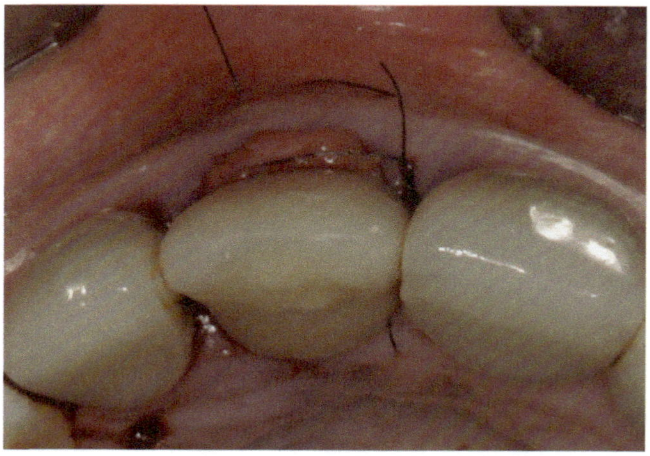
(h)

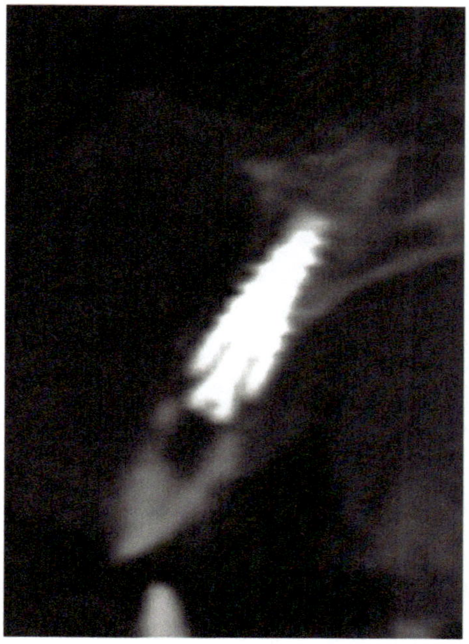
(i)

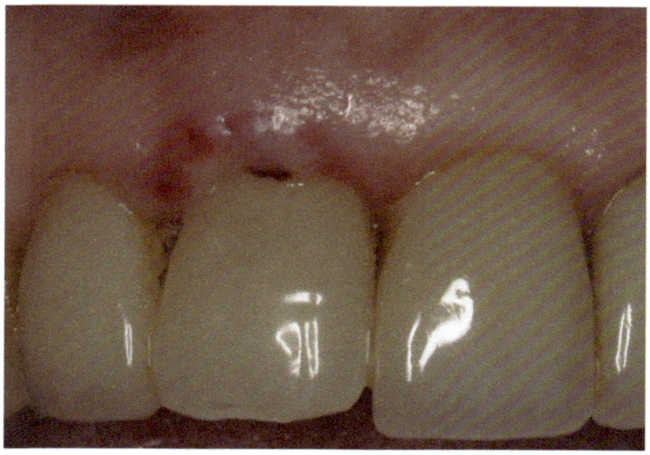
(j)

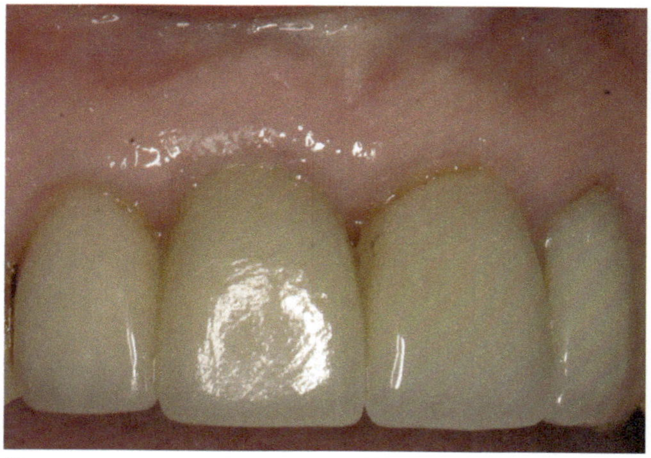
(k)

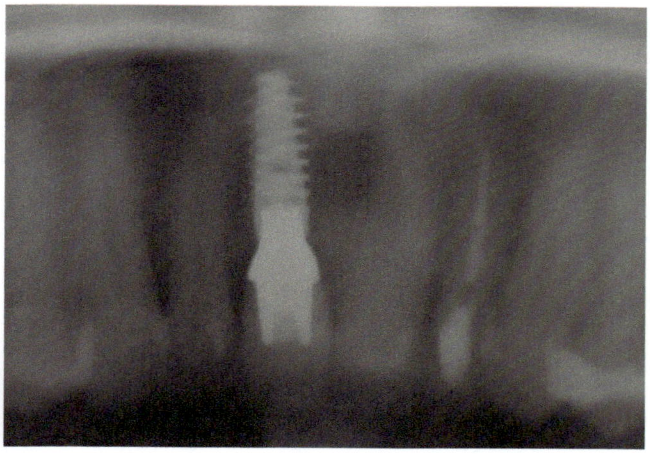
(l)

Figure 19.8 (Continued)
(g, h) An appropriately contoured graft was pulled into the pocket with a suture, and increased tissue thickness and vertical tissue height. 2.5 mm of tissue was left exposed on the facial aspect of the under-contoured provisional restoration. (i) The immediate post-op cross-sectional CBCT showed the facial bone volume after grafting of the buccal gap. (j) The maturing soft tissue graft and under-contoured non-functional restoration are seen here at 18 days. A final restoration image (k) and radiograph (l) show the coronal gingival position and bone levels. © Daniel R. Cullum

Alternately, a custom-shaped partial- or full-thickness graft from the tuberosity can be used to obturate a facial soft tissue gap enhancing tissue thickness (Figure 19.9a). The female patient shown in the figure can be seen after removal of a failing maxillary left central incisor and placement of an immediate implant and provisional restoration. The graft was trimmed to fit from the crestal bone level to fill the facial soft tissue gap and remain 1 mm coronal to the soft tissue margin. The graft was inserted with a horizontal mattress 6-0 nylon suture (Figure 19.9b and c). Figure 19.9d and e shows the pre-treatment and 13-month post-operative result with extended wear of the provisional restoration prior to definitive treatment.

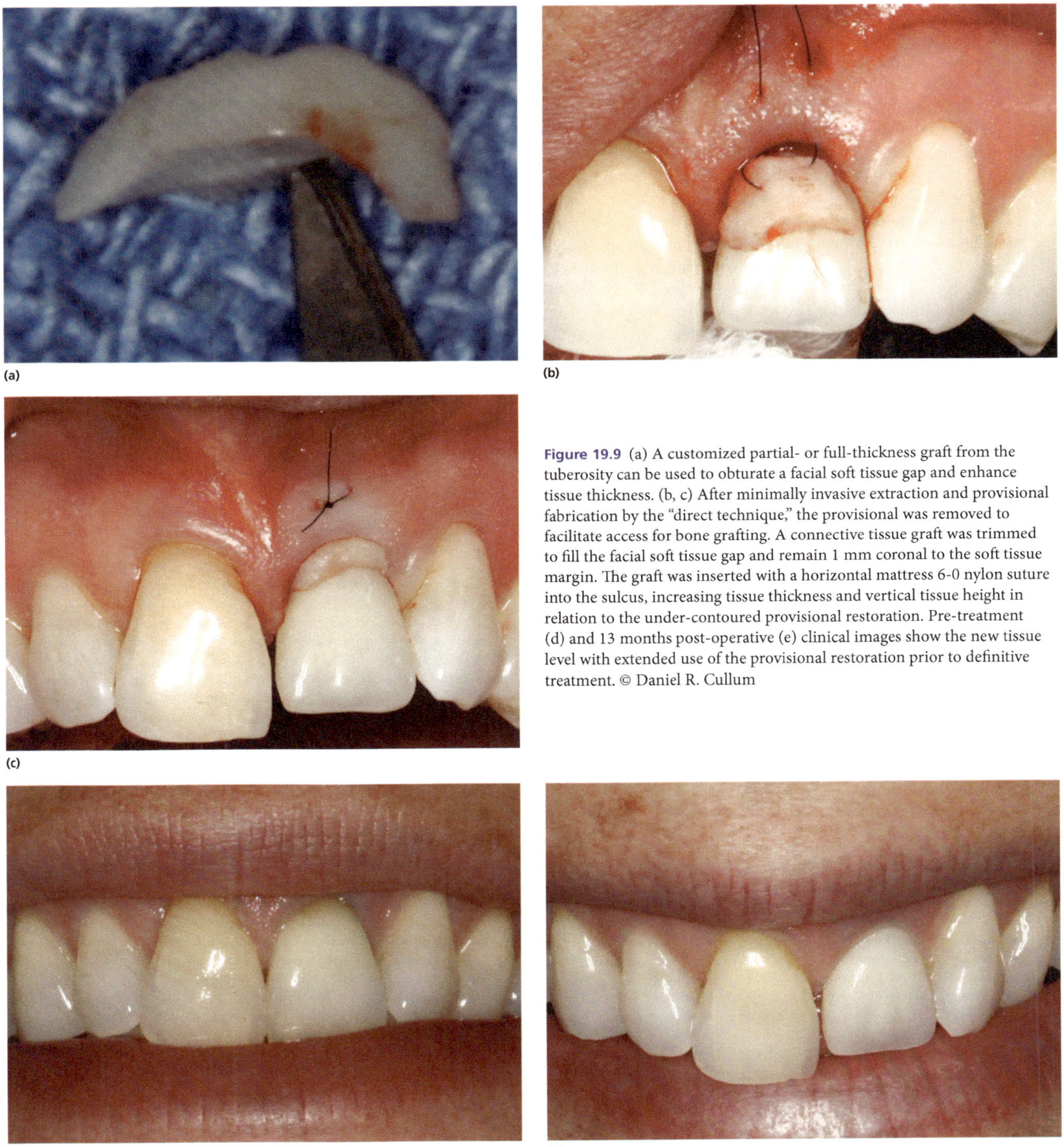

(a) (b) (c) (d) (e)

Figure 19.9 (a) A customized partial- or full-thickness graft from the tuberosity can be used to obturate a facial soft tissue gap and enhance tissue thickness. (b, c) After minimally invasive extraction and provisional fabrication by the "direct technique," the provisional was removed to facilitate access for bone grafting. A connective tissue graft was trimmed to fill the facial soft tissue gap and remain 1 mm coronal to the soft tissue margin. The graft was inserted with a horizontal mattress 6-0 nylon suture into the sulcus, increasing tissue thickness and vertical tissue height in relation to the under-contoured provisional restoration. Pre-treatment (d) and 13 months post-operative (e) clinical images show the new tissue level with extended use of the provisional restoration prior to definitive treatment. © Daniel R. Cullum

Conclusions

Achieving esthetically pleasing results when replacing a single missing anterior tooth with a dental implant requires application of the prosthetic and surgical principles discussed in this chapter. Utilizing flapless procedures for tooth extraction, grafting hard and soft tissues, and proper placement of the implant in three dimensions give the operator the best prospect of achieving immediate provisionalization. Immediate provisional restoration can maintain interproximal soft tissue support; however, the facial emergence profile should remain flat or concave during the initial healing interval. After osseointegration, peri-implant tissues can be further developed to the desired final restorative contours (see Chapter 4). Minimally invasive immediate implant placement with immediate provisional restoration provides a great service to the patient as it eliminates the need for a removable appliance. It is also a great benefit to the restorative dentist in maintaining near-normal gingival sulcus parameters, enhancing treatment outcomes significantly. Having an intact buccal plate has long been accepted as a prerequisite for immediate implant placement in order to achieve esthetic results. However, this requirement has been recently challenged as many have reported good results in this situation with palatal implant positioning, grafting of an adequate facial gap, and, if need be, simultaneous connective tissue grafting. Immediate implantation and provisional restoration are evidence-based treatments, but demand the highest levels of artistry, clinical skills, and perseverance. It has been the experience of both of us independently over 14 years of utilizing flapless placement and immediate provisional restoration that proper placement of the implant and with an under-contoured facial gingival margin are more critical to achieving good long-term esthetic results than having an intact buccal plate of bone.

References

1. Schulte W, Kleineikenscheidt H, Lindner K, et al. The Tübingen immediate implant in clinical studies. Dtsch Zahnarztl Z 1978; 33: 348–359 (in German).
2. De Rouck T, Collys K, Cosyn J. Immediate single-tooth implants in the anterior maxilla: a 1-year case cohort study on hard and soft tissue response. J Clin Periodontol 2008; 35: 649–657.
3. Grunder U. Stability of the mucosal topography around single-tooth implants and adjacent teeth: 1-year results. Int J Periodontics Restorative Dent 2000; 20: 11–17.
4. Palattella P, Toreslo F, Cordarro L. Two-year prospective clinical comparison of immediate replacement vs. immediate restoration of single tooth in the esthetic zone. Clin Oral Implants Res 2008; 19: 1148–1153.
5. Kan J, Rungcharassaeng K, Liddelow G, et al. Peri-implant tissue response following immediate provisional restoration of scalloped implants in the esthetic zone: a one-year pilot prospective multicenter study. J Prosthetic Dent 2007; 97: s109–s118.
6. Kan J, Rungcharasseang K, Lozada J, et al. Facial gingival tissue stability following immediate placement and provisionalization of maxillary anterior single implants: a 2- to-8-year follow-up. Int J Oral Maxillofac Implants 2011; 26: 179–187.
7. Chang M, Wennstrom J, Odman P, et al. Implant supported single-tooth replacement compared to contralateral natural teeth: crown and soft tissue dimensions. Clin Oral Implants Res 1999; 10: 185–194.
8. Small P, Tarnow D. Gingival recession around implants: a 1-year longitudinal prospective study. Int J Oral Maxillofac Implants 2000; 15: 527–532.
9. Hämmerle C, Chen S, Wilson T. Consensus statement and recommended clinical procedures regarding the placement of implants in extraction sockets. Int J Oral Maxillofac Implants 2004; 19(Suppl): 26–28.
10. Kan J, Rungcharassaeng K, Sclar A, et al. Effect of the facial osseous defect morphology on gingival dynamics after immediate tooth replacement and guided bone regeneration: 1-year results. J Oral Maxillofac Surg 2007; 65(Suppl 1): 13–19.
11. Kan J, Rungcharassaeng K, Lozada J. Immediate placement and provisionalization of maxillary anterior single implants: 1-year prospective study. Int J Oral Maxillofac Implants 2003; 18: 31–39.
12. Valentini P, Abensur D, Albertini J, et al. Immediate provisionalization of single extraction-site implants in the esthetic zone: a clinical evaluation. Int J Periodontics Restorative Dent 2010; 30: 41–51.
13. Huynh-Ba G, Pjetursson B, Sanz M, et al. Analysis of the socket wall dimensions in the upper maxilla in relation to immediate implant placement. Clin Oral Implants Res 2010; 21: 37–42.
14. Braut V, Bornstein M, Belser U, et al. Thickness of the anterior maxillary facial bone wall – a retrospective radiographic study using cone beam computed tomography. Int J Periodontics Restorative Dent 2011; 31: 125–131.
15. Vera C, De Kok I, Reinhold D, et al. Evaluation of buccal alveolar bone dimension of maxillary anterior and premolar teeth: a cone beam computed tomography investigation. Int J Maxillofac Implants 2012; 27: 1514–1519.
16. Januário A, Duarte W, Barriviera M, et al. Dimension of the facial bone wall in the anterior maxilla: a cone-beam computed tomography study. Clin Oral Implants Res 2011; 22: 1168–1171.
17. Park HH. A Chair-side Technique for Immediate Implant Placement with Immediate Provisionalization to Optimize Esthetic Outcome. Selected Readings in Oral and Maxillofacial Surgery. San Francisco, CA: Guild for Scientific Advancement in Oral and Maxillofacial Surgery, 2011, vol. 19, no. 2.
18. Adell R, Lekholm U, Rockler B, Brånemark P-I. A 15-year study of osseointegrated implants in the treatment of the edentulous jaw. Int J Oral Maxillofac Surg 1981; 10: 387–416.
19. Schnitman P, Wöhrle P, Rubenstein J. Immediate fixed interim prostheses supported by two-stage threaded implants: methodology and results. J Oral Implantol 1990; 16: 96–105.
20. Ericsson I, Nilson H, Lindh T, et al. Immediate functional loading of Brånemark single tooth implants. An 18 months' clinical pilot follow-up study. Clin Oral Implants Res 2000; 11: 26–33.
21. Wöhrle P. Single-tooth replacement in the aesthetic zone with immediate provisionalization: fourteen consecutive cases report. Pract Periodontics Aesthet Dent 1998; 10: 1107–1114.
22. Kan J, Rungcharassaeng K. Immediate placement and provisionalization of maxillary anterior single implants: a surgical and prosthodontic rationale. Pract Periodontics Aesthet Dent 2000; 12: 817–824.
23. Norton M. A short-term clinical evaluation of immediately restored maxillary TiOblast single-tooth implants. Int J Oral Maxillofac Implants 2004; 19: 274–281.
24. De Kok I, Chang S, Moriarty J, et al. A retrospective analysis of peri-implant tissue responses at immediate loaded/provisionalized micro-threaded implants. Int J Oral Maxillofac Implants 2006; 21: 405–412.
25. De Rouck T, Collys K, Cosyn J. Single-tooth replacement in the anterior maxilla by means of immediate implantation and provisionalization: a review. Int J Oral Maxillofac Implants 2008; 23: 897–904.
26. Crespi R, Capparé P, Gherlone E, et al. Immediate versus delayed loading of dental implants placed in fresh extraction sockets in the maxillary esthetic zone: a clinical comparative study. Int J Oral Maxillofac Implants 2008; 23: 753–758.
27. Cornelini R, Cangini F, Covani U, et al. Immediate restoration of implants placed into fresh extraction sockets for single-tooth replacement: a prospective clinical study. Int J Periodontics Restorative Dent 2005; 25: 439–447.
28. Groisman M, Frossard W, Ferreira H, et al. Single-tooth implants in the maxillary incisor region with immediate provisionalization: 2-year prospective study. Pract Proced Aesthet Dent 2003; 15: 115–122.
29. Grunder U, Gracis S, Capelli M. Influence of the 3-D bone-to-implant relationship on esthetics. Int J Periodontics Restorative Dent 2005; 25: 113–119.
30. Becker W, Hujoel P, Becker B. Effect of barrier membranes and autologous bone grafts on ridge width preservation around implants. Clin Implant Dent Relat Res 2002; 4: 143–149.
31. Chen S, Darby I, Adams G, et al. A prospective clinical study of bone augmentation techniques at immediate implants. Clin Oral Implants Res 2005; 16: 176–184.
32. Lee E, Gonzalez-Martin O, Fiorellini J. Lingualized flapless implant placement into fresh extraction sockets preserves buccal alveolar bone: a cone beam computed tomography study. Int J Periodontics Restorative Dent 2014; 34: 61–68.
33. Tsoukaki M, Kalpidis C, Sakellari D, et al. Clinical, radiographic, microbiological and immunological outcomes of flapped vs flapless dental implants: a prospective randomized controlled clinical trial. Clin Oral Implants Res 2013; 24: 969–976.
34. Crespi R, Cappare P, Gherlone E, Romanos G. Immediate provisionalization of dental implants placed in fresh extraction sockets using a flapless technique. Int J Periodontics Restorative Dent 2012; 32: 29–37.
35. De Carvalho B, de Carvalho E, Consani R. Flapless single-tooth immediate implant placement. Int J Oral Maxillofac Implants 2013; 28: 783–789.
36. Kan J, Morimoto T, Rungcharassaeng K. Gingival biotype assessment in the esthetic zone: visual versus direct measurement. Int J Periodontics Restorative Dent 2010; 30: 237–243.
37. Grunder U. Crestal ridge width changes when placing implants at the time of tooth extraction with and without soft tissue augmentation after a healing period of 6 months: report of 24 consecutive cases. Int J Periodontics Restorative Dent 2011; 31: 9–17.

38. Rungcharassaeng K, Kan J, Yoshino S, et al. Immediate implant placement and provisionalization with and without a connective tissue graft: an analysis of facial gingival tissue thickness. Int J Periodontics Restorative Dent 2012; 32: 657–663.
39. Lam R. Contour changes of the alveolar process following tooth extraction. An experimental study in the dog. J Clin Periodontol 1960; 10: 25–32.
40. Johnson K. A study of the dimensional changes occurring in the maxilla following tooth extraction. Aust Dent J 1969; 14: 241–244.
41. Schropp L, Kostopoulos L, Wenzel A. Bone healing following immediate versus delayed placement of titanium implants into extraction sockets – a prospective clinical study. Int J Oral Maxillofac Implants 2003; 18: 189–199.
42. Botticelli D, Berglundh T, Lindhe J. Hard-tissue alterations following immediate implant placement in extraction sites. J Clin Periodontol 2004; 31: 820–828.
43. Araújo M, Sukekava F, Wennstrom J, Lindhe J. Ridge alterations following implant placement in fresh extraction sockets: an experimental study in the dog. J Clin Periodontol 2005; 32: 645–652.
44. Araújo M, Sukekava F, Wennstrom J, Lindhe J. Tissue modeling following implant placement in fresh extraction sockets. Clin Oral Implants Res 2006; 17: 615–624.
45. Trombelli L, Farina R, Marzola A, et al. Modeling and remodeling of human extraction sockets. J Clin Periodontol 2008; 35: 630–639.
46. Qahash M, Susin C, Polimeni G, et al. Bone healing dynamics at buccal peri-implant sites. Clin Oral Implants Res 2008; 19: 166–172.
47. Spray J, Black C, Morris H, et al. The influence of bone thickness on facial marginal bone response: stage 1 placement through stage 2 uncovering. Ann Periodontol 2000; 5: 119–128.
48. De Rouck T, Collys K, Cosyn J. Immediate single-tooth implants in the anterior maxilla: a 1-year case cohort study on hard and soft tissue response. J Clin Periodontol 2008; 35: 649–657.
49. Evans C, Chen S. Esthetic outcomes of immediate implant placements. Clin Oral Implants Res 2007; 19: 73–80.
50. De Rouck T, Collys K, Wyn I, et al. Instant provisionalization of immediate single-tooth implants is essential to optimize esthetic treatment outcome. Clin Oral Implants Res 2008; 20: 566–570.
51. Lebene R, Glickman I. The response of alveolar bone to grinding with rotary diamond stones. J Periodontol 1963; 34: 105–119.
52. Caffesse R, Ramfjord S, Nasjleti C. Reverse bevel periodontal flaps in monkeys. J Periodontol 1968; 39: 219–235.
53. Wood D, Hoag P, Donnenfeld O, et al. Alveolar crest reduction following full and partial thickness flaps. J Periodontol 1973; 43: 141–144.
54. Blanco J, Nunez V, Aracil L, et al. Ridge alteration following immediate implant placement in the dog: flap versus flapless surgery. J Clin Periodontol 2008; 35: 640–648.
55. Chen S, Darby I, Reynolds E. A prospective clinical study of non-submerged immediate implants. Clin Oral Implants Res 2007; 18: 552–562.
56. Araújo M, Linder E, Lindhe J. Bio-Oss Collagen® in the buccal gap at immediate implants: a 6 months study in dog. Clin Oral Implant Res 2011; 22: 1–8.
57. Assaf J, Zanatta F, de Brito R Jr, et al. Computed tomographic evaluation of alterations of the buccolingual width of the alveolar ridge after immediate implant placement associated with the use of a synthetic bone substitute. Int J Oral Maxillofac Implants 2013; 28: 757–763.
58. Caneva M, Botticelli D, Rossi F, et al. Influence of implants with different sizes and configurations installed immediately into extraction sockets on peri-implant hard and soft tissues. An experimental study in dogs. Clin Oral Implants Res 2012; 23: 396–401.
59. Schroeder H. The Periodontium. Berlin: Springer Verlag, 1986.
60. Araújo M, Lindhe J. Dimensional ridge alterations following tooth extraction. An experimental study in the dog. J Clin Periodontol 2005; 32: 212–218.
61. Schulze R, Berndt D, d'Hoedt B. On cone-beam computed tomography artifacts induced by titanium implants. Clin Oral Implants Res 2010; 21: 100–107.
62. Naitoh M, Hayashi H, Tsukamoto N, et al. Labial bone assessment surrounding dental implant using cone-beam computed tomography: an *in vitro* study. Clin Oral Implants Res 2012; 23: 970–974.
63. Razavi T, Palmer R, Davies J, et al. Accuracy of measuring the cortical bone thickness adjacent to dental implants using cone beam computed tomography. Clin Oral Implants Res 2010; 21: 718–725.
64. Roe P, Kan J, Rungcharassaeng K, et al. Horizontal and vertical dimensional changes of peri-implant facial bone following immediate placement and provisionalization of maxillary anterior single implants: a 1-year cone beam computed tomography study. Int J Oral Maxillofac Implants 2012; 27: 393–400.
65. Benic G, Mokti M, Chen C, et al. Dimensions of buccal bone and mucosa at immediately placed implants after 7 years: a clinical and cone beam computed tomography study. Clin Oral Implants Res 2012; 23: 560–566.
66. Lau S, Chow J, Li W, et al. Classification of maxillary central incisors – implications for immediate implant in the esthetic zone. J Oral Maxillofac Surg 2011; 69: 142–153.
67. Salama H, Salama MA, Garber D, et al. The interproximal height of bone: a guidepost to predictable aesthetic strategic and soft tissue contours in anterior tooth replacement. Pract Periodontics Aesthet Dent 1998; 10: 1131–1141.
68. Grunder U. Stability of the mucosal topography around single-tooth implants and adjacent teeth: 1-year results. Int J Periodontics Restorative Dent 2000; 20: 11–17.
69. Choquet V, Hermans M, Adriaenssens P, et al. Clinical and radiographic evaluation of the papilla level adjacent to single-tooth dental implants. A retrospective study in the maxillary anterior region. J Periodontol 2001; 72: 1364–1371.
70. Kan J, Rungcharassaeng K. Inter-implant papilla preservation in the esthetic zone: a report of six consecutive cases. Int J Periodontics Restorative Dent 2003; 23: 249–259.
71. Jofre J, Valenzuela D, Quintana P, Asenjo-Lobos C. Protocol for immediate implant replacement of infected teeth. Implant Dent 2012; 21: 287–294.
72. Lang N, Pun L, Lau K, et al. A systematic review on survival and success rates of implants placed immediately into fresh extraction sockets after at least 1 year. Clin Oral Implants Res 2012; 23(Suppl 5): 39–66.
73. Pjetursson BE, Thoma D, Jung R, et al. A systematic review of the survival and complication rates of implant-supported fixed dental prostheses (FDPs) after a mean observation period of at least 5 years. Clin Oral Implants Res 2012; 23: 22–38.

SECTION VI

Comprehensive Applications of Minimally Invasive Surgery

CHAPTER 20

Skeletal Anchorage and Orthodontics in Implant Site Development

Michael P. Chaffee[1] **& Daniel R. Cullum**[2]
[1]Private Practice, Coeur d'Alene, ID, USA
[2]Private Practice, Coeur d'Alene, ID; Loma Linda University Department of OMS, Loma Linda, CA; UCLA Department of OMS, Los Angeles, CA, USA

Introduction

Eklund and Creekmore[1] first described the use of a bone screw for maxillary incisor intrusion, introducing skeletal anchorage to the field of orthodontics. Limitations of anchorage with conventional orthodontic mechanics are often addressed with surgical intervention or headgear appliances. While orthognathic surgery allows the practitioner to achieve optimal 3-D positioning, many patients choose not to pursue surgery due to cost and other reasons. Utilizing temporary anchorage devices (TADs) in many complex cases can help to achieve acceptable results without orthognathic surgical intervention.[2–4] Skeletal anchorage gives the capability of enhanced orthodontic control in all three planes of space.[5] The use of orthopedic bone screws and plates, mini-implants, and/or endosseous dental implants has been advocated to enhance orthodontic control in the vertical, horizontal, and transverse dimensions. Additionally, moving teeth through alveolar segments can optimize bone and soft tissue dimensions, correct asymmetry, and level occlusal plane. Minimally invasive dental implant surgery can be greatly facilitated by the skilled application of orthodontic treatment for site development and enhancement of occlusal, functional, and esthetic outcomes.

Temporary anchorage devices

TADs include surgical plates and micro-screw implants of many different designs. Modified surgical bone plates or plates specifically designed and fabricated for orthodontic purposes can be used (Figure 20.1a). These have the advantage of remote and monocortical screw placement, reducing the risk of damage to adjacent teeth. Micro-screw implants, also known as orthodontic mini-screws, come in a myriad of designs (Figure 20.1b). With rare exception, micro-screw implants have a machine-surfaced finish and are not designed to osseointegrate, with most being self-drilling (i.e. not requiring a pilot hole). They range in diameter from 1.2 to 2.0 mm with screw lengths from 4 to 12 mm. Head designs can vary significantly, and usually include an undercut, an opening, and/or a bracket slot. The length of the screw and head design should be chosen by the orthodontist based on the preferred orthodontic mechanics. Mini-plates and mini-screws are inserted with a limited surgical incision for access (Figure 20.1c and d) and irrigation during drilling, or using trans-mucosal placement for self-tapping designs (Figure 20.1a–f).

The anterior–posterior dimension

Orthodontic treatment mechanics can sometimes require maximum anterior–posterior (A–P) anchorage, which historically has been achieved extraorally using headgear appliances. However, patient compliance with headgear often is unpredictable and less than ideal, and obtaining absolute anchorage is difficult. Placement of standard endosseous dental implants, micro-screw implants, or bone plates can provide absolute anchorage, reducing compliance issues on the part of the patient.[6] Figure 20.2 demonstrates the pretreatment images for a patient with the use of micro-screw implants to achieve A–P anchorage.

An adolescent female presented with congenitally missing mandibular lateral incisors and a missing maxillary right second premolar (Figure 20.2). Treating the case using non-extraction in the lower arch would have caused both a significant increase in the lower inter-canine distance (shown to lead to instability) as well as excess proclination of the lower incisors. In addition, the patient would have incurred prosthetic costs to replace the missing teeth. Another approach to treat this class I skeletal case would have been to remove the remaining maxillary second premolar and over-retained right second primary molar. However, maximum maxillary anchorage was needed to prevent the mesial migration of the upper posterior teeth during space closure. Without complete anchorage, a class I molar relationship would not have been maintained, and patient compliance with headgear was also a concern. The chosen treatment plan included maxillary second premolar extraction and placement of bilateral micro-screw implants in the maxillary arch mesial to the first molars to achieve complete A–P control. Figure 20.3 shows the retraction mechanics associated with the TADs.

Minimally Invasive Dental Implant Surgery, First Edition. Edited by Daniel R. Cullum and Douglas Deporter.

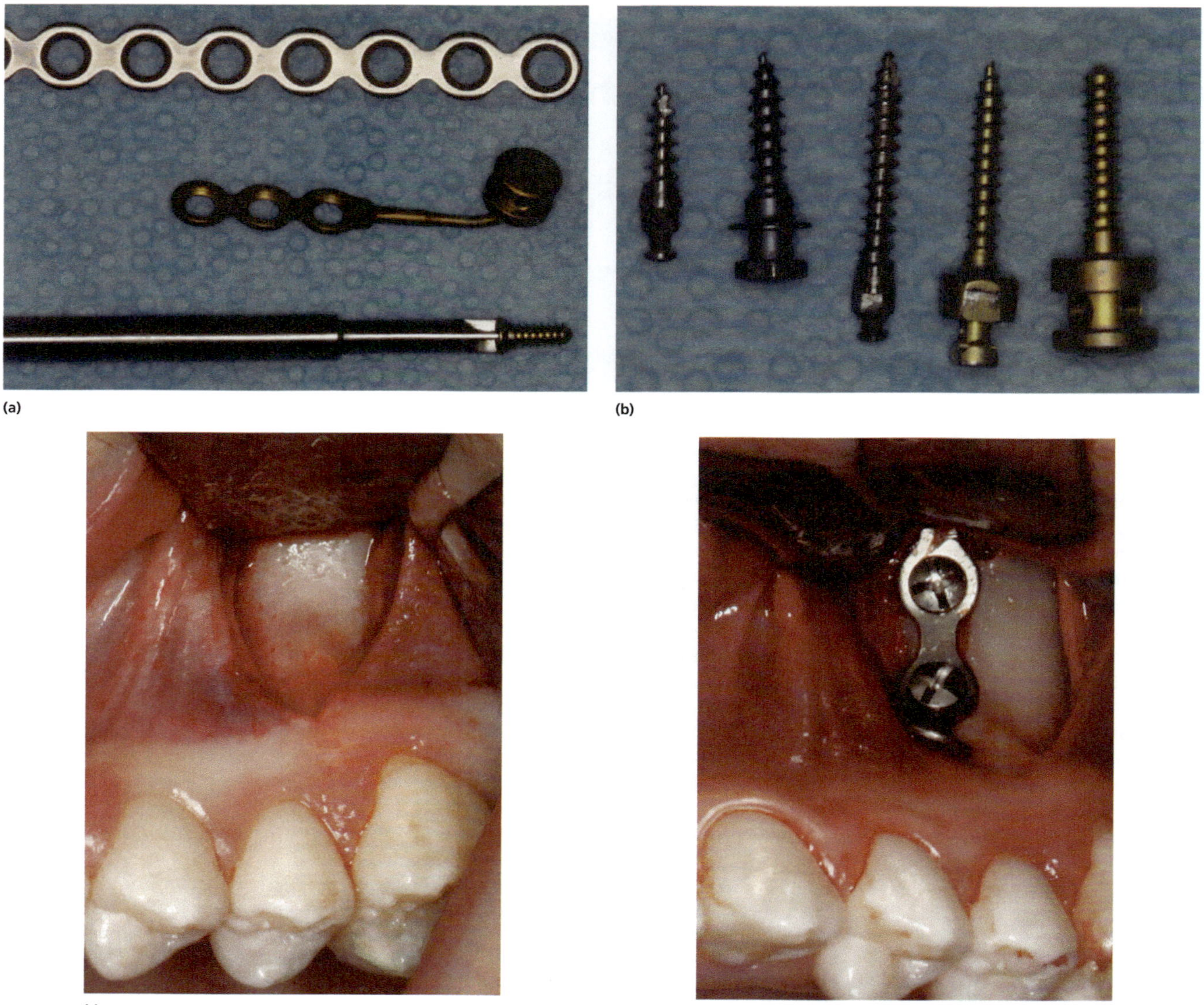

(a) (b) (c) (d)

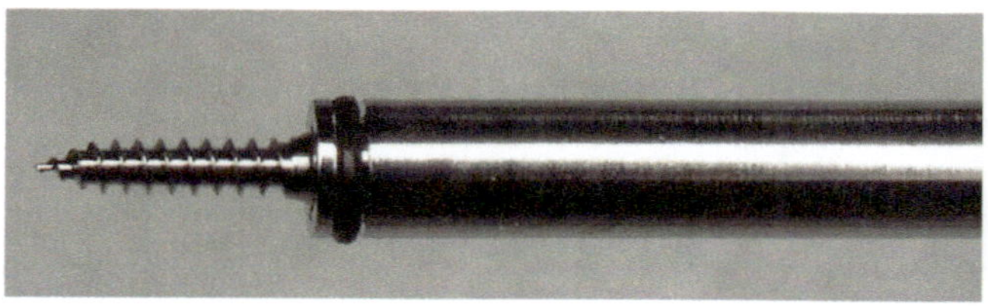

(e)

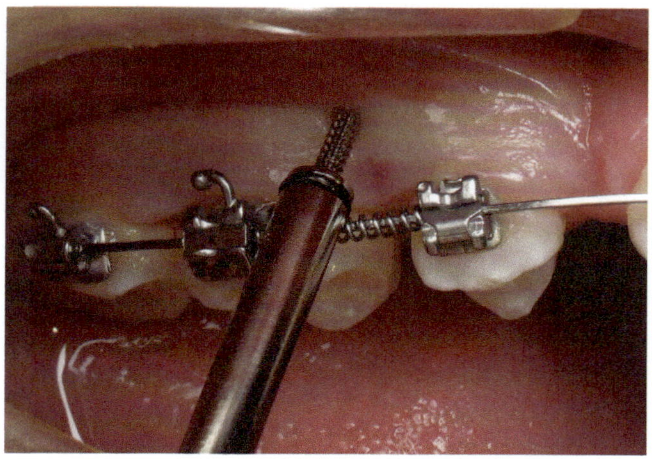

(f)

Figure 20.1 (a) Modified surgical bone plates or plates specifically designed and fabricated for orthodontics can be used for skeletal anchorage. (b) Orthodontic mini-screws range in diameter from 1.2 to 2.0 mm and lengths from 4 to 12 mm. Head designs can vary significantly and usually include an undercut, an opening, a bracket-like design, or a combination of these design features. (c, d) Minimal surgical access is necessary for mini-plate placement. (e, f) Alternatively, a self-tapping mini-screw can be placed in the driver and inserted trans-mucosally in the root interspace. *Source:* (a–d) © Daniel R. Cullum

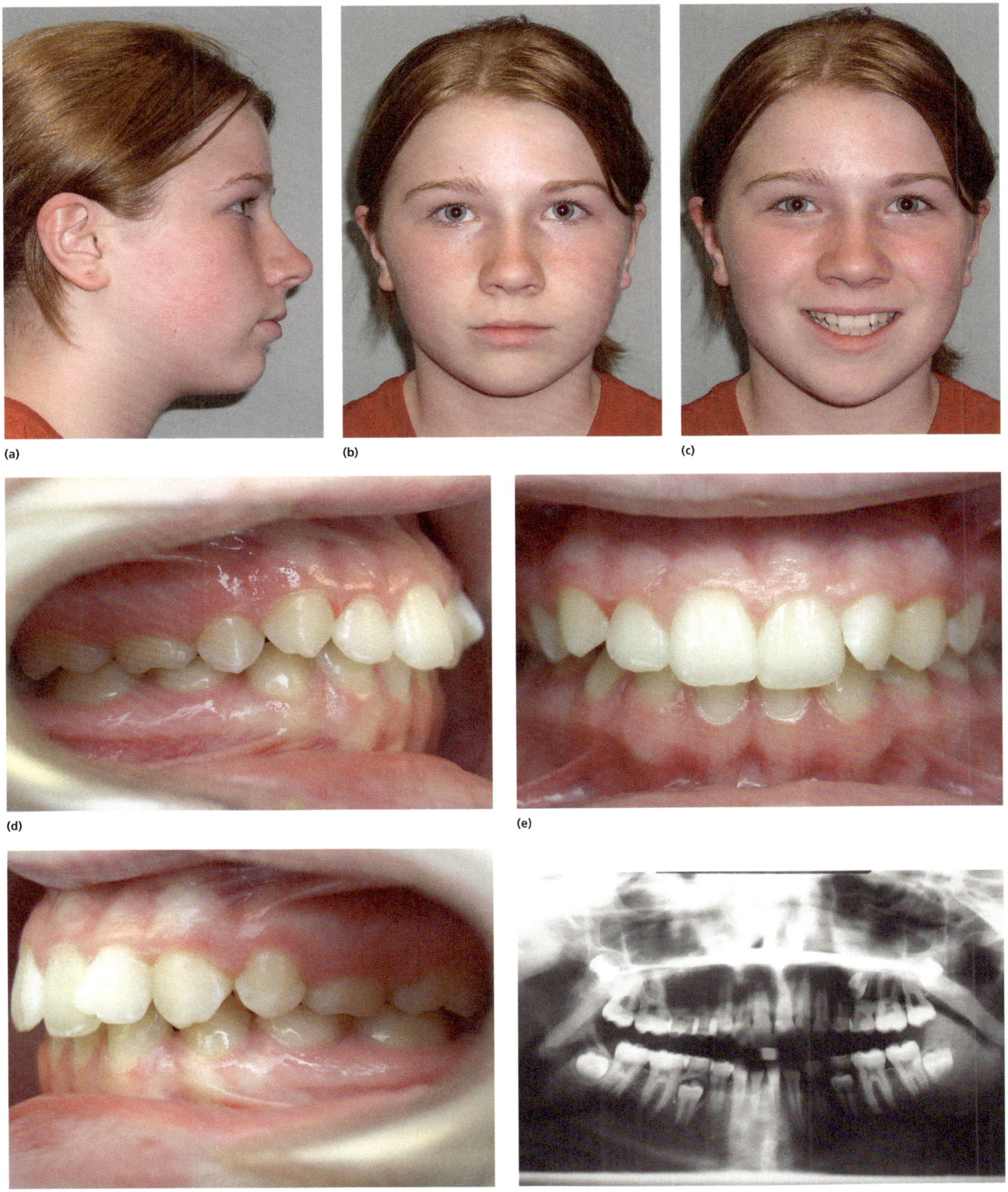

(a) (b) (c) (d) (e) (f) (g)

Figure 20.2 (a–g) Pretreatment photographs and panoramic radiograph showing class I malocclusion with missing mandibular lateral incisors.

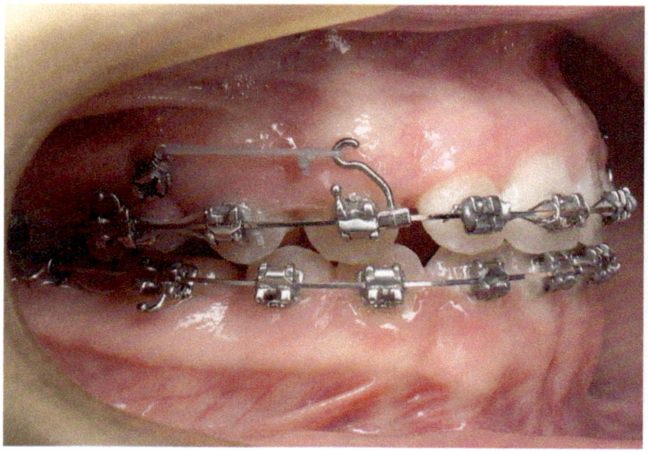

(a)

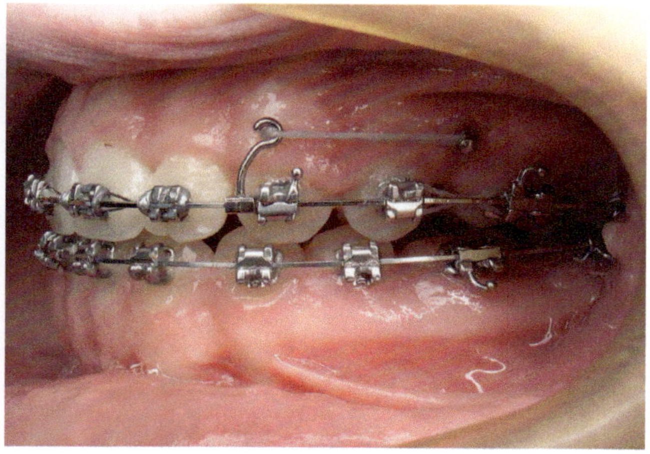

(b)

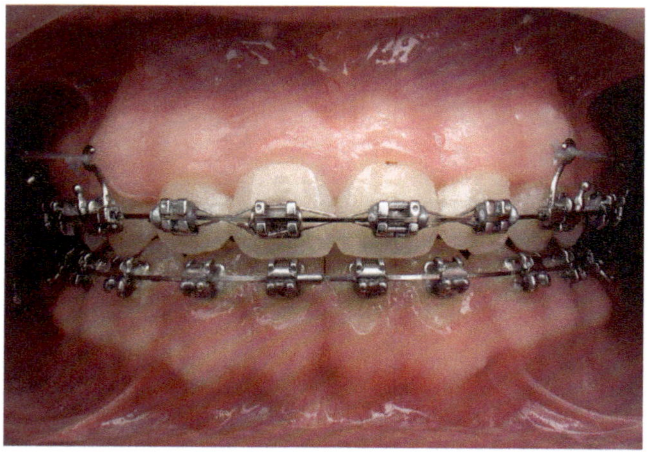

(c)

Figure 20.3 (a–c) Progress photographs demonstrating retraction mechanics to preserve anchorage.

Final facial and intraoral photographs demonstrate good facial esthetics and the resultant ideal class I occlusion with the maxillary canine teeth in function with mandibular first premolars (Figure 20.4a–f). The panoramic radiograph shows the patient on completion of orthodontic treatment (Figure 20.4g). The patient was able to avoid prosthetic replacement of the three missing teeth. The final lateral cephalometric radiograph and superimpositions seen in Figure 20.5 demonstrate complete maxillary space closure with incisor retraction and the maxillary molars maintained in position posterior to the extraction spaces, confirming that maximum A–P anchorage had been achieved.

The vertical dimension

The vertical dimension can be better controlled with skeletal anchorage compared with conventional orthodontic mechanotherapy. Maxillary or mandibular anterior teeth can be intruded to correct hyper-eruption and excessive gingival display. Figure 20.6 demonstrates the use of micro-screw implants at the bilateral canine and lateral incisor interspaces with intrusion mechanics. The pretreatment facial view demonstrates vertical maxillary excess with excess gingival display (Figure 20.6a). Intrusion of maxillary anterior teeth with micro-screw implants was completed to minimize the excessive gingival display (Figure 20.6b). A 4 mm intrusion of the maxillary incisors developed ideal incisor display and pleasing facial esthetics (Figure 20.6c).

On the contrary, patients with a high mandibular plane angle anterior open bite can have the proper amount of maxillary incisor display, but improper application of continuous archwire mechanics can result in excessive gingival display. The high-angle class I skeletal patient seen in Figures 20.7a–c and 20.8a presented with a significant anterior open bite. While the maxillary incisor display was acceptable, excessive gingival display could be seen in the premolar region. Three-piece maxillary impaction surgery was discussed as a treatment option, but was declined in favor of an alternative treatment plan using TADs. Treatment goals included prevention of extrusion of upper incisors, intrusion of the maxillary posterior teeth, and the resulting mandibular autorotation to close the anterior open bite and achieve proper anterior guidance. Segmental mechanics were utilized to prevent extrusion of the maxillary anterior teeth, which would have occurred if a continuous archwire had been applied early in treatment. Micro-screw implants were placed facially between maxillary first molars and second premolars, and on the palatal between first and second molars. Intrusion forces were applied with elastic thread (Figure 20.7d–f). Maxillary incisor brackets and mandibular brackets were not placed until the anterior open bite had been closed.

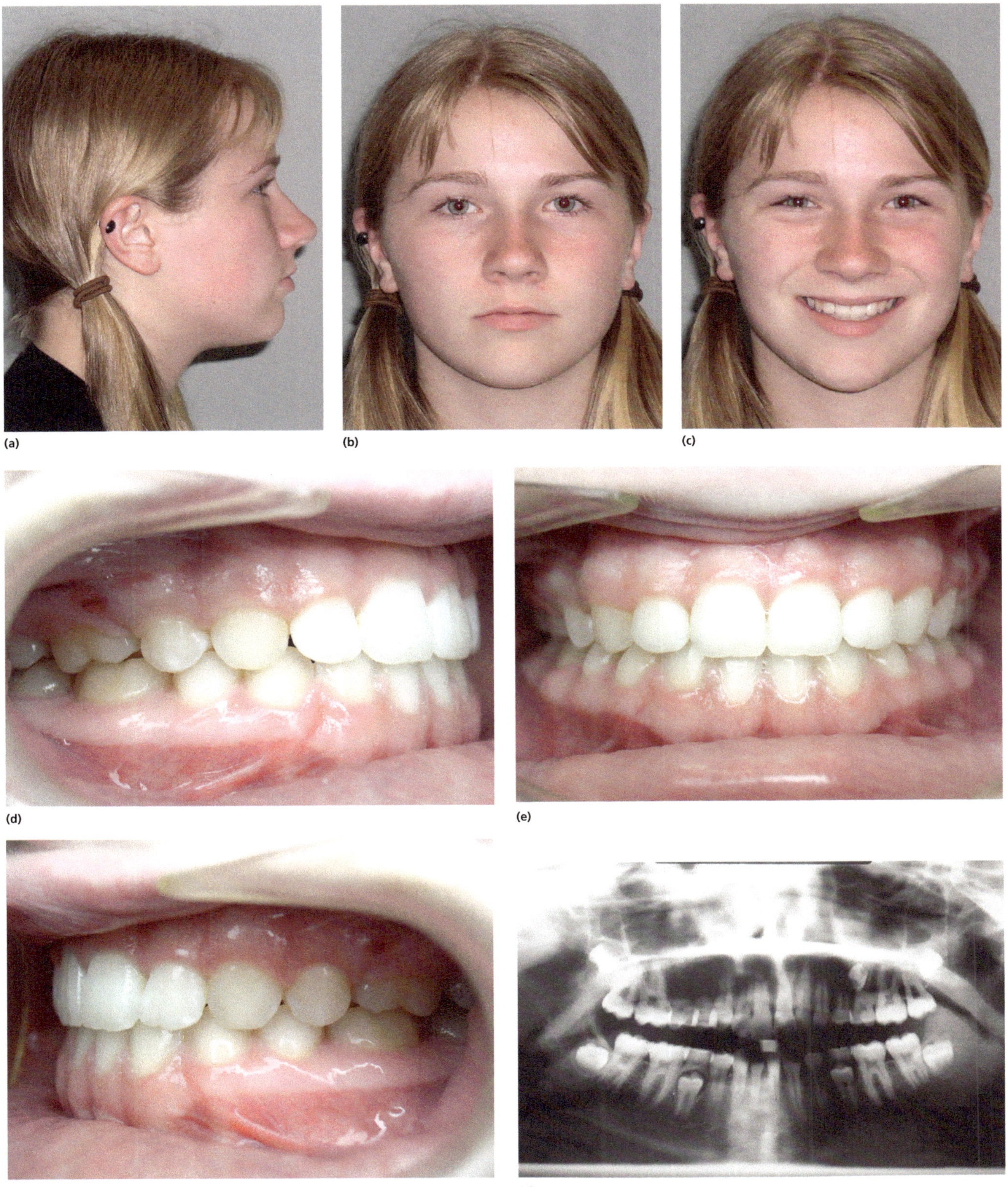

(a) (b) (c) (d) (e) (f) (g)

Figure 20.4 (a–g) Final facial and intraoral photographs and panoramic radiograph demonstrate good facial esthetics. Maxillary cuspids are functioning with mandibular first premolars and the patient was able to avoid prosthetic replacement of the congenitally missing teeth.

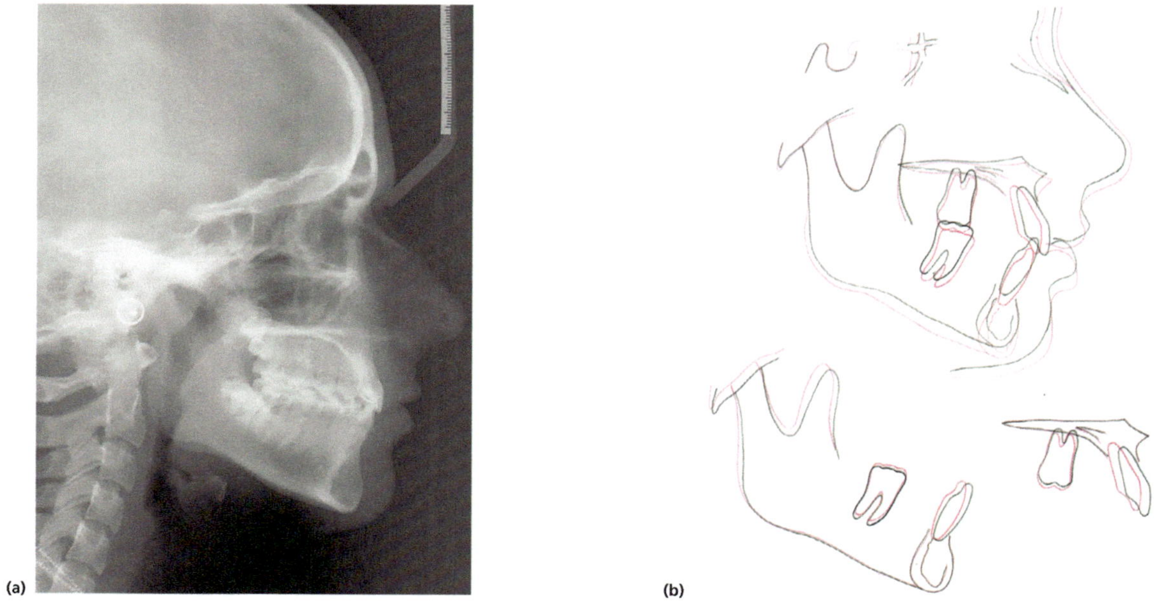

Figure 20.5 (a) Final lateral cephalometric radiograph and (b) superimposition tracings show maximum maxillary A–P anchorage.

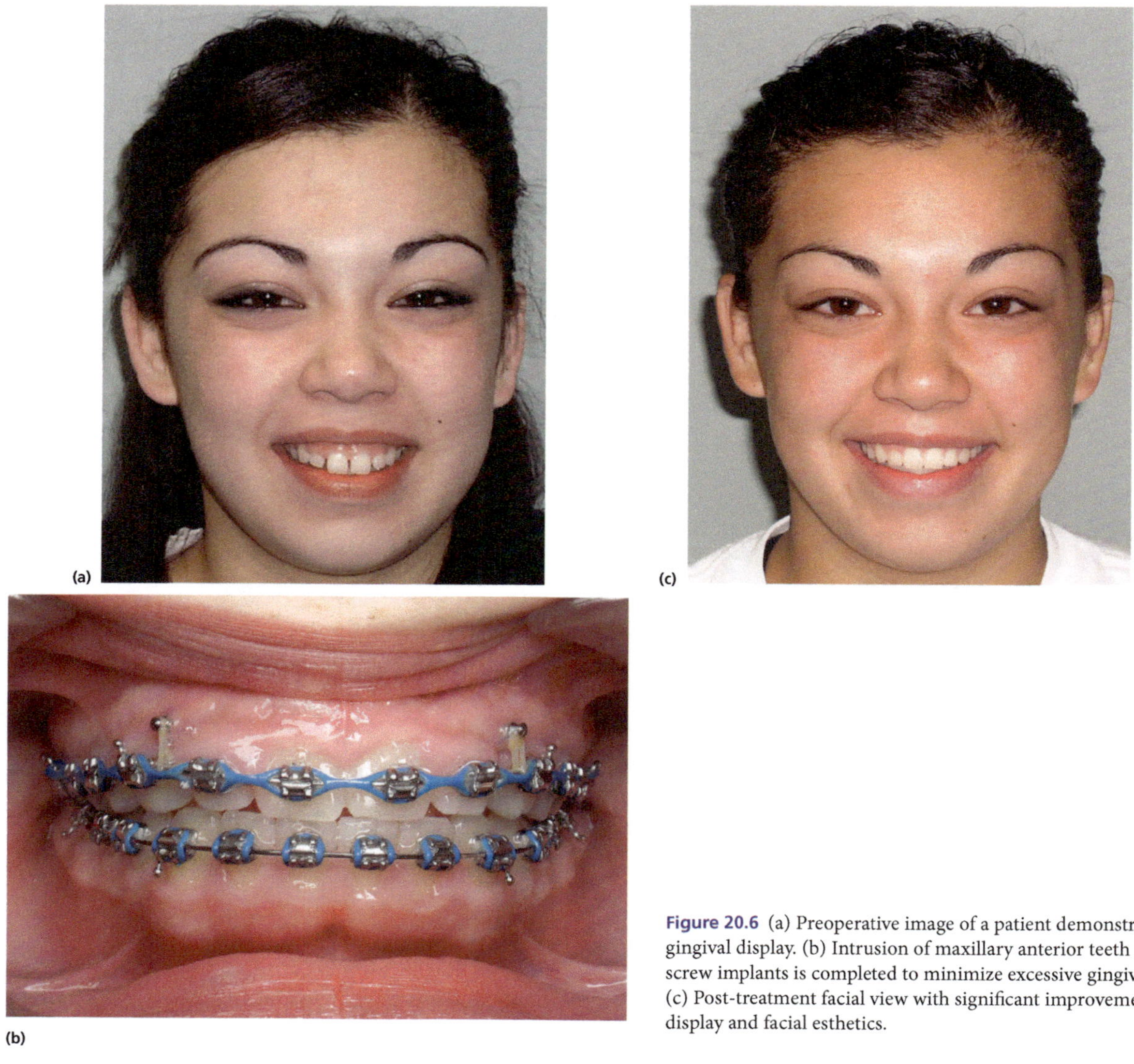

Figure 20.6 (a) Preoperative image of a patient demonstrating excess gingival display. (b) Intrusion of maxillary anterior teeth with micro-screw implants is completed to minimize excessive gingival display. (c) Post-treatment facial view with significant improvement in gingival display and facial esthetics.

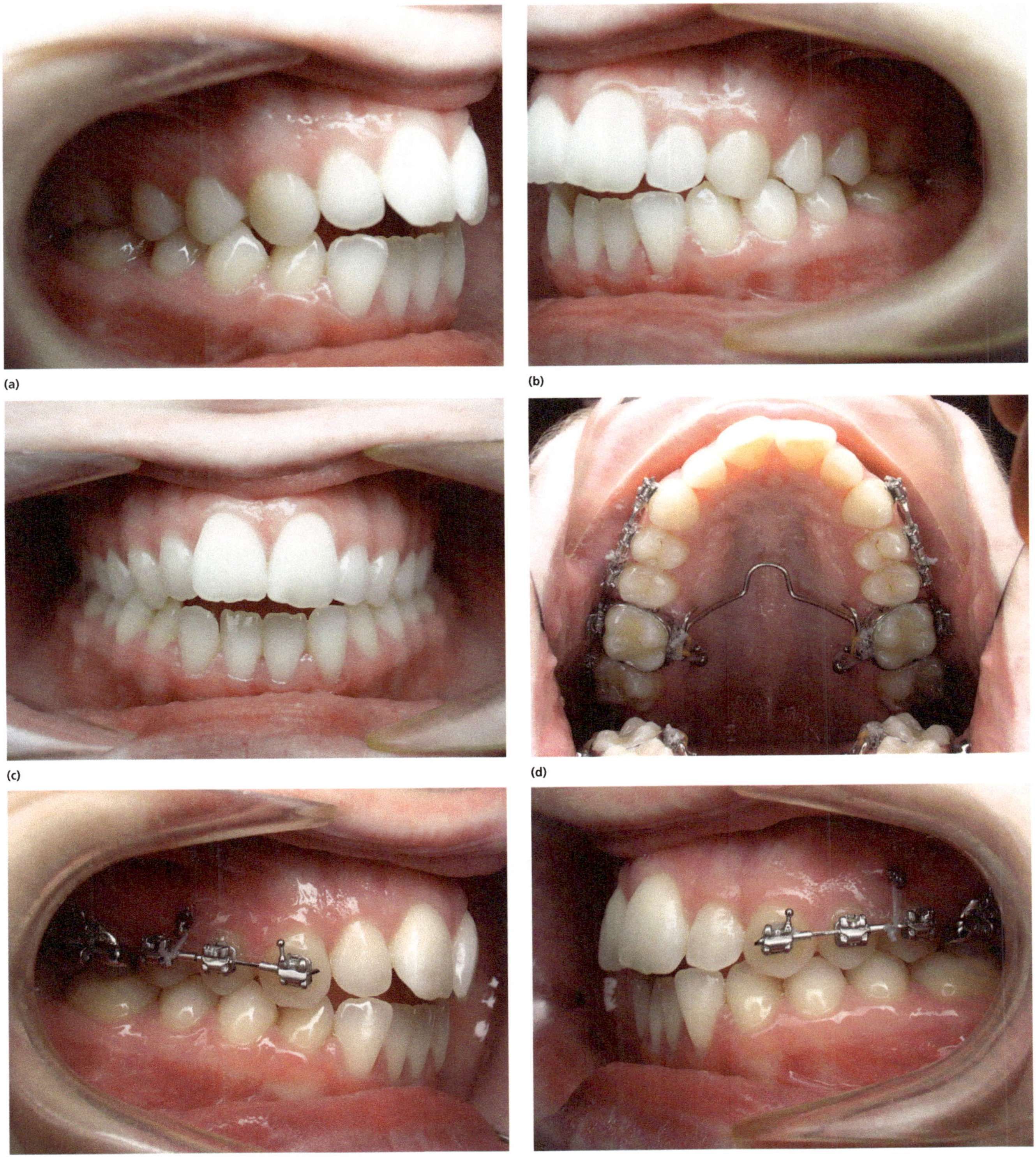

(a) (b) (c) (d) (e) (f)

Figure 20.7 (a–c) Preoperative images of a patient demonstrating excess gingival display and anterior open bite. (d–f) Segmental mechanics were applied to intrude posterior teeth and avoid extrusion of maxillary anterior teeth.

Figure 20.8 shows the improved facial esthetics with maxillary posterior excessive gingival display eliminated and the vertical position of the maxillary central incisors remaining unchanged. Control of the vertical dimension in a non-growing patient can also have a positive effect on the sagittal dimension, projecting the chin anteriorly. The cephalometric superimpositions following treatment show a closure of the mandibular plane angle with intrusion of the posterior teeth (Figure 20.9). The mandibular autorotation corrected the anterior open bite and achieved ideal intercuspation.

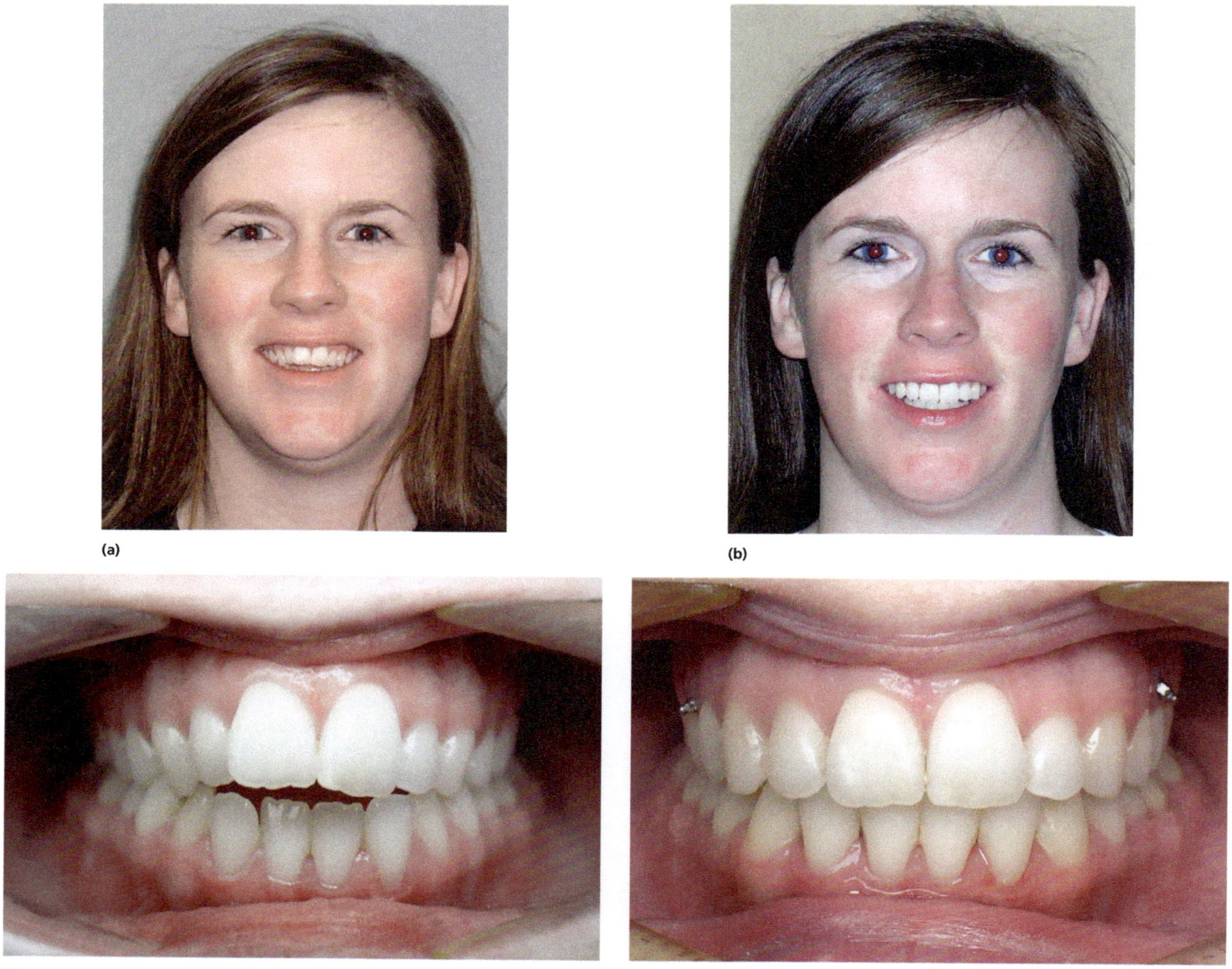

(a) (b) (c) (d)

Figure 20.8 (a-d) Pre- and post-treatment images with intrusion of posterior teeth using skeletal anchorage with TADs demonstrating; improved facial esthetics, elimination of the excess posterior gingival display, closure of the anterior open bite with ideal intercuspation and proper anterior guidance.

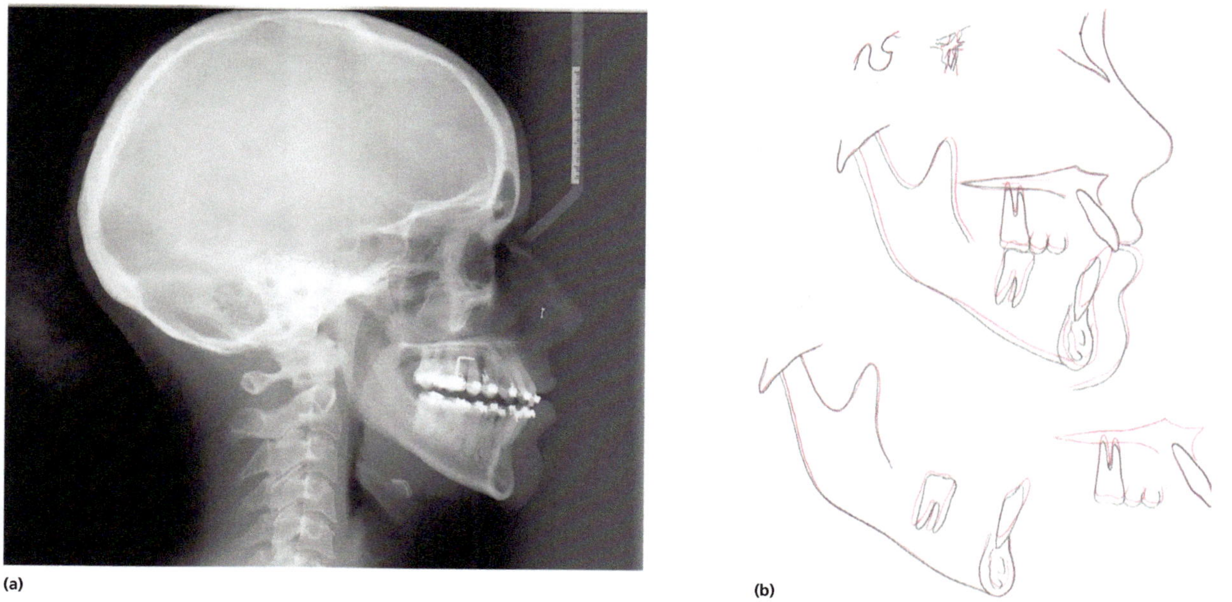

(a) (b)

Figure 20.9 (a) Progress cephalogram showing intentional overintrusion of the maxillary posterior teeth. (b) Cephalometric superimposition showing open bite closure from mandibular autorotation with chin projection, and reduction in lower facial height.

In growing class II adolescent patients, control of the vertical dimension via intrusion of posterior teeth can result in favorable A–P positioning of the mandible. Condylar growth and vertical facial growth are antagonists. Controlling two of the components of vertical facial growth (preventing eruption of the maxillary and mandibular posterior teeth), as described by Schudy[7,8] can result in counterclockwise rotation of the mandible and increased chin projection.

The transverse dimension

Indications for skeletal anchorage in the transverse dimension include correction of midline discrepancies that can be made more predictable using TADs. Figure 20.10 shows efficient midline correction with maxillary and mandibular micro-screw implants placed on the right side. Photographs were completed at 6-week intervals to demonstrate the interval changes.

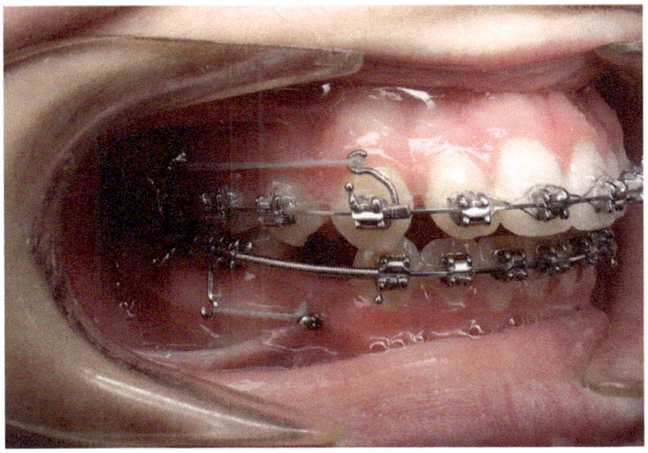

(a)

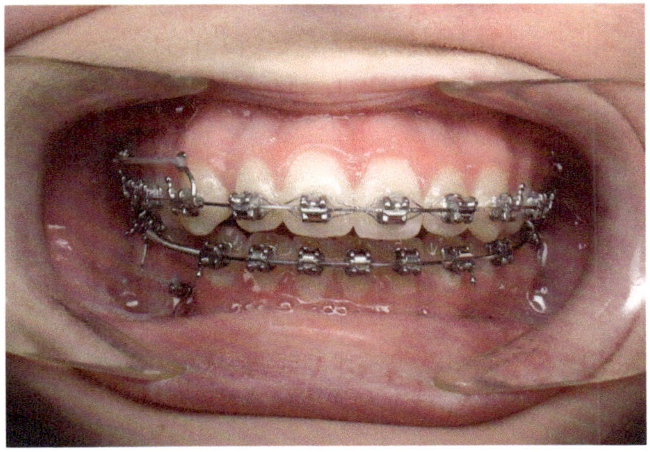

(b)

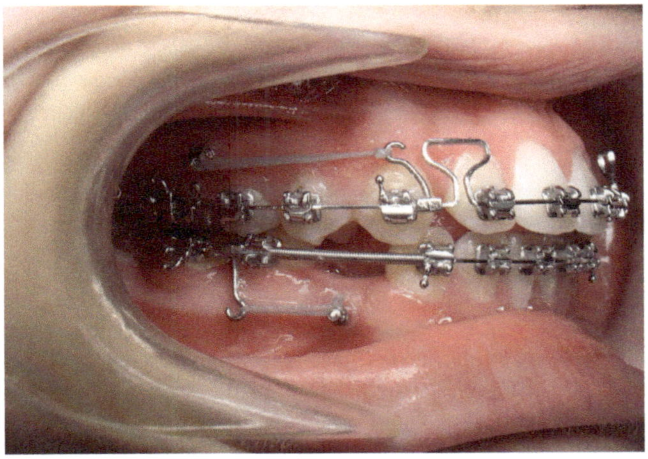

(c)

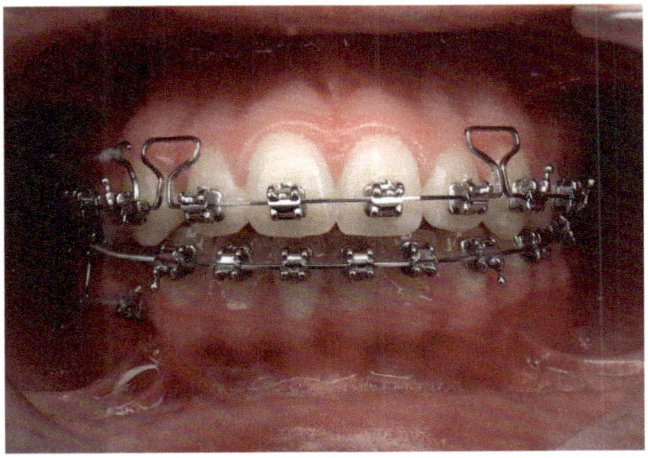

(d)

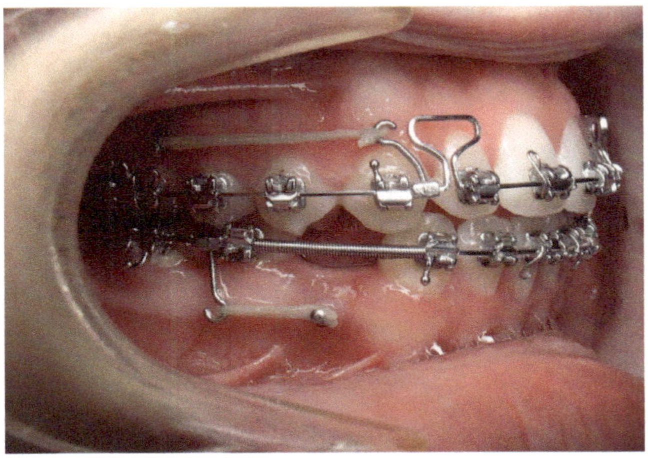

(e)

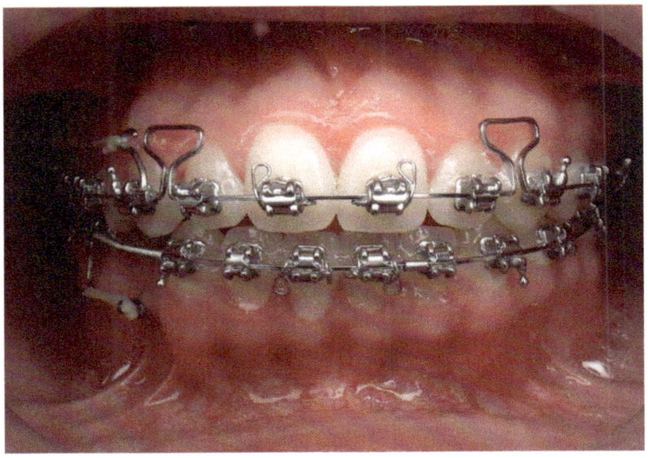

(f)

Figure 20.10 (a–f) Progress photographs taken at 6-week intervals showing efficient midline correction using TADs for simultaneous retraction of maxillary teeth and protraction of mandibular teeth.

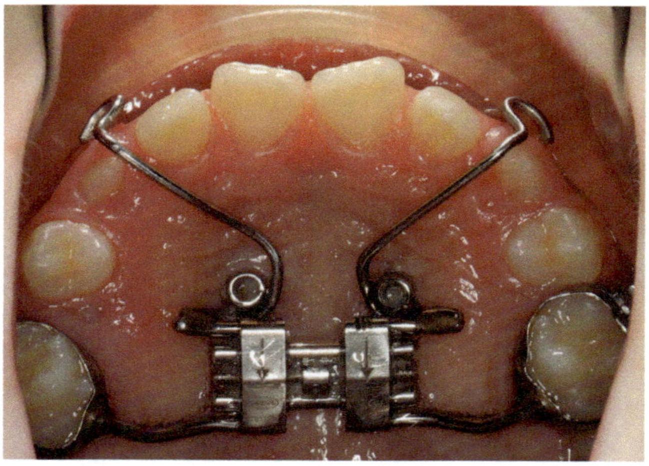

Figure 20.11 Skeletal rapid palatal expander incorporating two palatal TADs with pre-soldered abutments.

Maxillary expansion also can be enhanced using skeletal anchorage. Figure 20.11 demonstrates a Hyrax RPE appliance secured to the palate with two screws. Screw fixation on either side of the midline was used to facilitate skeletal expansion and limit the dental compensation that would have accompanied a conventional tooth-borne appliance.

Interdisciplinary treatment with orthodontic and implant site development

Application of orthodontic treatment principles and the mechanical advantages of TADs can be a significant advantage in treating patients with complex treatment needs. Prior to initiating dental implant treatment, significant correction of restorative, periodontal, and occclusal problems are often required. Congenitally missing teeth, extracted teeth, and severe caries can result in malocclusion, crowding, tipping, and/or extrusion of opposing teeth.

Case study 20.1

This shows a 21-year-old female referred for orthodontic evaluation of an anterior open bite and supereruption of the maxillary left first molar (Figure 20.12). The patient's medical history was non-contributory; however, she had a challenging dental history and dental phobia resulting in numerous non-restorable teeth and edentulous spaces. The patient wished to have comprehensive restorative treatment.

Diagnosis

The patient's main concern was a midline diastema and open bite. The supereruption of the maxillary first molar had resulted in inadequate inter-arch dimension for implant restoration in the mandibular left quadrant (Figure 20.13a). The patient was missing the maxillary right lateral incisor and mandibular left first molar. The maxillary right first and second molars and left second molar and the mandibular right and left second premolars and first molars were deemed non-restorable. Maxillary third molars were present, but incompletely erupted. The maxillary left lateral incisor had been endodontically treated and restored with a porcelain-fused-to-metal crown. Bilateral class I cuspid relationships were present. The anterior open bite measured 3 mm. A 3 mm maxillary midline diastema with a hyperplastic labial frenum was noted. The upper lip measured 20 mm, and the amount of maxillary incisor display at rest was 6 mm. The maxillary left first molar was hyper-erupted and was 2 mm from contacting the lower edentulous alveolar ridge on occlusion. Cephalometric analysis (Figure 20.13b) showed the patient had a mesocephalic class I skeletal relationship with mildly protrusive incisors (upper incisor to NA was +7 mm, lower incisor to APo was +6 mm). A skeletal anterior open bite was present with no occlusal contact from the right maxillary second premolar to the left canine (Figure 20.13).

Treatment options

Comprehensive dental and periodontal treatment with caries control and removal of non-restorable teeth was initiated. Orthodontic treatment with full fixed appliances was anticipated in combination with orthognathic surgery or TADs for skeletal anchorage. Orthognathic surgery would have required maxillary impaction with anterior open bite correction and developing adequate inter-arch dimension for restorative treatment in the mandibular left quadrant. Alternatively, TADs with skeletal anchorage could be used to intrude maxillary posterior teeth, closing the anterior open bite and providing adequate clearance for restorative treatment.

Treatment plan

Skeletal anchorage with TADs was chosen as the method of open bite closure, and the treatment plan was to restore the patient to first molar occlusion. The restorative treatment plan included a ceramo-metal crown for the maxillary left first molar, a provisional "bonded" pontic at the right maxillary lateral incisor position, and implant-supported restorations at the mandibular right and left first molar and second premolar sites.

Treatment sequence

Maxillary full bonded/banded 0.018″ self-ligation fixed appliances were placed. A trans-palatal arch from the maxillary right second bicuspid to the maxillary left first molar was placed in order to maintain torque control during the intrusion process. Extraction of the non-restorable teeth, frenectomy, and simultaneous TAD placement were completed. Open surgical mini-plates were placed facially and interproximally to the maxillary right first and second bicuspid and maxillary left second bicuspid and first molar teeth. Intrusion mechanics were initiated with elastic thread after subsequent placement of a rectangular archwire (Figure 20.14).

Posterior intrusion progressed well initially, but seemed too slow. It appeared as if the roots of the right maxillary second bicuspid after initial intrusion had contacted the inferior fixation screw, which had been placed in mono-cortical fashion. The coronal-most screw on the right mini-plate was removed (Figure 20.15a) and two palatal micro-screws (KLS Martin, Jacksonville, FL) placed distal to the maxillary right second premolar and left first molar (Figure 20.15b). Intrusion forces were re-established using elastic thread on the palatal and facial, and mandibular fixed appliances were placed (Figure 20.15c and d). Closing arch mechanics were then utilized to consolidate remaining maxillary spaces, and facial intrusion forces applied with some class III vector due to mandibular autorotation. Anterior vertical elastics were applied for a period of 6 weeks.

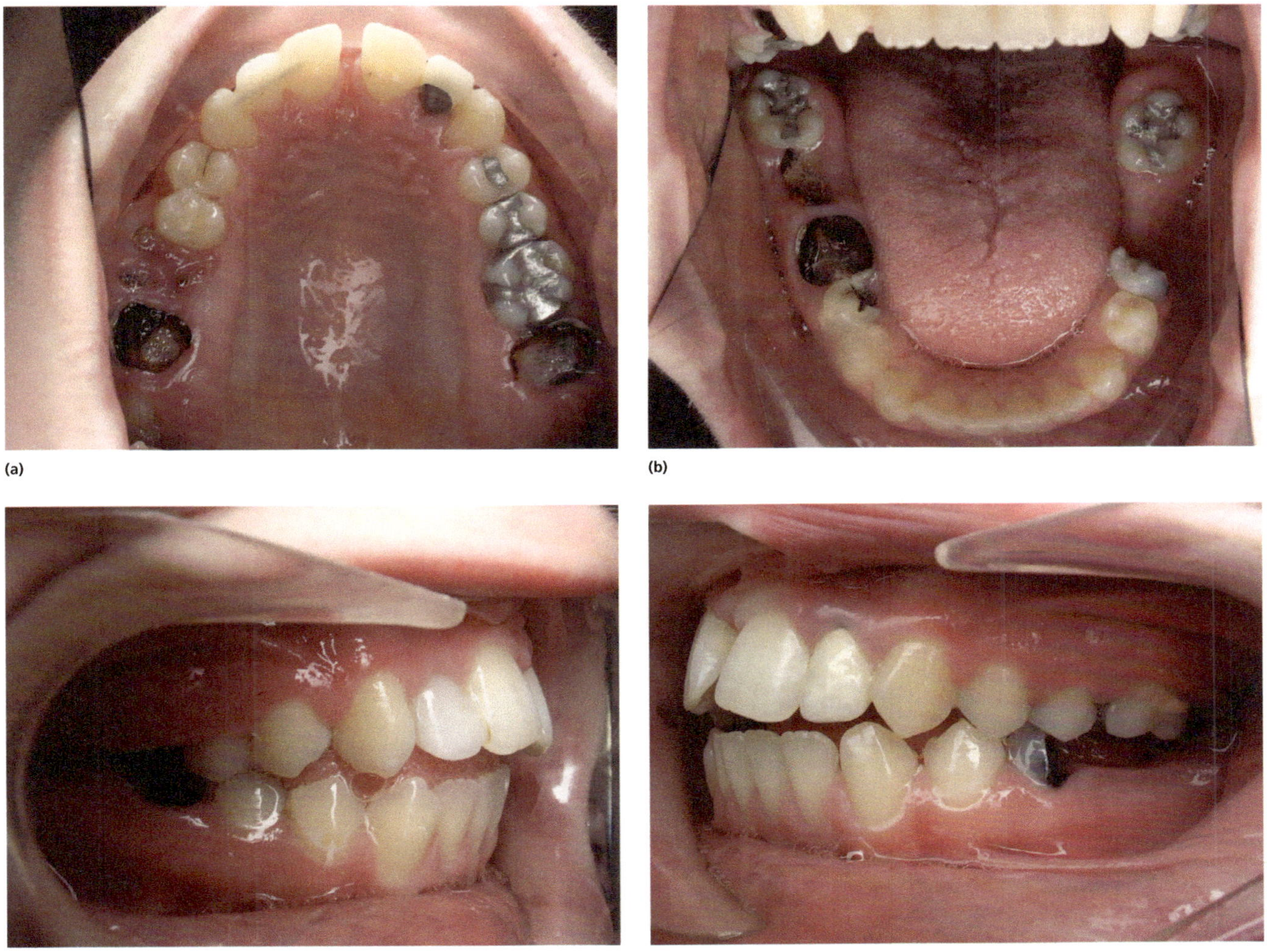

(a) (b) (c) (d)

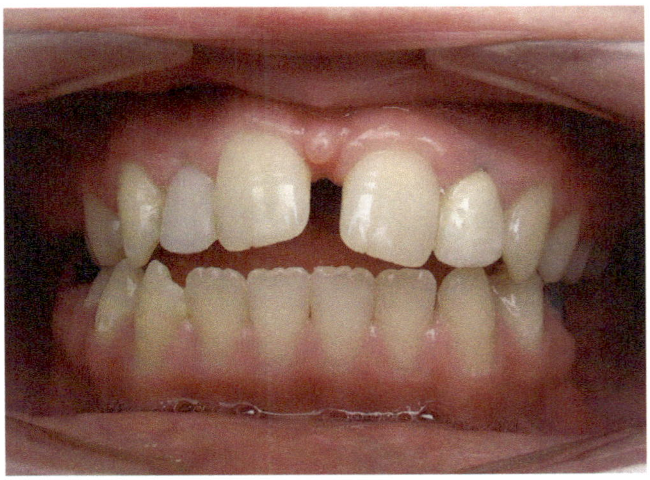

(e)

Figure 20.12 (a–e) Clinical images demonstrating several carious teeth, edentulous spaces, and orthodontic and occlusal concerns, including an anterior open bite and supereruption of #14.

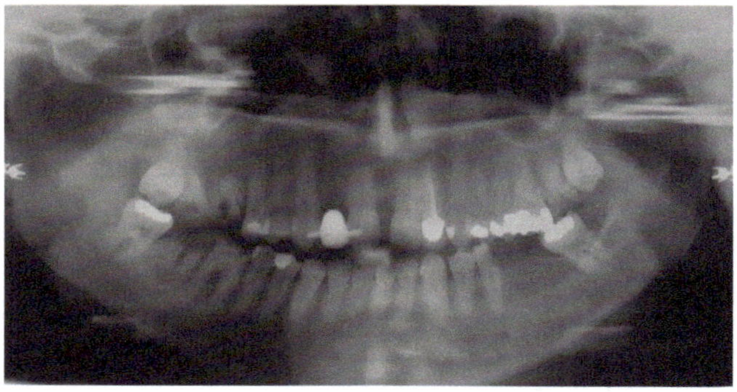

(a)

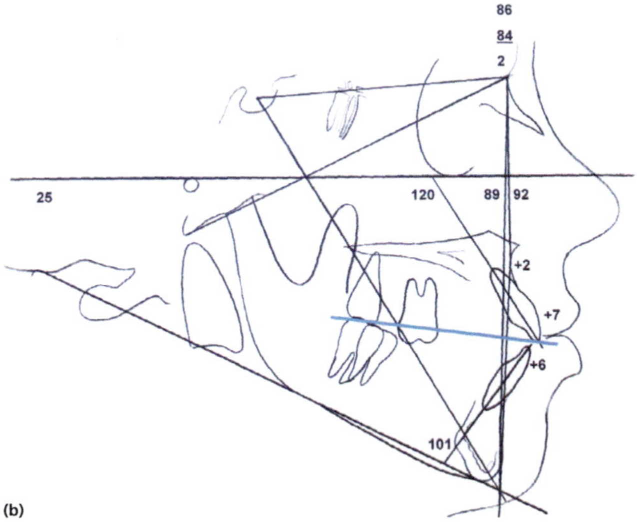

(b)

Figure 20.13 (a) Pretreatment panoramic radiograph and (b) cephalometric tracing.

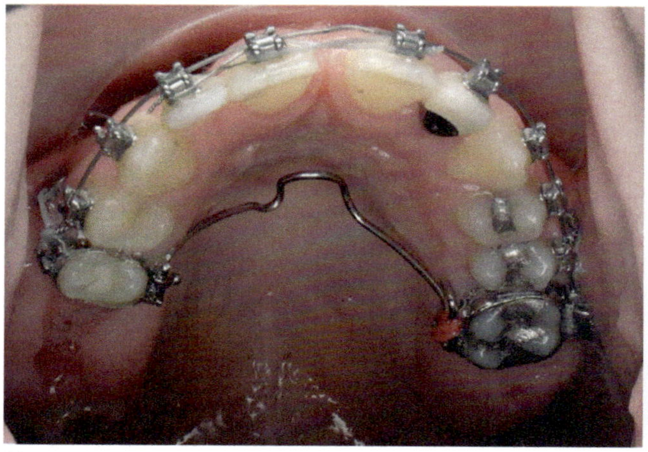

(a)

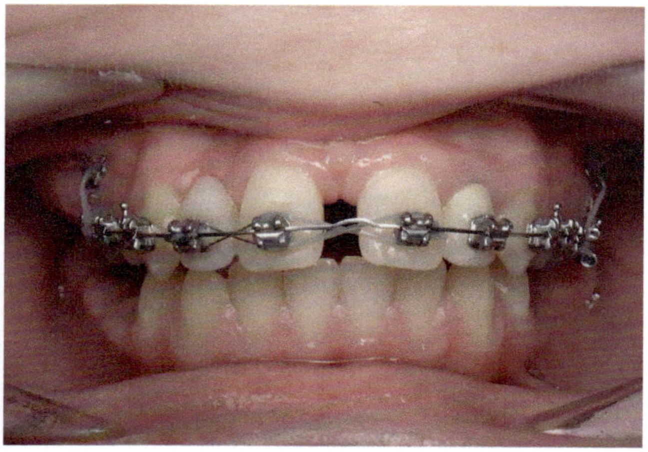

(b)

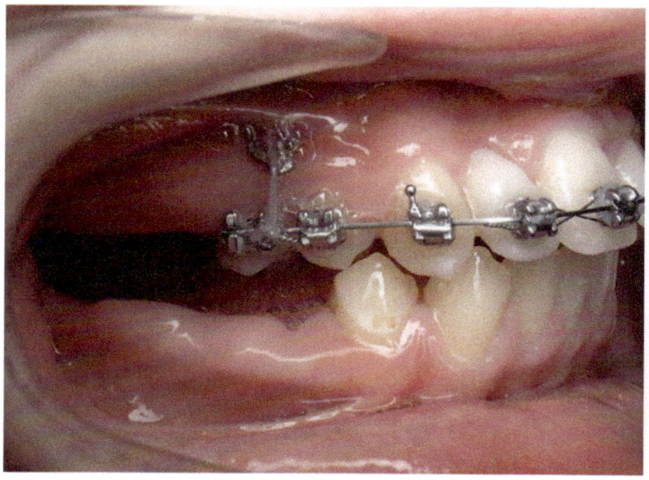

(c)

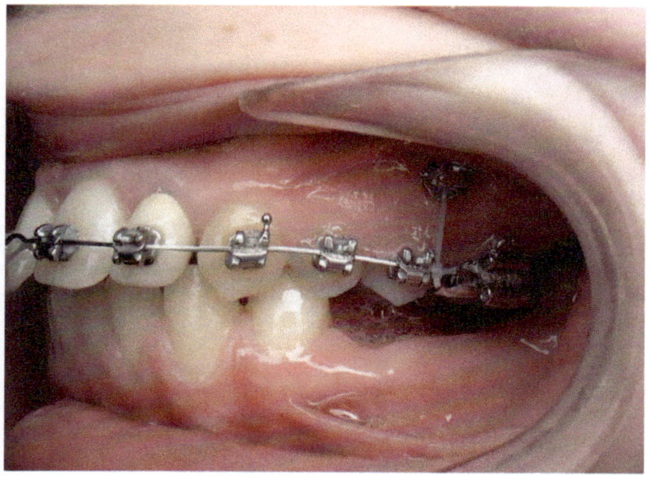

(d)

Figure 20.14 (a–d) Intrusive forces were applied to the posterior teeth with elastic thread tied from the bone plates to the archwire.

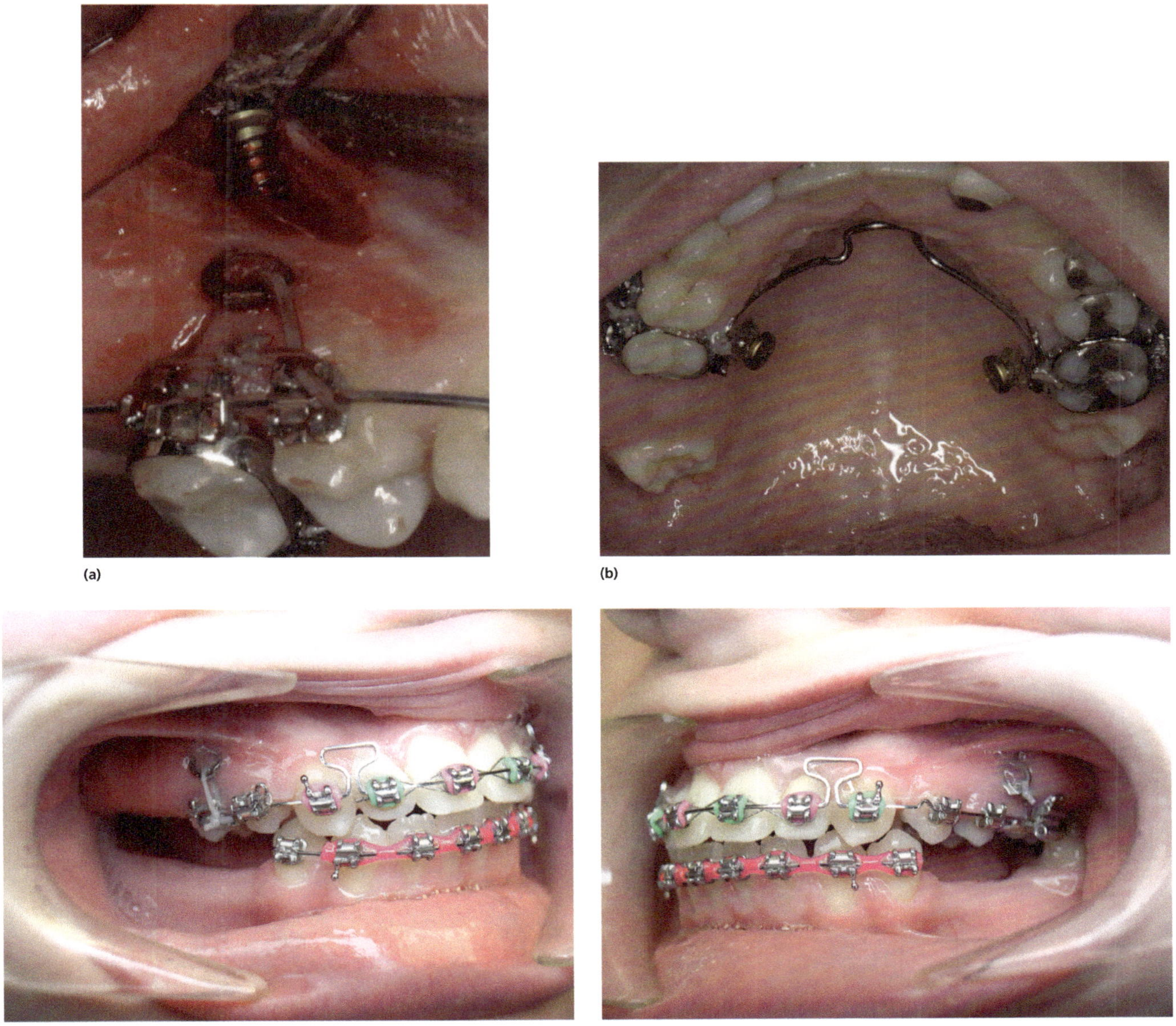

(a) (b) (c) (d)

Figure 20.15 (a–d) The coronal mono-cortical fixation screw was removed above the right second premolar and palatal TADs were placed and intrusion mechanics were continued. *Source:* (a,b) © Daniel R. Cullum

After debonding of the orthodontic appliances, the retention phase included bonded fixed retainers in both arches and a maxillary Essix® retainer (Raintree Essix, Sarasota, FL). Application of additional fixation was planned due to potential relapse of the maxillary left molar hyper-eruption over the course of the remaining implant and restorative treatments. A 330 carbide bur was used to convert the upper left mini-plate into an elastic hook. The Essix retainer was used nightly and twice weekly to secure an elastic across the occlusal surface of the Essix for further support.

Outcome

The patient's esthetics were remarkably improved, as seen on completion of the orthodontic phase (Figure 20.16a and b). The anterior open bite was successfully closed, avoiding maxillary incisor extrusion and possible increased gingival display (Figure 20.16c–e). The maxillary left first molar was intruded adequately to allow room for implant restoration of the mandibular left quadrant. Cephalometric evaluation confirmed significant mandibular autorotation with Pogonion advanced 3 mm and lower facial height decreased 4.5 mm (Figure 20.17). The maxillary left first molar was intruded 3.5 mm. No eruption of the lower incisors was seen. Slight advancement but no extrusion of the upper incisors was noted. The upper and lower third molars drifted mesially during the course of treatment.

The patient had sequential implant reconstruction of the multiple edentulous sites with stable bone and soft tissue. Figure 20.18 demonstrates the clinical and panoramic images of the patient after restoration. The maxillary lateral incisor implant was placed 3 years and the remaining implants over 7 years prior to these follow-up images.

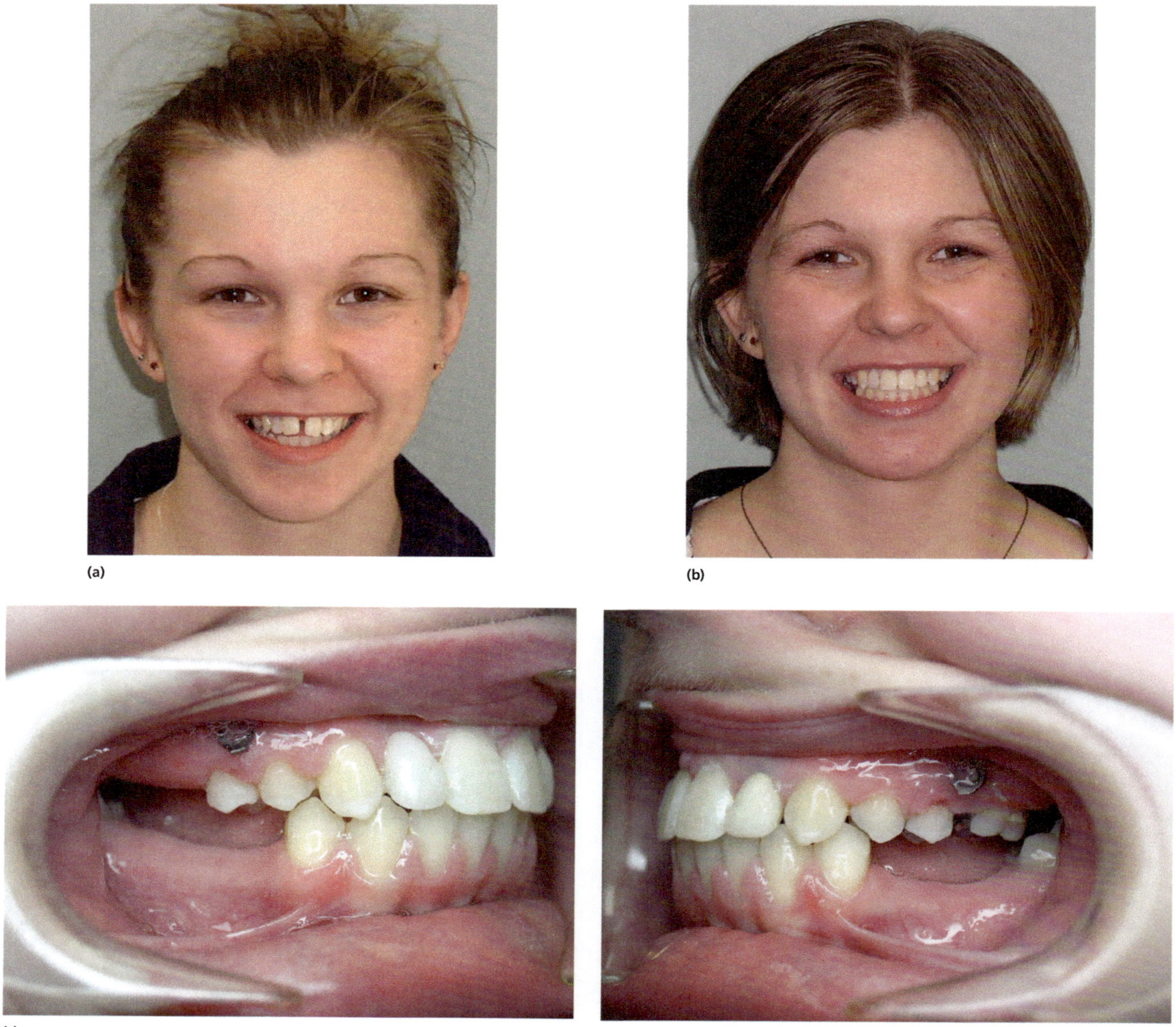

(a) (b) (c) (d)

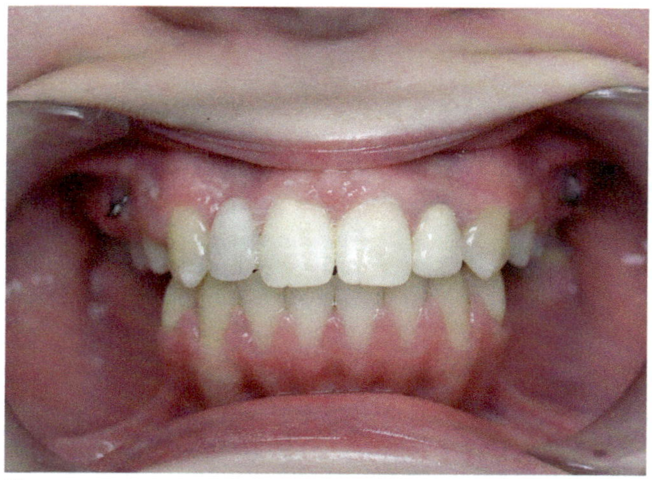

(e)

Figure 20.16 (a–e) Clinical images comparing facial views prior to treatment and after completion of the orthodontic phase with remarkably improved esthetics and an idealized occlusion. The anterior open bite was closed without any extrusion of maxillary incisors that would have led to an increase in gingival display. Increased vertical space was achieved for adequate restorative space for the planned implant restorations in the mandibular left quadrant.

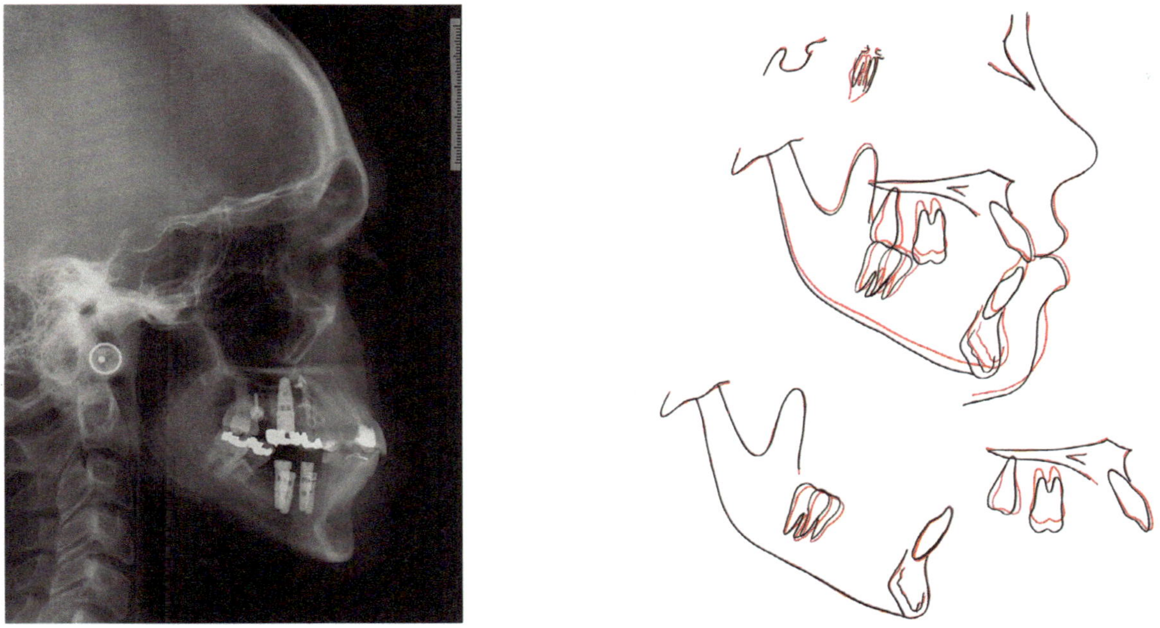

(a) (b)

Figure 20.17 (a) Post-orthodontic treatment lateral cephalogram and (b) cephalometric superimposition showing closure of anterior open bite by mandibular autorotation, without extrusion of maxillary anterior teeth.

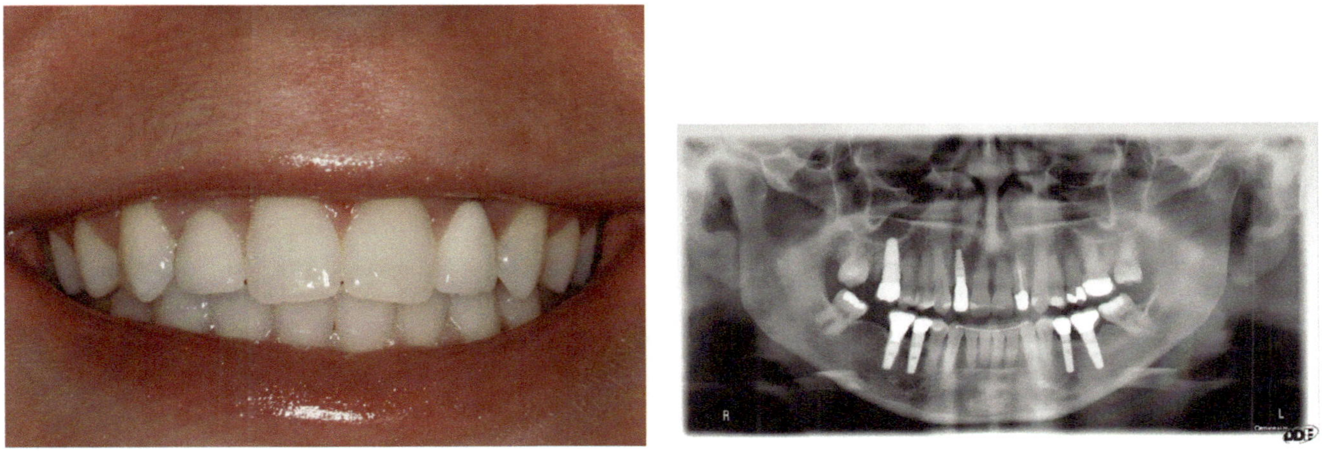

(a) (b)

Figure 20.18 (a) Clinical and (b) panoramic images of the patient 3 years after maxillary lateral incisor restoration and over 7 years since restoration of the previous implants. *Source:* (a) © Daniel R. Cullum

Case study 20.2

This case study presents a patient with bone and soft tissue loss in the esthetic zone, a great challenge in interdisciplinary dentistry. This 35-year-old female initially presented with a chief concern of "not liking the appearance of my smile" (Figure 20.19a).

Diagnosis

The patient described a history of trauma to the maxillary anterior teeth in childhood. The maxillary left canine had been endodontically-treated, including repair of a lateral perforation with amalgam, and now showed tremendous bone and soft tissue loss (Figure 20.19b and c). The patient was also missing the maxillary left lateral incisor and first premolar teeth. The left maxillary second premolar had endodontic treatment, and was restored with a post and core as the distal abutment of the failing five-unit bridge. Further evaluation revealed a canted maxillary anterior occlusal plane with excessive gingival display on the right side and excessive clinical crown length of the left cuspid restoration.

Treatment options

Full fixed orthodontic appliances were required in conjunction with orthognathic surgery or TADs for skeletal anchorage. It was felt that orthognathic surgery with maxillary impaction could correct the excessive gingival display on the right, and arch segmentation could assist with vertical repositioning to reduce the bone and

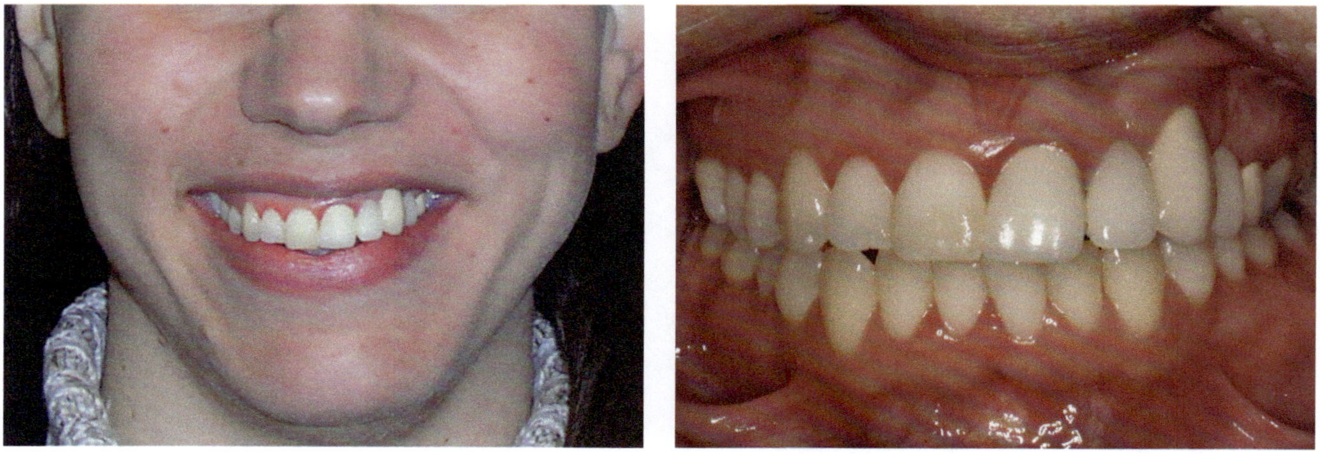

(a) (b)

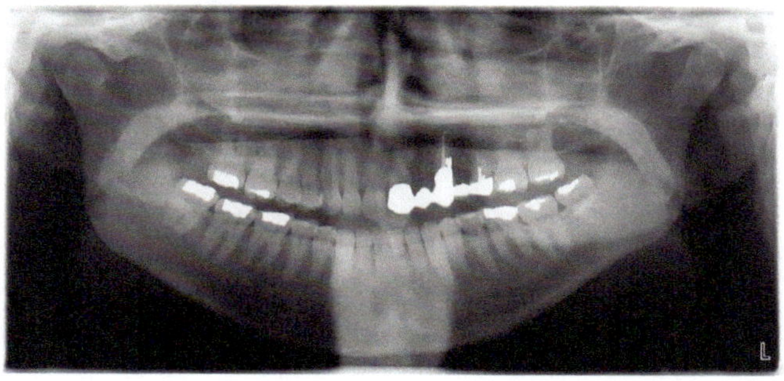

(c)

Figure 20.19 (a–c) Pretreatment facial and intraoral images and panoramic radiograph showing a canted maxillary occlusal plane and failing left maxillary fixed prosthesis. The canine demonstrated failing endodontic treatment, lateral perforation, and severe bone loss. *Source:* (c) © Daniel R. Cullum

soft tissue defect in the left cuspid area. Augmentation procedures to increase vertical bone and soft tissue height would have required multiple procedures. Alternatively, full fixed appliances with skeletal anchorage could be used to intrude maxillary right posterior teeth along with extrusion of the failing canine to develop bone and/or soft tissue, reducing or eliminating the need for bone augmentation.

Treatment plan

After comprehensive planning by the treatment team (a prosthodontist, orthodontist, and oral surgeon), the patient began orthodontic treatment with the primary goal of improving the occlusal plane cant by intrusion of the right maxillary teeth. Extrusion on the left maxillary teeth was also planned to increase the amount of vertical bone and soft tissue, and then to be followed by reassessment regarding the need for further implant site development.

Treatment sequence

Prior to orthodontic treatment, the prosthodontist placed provisional restorations on the failing bridge abutments. Maxillary full fixed orthodontic appliances were placed. A micro-screw implant was placed between the maxillary right first molar and second premolar teeth after 4 months of treatment. A second micro-screw was placed in the same area 3 months later to give additional anchorage for continued intrusion mechanics. Intrusive force was applied with elastic thread on the upper right side over a 12-month period, creating a planned posterior open bite that was maintained with indirect anchorage. Full-arch mandibular brackets were placed 9 months after beginning treatment, and used with posterior vertical elastics to close the posterior open bite by extruding the mandibular right posterior teeth, leveling the maxillary occlusal plane (Figure 20.20a and b).

Extrusion of the failing maxillary left cuspid was completed by use of an elastic thread tied to the archwire. (Figure 20.20c). This resulted in development of vertical bone and soft tissue. Comparison of the pretreatment and the progress reconstructed cone beam computed tomography images after 20 and 29 months showed more than 7 mm of vertical bone development and the regeneration of buccal–palatal dimension of the left cuspid site prior to its extraction and placement of an immediate implant (Figure 20.21).

After 27 months of active orthodontic treatment, immediate flapless 4.3 mm diameter, single-stage implants were placed in the left maxillary canine and second premolar sites (Figure 20.22). Pontics were placed on the archwire during the healing period, avoiding any contact with the implants or soft tissues (Figure 20.22a).

Outcome

As a result of the concurrent TAD-assisted right intrusion and left extrusion mechanics, dramatic esthetic changes occurred from the pretreatment presentation (Figure 20.23a). After implant integration, the maxillary orthodontic appliances were removed and an Essix retainer with pontics was inserted for interim esthetic management (Figure 20.23b).

Provisional restorations were placed with initiation of emergence profile development. A definitive restoration was completed at the left central incisor with the four-unit anterior cantilever provisional

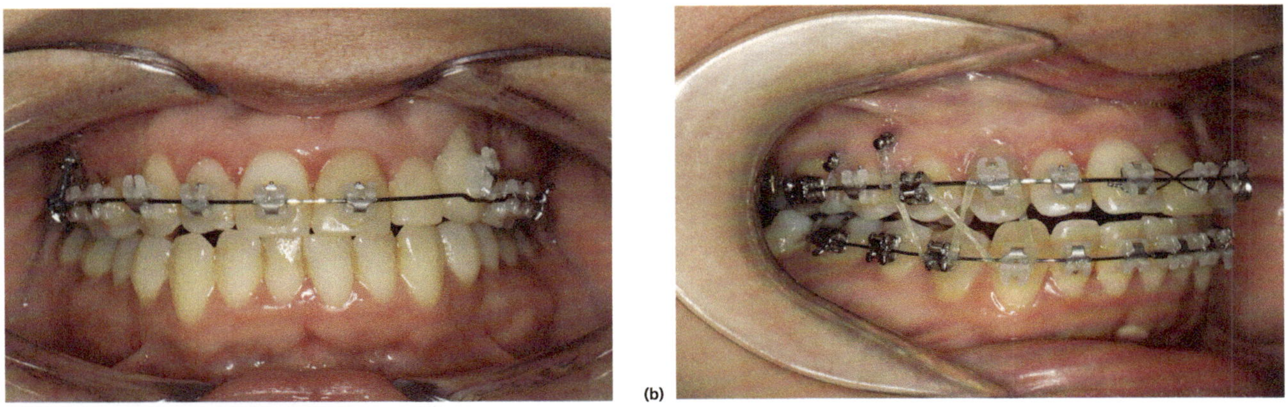

(a) (b)

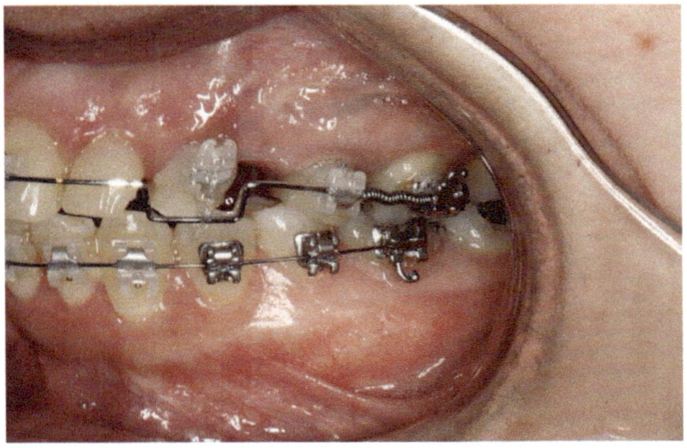

(c)

Figure 20.20 (a) Concurrent intrusion of the maxillary right posterior teeth along with extrusion of the failing maxillary left cuspid was completed. (b) Vertical elastics were used to close the posterior open bite that had resulted from intrusion of the maxillary right posterior teeth. (c) Extrusion of the left maxillary canine root was part of the pre-implant site development.

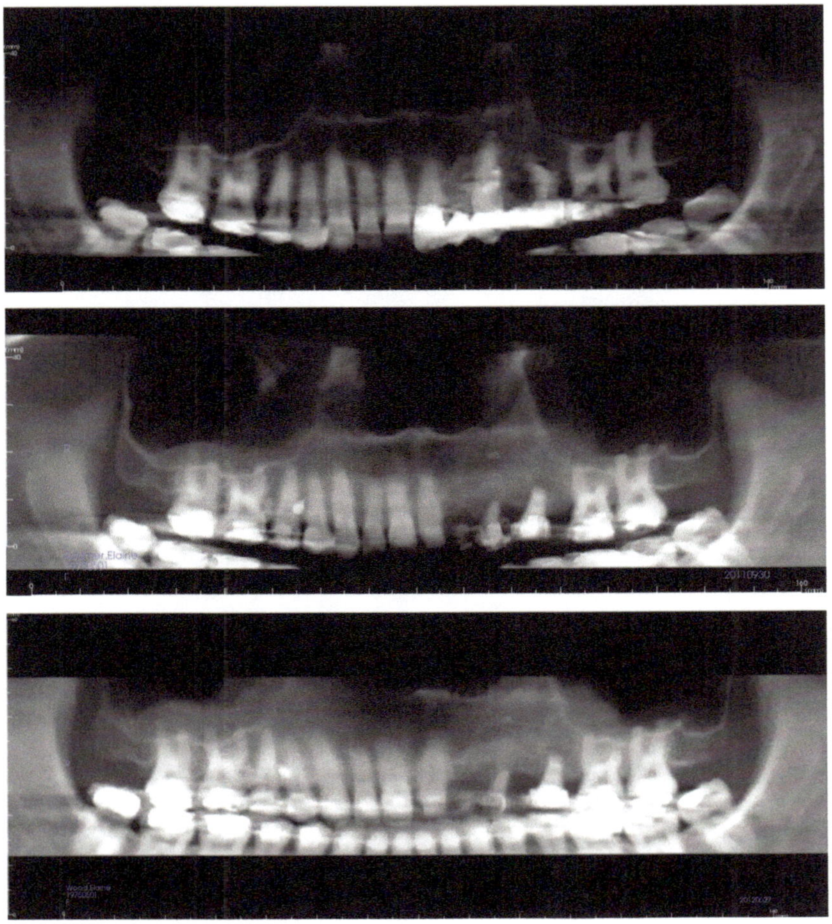

(a) (b) (c)

Figure 20.21 Cone beam computed tomography reconstructed panoramic images of (a) pretreatment, (b) 20 months, and (c) 29 months, demonstrate orthodontic site development with extrusion of the left maxillary cuspid. *(Continued)*

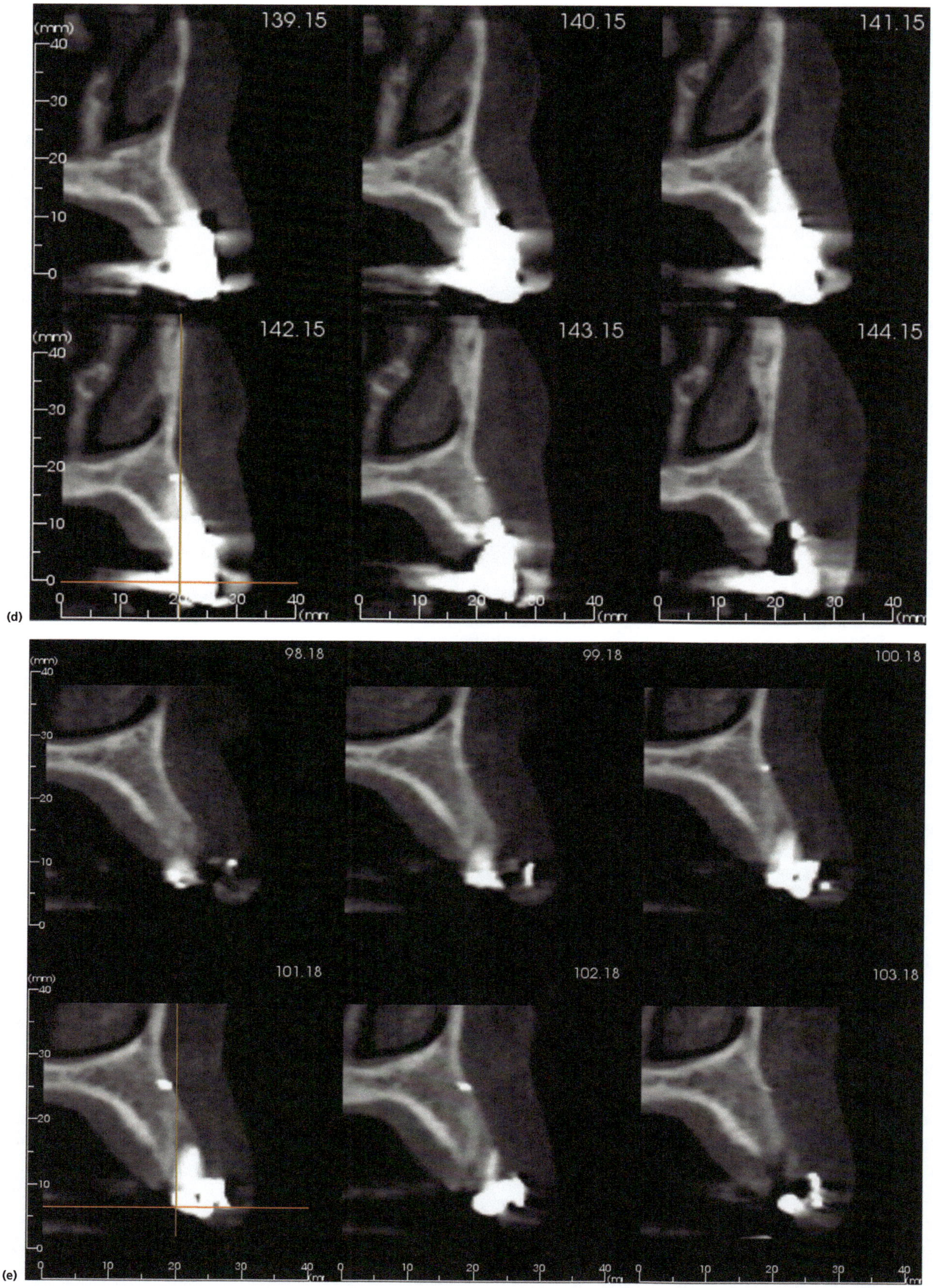

Figure 20.21 (Continued)
Cone beam computed tomography cross-sectional images of (d) pretreatment, and (e) 20 months.

(Continued)

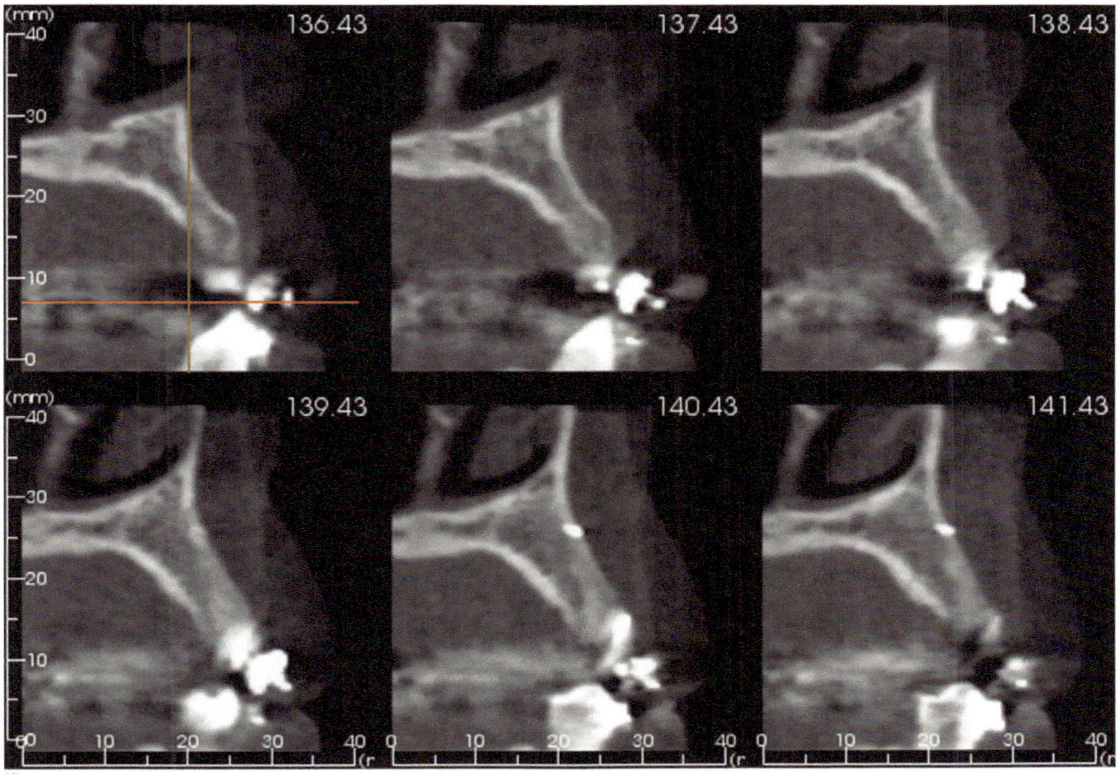

(f)

Figure 20.21 (Continued)
Cone beam computed tomography cross-sectional image (f) 29 months demonstrate orthodontic site development with extrusion of the left maxillary cuspid. © Daniel R. Cullum

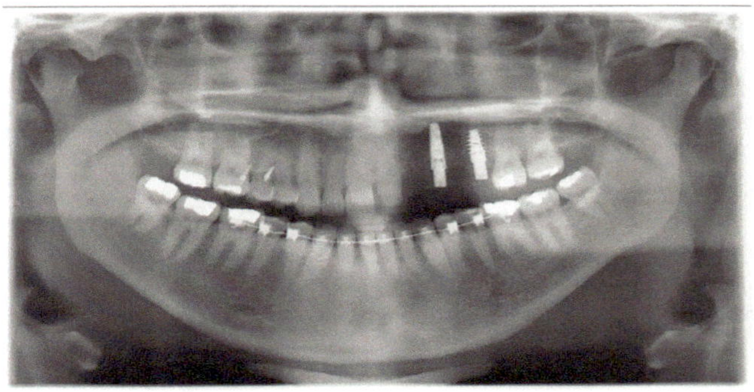

(a)

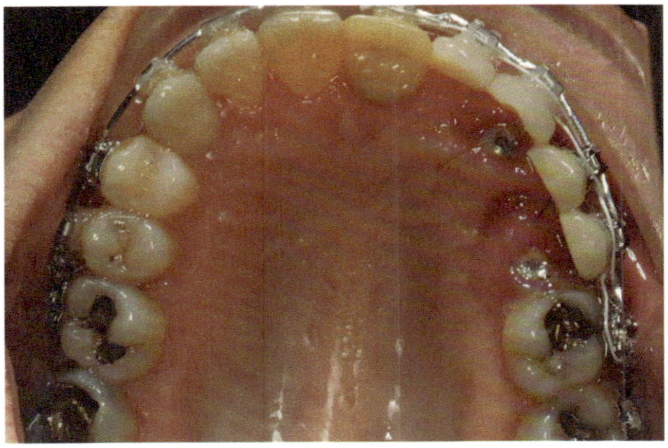

(b)

Figure 20.22 (a) Immediate post-implant placement panoramic image, 6 months prior to orthodontic debonding. (b) Clinical image 24 hours after implant placement. Pontics were placed on the archwire for interim esthetic management during the healing period. © Daniel R. Cullum

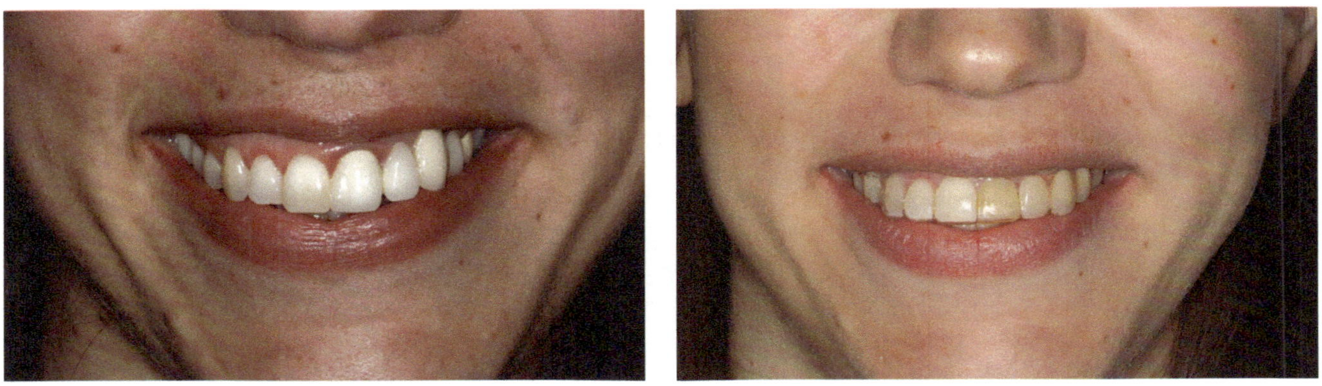

(a) (b)

Figure 20.23 (a) Pretreatment and (b) completed orthodontic treatment images demonstrate the changes in anterior occlusal plane cant; (b) shows the patient's smile with an Essix retainer and contoured pontics in place. © Daniel R. Cullum

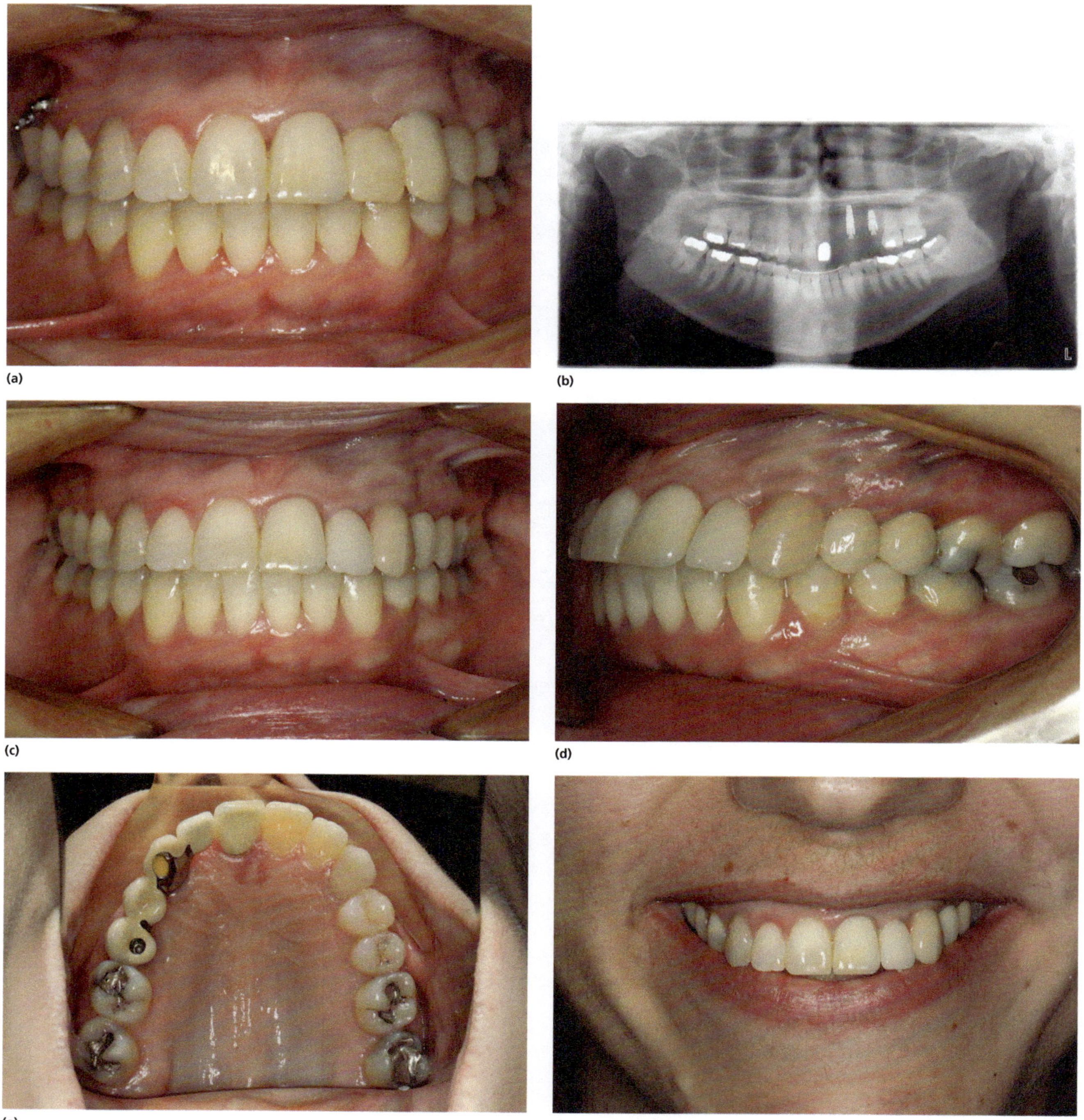

(a) (b) (c) (d) (e) (f)

Figure 20.24 (a–b) Provisional restorations were placed with initiation of emergence profile development. A definitive restoration was completed at the left central incisor with the four-unit anterior cantilever provisional restoration on implants at the left maxillary canine and second premolar. Significantly improved esthetic and stable results can be seen on clinical and panoramic images after 24 months. (c–f) Final restoration images can be seen with substantial improvement in gingival harmony and esthetics. Restorations Earl Ness DDS MSD. *Source:* (b) © Daniel R. Cullum

restoration in place for an extended period with images can be seen with substantial improvement in gingival harmony and esthetics (Figure 20.24c-f).

Case study 20.3

This case study presents a 46-year-old female who had had orthodontic treatment including four bicuspid extractions as an adolescent. She presented with an asymmetrical class II malocclusion. Her chief concern was her "crooked smile and small upper front teeth."

Diagnosis

This patient presented with an asymmetrical class II malocclusion. There was a full step class II molar relationship on the right and a class I molar relationship on the left. The asymmetry was limited to the maxillary arch (Figures 20.25 and 20.30a). Malformed "peg" maxillary lateral incisor teeth required post-treatment restorations for ideal esthetics. In addition to the A–P asymmetry, there was also a vertical asymmetry with a canted anterior occlusal plane. Gingival recession and root prominence were present on the maxillary left lateral incisor, cuspid, and bicuspid teeth.

Treatment options

This patient presented with a diagnostic and treatment planning dilemma. As a result of the previous bicuspid extractions, unilateral bicuspid extraction to resolve the maxillary asymmetry did not appear to be realistic. A non-extraction approach was an option, but effective distalization in this adult patient would be challenging. Orthognathic surgery was considered, with the ideal surgical treatment plan being maxillary and mandibular advancement to resolve both the A–P and vertical asymmetries. A compromised finish also was considered. Opening space adjacent to the lateral incisors for post-treatment restorations with asymmetry correction would result in excessive overjet.

Treatment plan

A surgical treatment plan was declined by the patient, who opted for extraction and skeletal anchorage. The maxillary right first molar was planned for extraction with trans-alveolar sinus elevation (see Chapter 15) sinus grafting and later placement of an endosseous implant, which would then provide anchorage for retraction of the right cuspid and bicuspid. A bicuspid crown was planned for the final implant restoration, with the final result being a second molar and two premolars in the maxillary right quadrant.

Treatment sequence

The maxillary right first molar was extracted with minimally invasive grafting using trans-alveolar sinus elevation. After healing, an endosseous implant was placed in the distal half of the extraction site and an immediate provisional bicuspid crown fabricated (Figure 20.26). After 8 weeks of site healing, the immediate provisional restoration was used to provide maximum A–P anchorage for retraction of the right cuspid and premolar teeth into a class I relationship

To correct the vertical asymmetry, a TAD was placed between the right maxillary cuspid and lateral incisor to intrude the teeth in that area and correct the occlusal cant (Figure 20.27). Following class I correction on the right side, spaces were opened adjacent to lateral incisors for post-orthodontic restoration.

Outcome

The canted maxillary occlusal plane was corrected with TAD-assisted intrusion of the maxillary right cuspid area. The

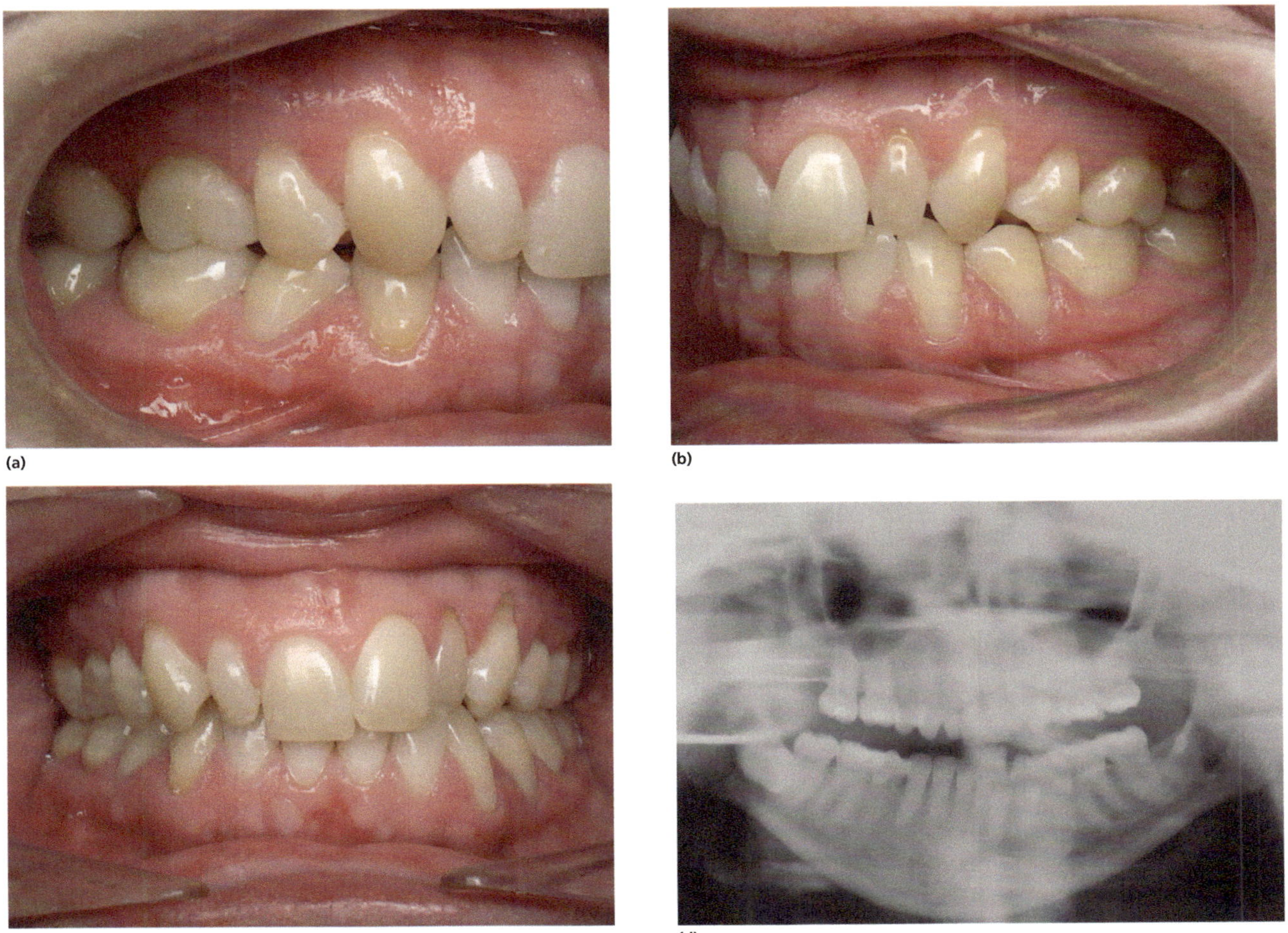

(a) (b) (c) (d)

Figure 20.25 (a–d) Pretreatment intraoral and panoramic radiographic views showed an asymmetric class II malocclusion with narrow maxillary lateral incisors.

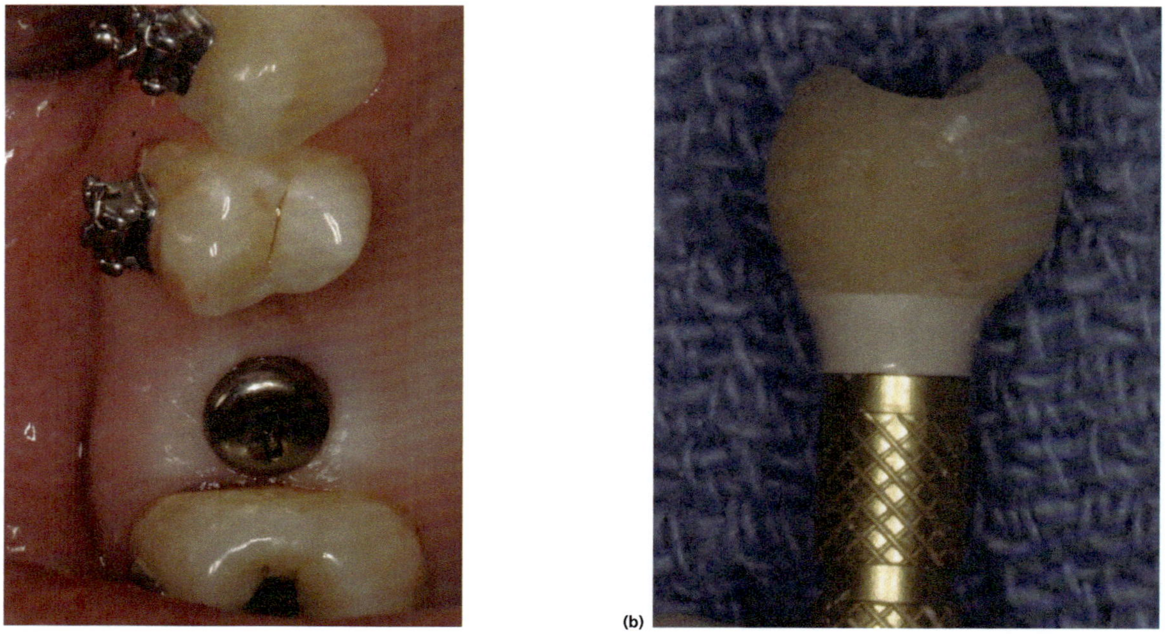

(a) (b)

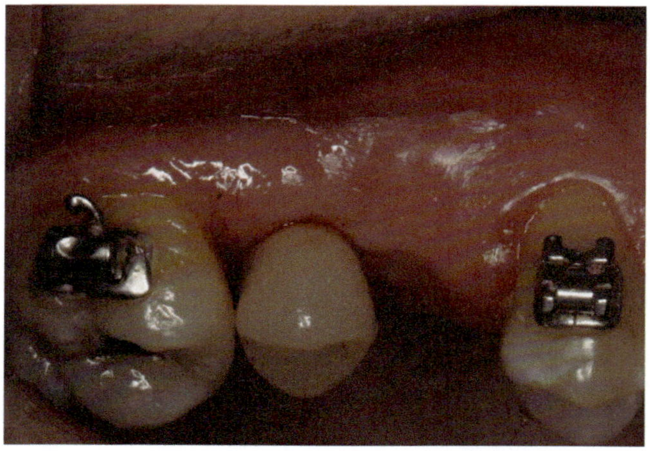

(c)

Figure 20.26 (a–c) Flapless immediate endosseous dental implant placement and immediate provisional restoration were completed for use in orthodontic anchorage. The implant was placed in distal half of the maxillary right first molar site and planned to support a final bicuspid restoration. © Daniel R. Cullum

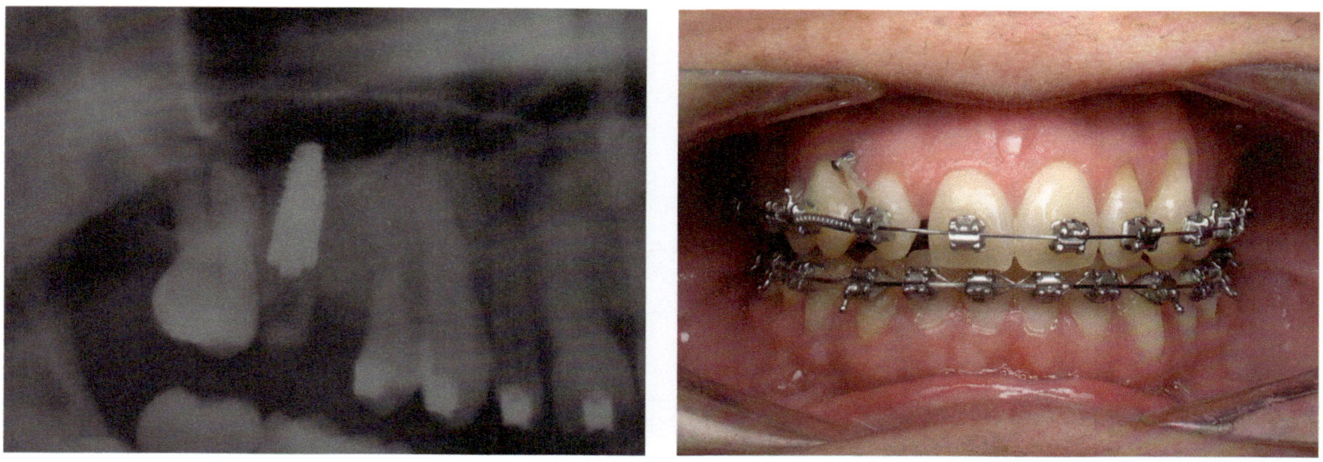

(a) (b)

Figure 20.27 (a) Panoramic and (b) clinical images after TAD placement between maxillary cuspid and lateral incisor and use for intrusion to level the anterior occlusal plane. *Source:* (a) © Daniel R. Cullum

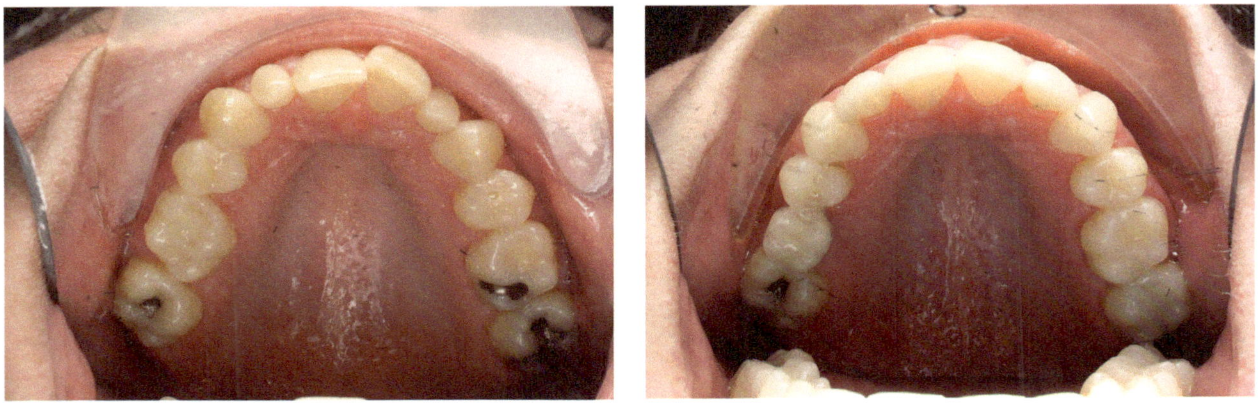

(a) (b)

Figure 20.28 (a) Pretreatment and (b) final orthodontic treatment occlusal views.

patient's esthetic outcome was idealized by providing the correct mesiodistal width of the maxillary lateral incisor sites with post-orthodontic restorations of these teeth (Figure 20.28). A class I cuspid relationship was established on the right side using the A–P anchorage from the endosseous implant. The initial treatment plan called for a premolar crown shape on the implant; however, restoration was with a primary molar crown form. The patient was extremely pleased with the outcome seen in the clinical and panoramic images in Figure 20.29.

A clinically stable and esthetic result can be seen comparing pretreatment and 8-year post-treatment facial views (Figure 20.30a and b) with a harmonious smile and the corrected anterior occlusal plane which parallels the patient's inter-pupillary line. Intraoral, smile, and panoramic radiographic views after 8 years can be seen in Figure 20.30c–g.

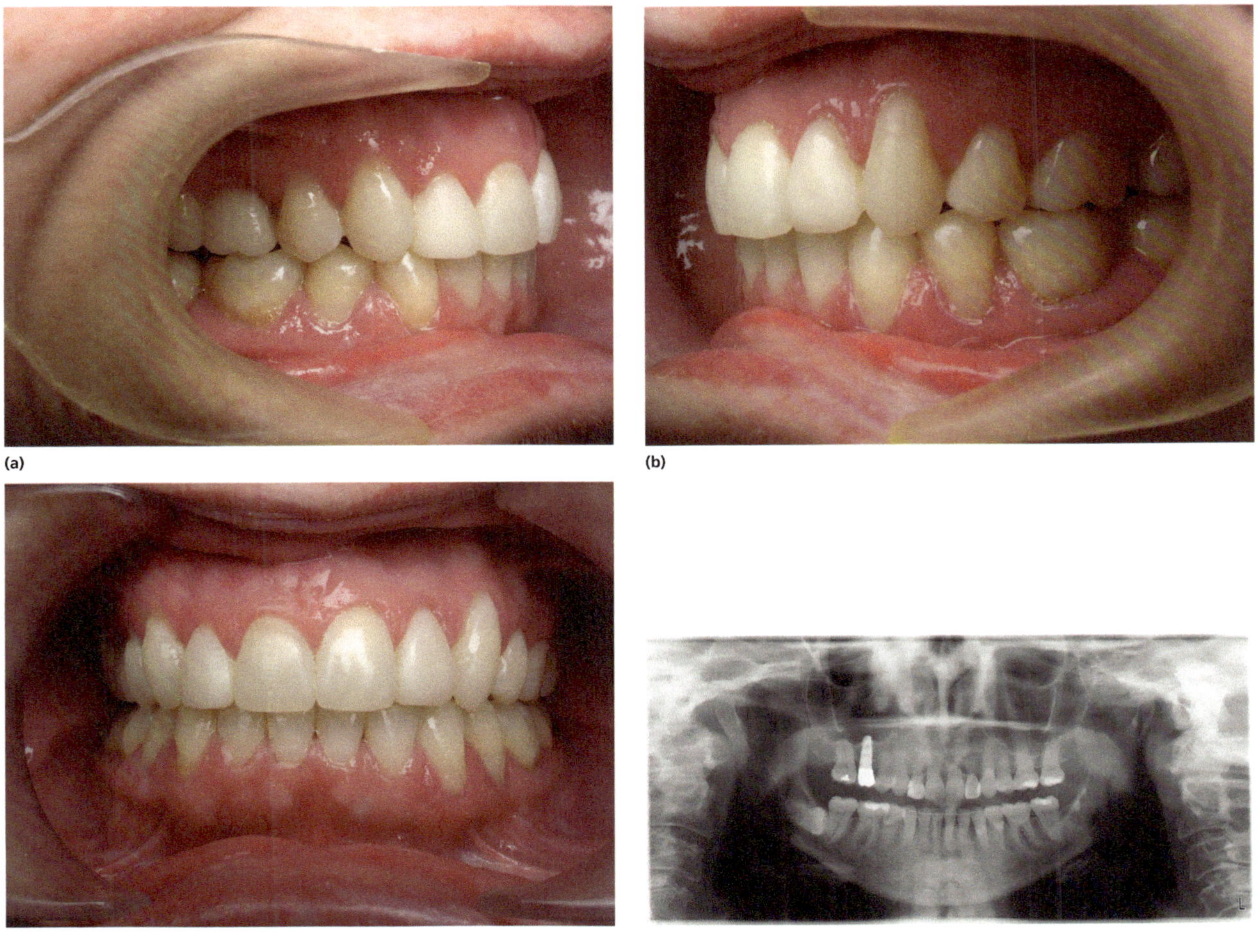

(a) (b) (c) (d)

Figure 20.29 (a–d) Final introral and panoramic radiograph views show the occlusion with its corrected anterior occlusal plane parallel to the patient's interpupillary line. A bilateral class I cuspid relationship and good proportions for the maxillary lateral incisors were achieved.

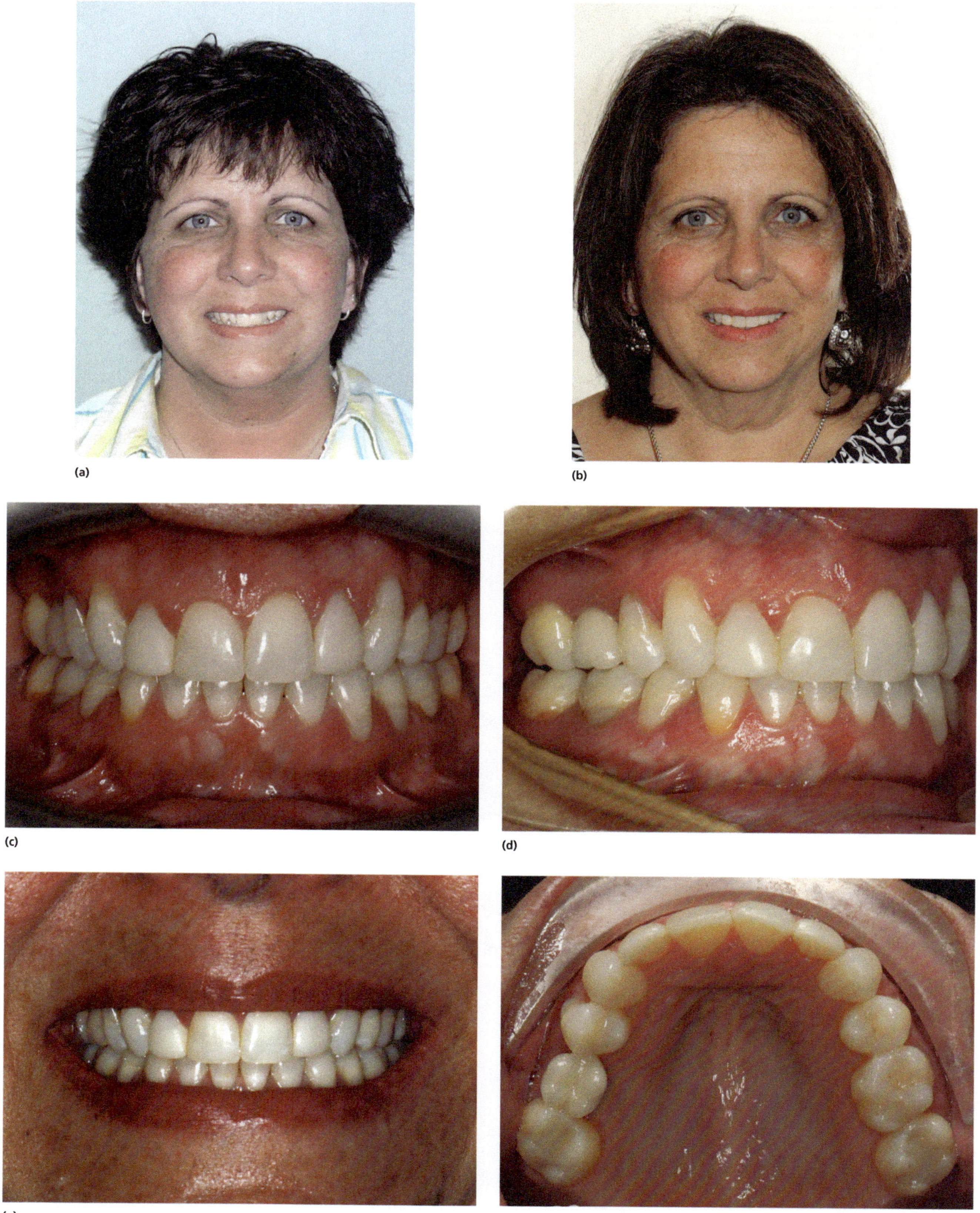

Figure 20.30 (a) Pretreatment and (b) 8-year post-treatment facial views showing a harmonious smile and the corrected anterior occlusal plane which parallels the patient's inter-pupillary line. (c–g) Intraoral, smile and panoramic radiographic views after eight years can be seen.
Source: (c,e,g) © Daniel R. Cullum

(*Continued*)

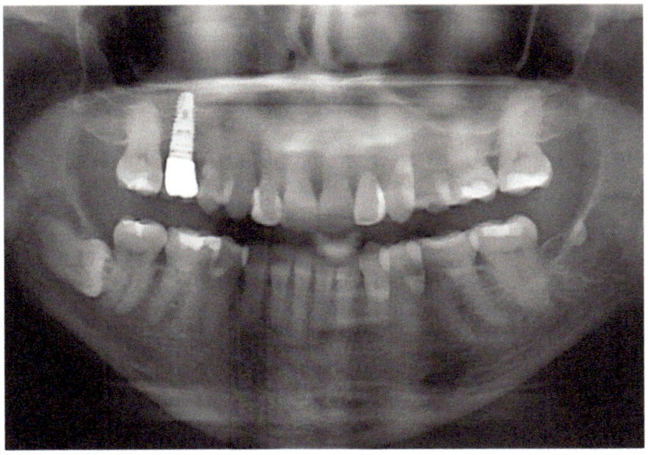

(g)
Figure 20.30 (Continued)

Conclusions

Application of orthodontic treatment using skeletal anchorage with TADs can have a profound influence on patient esthetics and function, as well as for implant site development. Appropriate diagnosis and interdisciplinary team management are necessary. All team members must continually be developing knowledge and skills in order to implement proper sequencing for an optimal treatment outcome. Minimally invasive dental implant surgery can facilitate, and is often enhanced with orthodontic treatment, including implant site development, as documented by the case studies presented.

References

1. Creekmore TD, Eklund MK. The possibility of skeletal anchorage. J Clin Orthod 1983; 17: 266–269.
2. Umemori M, Sugawara J, Mitani H, et al. Skeletal anchorage system for open-bite correction. Am J Orthod Dentofacial Orthop 1999; 115: 166–174.
3. Paik CH, Woo YJ, Boyd RL. Treatment of an adult patient with vertical maxillary excess using miniscrew fixation. J Clin Orthod 2003; 37: 423–428.
4. Sugawara J, Baik UB, Umemori M. Treatment and post-treatment dentoalveolar changes following intrusion of mandibular molars with application of a skeletal anchorage system (SAS) for open bite correction. Int J Adult Orthod Orthognath Surg 2002; 17: 243–253.
5. Lee, TC, Leung MT, Wong RW, Rabie AB. Versatility of skeletal anchorage in orthodontics. World J Orthod 2008; 9: 221–232.
6. Bae SM, Park HS, Kyung HM, et al. Clinical application of micro-implant anchorage. J Clin Orthod 2002; 5: 298–302.
7. Schudy FF. The rotation of the mandible resulting from growth – its implications in orthodontic treatment. Angle Orthod 1965; 35: 36–50.
8. Chaffee MP, Kim SH, Schudy GF. Skeletal anchorage for vertical control in extraction treatment of dolichofacial patients. J Clin Orthod 2009; 53: 749–762.

CHAPTER 21

Minimally Invasive Comprehensive Treatment: Case Studies

Daniel R. Cullum[1] & Earl Ness[2]

[1]Private Practice, Coeur d'Alene, ID; Loma Linda University Department of OMS, Loma Linda, CA; UCLA Department of OMS, Los Angeles, CA, USA

[2]Private Practice, Spokane, WA, USA

Outline of case studies

- Case study 21.1: a single-tooth implant in a site with a large apical defect.
- Case study 21.2: an anterior reconstruction with tunnel grafting and immediate provisionalization.
- Case study 21.3: immediate molar defects in a patient with multiple congenitally missing teeth.
- Case study 21.4: a multi-tooth defect staged with block bone and pedicle connective tissue grafting.
- Case study 21.5: failing short implants converted to an immediate "All-on-4"® with immediate provisional restoration.
- Case study 21.6: a full-arch immediate implant/immediate provisional reconstruction in mandible with delayed implant placement in maxilla using guided surgery with immediate provisional restoration.

Introduction

The purpose of this chapter is to demonstrate the clinical applications of minimally invasive surgery principles within the context of comprehensive prosthetic treatment. As introduced in Chapter 1, seldom does the patient present with a "simple" single-tooth problem. Treatment needs display varying complexity, budgets, and patient compliance. Many patients would benefit from interdisciplinary treatment, including orthodontics, as shown in Chapter 20. It is only through a careful and stepwise process of diagnosis and case planning that the problem list can be identified and treatment options developed. The following case series will demonstrate increasing complexity with multiple prosthetic and surgical challenges managed with minimally invasive surgical principles.

Case study 21.1

A healthy 41-year-old adult male presented with failing endodontic treatment at the maxillary left central incisor (Figure 21.1a and b). The tooth was injured in his youth with subsequent extensive restorative treatments. The patient's facial proportions were appropriate with a moderately low smile line on animation and mild incisal edge attrition (Figure 21.1c). The gingival zeniths were symmetric with good bone and soft tissue anatomy and no significant periodontal probing depths. The tooth had significant discoloration of the crown and moderate apical vestibular inflammation.

Diagnosis Fractured/non-restorable maxillary left central incisor with apical pathology and mild attrition.

Plan Extraction and grafting with staged implant reconstruction including a removable provisional restoration.

Treatment Surgical, minimally invasive removal of the residual root fragment was completed revealing a large apical bone defect. The defect was not accessible through the extraction socket. The crestal and interproximal bone and soft tissues were intact (Figure 21.1d). An apical semi-lunar incision was completed to allow for debridement of the apical pathology, while preserving the crestal bone bridge and soft tissue anatomy (Figure 21.1e). Particulate graft material was used to fill the socket and apical defect (Figure 21.1f). A collagen barrier (Cytoplast RTM®, Osteogenics, Lubbock, TX) was used to cover the apical site while a modified Bio-Col® technique was used crestally (Figure 21.1g). Both collagen products were saturated in rh-PDGF (off-label use of GEM 21S, Osteohealth, Shirley, NY) before being placed. Cone beam computed tomography (CBCT) images and clinical findings of the alveolar dimensions and healing after 6 months are seen in Figure 21.1h–j. There was good horizontal dimension and adequate soft tissue for implant placement.

A papilla-sparing, palatally-based incision was elevated with the intention of allowing apical positioning to enhance the gingival zenith height. Implant site development was completed with a 2 mm twist drill followed by osteotome expansion site development (ridge expansion osteotomy) (Figure 21.1k and l). The implant was placed using a non-submerged technique and a split-thickness dissection with beveled vertical incisions allowed apical flap positioning (Figure 21.1m and n). A removable provisional appliance was inserted after confirming no direct tissue contact (Figure 21.1o). After 4 months' healing, the bone and soft tissue contours showed excellent tissue volume and implant position (Figure 21.1p and q).

After site healing, a provisional restoration was prepared (Figure 21.1r), and followed by emergence profile development and tissue sculpting of the gingival zenith position (Figure 21.1s) The patient can be seen in Figure 21.1t–w, 1 year after the final restoration was inserted.

Minimally Invasive Dental Implant Surgery, First Edition. Edited by Daniel R. Cullum and Douglas Deporter.

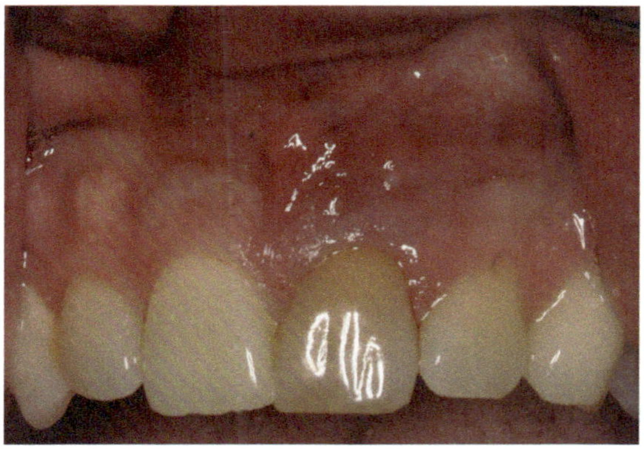

(a)

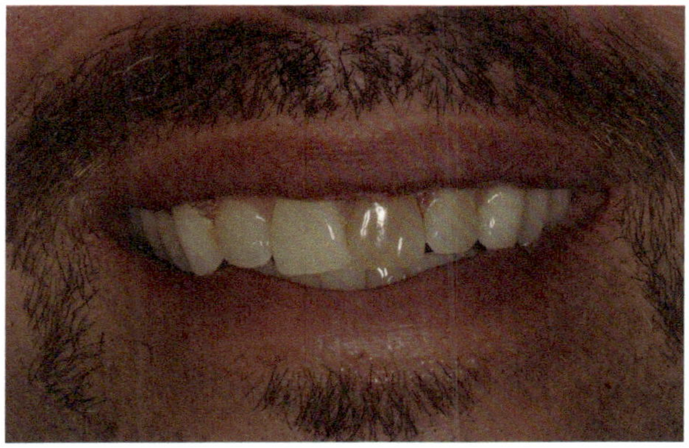

(b)

Figure 21.1 (a, b) A healthy adult male presented with a failing endodontically-treated maxillary left central incisor with a large apical radiolucency seen on the preop periapical radiograph. (c) The patient's facial proportions were appropriate with a moderately low smile line on animation; mild incisal edge attrition also was evident. (d) Minimally invasive surgical removal of the residual root fragment was completed revealing a large apical defect not accessible through the extraction socket. The crestal and interproximal bone and soft tissues were intact. (e) An apical semi-lunar incision was used to access the apical defect and complete site debridement, while preserving the crestal bone bridge and soft tissue anatomy. (f) Site grafting with particulate blended beta-tricalcium phosphate (beta-TCP; Cerasorb®, Curasan, RTP, NC), bovine HA (Osteograf N700®, Dentsply, Johnson City, TN), and recombinant human platelet-derived growth factor (rh-PDGF; GEM 21S®, Osteohealth, Shirley, NY) was completed from the apical and crestal aspects. (g) A collagen barrier (Cytoplast® RTM, Osteogenics, Lubbock, TX) was used to cover the apical site, while a modified Bio-Col® technique was used at the crest.

(Continued)

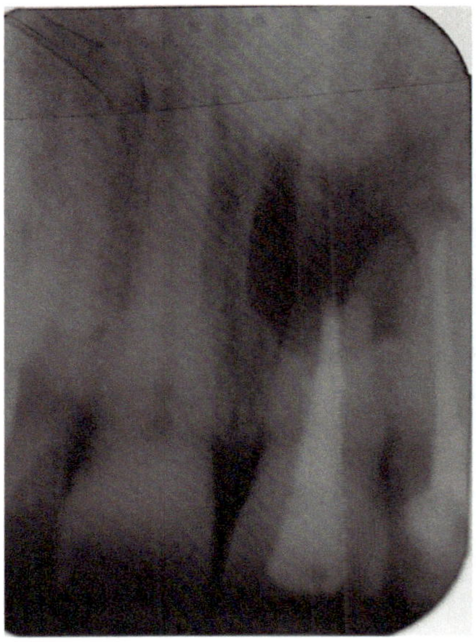

(c)

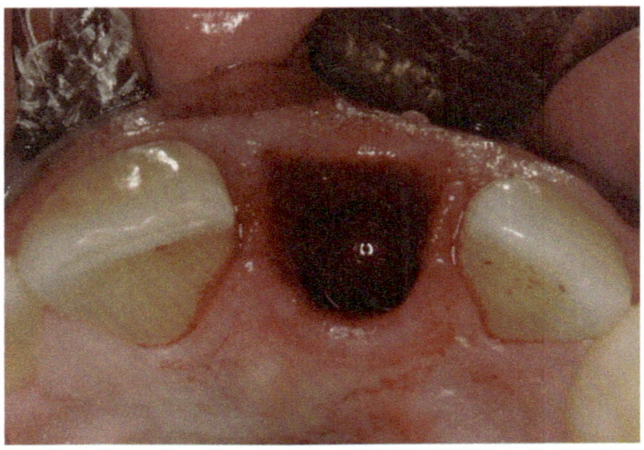

(d)

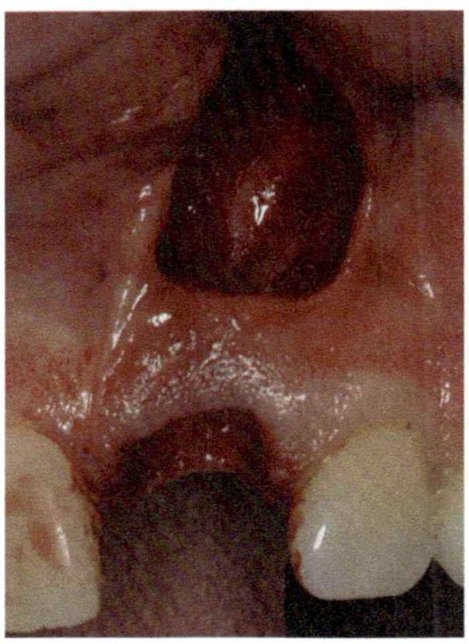

(e)

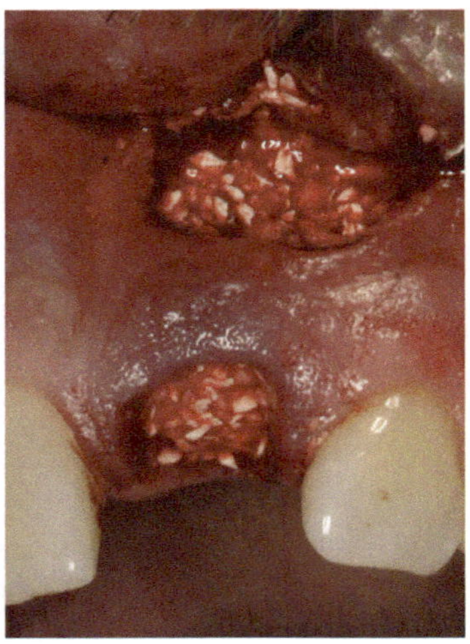

(f)

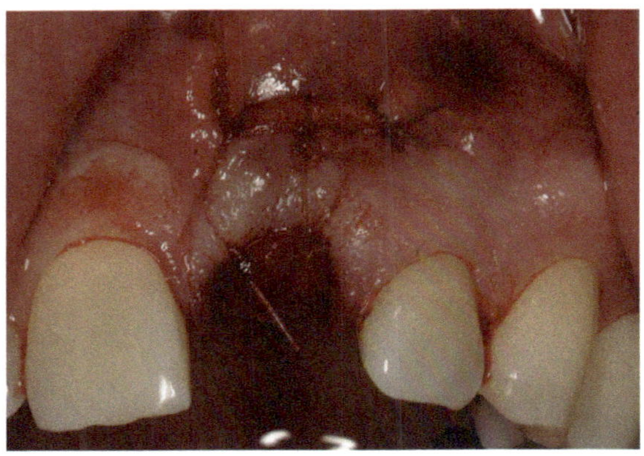

(g)

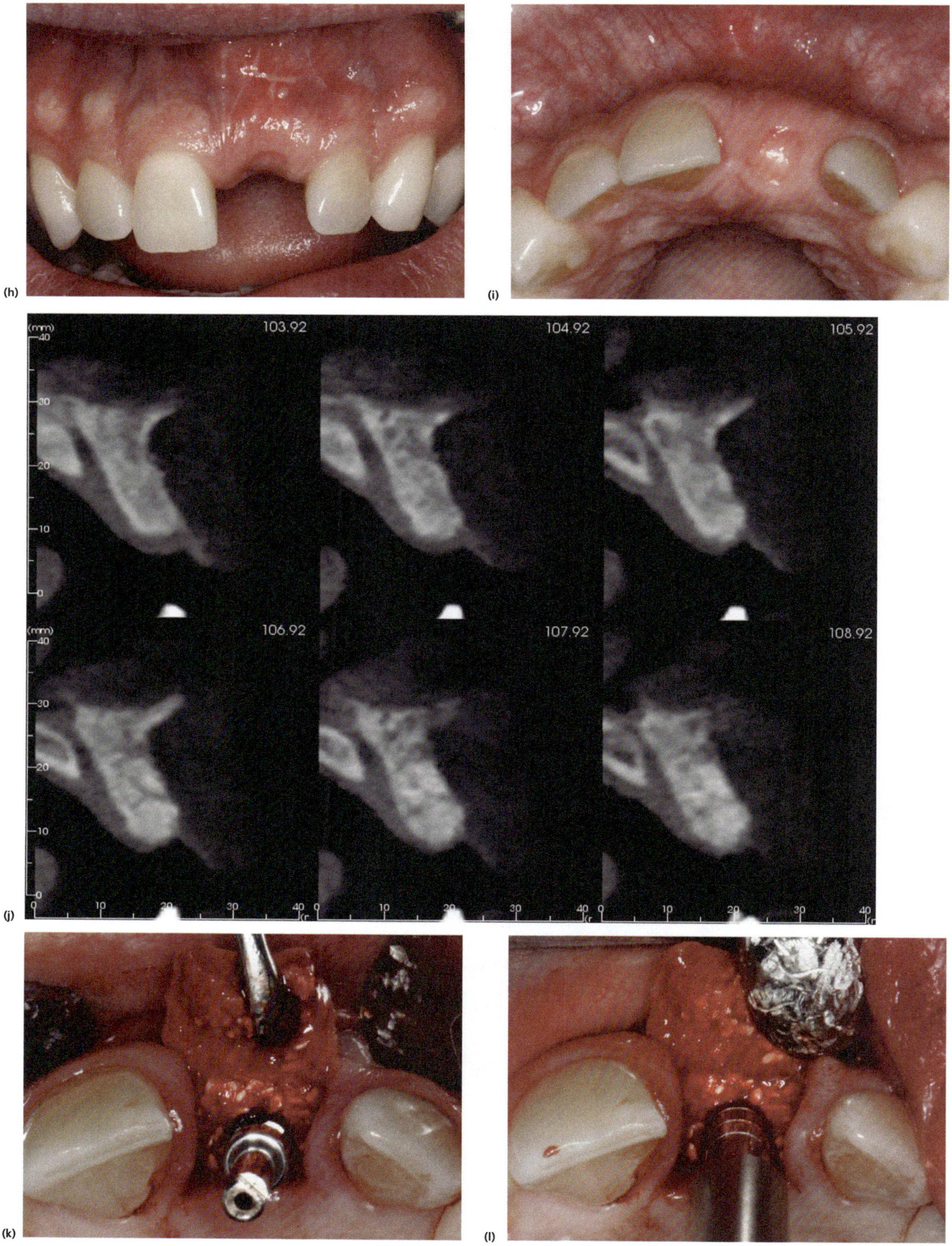

Figure 21.1 (Continued)
(h–j) CBCT and clinical images show the resulting alveolar dimensions after 6 months healing. (k, l) For implant placement, a papilla-sparing, palatally-based incision design was used. Following the use of a 2 mm diameter pilot drill to establish implant positioning, site development was completed using osteotomes.

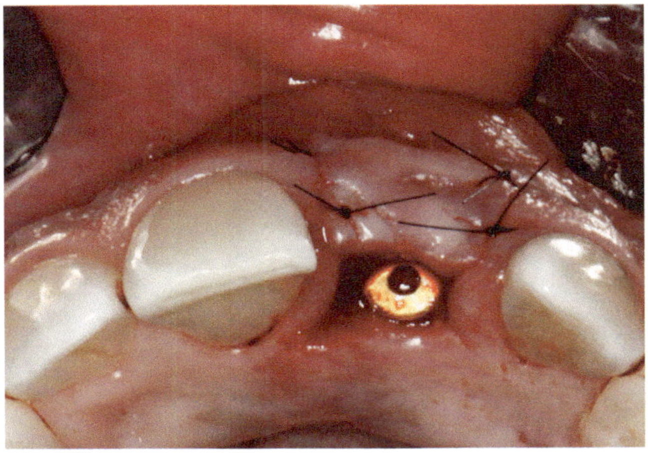
(m)

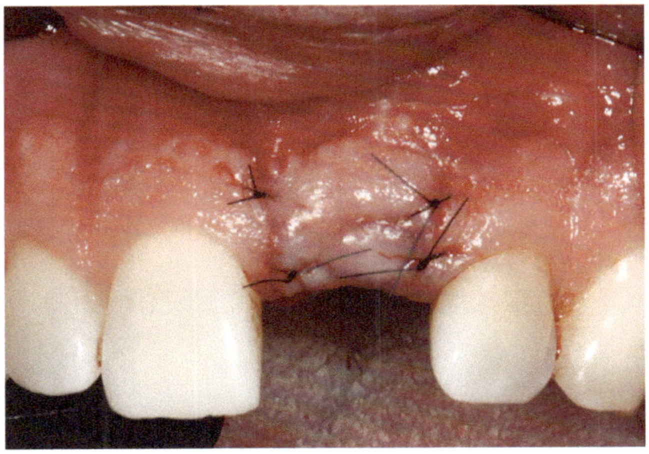
(n)

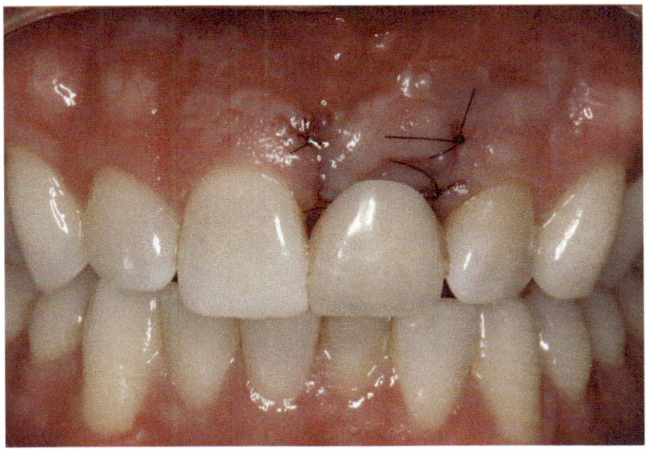
(o)

Figure 21.1 (Continued)
(m, n) Single-stage implant insertion was completed in association with a split-thickness buccal flap dissection to allow the facial soft tissues to be positioned apically. (o) A removable provisional appliance was inserted after confirming no direct tissue contact. (p, -q) After 4 months' healing, the bone and soft tissue contours showed excellent tissue volume.
(Continued)

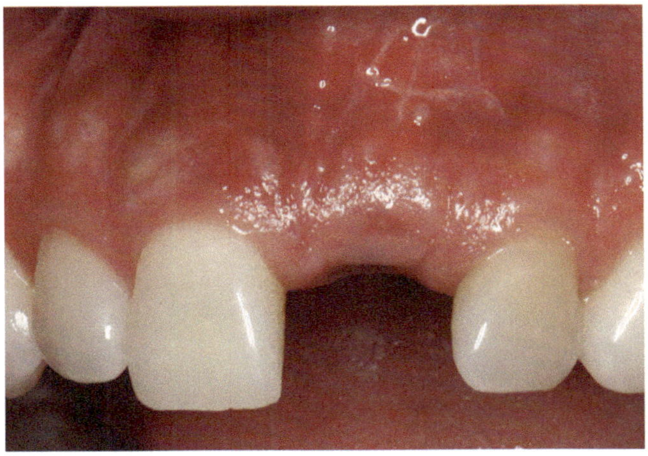
(p)

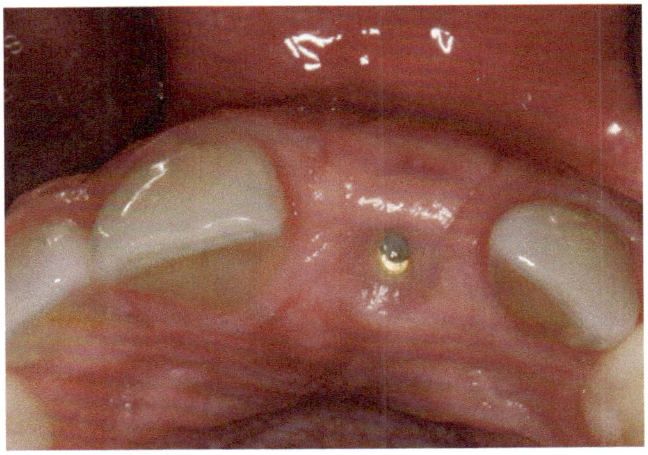
(q)

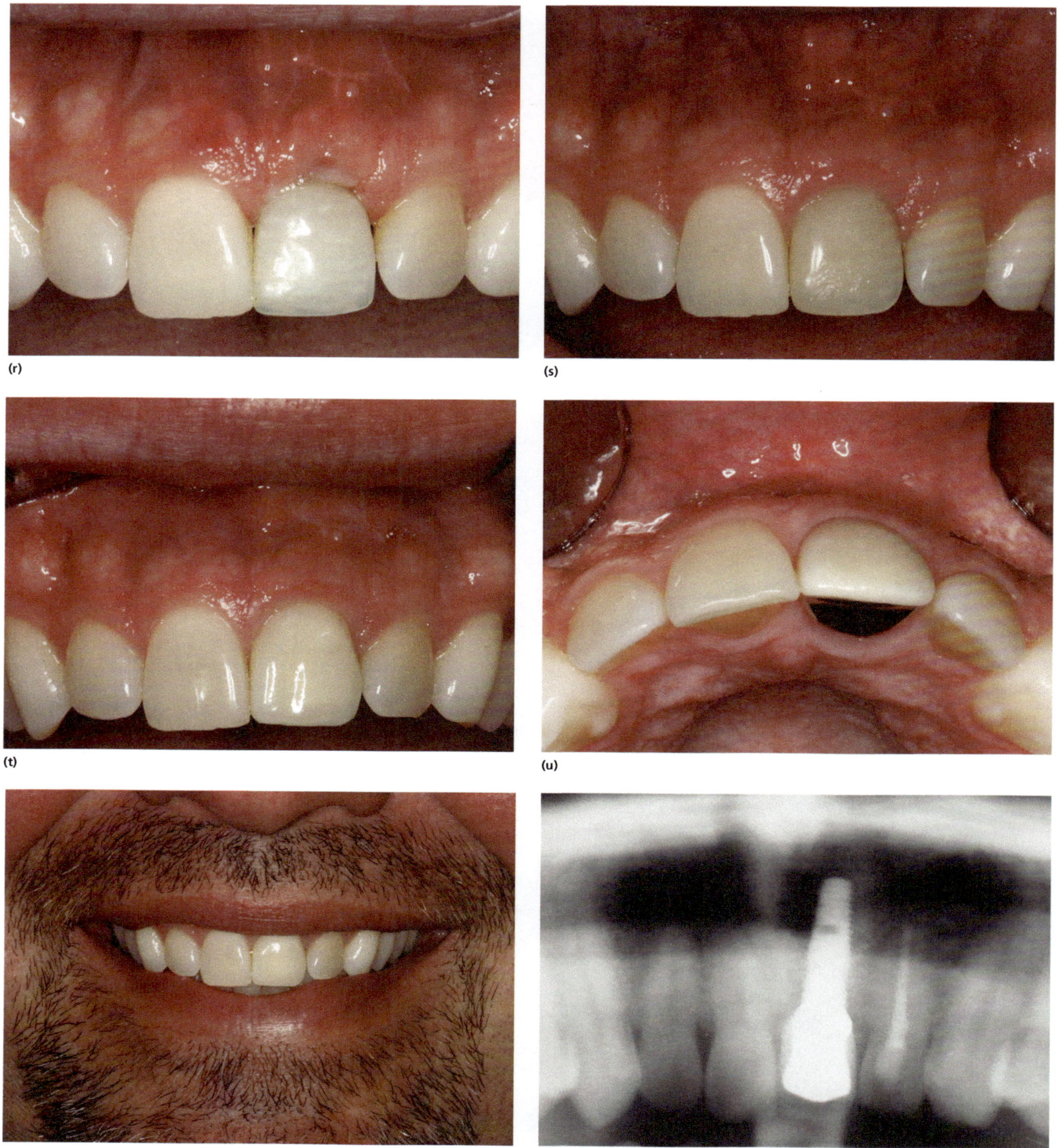

(r) (s) (t) (u) (v) (w)

Figure 21.1 (Continued)
(r, s) A provisional fixed restoration was completed, followed by emergence profile development and tissue sculpting to develop the gingival zenith position. (t–w) The patient can be seen here after 1 year post-restoration confirming excellent tissue contours. © Daniel R. Cullum.

Case study 21.2

A healthy 49-year-old adult male presented with a failing maxillary anterior fixed partial denture. The right lateral and left central incisors had failing endodontic treatments and were non-restorable (Figure 21.2a). The patient's facial proportions were appropriate with a low smile line on animation. There was moderate incisal edge attrition, a malposed lower left lateral incisor with poor incisal guidance, and fractured incisal edges on the failing bridge (Figure 21.2b). Panoramic and CBCT images were obtained to show the pretreatment alveolar dimensions (Figure 21.2c–f) After the patient was started on oral chlorhexidine rinses and an antibiotic, the condition of the soft tissues improved (Figure 21.2g). Figure 21.2h shows the treatment site after removal of the failed prosthesis. The gingival zenith was apical at the left central incisor and at the right lateral incisor with significant bone atrophy at the edentulous right central incisor site, gingival inflammation, a hyperplastic maxillary labial frenum, and no significant periodontal probing defects.

Diagnosis Failing maxillary anterior fixed partial denture and fractured non-restorable maxillary right lateral and left central incisors. Moderate attrition, a parafunctional habit, a malposed mandibular right lateral incisor, with alveolar atrophy at the edentulous right central incisor site, and a hyperplastic maxillary labial frenum.

Plan Extraction of the right lateral, left central and lateral incisor teeth with placement of an immediate implant-supported, non-functional fixed provisional restoration. Grafting of the lateral incisor implant buccal defects, socket grafting of the left central incisor site, and tunnel augmentation of the right central residual bone defect were determined to be appropriate. The immediate implant-supported provisional restoration was to be used for soft tissue contouring, emergence profile development, and soft tissue maturation after initial implant osseointegration. Re-contouring of the malposed crown of the mandibular right lateral incisor would be included in the final restorative phase.

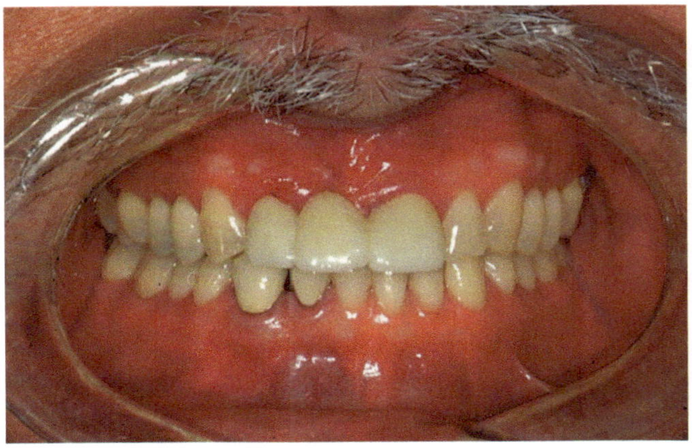

(a)

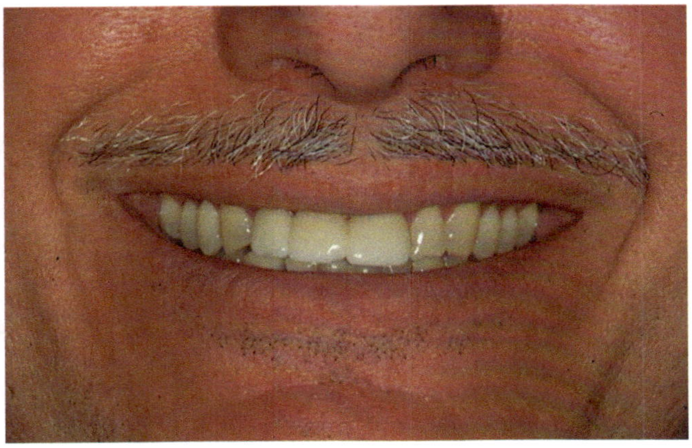

(b)

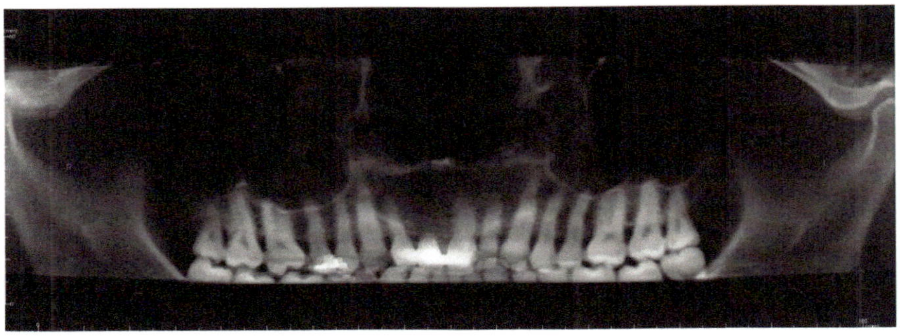

(c)

Figure 21.2 (a) A healthy 49-year-old adult male presented with a failing maxillary anterior fixed partial denture. The right lateral and left central incisors had failed endodontic treatments, and were non-restorable. Moderate incisal edge attrition and fractured incisal edges were present on the prosthesis, as well as the adjacent and opposing teeth. (b) Full smile view. (c–f) Pretreatment CBCT reconstructed panoramic and cross-sectional images demonstrated labial root proximity of the lateral incisors, apical radiolucency, and the existing bone volume.

(Continued)

(d)

(e)

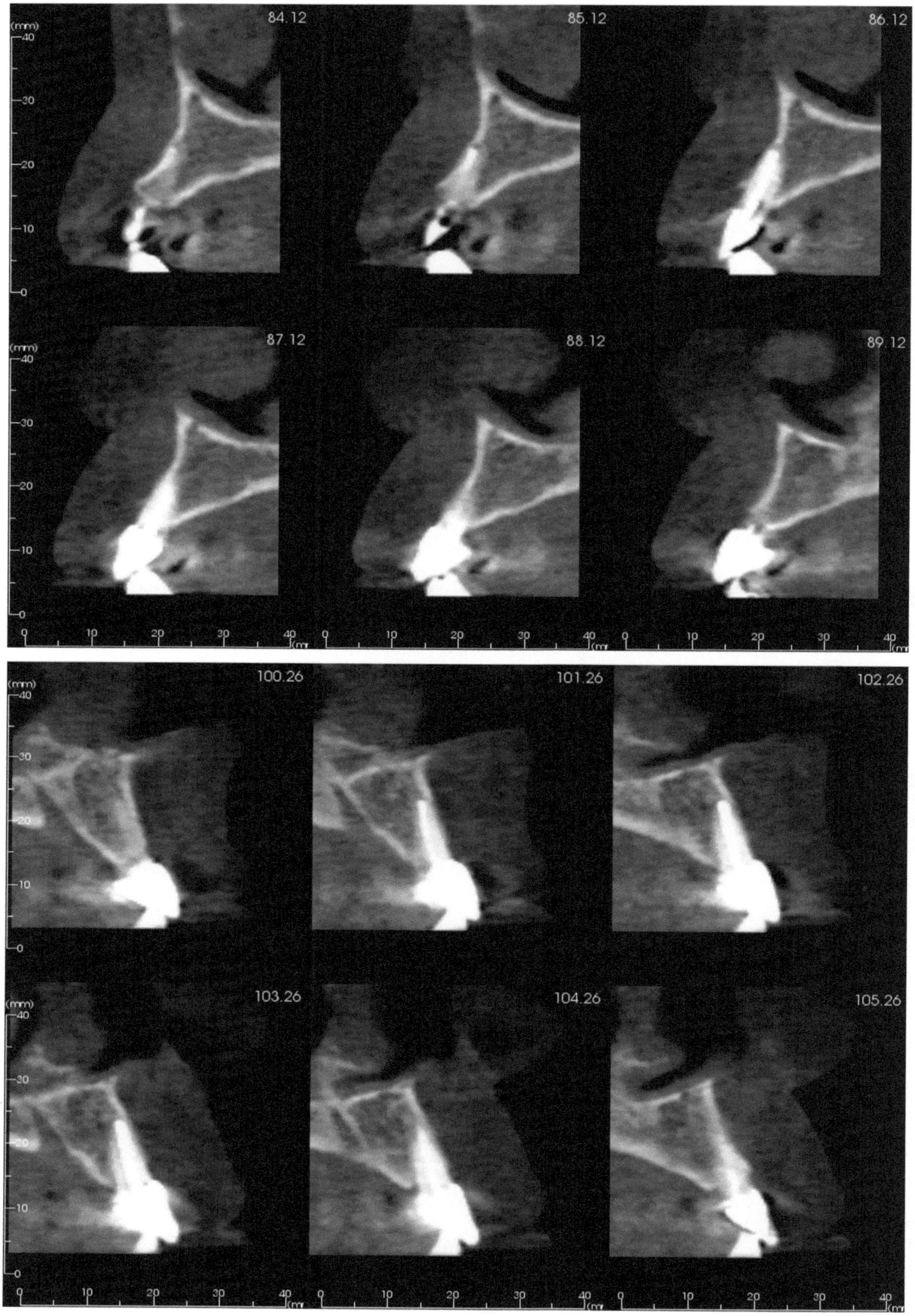

Figure 21.2 (Continued)

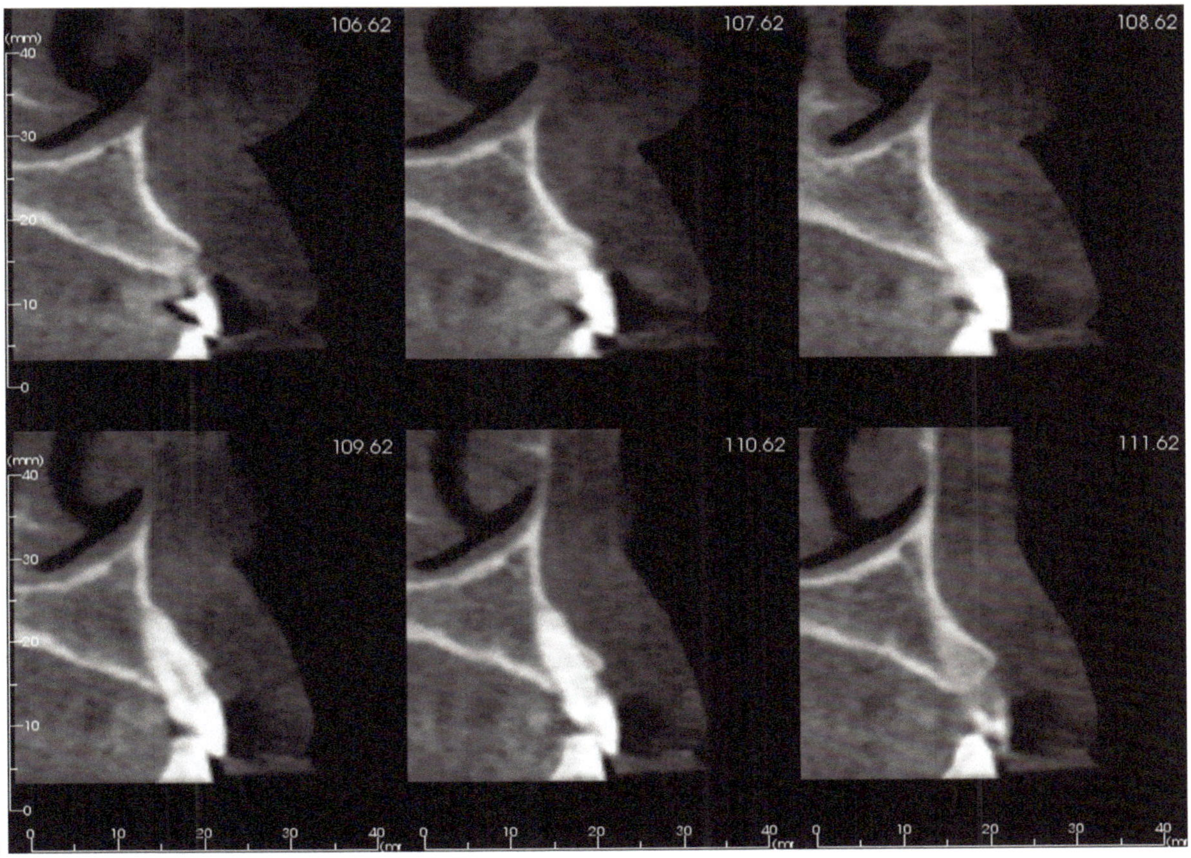

(f)

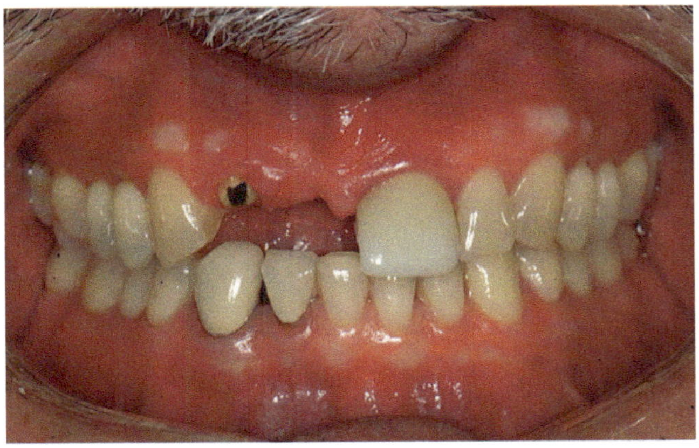

(g)

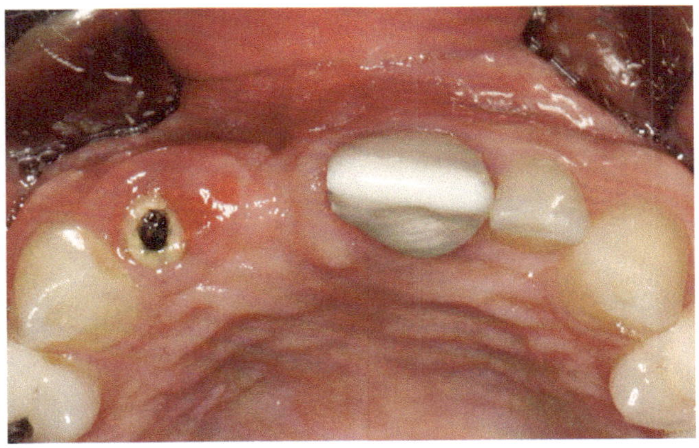

(h)

Figure 21.2 (Continued)
(g) Initial management with oral chlorhexidine rinses and an antibiotic led to reduced inflammation. (h) The soft tissue contours are seen here after prosthesis removal.

(Continued)

Treatment The residual root fragments were surgically removed using a minimally invasive technique (Figure 21.2i). The crestal/interproximal bone and soft tissues were intact except for a slight facial defect at the right lateral incisor site (Figure 21.2j). Implant site development was initiated with a 2 mm diameter twist drill ensuring palatal implant positioning (Figure 21.2k). Particulate grafting was used to close the residual peri-implant crestal bone gaps. A vertical midline incision was completed with laser excision (Figure 21.2l) to dissect the frenal connective tissue attachment from its underlying periosteum. The periosteum then was incised and elevated using tunneling to the crestal height both distally and coronally while preserving the soft tissue anatomy (Figure 21.2m). Tunnel grafting with particulate hydroxyapatite (HA) was completed (Figure 21.2n). Bovine collagen saturated in rh-PDGF was used to cover the apical site, while a modified Bio-Col technique was completed at the crestal bone and soft tissue gaps at the immediate implant and socket graft sites (Figure 21.2o). The patient was seen at the prosthodontist's office for placement of an immediate, screw-retained provisional restoration using direct pick-up technique on temporary plastic abutments. Early healing can be seen after 2 weeks and in a post-operative panoramic radiograph in Figure 21.2p–r. After 3 months' healing, the provisional restoration was modified to permit emergence profile development and soft tissue sculpting of the gingival zenith positions. The clinical and radiographic images can be seen after restoration in Figure 21.2s–v.

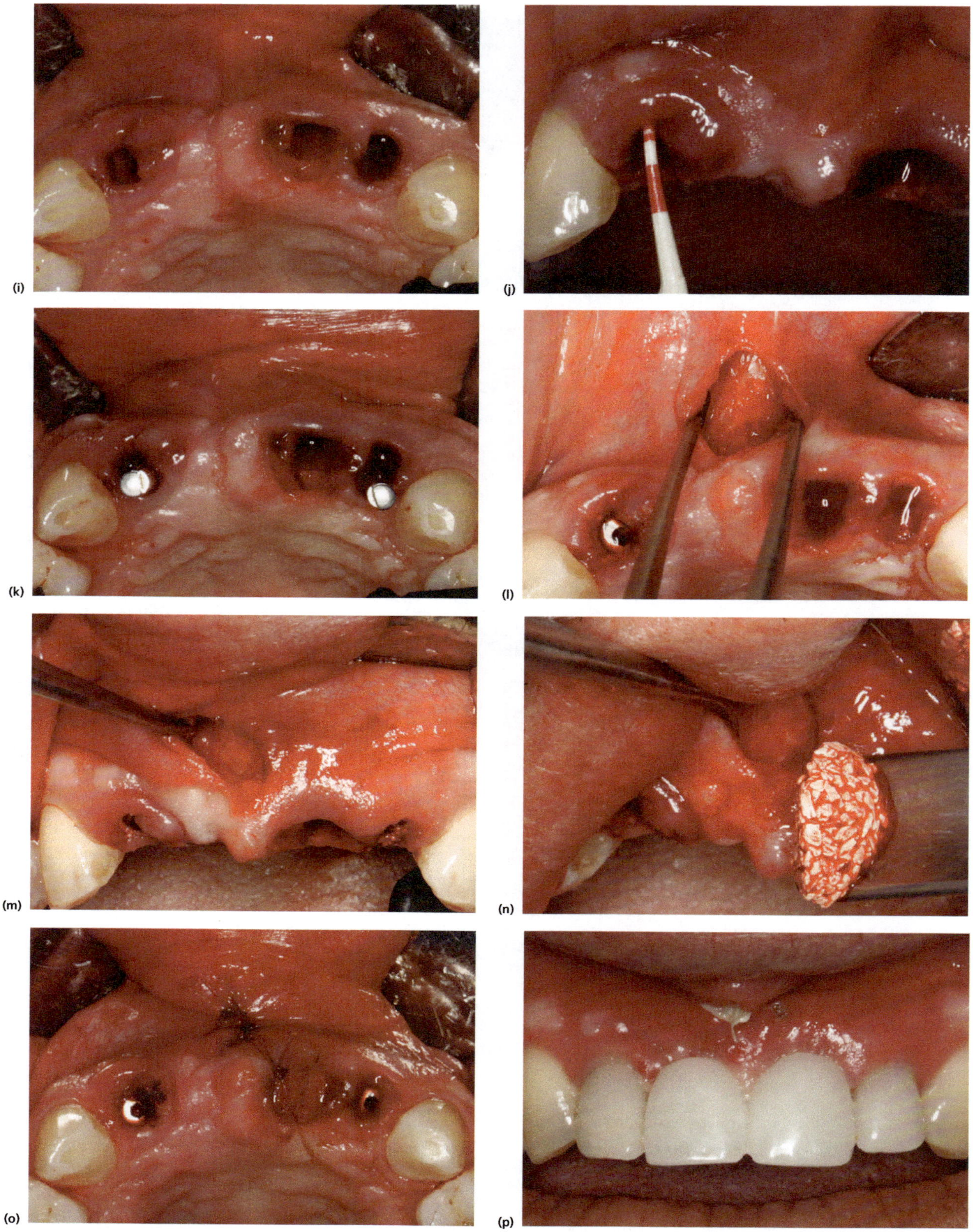

Figure 21.2 (Continued)

(i) An occlusal view after the removal of the teeth. (j) Probing of the residual defects confirmed intact interproximal bone and a slight mid-facial defect at the right central incisor. (k) Palatal implant positioning was established using a 2 mm diameter pilot drill. The implants were inserted and the residual buccal crestal bone gaps grafted. (l) The hyperplastic frenal attachment was excised down to periosteum using a laser. (m) The periosteum was incised and elevated distally and coronally with tunneling while preserving soft tissue anatomy. (n) Tunnel grafting was completed using particulate dense HA. (Osteograf N700®, Dentsply, Johnson City, TN). (o) A bovine collagen membrane was saturated with rh-PDGF (GEM 21S®, Osteohealth, Shirley, NY) and used to cover the apical site, while a modified Bio-Col® technique was used to manage the crestal bone and soft tissue gaps at the immediate implant and socket graft sites. (p, q) Early healing can be seen after 2 weeks.

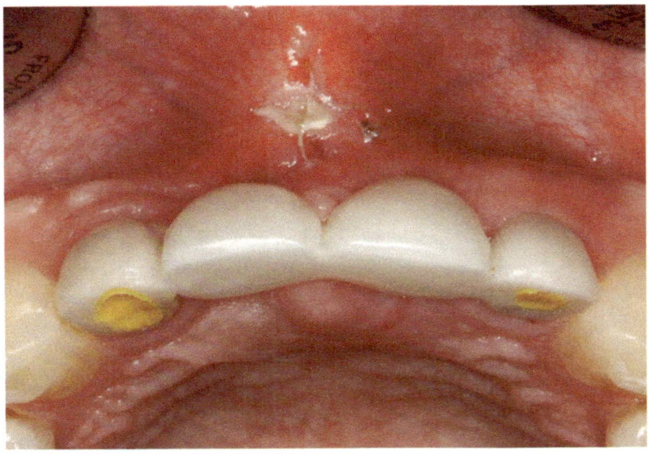
(q)

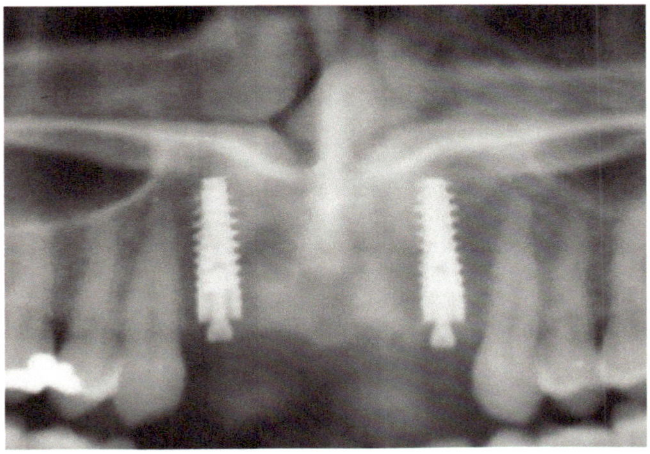
(r)

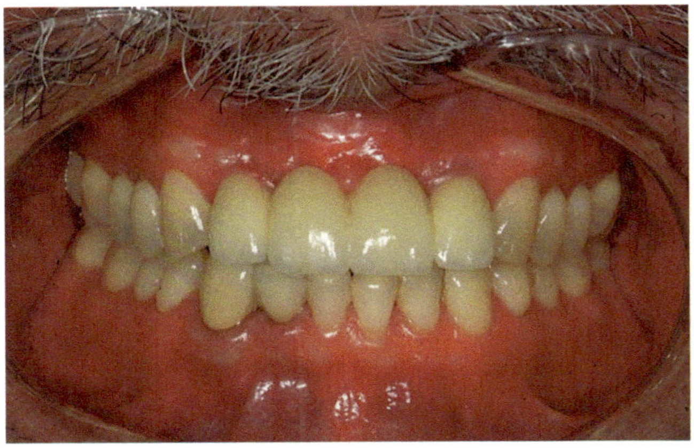
(s)

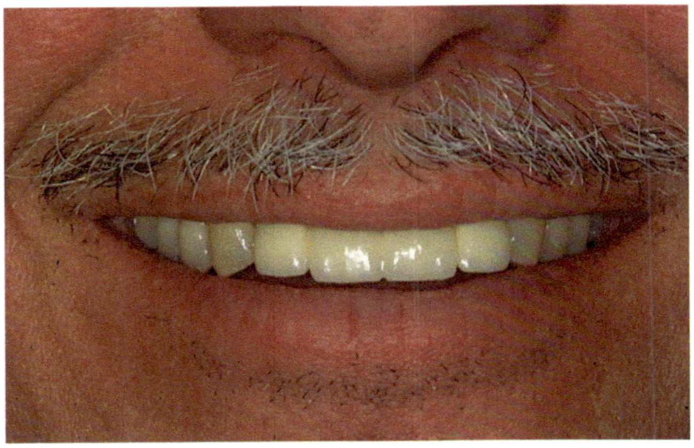
(t)

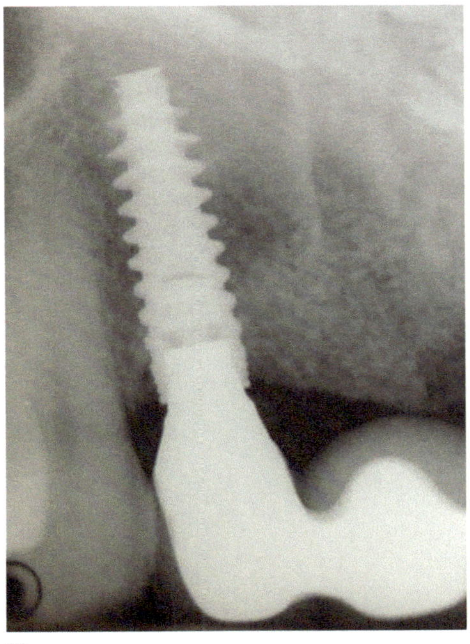
(u)

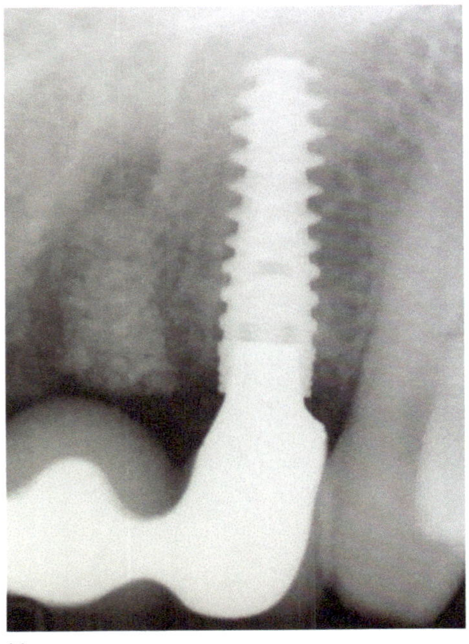
(v)

Figure 21.2 (Continued)
(r) A post-operative panoramic radiograph. (s–v) The clinical and periapical radiograph images after restoration. *Source:* (a–b, g, s–v) © Earl Ness. (c–f, h–r) © Daniel R. Cullum.

Case study 21.3

This 44-year-old female patient presented with bilateral congenitally missing maxillary lateral incisor and mandibular second premolar teeth (Figure 21.3a–g). The patient's facial proportions were appropriate with mild gingival display on animation, a 2 mm mandibular midline discrepancy to the left, and mild incisal edge attrition with adequate incisal guidance (Figure 21.3a and d). The mandibular first molars both showed soft tissue recession and inadequate attached tissue on the mesio-buccal roots. There also was a draining fistula secondary to a root fracture of the left first molar (Figure 21.3e and f). Cross-sectional CBCT images showed failing endodontic treatments with apical involvement on the right side and buccal root dehiscence of the left first molar (Figure 21.3h and i). The bilateral edentulous second premolar sites displayed moderate horizontal bone loss, as seen on the left in Figure 21.3i.

Diagnosis Congenitally missing maxillary lateral incisors and mandibular second premolars with non-restorable mandibular right and left first molars having recession defects and root dehiscences. Other findings included mild attrition, midline discrepancy, and moderate alveolar atrophy at the edentulous mandibular first premolar sites.

Plan Extraction of the right and left first molar teeth with single-stage, immediate implant placement and grafting. Ridge expansion site development with osteo-condensation at the first premolar sites (with overgrafting), apical soft tissue positioning, and single-stage implant placement. Osteotome expansion of the lateral incisor sites with single-stage implant placement and provisional restoration using a removable appliance.

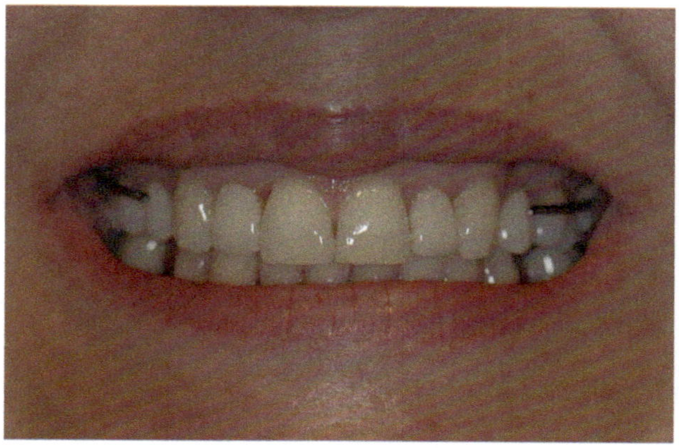
(a)

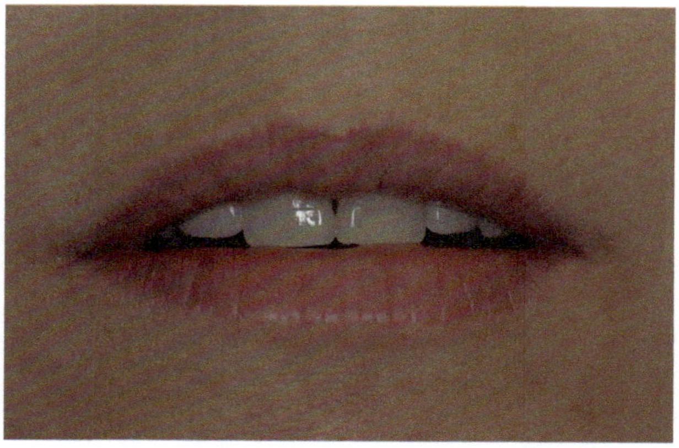
(b)

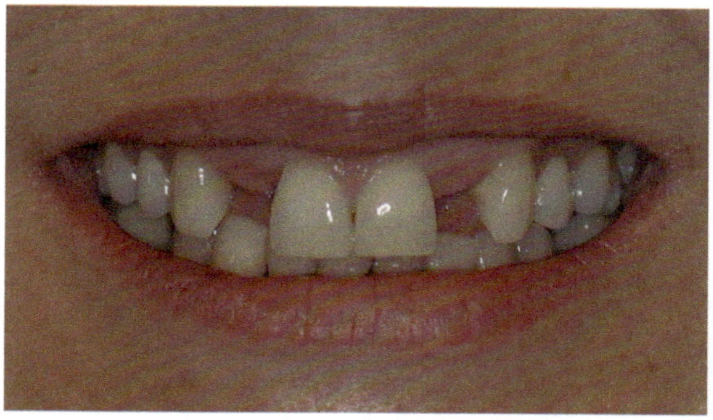
(c)

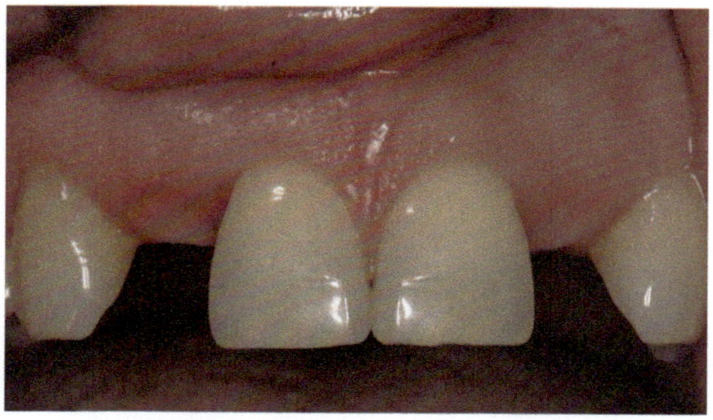
(d)

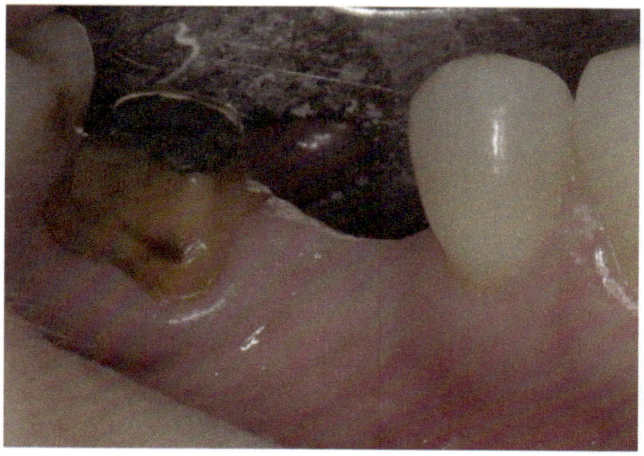
(e)

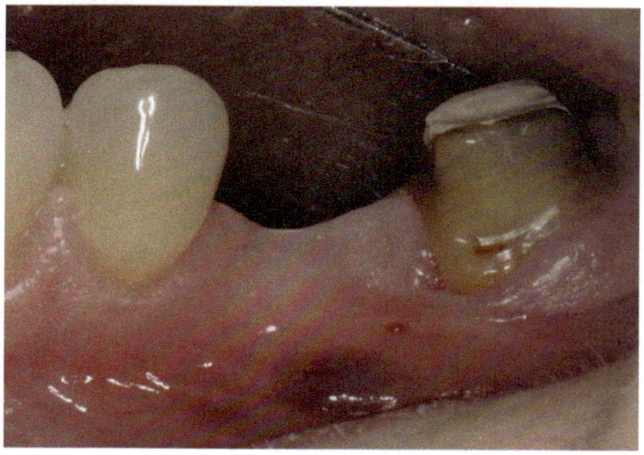
(f)

Figure 21.3 (a–d) This 44-year-old female patient presented with congenitally missing maxillary lateral incisors and mandibular second premolar teeth. The patient's facial proportions were appropriate with mild gingival display on animation, a 2 mm mandibular midline discrepancy to the left, and mild incisal edge attrition with good incisal guidance. (e, f) The mandibular first molars were failing with soft tissue recession, inadequate buccal attached tissue at the mesial root, and a draining fistula secondary to a root fracture on the left side.

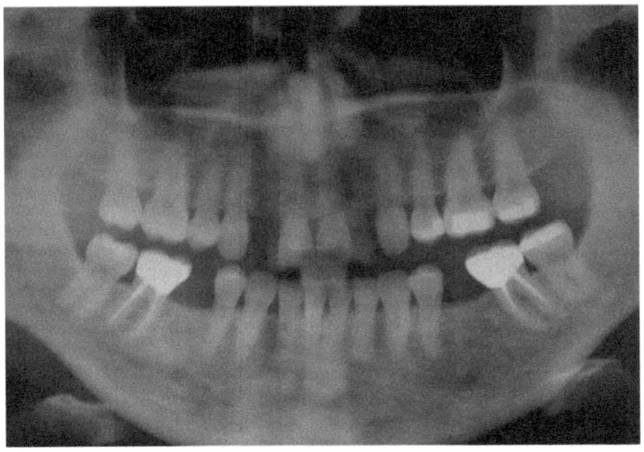

(g)

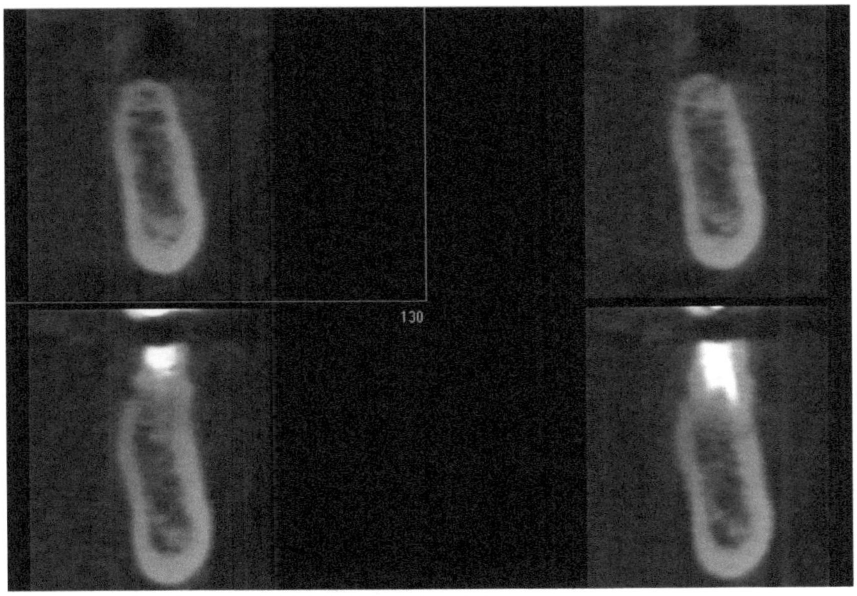

(h)

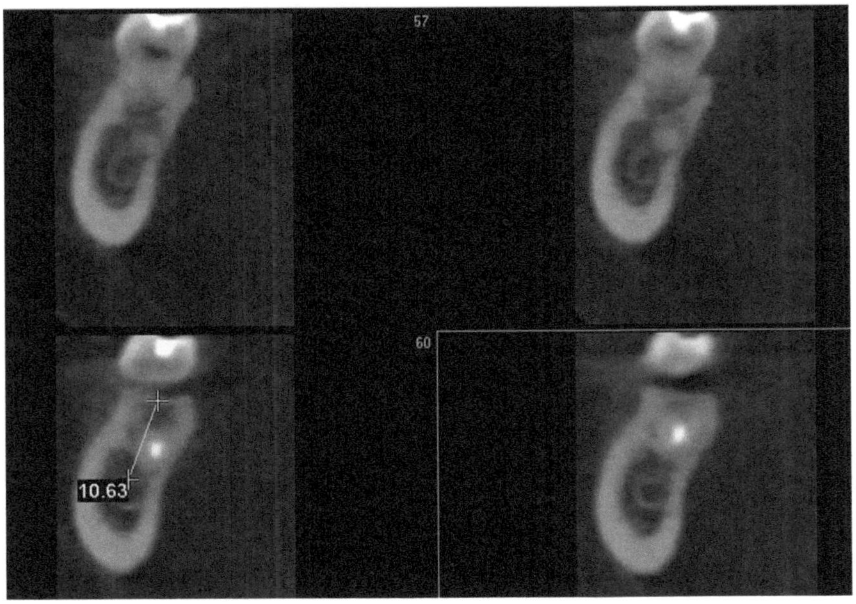

(i)

Figure 21.3 (Continued)

(g) The pretreatment panoramic image. (h) The CBCT cross-sectional image of the mandibular left first molar demonstrating a mesio-buccal root dehiscence. (i) The CBCT cross-sectional image of the mandibular left first molar demonstrated failed endodontic treatment with apical pathology. The residual bone height to the inferior alveolar nerve was about 11 mm.

(Continued)

Treatment Minimally invasive, surgical removal of the right and left mandibular molars was completed with debridement of the sites. A palatal full-thickness flap was extended anteriorly with the mesial papilla left intact at the premolar sites. The right mandibular sites had intact crestal and interproximal bone except for a 3 mm vertical facial dehiscence at the first molar and mild horizontal deficiency at the premolar (Figure 21.3j). Implant site development was initiated with a 2 mm diameter twist drill in the molar furcation and the premolar site (Figure 21.3j). Subsequently, piezoelectric bone surgery was used to asymmetrically develop the molar osteotomy towards the palatal aspect and the premolar site was expanded with screw expanders. Insertion of the implants toward the palatal aspect can be seen in Figure 21.2k. Insertion of healing caps, particulate grafting of the remaining bone defects, and crestal collagen seal (modified Bio-Col technique) of the soft tissue gaps were completed (Figure 21.2l).

Similar treatment was provided in the left mandible, but a much larger defect was present on the facial aspect at the site of the molar root fracture and fistula (Figure 21.3m). Use of a 5.0 mm diameter implant designed for apical engagement allowed adequate primary stability, leaving a large gap dimension and wound bed for particulate grafting (Figure 21.3n). The grafted defect was covered with a collagen barrier, the anterior flap was apically positioned, and the posterior flap extended with a marginal release at the mucogingival junction for anterior/lateral positioning. This allowed for a "v–y" closure at the previous vertical soft tissue defect at the molar to restore an adequate keratinized tissue margin. Initial passive closure of the repositioned flaps can be seen in Figure 21.3o. The sites were covered with light-cured periodontal dressing for 10 days.

The maxillary lateral incisor sites were treated with mini-flap exposure and osteotome site expansion after initial 2 mm drill positioning (Figure 21.3p). The immediate post-treatment panoramic radiograph can be seen in Figure 21.3q. Early healing of the mandibular molar sites showed maturing soft tissue and adequate width of keratinized tissue (Figure 21.3r and s). A long-term provisional restoration phase over 1 year was required (due to external circumstances), allowing emergence profile development and optimal esthetics (Figure 21.3t–x). The definitive restorations after more than 3 years are seen in Figure 21.4a–g and on a panoramic radiograph after 5 years in Figure 21.4h.

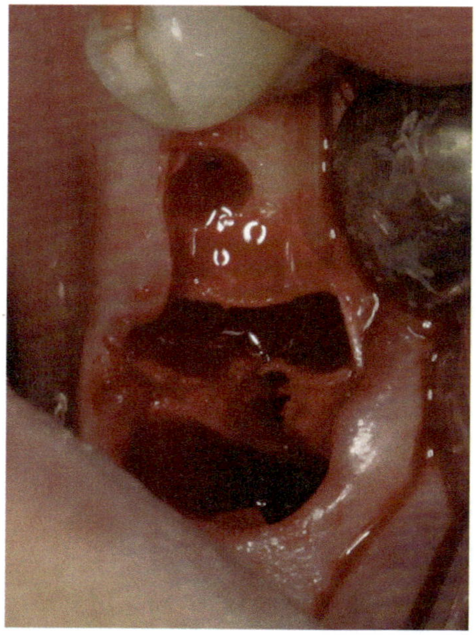

(j)

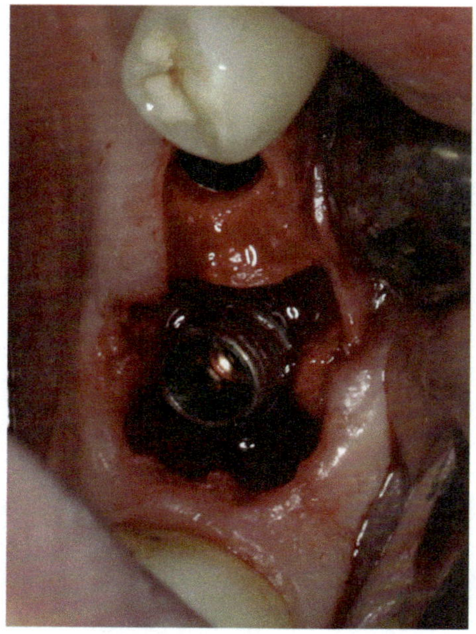

(k)

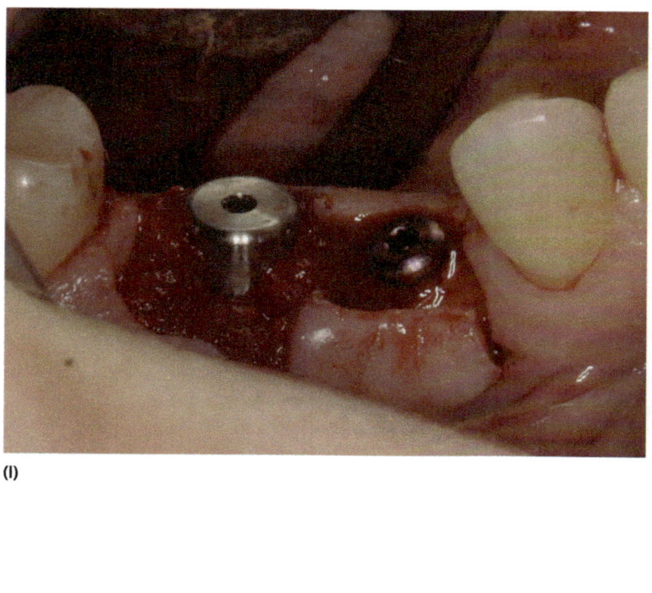

(l)

Figure 21.3 (Continued)

(j) The post-extraction situation in the right mandible showing the initial implant osteotomy in the furcation region, the mesio-buccal socket defect and the lingually incised, full-thickness flap exposing a screw expansion site being developed at the second premolar location. (k) Piezoelectric bone surgery was used to asymmetrically develop the molar towards the lingual aspect; the premolar site was expanded with screw expanders and implant insertion was completed toward the lingual aspect. (l) Healing caps were placed; mineralized particulate allograft closed the bone defects, while a crestal collagen seal of the soft tissue gaps using a modified Bio-Col® technique and passive apical positioning of the anterior flap; wound protection was achieved with a light-cured periodontal dressing.

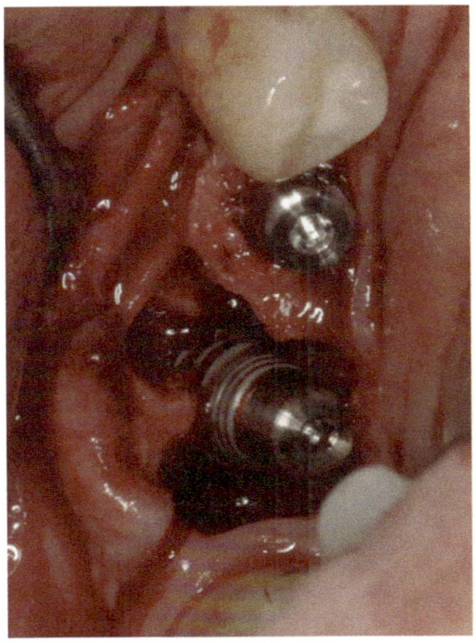

(m)

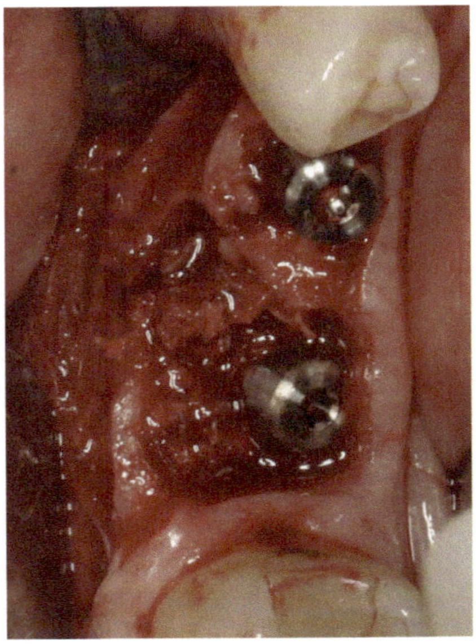

(n)

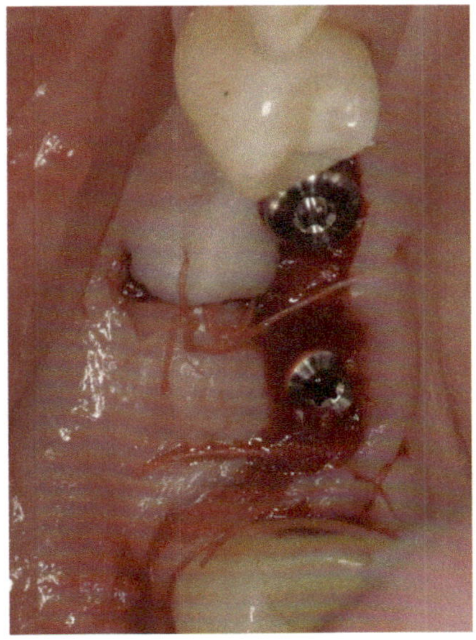

(o)

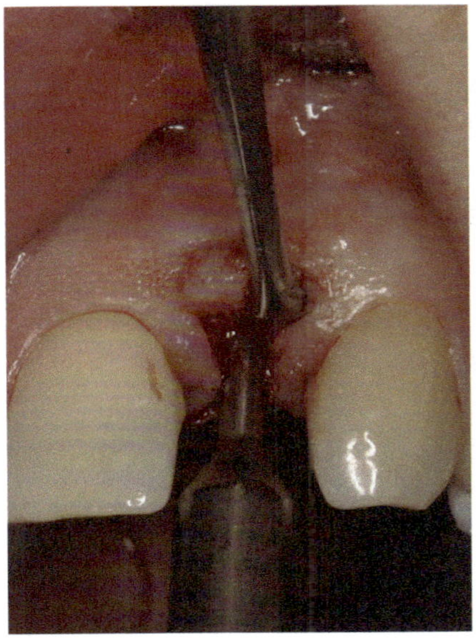

(p)

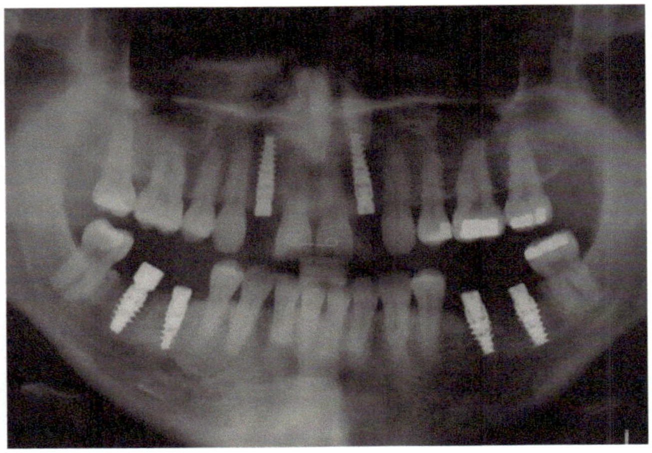

(q)

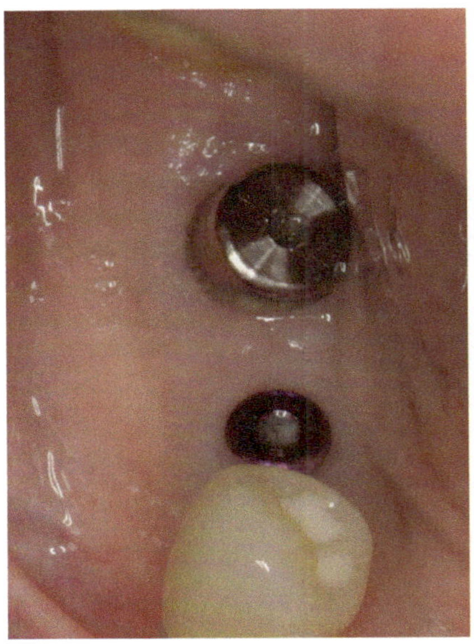

(r)

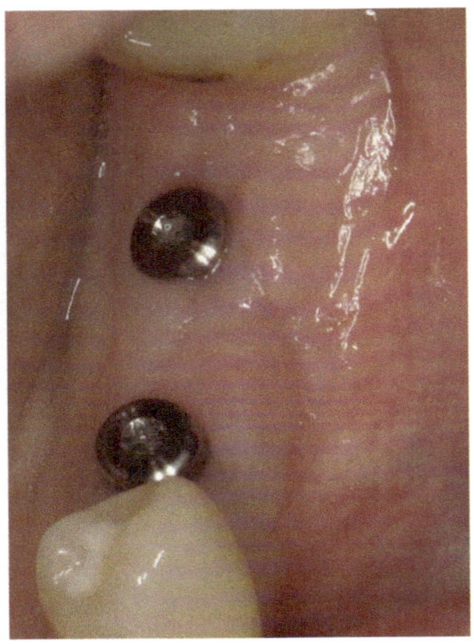

(s)

Figure 21.3 (Continued)
(m) The left mandible showed a large defect on the facial aspect at the site of the root fracture and fistula. (n) A 5.0 mm diameter implant was placed with apical engagement and good primary stability. A large gap dimension with lateral bone walls of 3.5–5 mm acted as an adequate wound bed for particulate grafting. The defect was grafted with mineralized particulate allograft and the posterior flap extended with a marginal release at the mucogingival junction for anterior/lateral positioning. (o) The wound was covered with a collagen barrier and the anterior flap apically positioned with a "v–y" closure at the previous vertical soft tissue defect of the first molar to restore adequate keratinized tissue margin. Initial passive closure of the repositioned flaps was assisted by collagen placed in the soft tissue gaps prior to final suturing and placement of light-cured periodontal dressing. (p) The maxillary lateral sites were exposed with a mini-flap, osteotome expansion was followed by implant and healing cap insertion. (q) The post-operative panoramic radiograph.(r, s) Early soft tissue healing at the mandibular sites showed good soft tissue contours and adequate keratinized tissue.

(Continued)

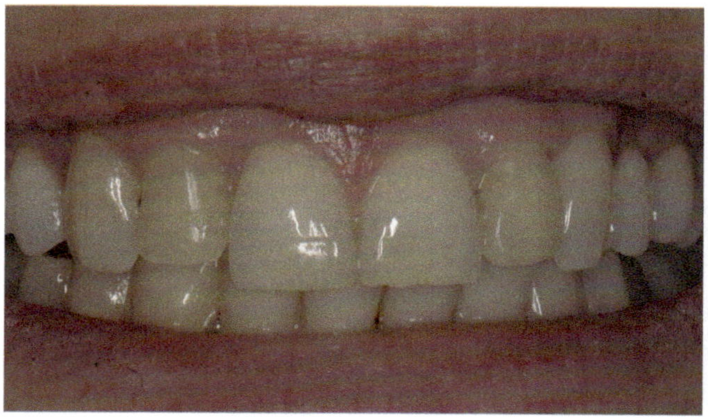

(t)

Figure 21.3 (Continued)
(t-x) A long-term provisional restoration was completed, allowing emergence profile development and optimal esthetics. © Daniel R. Cullum.

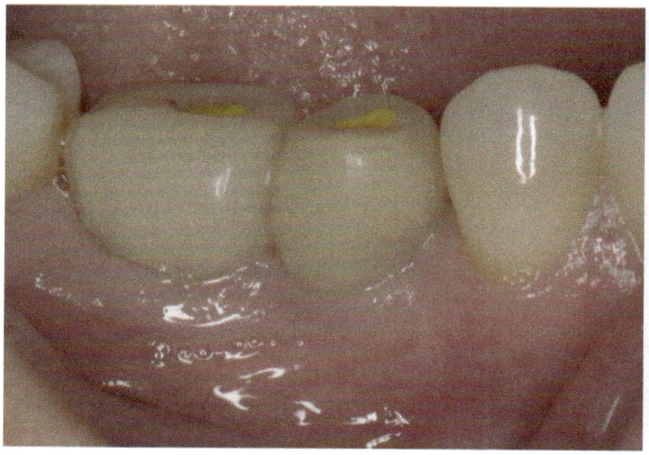

(u)

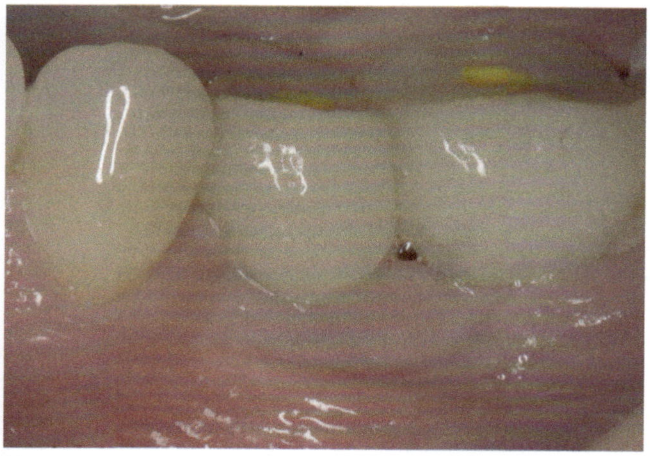

(v)

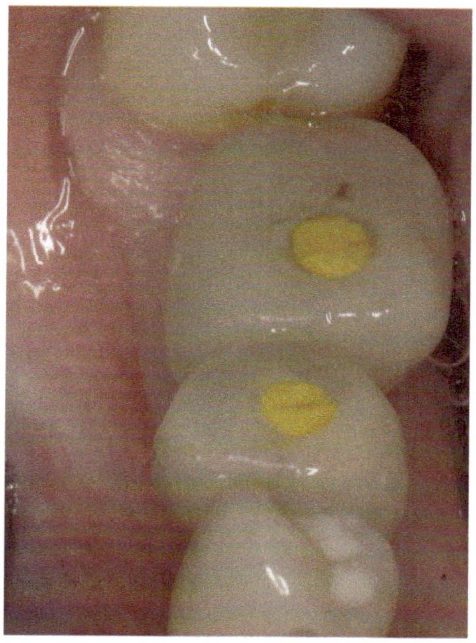

(w)

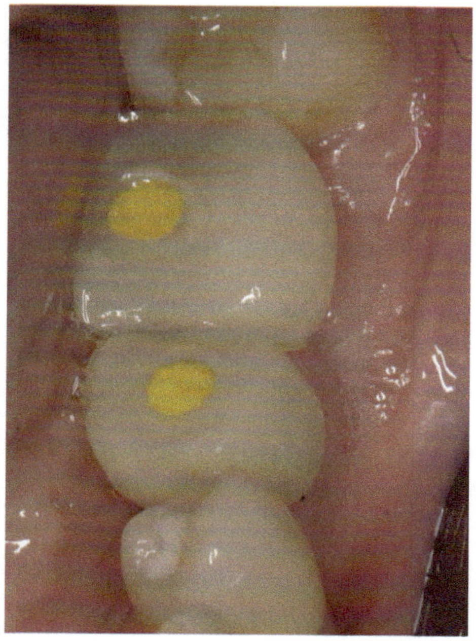

(x)

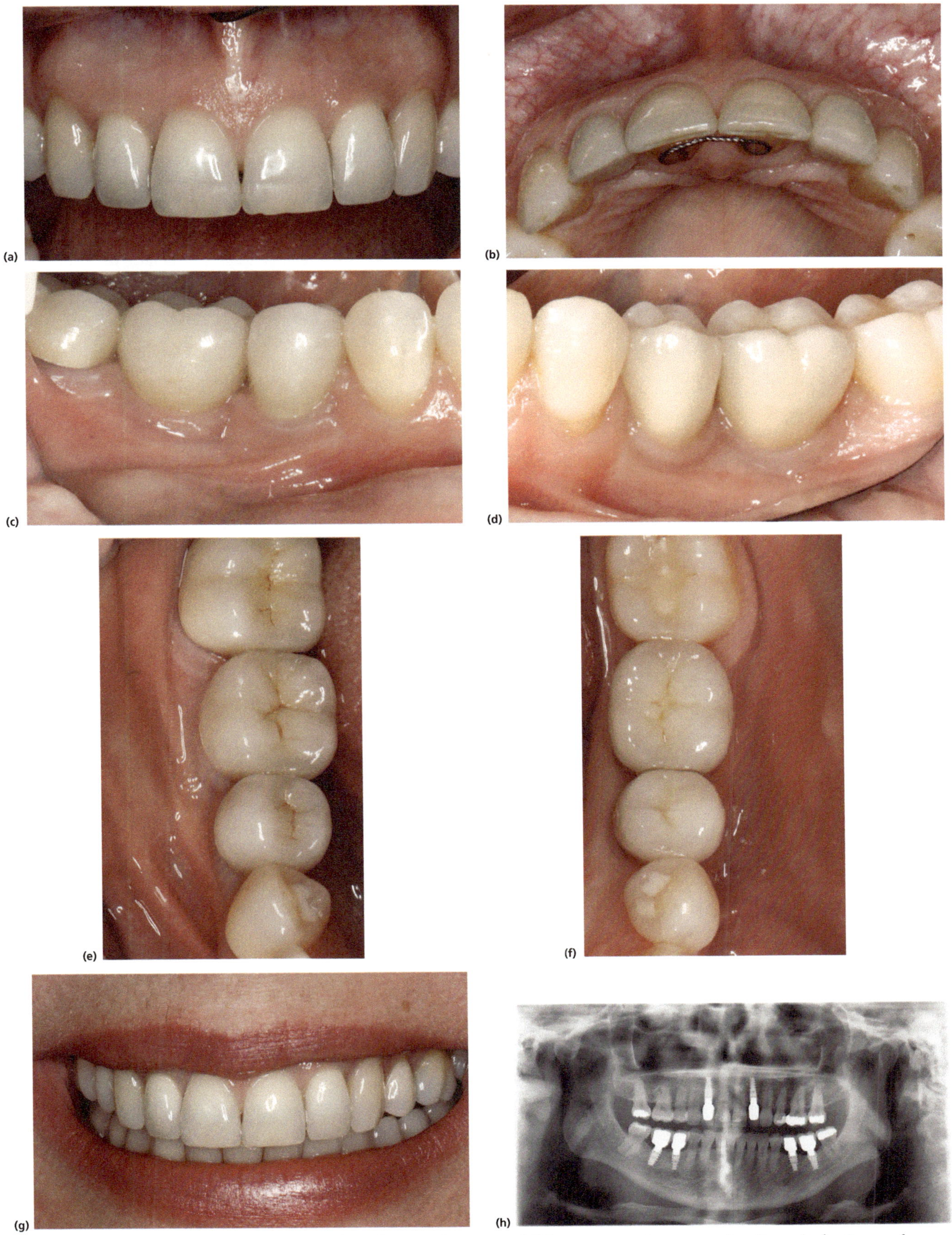

Figure 21.4 (a-g) The definitive restorations are seen here after more than 3 years. (h) The post-restoration panoramic radiograph after 5 years of function. © Daniel R. Cullum.

Case study 21.4

A healthy 54-year-old male patient presented with a failing right maxillary fixed prosthesis deemed to be non-restorable on clinical and radiographic evaluation (Figure 21.5a–c). A fixed provisional was fabricated and supported by the adjacent teeth. The patient demonstrated generalized gingival recession with exposed restorative margins and a significant recession defect on the fractured and non-restorable right maxillary canine.

Diagnosis Failing maxillary anterior fixed partial denture replacing the right first premolar, and a fractured non-restorable maxillary right canine. Moderate attrition, aging porcelain-fused-to-metal restorations, with alveolar atrophy at the edentulous right first premolar site and recession and root dehiscence at the right canine.

Plan *Phase 1:* Extraction of the right maxillary canine with onlay block graft reconstruction of the defect and connective tissue augmentation followed by an immediate tooth-supported, fixed provisional restoration.

Phase 2: Flapless minimally invasive, single-stage implant reconstruction with provisional restorative site development and definitive restoration in concert with restoration of adjacent natural teeth.

Treatment *Phase 1:* The residual root fragments were surgically removed using a minimally invasive technique (Figure 21.5d). The crestal/interproximal bone and soft tissues demonstrated a large facial vertical defect at the right canine and adjacent edentulous premolar site (Figure 21.5d and e). An epithelial–connective tissue dissection of the right palate was completed in continuity with a papilla-sparing buccally-based flap at the same depth through the edentulous site into the buccal vestibule (Figure 21.5f and g). An anterior pedicle (arrow) design for adequate tissue coverage over the planned augmentation is outlined with the solid line in Figure 21.5h. The incisions are completed and the flap is mobilized with the pedicle intact (Figure 21.5i and j). Figure 21.5k shows a block graft taken from mandible secured with fixation screws to reconstruct the buccal and vertical dimensions. The remaining defect was grafted with autologous bone and beta-TCP mixed with venous blood and covered with a collagen barrier (Figure 21.5l). The pedicle flap was rotated anteriorly and to the buccal to cover the graft, and sutured into position with 5-0 polyglycolic sutures (Figure 21.5m). The superficial flap from the edentulous site was laterally positioned in concert with the laterally and coronally positioned anterior flap for primary closure. This approach facilitated a double-layer closure over the rotated pedicle flap. The tooth-borne fixed provisional was re-inserted. After 6 months, panoramic imaging shows the healed, screw-retained block graft reconstruction (Figure 21.5o). The clinical situation and associated augmented crestal volume are seen in Figure 21.5p and q, before and after removal of the provisional restoration.

Phase 2: The fixation screws were removed via a 3 mm vertical incision over the screw heads. A papilla-sparing, palatally-based incision was used at the canine and first premolar sites for minimally invasive access and to maximize the facial keratinized tissue. Implant site development was completed with insertion of 3.5 mm diameter, conical connection platform-switched implants, done as a single-stage procedure (Figure 21.5r). The tooth-borne fixed provisional appliance was re-inserted after confirming no direct tissue contact. Following 4 months' healing, the bone and soft tissue contours appeared to be adequate, and provisional restoration of the teeth was completed. Long-term provisional restoration was requested by the patient, and was facilitated with the use of titanium abutments (Figure 21.5s and t). The patient can be seen with the definitive restoration 10 years after surgery in Figure 21.5u–w.

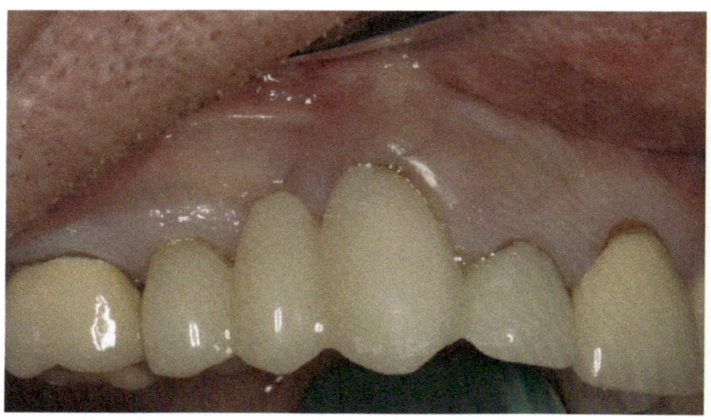
(a)

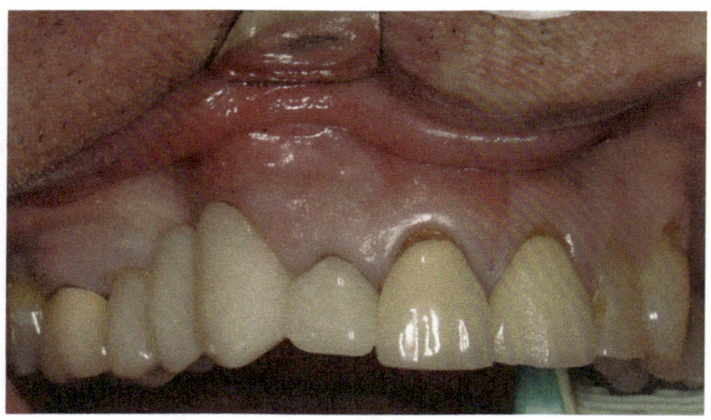
(b)

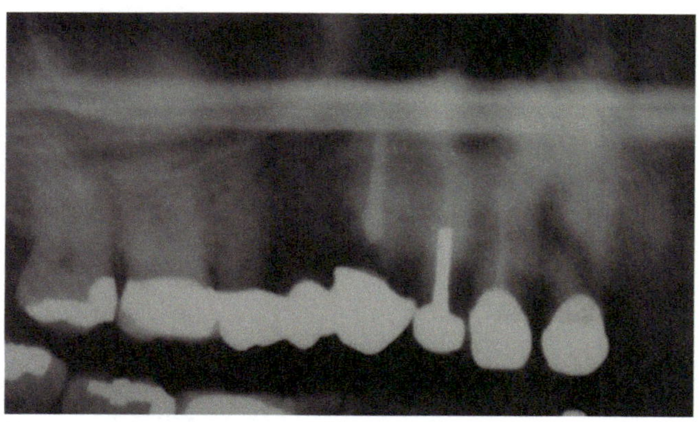
(c)

Figure 21.5 (a–c) Pretreatment clinical and radiographic images are seen here after insertion of a tooth-supported provisional restoration.

Figure 21.5 (Continued)

(d, e) *Phase 1*. Facial and vertical bone defects were found after the canine root extraction. (f, -g) An epithelial–connective tissue dissection of the right palate was completed in continuity with a papilla-sparing, buccally-based flap at the same depth in the edentulous site. (g) The underlying connective tissue–periosteum layer was left intact and allowed an incision design that maintained the connective tissue flap with a pedicle vascular supply for rhomboid rotation. (h) An anterior pedicle (arrow) design is indicated with by the solid line and planned to provide adequate tissue for coverage over the planned augmentation site. (i, j) The flap was mobilized, preserving the anterior pedicle, and rotated into the recipient position.

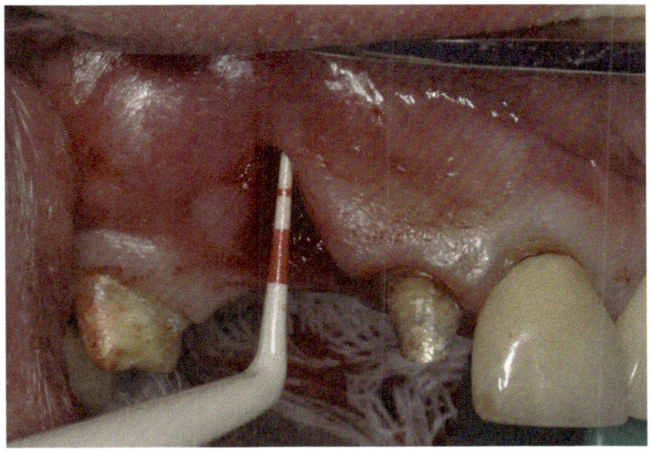

(d)

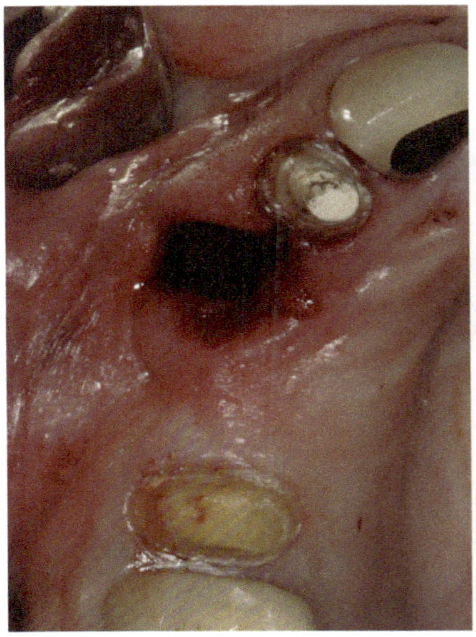

(e)

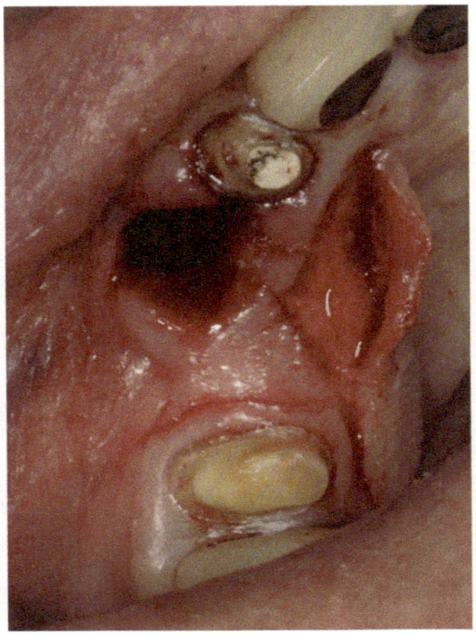

(f)

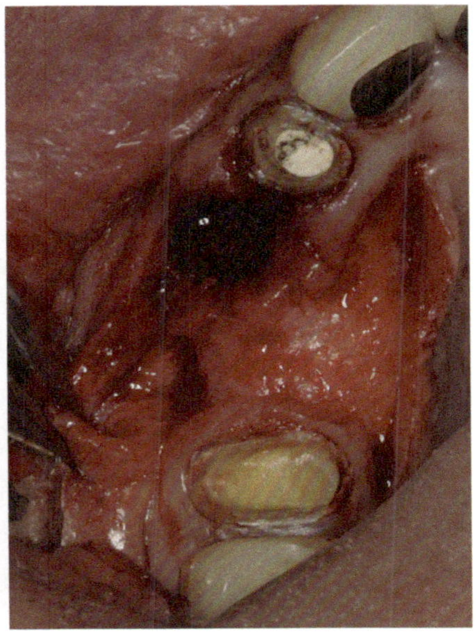

(g)

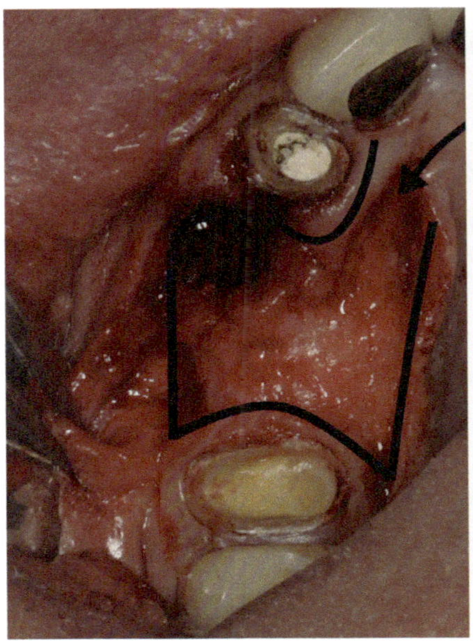

(h)

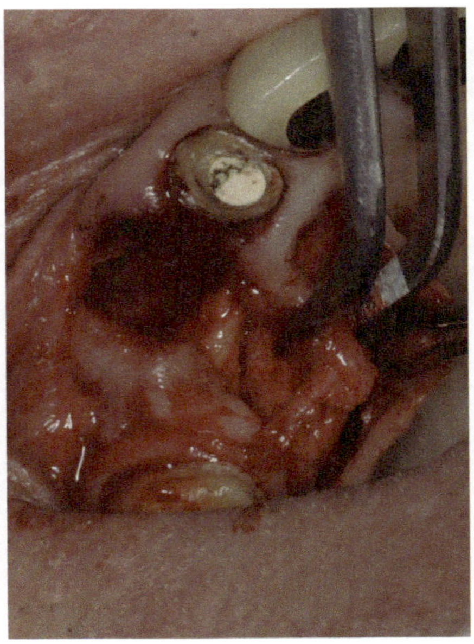

(i)

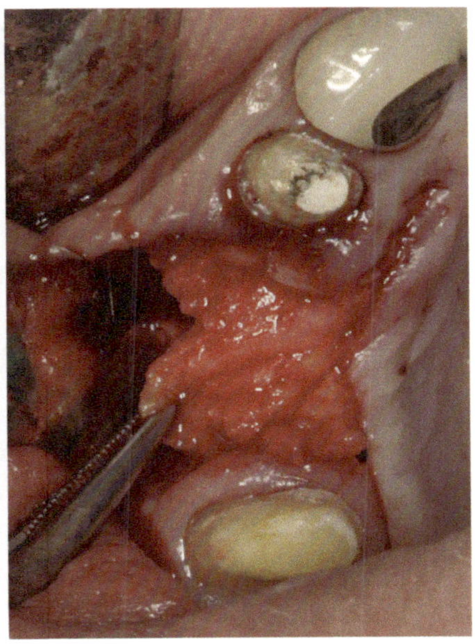

(j)

(Continued)

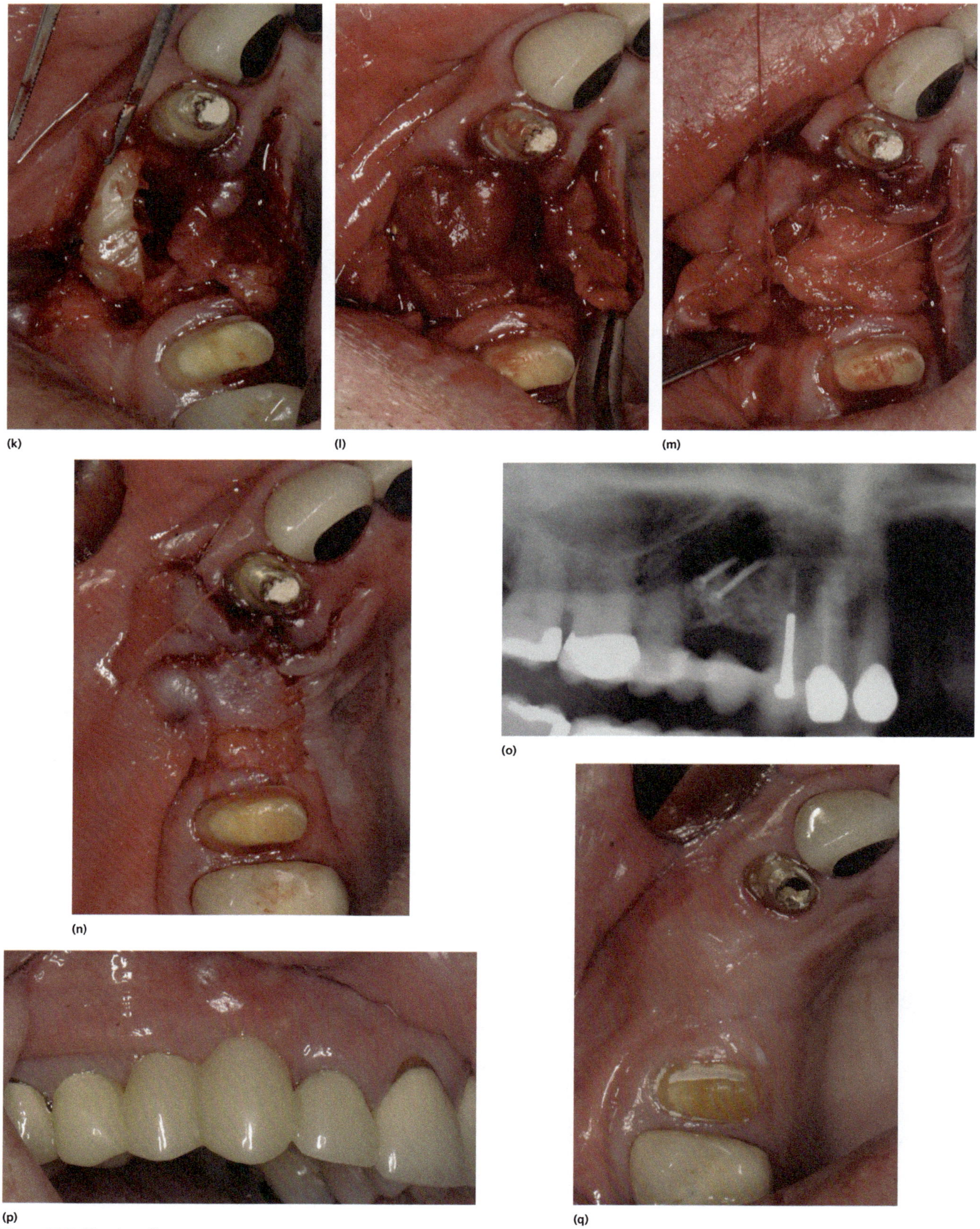

Figure 21.5 (Continued)
(k) A block graft harvested from the mandibular ramus was secured with screws and the remaining defect space grafted with autologous bone and beta-TCP mixed with venous heme. (l) A collagen barrier was placed over the graft. (m) The pedicle flap was rotated anteriorly and buccally to cover the graft, and sutured with 5-0 polyglycolic sutures. (n) The superficial flap from the edentulous site was laterally positioned in concert with the laterally and coronally positioned anterior flap to achieve primary closure over the rotated pedicle flap, facilitating a double-layer closure. The tooth-borne fixed provisional was re-inserted. (o) Post-operative panoramic imaging shows the screw-retained block graft reconstruction after 6 months. (p, q) The clinical situation is seen here after 6 months healing and after removal of the provisional restoration.

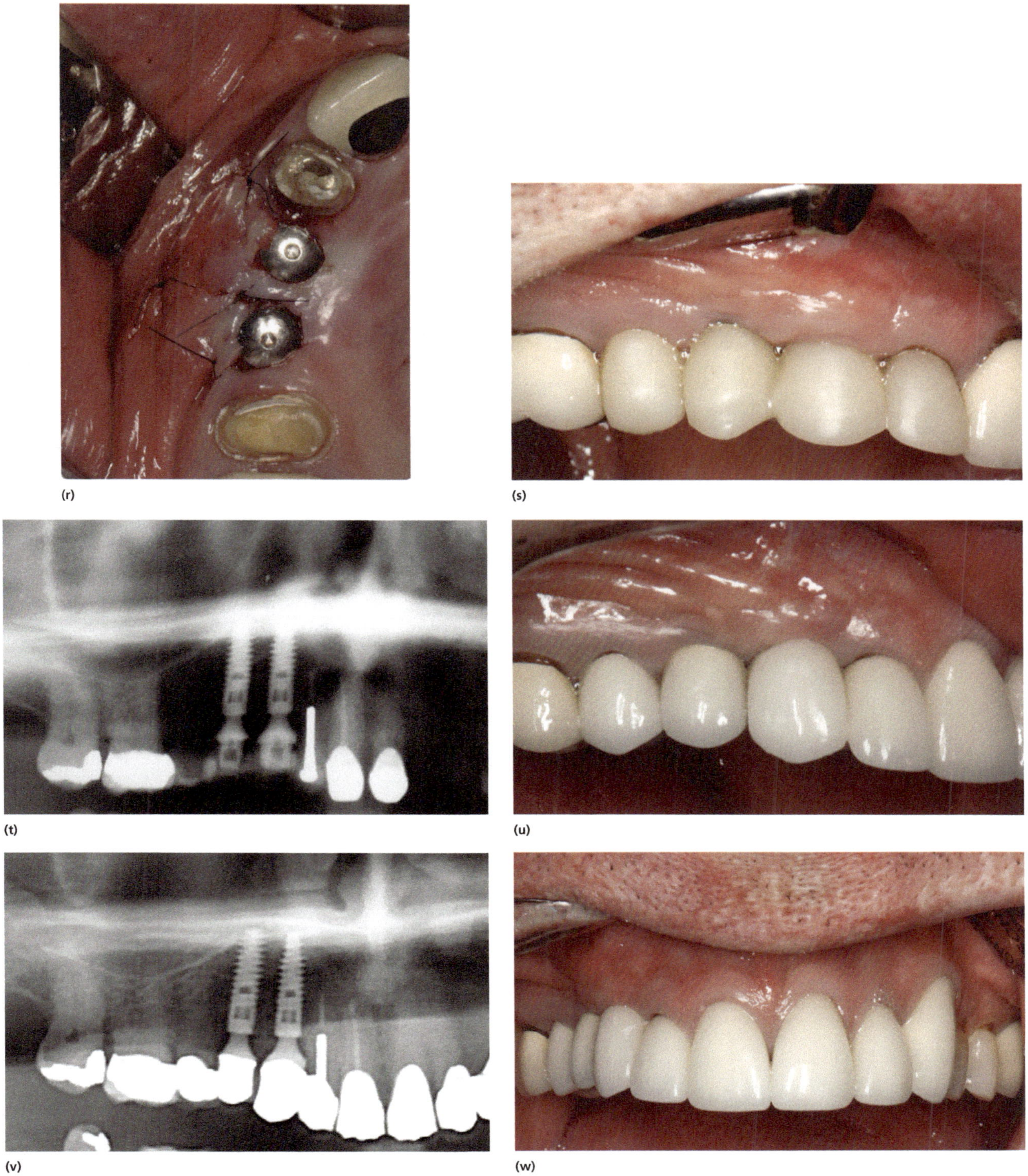

Figure 21.5 (Continued)

(r) *Phase 2.* This immediate post-operative view shows the outcome after minimally invasive, single-stage implant placement with a papilla-sparing incision and direct limited vestibular incision over the screws for their removal. (s, t) Provisional restoration was completed; however, the patient did not proceed with definitive restoration for some time. The patient is shown clinically here after 2 years with the provisional restoration, and in a panoramic radiograph. (u–w) The 10-year follow-up after final restoration and radiographic images. Restorative management by Dr Ron Forsberg, Sandpoint, ID. © Daniel R. Cullum.

Case study 21.5

A healthy 77-year-old female presented with a history of multiple implants placed over several years by several different surgeons. After an extended period with implant-supported provisional restorations in the lower arch, she lost confidence in her care providers and was referred for comprehensive evaluation and treatment. She was edentulous in the maxilla with a removable full denture (Figure 21.6a–e). The patient's facial proportions were appropriate with a full upper denture and moderate extrusion of her remaining mandibular teeth. On animation, she displayed a moderate to high smile line and a descending plane of occlusion. The panoramic radiograph showed horizontal bone loss of the mandibular implants, and the occlusal plane demonstrated extrusion of the anterior teeth with an excessive curve of Spee (Figure 21.6f).

Diagnosis Edentulous maxilla with a complete maxillary denture and extruded mandibular dentition with minimal bone volume in the inter-foraminal region of the anterior mandible. Failing/ailing mandibular implants with crestal bone loss.

Plan Extraction of the remaining mandibular teeth and compromised implants in conjunction with alveolectomy to level and reduce the anterior occlusal plane and create adequate prosthetic space for the fabrication of a new maxillary prosthesis to correct the esthetics and occlusion. The placement of four implants with angled

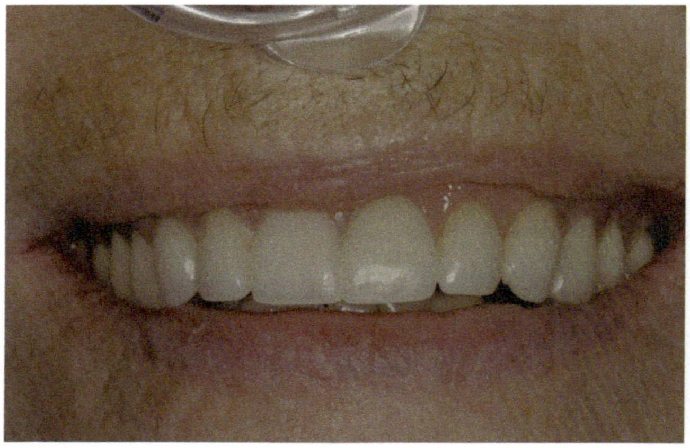

(a)

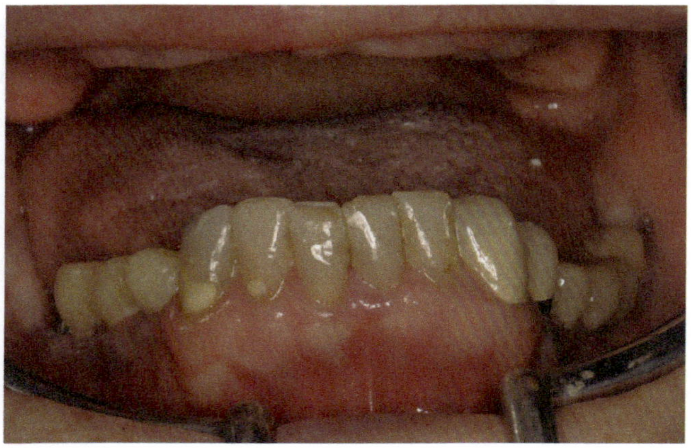

(b)

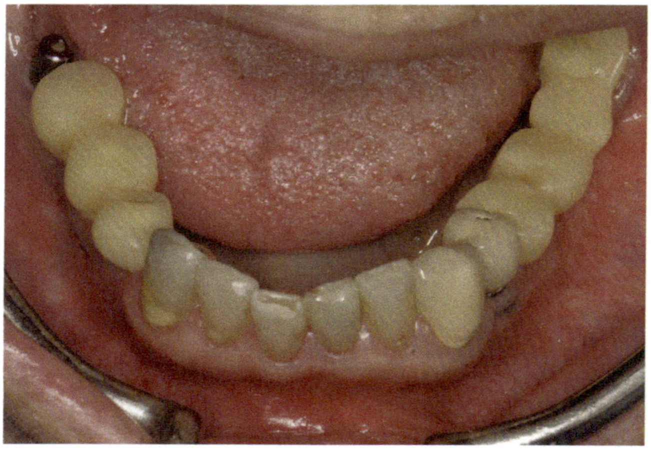

(c)

Figure 21.6 (a–e) Pretreatment clinical views of a failing partially dentate implant reconstruction showed an uneven occlusal plane, mandibular anterior extrusion, mucogingival problems, and an excessive curve of Spee.

(*Continued*)

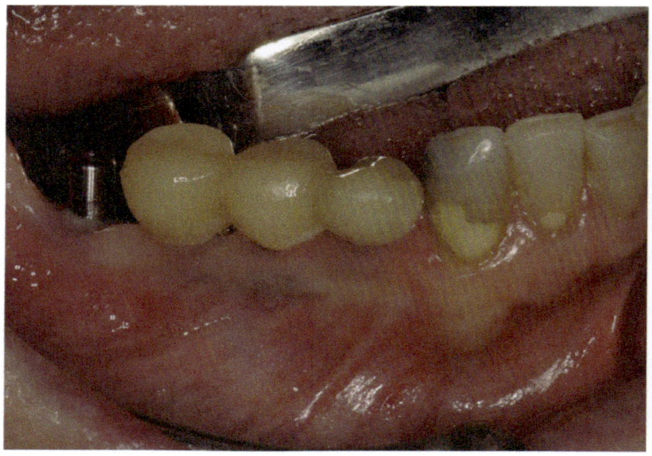

(d)

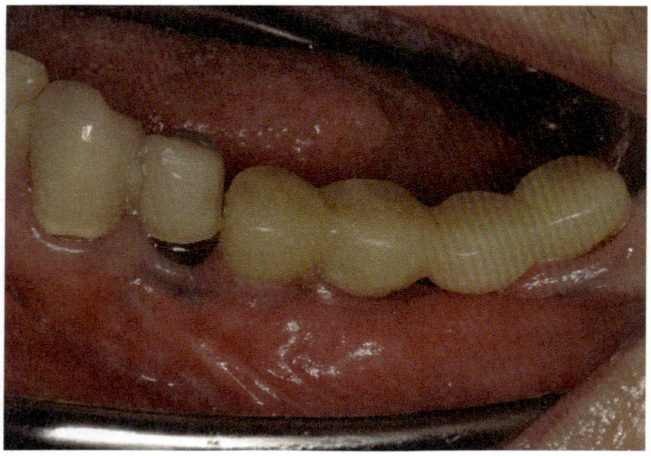

(e)

posterior fixtures was planned to provide adequate antero-posterior spread for an implant-supported, cross-arch-stabilized fixed immediate provisional restoration.

Treatment After prosthetic preparation for an interim, direct pick-up, cross-arch-stabilized prosthesis, the patient was seen for removal of the remaining mandibular teeth and compromised implants, and alveolectomy for leveling of the anterior occlusal plane and adequate prosthetic space (Figure 21.6g–i). Four implants were placed (Figure 21.6j–m), the posterior one on each side having angled positioning to maximize the antero-posterior spread. The patient was then provisionally restored with an implant-supported, fixed immediate provisional restoration (Figure 21.6n–p). The treatment outcome is seen in Figure 21.6q–u after 8 years, demonstrating a stable and long-term functional result. Figure 21.6v and w shows facial views to demonstrate the esthetic results after correction of tooth position.

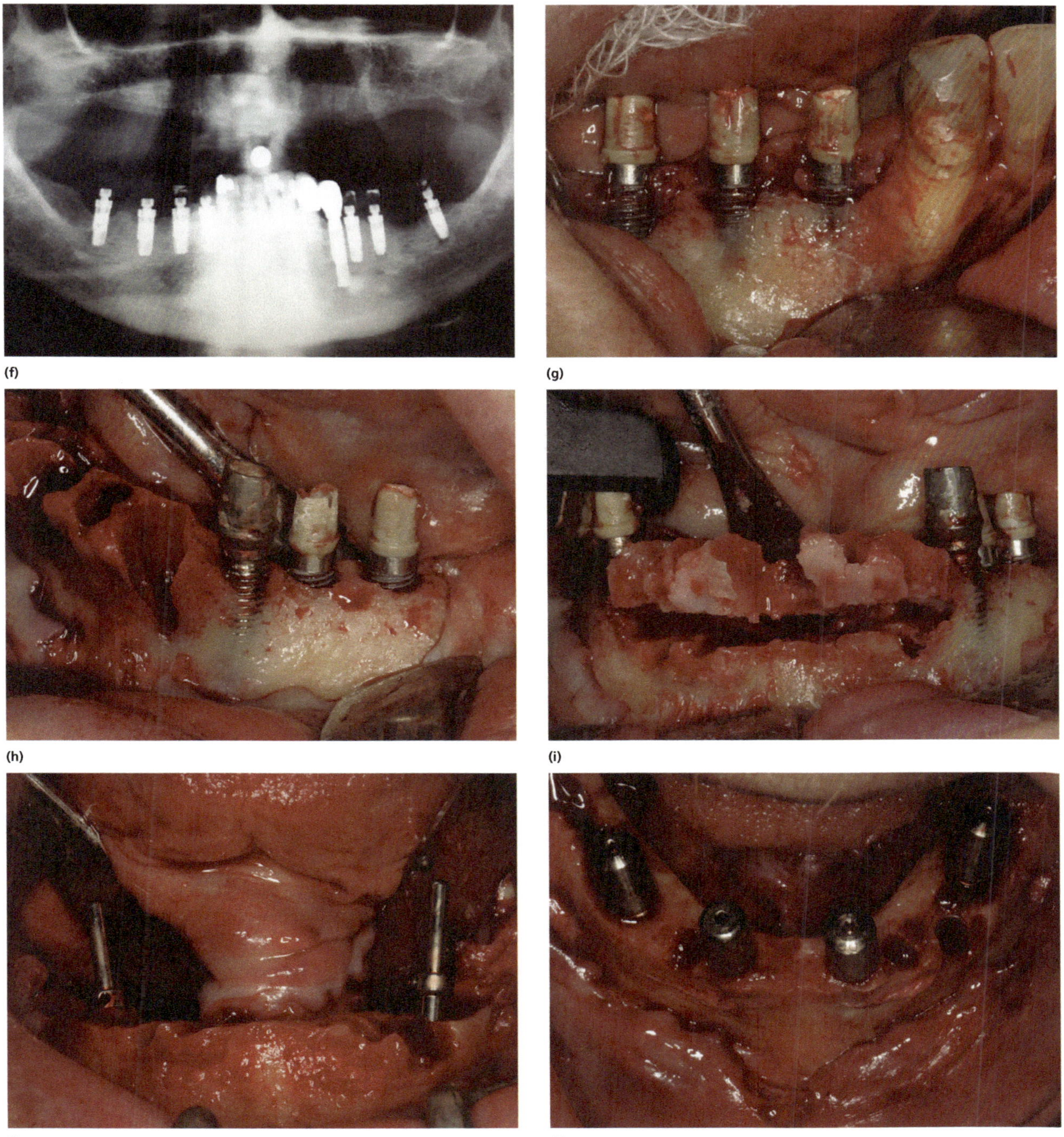

(f) (g) (h) (i) (j) (k)

Figure 21.6 (Continued)

(f) Pretreatment panoramic radiograph demonstrating crestal bone loss at multiple implant sites and extrusion of the anterior mandibular teeth. (g, h) Right and left surgical images after flap elevation show crestal bone loss, facial bone dehiscences affecting the remaining teeth, and implant platform height discrepancies with the residual crestal bone. (i) After extraction of the remaining teeth, an initial anterior alveolectomy of 10 mm was need to create prosthetic space. (j) Initial implant site assessment with direction indicators inserted at the two distally tilted implant sites. (k) The implants were placed using the "All-on-4®" concept with tall healing caps and good antero-posterior spread.

(Continued)

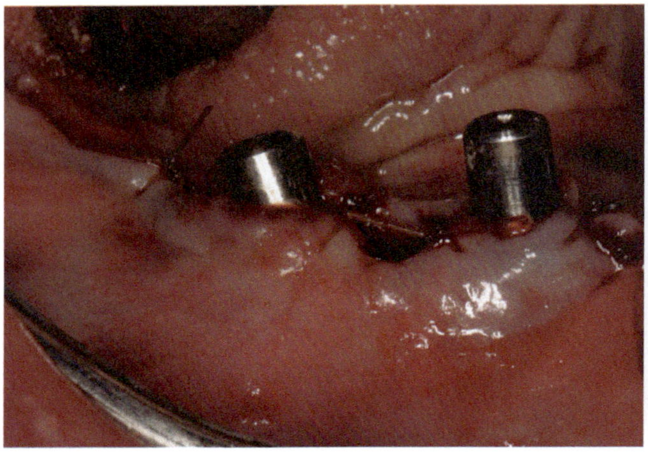

(l)

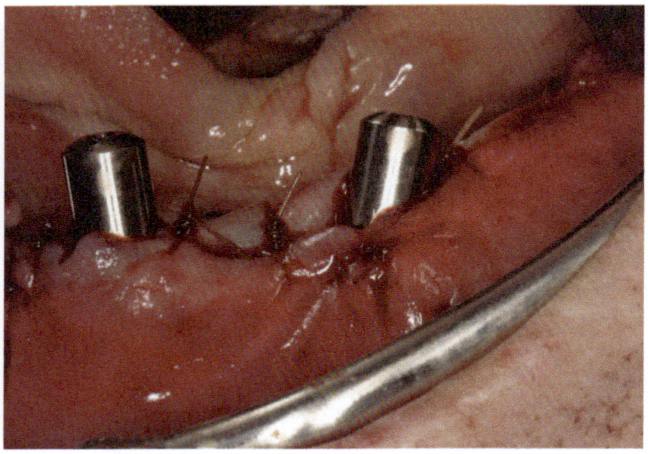

(m)

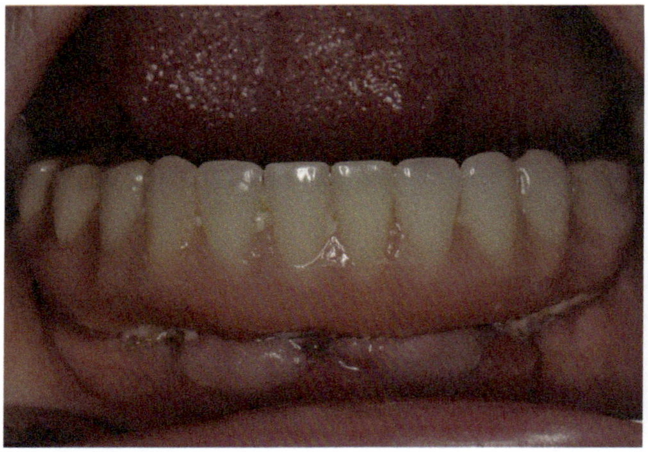

(n)

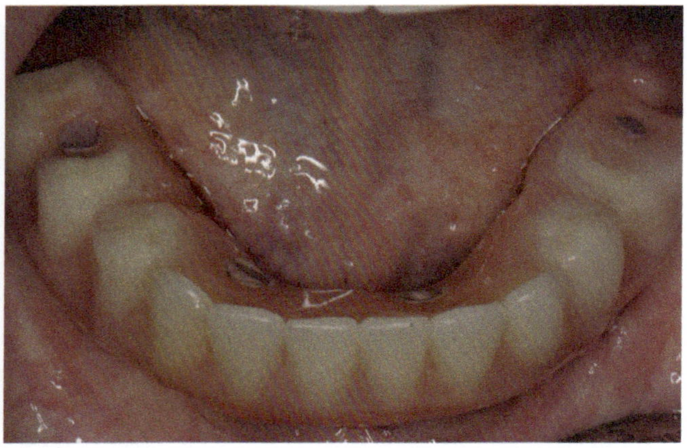

(o)

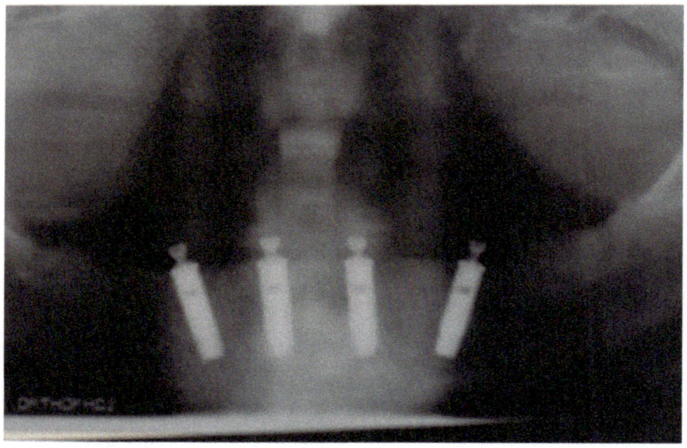

(p)

Figure 21.6 (Continued)

(l, m) Soft tissue closure and the right and left lateral views of the antero-posterior spread. The left view also shows a closure of the mesial and distal papillae to increase the height of the keratinized tissue lateral to the distal implant site. (n–p) Clinical and panoramic radiographic images showing the fabrication of an immediate direct pick-up, cross-arch-stabilized provisional prosthesis.

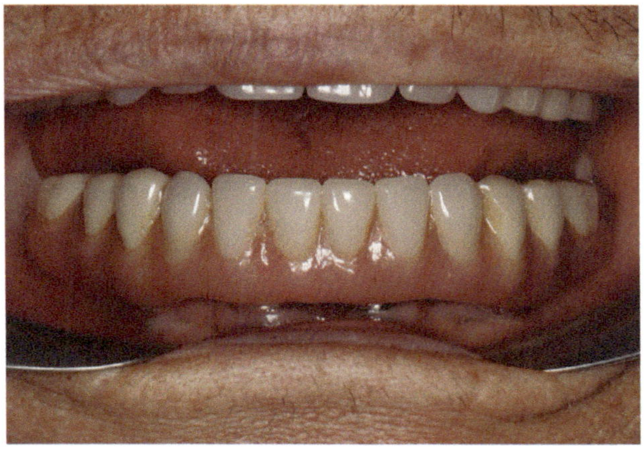
(q)

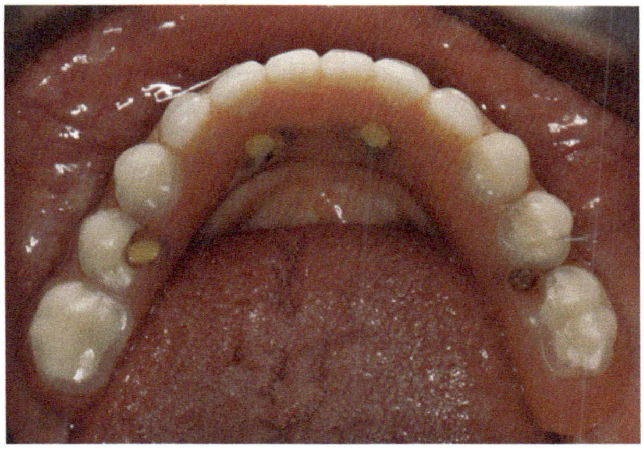
(r)

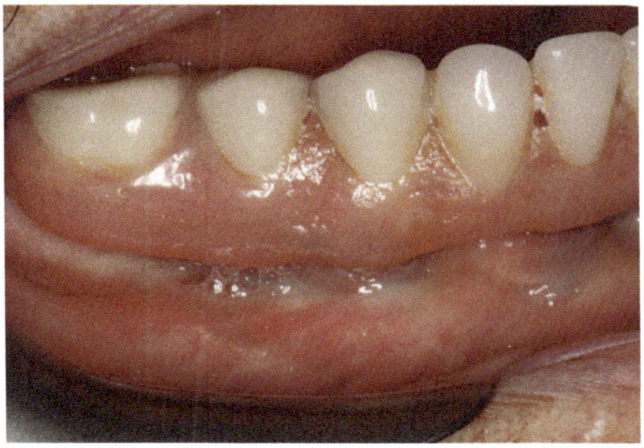
(s)

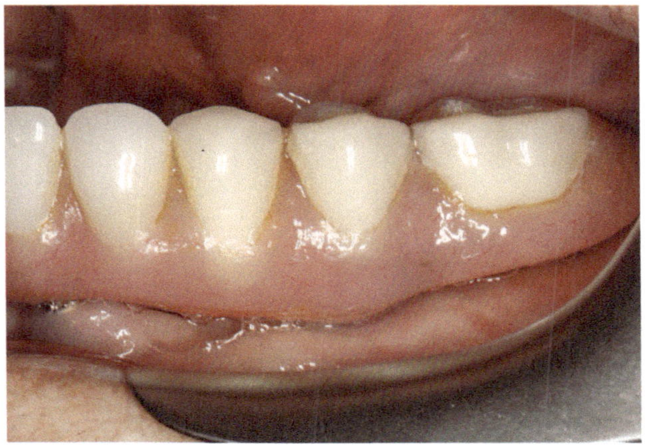
(t)

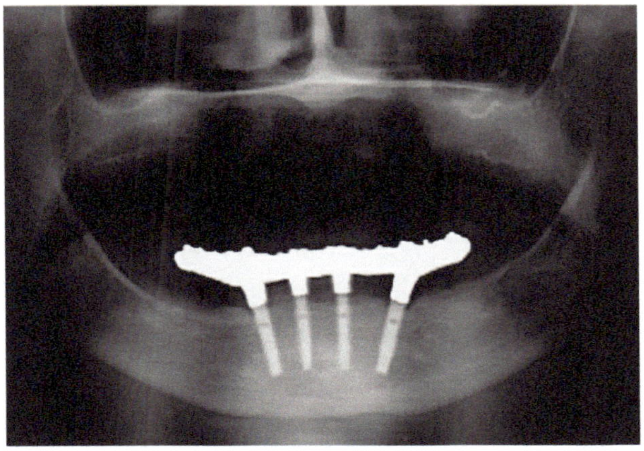
(u)

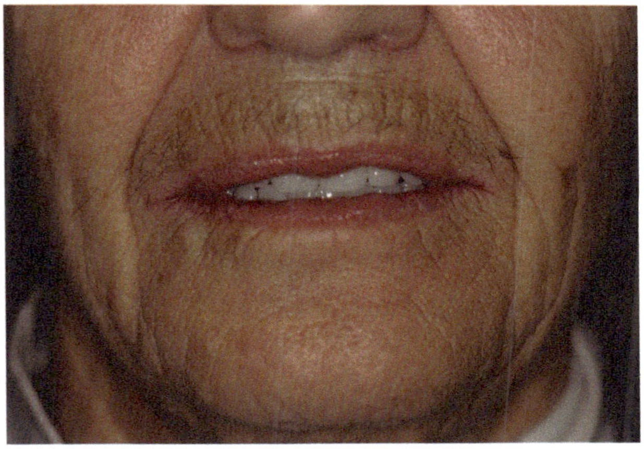
(v)

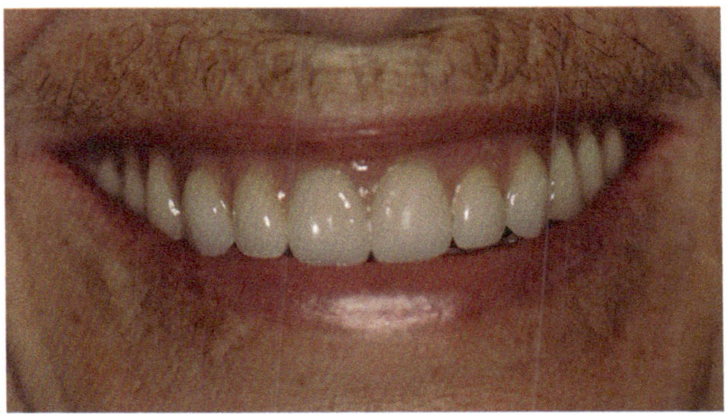
(w)

Figure 21.6 (Continued)
(q–u) The patient is shown here in clinical and radiographic images after 8 years, and demonstrating a stable and long-term functional result. (v, w) Facial views show the esthetic result. © Daniel R. Cullum.

(*Continued*)

Case study 21.6

A healthy 58-year-old female presented with a history of sinus grafting and removal of the posterior mandibular teeth. She was seeking comprehensive fixed implant reconstruction of both arches. The patient was wearing a maxillary full denture (Figure 21.7a). The patient's facial proportions were appropriate with a full upper denture and moderate extrusion of her remaining mandibular teeth (Figure 21.7b). On animation, she displayed a mid to low smile line and a slightly descending plane of occlusion (Figure 21.7c). The remaining mandibular teeth had horizontal bone loss and the anterior mandibular basal bone volume was compromised with narrow horizontal dimensions and undercuts (Figure 21.7d-j).

Diagnosis Edentulous maxilla with a removable denture and an extruded mandibular dentition with minimal anterior mandibular basal bone volume and undercut areas.

Plan *Phase 1:* Extraction of the remaining mandibular teeth with placement of an implant-supported, immediate, fixed provisional restoration. Six implants were planned because of the limited bone volume, which required the use of four narrow-diameter anterior implants and to maximize the A–P spread.

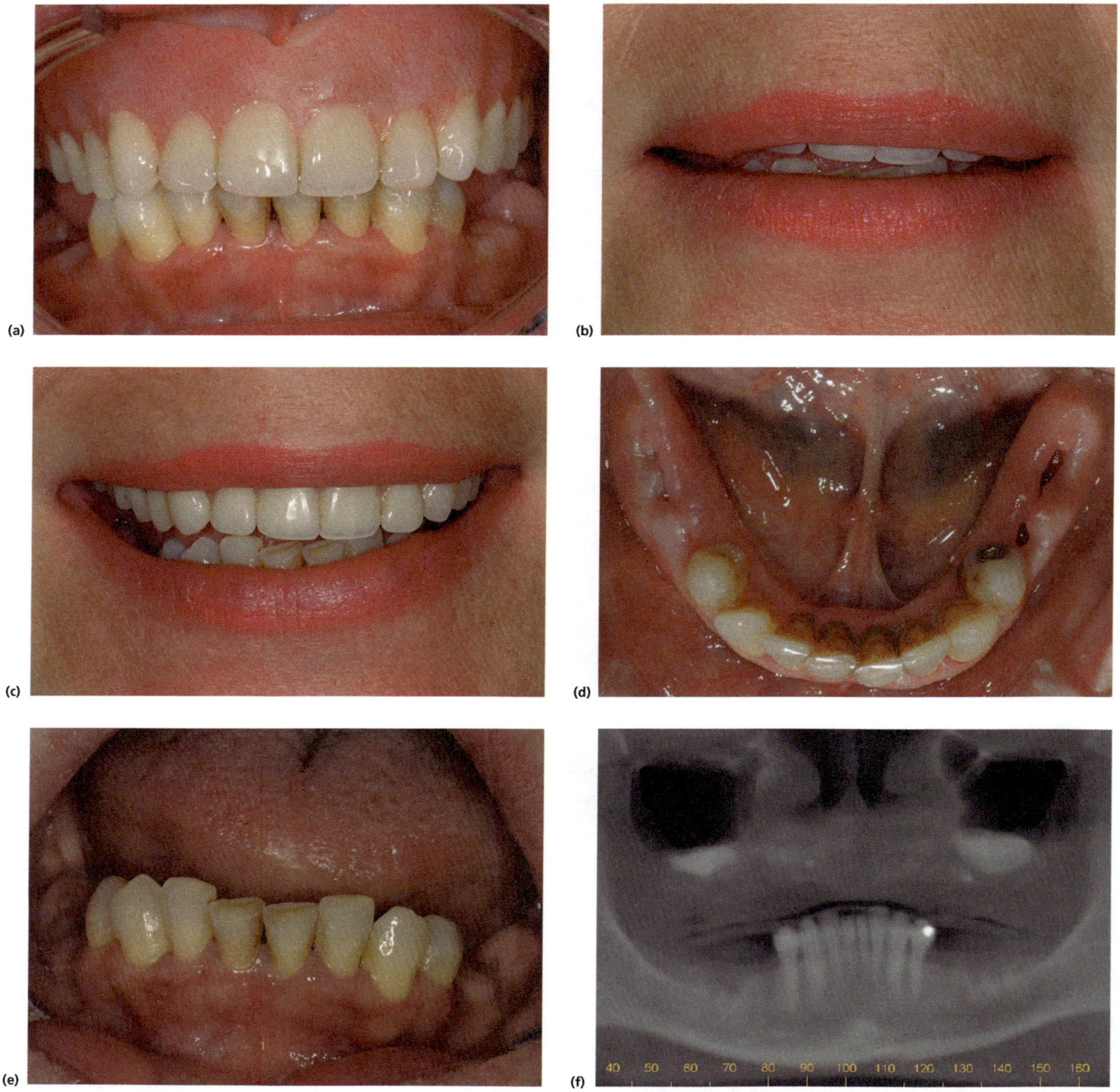

Figure 21.7 (a) The pretreatment intraoral view showed a complete maxillary denture and remaining anterior mandibular dentition. (b) The lip and tooth positions in repose. (c) The initial smile and tooth display. (d) The full arch mandibular occlusal view. (e) An anterior mandibular retracted view. (f) The 3-D reconstructed panoramic view of the arches showed extrusion of the anterior teeth, bone loss and an edentulous maxilla with healed bilateral sinus grafts.

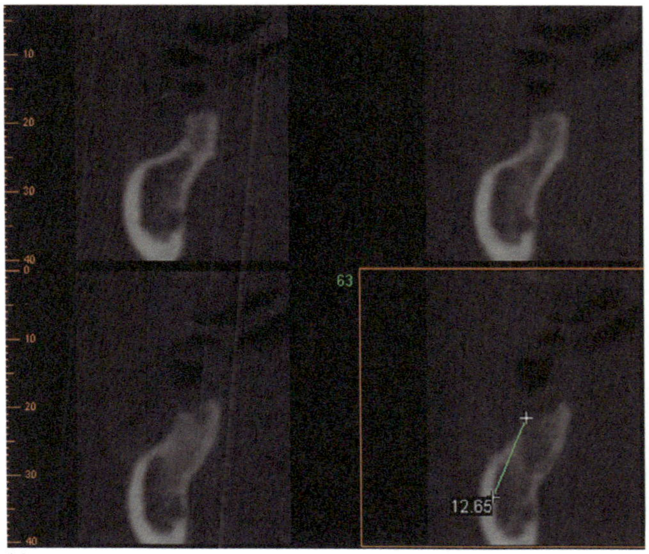

(g)

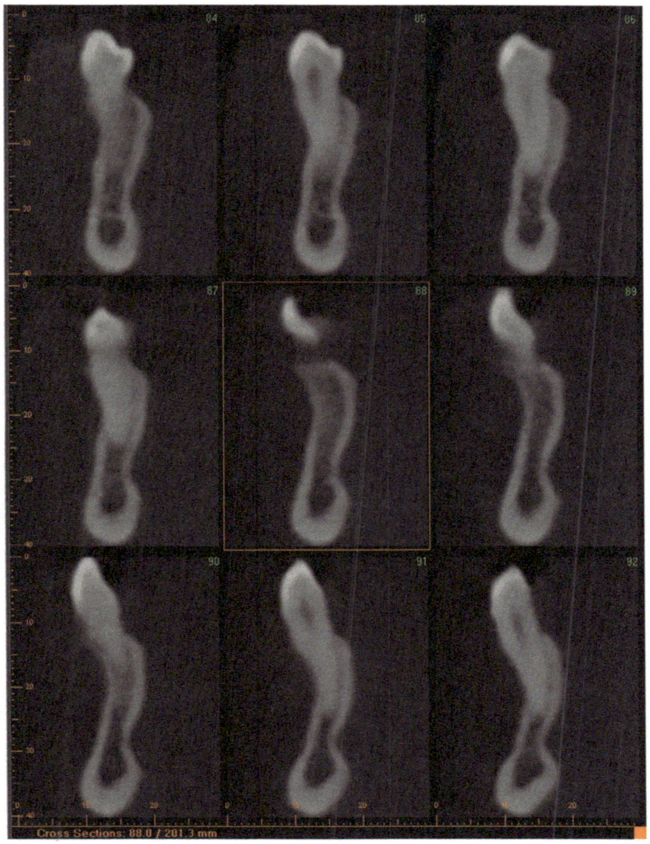

(h)

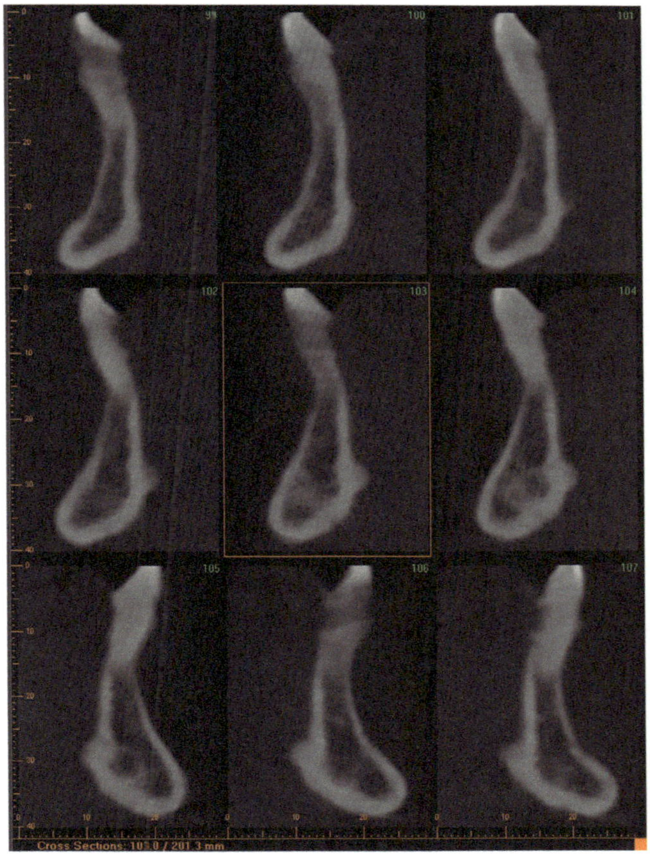

(i)

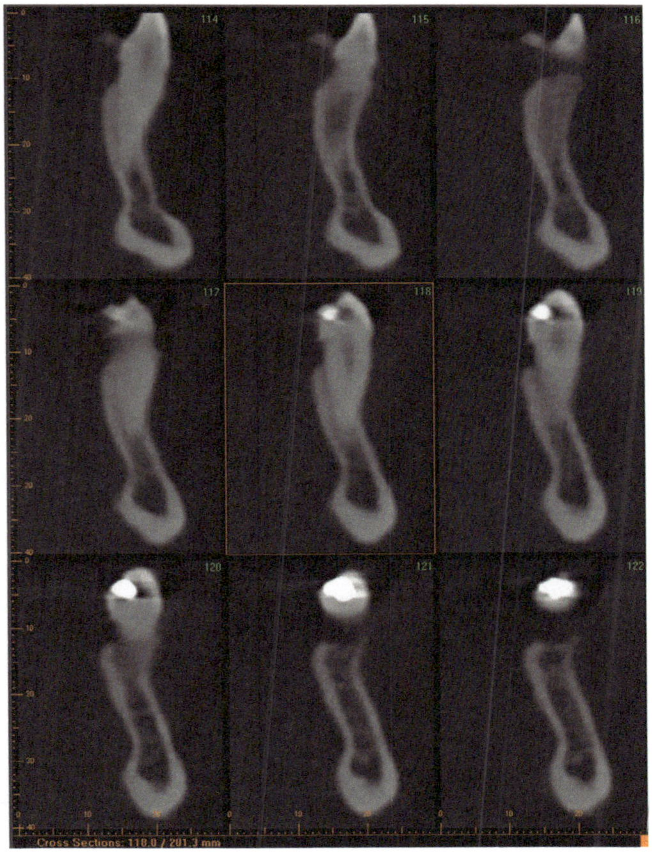

(j)

Figure 21.7 (Continued)
(g–j) The cross-sectional CBCT images showed the alveolar dimensions and lingual undercut.

(Continued)

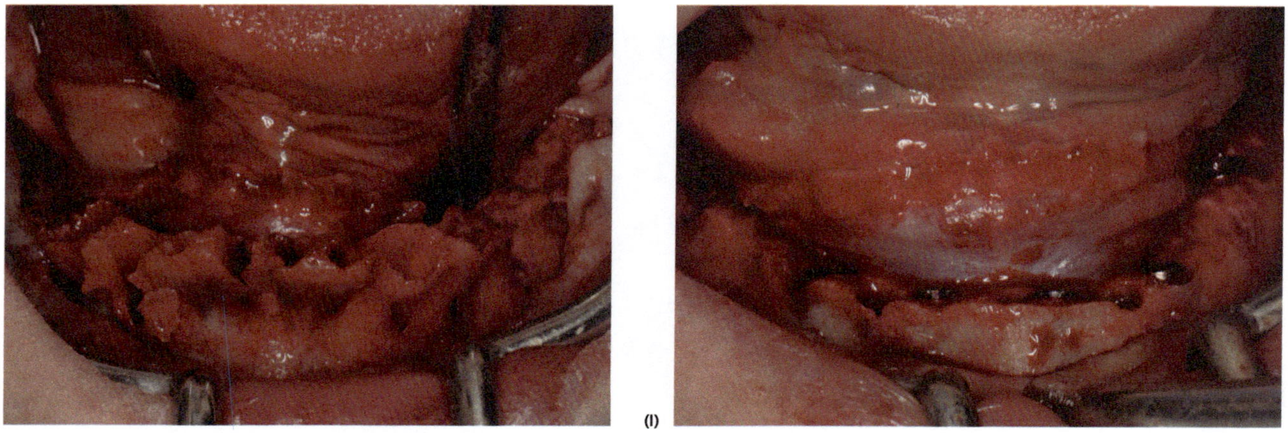

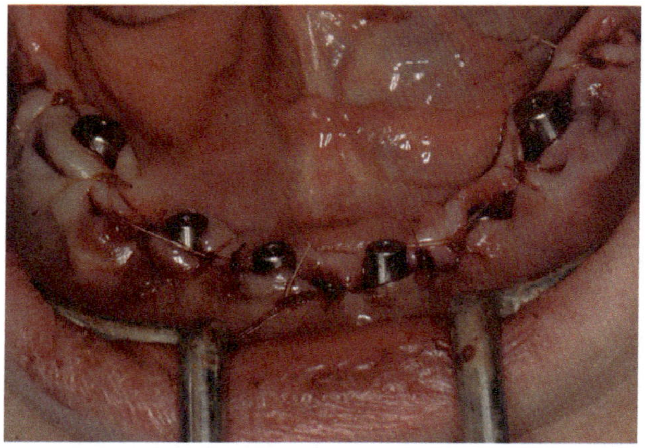

Figure 21.7 (Continued)
(k–m) The remaining mandibular teeth were removed and an alveolectomy performed to create adequate prosthetic space; thereafter six implants were placed with narrow platforms (3.5 mm diameter) in the anterior region. (n–q) The immediate prosthetic conversion to a fixed provisional restoration was completed. *Source:* (a–c) © Earl Ness. (e–q) © Daniel R. Cullum.

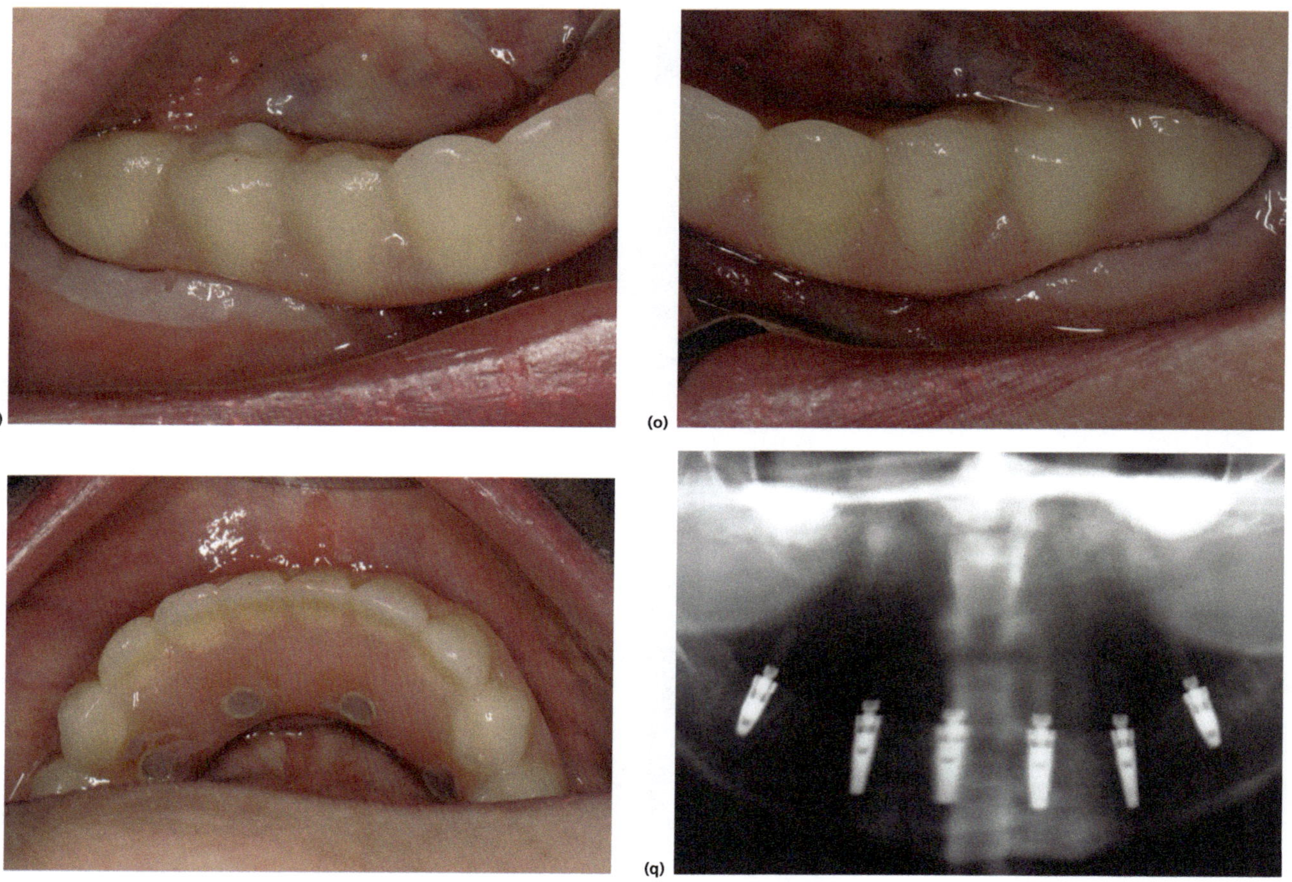

Phase 2: Guided surgery and implant placement were planned for the maxilla with maxillary guide fabrication and immediate direct provisional restoration (Figure 21.8a–f).

Treatment *Phase 1*: After preparation for an interim, direct pick-up prosthesis in the mandible, the patient was seen for removal of the remaining mandibular teeth, an alveolectomy, and placement of six narrow-diameter (3.5 mm) implants anteriorly (Figure 21.7k–m). Immediate prosthetic conversion of a fixed provisional restoration was completed with the immediate post-operative provisional as shown in Figure 21.7n–q.

Phase 2: After a suitable trial period with the mandibular restoration, the patient's maxillary reconstruction was undertaken with the placement of eight implants using guided surgery planning and CBCT/computer-aided manufacturing surgical guide fabrication (Figure 21.8a–h). Immediate direct conversion of the maxillary denture to a provisional fixed prosthesis was completed (Figure 21.6i–n). The patient was instructed to maintain a limited diet with the consistency of scrambled eggs, and to avoid direct chewing or clenching for the first 4 months after provisionalization. Following 4 months' healing, the definitive restoration process was undertaken with fabrication of maxillary and mandibular hybrid prostheses, as seen in Figure 21.8o–r.

The patient can be seen in Figure 21.8s and t on follow-up after 4 years. The retracted oral view and panoramic radiograph show an esthetic and stable clinical result.

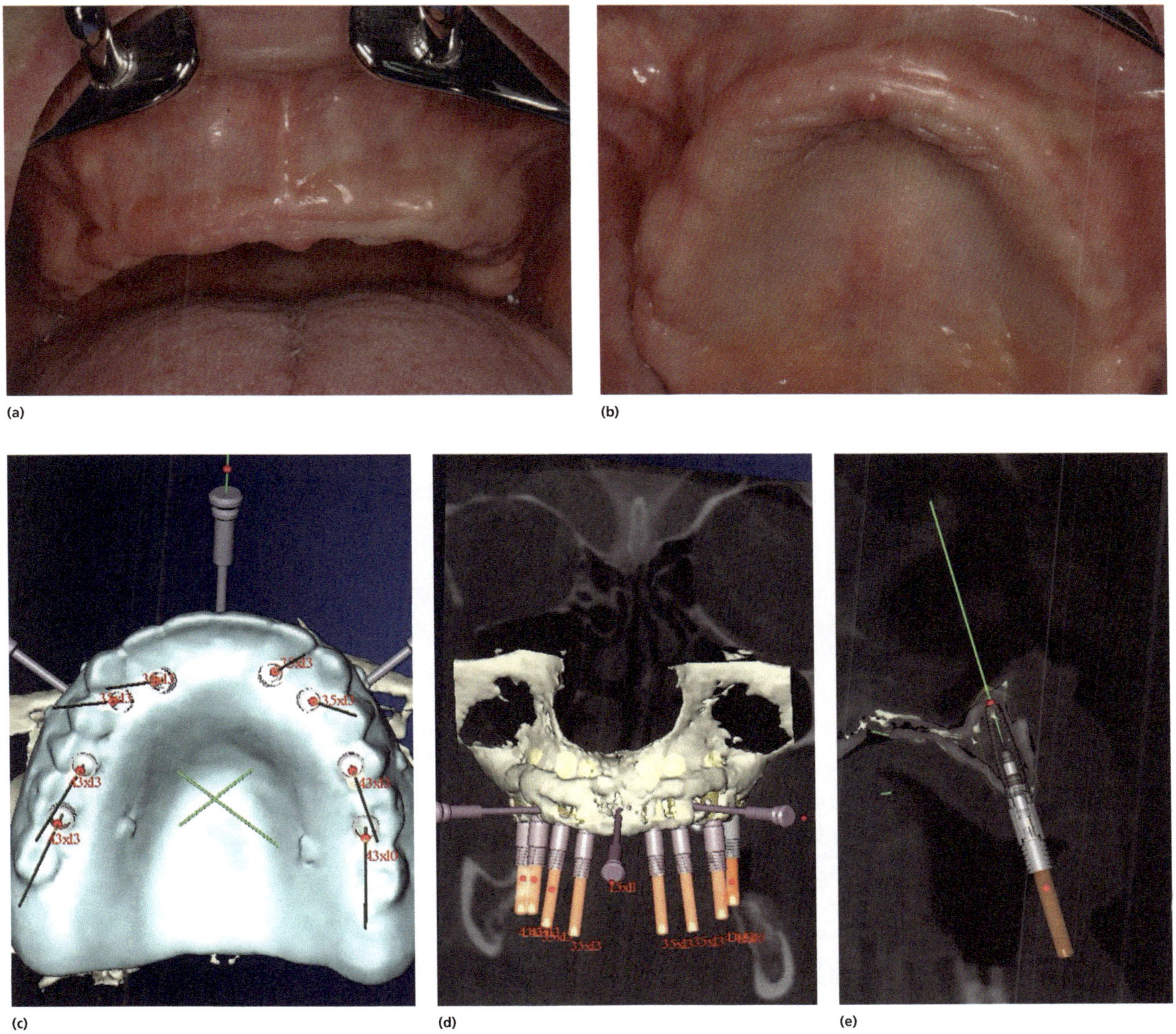

(a) (b) (c) (d) (e)

Figure 21.8 (a–f) Guided surgery was planned for the maxilla employing CBCT/computer-aided design maxillary guide fabrication and an immediate direct provisional restoration. (g, h) The implants are shown here in position after guided surgery. (i, j) Direct pick-up technique was used sequentially for provisional prosthesis fabrication using provisional plastic abutments. (k–m) The immediate provisional prosthesis.

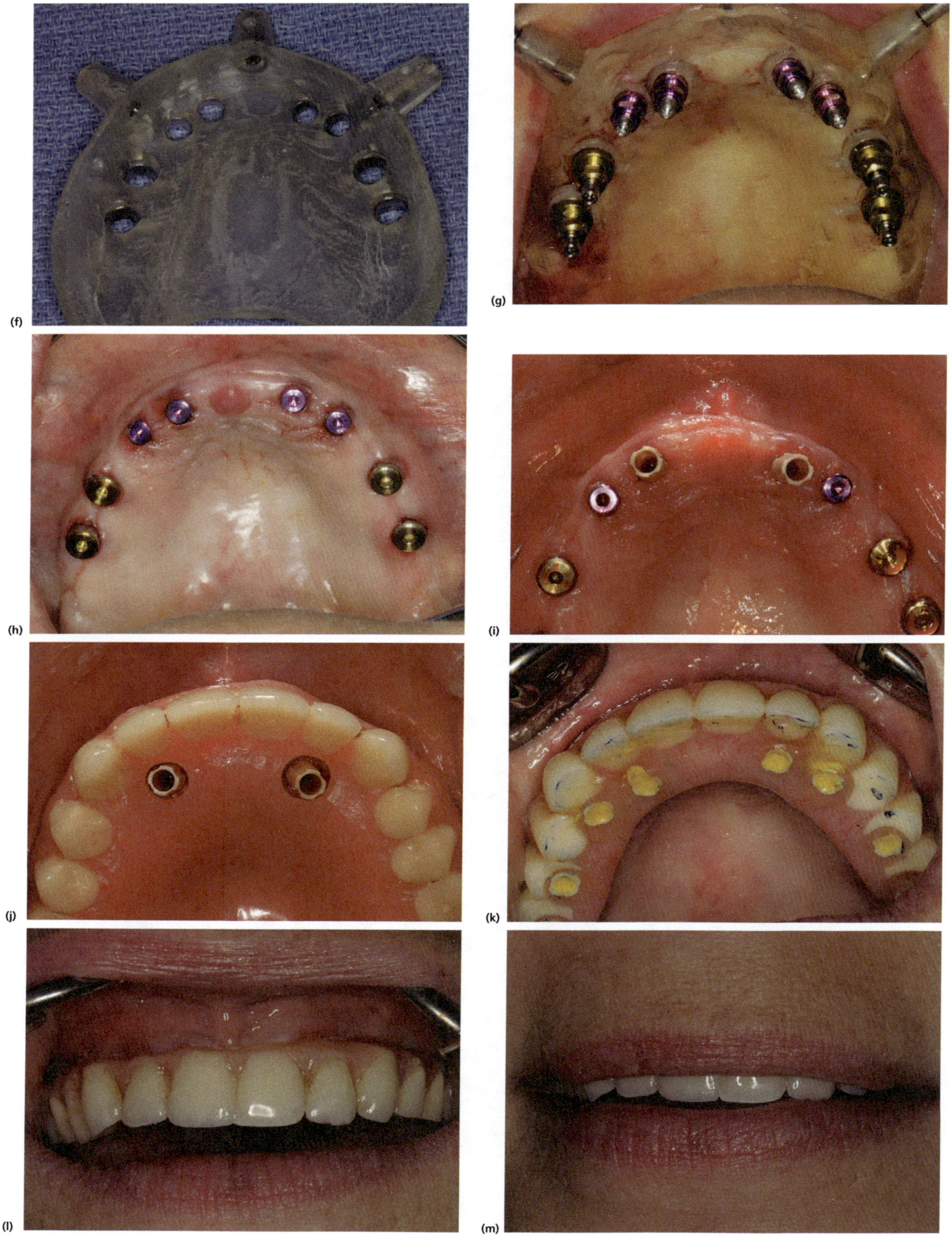

Figure 21.8 (Continued)

(Continued)

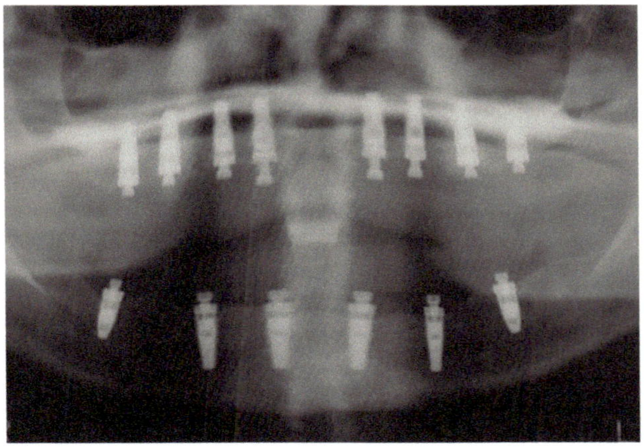
(n)

Figure 21.8 (Continued)

(n) A panoramic radiograph of the immediate maxillary prosthesis and the mandibular prosthesis described previously. (o, p) The definitive hybrid maxillary and mandibular prostheses are shown in clinical and panoramic radiographic images. (q, r) Facial views show an excellent esthetic result in repose and on full smile view. (s, t) Clinical and radiographic images demonstrate the definitive restoration after 4 years. *Source:* (i, j, o) © Earl Ness. (a–h, k–n, p–t) © Daniel R. Cullum.

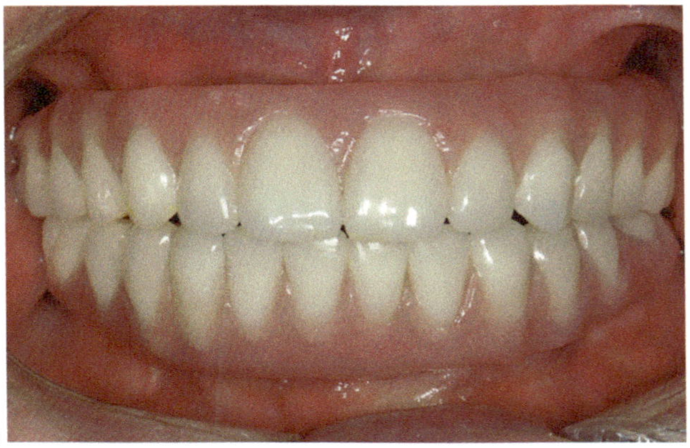
(o)

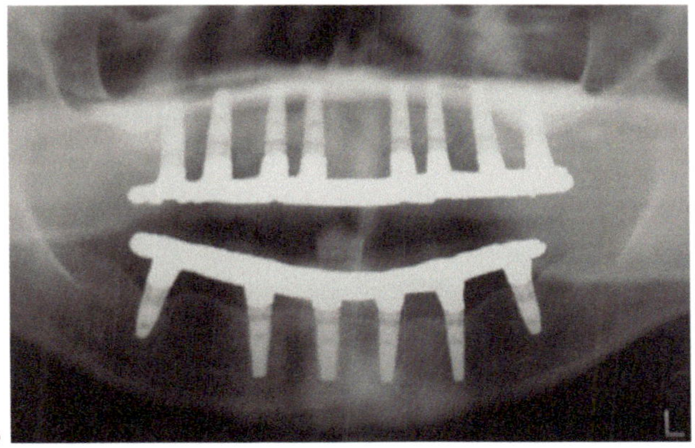
(p)

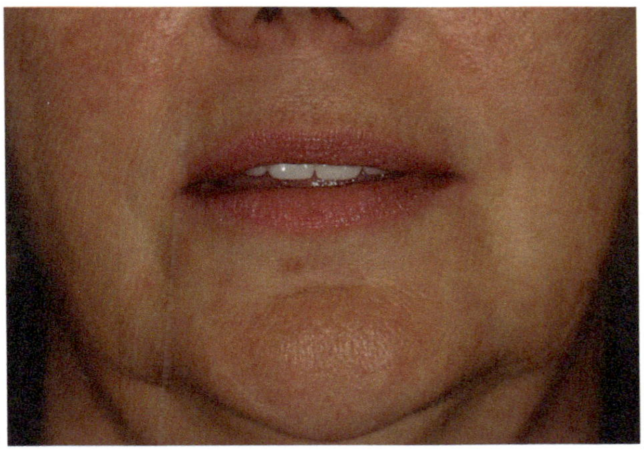
(q)

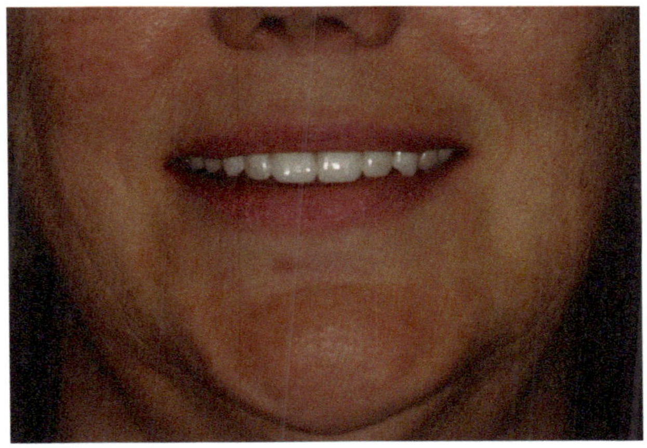
(r)

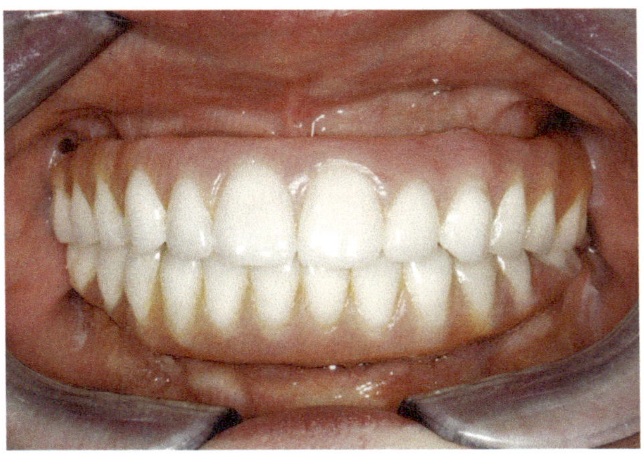
(s)

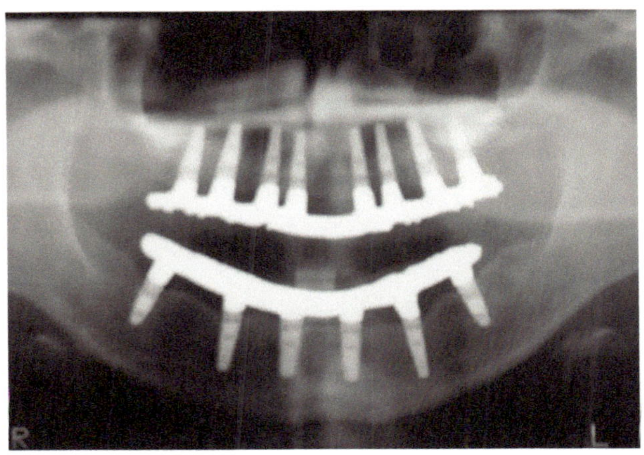
(t)

Index

Page numbers in *italic* refer to figures.
Sorting is letter-by-letter so that, for example, 'D osteotomes' comes after 'donor sites' and 'O-ring' comes after 'oral'.

A

absorbable collagen sponge (carrier for BMP), 119–120
  grafts for angled implants, 221
  technique, 120–127
abutments, *see also* healing abutments
  choice, 42
  platform switching, 58
  preparation, 45
  provisional, 69
    esthetic zone, 368–369, *371*, *373*
    PEEK polymer for, *71*, *80*
    titanium for, 69, 70, *73*, *81*
  screws for, *372*
acellular dermal matrix, 90, 150, *152*, *154*, 155, *156*
acid-etched surfaces, 193
acrylic burs, *372*, 374
adjacent implants
  BAOSFE, 266–268
  bone loss between, 57–58, 67–68
  narrow diameter, *214*
  plastic surgery for, 140
adjacent teeth
  endodontic treatment, 55
  extraction, 342–343
  immediate implant placement and, 369
age, on tooth display, 5
aging, removable prostheses, 22
allergies, 62
Alloderm® (acellular dermal matrix), 90, 150, *152*, *154*, 155, *156*
allografts *see* freeze-dried bone allografts
aluminum oxide dental implant, 337, *338*
alveolar crest, *see also entries beginning* crestal...
  height, bone anatomy, 8
  resorption, 36, *see also* crestal bone loss
alveolar defects, reconstruction, 13
alveolar mucosa, 137
alveolar ridge
  expansion
    narrow implants and, 213, *215–217*
    osteotome technique, 156, *157*
  maxilla, measurements, 33
  preservation, 89–106, 367–368
    bone grafting, 96–105, 120, 125–127
    flap design for 141
alveolectomy, *438*
anastomoses, endosseous, maxillary artery, 31
anatomic risk factors, 53–57
  ridge expansion, 289–290
angiogenesis, rhPDGF-BB on, 119, 135
angled implants
  complete arch treatment, 219–226
  numbers of, 221
angulated abutments, 42
anterior guidance, 12, 61
anterior incisal plane, 5f
anterior nasal spine, *175*
anterior open bite, correction, 393, 396–399, *400–401*
anterior–posterior anchorage, 387–390
anterior–posterior spread, 220–221, 433, *434*
antibiotics
  presurgical, 90, 100
  for rhBMP-2-ACS grafts, 120, 121, 125
antrum *see* maxillary sinus
apical positioned flaps, 142, 156
apico-coronal position, 14, 59
Arrestin® (minocycline), 55
asymmetry, 5, 6, 20
atraumatic technique, tooth extraction, 90–91
atrophy of bone *see* bone loss
augmentation procedures, 245–247, *see also* bone grafting; grafting *under* soft tissues
  esthetics, 13
  flap design for, 141
  immediate implant placement, 352–357, 378
  maxillary sinus and, 33–35
  rhBMP-2-ACS grafts with, 122
  simultaneous implant placement, 241
autogenous bone grafts, 122–123, 244–245
axial inclination, 8

B

barium appliances, 130, 170, *171*
barrier membranes, 90, 245, *see also* collagen barriers; hd-PTFE
  titanium mesh *vs*, 124
benign paroxysmal vertigo, 280, 291, 308–309
bi-cortical bone, ridge expansion and, 289, *290*
bicuspid teeth
  immediate implants, 337–338
  narrow implants, 211
bi-bevel osteotomes, *288*, *293*, 303, *304*, *306*
Bio-Col® technique, 91–96, 346
biologic width, 67, 107, 138, 140
  crestal bone loss, 201–202
  platform switching, 58–59, 68
bisphosphonates, 51
bisque bake try-in, 81, *83*
bite
  anterior open, 393, 396–399, *400–401*
  assessment, 4
  deep, 69
  inter-arch registration, 170, *179*, *182*
blade implants, 229, *see also* wedge implants
blanching of tissue, 70
block grafts, *185*, 428–431
  implant survival rates, 227
blood, autologous, 92
blood clotting, tooth extraction, 90
blood dyscrasias, 184–185
blood supply, ridge expansion, 313

Minimally Invasive Dental Implant Surgery, First Edition. Edited by Daniel R. Cullum and Douglas Deporter.

blood vessels
  lingual perforating vessels, 28
  maxillary artery, endosseous anastomoses, 31
  maxillary sinus, hemorrhage from, 61
bone
  required thickness, 66
  trabeculae, stress distribution, 203–204
bone-added osteotome sinus floor elevation, 251, 253–254, *255–256*, 256, *257*, 264–266, 282, 313
  immediate implant placement, 361–364
  perforation, 280
  ridge expansion with, 324–328
bone cysts, 127
bone-driven tissue transformation, 246–247
bone flaps, 285, 311
bone grafting, *see also* bovine xenograft
  alveolar ridge preservation, 96–105, 120, 125–127
  angled implants, 221
  augmentation procedures, 227
  autogenous, 122–123, 244–245
  buccal, 53
  flap design for, 141
  freeze-dried allografts
    demineralized, 119–120, 245
    mineralized, 120, 125–127, 245
  imaging for, 28
  materials, guided bone regeneration, 244–245
  maxillary sinus, 31, 33–35
  peri-implant defects, 337
  XXS Infuse® kit, 120–121
bone height, *see also* ridge height
  interproximal, on interdental papillae, 53, 66–67, 68
  trans-alveolar sinus elevation, 253, 282
bone loss, 67–68, 139–140, 184, *see also* bone remodeling; crestal bone loss; pneumatization of maxillary sinus
  augmentation procedures for, 13
  buccal plate, 367–368
    laser-ablated surfaces on, 108
  esthetic zone, 401–406
  imaging, 28
  immediate implants, 337–338
  immediate loading sites, 222
  implant positioning on, 57–58, *59*
  interproximal, 14
  from removable prostheses, 130, *132*
  ridge expansion and, 289
  smoking, 52
  tooth extraction, 120
bone morphogenetic protein-2, 119–136
  grafts for angled implants, 221
bone–periosteal flaps, 285, 311
bone quality
  growth factor-stimulated, 121, 125, 127, 135
  for ridge expansion, 289, *290*, 315
  short implants, 200, 204, 205
bone reduction, 24
bone regeneration *see* guided bone regeneration
bone remodeling, *see also* bone loss
  after tooth extraction, 89, 90
  interproximal, 14
  peri-implant, 139–140
bone spreading, 286, 311
bone-supported guides, 170
bone-to-implant contact, 337
bovine xenograft, 245
  Bio-Col® technique, 91–92, *93*
  carrier for rhPDGF-BB, 120
  deproteinized bovine bone mineral, 241
  mineralized bovine bone/collagen substitute, 129, *130*
bridges
  anterior mandible, immediate implant placement, 342–343
  cantilever bridges, failure, 219
bruxism, 52–53
  on prosthesis choice, 24
buccal bone grafting, 53
buccal fistula, *94*
buccal inclination
  excessive, ridge expansion and, 306–308, 331
buccal plate
  bone loss, 367–368
    laser-ablated surfaces on, 108
  fracture, 90–91, 306, 331–332
bucco-lingual angulation, 17, 247–248
bucco-lingual position, 14–17, 57
bucco-lingual width
  expansion, narrow implants and, 213, *215–217*
  loss after tooth extraction, 89
  wide-diameter implants, 198
bucco-palatal width, for osteo-mobilization, 315
burs, *see also* reamer burs
  acrylic, *372*, 374
  disposable, 199
  guided, 185
  Lindemann bur, 125, 370

C
Caldwell–Luc approach, 251
calibration, computer-guided technology, 172, *173*
cameras, digital, 4
cancellous bone, stress distribution, 203–204
canines
  fractures, 428–431
  immediate implant placement, 352, *353*, *377–378*
  ridge expansion at, 290
cantilever bridges, failure, 219
canting, occlusal plane, 402, *405*, 407
cardiovascular disease, 184–185
caries, tooth extraction, 98
casts, *see also* master casts
  diagnostic, 3
  stone casts, scanning, 43, 44
cavitation, ultrasonic bone surgery, 228
cement-retained prostheses, 45
  cement remnants, 67
  screw-retained prostheses *vs*, 58, 59
    imaging, 42–45
    provisional restorations, 69
cingulum bucco-lingual angulation, 247–248
circular fibers, implant–gingival complex, 138
classifications
  extraction sockets, 120
  immediate loading sites, 220, 222
  maxillary sinus septa, 33
  soft tissue recession, 140, 159
cleaning, extraction socket grafts, 100
clenching, on prosthesis choice, 24
collagen
  esthetic zone, 370
  laser-ablated surfaces on, 107, 112
collagen barriers
  immediate implant placement, 346
  palatal pedicle flaps, 163, *165*, *166*
  ridge split fractures, *307*
collagen membranes, 245
  alveolar ridge preservation, *98*, 99
    removal, 99, 100
  over mineralized particulate allografts, 241
collagen sponge, *see also* absorbable collagen sponge
  Bio-Col® technique, 92, *93*, *94*
  for maxillary sinus membrane tear, 281
CollaPlug®, 346
combination syndrome, 146
complete arch treatment, *see also* edentulous patients
  angled implants, 219–226
compliance *see* patient compliance
complications, 51–65, *see also specific procedures*
composite resin
  mock-ups, 10

provisional restorations, *372*, 374
soft tissue manipulation, *77*
compressive forces, wedge implants, 230
computed tomography *see* cone beam computed tomography
computer-guided technology, 169–189
indications, 173
condensation *see* osteo-condensation
cone beam computed tomography, 23–50, 169
barium appliances, 130, 170, *171*
buccal plate, 368
computer-guided technology, 170
extraction sites, *93*, *94*
immediate implant placement, 348
maxillary sinus, *252*, 253
for rhBMP-2-ACS grafts, 120, *121*
risk reduction, 61
congenital absence (teeth), 76–84, *176*, 246, 422–427
anatomic restriction, 173, *176*, *178*
narrow implants, 213
A–P anchorage, 387, *389*, 390, *391–392*
tissue manipulation, 36–41
connective tissue, *see also* alveolar mucosa
biologic width, 67, 107
grafting, 142–147
immediate implant placement, 356, 375, *379–380*, *381*
lateral repositioned pedicle flaps and, 161
from maxillary tuberosity, 152–154
ridge expansion, 303
tunnel flaps and, 152
laser-ablated surfaces on, 109–110, 111, 112–113
provisional matrix, 90
connector zones, multiple-unit restorations, cross-sectional areas, 12
consent, 4
contiguous sinus floor elevation (CSFE), 261–262, 272–276, *277*, *278–280*
after membrane tear, 281
ridge expansion with, 314, *316–318*, 328, *329–331*
contraindications, dental implants, 51
conversion prosthesis, dentures, 174
cooling, inadequate, 200
copings, for impressions, 74, *75*
coring drills, computer-guided technology, 172
coronal advanced flaps, 156–160
coronal diameter, implants, 368, 370
corono-apical position, 14, 59
corrosion, 62
cortical bone
fixation into, 219
ridge expansion and, 289, *290*
corticosteroids, for rhBMP-2-ACS grafts, 120, 121, 125
costs, computer-guided technology, 186
crestal bone loss, 67–68, 227
fracture risk, 62
narrow implants, 210
short implants and, 52, 201–203
tooth extraction, 53
wide-diameter implants, 198
crestal core elevation technique, 258
Crestal Lift Control® reamer bur, *257*
crestally initiated flaps, 141–142
crestal remodeling, 14
crest height, bone anatomy, 8
cross-arch stabilization 173–174, 433, *434*
cantilever bridges, 219
cross-sectional areas, multiple-unit restorations, connector zones, 12
cross-sectional views, radiography, 28, 35, 38
crowns, *371*, *373*, 374, *377*
crown-to-implant root ratios (*C/R*), short implants, 203
cumulative survival rates, immediate loading, 178
customization, abutment fabrication, 69, 368–369
cyanoacrylate, Bio-Col® technique, 92, 96
Cytoplast® hd-PTFE, alveolar ridge preservation, 96–105
Cytoplast® RTM™ *see* collagen barriers

D
data sets (DICOM), 28, 43–44, *see also* DICOM images
debridement, tooth extraction, 91, 99
deciduous teeth
extraction, 45
retained, 36–41
decortication, tooth sockets, 99
deep bite patients, 69
dehiscence
after open-barrier alveolar ridge preservation, 100
facial bones, 149–150
roots, 422–427
delayed implant placement, after ridge expansion, 320
demineralized freeze-dried bone allografts, 119–120, 245
DentaScan®, 169
dento-facial analysis, 5–6
dento-gingival analysis, 6
dentures, *see also* fixed partial dentures; overdentures; prostheses; removable prostheses
retro-fitting, 174
teeth, *372*
deproteinized bovine bone mineral (DBBM), 241
depth gauges, piezoelectric surgery, *232*, *233*
depth of insertion
bone stress *vs*, 208
in esthetic zone, 370
immediate implant placement, 352
dermis *see* acellular dermal matrix
designed intrabony length
crestal bone loss, 201–202
short implants, 193
deviation, surgical templates, 170–172
diabetes mellitus, 51
diagnosis, 3–4
diameter, *see also* narrow implants; wide-diameter implants
coronal, implants, 368, 370
failure of implants *vs*, 208
fracture risk *vs*, 210
diastemata, 10, 396–399
DICOM images, *see also* data sets
computer-guided technology, 170
digital dentistry, 43–44, *see also* computer-guided technology
digital photography, 3–4
displacement, dental implants, 61–62, 281, 368
disposable burs, 199
donor sites, autogenous bone grafts, 244–245
D osteotomes, *288*
ridge expansion, *293*, 303, *304*, 320
double-membrane technique, alveolar ridge preservation, 99
dressings *see* periodontal dressings
drilling
immediate implant placement, 352, *354*
esthetic zone, 369–370
trans-alveolar sinus elevation, 253, *254*
drilling guides, 170
drills, 185, *187*
coring drills, computer-guided technology, 172
drill-specific guide keys, 45
drug holidays, bisphosphonates, 51
durability, choice of restoration, 23–24
dysharmonies, gingival levels, 7f

E
edentulous patients, *see also* complete arch treatment
case studies, 367, 432–435, 436–441
treatment planning, 22–25
edge attrition (cases), 3–26, *413*, 417–419
edge position, incisal, 5–6
education of patients, computer-guided technology, 186
Elian classification, extraction sockets, 120
embrasures, incisal, 8–10
emergence profiles, 59, *60*, 368–369, 382
endodontic treatment, adjacent teeth, 55
endosseous anastomoses, maxillary artery, 31

epithelium, *see also* junctional epithelium
in connective tissue grafts, 146
laser-ablated surfaces on, 111, 112
Equimatrix® xenograft, 370
equine bone block, carrier for rhPDGF-BB, 120
error, surgical templates, 170–172
erythema, recombinant growth factors on, 135
Essix® appliances, 69, *98*, 99, *133*, 399
esthetic contour grafts, 241–250
esthetics, 12–13
plastic surgery for, 140–141
esthetic zone, 5, *see also* incisors; parasymphysis
evaluation, 12–13
immediate implant placement, 367–383
preoperative evaluation, 369
techniques, 369–370
incisions, 412, *413*
ridge expansion, 291–292
soft tissue and bone loss, 401–406
evidence, on blade implants, 229
examination, 4
periodontium, 3
expanded PTFE (porous PTFE), 90, *96*, 245
exposure (tooth display), 5
extraction of teeth
adjacent, 342–343
alveolar ridge preservation, 89–106
bone loss, 53
deciduous, 45
immediate implant placement after, 346, *347*, 369
technique, 90–91
virtual, *30*, 173, *177*
extraction sockets, 55, *56–57*, *see also* preservation *under* alveolar ridge
assessment for immediate implant placement, 340, 350
classification, 120
grafting, 100, 144–146
protection from saliva, 92, 96
extrusion
bone reduction, 24
in esthetic zone, 402, *403*
mandibular teeth (case), 432–435, *436*

F
fabrication
abutments, customization, 69, 368–369
guides, 170, *171*, 172
provisional restorations, 69–76
face, analysis, 4–6
facial displacement of implants, 368
Facilitate™ instrument tray, *186*
failing dentition, treatment planning, 22–25
failure of implants, 51, 172
allergy, 62
diameter *vs*, 208
endodontic treatment of adjacent teeth, 54
keratinized tissue width, 54
mini-implants, 146
narrow implants, 209, 210
overload, 204
short implants, 195, 199
smoking, 52
fibroblasts, laser-ablated surfaces on, 107, *109*
files, piezoelectric surgery, 230
fistula
buccal, *94*
from root fracture, 422–427
fixed partial dentures
cases of failure, 417–419, 428–431
narrow implants supporting, 210, 212, 213
flanges, prostheses, 13
flapless surgery, 169, 172
immediate implant placement, 338
narrow implants, 209
ridge expansion, 291–292, 295
flaps, *see also* pedicle flaps
bone, 285, 311
bone–periosteal, 285, 311
bone spreading, 286
full-thickness, ridge expansion, 296–300, 309, 320, *321–323*, 368
immediate implant placement, 352
mucoperiosteal, 61
open-book, *242*, 243, *244*, *246*
osteo-mobilization, 286–289
partial-thickness *see* partial-thickness flaps
plastic surgery, 141–152
primary closure, 90
rhBMP-2-ACS grafts and, 120, 125, 135
ridge expansion, 291–292, *293*, *294–295*, 296–297, 299–303
full-thickness, 296–300, 309, 320, *321–323*, 368
TASE and, 321
single-stage implant placement, 242–243
split-thickness *see* split-thickness flaps
tooth extraction, *97*, 98, 100, *101*
tunnel flaps, 141, 152–156, *420*
Food and Drug Administration, on blade implants, 229
forces on implants, 193, *194*, 230
foreign body effect, *157*
four-wall bony defects, creation, 311
fractures, *see also* greenstick fracture; up-fracture
buccal plate, 90–91, 306, 331–332
canines, 428–431
implants, 53
narrow diameter, 210
mandible, 62
micro-fractures, tooth extraction, 89
out-fractures, ridge splitting, 311–313
of provisional restorations, 374
at ridge expansion, 299, 306, 315, *316–317*, 331–332
ridge split fractures, 306, *307*
roots, 100, *103*
fistula, 422–427
Frankfort plane, *5*
free gingival grafts, 142
freeze-dried bone allografts, 150, 245
demineralized, 119–120, 245
mineralized, 120, 125–127, 245
frenum, excision, *420*
full arch treatment *see* complete arch treatment; edentulous patients
full-thickness flaps, ridge expansion, 296–300, 309, 320, *321–323*, 368
functional surface area, 193
future site development, crestal core elevation technique, 258

G
GC pattern resin, 74
GEM 21S® *see* platelet-derived growth factor
gingiva, 137–139, *see also* pink esthetics
alveolar mucosa *vs*, 137
analysis, 6, 7f
biotypes, 6, 66
computer-guided technology and, 172
deficiency, 53–54
display, 5–6
excess display, 390, *392*, *393*, *394*
free grafts, 142
immediate implant placement, 352, 369
narrow implants, 217
prostheses, 13
single missing tooth, 17, *18*
grafting, *see also* block grafts; bone grafting; connective tissue; freeze-dried bone allografts
acellular dermal matrix, 90, 150, *152*, *154*, 155, *156*
Bio-Col® technique, 91–96
with growth factors *see* recombinant human bone morphogenetic protein-2; recombinant human platelet-derived growth factor
immediate implant placement, 346, *347*, 356
esthetic zone, 375, 378, *379–380*, 381
molars, 357–361

maxillary sinus, 61, 251
open-barrier techniques, 99, 100, *103*
ridge expansion, 292, 295, 308, 331, 368, 370
single-stage implant placement, 241–250
soft tissues, 53, 141–152
treatment planning, 39
tunnel flaps and, 152
tunnel flaps, 141, 152–156, *420*
granulation tissue, 90, 91
greenstick fracture
osteo-mobilization, 285
out-fractures, ridge splitting, 311–313
grooves, laser-ablated surfaces, 107, 111
growth factors, *see also specific growth factors*
bone stimulated by, 121, 125, 127, 135
on erythema, 135
extraction site treatment, 92
guided bone regeneration (GBR), 90, 227
bone grafting, materials, 244–245
failure, 242
titanium mesh *vs*, 124
guides *see* templates

H
handles (for fabrication), *372*
harvesting, connective tissue grafts, 143–144, *147*, 152–154
hd-PTFE, alveolar ridge preservation, 96–105
head and neck, examination, 4
headgear appliances, 387
healing
bovine xenograft on, 245
diseases affecting, ridge expansion, 291
implant placement, 46
rhBMP-2-ACS grafts, 125, 135
submerged, short implants, 200
tooth extraction, 89–90, 100, *101*, *104*
trans-alveolar sinus elevation, 256
ultrasonic bone surgery, 228–229
healing abutments, 172, *183*, *see also* progressive early loading; provisional restorations
single-stage implant placement, 241
healing caps, 59, *60*
provisional restorations *vs*, 66–67
heat, computer-guided surgery, 172
height loss, alveolar ridge after tooth extraction, 89
hemorrhage, 61
high-density PTFE, alveolar ridge preservation, 96–105
historical aspects
computer-guided technology, 169
immediate implant placement, 337–338, 367–368
ultrasonic bone surgery, 227–228
history-taking, 3, 51
hopeless tooth, treatment planning, 17–20
hourglass mandible, angled implants, 221, 225
hybrid maxillary and mandibular prostheses, *441*
hydraulic pressure, trans-alveolar sinus elevation, 259
hydrodynamic piezoelectric internal sinus elevation, 259, *260*, 272, *273–274*
hydroxyapatite, bacterial colonization, 54
hypodontia, 125–127

I
illusions, esthetic, 10
ImageMaster-101® software, 169
imaging, 3, 28–50, *see also* cone beam computed tomography
immediate implant placement, 337–366, *see also* single-stage implant placement
esthetic zone, 367–383
preoperative evaluation, 369
techniques, 369–370
implant designs for, *349*
immediate loading, *see also* progressive early loading
after CT-guided placement, 173–180
angled implants, 221–222, 225
immediate implant placement, 338
narrow implants, 209
site classification, 220, 222
immediate restoration without loading (IRWL), narrow implants, 209
implant stability quotient, *see also* stability
esthetic zone, provisional restorations, 370
ultrasonic bone surgery, 229
units, 208
impressions, 69–76
incisal bucco-lingual angulation, 247–248
incisal edge, position, 5–6
incisal embrasures, 8–10
incisal plane, 5
incisions
after open-barrier alveolar ridge preservation, 100
apical positioned flaps, 156
coronal advanced flaps, 160
crestally initiated flaps, 141, 142
esthetic zone, 412, *413*
harvesting grafts, 143, 144
immediate implant placement, 350, 352
lateral repositioned pedicle flaps, 161, *162*
localized management of sinus floor, 313–314
minimally invasive, 61
open-book flap, 243, *244*
palatal pedicle flaps, 163, *165*
for rhBMP-2-ACS grafts, 120, 125
for rhPDGF-BB graft, 130, *133*
ridge expansion, *294–295*, 309
with BAOSFE, *325*
with CSFE, *316–318*
split-thickness, 292, *293*
with TASE, 319, *320*, 321
tunnel flaps, 152, *153*, 155
incisive canal, 35–36, *175*
incisors, *see also* esthetic zone
congenital absence *see* congenital absence (teeth)
failure, 130, *133–134*
immediate implant placement, 342–343
implants (case), 417–419
malformations, 407–409
narrow implants, 211, 212, 213
trauma, 412, *413*
infection, 61, 63, *see also* periodontitis
alveolar ridge preservation and, 96, 99, 100
guided bone regeneration and, 90
maxillary sinus, post-operative, 61, *62*
inferior alveolar nerve, *175*
avoidance, angled implants, 221
imaging, 28–29, *30*
inflammation
healing process, 90
laser-ablated surfaces on, 111, 112–113
narrow implants, 217
peri-implant, 54, *55*, 139
ultrasonic bone surgery, 229
informed consent, 4
Infuse® (Medtronic), 120–121, 123
insertion depth
bone stress *vs*, 208
in esthetic zone, 370
immediate implant placement, 352
insertion torques
early loading, 177–178
esthetic zone, 370
instruments, *see also* osteotomes; piezoelectric surgery; *specific instruments*
CSFE, 272, *275*, *317*, 318, 328
CT-guided surgery, 185, 186, *187*
graft placement, 90–91, 92
implant placement, 170, 172
osteo-condensation, *319*
osteo-mobilization, 301
insulin-like growth factor-1, 119
interactive virtual modeling, 41
inter-arch registration, bite, 170, *179*, *182*

inter-arch space, 10–12, 22–23
  reduced, 340
interdental papillae, 6
  adjustments for, 81–84
  immediate implant placement, 378
  between implants, 57–58
  interproximal bone height on, 53, 66–67, 68
  plastic surgery for, 140
  single-stage implant placement, 243
  tooth extraction and, 99
  v–y closure, *434*
inter-implant distance, 57–58, *60*
interproximal bone height, on interdental papillae, 53, 66–67, 68
interproximal papillae *see* interdental papillae
interproximal space, 14, 57
  narrow implants, 217
interpupillary plane, 5f
inter-radicular septa, immediate implant placement, 343, *344–346*, 349, 362, *363*
intraoral mock-ups, 10, *11*
intraoral optical scanners, 43
intra-osseous anastomoses, maxillary artery, 31
intrusion, orthodontics, 59, *60*, 390, *392*, *393*, 396, *398–399*, 402, *403*, 407–409
irrigation, tooth sockets, 369
ISQ *see* implant stability quotient; stability

J
jumping distances, 337
junctional epithelium (JE), 137–138
  laser-ablated surfaces on, 109, 110

K
keratinized tissue, 137, 247, 292

L
labial bone thickness, 247–248
labial bucco-lingual angulation, 247–248
labial inclination, excessive, *306*
laser-ablated implant surfaces, 107–111, 112–113, 138, 141
laser-assisted new attachment procedure (LANAP), 129–130
lateral repositioned pedicle flaps, 161–163
lateral window sinus grafting, 251
lichen planus, 54
light-cured periodontal dressings, 92
Lindemann bur, 125, 370
lingual perforating vessels, 28
lip-lift technique
  periapical radiography, 38
  virtual modeling, 41
lip support, 6
lithium disilicate restorations, dimensions required, 12
loading of implants, *see also* immediate loading; overloading
  after CT-guided placement, 172, 173–180
  progressive early loading, short implants, 200–201
  on soft tissues, 114, 115
local anesthesia, risk reduction by, 61
localized management of sinus floor (LMSF), 259, 313–314
long-term follow-up, narrow implants, 209–210
long-term provisional restorations, 424, *426*, 428

M
mallet (Rex®), *232*
malocclusion, 406–409, *see also* canting
mandible
  angled implants, 225
  fractures, 62
  imaging, 28–29
  molars
    immediate implant placement, *351*, 357–361
    narrow implants, 211–212
  parasymphysis, effect of strain, 219
manufacture *see* fabrication
manufacturers, computer-guided technology, 170
master casts, 70, *71–73*
  computer-guided technology, *179*, *182*
  stereolithography, 170, *172*
maxilla, *see also* tuberosity of maxilla
  expansion, 396
  molars, immediate implant placement, 361–364
  ridge expansion, 286–288, *289*
    TASE with, 311–333
  vascular canal, 33, *see also* endosseous anastomoses
maxillary artery, endosseous anastomoses, 31
maxillary central incisal edge, 5
maxillary central incisor position, 6
maxillary sinus, 251–253, *see also* Schneiderian membrane
  avoidance, angled implants, 221
  computer-guided technology, 173, *175*
  hemorrhage from blood supply, 61
  imaging, 29–34
  implant displacement into, 281
  post-operative infection, 61, *62*
  sloping floor, BAOSFE, 266–268
maxillary sinusitis, 281
mechanical expanders (rotary screw expanders), *287*, 292, *294–295*, 297, 298–299
mechanical overload *see* overloading
Mectron Piezosurgery® device, 230
medication-related osteonecrosis of the jaw (MRONJ), 51
membrane (maxillary sinus) *see* Schneiderian membrane
membranes, *see also* collagen membranes; double-membrane technique
  guided bone regeneration, 90
mental foramen, *30*, *31*, *175*
mesio-distal positioning, 57
mesio-distal size
  immediate implant placement, 342–343
  wedge implants, 230
metal restorations, dimensions required, 12
microcirculation, after tooth extraction, 90
micro-flap access, ridge expansion, 303–305
micro-fractures, tooth extraction, 89
microgap, 58, 67, *68*, 107, 203
micro-grooves, laser-ablated surfaces, 107, 111
micro-saws, piezoelectric surgery, 230, *231*
micro-screw implants, 387, *388*, 402
micro-threads, 202–203
midlines, 5
  correction, 395, 396–399
  diastemata, 10, 396–399
Miller classification, soft tissue recession, 140, 159
mineralization, after tooth extraction, 90
mineralized bovine bone/collagen substitute (MCBS), 129, *130*
mineralized freeze-dried bone allografts, 120, 125–127, 245
mineralized particulate allografts, single-stage implant placement, 241
Miner-Oss® mixed graft, 370
mini Beaver blade, ridge expansion, 302, *319*
mini-flap access, ridge expansion, 303–305
mini-implants (MDIs), 208
  failure, 146
mini-screws, orthodontic, 387, *388*, 402
minocycline (Arrestin®), 55
missing teeth, *see also* congenital absence; single missing tooth
  multiple, treatment planning, 20–22, 173
mobilization *see* osteo-mobilization
mock-ups, intraoral, 10, *11*
molars
  immediate implant placement, 338, 343, 349–350, *351*, 357–364
  malocclusion, 406–409
  mandible
    immediate implant placement, *351*, 357–361
    narrow implants, 211–212
  supereruption, 396, *397*
movement of natural teeth, *79*
Mucograft®, 146, *149*
mucoperiosteal flaps, 61
mucosa, alveolar, 137
mucosa-supported guides, 170
mucositis, peri-implant, 54, *55*

multiple missing teeth, treatment planning, 20–22, 173
multiple-unit restorations, connector zones, cross-sectional areas, 12
multi-rooted teeth *see* molars

N

narrow implants (NDIs), 208–218, *see also* blade implants
nasal crest cortex, vomer implants, 222–223, *224*
nasal floor, computer-guided technology, 173
natural teeth
  movement, *79*
  for provisional restorations, 374, *375–377*
Navigator® instrument tray, *186*
neovascularization, rhPDGF-BB on, 119, 135
nerves, *see also* inferior alveolar nerve
  computer-guided technology, *173*
  ultrasonic bone surgery, 228
night guards, 53
Nobel Biocare, drills, *187*
NobelGuide® technology, 169
  calibration device, 172, *173*
NobelReplace™ instrument tray, *186*
non-axis implants *see* angled implants
non-cutting apices, implants, 320
non-submerged implant placement, ridge expansion, 320
nose-blowing test, 254

O

occlusal design, 59–61
occlusal evaluation, 3
occlusal plane, 5
  canting, 402, *405*, 407
occlusal stability, 12
occlusal thickness, restorations, 10–12
occlusive barriers, *see also* barrier membranes
  guided bone regeneration, 90
  over rhBMP-2-ACS grafts, 124
off-angle implants *see* angled implants
off-axis access, 346
  immediate implant placement, *347*
  retention screws, 340
off-label applications
  Infuse® (Medtronic), 123
  rhPDGF-BB, 129–134, 146, *149*
Omnigrip® screw and driver, 340
one abutment, one time, 59
opacity *see* transparency
open-barrier techniques, alveolar ridge preservation, 96–105
open bite, correction, 393, 396–399, *400–401*
open-book flap, *242*, 243, *244*, *246*
optical scanners, 43
oral hygiene
  alveolar mucosa *vs* gingiva, 137
  narrow implants, 217
  problems, 52
  thin soft tissues, 140
O-ring configuration, implant–gingival complex, 138
orthodontics
  congenital absence of incisors, *79*
  intrusion, 59, *60*, 390, *392*, *393*, 396, *398–399*, 402, *403*, 407–409
  narrow implants and, 213, *215–217*
  skeletal anchorage, 387–411
  vertical dimension, 390–395
Ossix Plus® collagen membrane, 241
osteo-condensation, 285, 291, 292, 296–297, 311
osteo-mobilization, 285–286, 291, 292, *293*, 299–303, 311
  flaps, 286–289
  trans-alveolar sinus elevation with, 311–333
osteonecrosis of the jaw, medication-related (MRONJ), 51
osteoporosis
  drugs for, 51
  local, 53
osteotome ridge expansion technique, 156, *157*
osteotomes, *see also* D osteotomes
  bi-bevel, *288*, *293*, 303, *304*, *306*
  ridge expansion, *287–288*
  for short implants, 200
  spade, *287*, *293*, *303*
  trans-alveolar sinus elevation, 254
osteotome sinus floor elevation (OSFE), 251, 253, *254*, 262–263, 282, 313, *see also* bone-added osteotome sinus floor elevation
  ridge expansion with, 321–324
  Schneiderian membrane, 254, 256, 258, 259, *260*, 261–282
  short implants, 256, *257*
osteotomies, *see also* ultrasonic bone surgery
  ridge expansion, 253, 285
  short implants, 199–200
  trans-alveolar sinus elevation, 253
  wedge implants, 230
ostiomeatal complex, imaging, 31
out-fractures, ridge splitting, 311–313
overdentures, narrow implants supporting, 209, 210–211
overloading, 60–61
  short implants, 203–205
over-seating, immediate implants, 337

P

Palacci, P., papilla regeneration technique, 243, *244*
Palacci, P, and Nowzari, H., lateral repositioned pedicle flaps, 161, *162*
palatal bone, esthetic zone, 369
palatal pedicle flaps, 163, *164–166*
papillae *see* interdental papillae
paranasal sinuses *see* maxillary sinus
parasymphysis, *see also* esthetic zone
  mandible, effect of strain, 219
partial-thickness flaps, *see also* split-thickness flaps
  ridge expansion, 311
    BAOSFE with, 324
particle-blasted surfaces, 193, 199
particulate allografts, *see also specific types*
  mineralized, single-stage implant placement, 241
patient acceptability, angled implants, 221
patient compliance
  headgear appliances, 387
  ridge expansion with TASE, 332
pedicle flaps, 142, 156–166, 428–431
  immediate implant placement, 350–352
    single-rooted teeth, 352–356
PEEK polymer, *71*, *80*
percussion, osteotomy, 253
perforating vessels, lingual, 28
perforation
  for rhBMP-2-ACS grafts, 125
  single-stage implant placement, 243
perforation (accidental)
  ridge expansion and, 303
  by screws, 42, 43
  TASE, 33, 61, 254–256, 280–281
periapical radiography, 38
peri-implant bone remodeling, 139–140
peri-implant defects, 337–338, 346
peri-implantitis, 54–55, *56*
  narrow implants, 209
  smoking, 52
peri-implant mucositis, 54, *55*
peri-implant surgery *see* plastic surgery
periodontal dressings
  light-cured, 92
  ridge expansion, 295–296
periodontal pockets, 55
periodontitis, 52, 63
periodontium, 137
  examination, 3
  plastic surgery, 137–168
periosteum, single-stage implant placement, 243
petroleum jelly, *72*
phonetics, evaluation, 12
photography, digital, 3–4

piezoelectric surgery, 228–237
  esthetic zone, 370
  hydrodynamic internal sinus elevation, 259, *260*, 272, *273–274*
  ridge expansion, 291, *294–295*, 298, *319*, 321
  TASE, 259, *260*, *319*, 321
pilot holes, narrow implants, 210
pink esthetics, 12–13
plane of occlusion *see* occlusal plane
planning, 4, 17–26, *see also* computer-guided technology; radiography
  for multiple missing teeth, 173
  position of implant, 14–17
  restorative driven, 57
  software, 28, 39–41
    SimPlant®, 169, 170, *171*
  for trauma, 184
plastics, for provisional abutments, 69
plastic surgery, 137–168
  before ridge expansion, 289
platelet-derived growth factor, 92, 119–121, 129–134
  Mucograft® with, 146, *151*
platelet-rich plasma, 125
plates, for skeletal anchorage, 387, *388*
platform switching, 58–59, 68, 141, 203
  esthetic zone, 368, 369
pneumatization of maxillary sinus, 251, 311, *312*
  immediate implant placement, 361–364
  immediate loading sites and, 222
polyethylene mesh, in rhBMP-2-ACS grafts, 123–124
polytetrafluoroethylene *see* hd-PTFE; PTFE
pontics, interproximal bone height and, 67
porcelain-fused-to-metal restorations, dimensions required, 12
porcine dermal matrix xenograft, 146, *149*
porous PTFE, 90, *96*, 245
position of implant, 247–248
  planning, 14–17
  risk factors, 57–59
posterior occlusal plane, 5f
posts, for impressions, 70–74, *75*
povidone iodine, 91
premature occlusal contacts, 61
premolars, congenital absence, 387, *389*, 390, *391–392*, 422–427
primary closure, with flaps, 90
progressive early loading, short implants, 200–201
proportions
  face, 4
  teeth, 6–8
proprioception, 60
prostheses
  bruxism on choice, 24
  cement-retained *see* cement-retained prostheses
  crowns, *371*, *373*, 374, *377*
  gingival, 13
  hybrid maxillary and mandibular, *441*
  implant-supported, 4, 22
  overdentures, narrow implants supporting, 209, 210–211
  removable *see* removable prostheses
  retro-fitting, 174
  risk factors, 57–61
  scan prostheses, 170
  screw-retained *see* screw-retained prostheses
  transitional *see* provisional restorations
  tunnel allografts for, 155, *156*
provisional matrix, connective tissue, 90
provisional restorations, 66–85, *see also* healing abutments; progressive early loading
  after CT-guided implant placement, 172
  esthetic zone, 367, 370–381
    abutment design, 368–369
  immediate, 174–177, 350
  over rhBMP-2-ACS grafts, 121
Proximator® instruments, 90–91, 92
psycho-social factors, immediate loading, 221–222
pterygoid process, angled implants, 223, *224*
PTFE
  barrier membranes, 245
  hd-PTFE, alveolar ridge preservation, 96–105
  porous, 90, *96*, 245
punches, computer-guided technology, 172
Puros® Cancellous mineralized particulate allograft, 241

R
radiography, 3, 28–50
radiotherapy, 184
RANK-L inhibitors, 51
rapid palatal expanders (RPE), 396
reamer burs
  BAOSFE, 266–272
  trans-alveolar sinus elevation, 256–258
recession of soft tissues, 139, 140, 159
  immediate implant placement, 352, 367, 378, *379*
recombinant human bone morphogenetic protein-2, 119–136
  grafts for angled implants, 221
recombinant human platelet-derived growth factor, 92, 119–121, 129–134
  Mucograft® with, 146, *151*
reconstruction (images), 39–41
  immediate implant placement and, 338, *339*, 348
regeneration *see* guided bone regeneration
removable prostheses, *see also* dentures
  causing bone resorption, 130, *132*
  implant-supported, 22
  provisional, 69
reparability, choice of restoration, 23–24
resins, *see also* composite resin
  GC pattern resin, 74
  provisional restorations, 70
resistance form, angled implants, 221
resorption
  alveolar crest, 36, *see also* crestal bone loss
  roots, 37
retraction mechanics, temporary anchorage devices, *390*
retro-fitting, dentures, 174
Rex® mallet, *232*
Rex® wedge implant, 230, *233*, *234*, 235
ridge expansion, 285–310, *see also* expansion *under* bucco-lingual width
  complications, 306–309
  full-thickness flaps, 296–300, 309, 320, *321–323*, 368
  grafting, 292, 295, 308, 331, 368, 370
  osteotome technique, 156, *157*
  TASE with, 311–333
    complications, 331–332
ridge expansion osteotomy, 253, 285
ridge height, *see also* bone height
  for osteo-mobilization with TASE, 315
ridge split fractures, 306, *307*
ridge splitting, 285, 311–313, 320
risks, 51–65
  ridge expansion, 289–290
roots
  fractures, 100, *103*, 422–427
  pathology, preoperative evaluation, 369
  resorption, 37
  tooth extraction, 90–91
rotary screw expanders, *287*, 292, *294–295*, 297, 298–299
roughness of implant surfaces, 193–195
  bacterial colonization, 54
  narrow implants, 209
rounding of teeth, 9
running room, 59

S
SACT (sinus alveolar crest tenting), TASE, 259–261
saliva, protection of extraction sockets, 92, 96
scanning appliances, 43–44, *178–181*
scan prostheses, 170
scarring, after tooth extraction, 89
Schneiderian membrane
  OSFE, 254, 256, 258, 259, *260*, 261–282
  tears, 33, 61, 254–256
screwdrivers, *372*, 374

screw expanders, *287*, 292, *294–295*, 297, 298–299
screw-retained prostheses, 13, 18–20
bucco-lingual angulation, 17
cement-retained prostheses *vs*, 58, 59
imaging, 42–45
provisional restorations, 69
provisional, esthetic zone, 369, 370–371
screw retention, immediate implant placement, 338–340
segmentation (software sensitivity), 173, *176*, *see also* transparency
self-threading implants, TASE, 254
semi-lunar vestibular incision, 61
septa of maxillary sinus, 33
BAOSFE, 266
CSFE, *278*
sequential implant restorations, 22
shade guides, *372*
shape of teeth, 8
Sharpey's fibers, 107, 138
shear forces, wedge implants, 230
short implants, 52, 193–207
OSFE, 253, *254*, 256, *257*
side-cutting reamer burs *see* reamer burs
SimPlant® (software), 169, 170, *171*
simulation of implant, software, 38, *39*, 40–41
single missing tooth, *see also* congenital absence
treatment planning, 17, *18*
single-rooted teeth, immediate implant placement, 352–356
single-stage implant placement, 241–250, *see also* immediate implant placement
ridge expansion and, 295
sintered porous-surfaced press-fit implants, 195, *196*, *197*, *198*, *201*
osteotome sinus floor elevation, 253, *254*
sinus alveolar crest tenting (SACT), TASE, 259–261
sinuses
paranasal *see* maxillary sinus
sinus floor elevation, 251–284, *see also* bone-added osteotome sinus floor elevation; contiguous sinus floor elevation; osteotome sinus floor elevation
size of implant, 17
mesio-distal, wedge implants, 230, 342–343
skeletal anchorage, 387–411
SLA® Straumann implants, 198–199
sloping floor of maxillary sinus, BAOSFE, 266–268
smoking, 52, 195
maxillary sinus infection, 61
narrow implants, 210
smoothing chisels, piezoelectric surgery, 230, *232*
soft tissues, *see also* connective tissue; recession of soft tissues; thin *vs* thick biotypes
after tooth extraction, 89
esthetics, 12–13
esthetic zone, loss, 401–406
grafting, 53, 141–152
treatment planning, 39
tunnel flaps and, 152
healing, 46
loading of implants on, 114, 115
manipulation, 76–84
platform switching on, 58–59
surgery *see* plastic surgery
thickness *vs* implant position, 247–248
software, 28, 39–41, 169–172, *see also* virtual teeth
implant simulation, 38, *39*, 40–41
3-D Dental, 169, *339*
sound, osteotomy, 253
spade osteotomes, *287*, *293*, *303*
speech, evaluation, 12
splinting, 199, 203
split grafts, ridge expansion, 292
split-thickness dissection, *148*
split-thickness flaps, 141, 142, 149–150, *151*, *see also* partial-thickness flaps
ridge expansion, 289, 301–303, 315, *316–318*, 319–320, 321
CSFE with, *329–331*
split-thickness incisions, ridge expansion, 292, *293*
stability, *see also* insertion torques
diameter *vs*, 208
occlusal, 12
provisional restorations, esthetic zone, 370
short implants, 200
ultrasonic bone surgery, 229
Standard Tessellation Language, 43
stepped technique, CSFE, *261*, 272, *275*
stereolithography, 43
guide fabrication, 170, 172
stone casts, scanning, 43, 44
Straumann guided surgery instrument tray, *186*
stress
loading of implants, 115, *194*
narrow implants, 208
short implants, 203–204
wide-diameter implants, 196
subepithelial tunnel grafting, ridge expansion, 303
sublingual hematoma, 61
submerged healing, short implants, 200
suction, for maxillary sinus membrane tear, 281
supereruption, molars, 396, *397*
superficial-layer split-thickness flaps, 141, 149–150, *151*
supraperiosteal pouch, grafts in, 378, *379–380*
supraperiosteal tunneling, ridge expansion, 303
surface rendering, from DICOM images, 170
surfaces of implants, *see also* roughness of implant surfaces
acid-etched, 193
laser ablation, 107–113, 138, 141
particle-blasted, 199
surface topography of implants, 193–195, *see also* roughness of implant surfaces
SurgiGuide® technology, 169
survival rates (cumulative), immediate loading, 178
sutures
Bio-Col® technique, 92, *93*, *94*
grafting, immediate implant placement, 378, *381*
lateral repositioned pedicle flaps, 161
open-barrier techniques, 99, 100
tunnel flaps, 152, 155

T
tapered implants
immediate implant placement, 364
ridge expansion, 290, 292, 308, 320, 331–332
trans-alveolar sinus elevation, 256
tapered internal connections, *59*, *68*, 141
TASE *see* trans-alveolar sinus elevation
templates, 45, 169–170, *171*
error, 170–172
esthetic zone, 369
vacuform, *72*, *74*, 169–170
temporary anchorage devices, 387, *393*, *395*
case of malocclusion, *408*
retraction mechanics, *390*
temporary restorations, *46*
tensile forces, wedge implants, 230
tension-free closure, single-stage implant placement, 243
tension-free suturing, extraction socket grafts, 100
tenting screws, 130, *132*
thickened oxide layers, 193
thin *vs* thick biotypes, 137, 139–140, 245–246
flap design, 141
immediate implant placement, 352, 368
3-D Dental software, 169, *339*
3-D imaging *see* cone beam computed tomography
tissue engineering, 119
tissue punches, computer-guided technology, 172
titanium
allergy, 62
provisional abutments, 69, 70, *73*, 81
provisional restorations, 70, *77*, *80*
titanium mesh, in rhBMP-2-ACS grafts, 123–124, 125–129
titanium plasma spray-coated surfaces, 193, 195
narrow implants, 209
tooth display, 5
tooth-supported guides, 170–172
torque *see* insertion torques

trabeculae, stress distribution, 203–204
trans-alveolar sinus elevation (TASE), 251–284, 401–406
advanced techniques, 259–262
case of malocclusion, 407
complications, 280–282
immediate implant placement with, 361–364
ridge expansion with, 311–333
complications, 331–332
specific procedures, 262–280
technique, 253–258
transcrestal sinus floor elevation, 261
transitional prostheses *see* provisional restorations
transition lines, soft tissues and prostheses, 13
transparency, *see also* segmentation
selective, *31*, 40, *41*
trans-sinus implant placement, 221
transverse dimension, orthodontics, 395–396
trauma
esthetic zone, 401
incisors, 412, *413*
reconstruction, 13
treatment planning, 17, *18*, 184
trephines, crestal core elevation technique, 258
Triad® resin, 70
trial length, trans-alveolar sinus elevation, 253, *254*
triangle of bone concept, 35, 38–40, 42
trifurcation of roots, molars, 343
tuberosity of maxilla
angled implants, 223, *224*
grafts from, 144, *147*, 152–154, 381
tunnel flaps, 141, 152–156, *420*

U
ultrashort implants, 197–198, 204–205
ultrasonic bone surgery, 227–229, *see also* piezoelectric surgery
hydrodynamic piezoelectric internal sinus elevation, 259, *260*, 272, *273–274*
trans-alveolar sinus elevation, 259
ultra-wide implants, 197
immediate placement for molars, 349, *351*
undercuts
imaging, 29, *30*
immediate implant placement and, 338–340, *341*, *353–354*
ridge expansion and, 289, *290*, *292*, 303, 308
up-fracture, 253
future site development, 258
upright position, assessment of patient, 4

V
vacuform templates, *72*, *74*, 169–170
vascular canal, maxilla, 33, *see also* endosseous anastomoses
vertical anterior osteoplasty, angled implants and, 222, *223*
vertical dimension, orthodontics, 390–395
vertical space *see* inter-arch space
vertigo (benign paroxysmal), 280, 291, 308–309
vestibular incision, 61
virtual implants, 169, 170, *171*
virtual teeth, 41, *42*
extraction, *30*, 173, *177*
vomer implants, 222–223, *224*
v–y closure, 424, *425*, *434*

W
walls, number in bone defects, 242
wax fill-ins, 10
wax-ups, 4
for rhBMP-2-ACS grafts, 125
wedge implants, 230–237, *see also* blade implants
white esthetics, 12–13
wide-diameter implants, 195–199
immediate implant placement for molars, 349, *351*
width to length ratios, teeth, 8

X
xenografts, *see also* bovine xenograft
carrier for rhPDGF-BB, 120
esthetic zone, 370
mineralized bovine bone/collagen substitute (MCBS), 129, *130*
peri-implant defects, 337
porcine dermal matrix, 146, *149*
XXS Infuse® bone graft kit, 120–121

Z
zirconium restorations, dimensions required, 12
zygoma, angled implants, 223

Printed in the USA/Agawam, MA
September 17, 2026

910661.052